American Medical Association
Physicians dedicated to the health of America

Second Edition

CLINICAL
PREVENTIVE
MEDICINE

Richard S. Lang, MD, MPH, FACP
Chairman, Department of General Internal Medicine
Head, Section of Preventive Medicine
The Cleveland Clinic Foundation
Cleveland, Ohio

Donald D. Hensrud, MD, MPH, FACP
Associate Professor of Preventive Medicine and Nutrition,
Mayo Clinic College of Medicine
Director, Executive Health Program, Mayo Clinic
Rochester, Minnesota

Illustrated

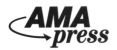

AMA Press

Tony J. Frankos, Vice President,
   Business Products
Mike Desposito, Publisher
Jean Roberts, Director, Production and
   Manufacturing
Barry Bowlus, Senior Acquisitions Editor
Reg Schmidt, Marketing Manager
Amy Postlewait, Marketing Manager
Rosalyn Carlton, Senior Production
   Coordinator
Boon Ai Tan, Senior Production Coordinator
Ronnie Summers, Senior Print Coordinator
Pat Lee, Technical Developmental Editor
Katharine Dvorak, Developmental Editor

Carol Brockman, Project Manager
Mary Ann Albanese, Art Editor
Benita Ezerins, Administrative Assistant
Coralee Montez, Administrative Secretary

CPT Research and Development Staff

Consultants

Kathy Louden, Copy Editor
Jane Piro, Developmental Editor
Mary Kay Kozyra, Proofreader
Linda Herr Hallinger, Indexer

GAC, Designer/Compositor

Clinical Preventive Medicine
Second Edition

Internet address: www.amapress.org

First edition published by Mosby-Year Book, Inc. ©1993.

Additional copies of this book may be ordered by calling 800 621-8335.
Secure on-line orders can be taken at www.amapress.com.
Mention product number OP088404.

ISBN 1-57947-417-9

BP57:03-P-082:04/04

Library of Congress Cataloging-in-Publication Data

Clinical preventive medicine / [edited by] Richard S. Lang, Donald D. Hensrud. —2nd ed.
   p. ; cm.
Includes bibliographical references and index.
ISBN 1-57947-417-9
1. Medicine, Preventive.
[DNLM: 1. Preventive Medicine. WA 108 C641 2004] I. Lang, Richard S. II. Hensrud, Donald D.

RA427.9.C55 2004
613—dc22

2004001807

DEDICATION

The publisher and editors of *Clinical Preventive Medicine, Second Edition,* wish to dedicate this book to Richard N. Matzen, Sr, MD, for his significant contribution within the field of prevention and to the first edition. Without his initial vision and resolve, this second edition would not have been possible.

We also thank him for all of his efforts and hard work for this second edition, and for his high standards and drive toward quality to help make this book more valuable to an ever-increasing audience.

CONTRIBUTORS

Oluranti Aladesanmi, MD, MPH
Department of General Internal Medicine
The Cleveland Clinic Foundation
Cleveland, Ohio

Benjamin J. Ansell, MD, FACP
Associate Professor of Medicine
Director, UCLA Comprehensive
    Health Program
Department of Medicine
David Geffen School of Medicine at UCLA
Los Angeles, California

Kathleen R. Ashton, PhD
Department of Psychiatry and Psychology
The Cleveland Clinic Foundation
Cleveland, Ohio

J. Michael Bacharach, MPH, MD, FACC
Clinical Assistant Professor
University of South Dakota School of Medicine
North Central Heart Institute
Heart Hospital of South Dakota
Sioux Falls, South Dakota

David R. Baines, MD
Faculty Physician
Alaska Family Practice Residency
Anchorage, Alaska
Assistant Professor of Medicine
University of Washington, School of Medicine
Seattle, Washington

Patrick T. Baker, MSHS, OTR/L, CDRS
Department of Physical Medicine
    and Rehabilitation
The Cleveland Clinic Foundation
Cleveland, Ohio

Patricia A. Barrier, MD, MPH
Associate Dean for Student Affairs
Assistant Professor
Preventive Medicine
Mayo Clinic College of Medicine
Rochester, Minnesota

Pelin Batur, MD
Associate Staff
Cleveland Clinic Independence
    Family Health Center
Independence, Ohio
Department of General Internal Medicine and
    Women's Health Center, Gault Women's
    Health and Breast Pavilion
The Cleveland Clinic Foundation
Cleveland, Ohio

Brent A. Bauer, MD
Director, Complementary and Integrative
    Medicine Program
Mayo Clinic
Rochester, Minnesota

Carol E. Blixen, PhD, RN
Associate Staff
Division of Clinical Research
Associate Director
Clinical Investigator Development Program
The Cleveland Clinic Foundation
Cleveland, Ohio

Amy Bode, MD, MSPH
University of Colorado School of Medicine
Denver, Colorado

Carol A. Burke, MD, FACG, FACP
Director, Center for Colon Polyp and Cancer
    Prevention
Department of Gastroenterology
    and Hepatology
The Cleveland Clinic Foundation
Cleveland, Ohio

Tim Byers, MD, MPH
Department of Preventive Medicine
    and Biometrics
University of Colorado School of Medicine
Denver, Colorado

John P. Campbell, MD, FACP
Section of Preventive Medicine
Department of General Internal Medicine
The Cleveland Clinic Foundation
Cleveland, Ohio

Rajeev Chaudhry, MD, MPH
Consultant and Practice Chair
Division of Community and Internal Medicine
Mayo Clinic
Rochester, Minnesota

Matthew M. Clark, PhD, ABPP
Associate Professor
Department of Psychiatry and Psychology
Mayo Clinic
Rochester, Minnesota

Gregory B. Collins, MD
Section Head
Alcohol and Drug Recovery Center
Department of Psychiatry and Psychology
The Cleveland Clinic Foundation
Cleveland, Ohio

Clayton T. Cowl, MD, MS
Associate Professor of Medicine
Division of Preventive &
    Occupational Medicine
Division of Pulmonary & Critical Care Medicine
Mayo Clinic and Mayo College of Medicine
Rochester, Minnesota

Robert J. Dimeff, MD
Medical Director
Section of Sports Medicine
Department of Orthopaedic Surgery
The Cleveland Clinic Foundation
Cleveland, Ohio

Julie A. Elder, DO
Associate Staff
Cleveland Clinic Willoughby
    Family Health Center
Willoughby Hills, Ohio
Department of General Internal Medicine and
    Women's Health Center, Gault Women's
    Health and Breast Pavilion
The Cleveland Clinic Foundation
Cleveland, Ohio

Stephen B. Erickson, MD, FACP
Assistant Professor of Medicine
Mayo Clinic College of Medicine
Consultant, Mayo Clinic and Mayo Foundation
Rochester, Minnesota

Vahab Fatourechi, MD, FACP
Professor of Medicine
Mayo Clinic College of Medicine
Chair, Thyroid Group
Consultant, Division of Endocrinology
    and Metabolism
Mayo Clinic
Rochester, Minnesota

Adele Fowler, MD
Associate Staff
Department of General Internal Medicine
The Cleveland Clinic Foundation
Cleveland, Ohio

Gita P. Gidwani, MD
Consultant, Departments of Obstetrics,
    Gynecology, and Pediatrics
Women's Health Center, Gault Women's
    Health and Breast Pavilion
The Cleveland Clinic Foundation
Cleveland, Ohio

Lilian Gonsalves, MD
Vice Chair, Department of Psychiatry
    and Psychology
Women's Health Center, Gault Women's
    Health and Breast Pavilion
The Cleveland Clinic Foundation
Cleveland, Ohio

Bobbie S. Gostout, MD
Assistant Professor of Obstetrics
    and Gynecology
Mayo Clinic
Rochester, Minnesota

Vladimir Hachinksi, MD, FRCPC, DSc
Professor, Department of Clinical
    Neurological Sciences
University of Western Ontario
London Health Sciences Centre
London, Ontario, Canada

Philip T. Hagen, MD, FACPM
Vice Chair, Clinical Preventive Medicine
Division of Preventive and
    Occupational Medicine
Mayo Clinic
Rochester, Minnesota

Milt Hammerly, MD
Director, Medical Operations and
    Integrative Medicine
Catholic Health Initiatives
Senior Clinical Instructor
Health Sciences Center
University of Colorado
Boulder, Colorado

Stephen P. Hayden, MD, FACP
Department of General Internal Medicine
The Cleveland Clinic Foundation
Cleveland, Ohio

J. Taylor Hays, MD
Associate Director
Nicotine Dependence Center
Mayo Clinic
Rochester, Minnesota

Catherine A. Henry, MD, FACP
Section of Preventive Medicine
Department of General Internal Medicine
Head and Neck Institute
The Cleveland Clinic Foundation
Cleveland, Ohio

Donald D. Hensrud, MD, MPH, FACP
Associate Professor of Preventive
    Medicine and Nutrition
Mayo Clinic College of Medicine
Director, Executive Health Program
Mayo Clinic
Rochester, Minnesota

Julie C. Huang, MD
Department of Cardiovascular Medicine
Cleveland Clinic Foundation
Cleveland, Ohio

Gordon L. Jensen, MD, PhD
Professor of Medicine
Vanderbilt University Medical Center
Director
Vanderbilt Center for Human Nutrition
Nashville, Tennessee

Xian Wen Jin, MD, PhD, FACP
Department of General Internal Medicine
The Cleveland Clinic Foundation
Cleveland, Ohio

Mary Jo Kasten, MD
Assistant Professor of Medicine
Mayo Clinic College of Medicine
Consultant
Divisions of General Internal Medicine
    and Infectious Diseases
Mayo Clinic
Rochester, Minnesota

J. Anthony Kendrick, MS
Public Relations Consultant
Medical Writer/Editor
Gaithersburg, Maryland

Donald T. Kirkendall, PhD
Clinical Assistant Professor
Department of Orthopaedics
University of North Carolina
Chapel Hill, North Carolina

Eric A. Klein, MD
Head, Section of Urologic Oncology
Glickman Urological Institute
The Cleveland Clinic Foundation
Cleveland, Ohio

Shakuntala Kothari, MD
Department of General Internal Medicine
Women's Health Center, Gault Women's
    Health and Breast Pavilion
The Cleveland Clinic Foundation
Cleveland, Ohio

Lois E. Krahn, MD
Associate Professor of Psychiatry
Chair, Department of Psychiatry
    and Psychology
Mayo Clinic
Scottsdale, Arizona

Richard Kring, MS, PT
Department of Sports Health and
    Orthopedic Rehabilitation
The Cleveland Clinic Foundation
Cleveland, Ohio

Richard S. Lang, MD, MPH, FACP
Chairman, Department of General
    Internal Medicine
Head, Section of Preventive Medicine
The Cleveland Clinic Foundation
Cleveland, Ohio

Philip L. Lartey, MD
Resident, Adult Psychiatry
The Cleveland Clinic Foundation
Cleveland, Ohio

Mandy C. Leonard, PharmD, BCPS
Department of Pharmacy
The Cleveland Clinic Foundation
Cleveland, Ohio

Leonid E. Lerner, MD, PhD
Cole Eye Institute and Division of
    Ophthalmology
The Cleveland Clinic Foundation
Cleveland, Ohio

Hilel Lewis, MD
Chairman
Cole Eye Institute and Division of Ophthalmology
The Cleveland Clinic Foundation
Cleveland, Ohio

Donald A. Malone, Jr, MD
Section Head, Adult Primary Services
Department of Psychiatry and Psychology
The Cleveland Clinic Foundation
Cleveland, Ohio

Anjli Maroo, MD
Department of Cardiovascular Medicine
Cleveland Clinic Foundation
Cleveland, Ohio

Richard N. Matzen, Sr, MD
Emeritus Physician in Residence
First and Former Chairman
Department of Preventive Medicine,
    Emil Buehler Scholar in Preventive
    and Aviation Medicine
The Cleveland Clinic Foundation
Cleveland, Ohio

Mark E. Mayer, MD
Director of Education Programs
Department of General Internal Medicine
The Cleveland Clinic Foundation
Cleveland, Ohio

Daniel J. Mazanec, MD
Head, Section of Spine Medicine
Vice Chairman, The Cleveland Clinic
    Spine Institute
The Cleveland Clinic Foundation
Cleveland, Ohio

Michael G. McKee, PhD
Head, Section of General and
    Health Psychology
Vice Chair, Department of Psychiatry
    and Psychology
The Cleveland Clinic Foundation
Cleveland, Ohio

José G. Merino, MD, MPhil
Assistant Professor
Department of Neurology
University of Florida
Jacksonville, Florida

**Barbara J. Messinger-Rapport, MD,
    PhD, FACP**
Assistant Professor of Medicine
Case Western Reserve University
Cleveland, Ohio
Section of Geriatric Medicine
Department of General Internal Medicine
The Cleveland Clinic Foundation
Cleveland, Ohio

Anita D. Misra-Hebert, MD
Associate Staff
Department of General Internal Medicine
The Cleveland Clinic Foundation
Cleveland, Ohio

Michael T. Modic, MD
Chairman
Division of Radiology
The Cleveland Clinic Foundation
Cleveland, Ohio

Robin G. Molella, MD, MPH
Division of Preventive and
    Occupational Medicine
Mayo Clinic
Rochester, Minnesota

James L. Mulshine, MD
Head, Experimental Intervention Section
Cell and Cancer Biology Branch
Upper Aerodigestive Research Faculty
Center for Cancer Research
National Cancer Institute, National
 Institutes for Health
Department of Health and Human Services
Bethesda, Maryland

Felipe Navarro, MD, FACC, FACP
Clinical Assistant Professor, University of
 South Dakota School of Medicine
North Central Heart Institute
Heart Hospital of South Dakota
Sioux Falls, South Dakota

Nancy A. Obuchowski, PhD
Associate Staff
Department of Biostatistics and Epidemiology
 and the Division of Radiology
The Cleveland Clinic Foundation
Cleveland, Ohio

Robert Orenstein, DO, FACP
Assistant Professor
Mayo Clinic College of Medicine
Divisions of General Internal Medicine
 and Infectious Diseases
Mayo Clinic
Rochester, Minnesota

Robert M. Palmer, MD, MPH
Head, Section of Geriatrics
Department of General Internal Medicine
The Cleveland Clinic Foundation
Cleveland, Ohio

Gregory A. Poland, MD
Mayo Vaccine Research Group
Mayo Clinic
Rochester, Minnesota

Michael B. Rocco, MD
Staff Cardiologist; Sections of Clinical
 Cardiology and Preventive Cardiology
The Cleveland Clinic Foundation
Cleveland, Ohio
Assistant Professor of Medicine
Case Western Reserve University
Cleveland, Ohio

Randall K. Roenigk, MD
Professor and Chair
Department of Dermatology
Mayo Clinic
Rochester, Minnesota

Douglas G. Rogers, MD
Section Head, Pediatric Endocrinology
Department of Endocrinology, Diabetes,
 and Metabolism
The Cleveland Clinic Foundation
Cleveland, Ohio

Ellen S. Rome, MD, MPH
Head, Section of Adolescent Medicine
The Children's Hospital at the Cleveland
 Clinic Foundation
Cleveland, Ohio

Anne M. Rosenberg, MD
Division of Endocrinology and Metabolism
Mayo Clinic
Rochester, Minnesota

Marie-Andree Roy, MSc
Vanderbilt Center for Human Nutrition
Vanderbilt University
Nashville, Tennessee

Howard M. Saal, MD
Professor of Clinical Pediatrics
Division of Human Genetics
Head, Clinical Genetics
Cincinnati Children's Hospital Medical Center
University of Cincinnati College of Medicine
Cincinnati, Ohio

Priya Sampathkumar, MD
Division of Infectious Diseases
Mayo Clinic
Rochester, Minnesota

John A. Schaffner, MD
Division of Gastroenterology
Mayo Clinic
Rochester, Minnesota

Sidna M. Scheitel, MD, MPH
Consultant
Division of Community Internal Medicine
Mayo Clinic
Assistant Professor of Medicine
Mayo Clinic College of Medicine
Rochester, Minnesota

David B. Schowalter, MD, PhD
Assistant Professor, Medical Genetics
Mayo Clinic College of Medicine
Rochester, Minnesota

Raul J. Seballos, MD, FACP
Section of Preventive Medicine
Department of General Internal Medicine
The Cleveland Clinic Foundation
Cleveland, Ohio

Kenneth J. Serio, MD
Assistant Professor of Medicine
Department of Medicine
VA San Diego Healthcare System
University of California
San Diego, California

Andrea L. Sikon, MD
Associate Staff
Department of General Internal Medicine
Women's Health Center, Gault Women's
    Health and Breast Pavilion
The Cleveland Clinic Foundation
Cleveland, Ohio

Peter Sinks, MD
Clinical Associate
Center for the Spine
The Cleveland Clinic Foundation
Cleveland, Ohio

Glen D. Solomon, MD, FACP
Chairman, Department of Medicine
Lutheran General Hospital
Park Ridge, Illinois
Professor and Associate Chair of Medicine
The Chicago Medical School
North Chicago, Illinois

Dennis L. Sprecher, MD
Adjunct Professor, University of Pennsylvania
Department of Medicine
Director, Atherosclerosis/Dyslipidemia
Discovery Medicine
GlaxoSmithKline

Paul V. Targonski, MD, PHD
Assistant Professor of Medicine and
Senior Associate Consultant
Division of Community Internal Medicine
Mayo Clinic
Rochester, Minnesota

Holly L. Thacker, MD, FACP
Director, Women's Health Center
Gault Women's Health and Breast Pavilion
Department of General Internal Medicine
Department of Obstetrics and Gynecology
The Cleveland Clinic Foundation
Cleveland, Ohio

Brad T. Tinkle, MD, PhD
Medical Genetics Resident
Division of Human Genetics
Department of Pediatrics
Cincinnati Children's Hospital Medical Center
University of Cincinnati College of Medicine
Cincinnati, Ohio

Michael H. Trujillo, MD, MPH, MS
Associate Professor
University of New Mexico Health Sciences Center
Department of Family and Community Medicine
Assistant Surgeon General/RADM (ret)
Former Director of Indian Health Service
Albuquerque, New Mexico

Frederick Van Lente, PhD
Vice-Chairman
Department of Clinical Pathology
The Cleveland Clinic Foundation
Cleveland, Ohio

Prathibha Varkey, MD, MPH
Assistant Professor in Preventive Medicine
    and Internal Medicine
Division of Preventive and
    Occupational Medicine
Department of Internal Medicine
Mayo Clinic
Rochester, Minnesota

Kristin S. Vickers, PhD
Assistant Professor of Psychology
Department of Psychiatry and Psychology
Mayo Clinic College of Medicine
Rochester, Minnesota

Abinash Virk, MD, DTMH
Assistant Professor of Medicine
Director
Travel and Geographic Medicine Clinic
Mayo Clinic
Rochester, Minnesota

Elizabeth E. Warner, MD
Cell and Cancer Biology Branch
Center for Cancer Research
National Cancer Institute
National Institutes for Health
Department of Health and Human Services
Bethesda, Maryland

Alan M. Weiss, MD, MBA
Associate Staff
Department of General Internal Medicine
The Cleveland Clinic Foundation
Cleveland, Ohio

Carolyn Welty, MD
Associate Clinical Professor
Department of Medicine
Division of Geriatrics
University of California
San Francisco, School of Medicine
San Francisco, California

Jaeyoung Yoon, MD, PhD
Assistant Professor
Department of Dermatology
Mayo Clinic
Rochester, Minnesota

REVIEWERS

Roger S. Blumenthal, MD, FACC
Associate Professor of Medicine
Director, The Johns Hopkins Ciccarone Center
    for the Prevention of Heart Disease
Associate Professor of Medicine/Cardiology
Johns Hopkins Medical Institutions
Baltimore, Maryland

Terry Mahan Buttaro, MS, APRN, BC
Instructor, Simmons College School
    for Health Studies
Beth Israel Deaconess Medical Center North
Boston, Massachusetts

Jennifer Eng-Wong, MD, MPH
Staff Clinician
Medical Oncology Clinical Research Unit
National Cancer Institute
Bethesda, Maryland

Eric V. Granowitz, MD
Assistant Professor of Medicine
Tufts University School of Medicine
Baystate Medical Center
Boston, Massachusetts

Douglas C. Heimburger, MD
Professor of Nutrition Sciences & Medicine
University of Alabama at Birmingham
Birmingham, Alabama

Tom Houston, MD
Professor of Public Health and Family Medicine
Jim Finks Chair in Health Promotion
Louisiana State University School
    of Public Health
New Orleans, Louisiana

Pasi A. Jänne, MD, PhD
Lowe Center for Thoracic Oncology
Dana Farber Cancer Institute
Department of Medicine, Brigham
    and Women's Hospital
Boston, Massachusetts

Robert Kushner, MD
Medical Director
Wellness Institute
Northwestern Memorial Hospital
Professor of Medicine
Feinberg School of Medicine
Northwestern University
Chicago, Illinois

Andrew J. Saxon, MD
Professor, Department of Psychiatry
    and Behavioral Sciences
University of Washington
Seattle, Washington

The mission the editors of this book have assumed is to provide a practical handbook and reference to the acquisition of knowledge in preventive medicine and its appropriate delivery for fellow practitioners (or physicians in training) whether they be primary care physicians or specialists. Nurses, physician assistants, nurse practitioners, or clinical assistants—important partners in the physician's office team—will find many parts of this text eminently useful in their tasks, and would do well to have such a reference at hand. Such personnel can be invaluable in the physician's evaluation of risk, need and delivery of preventive care. I believe those who use the text will agree the editors and the selected chapter authors in various disciplines, have done a notable service.

In the title, CLINICAL is the key word. Appropriately the editors have recruited authors with strong credentials in clinical medicine and vested interests in preventive medicine and the delivery of care in their specialties and have an ethos and awareness of each patient's propensities to particular disabilities and/or illness. In order to succeed in delivering preventive medicine effectively, it is the doctor in practice who daily sees patients who must be counted on to achieve the goals of preventive health care. This cannot be overemphasized.

The awareness of the contribution prevention can be to the future health of all patients is generally accepted. The development of the preventive mind-set per force precedes the consistent effective routine application of prevention. Eventually it becomes an unconscious part of the physician's care. This book is one tool that can be used in the acquisition of such skills. This book, by clinicians and for clinicians, is suited for office use and medical school faculty in teaching clinical medicine.

How does this book's approach to the subject matter differ from other books? It continues and improves on the motif established in the first edition, of not only identifying specific disease predispositions of the individual (and why) but then, through the individual, identifies the patient's familial group at risk for that disease, for example renal calculi or diabetes. In addition (and in contrast to the study of the individual and a single disease), large ethnic, racial and geographic populations and gender are profiled and described for predispositions to any and all illnesses and disorders to which this population is particularly prone, whether it be of genetic, cultural, environmental or dietary causation. This is helpful both to the practitioner with a homogenous practice and to one with a heterogeneous urban practice.

The text also examines specific tools commonly used preventively, such as diet and exercise, and evaluates each preventive tool as to what it can do, what can and cannot be expected of it, and when it is appropriate or when not.

To find all the above comprehensively covered in one text with the addition of seasoning such as alternative medicines and genetics to the usual clinical concerns of the doctor is unique in my view.

Richard N. Matzen, Sr, MD

A paradigm shift is occurring in medicine in which the focus is turning away from reparative medical and surgical care and toward a greater emphasis on prevention. This shift has been influenced by physicians having a more thorough understanding of the natural histories of diseases and the factors influencing them. Also, we now have greater knowledge of both how and when to intervene in these natural histories.

New and improved medical technology is racing forward at an astounding pace enabling the detection of medical conditions earlier. Genetic codes are being unraveled and the ability to intervene through genetic testing and altering the genes themselves to improve outcomes is developing.

At the same time, computer technology and advances in information transfer have led to better informed health care consumers who are taking more ownership of their personal health and well being. They are keenly aware that premature death and disability are influenced by choices of diet, exercise, personal habits, safety risks, and preventive interventions. Medical professionals are confronted each day with more and more questions from health care consumers educated by their own internet searches or the media's reporting of medical advances. In addition, health care providers are being significantly influenced by the marketing and advertisement of products, including over-the-counter pharmaceuticals and prescription medications.

Clinical Preventive Medicine, Second Edition, is organized to provide the medical professional with a useful framework to better understand and answer these preventive health questions. This book first fosters a basic understanding of preventive concepts and then considers prevention in specific contexts: behavioral and psychological influences; physical activities; nutrition including supplements, vitamins, hormones, herbal products and performance enhancers; complementary and alternative medicine; age, gender, and race; and finally common conditions that cause significant morbidity and mortality. *Clinical Preventive Medicine, Second Edition,* aims to guide the clinician in the use of counseling, screening, chemoprevention, vaccinations, and personal safety equipment, and to provide a better understanding of diet, exercise, and the interaction of mind and body in the prevention of disease. An additional reference tool is the appendix, which contains the Current Procedural Terminology (CPT®) 2004 codes that apply to preventive medicine.

The first edition of *Clinical Preventive Medicine,* published 10 years ago, was timely and well received. As in the first edition, practicing clinicians recognized for their expertise and scientific experts and leaders in their respective fields contributed to this second edition.

This book is written and designed to be a resource for medical students, primary care physicians, nurses, and allied health professionals, as well as subspecialists who also need to understand the practical aspects of clinical preventive medicine. No doubt, interested health care consumers will also find this edition enlightening and informative.

We hope that *Clinical Preventive Medicine, Second Edition,* will prompt discussion and debate and foster novel directions in the stimulation of new knowledge. We are confident that ultimately, this book will help health care consumers make positive choices in their preventive health initiatives enabling them to live longer, healthier, and happier lives.

Richard S. Lang and Donald D. Hensrud

The successful completion of a book of this magnitude involves and depends on the efforts of many individuals. We wholeheartedly thank all of these persons, our colleagues, and our contributors for their creativity and abilities that helped to bring this book together.

We extend our most sincere appreciation and gratitude to Pat Lee, Eileen Lynch, Barry Bowlus, and to all of the talented editors and assistants of AMA Press. Also, we would like to recognize our secretarial staff Theresa Bloom, Jane Gould, and Leslie Tuohy for their support, understanding and hard work.

Most importantly, we thank our spouses—Lisa R. Kraemer and Natasha Matt-Hensrud, and our children—Jonathan, Katherine, William, and Daniel, and Gabrielle, Alexandra, and Isaac. They offered us their love, encouragement, and understanding during the long hours.

Finally, we offer this book in appreciation of our mothers, Margaret and Janet, our extended families, our friends, and our patients with the hope of their enjoying long, happy, and healthy lives.

Richard S. Lang, MD
Donald D. Hensrud, MD

CONTENTS

Principles of Preventive Medicine and Clinical Prevention

Preventive Medicine: Definition and Application

Richard N. Matzen, Sr, MD

DEFINITION OF CLINICAL PREVENTIVE MEDICINE

A definition of clinical preventive medicine (CPM) was deliberated on and proposed in Atlanta, Georgia, at the Carter Center in January 1989 at a special meeting of the House of Delegates of the American Medical Association.[1] The deliberating body was composed of representatives of the American College of Preventive Medicine (ACPM), the Aerospace Medical Association, the American College of Occupational Medicine, the American Association of Public Health Physicians, and the Association of Preventive Medicine Residents. The definition was based on a CPM survey conducted by the American Board of Preventive Medicine (ABPM) and the proposed definition was forwarded to that Board. The ABPM examines and certifies candidates in aerospace medicine, occupational medicine, public health, and general preventive medicine (PM). After completing the required training, a candidate may take 1 or more of these board examinations.

The whole of the definition proposed is as follows:

Clinical preventive medicine (CPM) is an integral part of preventive medicine concerned with the maintenance and promotion of health and the reduction of risk factors which result in injury and disease. CPM is practiced in the clinical setting through the assessment of risk factors to disease and injury and the application of preventive interventions. The CPM practitioner may be involved in risk reduction programs for individuals, communities, employees, or other populations.

Clinical preventive medicine specialists have the knowledge and skills necessary to accomplish the following:

A. Assess risk of individuals for disease, using techniques such as screening and health risk assessment tools.

B. Implement interventions to modify or eliminate individuals' risk for disease/injury, using biologic, behavioral, and environmental approaches.

C. Organize and manage practice settings to facilitate the integration and monitoring of personal preventive services and be an advocate for health promotion activities for the individual.

D. Apply risk assessment, risk reductions, and media techniques to communities and populations including employee groups: be an advocate for health promotion and a resource for information about prevention strategies in the community.

E. Evaluate the effectiveness of individual and community risk reduction techniques and be a consultant to physicians, industry, and government for program development and evaluation.[1]

Definition reprinted by permission of the ACPM.

The definition quoted through item C could be used for CPM as it pertains to the practice of PM by non-PM specialists (eg, family practitioner, internist, pediatrician) and application of PM in the clinician's office. Items D and E pertain to the community and complete the definition as it defines the role of CPM in the specialty practice of general PM and its related boards.

Primary, Secondary, and Tertiary Prevention

Prevention is the act of hindering or averting the occurrences of a disease or injury. There are 3 levels of positive interference in the evolution of a morbid state or disease: primary, secondary, and tertiary prevention.

Primary prevention

The reduction of risk factors before occurrence of a disease, condition, or injury has occurred. Examples: the use of polio or measles vaccine; the control of pollution or exposures that would result in morbidity.

Secondary prevention

The early detection of the potential for the development of a disease or condition or the existence of a disease while asymptomatic, to allow positive interference to prevent, postpone, or attenuate the symptomatic clinical state. Example: the prophylactic use of isoniazid in a person recently converted to a tuberculin-positive state.

Tertiary prevention

The treatment of an existing symptomatic disease process or condition to ameliorate its effects, delay or prevent its progress. Example: the close control of diabetes to prevent its complications.

Generally, prevention is thought of in terms of primary prevention and discovery through screening. In fact, prevention should be thought of throughout the time line of a disease, so as to preclude or ameliorate secondary or tertiary states in the life cycle of the disease or morbid state.

Inherent in the goals of clinical prevention is the concept of *health:* a state of complete physical, mental, and social well-being, not merely the absence of disease and infirmity. The primary health care provider addresses some aspect of all of these areas during interactions with patients. For a variety of reasons, the traditional primary care doctor-patient interaction has often emphasized the physical aspect of this definition more than the mental and social. Primary prevention by way of health education and health promotion helps to address the mental and social aspects of maintaining "health." *Health education* refers to those "learning experiences designed to predispose, enable, and reinforce voluntary adaptations of individual or collective behavior conducive to health." *Health promotion* is the "combination of health education and related organizational, economic, and environmental supports for behavior conducive to health."[2] In the broad sense, health promotion is those activities designed to alter behavior, environment, or heredity to improve health.

The concept of the well individual causes difficulty for many practitioners because perceptions vary. Patient and physician (observer) perceptions differ regarding what wellness is and how complaints or concerns are expressed. Patients run the spectrum from the stoic individual to the chronic complainer or hypochondriac. The stoic individual may be seen as asymptomatic when, in fact, symptoms are present but disregarded. The chronic complainer may be judged symptomatic when, in fact, he or she is experiencing his or her own normal state of health. Similarly, physicians define health, wellness, or symptoms in the framework of their own perceptions and biases. These variations in perceptions and expression cloud the concept of the periodic health examination for the practitioner. Other problems arise from the anecdotal experience of physicians. The practitioner may tend to "overscreen" future patients for the condition he or she overlooked in an earlier patient, disregarding screening guidelines and the scientific evidence pertaining to them. Conversely, lack of knowledge about a disease process or techniques of prevention for that disease may cause a physician to overlook a given test or intervention and "underscreen" an individual. The periodic health examination properly done can provide an important framework for physicians in their approach to the variety of patients who enter the office on any given day and can assist in overcoming these problems of perception, bias, anecdote, and lack of knowledge.

The foundation of the periodic health examination is based on the following precepts:[3]

1. Patients without symptoms can harbor organic disease.
2. Disease can be detected at an "early" stage.
3. Discovery of disease can lead to arrest, reversal, retardation, or cure of that disease and thereby reduce morbidity and/or mortality.

Delivery of Preventive Health Care

To effectively reach and affect the entire population and to achieve goals such as those set forth in *Healthy People 2010*[4] preventive medicine must be available to all patients and practiced in the offices of all physicians, in particular those of primary care doctors. This statement is amply supported by the fact that all issues of the *Guide to Clinical Preventive Services*[5] (the book of reports of the US Preventive Services Task Force) and *Clinician's Handbook of Preventive Services*[6] (a publication of the US Public Health Service "Put Prevention Into Practice" campaign) have stated that the books are aimed at physicians in the primary care specialties and at supportive clinical personnel. A representative example is found in the introduction to the 1989 edition of the *Guide*[5] as follows: "This report is intended for primary care clinicians: physicians, nurses, nurse practitioners, physician assistants, other allied health professionals, and students." Knowledge of preventive medicine, and the tools it employs should be a part of the training, not only of the physician but also the nurse, nurse practitioner, physician assistant, and all allied health personnel.

TRAINING IN CPM FOR NON-PM SPECIALISTS

The training alluded to earlier must, of course, be carried out in the nation's medical and nursing schools, residency programs, and other health personnel training facilities. Unfortunately, neither uniformity to this training or an organized basis exists in all training programs. To accomplish that goal will require encouragement and/or action by the American Association of Medical Colleges, requirements of the various boards, and other formal professional groups that can influence medical curriculum and/or training. This statement applies to nursing and physician assistant training as well.

At a July 2002 meeting of the Preventive Medical Leadership Forum, medical directors were identified as being able to play a major role in developing preventive medical electives for medical students, not just by faculty but also by the majority of CPM and PM physicians who practice in a community setting. Clinical preventive medicine electives and formal lecture series for medical students can be offered in schools with a CPM/PM faculty or residency, or in an associated school of public health. However, most schools do not sponsor PM residencies or have an associated public health school. These institutions can, however, through a liaison with community CPM and PM practitioners, offer students electives in this discipline.[7]

In April 2001, Dickey and Tran[8] published a study on the amount of time devoted to the teaching of PM at the University of California, San Francisco School of Medicine for the years 1996–1997 dividing the study into preclinical and clinical years. They noted that PM was taught as a dedicated required course at only 24 of 126 schools. They also reported that the organized, consistent teaching of PM as a crosscutting subject taught in and by various departments presents very real practical problems as to content, emphasis, effectiveness, and oversight. Only a modest amount of time was found to be devoted to the subject, with a highly variable retention rate by students. Both students and faculty agreed that more time was needed in the curriculum for CPM. Preference by the student as to how the subject was taught ranked, in descending order, working up patient cases, lecture, and discussion with house staff. Learning by self-acquisition was the very last preference, at 1.2%.

In the "Commentary" section of the *American Journal of Preventive Medicine,* Rahman[9] observed that "the teaching of CPM has been relegated to a second-class status in many medical schools" and that there appears to be little disagreement that CPM is inadequately taught at both undergraduate and postgraduate levels. Many approaches, styles, and content differences in the teaching of CPM exist. At Ohio State University College of Medicine, where there is a Department of Preventive Medicine,[10] the program is more unilateral, in contrast to the University of California, San Francisco, where a cross-sectional multidisciplinary approach is applied.

EDUCATIONAL RESOURCES AND PRACTICAL APPLICATION OF CPM FOR PHYSICIANS IN PRACTICE

Physicians already in practice must depend on their own interest and resolution to introduce consistent CPM into their practice. Postgraduate short courses and Web sites from ACPM and the related boards of general PM are available as resources. The governmental Agency for Healthcare Research and Quality (AHRQ) carries the recommendations of the US Preventive Services Task Force. The evidence-based recommendations of the first

US Preventive Services Task Force addressed 60 different illnesses and conditions and 169 interventions to prevent them, delay the onset of a clinically morbid state, or otherwise favorably modify their course. This guide was issued in 1989 under the title, *A Guide to Clinical Preventive Services.*[6] The second US Preventive Services Task Force updated, expanded, and modified the recommendations of the first guide and proceeded to address other illnesses and conditions. This resulted in the publication of the *Guide to Clinical Preventive Services, Second Edition*, published in 1998.[11] The third task force released its first recommendations in a supplement to the April 2001 issue of the *American Journal of Preventive Medicine.*[8] In addition to its first 4 recommendations, the history of the task forces, the methodology used to arrive at recommendations, cost-effectiveness of the application of CPM, and other related subjects were concisely presented. These recommendations are now released on the AHRQ Web site and in selected journals. These position papers may be found upon their completion in the *American Journal of Preventive Medicine* and the specialty journals of internal medicine. Changing to a journal-based rather than book-based format allows the task force to make position statements available immediately rather than waiting until an aggregate makes a volume publication feasible. This change was inaugurated by the publication of a supplement to the *American Journal of Preventive Medicine* in April 2001 titled "The Third US Task Force: Background, Methods, and First Recommendations." The first 4 recommendations contained in this issue were on the evidence for the effectiveness of screening for skin cancer, bacterial vaginosis during pregnancy, lipid disorders in adults, and chlamydia.[12] Other position statements and recommendations have followed.

The American Academy of Family Practice (AAFP) has been active in prevention and is a good source of material. "Prevention" was adopted as its theme and annual clinical focus for the 2003 annual meeting. The focus addressed primary, secondary, and tertiary prevention and the prevention of medical errors. The program included two keynote addresses: "What's New from the US Task Force," by Dr Alfred O. Berg, task force chairman, and "Primary, Secondary, and Tertiary Prevention in Minority Populations," by Dr Denise Rogers. The AAFP annual meeting program included:

- annual meeting sessions on prevention;
- American Family Physician monographs on tertiary prevention of cardiovascular disease, asthma, and diabetes;
- handouts of PM articles that have appeared in the AAFP publications;
- Web-based links to cooperating partners along with a Web-based "Prevention Resources Guide" to include resources from AAFP and cooperating partners; and

■ a video CME program, "Prevention Strategies in Family Practice," focusing on early prevention risk factors and detection of, among others, depression, obesity, and cancer screening and the use of diet, nutrition, smoking cessation, and exercise in the PM strategies of disease prevention and the prevention of secondary and tertiary stages of a morbid condition.[13]

Put Prevention into Practice (PPIP) is a kit of office-based tools for the implementation and facilitation of offering preventive services through office-based providers.[14] To be effective, PPIP requires introduction into a practice and also maintenance. A study of the introduction, success, and performance of this tool was conducted at 5 primary care clinic sites funded by the Texas Department of Health over 6 years.[15] The program was maintained throughout at 5 of the 6 sites. A site's effectiveness and functioning over time was found not to depend on how successfully the program was implemented, but on institutional strength and the integration of the program into the systems used. Support by a person in the mid- or upper level of an organization, and a stable organization were identified as keys to success. (PPIP is available through the AHRQ Web site.)

Much information regarding medical, social, family, and occupational history to establish or evaluate health risks may be obtained via written or computer-based health risk appraisal tools and instruments. The more time-consuming delivery of preventive care education and instruction may be aided by similar tools but is optimized by employment of well-trained support personnel. Delivery of these services is covered in Chapter 3.

SCREENING FOR PREVENTABLE CONDITIONS

Prevention often implies detection of a condition, disease, or risk factor. Screening is the application of a test to determine those with or likely to have a condition or disease. Screening may be done on an individual basis over a period of years, tailoring the screening to the particular needs of the individual patient. Screening may be done with a subset of patients with similar characteristics and risks or on a practice-wide basis, or it may address units of population (so-called mass screening). Whatever the need or the case, certain principles should be applied to the planning of that screening. These principles were outlined in a World Health Organization (WHO) recommendation, written by Wilson and Jungner[16] in 1968.

World Health Organization Definition

1. The condition sought should be an important health problem.
2. There should be an accepted treatment for patients with recognized disease.
3. Facilities for diagnosis and treatment should be available.
4. There should be a recognizable latent or early symptomatic stage.
5. There should be a suitable test or examination.
6. The test should be acceptable to the population.
7. The natural history of the condition, including development from latent to declared disease, should be adequately understood.
8. There should be an agreed policy on whom to treat as patients.
9. The cost of case-finding (including diagnosis and treatment of patients diagnosed) should be economically balanced in relation to possible expenditure on medical care as a whole.
10. Case-finding should be a continuing process and not a "once-and-for-all" project.

Put Prevention into Practice: The Clinician's Handbook of Preventive Services, Second Edition, discusses sensitivity, specificity, and positive predictive values, frequency, and magnitude of screening, etc, all of which must be considered in setting up a screening program.

Selective vs Mass Screening

Selective or targeted screening is more desirable than mass screening. An example of this superiority is the National Tuberculosis Association's (NTA's) use of the mobile chest X-ray screening program as a mass screening method in the first half of the 20th century. The goal of the NTA was to eradicate tuberculosis in our society by finding cases to isolate and treat, and thus remove the risk of further communication of the disease. Along with the patch testing in schools, mobile vans with X-ray equipment were stationed at target locations and brought to businesses for screening. Annual X-ray examinations were encouraged, and the association waged an effective and massive campaign of public education about the disease over many decades. In its early years, by most measures, the program appeared to be cost effective.

As nutrition, sanitary conditions, housing, and effective treatment improved, especially after World War II, when modern antituberculous antibiotics became available, cases became more infrequent. In the 1960s, the NTA found that the yield of this program was minimal and the cost appreciable, but there were pockets of people in the general population where the disease still existed to a greater degree. The mass screening of the mobile van was abandoned in favor of selective or targeted screening of population subsets, such as in prisons and city hospitals serving the poor, where the disease was found to be most common. The mobile unit X-ray program was eventually abandoned.

Each practicing physician should examine and apply selective screening to his or her patient population with discrimination. One physician's needs may differ considerably from his or her colleague's practice and needs in the same city. A target subset within a practice may differ by age or race and thereby influence appropriateness of screening. For example, a practice may have an international subset of patients predisposed to a certain condition for which screening may be indicated that is not generally considered for the average patient. As the world gets "smaller," not only an awareness but also a knowledge of geographic, ethnic, and racial predispositions are becoming necessities to practice medicine well.

Private clinical practice also provides a setting for making good decisions about cost-effectiveness to the individual. The excellent and authoritative *Guide to Clinical Preventive Services*[11] and the recommendations of the US Preventive Services Task Force should in most cases be taken into account, and serve as a guide to screening and preventive intervention. Using this information, the practitioner can best determine how a patient, by virtue of genetic makeup, personality, stresses, behavioral characteristics, and financial resources, is best served with particular interval screening procedures. Ideally, the physician will not only advise patients about the continuing screening process but also ask the patients for input and their perceptions of needs.

Cost-effectiveness becomes a critical issue when the common good is considered in our time of shrinking resources. Many practitioners therefore use the random care visit to address a preventive care concern, often without charge. Screening must be done with circumspection and logic, weighed not only for cost but also for effectiveness. Has the proposed screening method proved to be of worth in your experience for the particular use to which you wish to put it?

Preventive Medicine as a Specialty

The role of the clinician is vital to the delivery of CPM. The specialty of PM is equally important to the health of the nation and the public good. The chief role of the specialty of PM is to address the preventive health needs of larger population groups than the clinician does, and to provide information *to* and a research base *for* the practitioners so they may better the delivery of CPM to the individual. The clinical activities of the specialty are best illuminated by exploring the specialty itself.

Physicians in PM have served as health planners and administrators, biostatisticians and statistical analysts, teachers of PM, researchers, and clinicians applying PM in the health care system. The American Board of Preventive Medicine (ABPM) has examined and certified physicians in this field since 1949. Board certification requires 3 years of specialty training: a clinical year, an academic year and a 1-year practicum. Program requirements for PM training are described in detail in the *Graduate Medical Education Directory* 2002-2003 published by the American Medical Association (AMA).[17] The directory also describes a 2-year program in "Medical Toxicology (Preventive Medicine)" which may be incorporated with an accredited residency in PM. The

ABPM should be consulted regarding eligibility for subspecialty certification in such a program. This book also contains the programs in PM accredited by the Council for Graduate Medical Education (ACGME). The board examinations may be taken after completion of the 3 years of accredited training and after a fourth year of training, teaching, research, or practice.

Preventive medicine is composed of 4 specialties: general PM, public health, occupational medicine, and aerospace medicine. However, there are only 3 board examinations, with general PM and public health combined as 1 examination.

"1. Aerospace medicine focuses on the health of the operating crews and passengers of air and space vehicles, together with the support personnel who are required to operate such vehicles. Segments of this population often work and live in remote, isolated and sometimes closed environments under conditions of physical and psychological stress.

2. Occupational medicine focuses on the health of workers, including the ability to perform work; the physical, chemical, biological and social environments of the workplace; and the health outcome of environmental exposures. Practitioners in this field diagnose, treat, and prevent morbid conditions caused by environmental exposures and stressors. They recognize that work and the environment in which work is performed can have favorable or adverse effects upon the health of workers as well as of other populations; that the nature or circumstances of work can be arranged to protect worker health; and that health and well-being at the workplace are promoted when worker's physical attributes or limitations are accommodated in job placement.

3. Public health and general PM focuses on promoting health, preventing disease, and managing the health of communities and defined populations. These practitioners combine population-based public health skills with knowledge of primary, secondary, and tertiary prevention-oriented clinical practice in a wide range of settings."[17]

A shortage in preventive medical specialists in the United States[18] was reported 10 years ago and this situation seems to have changed little in the past decade. The ACPM recently noted that the number of newly board-certified PM physicians is declining and the number of enrollees in PM residency programs is decreasing.[19] The number of physicians in the practice of PM and its branches in 2001 and the professional activities of these physicians were compiled by the AMA and are outlined in Table 1-1 and Table 1-2.[20]

Other PM specialists include physicians who are board eligible but not yet certified, public health specialists and toxicologists with a PhD degree, and physicians and other professionals who have completed the postgraduate work to obtain a master of public health (MPH) degree.

SUMMARY

Taken in total, the number of professionals in the field of PM still remains small. At the same time, the need for specialists trained in PM and its subspecialties increases as we face the hazards of bioterrorism, the epidemic of acquired immunodeficiency syndrome (AIDS), the emergence and spread of other viral diseases such as the Ebola and West Nile viruses, and antibiotic drug resistance. Greater understanding of disease causation and the unraveling and application of human genetics further increases the need for such specialists.

TABLE 1-1

Total Physicians by Specialty, 2001

Specialty	No.
Aerospace medicine	488
General preventive medicine	1851
Occupational medicine	2860
Public health	1785
Total	**6984**

*Data are from *Physician Characteristics and Distribution in the US,* tables 1.2 and 1.8.[20]

TABLE 1-2

Major Professional Activity*

Specialty	Patient Care	Admin	Teaching	Research	Other
Aerospace	285	148	8	29	18
Internal PM	13	0	0	0	0
Occupational medicine	2016	602	41	95	106
Public health, general PM	377	908	71	324	105
General PM	1369	231	34	135	34
Total	**4060**	**1889**	**154**	**583**	**263**

*Data are from *Physician Characteristics and Distribution in the US,* tables 1.2 and 1.8.[20]
Admin indicates administration; and PM, preventive medicine.

REFERENCES

1. *ACPM News,* The Newsletter of the American College of Preventive Medicine. 1989;1:3.

2. Green LW. Prevention and health education. In: *Maxcy-Rosenau Public Health and Preventive Medicine.* Norwalk, Conn: Appleton-Century-Crofts; 1986:1089–1090.

3. Charap MH. The periodic health examination: genesis of a myth. *Ann Intern Med.* 1981;95:733–735.

4. U.S. Department of Health and Human Services. *Healthy People 2010.* McLean, Va: International Medical Publishing, Inc; 2000.

5. Report of the U.S. Preventive Services Task Force. *Guide to Clinical Preventive Services.* Baltimore, Md: Williams & Wilkins; 1989:xix.

6. *Put Prevention into Practice: The Clinician's Handbook of Preventive Services, Second Edition.* US Government Printing Office, Washington, DC, 1998.

7. Applegate M. From the Joint Council of Medical Directors. Preventive medicine electives for medical students. *ACPM News,* The Newsletter of the American College of Preventive Medicine. Winter 2002;42:14–15.

8. Dickey LL, Tran K. Evaluating the teaching of clinical preventive medicine: a multi-dimensional approach. *AJPM.* 2001;20:190–195.

9. Rahman MI. Training preventive medicine residents to put prevention into practice (commentary). *AJPM.* 1996;12:221–224.

10. Keller MD. Teaching preventive medicine. In: Matzen RN, Lang RS, eds. *Clinical Preventive Medicine.* St. Louis, Mo: Mosby-Year Book, Inc.; 1993:32–40.

11. Report of the U.S. Preventive Services Task Force. *Guide to Clinical Preventive Services, Second Edition.* McLean, Va: International Medical Publishers.

12. Atkins D, Best D, Shapiro EN. *The Third U.S. Preventive Services Task Force: Background, Methods, and First Recommendations. AJPM.* 2001; 20(suppl):44–107.

13. ACPM to support AAFP focus on prevention. *ACPM News;* The Newsletter of the American College of Preventive Medicine. Fall 2002;42:4–5.

14. Berg AO, Allan JD. Introducing the Third U.S. Preventive Services Task Force. In: Atkins D, Best D, Shapiro EN, eds. *The Third U.S. Preventive Services Task Force: Background, Methods, and First Recommendations. AJPM.* 20(suppl):3–4.

15. Goodson P, Smith MM, Evans A, Meyer B, Gottlieb NH. Maintaining prevention in practice: survival of PPIP in primary care settings. *AJPM.* 2001;20:184–189.

16. Wilson JMB, Jungner G. *Principles and Practice in Screening for Disease.* Geneva, Switzerland (printed in France); The World Health Organization; 1968.

17. *Graduate Medical Education Directory 2002–2003.* Chicago, Ill: AMA Press; 2002:298–309.

18. Matzen R. Preventive medicine today: definition, mission, and manpower. In: Matzen RN, Lang RS, eds. *Clinical Preventive Medicine.* St Louis, Mo: Mosby-Year Book, Inc.; 1993:3–19.

19. ACPM report card. ACPM News: the Newsletter of the American College of Preventive Medicine. Winter 2002;42:1–8.

20. Pasko T, Smart DR. *Physician Characteristics in the US 2003–2004 Edition.* Chicago, Ill: AMA Press; 2003:9,15–19.

chapter 2

Principles of Biostatistics and Epidemiology in Clinical Preventive Medicine

Prathibha Varkey, MD, MPH, and Philip T. Hagen, MD

INTRODUCTION

Epidemiology and biostatistics are the "basic sciences" behind prevention. In clinical preventive medicine (CPM), the evidence from this science is applied to the individual. The rigorous weighing of evidence from studies, including analyzing the validity and strengths of study results, determining to whom it is most appropriate to apply the results, and balancing conflicting evidence regarding risks and benefits, has long been the goal of the careful clinician. The systematic teaching and practice of this approach have come to be known as evidence-based medicine.

In this chapter, we will focus on the basic principles of epidemiology, biostatistics, and evidence-based medicine. We hope to arm the clinician with enough knowledge to understand the role of each in preventive medicine and to stimulate further inquiry.

EPIDEMIOLOGY AND BIOSTATISTICS

The word *epidemiology* has its origins in Greek; *epi* means "upon," *demos* means "population," and *logy* means "study of." Epidemiology is the study of factors that determine the occurrence and distribution of disease in a population. Clinical epidemiology focuses on factors that affect the screening, diagnosis, treatment, and outcomes of diseases in patient care. The methods of epidemiology allow a valid study to be designed to describe or answer a question about disease and disease factors in populations. *Biostatistics,* on the other hand, is the tabulation and analysis of biological and medical data. It allows inferences to be made from the data in a valid way based on the nature of the data.

Epidemiology and biostatistics are useful for many purposes, including clinical decision making, health services research, the investigation of outbreaks, prioritizing public health resource allocation, evaluation of community or individual health interventions, and the investigation of the frequency, natural history, and biological spectrum of a disease.

EPIDEMIOLOGIC MEASUREMENTS

The frequency of a disease or disease-related factor in a population can be defined in a number of ways. Two important descriptions of frequency include incidence and prevalence.

Incidence is the frequency or number of new events (diseases, deaths, or injuries) that occur during a specified period in a defined population. *Cumulative incidence* is the number of new events that occur during a specified period in a population that is at risk (eg, incidence of new cases of acquired immunodeficiency syndrome, or AIDS, in a given population in a given period). Scientists use it as roughly synonymous with attack rate, risk of disease, or probability of getting the disease. *Incidence density* is the number of new events of a disease occurring in a specified time period per person time-at-risk during the period. Incidence density is especially useful when the event of interest may occur more than once in an individual during the period of the study (eg, incidence density of acute exacerbations of chronic obstructive lung disease per year).

Prevalence is the number of cases of a specified disease or condition in a defined population at a particular point in time (*point prevalence*) or during a specified period of time (*period prevalence*). If the incidence of disease and its duration in affected individuals are stable over time, the relationship between prevalence and incidence may be expressed as follows:

$$\text{Prevalence} = \text{Incidence} \times \text{Average Duration}$$

The frequency of new events that occur in a defined time period expressed as a fraction of the average population at risk is often expressed in terms of *rates*. Commonly used rates[1] in population data are shown in Table 2-1. Please note that prevalence in common usage (point prevalence) is not a rate, although it often is expressed this way.

TABLE 2-1

Equations for Commonly Used Rates*

(1) Crude Birth Rate $=$ $\dfrac{\text{Number of Live Births (Defined Place and Time Period)}}{\text{Midperiod Population (Same Place and Time Period)}} \times 1000$

(2) Crude Death Rate $=$ $\dfrac{\text{Number of Deaths (Defined Place and Time Period)}}{\text{Midperiod Population (Same Place and Time Period)}} \times 1000$

(3) Age-specific Death Rate $=$ $\dfrac{\substack{\text{Number of Deaths to People in a Particular Age Group} \\ \text{(Defined Place and Time Period)}}}{\text{Midperiod Population (Same Age Group, Place, and Time Period)}} \times 1000$

(4) Cause-specific Death Rate $=$ $\dfrac{\substack{\text{Number of Deaths due to a Particular Cause} \\ \text{(Defined Place and Time Period)}}}{\text{Midperiod Population (Same Place and Time Period)}} \times 1000$

(5) Case-Fatality Rate $=$ $\dfrac{\substack{\text{Number of People Who Die of a Disease} \\ \text{(Defined Time and Place)}}}{\text{Total Number of People Who Get the Disease}}$

(6) Proportional Mortality Rate $=$ $\dfrac{\substack{\text{Number of Deaths due to a Specific Disease} \\ \text{in a Specified Time Period}}}{\text{Total Number of Deaths During That Time Period}}$

(7) Infant Mortality Rate $=$ $\dfrac{\substack{\text{Number of Deaths to Infants Under 1 Year of Age} \\ \text{(Defined Place and Time Period)}}}{\text{Number of Live Births (Same Place and Time Period)}} \times 1000$

(8) Neonatal Mortality Rate $=$ $\dfrac{\substack{\text{Number of Deaths to Infants Under 28 Days of Age} \\ \text{(Defined Place and Time Period)}}}{\text{Number of Live Births (Same Place and Time Period)}} \times 1000$

(9) Postneonatal Mortality Rate $=$ $\dfrac{\substack{\text{Number of Deaths to Infants Between 28 and 365 Days of Age} \\ \text{(Defined Place and Time Period)}}}{\substack{\text{Number of Live Births (Same Place and Time Period)} \\ -\text{ Number of Neonatal Deaths (Same Place and Time Period)}}} \times 1000$

(10) Perinatal Mortality Rate $=$ $\dfrac{\substack{\text{Number of Stillbirths (Defined Place and Time Period)} \\ +\text{ Number of Deaths to Infants Under 7 Days of Age} \\ \text{(Same Place and Time Period)}}}{\substack{\text{Number of Stillbirths (Same Place and Time Period)} \\ +\text{ Number of Live Births (Same Place and Time Period)}}} \times 1000$

(11) Maternal Mortality Rate $=$ $\dfrac{\substack{\text{Number of Pregnancy-Related Deaths} \\ \text{(Defined Place and Time Period)}}}{\text{Number of Live Births (Same Place and Time Period)}} \times 100{,}000$

*Adapted from Jekel J, Katz DL, Elmore JG. Epidemiologic data sources and measurements. Box 2-5, page 38. In *Epidemiology, Biostatistics, and Preventive Medicine.* 2nd ed. Philadelphia, Pa: WB Saunders Co; 2001.

CAUSE vs ASSOCIATION

Causative agents may be single, as in the infectious disease model, or a complex cascade of multiple agents, as in chronic disease. Coronary artery disease is a good example of the latter. Smoking, hypertension, diabetes, and hypercholesterolemia all appear to have an important causal role in heart disease. Yet, none appear necessary. This complex "web" of causal factors may prove difficult to untangle, but understanding it is critical to intervention and prevention of disease.

A statistical association of an agent with a disease does not establish it as the cause of the disease. Several criteria increase the probability of a statistical association being causal. Several authors have contributed to these criteria. The criteria include the following:

- *Strength of the association:* This is usually measured in terms of relative risk. Thus, the higher the relative risk of a disease after exposure to an agent, the higher the likelihood of the agent being a cause of the disease.
- *Consistency of the association:* Studies in different populations should demonstrate similar associations between an agent and disease.
- *Specificity of the association:* Absence of exposure to a causal agent should prevent or significantly reduce the occurrence of disease.
- *Biological plausibility:* The association of the risk factor or agent and the disease must make sense based on the natural history of the disease and what is known of the biological activity of the agent.
- *Presence of a dose-response relationship:* Risk of disease is greater with stronger exposure to the risk factor.

In addition, when it is possible to study the temporal relationship of factors or agents, exposure to a causal factor must, logically, precede the disease.

BIAS

Much of what is done in the design of analytic studies is done to avoid *bias*.[2] Bias can be defined as an error in the design or conduct of a study that causes a systematic deviation of the observed result from the true result. Also known as differential or nonrandom error, bias occurs when there is a distortion of a test result that leads to a unidirectional deviation from the mean that cannot be corrected by statistical manipulation. Some of the more common biases are discussed in the following section.

Selection Bias

Selection bias occurs when a treatment population is consistently selected in such a way as to be different from the comparison population before the treatment is carried out. This is illustrated in the randomized clinical trial by Woolf et al,[3] which compares ambulatory patients who consent and do not consent to participate in clinical trials. This study concluded that patients who consented to release personal information for health services research differed significantly from those who did not, thus leading to misinterpretation of outcomes for the general population.

Some common forms of selection bias are Berkson bias and the healthy worker effect.

Berkson bias

First recognized by Berkson[4] in 1946, this bias has been best described where hospital controls are used in a case-control study. If the controls are hospitalized due to an exposure that is also related to the disease under study, then the measure of effect may be weakened.

Healthy worker effect

People who are working are healthier than are people who are not working. Therefore, in case-control studies in which cases are workers, controls should also be workers; otherwise, the association between an exposure and a disease will tend to be biased to the null.

Information (Misclassification) Bias

Information bias occurs when the method of data collection or measurement of variables causes the groups being compared to differ systematically. Some common forms of information bias are recall, measurement, and unacceptability biases.

Recall bias

The problem of recall bias is encountered in case-control studies in which the recall of exposure may differ between cases and controls. An example is a study in which mothers who give birth to babies with congenital anomalies are more likely to remember exposure to medications, infections, and injuries during pregnancy.

Measurement bias

Measurement bias results from incorrect collection of baseline or follow-up measurements. An example is the misclassification of patients based on results of blood pressure machines across different sites that are not calibrated.

Unacceptability bias

An unacceptability bias occurs when patients give what they think will be desirable answers to interviewer's questions. This often is encountered in studies with survey questions related to dietary, exercise, behavioral, and recreational habits.

CONFOUNDING

A variable that has an association with both the disease and the risk factor under study is called a confounding variable. A classic example is that of alcohol, which is a confounding variable in a case-control study evaluating the relationship between smoking and lung cancer. Because people who drink alcohol tend to smoke more, they would also have higher rates of lung cancer. However, alcohol has no causal relationship to lung cancer. It is important to recognize that a confounding variable in a research study may be responsible for part or all of the effect of an alleged variable.

EPIDEMIOLOGIC RESEARCH DESIGN

Study design may depend on many factors, including cost, time for completion, access to medical records, the intent, or the question to be answered. Scientists have developed a rich armamentarium of study designs. They fall into 2 major classes: *observational* studies for generating and testing hypotheses, and *experimental* studies for testing hypotheses.[5]

In an observational study, individuals are observed in their natural state, whereas in an experimental study the investigator has control over an individual's exposure to an intervention or risk factor. Table 2-2 lists the US Preventive Services Task Force system of rating scientific evidence based on outcomes from the various types of studies. Table 2-3 summarizes the advantages and disadvantages of common types of studies.

Observational Studies

The 3 classes of observational studies are the cross-sectional, cohort, and case-control studies.

Cross-sectional study

The cross-sectional study is a descriptive study of a population at a single point in time. If cross-sectional studies are repeated in different groups of individuals, some evidence of temporal changes can be found. This study design has the advantage of being quick and relatively easy to perform. The primary summary measures derived from a cross-sectional study are prevalence of risk factors and diseases. Cross-sectional studies are also particularly suited to measure the health status, needs, and attitudes of a population. The representative samples of the US population chosen for the national surveys conducted by the National Center for Health Statistics[6] (the National Health Interview Survey and the National Health and Nutrition Examination Survey) are examples of cross-sectional studies.

Cross-sectional studies can give estimates of association between diseases or between risk factors and diseases. If the risk factor does not change over time (eg, a person's sex), the cross-sectional survey can provide a valid estimate of the statistical association between the factor and disease. For a risk (exposure) factor that changes over time, the cross-sectional study may not be able to determine the temporal relationship between the exposure and the disease. Another disadvantage is that the cross-sectional study selects for longer-lasting and more indolent cases. This phenomenon, also known as *Neyman* or *late-look bias,* occurs because severe diseases that tend to be rapidly fatal are less likely to be found in a cross-sectional survey.

Prospective cohort study

In a prospective cohort study, the investigator follows a group of individuals without disease until they develop disease or the study ends. Depending on the study question, a prospective study also may begin with individuals who already have disease and follow them until they reach an outcome, such as death. The prospective cohort study is most useful to define risk factors or to describe the natural history of the disease process. A classic example of a prospective cohort study is the Framingham Heart Study, which selected a sample of 5127 men and women from Framingham, Mass, who were free of coronary heart disease in 1952.[7] These individuals have been periodically reexamined since that time.

Retrospective cohort study

In a retrospective cohort study, the investigator examines data, disease, or outcome occurrence in individuals who have had a particular exposure or etiologic characteristic of interest.[8] In this case, the investigator goes back into historical records to select individuals based on their exposure status or the absence or presence of risk factors. An example is a retrospective study comparing mortality rates of lung cancer among asbestos workers and cotton textile workers.[9] The study populations were identified from tax forms that were filed between 1948 and 1951.

TABLE 2-2

USPSTF Rating System of Quality of Scientific Evidence*

I.	Evidence from at least one well-designed randomized controlled trial
II-1.	Evidence from well-designed controlled trials without randomization
II-2.	Evidence from well-designed cohort or case-control studies
II-3.	Evidence from multiple time series with or without intervention, or dramatic results in uncontrolled experiments
III.	Descriptive studies, expert opinion, expert panel consensus

*Adapted from *The Clinician's Handbook of Preventive Services.* 2nd ed. Rockville, Md: Dept of Health and Human Services, US Public Health Service; 1998. USPSTF indicates US Preventive Services Task Force.

Case-control study

In case-control studies, individuals are classified by their disease status or condition (cases have disease; controls do not have disease). The investigator then examines if the cases and controls differ with respect to a given exposure or etiologic characteristic.[10] An example is a study examining the association of the measles-mumps-rubella vaccination and the subsequent development of autism.[11] In carrying out a case-control study, several important issues must be considered, including selection of cases, selection of controls, and measurement of the risk factors, as all of these can be sources of bias.

A special category of case-control studies is the *nested case-control study.* Once sufficient outcomes have accrued in a cohort study, diseased individuals can be compared with those free from disease (cases compared with controls), and exposure status of both cases and controls can be compared. Nested studies are most often used when a potential confounder is identified in the initial analysis as an important determinant of excess disease risk. An example is a study demonstrating consistent high viral load of human papilloma virus 16 as a risk of developing cervical carcinoma in situ.[12]

Experimental Studies

The best way to avoid many biases, both known and unknown, is to use concurrent controls whereby patients are randomized to receive either the new treatment or no treatment ("usual care"). This type of study is called a *randomized, controlled clinical trial.*[13-16] Careful randomization with adequate numbers of subjects should create 2 or more groups with the same underlying characteristics, thereby reducing the likelihood of bias by ensuring that the only difference between the groups is the variable of interest (eg, the treatment under study).

Another feature of the randomized study that can help avoid biases is blinding or masking. In a *double-blind study,* neither the investigator nor the patient knows the assignment of the intervention. This approach is often possible in drug trials in which placebo pills can be given to patients but is less feasible with surgical or nutritional interventions. In a *single-blind study,* the investigator alone knows the treatment assignment.

In many real-world studies, people randomized to the treatment arm may not follow through with some or all of the treatments, potentially making an effective

T A B L E 2-3

Comparison of Different Study Designs*

Type of Study	Advantages	Disadvantages
Cohort study	Evaluate temporal relationships Direct measurement of disease and risks Necessary if incidence rates are needed from the study Minimizes bias in determining exposure Valuable when exposure or risk factor is rare Valuable for evaluation of multiple outcomes	Large sample size Lengthy follow-up may be necessary Loss of follow-up can bias results May be expensive to conduct Cannot control for unmeasured confounding
Case-control study	Small sample size Less expensive Useful when disease is rare or has long latent period Ability to evaluate multiple etiologic factors for a single disease	Bias in measurement of risk factors Choice of controls is difficult Only 1 endpoint or outcome Temporal relationship difficult to establish Evaluation of only a few risk factors
Randomized, controlled trial	Gold standard of research design Maximizes internal validity Equal distribution of potential confounders in study groups	Generally lengthy and expensive Blinding may be difficult Ascertainment bias Loss of subjects due to follow-up, dropouts, and crossover may influence study results Ethical and legal issues External validity may not be strong

*Adapted from Beck GJ. The clinical application of epidemiology and the interpretation of diagnostic tests. In: Matzen RN, Lang RS, eds. *Clinical Preventive Medicine.* St Louis, Mo: Mosby; 1993:97–108.

investigational treatment appear less so. Nevertheless, when an investigator includes all of the subjects in the group to which they were randomly assigned, whether or not they completed treatment, the analysis is said to be carried out by *intention to treat.* This is considered more intellectually rigorous and a better reflection of the net benefit of applying a new treatment to a whole population.

A modification of the randomized controlled trial is the *crossover design,* in which each person acts as his or her own control by receiving both the intervention and control arms of the study, but at different time points in time.[17] This type of study is particularly useful when outcome is measured by subjective symptoms (eg, relief of pain from analgesics). The order in which treatment is given is randomized so that patients receive it in different sequence. Outcome is measured at the end of each period of treatment. This study design is feasible only if the outcome is immediate and there is no carry-over effect from having received an intervention.

In a *quasi-experimental study,* the investigator controls the assignment of the intervention or treatment to a particular study arm. Because the assignment is not random, these studies have problems with potential selection bias and confounding. Examples of quasi-experimental studies include preintervention and postintervention trials.

Other special study designs include the factorial design and meta-analysis. In a *factorial design study,* a simultaneous study of more than one type of treatment or intervention is conducted.[18,19] The primary advantage of a factorial design is that 2 hypotheses can be addressed at once. However, if an unknown interaction exists between the 2 factors or the factors and disease being studied, the results may be misleading or not useful.

Another study that has become popular in the past decade is the *meta-analysis.*[20] It is useful in summarizing information obtained in multiple single studies on one topic. The researcher identifies all studies of similar design on a subject for which data on the characteristics of participants and endpoints are published. The data are combined and analyzed quantitatively as if they were all 1 study. If properly done, the meta-analysis may have substantially more power to answer a research question than do any of the individual studies. Meta-analyses can be helpful in studies of cost-effectiveness and decision analysis for clinical or policy decisions.

RISK

Risk is the characteristic of a disease that is often most important in prevention. Fundamental assessment of risk in epidemiologic studies can be understood by means of a 2×2 table. This table, which relates exposure status to disease status, is depicted in Table 2-4. In this table, $a + b$ represents individuals who are exposed or have the risk factor and $c + d$ represents individuals without exposure. Thus, the incidence of disease in exposed individuals is $a/(a + b)$, and that in the unexposed group is $c/(c + d)$. In case-control studies, risk ratios (relative risk) cannot be calculated directly but must be estimated from the odds ratio, whereas cohort and randomized controlled trials allow calculation of both relative and absolute risk.

Relative risk, or risk ratio, is the ratio of the incidence of the disease or other outcome of interest in subjects exposed to a particular risk factor, to the incidence of the outcome among subjects who were not exposed to the risk factor. If the relative risk is less than 1, the exposure reduces the risk of disease (ie, it is protective). The equations for relative risk and other risk calculations are given in Table 2-5.

Odds ratio is the odds of exposure in the disease group divided by the odds of exposure in the nondiseased group. When the disease is rare (affecting <5% of the population), the odds ratio is a good estimate of the relative risk. Similar to the relative risk, an odds ratio equal to 1 indicates that there is no association between the exposure (or risk factor) and the disease or outcome. Values greater than 1 indicate an increased risk of disease with exposure, and values less than 1 indicate a decreased risk of disease with exposure.

Attributable risk is the difference between the incidence of disease in the individuals with the risk factor (exposed) and those without (unexposed). Attributable risk is of particular interest to the health planner, as it gives the absolute percentage of individuals in whom the disease develops after exposure. This measure accounts for the baseline incidence of disease and calculates the absolute amount of excess risk in an individual. It is also useful in CPM, health promotion, and preventive counseling, to demonstrate how much modifying a risk factor may reduce risk of disease. The reciprocal of attributable risk is called the *number needed to treat* and provides a useful measure of the number of people that would need to be treated (or number in whom a risk factor

TABLE 2-4

Two-by-Two Table for Computation of Risk*

		Disease	
		Present	Absent
Risk	Present	a	b
factor	Absent	c	d

*a indicates subjects with both the risk factor and the disease;
b, individuals with the risk factor, but not the disease;
c, individuals with the disease but not the risk factor; and
d, individuals with neither the risk factor nor the disease.

would need to be modified) to gain 1 additional outcome (typically a life saved or a disease avoided).

Other useful measures of risk include the *attributable risk percent,* which is the proportion of disease among the individuals with the risk factor (exposed) that is due to the risk factor. In other words, if the exposure could be discontinued, the risk of disease would be reduced by this percent. The *population attributable risk* is the rate of disease in the population that is due to the exposure to the risk factor, and the *population attributable risk percent* is the proportion of cases of disease that is due to a certain risk factor. Thus, it is the amount of disease that would be prevented if the risk factor could be eliminated from the population. By using the population attributable risk percent, health services policy analysts are able to calculate the impact of preventive policies. Once the costs and benefits are known, optimal allocation of resources can be determined using cost-benefit and cost-effectiveness analyses.

CHARACTERISTICS OF TESTS

Tests are part of the day-to-day practice of CPM. How well a test performs and how well it is used has much to do with the user understanding its characteristics. The *accuracy* of a screening or diagnostic test relates to its ability in correctly identifying the presence or absence of disease. *Precision (reproducibility or reliability)* is the ability of a test to give the same result or a very similar result with repeated measurements at the same time or on the same sample. Because some individuals may be classified as having or not having the disease on the basis of the diagnostic test, it is crucial to reduce the rate of misclassifications or errors. *Type 1 error* (false-positive or alpha error) occurs when data indicate the presence of disease when, in fact, there is none. *Type II error* (false-negative or beta error) occurs when data indicate the absence of disease when there is disease.

Validity is the extent to which a test measures what it is designed to measure. Validity has 2 important components. The first is *sensitivity,* which is the ability of a test to correctly identify individuals with a specific disease or outcome of interest. The second is *specificity,* which is the measure of the ability of a test to correctly identify individuals who do not have the disease or outcome of interest. Other measures that are important include the *false-positive rate,* which is the proportion of individuals who do not have the disease but test positive for it; and the *false-negative rate,* which is defined as the proportion of individuals who have the disease yet test

T A B L E   2-5

Risk Calculations

Relative Risk	$= \dfrac{\text{Incidence in Exposed Persons}}{\text{Incidence in Unexposed Persons}}$	$= \dfrac{\frac{a}{(a+b)}}{\frac{c}{(c+d)}}$
Odds Ratio (OR)	$= \dfrac{\frac{a}{b}}{\frac{c}{d}}$	$= \dfrac{ad}{bc}$
Attributable Risk	$= \text{Incidence in Exposed} - \text{Incidence in Unexposed}$	$= \dfrac{a}{(a+b)} - \dfrac{c}{(c+d)}$
Number Needed to Treat	$= \dfrac{1}{\text{Attributable Risk}}$	
Attributable Risk Percent	$= \dfrac{\text{Incidence in Exposed} - \text{Incidence in Unexposed}}{\text{Incidence in Exposed}}$	$= \dfrac{\frac{a}{(a+b)} - \frac{c}{(c+d)}}{\frac{a}{(a+b)}}$
Population Attributable Risk	$= \text{Total Incidence} - \text{Incidence in Unexposed}$	$= \dfrac{(a+c)}{(a+b+c+d)} - \dfrac{c}{(c+d)}$
Population Attributable Risk Percent	$= \dfrac{\text{Total Incidence} - \text{Incidence in Unexposed}}{\text{Total Incidence}}$	$= \dfrac{\frac{(a+c)}{(a+b+c+d)} - \frac{c}{(c+d)}}{\frac{a+c}{(a+b+c+d)}}$
or	$= \dfrac{OR - 1}{OR} \times \dfrac{a}{(a+c)}$	

negative for it. The calculations and interrelationships of these test characteristics are shown in Table 2-6.

Many diagnostic tests are based on a continuous measurement, such as serum prostate-specific antigen (PSA) or serum glucose level. In such cases, there is need for a single value that would best separate disease from no disease or abnormal from normal. Figure 2-1 illustrates the effect of the cutoff point as well as sensitivity, specificity, and false-positive and false-negative rates for a diagnostic test. The 2 curves in the figure represent the frequency distribution of the test value in the populations with the disease and without the disease. Few tests perfectly discriminate between normal and abnormal, and hence there is overlap between the 2 graphs. If the cutoff point is moved to the left (lower test value), the sensitivity of the test would be increased but the specificity would be decreased, and vice versa. This points out the limitations of using a single diagnostic test for making a definitive diagnosis.[21] In general, pairing a test with high sensitivity (a high true-positive rate) to screen and a test with high specificity (a high true-negative rate) to confirm is desirable.

Receiver Operating Characteristic Curve

The *receiver operating characteristic (ROC) curve*[22-24] is used by investigators to summarize the overall accuracy of a test regardless of the cutoff point. The true-positive probability is plotted on the y-axis, and the false-positive probability that arises from every possible cutoff point is plotted on the x-axis (Fig 2-2). If the diagnostic test is no better than chance in determining disease (ie, the true-positive rate equals the false-positive rate), the ROC curve would follow the "no benefit line" and the area under the curve would be equal to 0.5. For a test, it is desirable that the true-positive rate is close to 1 and the false-positive rate is very small. In this case, the ROC curve would rise steeply toward the upper left hand corner, as shown in the graph. Perfect accuracy would be depicted if the area under the curve were equal to 1. Thus, the area under the curve can be used as a basis for comparing 2 different diagnostic tests on their ability to discriminate between those with and without disease. An example of the use of ROC curves has been well described in radiologic imaging.[25]

Predictive Value of a Test

The most important feature of a test to a clinician is often how good the test is in predicting the true outcome of interest in the absence of the knowledge regarding the true disease status. The *positive predictive value* (PPV) of a test is the probability that the individual really has disease when the test result is positive, or abnormal. The *negative predictive value* (NPV) of a test is the probability that the individual truly does not have disease

TABLE 2-6

Two-by-Two Table for Hypothesis Testing*

Test		Disease	
		Present	Absent
	Positive	a	b
	Negative	c	d

Sensitivity $= \dfrac{a}{(a + c)}$

Specificity $= \dfrac{d}{(b + d)}$

False-positive rate $= \dfrac{b}{(b + d)}$

False-negative rate $= \dfrac{c}{(a + c)}$

Sensitivity $= 1 - \text{false negative rate}$

Specificity $= 1 - \text{false positive rate}$

Positive predictive value $= \dfrac{a}{(a + b)}$

Negative predictive value $= \dfrac{d}{(b + d)}$

Prevalence $= \dfrac{(a + c)}{(a + b + c + d)}$

Accuracy $= \dfrac{(a + d)}{(a + b + c + d)}$

*a indicates individuals with a true-positive result; b, individuals with a false-positive test result; c, individuals with a false-negative test result; and d, individuals with a true-negative test result.

if the test result is negative, or normal. The predictive value of a test depends on the sensitivity and specificity as well as the prevalence of disease in the population to which the test is being applied. If the population has a high disease prevalence (assuming a high sensitivity and specificity), the positive predictive value approaches 100% and the negative predictive value approaches 0. The reverse is true if the disease prevalence is low. The relationship between predictive value and sensitivity, specificity, and prevalence is derived from Bayes theorem and is shown below.

$$PPV = \frac{(\text{Prevalence})(\text{Sensitivity})}{(\text{Prevalence})(\text{Sensitivity}) + (1 - \text{Prevalence})(1 - \text{Specificity})}$$

$$NPV = \frac{(\text{Prevalence})(\text{Sensitivity})}{(1 - \text{Prevalence})(\text{Sensitivity}) + (\text{Prevalence})(1 - \text{Specificity})}$$

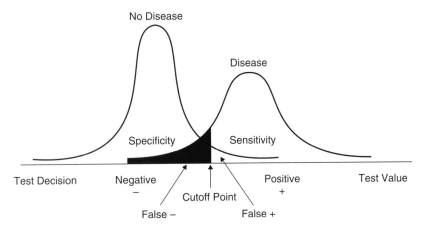

F I G U R E 2-1

Validity of test and its relationship to cutoff point.

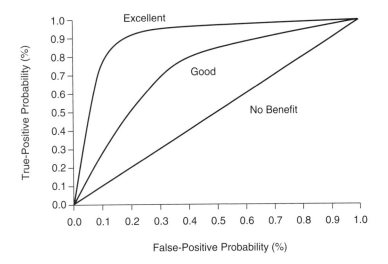

F I G U R E 2-2

Receiver operating characteristic, or ROC, curve.

Thus, the positive predictive value of a test can be increased by increasing the specificity. Negative predictive value, on the other hand, can be increased by increasing the sensitivity. These relationships are important in interpreting the results of a diagnostic test or implementing a screening program. Increasing disease prevalence by screening higher risk individuals or using a very sensitive screening test to "enrich the prevalence" will improve the positive predictive value.

SAMPLING

It is usually difficult and unnecessary to study a whole population to obtain useful and valid information about the population. The investigation of a sample from the population reduces the number of individuals who have to be investigated. However, it is important to ensure adequate sample size and choose a sample that is representative of the parent population. Some commonly

used sampling methods are the simple random sample, systematic sample, and cluster sampling.

Simple Random Sample

Each individual in the study population has an equal chance of being selected in a simple random sample. Computer-generated random numbers can be used to decide which individuals should be included.

Systematic Sample

Individuals are selected at regular intervals from a list of the total population in a systematic sample. For example, every fifth patient visiting a particular preventive medicine clinic in March is selected for a pertinent study. This type of sampling is easier and more convenient for individuals performing the investigation but is slightly more prone to bias than randomized sampling.

Cluster Sampling

In cluster sampling, groups are selected for sampling as opposed to individuals. This is particularly useful to ensure that small subgroups of particular interest to the investigator are adequately represented. The subgroup is identified and sampled at a predetermined rate different from other subgroups. Cluster sampling may be used to study the effects of an intervention applied to a group, such as community education in a particular neighborhood.

HYPOTHESIS TESTING

One of the most important concepts in biostatistics is hypothesis testing. Based on results obtained from sample studies and by means of hypothesis testing, a scientist can make inferences about a variable of interest in a population. By convention, the *null hypothesis* states that there is no association between the variables under study. Also, by convention, the existence of a meaningful association between the variables under study is considered the *alternate hypothesis.* Tests of significance are used to reject or not reject the null hypothesis. If the tests of significance suggest that a difference is real and not due to chance, the null hypothesis is rejected. The significance of the test of the null hypothesis is summarized in the P value. The P *value* is the probability that the observed difference in outcome is obtained by chance. For more details on the P value, refer to the book by Ingelfinger et al.[26]

The 2 important principles regarding the P value are as follows:

1. If $P<0.05$, the null hypothesis is rejected. This means that the data suggest a strong evidence against the null hypothesis. Traditionally, scientists have been willing to accept a false positive error rate of 5%, ie, when $P<0.05$, there is a 5% risk of rejecting the null hypothesis when it is true.

2. If $P>0.05$, null hypothesis is not rejected, suggesting that there is no strong evidence in the data against the null hypothesis. This could reflect the lack of a true relationship between the variables under study as suggested by the null hypothesis. However, it may also simply reflect that the study does not have enough power (small sample size).

The second method of evaluating the significance of a test is by calculating a *confidence interval* on the relative risk or the odds ratio.[27,28] The size of the confidence interval gives a measure of the estimate of the relative risk or odds ratio that is consistent with the data. If the confidence interval includes the value 1.0, it implies that there is no statistically significant association between the 2 variables being studied; that is, the null hypothesis is not rejected.

The probability that a study will detect a defined difference if it truly exists is called *power.* Commonly, a power of 80% is acceptable and is used to determine the size of the sample needed in the study. It is important to understand that if the sample size is too small, no statistical significance may be found even in the presence of a clinically significant association. On the other hand, if the sample size is too large, a very small statistically significant (but clinically insignificant) association could be detected.

NORMAL DISTRIBUTION

The *normal* or *gaussian distribution* is a theoretical probability distribution. It is represented by an idealized bell shape, called a normal curve, which is symmetrical about the same point represented by the mean, median, and mode and extends to infinity in both directions. The dispersion from the mean or spread is represented by the standard deviation (SD). Sixty-eight percent of the data fall within 1 SD of the mean, 95% of the data within 2 SDs of the mean, and 99% of the data within 3 SDs of the mean (Fig 2-3).

Commonly used statistical tests of significance vary by the type of variable under consideration. *Nominal variables* are named or categorical variables that do not have a measurement scale (eg, ethnicity, blood group). *Ordinal variables* are variables that can be ranked, but are not measured on a continuous measurement scale (eg, satisfaction with an episode of care). *Dichotomous variables* are variables that can have only two outcomes (eg, success/failure). Continuous variables are variables in which data can be measured over the range of an uninterrupted scale (eg, height, weight). Commonly used tests of statistical significance as well as their uses are listed in Table 2-7.

EVIDENCE-BASED MEDICINE

In the 1980s, the practice of evidence-based medicine as a new paradigm took shape. In 1992, the Evidence-Based Medicine Working Group published a description of this practice.[29] They outlined a set of skills that required the following:

- An understanding of basic pathophysiologic mechanisms of disease
- Clinical experience and skills
- Caution regarding a practice based only on experience, expert opinion, or pathophysiologic understanding of disease in the absence of systematic observation
- Efficient literature-searching skills
- Application of formal rules of evidence in critical appraisal of the literature

In clinical medicine, this practice follows a process of:

1. Defining a patient-centered problem—for example, should this patient have PSA blood testing?
2. Performing an efficient literature search
3. Selecting the best and most applicable articles

4. Applying critical analysis skills to the studies to see whether they provide valid evidence to apply to a specific patient

5. Applying the evidence gathered from the literature in combination with clinical experience and knowledge

6. Communicating this information empathically to the patient

7. Making a clinical decision

This new paradigm for practice was enabled by a combination of factors, including the increased recognition and use of the randomized controlled clinical trials and the advent of computerized literature searching. Its growth and acceptance are fueled by an increasingly educated patient population interested in being actively involved in their own health care decision making. The practice of evidence-based medicine has been substantially aided by systematic efforts at critical appraisal of the literature on a specific question, such as the Cochrane Database of Systematic Reviews produced by the Cochrane Collaboration.[30]

REFERENCES

1. Jekel J, Katz DL, Elmore JG. Epidemiologic data source and measurements. In: *Epidemiology, Biostatistics, and Preventive Medicine.* 2nd ed. Philadelphia, Pa: WB Saunders Co; 2001:20–42.

2. Fletcher RH, Fletcher SW, Wagner EH. Chapter 1: Introduction. In: Fletcher RH, Fletcher SW, Wagner EH,

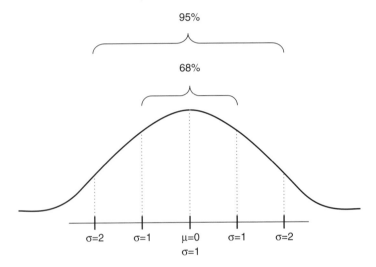

FIGURE 2-3

Normal curve.

TABLE 2-7

Indications for specific tests of significance*

Variables to be tested		Test of Significance
Continuous	Continuous	Pearson correlation coefficient; linear regression
Continuous	Ordinal	Spearman's correlation coefficient
Continuous	Dichotomous unpaired	Student's t test
Continuous	Dichotomous paired	Paired t test
Continuous	Nominal	ANOVA (analysis of variance)
Ordinal	Ordinal	Spearman's correlation coefficient; Kendall correlation coefficient
Ordinal	Dichotomous unpaired	Mann-Whitney U test
Ordinal	Dichotomous paired	Wilcoxon matched pairs, signed rank tests
Ordinal	Nominal	Kruskal-Wallis test
Dichotomous	Dichotomous unpaired	Chi-square test; Fischer's exact test
Dichotomous	Dichotomous paired	McNemar chi-square test
Dichotomous	Nominal	Chi-square test
Nominal	Nominal	Chi-square test

*Adapted from Jekel J, Katz DL, Elmore JG. Bivariate Analysis. Table 11-1, page 173. In *Epidemiology, Biostatistics, and Preventive Medicine.* 2nd edition. 2001; W.B. Saunders eds. *Clinical Epidemiology: the essentials.* 3rd ed. Baltimore, Md: Williams & Wilkins; 1996:1–18

3. Woolf SH, Rothemich SF, Johnson RE, Marsland DW. Selection bias from requiring patients to give consent to examine data for health services research. *Arch Fam Med.* 2000;9:1111–1118.

4. Berkson J. Limitations of the application of a fourfold table analysis to hospital data. *Biometrics Bull.* 1946;2:47–53.

5. Szklo M, Nieto FJ. *Basic Study Designs in Analytical Epidemiology: Epidemiology Beyond the Basics.* New York, NY: Aspen Publishers; 2000:3–53.

6. Centers for Disease Control and Prevention. National Center for Health Statistics Web site. Available at: www.cdc.gov/nchs/. Accessed April 14, 2003.

7. Dawber TR. *The Framingham Study: The Epidemiology of Atherosclerotic Disease.* Cambridge, Mass: Harvard University Press; 1980.

8. Hennekens CH, Buring JE. *Epidemiology in Medicine.* Boston, Mass: Little Brown & Co; 1987.

9. Enterline PE. Mortality among asbestos product workers in the US. *Ann NY Acad Sci.* 1965;132:156.

10. Schlesselman JJ. *Case-controlled Studies: Design, Conduct, Analysis.* New York, NY: Oxford University Press; 1982.

11. Smeeth L, Hall AJ, Rodrigues LC, Huang X, Smith PG, Fombonne E. A case-control study of autism and mumps-measles-rubella vaccination using the general practice research database: design and methodology. *BMC Public Health.* 2001;1:2.

12. Ylitalo N, Sorensen P, Josefsson AM, et al. Consistent high viral load of human papillomavirus 16 and risk of cervical carcinoma in situ. A nested case-control study. *Lancet.* 2000;355:2194–2198.

13. Friedman LM, Furberg CD, DeMets DL. *Fundamentals of Clinical Trials.* 2nd ed. Littleton, Mass: PSG Publishing Co; 1985.

14. Meiner CL. *Clinical Trials: Design, Conduct and Analysis.* New York, NY: Oxford University Press; 1989.

15. Peto R, Pike MC, Armitage P, Breslow NE, Cox DR, Howard SV, Mantel N, McPherson K, Peto J, Smith PG. Design and analysis of randomized clinical trials requiring prolonged observation of each patient. I. Introduction and design. *Br J Cancer.* 1976;34:585–612.

16. Peto R, Pike MC, Armitage P, Breslow NE, Cox DR, Howard SV, Mantel N, McPherson K, Peto J, Smith PG. Design and analysis of randomized clinical trials requiring prolonged observation of each patient. II. Analysis and Examples. *Br J Cancer.* 1977;35:1–39.

17. Louis TA, Lavori PW, Bailar JC III, Polansky M. Crossover and self-controlled designs in clinical research. *N Engl J Med.* 1984;310:24–31.

18. Brittian E, Wittes J. Factorial designs in clinical trials: the effects of non-compliance and subadditivity. *Stat Med.* 1989;8:161–171.

19. Hung HMJ. Evaluation of a combination drug with multiple doses in unbalanced factorial design clinical trial. *Stat Med.* 2000 Aug 30;19(16):2079–87.

20. Stroup DF, Berlin JA, Morton SC, et al. Meta-analysis of observational studies in epidemiology. *JAMA.* 2000;283:2008–2012.

21. Beck GJ. The clinical application of epidemiology and the interpretation of diagnostic tests. In: Matzen RN, Lang RS, eds. *Clinical Preventive Medicine.* St Louis, Mo: Mosby; 1993:97–108.

22. Erdreich LS, Lee ET. Use of relative operating characteristic analysis in epidemiology. *Am J Epidemiol.* 1981;114:649–662.

23. Metz CE. Basic principles of ROC analysis. *Semin Nucl Med.* 1978;8:283–298.

24. Sackett DL, Haynes RB, Guyatt GH, Tugwell P. The interpretation of diagnostic data. In: Sackett DL, Haynes RB, Guyatt GH, Tugwell P, eds. *Clinical Epidemiology: A Basic Science for Clinical Medicine.* Boston: Little, Brown; 1991:69–152

25. Swets JA. ROC analysis applied to the evaluation of medical imaging techniques. *Invest Radiol.* 1979;4:109–121.

26. Ingelfinger JA, Mosteller F, Thibodeau LA, Ware JH. *Biostatistics in Clinical Medicine.* 2nd ed. New York, NY: Macmillan Publishing Co Inc; 1987.

27. Kahn HA, Sempos CT. *Statistical Methods in Epidemiology.* New York, NY: Oxford University Press; 1989.

28. Norman GR, Streiner DL. Statistical interference. In: Norman GR, Streiner DL, eds. *PDQ Statistics.* BC Decker Inc, Hamilton, Ontario and Philadelphia; 1986:27–41.

29. Evidence-Based Medicine Working Group. Evidence-based medicine. *JAMA.* 1992;268:2420–2425.

30. The Cochrane Collaboration Web site. Available at: www.cochrane.org. Accessed April 14, 2003.

RESOURCES

Fletcher RH, Fletcher SW, Wagner EH. *Clinical epidemiology: the essentials.* 3rd ed. Baltimore, Md: Williams & Wilkins; 1996.

Jekel J, Katz DL, Elmore JG. *Epidemiology, Biostatistics, and Preventive Medicine.* 2nd ed. Philadelphia, Pa: WB Saunders; 2001.

Ingelfinger JA, et al: *Biostatistics in clinical medicine.* 2nd ed. New York: Macmillan; 1987.

Centers for Disease Control
www.cdc.gov/nchs/

The Cochrane Collaboration
www.cochrane.org/

chapter 3

Practical Office-Based Preventive Medicine and Delivery Systems

Sidna M. Scheitel, MD, MPH, and Rajeev Chaudhry, MD, MPH

INTRODUCTION

Primary care physicians usually agree that delivery of preventive services is important for their patients.[1] However, they have not been successful in fully implementing published guidelines into their clinical practices.[2-4] The reported delivery rates of adult preventive services range from 20% to 70%.[1,5] There are 140,000 new cases of colorectal cancer and 56,700 deaths in the United States annually,[6] but only 25% to 35% of eligible patients receive colon cancer screening.[7] Not having enough time during busy clinical encounters is an important reason cited by physicians for their inability to deliver preventive services.[8,9] However, some primary care physicians have been able to deliver preventive services during busy encounters when they have implemented systems to ensure that the patients are offered preventive services.[10]

This chapter discusses barriers to delivering preventive services and introduces the Chronic Care Model as a framework for improving the delivery of preventive services. Individual components of the Chronic Care Model are reviewed: community resources and policies, self-management support, design of delivery systems, decision support, and clinical information systems. At the end of the chapter, a nonrandomized case study from Austin Medical Center, "Project 90 by 2000," is reviewed as an example of using some of the concepts discussed in the chapter to improve preventive services.

BARRIERS TO DELIVERING PREVENTIVE HEALTH CARE

Many barriers interfere with the delivery of preventive care. In one study, physicians indicated that the reasons for noncompliance with appropriate office reminders were the physician's lack of time and the patient's beliefs about the need for preventive care or the patient's fear of preventive care.[11] "Competing Demands of Primary Care" is a model proposed by Jaén and colleagues[12] to illustrate the barriers to delivering clinical preventive services. A similar model was described by Frame[13] in 1992. Both models categorize barriers into 3 subsets: (1) physician, (2) patient, and (3) practice environment or health system barriers (Fig 3-1). The existence of these barriers stresses the need for the development of a new model of care to improve the delivery of preventive services.

CHRONIC CARE MODEL

The model for the delivery of health care remained fairly consistent throughout the 20th century. The current model was developed and organized around the diagnosis and treatment of acute conditions and symptoms, but it is not optimal for the delivery of preventive services. Instead, the Chronic Care Model was proposed as a framework to improve the delivery of both chronic disease management and preventive services by providing evidence-based, population-based, patient-centered care (Fig 3-2).[14]

The interactions between patients and clinicians that are required for improving the delivery of preventive services are similar to those required for improving the management of chronic diseases. In the Chronic Care Model, "productive interactions" lead to (1) patients receiving interventions that are effective and (2) patients and families receiving the information, behavioral support, and continuity of care that they need. Before these interactions can be productive, however, patients must be informed and "activated." They must be able to manage their health confidently and know how to use the health care system. Similarly, clinicians and their practice teams must be prepared and proactive. They must have the information, resources, and time to provide effective interventions.

The model is divided into community and health system interventions because social-environmental factors influence lifestyle. Community interventions include the use of resources to remove barriers that prevent community members from receiving preventive care and to influence the long-term success of preventive care

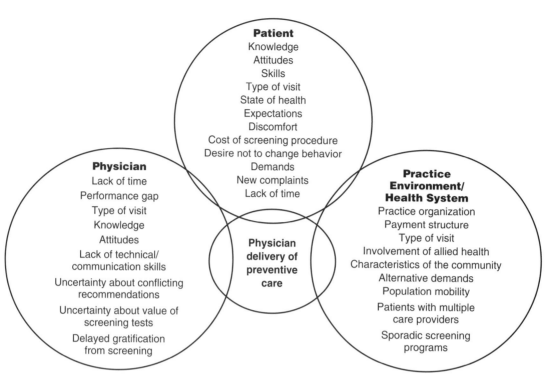

F IGURE 3-1

Barriers to clinical prevention. Modified from Jaén et al[12] and Frame.[13] By permission of Dowden Health Media and the American Academy of Family Physicians.

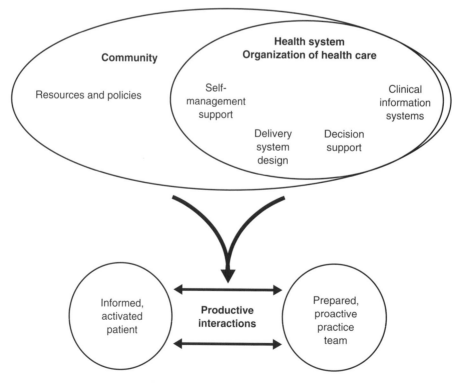

Functional and clinical outcomes

F IGURE 3-2

Components of Chronic Care Model. From Glasgow et al.[14] By permission of Milbank Memorial Fund.

programs by changing social-environmental factors. Health system interventions include the following elements:

1. Self-management support refers to helping patients understand that they are part of the process. They need to understand that their participation is crucial in establishing attainable, worthwhile goals.

2. The practice team must have clinical information systems, which give members of the team access to patient-specific information.

3. The practice team must also have decision support—that is, relevant clinical knowledge.

4. Delivery system design refers to how information is used. A practice team needs more than knowledge and patient data. The team must work within a system that is designed to improve the performance of the team by improving, for example, the appointment system and the mechanisms for ensuring continuity of care.

5. Ultimately, the health system infrastructure relies on the support of the health care organization's leadership.

INTERVENTIONS FOR IMPROVING DELIVERY OF PREVENTIVE SERVICES

The following section reviews effective interventions for improving the delivery of preventive services. In addition, practical advice is available in a comprehensive manual, *Clinician's Handbook of Preventive Services: Put Prevention Into Practice.*[15]

Community Resources and Policies

Let us consider 2 vantage points that societies have used to address health and disease: (1) to provide healers to care for the sick and (2) to prevent disease from occurring. Traditionally, the healers consisted of physicians, and the promotion of healthful conditions in the community was spearheaded by public health agencies.[16] In the past decade, the activities of the medical and public health sectors have merged for the following reasons:

1. It is generally recognized that tobacco use, unhealthful diet and physical activity patterns, alcohol abuse, high-risk sexual behaviors, motor vehicle crashes, and illicit use of drugs are responsible for up to 50% of premature deaths.[17]

2. Expanded coverage for clinical preventive services has been provided by private and federal insurance programs.

3. Purchasers of health care services for organizations require reports on quality indicators that are mostly composed of clinical preventive services.[18]

4. Physicians have shifted from solo practices to group practices and networks that can devote resources to preventive services during clinical encounters. This also has reduced the number of independent medical practitioners with whom a public health agency interacts.[19]

A strategy for successful community health initiatives is summarized in the following 8 steps:

1. Assess data to recognize opportunities for improvement.

2. Organize a multidisciplinary team.

3. Launch a media campaign to educate the public.

4. Reorganize clinical practice to facilitate delivery of preventive services and improve access.

5. Establish reward systems to provide incentives for health promotion.

6. Influence health system policy to provide financial resources for preventive services and encourage healthy lifestyles.

7. Analyze the results and consider again the initiatives (as part of the "plan, do, study, act" cycle).

8. Report successful strategies.

The third step, launching a community media campaign, is especially important. For every prevention initiative to succeed, public education is critical. Education may emphasize topics related to personal behavior, such as smoking, illicit drug or alcohol use, diet and activity, injury prevention (eg, wearing a helmet while biking), not driving while under the influence of alcohol, and sexual activity. Cancer screenings and immunizations may also be topics in the campaigns. The spokesperson is usually a public health official, celebrity, or respected practicing physician whose recommendations the public trusts. The message usually is delivered in newspaper articles, on radio and television talk shows, and by flyers and posters at workplaces, grocery stores, schools, and churches. The message should advise not only about personal behavior but also about how to access services such as cancer screening or immunization. Web-based sites are increasingly important, relatively inexpensive tools in media campaigns.

Self-Management Support

Before a preventive medicine plan can be effective, the process of "patient activation" must occur; patients must understand that they need preventive services and must seek the services.[20] Their behavior toward preventive screening is a product of tangible and attitudinal variables. The tangible variables include available information, prompts that they receive, access to care, and affordability of care. The attitudinal variables include the patient's perception of the information, the task required to accomplish the goal, and the patient's abilities to accomplish the task.

The Health Belief Model, which addresses factors influencing health behaviors,[21] is based on the following principles of social learning theory:

1. Perceptions influence behavior.
2. Perceptions can be changed by new input.
3. Changes in perceptions can lead to changes in behavior.

In this model, patients decide to act on preventive health recommendations because of perceptions called health beliefs. These health beliefs include whether patients are concerned about their health and believe that they have control over health outcomes. Health beliefs also include whether patients believe any of the following: (1) the information about the disease is valid, (2) they are susceptible to the disease, (3) the severity of the disease is great enough to warrant overcoming any barriers to taking action, and (4) the action would be beneficial. Patients are most likely to take preventive action if they have the combination of health beliefs described in Table 3-1. Compliance was higher for breast cancer screening by mammography when patients received an intervention including information about mammography and individually tailored belief counseling.[22]

Various patient education materials are available. For example, posters were placed in examination rooms and restrooms in our primary care ambulatory practices at Mayo Clinic in Rochester, Minnesota. The messages on the posters (approved by our colleagues) included recommendations for preventive service. After the posters were displayed, patients began asking their physicians about preventive services. Additional educational materials included informational brochures on screening tests, immunizations, and lifestyle and behavior changes, and classes and videos about developing the skill of breast self-examination.

People in many types of roles can educate patients about preventive services. Studies show that a physician's suggestions for screening are extremely beneficial.[23,24] Use of the entire office staff as educators has additional benefit. Specifically, the use of trained lay health workers (people who have not had any formal medical education) has improved participation in mammography screening and clinical breast examination among low-income, inner-city African American women.[25]

One study showed that when patients carry reminder cards for health maintenance procedures, the delivery of preventive services improves.[26] The comparison was between the use of a patient reminder card for health maintenance procedures along with a computer-generated prompt for physicians and the use of only a computer-generated prompt. The receptionist gave the reminder cards to the patients (Fig 3-3). Each patient was instructed to keep the card, bring it to all appointments, and show it to the physician.

Design of Delivery Systems

Reminders for clinicians

Both computer-generated and manually generated reminders are effective for most preventive services.[27] The reminders generally consist of a summary of the preventive services the patient has received each year (Fig 3-4). Computer-generated reminders also help clinicians by presenting previous results from preventive care tests. These reminders are most useful for vaccinations, less useful for colorectal cancer screening and cardiovascular risk reduction, and least useful for breast and cervical cancer screening. Delivered at the point of care, these reminders have little or no effect on cervical cancer screening.[27,28] Clinician compliance with reminder recommendations is more effective for ordering a test than for performing a procedure.

The use of a preventive service summary or flow sheet alone will not necessarily improve delivery of preventive services.[29,30] Not all clinicians are motivated to review the summary or flow sheet. Improvements in the delivery of service are more likely to occur if additional system changes are made. For example, the responsibilities of nursing or other office staff members could be expanded to include reviewing the patient summary or flow sheet and identifying services that are due. Another system change would be to use a computer information system to automatically order services as indicated on the preventive service summary.

Health Beliefs Favoring Use of Screening According to Health Belief Model*

Belief	Probability of Taking Preventive Action
Cues (exposure to information about the disease and prevention)	High
Risk (perception of personal susceptibility to the disease)	High
Severity (perception of negative symptoms and consequences)	High
Barriers to taking action (includes perceived cost, accessibility, doubt, fear, embarrassment, level of difficulty)	Low
Benefits of taking action (perceived advantages and positive effects)	High

*Adapted from Plaskon PP, Fadden MI. Cancer screening utilization: is there a role for social work in cancer prevention? *Soc Work Health Care.* 21:59–70, 1995. By permission of Haworth Press.

Heath Maintenance Project
DEPARTMENT OF MEDICINE. ECU SCHOOL OF MEDICINE

NAME: _____

	DATE PERFORMED		
1) Breast exam yearly after age 40			
2) Pap smear after 2 negative smears every three years			
3) Mammography yearly after age 50			
4) Stool for occult blood yearly after age 50			
5) Influenza vaccine yearly after age 65 or younger with chronic disease			
6) Pneumococcal vaccine once to those over 65 or younger with chronic disease			

Heath Maintenance Project
DEPARTMENT OF MEDICINE. ECU SCHOOL OF MEDICINE

NAME: _____

	DATE PERFORMED		
1) Stool for occult blood yearly after age 50			
2) Influenza vaccine yearly after age 65 or younger with chronic disease			
3) Pneumococcal vaccine once to those over 65 or younger with chronic disease			

FIGURE 3-3

Health maintenance cards used in study at East Carolina University (ECU) School of Medicine. *Top,* Card for women. *Bottom,* Card for men. From Turner et al.[26] By permission of the American Medical Association.

An effective prompt is to include smoking status with the data about vital signs. Fiore et al[31] initiated a simple intervention by making smoking status part of the vital signs assessment that was completed by the medical assistant before the physician saw the patient. The medical assistant inquired about smoking status ("current," "former," or "never") and documented the patient's response (Fig 3-5). Use of the vital-signs intervention increased the rate of identifying smokers. Of all patients surveyed (smokers and nonsmokers), 57.7% at baseline and 80.8% during the intervention phase reported that a clinician or nonclinician had asked that day whether they smoked. Use of the vital sign intervention also increased the rates that physicians advised their patients to quit smoking and provided specific advice or suggestions on how to stop smoking.

In one study, the use of reminders for physicians was enhanced by requiring physicians to explain why recommended preventive services were not ordered.[11] This intervention was tested for ordering fecal occult blood tests, mammograms, and Papanicolaou tests. The physicians were asked to circle one of the following responses: (1) done/ordered today, (2) not applicable, (3) patient refused, or (4) next visit. If any response other than "done/ordered today" was circled, the physician was directed to complete an additional form, called the preventive care sheet, which asked for an explanation

Preventive Services (Adult)

Sheet Number [ ]

Number (Above) and Name _____

Indicate in the boxes below the last date (mo./yr.) each test was completed (or refused) and if applicable, use the following codes to indicate status: N=neg/normal; AB= abnormal; R= refused and E = completed elsewhere and results (N/AB)

Date		1995	1996	1997	1998	1999	2000	2001	2002
Mammogram									
Pap smear									
Cholesterol screening									
Colorectal cancer screening									
Flexible sigmoidoscopy/procto									
Barium enema									
Colonoscopy									
TD (tetanus) vaccination									
Influenza vaccination									
Pneumococcal vacc.									

FIGURE 3-4

Summary sheet used at Mayo Clinic, Rochester, Minnesota, for preventive services. Procto indicates proctoscopy; vacc, vaccination. By permission of Mayo Foundation for Medical Education and Research.

why a preventive health test was considered but not performed.

Expanding access to care

By expanding access to health care services, health care organizations increase their opportunities to deliver preventive services. Access can be expanded in various ways, including the following.

1. With increasing numbers of patients employed outside the home, changing the hours of appointment availability should be considered.

2. Some preventive services can be provided in clinical settings in which they are not already provided, such as primary care visits for acute problems and emergency departments, inpatient units, and subspecialty clinics. The opportunity exists to assess, advise, and deliver preventive services at every health care encounter.

3. Drop-in clinics and home visits have been used for the delivery of vaccinations.

4. The use of group outpatient visits is another strategy. Compared with the traditional physician-patient visits among older, chronically ill members of health maintenance organizations, group outpatient visits improved delivery of both pneumococcal and influenza vaccinations.[32] These group visits consisted of a socialization period, an educational presentation, a review of health maintenance needs, and an assessment of acute care needs.

5. Provision of transportation to the clinic may help patients.

Independent clinics

The Breast Cancer Screening Program at the Group Health Cooperative in Seattle, Washington, is an example of an effective mammography program that is delivered

```
Blood pressure: _____

Pulse: _____    Weight: _____

Temperature: _____

Respiratory rate: _____

Smoking:      Current     Former     Never
                       (circle one)
```

FIGURE 3-5

Vital signs stamp, which includes smoking status. From Fiore MC. The new vital sign: assessing and documenting smoking status. *JAMA*. 1991;266:3183–3184. By permission of the American Medical Association.

in regional centers. The program improved annual mammography screening rates from 65% to 78% in women aged 52 to 69 years.[33]

Belcher[30] found that, in a patient population at a Veterans Affairs Medical Center, a health promotion clinic staffed by 2 nurse practitioners improved the rates of blood pressure screening, tobacco counseling, alcohol counseling, and colorectal cancer screening, compared with the rates in 2 enhanced "usual care" models. One enhanced usual care model consisted of providing a patient summary of preventive services, training sessions, and annual assessment of audit results to the clinicians. In the other enhanced usual care model, educational materials and a wallet-sized pocket guide were mailed to the patients in addition to the clinical interventions. Only 25% of the patients received care from a general internist. The remainder of the patients received care from a specialist, surgeon, or psychiatrist.

An independent clinic can provide an opportunity for the systematic delivery of preventive services. This is particularly important if access to primary care is limited.

Team approach

Delivering preventive care requires a team approach.[34,35] Nonphysician care providers, such as nurses, play a major role in implementing health promotion practices in the clinical setting. Expanding nursing roles to decrease the reliance on physicians can greatly improve the delivery of preventive services. One common approach is to have a registered nurse or a licensed practical nurse review the patient's chart before the patient-physician encounter. This activity is called visit planning. Any preventive services not done are marked on a preventive services sheet (see Fig 3-4) or flow sheet, and a friendly reminder is placed on the front of the record. Gonzalez et al[36] implemented this strategy in an internal medicine residents' clinic. Mean improvement in delivery of preventive services was 31% in the intervention group and only 4% in the control group. Nurses have also assisted in mailing reminders to patients.[29]

When the responsibilities of receptionists were redefined, breast cancer screening rates improved from 4% to 9% in an ethnically diverse population in Newham, England, an inner-city borough of London.[37] The receptionists in the intervention group participated in a 2-hour group training session. They were informed about the breast screening program and women's concerns, and they were asked to contact all women on their practice list of nonattendees by telephone, if possible, or by sending them a standard letter from their general practitioner.

Kottke et al[38] tested a clinic-wide teamwork approach to delivering preventive services in 10 clinics at 29 sites in Minnesota. Responsibility was spread among the staff for identifying smokers, assessing their smoking habits, advising them to quit, negotiating action, and providing follow-up counseling. Of the 466 patients reporting from these sites, 40.5% said that they had been counseled about smoking, compared with 26.4% of the 507 patients at the sites that did not deliver preventive care.

Standing orders involve programs in which nonphysician medical personnel prescribe or deliver services to patients without direct physician involvement at the time of the visit. On the basis of its systematic review of published studies, the Task Force on Community Preventive Services (in coordination with the Centers for Disease Control and Prevention) recommended that standing orders be used to improve vaccination coverage among adults.[39] Eight studies of standing-orders programs to improve vaccination coverage rates among adults showed a median increase in coverage of 28%. There was not enough evidence to determine whether standing orders are effective in increasing coverage among children. Studies indicate that standing orders are particularly effective in improving the delivery of vaccinations for influenza and pneumonia.

Reminders and recalls for patients

Reminders and recalls inform patients that they are due (reminders) or overdue (recalls) for specific preventive services. The manner in which reminders or recalls are delivered, such as by computer, mail, or telephone, may vary. The content of reminders can be either specific or general. Patients' responsiveness to mailed reminders for preventive services requires that the reminder letter be distinguished from a bill, convey a personally relevant message, and address logistical barriers to preventive services.[40] Information about appointment scheduling and payment options may be helpful.

Reminders that explain the importance of prevention are the most effective. In a study of influenza vaccination, patients who received a postcard reminder that emphasized elements of the Health Belief Model had higher vaccination rates (51.4%) than did patients who received no postcard (20.2%), a neutral postcard (25.0%), or a personal postcard (41.0%) (Fig 3-6).[41]

In one study, telephone reminders were more effective than reminder letters to increase influenza vaccination rates among high-risk patients.[42] However, the message delivered by telephone was personalized by including the patient's high-risk diagnosis and mentioning the patient's physician by name as the person recommending the vaccination. The letter was a standard form letter without a diagnosis or a physician's name. One disadvantage of telephone reminders is the cost. Often multiple attempts to reach the patient are necessary.

Support of the health care organization

For a preventive services program to succeed, it must have the support of the health care organization's leadership. At Mayo Clinic, the delivery of preventive

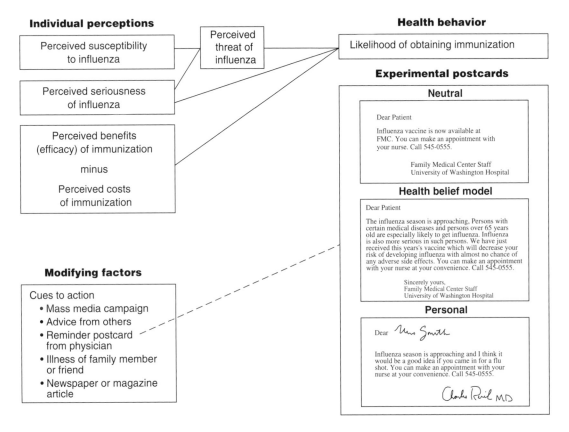

Health Belief Model and experimental postcards. From Larson et al.[41] By permission of Lippincott Williams & Wilkins.

services is one of the primary care performance measures reviewed by the board of governors. The systems in primary care are continually redesigned to improve the delivery of preventive services. The redesign process is led by physicians in various primary care departments and divisions, and the institutional leadership provides support for these activities. Each primary care clinical work site has a guideline implementation team that meets twice monthly. Membership on these teams is multidisciplinary, consisting of a nurse, secretary, receptionist, facilitator, and physician. Both the physician and the facilitator are given dedicated time to work on the project. In addition, technical support is available from analysts, programmers, and statisticians.

Decision Support

Clinician assessment and feedback

Clinician assessment and feedback are used to improve delivery of preventive services. In this technique, clinicians receive evaluations on how well they have delivered specific preventive services to their patients. Assessment and feedback interventions are sometimes compared with a goal or a standard (benchmarking). Sometimes incentives are used. Assessment and feedback may improve the delivery of preventive services by changing provider knowledge, attitudes, and behavior, or features of the delivery system for preventive services. With clinician assessment and feedback, vaccination coverage has increased by a median of 16% (range, 9% to 41%).[43] In another study, when residents received a histogram showing a blinded comparison of the frequency of mammography among their peers on a monthly basis, the mammography rate for women 50 to 74 years old increased 26%.[44]

Sources for guidelines

For effective delivery of preventive services, clinicians must have the knowledge required for optimal patient care. There are many sources for preventive services guidelines (see "Resources" at the end of the chapter).

The development and maintenance of guidelines are extremely time-consuming. At Mayo Clinic, guideline development and maintenance are done collaboratively through the Institute for Clinical Systems Improvement. The institute is a not-for-profit organization in Bloomington, Minnesota, which assists in developing and maintaining guideline and technology assessment reports and in implementing guidelines. The member organizations consist of 30 medical groups and 6 health plans from Minnesota that collaborate by providing content experts for guideline development. Guideline recommendations are based on the best existing evidence, which is graded to indicate the level of evidence. After a guideline is developed, it is circulated widely for critical review by all the member organizations.

Education of clinicians

Through education, clinicians gain not only more knowledge but also new insights that may affect their attitudes. This information may be delivered in written materials, videotapes, lectures, continuing medical education programs, and computer software. However, simply educating clinicians about guidelines does little to change prevention practice behaviors.[45] In a study in which a complete set of annotated recommendations (point-of-care education) was combined with a history and physical examination form in a resident continuity clinic, the rate of delivery of appropriate preventive services improved.[46] In another study, a combined approach of provider education and collaborative problem solving improved the rate of influenza vaccination by 34% compared with a control group.[47] Therefore, although provider education is necessary, it alone is not sufficient to improve the delivery of preventive services. In addition to provider education, system prompts and reminders are needed to translate guidelines and education into practice.

Clinical Information Systems

There is a great need for clinical information systems in medical practice. Information is collected from patients and diagnostic evaluations to make medical decisions. In addition, information is used to communicate with patients, to educate patients, and to document patient care for audiences inside and outside of medical facilities. However, health care organizations spend less on information technology (about 2.6% of their operating budgets) than do banking organizations (which spend 8% to 9% of their operating budgets).[48]

Clinical information systems assist in displaying important information in a useful format, providing physician and patient reminder prompts, gathering patient data, and providing patient education. The traditional clinical chart contains an extensive amount of information that is not readily available in a format that supports the delivery of preventive services during the amount of time typically given for an office visit.[49] Patient summaries or flow sheets contain the relevant information for the particular clinical decision that is needed (Fig 3-7). These data are abstracted from the mass of data in the medical record by a clinical information system. In addition, patient summaries may be combined with "physician alert" reminders or patient reminders that services are due. Compared with an appointment-triggered, manual tracking system based on flow sheet data, a computer-based health maintenance tracking system that generated annual provider and patient reminders for all patients, regardless of appointment status, was more effective and less expensive in improving delivery of preventive services.[50]

Stanford Health-Net is a computer network for health promotion that emphasizes specific self-care and preventive strategies. In a randomized, controlled, prospective study testing the efficacy of Health-Net among graduate and undergraduate students, the results showed a decrease in ambulatory medical visits and an increase in understanding how to prevent the acquisition of sexually transmitted diseases.[51] Health-Net contains 4 components: an electronic mail system, an electronic bulletin board, information and referral listings, and a self-help health information library.

Tobacco use, alcohol and drug abuse, diet, physical activity patterns, firearm use, sexual behavior, and motor vehicle injuries contribute greatly to mortality, as mentioned earlier.[17] Assessment and counseling for these health risk behaviors are extremely important in primary care practice. Health care organizations and employer groups are also increasingly interested in profiling the health risk behaviors of their enrollees. Assessment of health risk behaviors during in-person interviews at a visit to a physician may be time-consuming. Alternatively, assessment may be undertaken by use of telephone surveys or mailed surveys.[52] At Mayo Clinic, physical activity patterns; fruit and vegetable intake; risk factors for sexual diseases; and tobacco, alcohol, and caffeine use are assessed every year for established and new patients by a mailed survey that patients complete before their visit. This helps physicians advise patients about healthy lifestyles during clinical encounters. (A more detailed discussion of assessment of health risk behaviors appears in Chapter 41.)

The health risk appraisal, a computer-scored lifestyle analysis questionnaire, is an electronic tool used to obtain patient information and provide feedback and education to the patient. It was developed in the 1970s by the Centers for Disease Control as a tool for health promotion.[53] With the use of actuarial estimates of the mean probability of dying within the next 10 years, according to a participant's age, sex, and race, the health risk appraisal analyzes the participant's lifestyle and calculates a "health age" on the basis of the individual's risk estimates.[54]

CASE STUDY: "PROJECT 90 BY 2000"

In 1997 in a community of 22,000 in southeastern Minnesota, Austin Medical Center-Mayo Health System launched a community health initiative in collaboration with the county public health office to improve the delivery of adult preventive services. The goal, to be reached by the end of 2000, was for community residents to receive at least 90% of all screenings for which they were eligible for lipid levels, immunizations (tetanus, influenza, and pneumococcal), cancer (colorectal, breast, and cervical), hypertension, and tobacco use.

A multidisciplinary team oversaw the project, and quality improvement teams were established for specific preventive services. Baseline rates were assessed, current processes were diagrammed on flowcharts, and variations were identified. Practice guidelines of the Institute for Clinical Systems Improvement were followed. Tools provided for the clinical practice were past history forms, pocket card guides, and standing orders for the

Health Maintenance Status Physician Reminder

Office: Dansville		Months Override:			Physician		
Patient Name:			Guarantor:				
Date of Birth:			Sex:				
Date of Report:			Age:				

Procedure	Previously Done	Code	Last Done	Code	Overdue	Next Due	Done in Interim
History of tobacco use	/ /		06/22/92	D		/ /	___ ___/___
Blood pressure	05/10/90	D	06/22/92	D		06/22/94	___ ___/___
Serum cholesterol	/ /		06/22/89	D	YES	*NOW*	___ ___/___
Fecal occult blood test for colon	05/10/90	D	06/22/92	D		06/22/94	___ ___/___
Weight	/ /		06/22/92	X		06/22/96	___ ___/___
Tetanus-diphtheria immunization	/ /		06/22/83	D	YES	*NOW*	___ ___/___
Teach self-examination for lumps	/ /		05/10/90	D		05/10/94	___ ___/___
Papanicolaou test	/ /		01/29/93	E		01/29/95	___ ___/___
Physician breast examination	/ /		01/29/93	E		01/29/95	___ ___/___
Evaluate for osteoporosis risk	/ /		/ /		YES	*NOW*	___ ___/___

FIGURE 3-7

Example of computer-generated patient summary. D indicates procedure done and results were normal; E, procedure done elsewhere; and X, procedure done but results were abnormal. From Frame et al.[50] By permission of the American Medical Association.

nursing staff to facilitate assessment and delivery of preventive services. Education of physicians and nurses was provided to standardize the use of guidelines. Education of the public was provided by posters placed in examination rooms, hallways, waiting areas, grocery stores, nursing homes, schools, and pharmacies. Radio talk shows, newspaper articles, and advertisements in the newspaper also provided educational messages. Rates of

preventive service delivery were monitored quarterly, and feedback to physicians and nurses was provided. Incentives also were developed for physicians and nurses.

The project was a success. By the end of 2000, community residents had received 94% of all preventive services for which they were eligible. The results were most remarkable for adult immunizations (Fig 3-8).

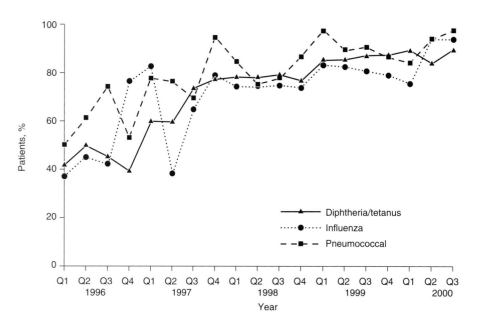

FIGURE 3-8.a

Percentage of all adult patients with current influenza, pneumococcal, and diphtheria/tetanus vaccinations.

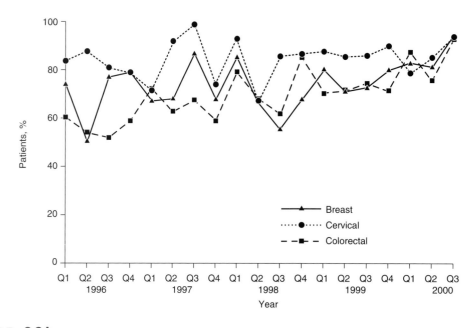

FIGURE 3-8.b

Breast, cervical, and colorectal cancer screening rates for eligible adult patients.

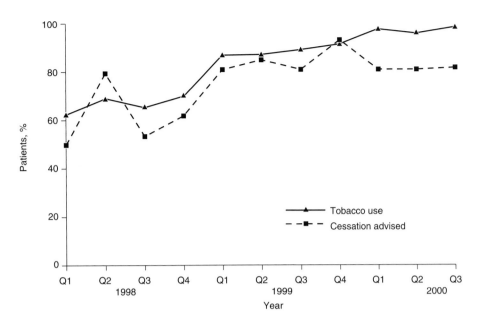

FIGURE **3-8.c**

Tobacco use screening for eligible adult patients and cessation advice for all users.

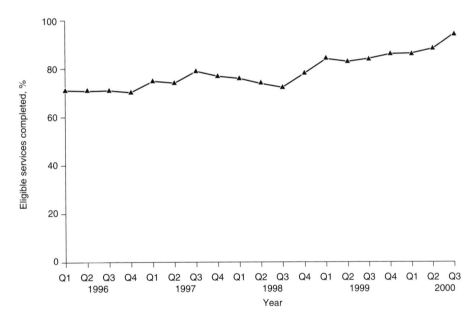

FIGURE **3-8.d**

Percentage of eligible services completed among all patients aged 18 to 80 years. Q indicates quarter.

SUMMARY

Results from decades of thoughtful studies aimed at improving the delivery of preventive services show that multiple interventions are effective. The tools exist to redesign medical practices to consistently deliver preventive services. Health system interventions consisting of self-management support, development of clinical information systems, decision support, redesign of delivery systems, and leadership support, in concert with optimizing community resources, provide a model for delivery of preventive services.

REFERENCES

1. Kottke TE, Solberg LI, Brekke ML, Cabrera A, Marquez MA. Delivery rates for preventive services in 44 midwestern clinics. *Mayo Clin Proc.* 1997;72:515–523.

2. US Department of Health and Human Services, Public Health Service. *Healthy People 2000: National Health Promotion and Disease Prevention Objectives.* Washington, DC: US Government Printing Office; 1991. DHHS Publication PHS 91–50212.

3. US Preventive Services Task Force. *Guide to Clinical Preventive Services.* 3rd ed. Rockville, Md: US Department of Health and Human Services; 2000–2003. Available at: www.ahcpr.gov/clinic/uspstfix.htm. Accessed January 20, 2003.

4. US Department of Health and Human Services, Public Health Service. *Healthy People 2000: Midcourse Review and 1995 Revisions.* Washington, DC: US Government Printing Office; 1995.

5. Lewis CE. Disease prevention and health promotion practices of primary care physicians in the United States. *Am J Prev Med.* 1988;4:9–16.

6. American Cancer Society. *Cancer Facts & Figures 2001.* Atlanta, Ga: American Cancer Society; 2001.

7. Vernon SW. Participation in colorectal cancer screening: a review. *J Natl Cancer Inst.* 1997;89:1406–1422.

8. Kottke TE, Brekke ML, Solberg LI. Making 'time' for preventive services. *Mayo Clin Proc.* 1993;68:785–791.

9. Gemson DH, Elinson J. Cancer screening and prevention: knowledge, attitudes, and practices of New York City physicians. *N Y State J Med.* 1987;87:643–645.

10. Chaudhry R, Kottke TE, Naessens JM, et al. Busy physicians and preventive services for adults. *Mayo Clin Proc.* 2000;75:156–162.

11. Litzelman DK, Dittus RS, Miller ME, Tierney WM. Requiring physicians to respond to computerized reminders improves their compliance with preventive care protocols. *J Gen Intern Med.* 1993;8:311–317.

12. Jaén CR, Stange KC, Nutting PA. Competing demands of primary care: a model for the delivery of clinical preventive services. *J Fam Pract.* 1994;38:166–171.

13. Frame PS. Health maintenance in clinical practice: strategies and barriers. *Am Fam Physician.* 1992;45:1192–1200.

14. Glasgow RE, Orleans CT, Wagner EH. Does the chronic care model serve also as a template for improving prevention? *Milbank Q.* 2001;79:579–612.

15. *Clinician's Handbook of Preventive Services: Put Prevention Into Practice.* 2nd ed. Washington, DC: Office of Public Health and Science, Office of Disease Prevention and Health Promotion, US Department of Health and Human Services, Public Health Service; 1998.

16. Lasker RD and the Committee on Medicine and Public Health. *Medicine & Public Health: The Power of Collaboration.* New York, NY: New York Academy of Medicine; 1997.

17. McGinnis JM, Foege WH. Actual causes of death in the United States. *JAMA.* 1993;270:2207–2212.

18. National Committee for Quality Assurance. *HEDIS-Health Plan Employer Data and Information Set. Specifications for CAHPS 3.0H.* Vol 3 (PPO Version). Washington, DC: National Committee for Quality Assurance; 2003.

19. Rosenbaum S, Richards TB. Medicaid managed care and public health policy. *J Public Health Manage Pract.* 1996;2:76–82.

20. Solberg LI, Kottke TE, Brekke ML, Conn SA, Magnan S, Amundson G. The case of the missing clinical preventive services systems. *Effective Clin Pract.* 1998;1:33–38.

21. Becker MH, ed. The health belief model and personal health behavior. *Health Education Monogr.* 1974;2(suppl):323–473.

22. Champion VL. Strategies to increase mammography utilization. *Med Care.* 1994;32:118–129.

23. Rimer BK, King E. Why aren't older women getting mammograms and clinical breast exams? *Womens Health Issues.* 1992;2:94–100.

24. Fox SA, Stein JA. The effect of physician-patient communication on mammography utilization by different ethnic groups. *Med Care.* 1991;29:1065–1082.

25. Sung JF, Blumenthal DS, Coates RJ, Williams JE, Alema-Mensah E, Liff JM. Effect of a cancer screening intervention conducted by lay health workers among inner-city women. *Am J Prev Med.* 1997;13:51–57.

26. Turner RC, Waivers LE, O'Brien K. The effect of patient-carried reminder cards on the performance of health maintenance measures. *Arch Intern Med.* 1990;150:645–647.

27. Shea S, DuMouchel W, Bahamonde L. A meta-analysis of 16 randomized controlled trials to evaluate computer-based clinical reminder systems for preventive care in the ambulatory setting. *J Am Med Inf Assoc.* 1996;3:399–409.

28. Austin SM, Balas EA, Mitchell JA, Ewigman BG. Effect of physician reminders on preventive care: meta-analysis of randomized clinical trials. *Proc Ann Symp Comput Appl Med Care.* 1994;121–124.

29. Robson J, Boomla K, Fitzpatrick S, et al. Using nurses for preventive activities with computer assisted follow up: a randomised controlled trial. *Br Med J.* 1989;298:433–436.

30. Belcher DW. Implementing preventive services: success and failure in an outpatient trial. *Arch Intern Med.* 1990;150:2533–2541.

31. Fiore MC, Jorenby DE, Schensky AE, Smith SS, Bauer RR, Baker TB. Smoking status as the new vital sign: effect on assessment and intervention in patients who smoke. *Mayo Clin Proc.* 1995;70:209–213.

32. Beck A, Scott J, Williams P, et al. A randomized trial of group outpatient visits for chronically ill older HMO members: the Cooperative Health Care Clinic. *J Am Geriatr Soc.* 1997;45:543–549.

33. Potosky AL, Merrill RM, Riley GF, et al. Breast cancer survival and treatment in health maintenance organization and fee-for-service settings. *J Natl Cancer Inst.* 1997;89:1683–1691.

34. Frame PS, Carlson SJ. A critical review of periodic health screening using specific screening criteria: III. Selected diseases of the genitourinary system. *J Fam Pract.* 1975;2:189–194.

35. Canadian Task Force on the Periodic Health Examination. The periodic health examination. *Can Med Assoc J.* 1979;121:1193–1254.

36. Gonzalez JJ, Ranney J, West J. Nurse-initiated health promotion prompting system in an internal medicine residents' clinic. *South Med J.* 1989;82:342–344.

37. Atri J, Falshaw M, Gregg R, Robson J, Omar RZ, Dixon S. Improving uptake of breast screening in multiethnic populations: a randomised controlled trial using practice reception staff to contact non-attenders. *Br Med J.* 1997;315:1356–1359.

38. Kottke TE, Solberg LI, Brekke ML, Conn SA, Maxwell P, Brekke MJ. A controlled trial to integrate smoking cessation advice into primary care practice: Doctors Helping Smokers, Round III. *J Fam Pract.* 1992;34:701–708.

39. Centers for Disease Control and Prevention. Vaccine-preventable diseases: improving vaccination coverage in children, adolescents, and adults: a report on recommendations of the Task Force on Community Preventive Services. *MMWR Morb Mortal Wkly Rep.* 1999;48(RR-8):1–15.

40. Ornstein SM, Musham C, Reid A, Jenkins RG, Zemp LD, Garr DR. Barriers to adherence to preventive services reminder letters: the patient's perspective. *J Fam Pract.* 1993;36:195–200.

41. Larson EB, Bergman J, Heidrich F, Alvin BL, Schneeweiss R. Do postcard reminders improve influenza compliance? A prospective trial of different postcard 'cues.' *Med Care.* 1982;20:639–648.

42. Brimberry R. Vaccination of high-risk patients for influenza: a comparison of telephone and mail reminder methods. *J Fam Pract.* 1988;26:397–400.

43. Briss PA, Rodewald LE, Hinman AR, et al and the Task Force on Community Preventive Services. Reviews of evidence regarding interventions to improve vaccination coverage in children, adolescents, and adults. *Am J Prev Med.* 2000;18(suppl):97–140.

44. Nattinger AB, Panzer RJ, Janus J. Improving the utilization of screening mammography in primary care practices. *Arch Intern Med.* 1989;149:2087–2092.

45. Anderson RM, Funnell MM, Butler PM, Arnold MS, Fitzgerald JT, Feste CC. Patient empowerment: results of a randomized controlled trial. *Diabetes Care.* 1995;18:943–949.

46. Shannon KC, Sinacore JM, Bennett SG, Joshi AM, Sherin KM, Deitrich A. Improving delivery of preventive health care with the comprehensive annotated reminder tool (CART). *J Fam Pract.* 2001;50:767–771.

47. Karuza J, Calkins E, Feather J, Hershey CO, Katz L, Majeroni B. Enhancing physician adoption of practice guidelines: dissemination of influenza vaccination guideline using a small-group consensus process. *Arch Intern Med.* 1995;155:625–632.

48. Smith L. The coming health care shakeout. *Fortune.* 1993;127:70–75.

49. McDonald CJ. Protocol-based computer reminders, the quality of care and the non-perfectability of man. *N Engl J Med.* 1976;295:1351–1355.

50. Frame PS, Zimmer JG, Werth PL, Hall WJ, Eberly SW. Computer-based vs manual health maintenance tracking: a controlled trial. *Arch Fam Med.* 1994;3:581–588.

51. Robinson TN. Community health behavior change through computer network health promotion: preliminary findings from Stanford Health-Net. *Comput Methods Programs Biomed.* 1989;30:137–144.

52. Thompson BL, Nelson DE, Caldwell B, Harris JR. Assessment of health risk behaviors. *Am J Prev Med.* 1998;16:48–58.

53. Health risk appraisal: United States. *MMWR Morb Mortal Wkly Rep.* 1981;30:133–135.

54. Goetz AA, Duff JF, Bernstein JE. Health risk appraisal: the estimation of risk. *Public Health Rep.* 1980;95:119–126.

RESOURCES

The following are online sources for preventive service guidelines:

American College of Physicians-American Society of Internal Medicine
(www.acponline.org/sci-policy/guidelines)

Canadian Task Force on Preventive Health Care
(www.ctfphc.org)

Institute for Clinical Systems Improvement
(www.icsi.org)

National Cholesterol Education Program
(www.nhlbi.nih.gov/guidelines/cholesterol/index.htm)

National Guideline Clearinghouse
(www.guideline.gov)

The Seventh Report of the Joint National Committee on Prevention, Detection, Evaluation, and Treatment of High Blood Pressure
(www.nhlbi.nih.gov/guidelines/hypertension/)

US Department of Health and Human Services
(www.hhs.gov/policies/index.shtm/#policies)

US Preventive Services Task Force
(www.ahcpr.gov/clinic/uspstfix.htm)

chapter 4

Laboratory Screening

Frederick Van Lente, PhD

INTRODUCTION

There are 2 major goals of the clinical laboratory in the practice of preventive medicine (PM): (1) to assess the risk of future disease and (2) to detect occult disease not evident by history or physical examination. Smaller yet important roles are the confirmation of suspected disease and the monitoring of chronic disease and the medications used to treat them.

The correct assessment of a laboratory test performance requires a review of the statistical tools used to quantify test diagnostic efficiency and the concepts of informational content. These concepts will enhance any rational approach to the use of laboratory resources.

TEST PERFORMANCE CRITERIA

The ability of a given laboratory test to effectively yield the diagnostic information asked of it varies dramatically by test, disease, and clinical setting. The 5 principal concepts involved are:

1. sensitivity—the positivity or abnormality of a test result in the presence of the disease under consideration
2. specificity—the negativity or normality of a test result in the absence of the disease under consideration
3. positive predictive value—the probability that a positive or abnormal test result indicates that the patient has the disease under consideration
4. negative predictive value—the probability that a negative or normal test result indicates that the patient does not have the disease under consideration
5. efficiency—the percentage or fraction of test results that correctly indicates the presence or absence of disease

These concepts have become central to any discussion of the value of a given laboratory test and are particularly important when tests are used in screening and outpatient settings. Clearly, it is desirable for a test to be both sensitive (able to detect all cases of a disease that it is meant to signal) and specific to that disease and thus not confusing or confounding. The corresponding predictive values are derived from sensitivity and specificity:

$$\text{Positive Predictive Value} = \frac{\text{True-Positives}}{\text{True-Positives} + \text{False-Positives}}$$

$$\text{Negative Predictive Value} = \frac{\text{True-Negatives}}{\text{True-Negatives} + \text{False-Negatives}}$$

These equations introduce another factor: prevalence. Prevalence refers to the actual prevalence of the disease in question in the population being tested, that is, the ratio of the sum of true-positives and false-negatives to the total number of individuals tested.

The prevalence of disease is the major determinant of test effectiveness when laboratory analyses are used in the outpatient or preventive health setting. This point cannot be overemphasized because many users of laboratory tests do not distinguish the various testing environments, such as outpatient symptomatic, outpatient asymptomatic, elective surgery screen, or emergent. It would seem both obvious and highly desirable to use different test batteries in various populations depending on their characteristics.

The prevalence of disease in the preventive health setting is naturally low and in some cases extremely low. This testing is equivalent to finding the "needle in the haystack." Despite some variation in these prevalence rates by location and ethnicity, they still more than suffice as guides.

The influence of prevalence on the effectiveness of laboratory tests is best illustrated by example. Let us assume that a given laboratory test exhibits both a sensitivity and specificity of 0.95 for detecting disease D when the test value is above the upper limit of the reference interval (normal range). This type of evaluation is actually a simple 2×2 table. Table 4-1.A shows these results at a prevalence of disease of 0.5. That is, half of the patients who were tested suffer from the disease. It can be seen that of the positive results, 475 are true-positives but 25 are false-positive results.

This test also failed to detect the disease in 25 patients. A patient who presents with a test value above our discriminating limit, as shown in the table, will have a 0.95 probability of having the disease in question, whereas an individual with a normal result will have a 0.95 probability of not having the disease. These numbers do not appear unreasonable and show the equivalency of sensitivity and predictive value when the disease prevalence equals 0.5.

Table 4-1.B illustrates the use of the same test and interpretations used in Table 4-1.A with the exception that the prevalence of disease in the tested clinical population has decreased to 1%. Here it can be seen that of the total 59 positive or abnormal results, 9 are true-positives and 50 are false-positives. Thus, only 15% of the abnormal results indicate disease. If the prevalence of disease decreases to 0.1%, then only 2% of abnormal results are true-positives. The percentage of abnormal results that are true-positives is the predictive value of that test result.

The preceding examples illustrate the devastating effect that low disease prevalence has on the true effectiveness of laboratory testing at a given degree of sensitivity and specificity. This effect is dominated by the effect of specificity. That is, specificity is the dominant concern in most situations where laboratory tests are used to screen for major disease, especially cancer. Table 4-2 illustrates the effect of specificity on predictive value at a given prevalence rate of 1%. As disease prevalences approach those seen in the PM setting, the test specificity must approach perfection (1.0) before predictive values approach useful levels. This concept will be developed later in this chapter when specific tests and screening programs are discussed.

The information contained in the laboratory test results obtained in the preventive health setting can be improved by other means as well. These intuitive approaches, used by many clinical practices, are still underemphasized in formal treatments of the subject. They include the strength of the signal, confirmatory testing, and pattern analysis.

When a patient presents with a given laboratory test result, it is often interpreted on an "asterisk basis," that is, normal or abnormal (positive or negative). In fact, most of the predictive value concepts just reviewed are actually designed for qualitative, positive or negative, binary classification of results. Most laboratory results, however, are continuous and can demonstrate a strength of signal. Thus, some test results are worse or more abnormal than others. Stated another way, the sensitivity, specificity, and predictive value of laboratory results change with the degree of abnormality. Table 4-3 shows the predictive value (probability) of a patient having suffered a myocardial infarction at presentation at the emergency room as a function of the peak troponin T value obtained within the first 12 hours after presentation. It can be seen clearly that the likelihood of disease increases significantly as the laboratory "signal" for infarction increases. This same relationship exists for most laboratory tests in most circumstances. In particular, test results that reflect pathological alteration of, or release from, reserves can signal the severity of disease by their degree of change from normality. This pattern holds true for enzymes, hemoglobin, and electrolytes.

The lack of specificity of a relatively sensitive test can be overcome by efficient confirmation by a relatively specific test. This approach to "combination testing" is a variation on combining probabilities; as more indicators become "positive," the likelihood of diseases increases. This concept is illustrated in Table 4-4 using a hypothetical screening test with a sensitivity and specificity of 0.99 and 0.80, respectively; a confirming test with a sensitivity/specificity of 0.80/0.99, respectively; and a disease prevalence of 0.01, or 1%. The probability that a patient with positive results of the screening test has a given disease is 0.048, but climbs to 0.80 if the result of the confirmatory test is also positive. This approach fails to detect disease in 2 individuals while correctly classifying 196 initial positive results as normal (healthy individuals).

The preceding discussion raises the question of why both tests are not performed simultaneously in this type of situation. The answer is multifactorial. First, the confirmatory test is often elaborate, expensive, and inaccessible. The cited criteria for testing in a screening context will be

TABLE 4-1

Effect of Prevalence in Effectiveness of Laboratory Tests

Disease Status	Test Result		
	Positive	**Negative**	**Total**
A			
Diseased	475	25	500
Nondiseased	25	475	500
Total	**500**	**500**	**1000**
B			
Diseased	9	1	10
Nondiseased	50	940	990
Total	**59**	**941**	**1000**

TABLE 4-2

Effect of Specificity on Predictive Value*

Specificity	**Predictive Value**
0.900	0.100
0.950	0.180
0.975	0.300
0.990	0.500
0.995	0.700
1.000	1.000

*Prevalence of disease = 0.01; test sensitivity = 0.95.

TABLE 4-3

Predictive Value of Troponin T for Myocardial Infarction as Function of Signal

Troponin T (μg/L)	Predictive Value
0.00–0.09	0.01
0.10–0.19	0.08
0.20–0.90	0.38
1.00–1.99	0.79
2.00–9.99	0.83
>10.00	1.00

TABLE 4-4

Combination Testing: Effect on Predictability of Test Results*

Disease Status	Positive	Negative	Total
Diseased	10	0	10
Nondiseased	198	792	990
Total	**208**	**792**	**1000**

	Both Tests Positive	Second Test Negative	Total
Diseased	8	2	10
Nondiseased	2	196	198
Total	**10**	**198**	**208**

*Confirmatory test sensitivity/specificity = 0.80/0.99; screening test sensitivity/specificity = 0.99/0.80

Number of individuals = 1000

Prevalence of disease = 0.01

discussed in further detail later, but economics and logistics are major factors. The delay in availability of results can also adversely affect the medical decision-making process. If the laboratory test is used to detect a major disease, such as cancer, knowledge of an initial false-positive result before knowledge of a subsequent true-negative confirmatory result can cause great anxiety for the patient. These issues are currently paramount in certain screening contexts and will be discussed later in this chapter.

Another variation of combination testing is the use of multiple organ- or system-specific test results to arrive at a more specific diagnosis. This constellation of findings is often referred to as a pattern of results that is consistent with a certain disease state. This approach was promulgated in the late 1960s by advocates of the multi-test automated clinical laboratory analyzers now in general use in both clinical chemistry and hematology. As will be discussed later, it remains doubtful if this modality is really useful in the asymptomatic patients using one test panel other than in the differential diagnosis of anemia. Nonetheless, some of these patterns have become part of the medical jargon, including "microcytic anemia" or "macrocytic anemia."

NORMAL RANGE

Much of what has been discussed in the previous section assumed that a given laboratory result was compared with a reference limit of values given for apparently healthy individuals. The adequacy of the normal range concept is often criticized. Several factors affect the accuracy of these ranges as provided by many laboratories. They are often gleaned from textbooks or manufacturer's information sheets by laboratories without the resources to validate their own ranges. This practice may be restricted by new federal laboratory regulations. They also may have been derived from populations with markedly different demographics than the population being tested. They may not be current with respect to the laboratory methods in use (ie, historical ranges). Finally, they may have been derived using the wrong statistical tools.

There seem to be no rules for derivation of normal ranges. In the first place, who is actually normal? There

are elegant lists of multiple definitions for normal, even in the medical context, but these are not totally satisfying when trying to decide the correct application of laboratory tests in a preventive health setting. In fact, in this context, the use of the word *normal* is entirely misplaced because individuals of similar health status are often used to generate the ranges in the first place. Most experts have advocated the use of the term *reference interval* instead of *normal range*. In the outpatient setting this is quite appropriate, because in the absence of overt disease detected independently, the screening population's inherent distribution of laboratory test results is used to identify those individuals whose results are unusual. These *outliers* are just that, and their results have little to do with the detection of disease in their cohort population. Instead, the possibility of existent disease is inferred from other cohort populations who have a higher prevalence of disease. Sometimes this works; sometimes it doesn't.

The distribution of laboratory results obtained in individuals without disease depends on several factors. The clinician using the clinical laboratory should be aware of these factors to initiate informed dialogue with the service provider when questions arise regarding these ranges. The most important factors, age and sex, strongly influence many metabolic parameters, such as hemoglobin, uric acid, phosphorus, bilirubin, alkaline phosphatase, urea nitrogen, creatinine, and creatinine clearance. Genetics may influence other parameters, often between ethnic groups.

The adequate delineation of reference intervals into even age and sex groups is rare outside of the largest laboratory facilities. The reason is simple. It requires an extremely large population and database to establish ranges with confidence (150 or more individuals) when categorizing many sex and age decades (27,000 results). Even these numbers would not suffice for the pediatric population when substantial changes occur within decades. It is not surprising, therefore, that these ranges are often estimations at best.

The distribution of data in reference populations and, therefore, in health maintenance populations exhibits many forms. Occasionally, data conform to the infamous normal (gaussian) distribution and usually reflect passive forces that dictate the usual values found in individuals. Examples include many diet-dependent analytes such as potassium. More often, the distribution is either kurtotic (peaked) or skewed (trailing) because of various factors.

Data distributions can greatly affect the use of laboratory tests in the outpatient setting when the upper limit of normal is not established properly. The "infamous" range of mean ±2 SD (parametric method) is only accurate for normally distributed data. If, for example, the data are strongly skewed to higher values and parametric methods are used to set the upper limit, then an inordinate number of healthy individuals will be classified by testing as abnormal because the statistical method will underestimate the upper limit. Only ranking (nonparametric) methods should be used whenever the distribution of values in the reference population is unusual.

What does the reference range dictate about the other individuals who are tested by the same method and whose data are compared with the original distribution? The answer depends on what the range describes (or is thought to describe). The apparent absolute standard is that because the range was calculated as mean ±2 SD, the range encompasses the central 95% of the population. Thus, 2.5% of the population must be not sick above and below this range. This criterion automatically results in a test specificity of not greater than 0.975 when the upper limit of this range is used to discriminate diseased from nondiseased patients. This statistical fact has led to the widely accepted practice of ignoring slightly abnormal test results. In addition, individuals exhibiting initial laboratory values at or near the limit of the reference range will often retest within the range.[1] This phenomenon is also well known and results from both the imprecision of the method and the statistical reality of regression to the mean.

A more controversial concept is the potential value of the normal result in many clinical settings. To the extent that a laboratory test has an acceptable diagnostic sensitivity and, therefore, an acceptable negative predictive value, this concept has merit. In this interpretation of normal or negative laboratory results, the probability of disease is low, which allows the physician to make more effective medical decisions, especially if faced with multiple problems or possible diagnoses. In other words, the normal result can allow ruling out and focus.

LABORATORY-DERIVED RISK ASSESSMENT

A large number of laboratory tests used in health maintenance and PM are risk factors for future diseases. The burden of chronic disease is great, and these tests are part of the armamentarium of disease prevention. They work in concert with clinical and pharmacologic risk modifiers. What is important about risk factor result assessment is that nobody is truly "normal." Everyone is at some finite risk of future development of disease. Risk factor interpretations are usually evidence-based and supported by large and repeated longitudinal clinical studies. Pertinent examples of these include the Framingham Study, the Physicians' Health Study, and the Nurses' Health Study.

The results of tests such as the total cholesterol/high-density lipoprotein cholesterol (HDL-C) ratio and high-sensitivity C-reactive protein (hsCRP) are often expressed as "relative risks." One therefore needs to ascertain relative to what? As a rule, the risk is relative to those individuals who are in the lowest part of the absolute risk distribution of test results. These values (it is always a range of values) can be assigned a relative risk of 1.0. The remaining result ranges are then assigned a risk relative to the lowest risk group. Therefore, it is important to remember that a test result associated with a relative risk of some condition equal to 1.0 does not imply the absence of risk but rather the lowest risk found in the population. The determination of what that risk might be usually requires review of the published clinical study and has not been routinely included in the laboratory reporting of these tests.

STANDARD LABORATORY INVESTIGATIONS

The evolution of the standard practice in most current medical situations has resulted in the widespread application of well-accepted panels of laboratory tests, a process aided immensely by the development of medical technology. The commonly available test groupings used in general outpatient testing environments include the ubiquitous chemistry panels, the complete blood cell (CBC) count, and urinalysis. These tests are often used in an unselective, surveillance manner in populations where the prevalence of most diseases is quite low. Given the previous discussion of test efficiency, it is worthwhile to extend these principles to the specific application of multicomponent, chemistry test panels. It has been stated that if the normal range for a component of a test panel has been established using a central 95th percentile technique (mean ±2 SD), then 5% of healthy individuals will be outside this range or abnormal. If no tests in a panel are assumed to be statistically independent, the probability that a normal person will exhibit at least one abnormality is $1 - (0.95)^n$. This statistical fact can have dramatic results. On a 6-test panel, the probability is 26%. In other words, the more tests performed, the greater the chance of a false-positive result. For this reason, unnecessary tests should not be performed regardless of the economics. The fact that this effect may not be as evident is a reflection of the application of wider normal ranges and the fact that not all analytes behave randomly.

The use of these test panels in a screening mode is assumed to be valuable to detect physiologic aberrations that signal pathological conditions. This approach, however, should satisfy effectiveness criteria, including the detection of otherwise latent disease, cost-effectiveness, effectiveness of early treatment, cost and risk of misclassification, and the societal burden of targeted diseases.[2]

These concerns should be kept in mind during the following discussion, which considers that value of testing an ambulatory asymptomatic population. Although the rationale and problems associated with selected examples of components of these standard test packages are described, an exhaustive discussion of all possible test components will not be attempted.

Medical Necessity

Medicare rules for utilization of laboratory tests have had a major impact on the way clinical laboratories provide services. Contrary to the mission of PM, in a stance criticized by many, the Center for Medicare Services (CMS) severely restricted use of laboratory tests for screening purposes. Use of many laboratory tests is guided by edicts known as National Coverage Decisions (NCD). Central to these rules was the promulgation of the concept of medical necessity. A physician advisory panel determines which working symptoms or diagnoses are acceptable justifications for ordering a certain laboratory test. Once these recommendations are accepted, Medicare will reimburse for the test only in those scenarios. Medicare will also consider consistent use of the laboratory test in other circumstances abusive, and possibly, fraudulent practices.

The discussions of specific tests in this chapter will include pertinent reference to the Medicare rules and guidelines. These tend to mold laboratory practices in most outpatient settings regardless of insurance coverage. Medicare requires that an "Advanced Beneficiary Notification" be signed by a patient whose laboratory tests may not be covered under their guidelines. The NCD are listed in Table 4-5.

Automated Chemistry Profile

Chemistry panels have undergone a major overhaul in the last decade. Initially any number of tests in almost any combination were available, particularly from independent, commercial laboratories. The government,

however, uncovered widespread fraud and abuse relative to use of these large panels and improper billing to Medicare. This led to major reduction in the number of tests in these panels and the development of an "approved" set of components for a small number of panels. Currently, there are 5 approved chemistry panels: electrolyte panel, basic metabolic panel, comprehensive metabolic panel, hepatic function panel, and renal function panel. The presumed relationship between the component tests and the organ system are shown in Table 4-6.

The use of multicomponent chemistry panels is most commonly applied to a "rule-out" approach. The essence of its utility is the finding of all normal results. The problem is that when the frequency of abnormality approaches that seen in the reference population, the justification for the testing program becomes difficult. It can still be argued that a disease in question, for example, myeloma, is serious enough that the single case found could justify the testing of thousands of nondiseased individuals if it led to an improved outcome, financial considerations notwithstanding. In any event, the discovery of an abnormal result without any clinical correlation always presents a dilemma. Is the result clinically significant, is there a laboratory problem, or is the reference interval inappropriate?

TABLE 4-5

Medicare National Coverage Decisions (NCD)

α-Fetoprotein
Blood cell counts
Carcinoembryonic antigen (CEA)
Collagen cross-links
Digoxin
Fecal occult blood
γ-Glutamyltransferase (GGT)
Glucose
Glycated hemoglobin
Hepatitis panel
Human immunodeficiency (HIV) diagnostic testing
HIV monitoring testing
Human chorionic gonadotropin (HCG)
Ionized calcium
Iron studies
Lipid testing
Prostate-specific antigen (PSA)
Partial thromboplastin time (PTT)
Thyroid testing
Cancer antigen 125 (CA 125)
CA 15-3/27.29
CA 19-9
Urine culture

Aspartate Aminotransferase and Alanine Aminotransferase

The prevalence of fatty liver changes is high. These changes may occur as a result of alcoholic liver disease or nonalcoholic steatohepatitis. The first indication that the liver enzymes aspartate aminotransferase (AST) and alanine aminotransferase (ALT) may indicate fatty liver changes was the testing of blood donors to screen for what is now known to be hepatitis C. The data obtained from these programs indicated a significant tail in the upper portion of the distribution of values from "normal" individuals. This is a prime example of the shortcomings of some "normal" reference intervals for laboratory test results. It was subsequently found that these individuals were overweight and the increased enzyme activities were probably reflecting fatty liver changes. Some authors have suggested that the upper limit of normal for ALT be lowered to improve case finding of occult liver disease.[3] Therefore, these tests do serve a screening function on the standard metabolic chemistry panels.

The finding of an unexpected abnormality, particularly one less than 2 times the upper limit of normal, may be consistent with subclinical hepatic dysfunction. This may indicate fatty changes in the liver due to the metabolic syndrome (see the next section), alcohol abuse, or viral hepatitis. Prudent follow-up in the absence of an increased body mass index or hypertriglyceridemia would include serologic testing for viral hepatitis serologies. Various tests have been forwarded as screening markers for alcohol abuse, but none has been found extremely useful. An increased γ-glutamyltransferase (GGT) activity may be present but would not add any useful information in the context of an increased AST or ALT value unless the latter were due to substantial muscle lysis. In that case, the GGT would likely be within the reference interval.

Glucose and Hemoglobin A$_{1c}$

The definition of diabetes mellitus and the recommendations for laboratory screening have undergone several iterations over the years; however, the diagnosis of this condition is made exclusively by the determination of hyperglycemia. The hyperglycemic state may or may not be associated with the classic symptoms of diabetes. The most recent recommendations for use of the serum or plasma glucose value in reaching the diagnosis of diabetes were established by the American Diabetes Association in 1997.[4] They are as follows:

- Symptoms of diabetes and casual (any time of day) glucose value of 200 mg/L or greater
- Fasting glucose value greater than or equal to 126 mg/dL
- 2-hour post-glucose-load glucose value greater than or equal to 200 mg/dL

If any one of these criteria is met, confirmation testing should be performed on a subsequent day. It should be emphasized that these laboratory criteria work best in the context of adequate diet and fasting times of at least 8 hours.

The American Diabetes Association recommends that the fasting blood glucose level be measured in all asymptomatic persons aged 45 years or more. If results are less than 110 mg/dL, testing should be repeated at least every 3 years. Screening of individuals at increased risk of diabetes is indicated at 10 years of age and should be repeated every 2 years. The presence of family history,

TABLE 4-6

Common Components of Chemistry Panels*

Test	System
Total protein	Plasma cell
Albumin	Liver/kidney
Bilirubin	RBC/liver
Urea nitrogen	Vascular/kidney
Creatinine	Kidney
Calcium	Kidney/bone/hormonal
Electrolytes	Kidney/hormonal
Sodium	
Potassium	
Carbon dioxide	
Chloride	
Enzymes	
AST	Muscle, liver
ALT	Liver
Alkaline phosphatase	Liver/bone

*RBC indicates red blood cells; AST, aspartate aminotransferase; and ALT, alanine aminotransferase.

TABLE 4-7

Total, HDL, and LDL Cholesterol Risk Ratios*

CAD Risk	TC/HDL-C Ratio	LDL/HDL-C Ratio
Men		
½ Average	3.43	1.00
Average	4.97	3.55
2× Average	9.55	6.25
3× Average	23.99	7.99
Women		
½ Average	3.27	1.47
Average	4.44	3.22
2× Average	7.05	5.03
3× Average	11.04	6.14

*HDL indicates high-density lipoprotein; LDL, low-density lipoprotein; CAD, coronary artery disease; TC, total cholesterol; HDL-C indicates high-density lipoprotein cholesterol; and LDL-C, low-density lipoprotein cholesterol. Ratios are from the Framingham Study.

overweight, and insulin-resistance are all considered risk factors. In addition to the well-known association of type 2 diabetes with the cardiovascular risk in the context of the "metabolic syndrome," it has been suggested recently that individuals with impaired glucose tolerance be considered in the same light. That is, normalization of the fasting glucose is central to the treatment goal. Individuals with impaired glucose tolerance have an increased risk of progression to overt type 2 diabetes and should be identified and treated.[5]

The use of hemoglobin A_{1c} in the screening or diagnosis of type 2 diabetes remains controversial. This test is well established as the primary laboratory means to assess glycemic control in patients with both type 1 and type 2 diabetes. This parameter reflects the mean ambient blood glucose concentration over the previous several months. It has been suggested that glycated hemoglobin may serve as an adjunct for screening for type 2 diabetes, as the finding of a value above the upper limit of normal is suggestive of significant severe glucose intolerance.[6]

Medicare does not support screening using fasting glucose in the absence of suggestive symptoms or the presence of abnormal blood chemistry findings implying hyperglycemia. Medicare also supports use of hemoglobin A_{1c} in monitoring of diabetics at the rate of no more than 4 times per year.

Lipid Evaluations

The laboratory assessment of lipid-associated atherosclerotic risk has become a part of the standard group of laboratory tests used in health maintenance. The recommended tests and their use in risk factor modulation have been guided by the National Cholesterol Education Panel.[7] The basis of these recommendations is the lipid paradigm. Increased circulating cholesterol concentrations imply increased levels of low-density lipoprotein (LDL). The LDL, in turn, cannot be taken up effectively by the LDL-receptor in peripheral tissue, leading to increased modification of LDL during its resident time in the circulation. The modified LDL is taken up by the scavenger receptor of macrophages in the vascular endothelium, leading to atheroma development and subsequent atherosclerosis. High-density lipoprotein (HDL) is directly involved in "reverse" cholesterol transport from peripheral tissue back to the liver and has been shown to be protective against coronary artery disease (CAD).

The commonly accepted "lipid panel" includes measurement of total cholesterol, triglycerides, and HDL-C. The distribution of cholesterol among the other 2 major lipoprotein types is usually estimated by calculation:

$$\text{Very-low-density Lipoprotein Cholesterol (VLDL-C)} = \frac{\text{Triglycerides}}{5}$$

$$\text{Low-density Lipoprotein Cholesterol (VLDL-C)} = \text{Total Cholesterol} - (\text{VLDL-C} + \text{HDL-C})$$

These calculated values are considered reasonable estimations as long as the triglyceride levels concentrations are less than 400 mg/dL. When triglyceride levels are greater than 400 mg/dL, the assumptions of triglyceride distribution among lipoproteins no longer hold and the calculated values will demonstrate significant deviation from their actual concentrations. In this situation the LDL-C should be directly measured and the VLDL-C calculated:

$$\text{VLDL-C} = \text{Total Cholesterol} - (\text{HCL-C} + \text{LDL-C}).$$

From these values, ratios can be easily calculated to enhance risk assessment. These include the total cholesterol/HDL-C ratio and the LDL-C/HDL-C ratio. The risks of CAD associated with these ratios as derived from the Framingham Study are shown in Table 4-7.

The Adult Treatment Panel III of the National Cholesterol Education Panel released new guidelines in May 2001.[8] These guidelines support measurement of the 3 major components of the lipid profile discussed above, and they introduced new treatment thresholds based on the 10-year coronary risk tool. A new classification of cholesterol distribution was also promulgated, non-HDL-C. This is based on the view that all non-HDL lipoprotein particles are probably potentially atherogenic. It is simply calculated as follows:

$$\text{Non-HDL-C} = \text{Total Cholesterol} - \text{HDL-C}$$

Non-HDL-C represents a broad category of lipoprotein particles, including LDL, lipoprotein(a), VLDL, and triglyceride-rich remnant particles. When fasting triglyceride levels are greater than 200 mg/dL after the recommended LDL goal is reached, a secondary goal is set 30 mg/dL higher than the LDL goal.

The Adult Treatment Panel III also focused on the so-called metabolic syndrome, in which laboratory test results are inherent. This secondary target of therapy is a constellation of findings that includes abdominal obesity, increased triglyceride levels ($\geq$150 mg/dL), low HDL-C (<40 mg/dL in men or <50 mg/dL in women), and increased blood pressure and fasting glucose level of 110 mg/dL or greater. Although there have been several studies looking directly at indexes of insulin resistance as predictors of CAD risk, no general recommendation for testing of apparently overweight individuals has been forthcoming.

Additional lipid laboratory determinants of CAD risk include apolipoproteins, lipoprotein(a), and particle sizing. The major apolipoprotein components of LDL— apolipoprotein B and HDL, apolipoprotein A can be measured directly using immunoassays. They tend to provide the same information as the cholesterol content of these particles, and although some have argued that these measurements are superior, there has been no general recommendation for their use. Lipoprotein (a) is a close relative to LDL, consisting of an LDL with an extra apolipoprotein, apolipoprotein(a) attached. This lipoprotein appears to fluctuate primarily due to heredity, and a value greater than 0.3 g/L (30 mg/dL) is associated with increased risk of CAD.[9] Whether this test offers major contribution to the overall risk evaluation of the general population remains open to question.

Several large cohort studies have shown that small, dense LDL particles are strongly associated with increased risk of development of CAD.[10] Whether this finding is truly independent of total LDL concentration and other lipid risk predictors is still somewhat open to question in the general screening population cohort. The laboratory determination of LDL particle size requires special methods, such as electrophoresis and nuclear magnetic resonance spectroscopy, and is therefore not easily integrated with the primary panel of lipid measurements. Particle sizing methods can determine the relative concentrations of large LDL, intermediate LDL, small LDL, and intermediate-density lipoprotein. These measurements have yet to be established as part of the mainstream CAD screening profile.

Medicare supports use of the lipid panel up to 2 times a year, and up to 6 times per year for any component when a diagnosis supports the medical necessity. This includes obesity, alcoholism, abnormal chemistry panel findings, and *disorders of lipid metabolism.*

C-reactive Protein and Inflammatory Markers

It has been well known that the lipid-related markers of CAD risk account for only some of the total risk of this widespread disease. During the 1990s several large cohort studies established a link between circulating concentrations of C-reactive protein (CRP) within the previously "normal" range of values and the future risk of coronary disease.[11,12] Interestingly, a similar association was found between CRP and outcomes in separate cohorts of patients with established CAD. These discoveries led to the new inflammatory paradigm component of the CAD pathogenesis model. C-reactive protein is a nonspecific acute-phase protein produced by the liver in response to cytokine signals. It has been used for decades to monitor the acute-phase reaction associated with inflammatory conditions such as rheumatoid arthritis. C-reactive protein concentrations increased above 0.3 mg/dL are associated with many clinical inflammatory scenarios, and values may reach 30.0 mg/dL in severe sepsis or disseminated malignancies. The range of values found in the general population holds fairly constant below 0.3 mg/dL in the absence of major illness, and it is these values that predict CAD risk. Because appropriate analytical performance is required to assess CRP concentrations in this lower range, a modified assay widely called high-sensitivity CRP (hsCRP) is required for adequate determinations.

The ability of CRP values to predict risk of CAD was found to be mostly independent of and complementary to established risk parameters. The outstanding question is, What is the appropriate treatment regimen for individuals who are at increased risk due to relatively high CRP values? There is early promise that statins may provide a double dose of treatment by reducing cholesterol and LDL-C as well as CRP; however, this finding awaits confirmation by prospective, well-controlled studies.[13] This should provide the basis for testing, interpretation, and treatment recommendations and guidelines.

In early 2003 a panel of the Centers for Disease Control and Prevention and the American Heart Association published guidelines for use of hsCRP in the assessment of CAD risk.[14] Members of the panel recommended that measurement of hsCRP would be of value in patients at an intermediate, 10-year risk of disease. Individuals with a predetermined 10-year risk of 10% to 20% would benefit from this measurement, and the information should help guide treatment and modification of lifestyle. Panel members also determined that hsCRP should not replace, but rather augment, assessment of the traditional risk factors. They recommended that 2 measurements be made at least 2 weeks apart and the results averaged. The relative risk categories to be used in interpretation of the measurements are as follows: low risk, less than 1.0 mg/L of hsCRP; average risk, 1.0 to 3.0 mg/L of hsCRP; and high risk, greater than 3.0 mg/L of hsCRP. Individuals with values greater than 10 mg/L should be evaluated for acute inflammation or infection.

There has been considerable investigation of other "inflammatory" markers associated with the acute-phase response. These include a variety of parameters, including interleukin-6, albumin, proteinuria, procoagulant factors, and leukocytosis. Although both retrospective and prospective studies have evaluated many inflammatory and traditional markers for interdependence, few have included a complete list. Laboratory tests for markers of oxidative stress also have received interest and may be an extension or component of the inflammatory model. This may be due, in part, to the involvement of leukocytes in the inflammatory response. Neutrophils are especially capable of mobilizing their oxidative metabolites when activated. One of the most promising laboratory tests for cellular oxidative activity is myeloperoxidase activity in blood.[15] This has been shown to be significantly higher in patients with CAD and may provide additional risk assessment in the health maintenance setting. This marker also awaits validation by appropriate longitudinal study.

Homocysteine

Homocysteine is a metabolic amino acid intermediate whose concentration is controlled by the action of several enzymes involved in metabolism of sulfur amino acid B_{12}. Its circulating concentration is highly dependent on body stores (status) of vitamins B_{12} and B_6, and folate. The interest in serum homocysteine concentrations derived from the long-standing knowledge that patients with hereditary homocystinuria demonstrated premature CAD.

Early studies showed increased homocysteine concentrations in patients with established CAD.[16] There has also been considerable interest in genetic variation of one of the enzymes that affect homocysteine concentrations, methylene tetrahydrofolate reductase (*MTHFR*). However, the determination of *MTHFR* genotype is not particularly useful. Those individuals homozygous for the high-risk thermolabile variant of *MTHFR* have only a 16% greater risk of development of CAD.[17]

Recent studies have shown that the association of plasma homocysteine values and risk of CAD is not as strong as initially thought.[19] Many early studies were conducted before the increased fortification of cereal with folate to reduce the incidence of birth defects. This fortification has improved the general folate status of the American population that, in turn, may have altered the significance of the findings of later studies. In addition, it has been estimated that the nongenetic population-based risk for individuals of European descent may be as little as 2%. The nutrition committee of the American Heart Association has recommended that population screening for increased homocysteine is not warranted.[18]

Nonetheless, a finding of a serum homocysteine value of greater than 10.00 μmol/L should be considered less than optimal considering the low cost and relative safety of vitamin supplementation. Determination of homocysteine status is more indicated in individuals with a strong history of heart disease without hyperlipidemia and in individuals with renal insufficiency.

Brain Natriuretic Peptide

The natriuretic peptides are hormones that regulate electrolyte balance, fluid volume, and blood pressure. Brain (B)-type natriuretic peptide (BNP) is secreted by the heart ventricles. Under conditions of sustained ventricular expansion and overload, BNP and its related peptide, N-terminal proBNP are released into the circulation. Their concentrations can be dramatically increased in severe congestive heart failure. Because plasma BNP concentrations increase relative to the degree of heart failure, this marker has generated a great deal of interest in its potential role as an objective indicator of the severity of heart failure as well as a diagnostic tool in individuals with shortness of breath.

Asymptomatic left ventricular dysfunction is a treatable precursor of heart failure. B-type natriuretic factor has been evaluated as a potential marker for this condition obviating the need for expensive echocardiography. The concentrations of BNP are increased in these patients above what is usually seen in normal individuals. A community-based study of the Framingham Study cohort demonstrated that measurement of BNP was not particularly useful in identifying individuals with left ventricular hypertrophy and systolic dysfunction.[19] Discrimination limits set for 0.95 specificity of the assay showed sensitivities of 0.27 for men and 0.13 for women.

Obviously, decreasing the test discrimination threshold would rapidly increase the rate of false-positives in this group. Therefore, there is little evidence to suggest that measurement of BNP in the general population will be a useful screening tool for left ventricular hypertrophy.

Iron Function Tests

Classic hereditary hemochromatosis is the most prevalent monoallelic genetic disease in Europeans. Individuals affected with this inborn error carry a unique nonsense mutation (C282Y) that alters a major—histocompatibility complex class I-like protein known as HFE. It is estimated that as many as 1 in 10 white Americans carries at least one allele with this mutation. This makes heritable iron overload potentially one of the most common occult diseases. Several other mutations in HFE, including H63D, have been identified, but their clinical significance is not as clear. Although the C282Y mutation clearly can result in hematochromatosis, there is a great variation in the clinical manifestation of this condition.[20] Some individuals homozygous for the C282Y mutation have no clinical or biochemical evidence of iron overload.

The availability of genetic testing for hemochromatosis has generated substantial interest in its use as a screen for inherited risk of iron overload. The test is straightforward, and the disease is very prevalent and treatable. Once again, there are concerns regarding what questions the test result answers. Some individuals who are homozygous or mixed-heterozygous for mutations apparently do not suffer the adverse effects resulting from iron overload, whereas many patients with overt iron overload carry no hemochromatosis mutation. A large cohort study showed that only 1 of 152 subjects who were homozygous for C282Y had symptoms of hereditary hemochromatosis.[21] There is also a subgroup of individuals who have hereditary hemochromatosis due to mutations other than those identified in HFE. Genetic testing for phenotypic iron overload, therefore, remains problematic. An expert panel of the Centers for Disease Control and Prevention and the National Human Genome Research Institute concluded that genetic screening could not be recommended for hemochromatosis.[22]

There have been several guidelines promulgated for laboratory screening for iron overload. Measurement of serum iron, iron-binding capacity (transferrin), and degree of transferrin saturation are simple and relatively inexpensive tests that can be used for this purpose.[23] Normal iron saturation levels on 2 occasions in adult life are sufficient to exclude hereditary hemochromatosis. When the transferrin saturation exceeds 60%, iron overload must be considered. An increased concentration of serum ferritin (the iron storage protein) confirms the presence of iron overload. If the serum ferritin concentration is within normal limits, testing should be repeated every several years. Genetic testing may be performed to ascertain the hereditary nature of the iron overload.

Thyroid Function Tests

Laboratory screening for thyroid dysfunction is dominated by the use of thyroid-stimulating hormone, or thyrotropin (TSH). The prevalence of both hypothyroidism and hyperthyroidism is estimated to be 2% to almost 10% in the general population, and appropriate therapeutic approaches are available. Laboratory assays for TSH have evolved to the point where they are extremely sensitive ("third generation" or higher) and can easily detect the suppressed pituitary output in reaction to thyroid hyperfunction. Assays for TSH are now of sufficient quality and performance that they are capable of detecting apparent dysfunction in clinically asymptomatic individuals. Much of the discussion of appropriate response to studies of thyroid function centers on recommendations for appropriate response to such subclinical disease.

A generally accepted algorithm for thyroid screening includes measurement of TSH periodically, particularly in older women.[24] A finding of a "normal" TSH concentration has a relatively high negative predictive value in ruling out primary thyroid disease. Once again, however, we have a conundrum regarding what is "normal," since subclinical disease is known to exist. For example, many laboratories use a reference interval for TSH that is approximately 0.5 to 5.5 mU/L, but longitudinal studies have shown that an individual whose TSH is greater than 2.0 mU/L is at increased risk of the development of overt hypothyroidism over the next 20 years.[25] If only individuals shown to have a negative reaction for thyroid peroxidase autoantibodies are included in the reference population, the 95% reference interval becomes about 0.5 to 3.6 mU/L.[26] It would be useful for practitioners to establish their specific laboratory-determined reference interval for TSH.

The measurement of the primary thyroid hormones total thyroxine (T_4), free thyroxine (fT_4), and free thyronine (fT_3) is best used in follow-up testing once an abnormal TSH value is revealed.

Prostate-Specific Antigen

Prostate-specific antigen (PSA) is a metalloproteinase derived from the prostate gland that is increased in conditions of prostate dysfunction, both benign and malignant. Originally designed and approved as a tumor marker for monitoring treatment and recurrence of prostate adenocarcinoma, PSA testing in the general male population has increased steadily throughout the last decade. Free PSA screenings are not uncommon. Prostate-specific antigen testing has been shown to be more sensitive than the digital rectal examination for detecting prostate cancer. The upper reference level for PSA is generally 4.0 ng/mL, but at this threshold 10% to 20% of early prostate cancers will be missed by PSA testing alone.[27] In addition, PSA values can be increased above this level in prostatitis and benign prostatic hypertrophy. The yield of PSA screening increases substantially with repeated annual testing.

Prostate-specific antigen is present in the blood circulation in multiple forms. These forms tend to be present in different proportions in malignant and benign conditions. As a proteinase, PSA is greatly bound to antiproteinases and, therefore, is present in both the free and complex forms. Immunoassays currently in use should be able to detect both the free and bound forms and yield an accurate total PSA value. Free-PSA assays are also widely available, which measure only the free, unbound PSA in blood. A complexed PSA assay is also available. The proportion of the total PSA concentration that remains free is much higher in benign prostate disease (>25%) than is the case with adenocarcinoma (<8%).[28] The recommended use for free-PSA testing is to assess patients whose initial total PSA value is in the range above the reference interval of 4.0 ng/mL but less than the 10.0 ng/mL level above which cancer is likely to be present.[28] In this group, free PSA can rule in or rule out benign and malignant disease, obviating the need for some biopsies.

Medicare allows 1 PSA test for screening purposes every 11 months for men over the age of 50 years.

Urinalysis

Urinalysis is one of the major groups of laboratory tests, ranking behind only chemistry profiles and CBC counts in the number of tests performed annually in the United States. These urine parameters, measured easily by the "dipstick" method, provide information about the status of the genitourinary system.

Urine is a complex biologic fluid whose composition depends on many factors, some of which are totally unrelated to the presence or risk of disease. The contents of urine in both healthy and diseased individuals depend on body mass, fluid intake, dietary intake, exercise status, and time of day. Therefore, knowledge of the individual's habits just before collection of either a random or morning-void specimen is helpful in interpreting results.

The laboratory examination of urine may now be performed using a wide variety of techniques. These vary from the historical manual techniques of dipstick, centrifuge, and microscope to totally automated, computer-controlled instruments; the latter methods are used in most large laboratories. The diagnostic and surveillance uses of urinalysis in the preventive care setting focus on urinary tract infections, hematuria, and proteinuria.

Urinary tract infection

Up to 6% of women are affected by urinary tract infections each year.[29] The first line of evaluation is often urinalysis. If the infection is suspected clinically, the patient should be instructed to collect a midstream, clean-voided specimen for which appropriate supplies are readily available. The microscopic confirmation of infection includes the presence of red or white blood cells and bacteria seen under the high-power microscopic field.

The finding of bacteria in this examination corresponds to more than 10 organisms per milliliter of urine upon culturing of the urine, which is the obvious confirmation test procedure.

The screening of asymptomatic individuals for urinary tract infections can be more problematic. A recent review noted that school-aged boys and girls exhibit an incidence of bacteriuria of 0.03% and 1% to 2%, respectively. During midlife, these prevalences rise to 3% to 4% for women and increase further to as high as 10% at age 50 years. Older patients may have an even higher incidence due to prostate and bladder dysfunction, with an incidence approaching 20% after age 65. These disease prevalences are substantially higher than many that are "screened" by other laboratory tests discussed in this chapter.

Hematuria

Although the presence of as few as 10 red blood cells in urine can signal clinically significant conditions, their presence also can result just from exercise. In children, up to 22% of cases of hematuria are without apparent cause; in adults, up to 50% of cases are without apparent cause. Conditions associated with the presence of hematuria include neoplasm, stones, inflammation, and benign prostatic hypertrophy.[30]

The evaluation of hematuria should be accompanied by a thorough history and physical examination to rule out specific causes, such as acute glomerulonephritis and abdominal and pelvic masses. One note of caution is that the determination of slight hematuria requires a freshly voided specimen, particularly if the urine has a relatively low specific gravity. If these specimens are stored or transported so that many hours pass before analysis, the blood cells are likely to disintegrate and render the dipstick findings negative. This effect is due to dilution of the hemoglobin released from the red blood cells in the total volume of the urine specimen.

Proteinuria

Healthy adults excrete up to 150 mg of urinary protein each day. About 60% are derived from normal plasma proteins, and the remaining 40% are derived from the kidney and genitourinary tract. A variety of proteins are in the urine, including albumin, transferrin, amylase, urokinase, immunoglobin, and mucoprotein. The major components are albumin, mucoprotein, and immunoglobins, which account for about 95% of the total.[31]

The presence of excessive proteinuria must be distinguished from the transient proteinuria that results from strenuous exercise, stress, and hypothermia. As implied by its name, transient proteinuria resolves in the absence of the insult. Persistent proteinuria, which may result from either tubular or glomerular renal disease, should be evaluated completely.

The initial finding of proteinuria in the health maintenance setting should be investigated, especially if the individual is asymptomatic. Repeated urinalysis is indicated to determine whether the proteinuria is transient. If proteinuria is persistent and nonorthostatic, further testing is warranted. Presumably, a patient with substantial decrement of plasma albumin would not present as an outpatient, but this result is often readily available and can be checked easily. It is also likely that plasma urea and creatinine concentrations are available for review to assess grossly the patient's renal function. Additional laboratory tests can be performed to assess the nature of the proteinuria more precisely. These tests include urine protein electrophoresis and urinary light chains; the latter should always be evaluated when an individual also exhibits an increased serum total protein concentration and proteinuria. A 24-hour urine collection to determine both total daily protein output and creatinine clearance is more useful than the initial random or morning-void specimen measurements.

Microalbuminuria

In diabetic patients, the best test for evaluating early-onset proteinuria is quantification of urine albumin using immunoassays. These tests are more sensitive to the initial increases in albuminuria associated with diabetic nephropathy. In general, microalbuminuria is considered present when excretion exceeds 30 mg/g creatinine.

Complete Blood Cell Count

Hematology panels that show the CBC count are similar to chemistry panels, as they are most useful for ruling out abnormalities. Again, it is important to keep in mind the diagnostic goals in a population with a low prevalence of disease. The usual expected outcome is the detection of anemia, particularly nutritional anemias, and inflammatory processes. The salient parameters evaluated to achieve these goals are the erythrocyte and leukocyte counts, hemoglobin concentration, and red blood cell indexes.

In a health maintenance population, neither the white blood cell count (WBC) nor the mean corpuscular value (MCV) exhibits a statistically significant incidence of abnormal results.[32] Although 75% of cases of decreased MCV usually represent either thalassemia or iron deficiency, only 15% of cases of increased MCV represent megaloblastic anemias. It would appear that the remainder of cases is a result of toxic changes secondary to alcohol intake or drug regimens. The experience in the preventive health setting is that the entry for investigation of the CBC count was more often triggered by a clear abnormality of the MCV because a marked decrease in hemoglobin was rarely seen in an asymptomatic population.

Medicare does not support testing the CBC count, or its components, for screening purposes and will deny payment for such use.

REFERENCES

1. Koch DD, Hassemer DJ, Wiebe DA, Laessig RH. Testing cholesterol accuracy. *JAMA*. 1988;260:2252–2259.

2. Cebul RD, Beck JR. Biochemical profiles. In: Sox HC, ed. *Common Diagnostic Tests*. Philadelphia, Pa: American College of Physicians; 1987;277–304.

3. Prati D, Taioli E, Zanella A, et al. Updated definitions of healthy ranges for serum alanine aminotransferase levels. *Ann Intern Med*. 2002;137:1–9.

4. American Diabetes Association. Report of the expert committee on the diagnosis and classification of diabetes mellitus. *Diabetes Care*. 1997;20:1183–1197.

5. Sinha R, Fisch G, Teague B, et al. Prevalence of impaired glucose tolerance among children and adolescents with marked obesity. *N Engl J Med*. 2002;346:802–810.

6. Barr RG, Nathan DM, Meigs JB, Singer DE. Tests of glycemia for the diagnosis of Type 2 diabetes mellitus. *Ann Intern Med*. 2002;137:263–272.

7. National Cholesterol Education Program. Second report of the Expert Panel on Detection, Evaluation and Treatment of High Blood Cholesterol in Adults (Adult Treatment Panel II). *Circulation*. 1994;89:2486–2497.

8. Expert Panel on Detection, Evaluation, and Treatment of High Blood Cholesterol in Adults (Adult Treatment Panel III): executive summary of third report of the National Cholesterol Education Program (NCEP) Expert Panel on Detection, Evaluation and Treatment of High Blood Cholesterol in Adults. *JAMA*. 2001;285:2468–2497.

9. Shlipak MG, Simon JA, Vittinghoff E, et al. Estrogen and progestin, lipoprotein(a) and the risk of recurrent coronary heart disease events after menopause. *JAMA*. 2000;283:1845–1852.

10. Blake GJ, Otvos JD, Rafai N, Ridker PM. Low-density lipoprotein particle concentration and size as determined by nuclear magnetic resonance spectroscopy as predictors of cardiovascular risk in women. *Circulation*. 2002;106:1930–1937.

11. Ridker PM, Cushman M, Stampfer MJ, Tracy RP, Hennekens CH. Inflammation, aspirin, and the risk of cardiovascular disease in apparently healthy men. *N Engl J Med*. 1997;336:973–979.

12. Ridker PM, Rifai N, Rose L, Buring JE, Cook NR. Comparison of C-reactive protein and low-density lipoprotein cholesterol levels in the prediction of first cardiovascular events. *N Engl J Med*. 2002;347:1557–1565.

13. Vorchheimer DA, Fuster V. Inflammatory markers in coronary artery disease: let prevention douse the flames. *JAMA*. 2001;286:2154–2156.

14. Pearson TA, Mensah GA, Alexander RW, et al. Markers of inflammation and cardiovascular disease: application to clinical and public health practice: a statement for healthcare professionals from the Centers for Disease Control and Prevention and the American Heart Association. *Circulation*. 2003;107:499–511.

15. Zhang R, Brennan M-L, Fu X. Association between myeloperoxidase levels and risk of coronary artery disease. *JAMA*. 2001;286:2136–2142.

16. Malinow MR, Bostom AG, Krauss RM. Homocyst(e)ine, diet and cardiovascular diseases: a statement for healthcare professionals from the Nutrition Committee, American Heart Association. *Circulation*. 1999;99:178–182.

17. Klerk M, Verhoef P, Clarke R, Blom HJ, Kok FJ, Schouten EG, and the MTHFR Studies Collaboration Group. MTHFR 677C→T polymorphism and risk of coronary heart disease: a meta-analysis. *JAMA*. 2002;288:2023–2031.

18. Wilson PWF. Homocysteine and coronary heart disease: how great is the hazard? *JAMA*. 2002;288:2042–2043.

19. Vasan RS, Benjamin EJ, Larson MG, et al. Plasma natriuretic peptides for community screening for left ventricular hypertrophy and systolic dysfunction: the Framingham Study. *JAMA*. 2002;288:1252–1259.

20. Khoury MJ, McCabe LL, McCabe ERB. Population screening in the age of genomic medicine. *N Engl J Med*. 2003;348:50–58.

21. Beutler E, Felitti VJ, Koziol JA, Ho NJ, Gelbart T. Penetrance of 845G-A (C282Y) HFE hereditary haemochromatosis mutation in the USA. *Lancet*. 2002;359:211–218.

22. Cogswell ME, Burke W, McDonnell SM, Franks AL. Screening for hemochromatosis: a public health perspective. *Am J Prev Med*. 1999;16:134–140.

23. Andrews NC. Disorders of iron metabolism. *N Engl J Med*. 1999;341:1986–1994.

24. Stockigt JR. Case finding and screening strategies for thyroid dysfunction. *Clin Chim Acta*. 2002;315:111–124.

25. Vanderpump MPJ, Tunbridge WMG, French JM. The incidence of thyroid disorders in the community: a twenty-year follow-up of the Whickham Survey. *Clin Endocrinol*. 1995;43:55–68.

26. Bjoro T, Holmen J, Kruger O. Prevalence of thyroid disease, thyroid dysfunction and thyroid peroxidase antibodies in a large, unselected population: the Health Study of Nord-Trondelag (HUNT). *Eur J Endocrinol*. 2000;143:639–647.

27. Harris R, Lohr KN. Screening for prostate cancer: an update of the evidence for the U.S. Preventive Services Task Force. *Ann Intern Med*. 2002;137:917–929.

28. Catalona WJ, Partin AW, Slawin KM, Brawer MK, Flanigan RC, Patel A. Use of the percentage of free prostate-specific antigen to enhance differentiation of prostate cancer from benign prostatic disease: a prospective multicenter clinical trial. *JAMA*. 1998;279:1542–1547.

29. Fang LST. Urinalysis in the diagnosis of urinary tract infections. *Clin Lab Med*. 1988;8:567–576.

30. Bloom JK. An algorithm for hematuria. *Clin Lab Med*. 1988;8:577–581.

31. Kim MS. Proteinuria. *Clin Lab Med*. 1988;8:527–533.

32. Van Lente F, Castellani W, Chou, D, Matsen RN, Galen RS. Application of the EXPERT consultation system to accelerated laboratory investigation. *Clin Chem*. 1986;32:1719–1724.

chapter 5

Imaging as a Screening Tool

Michael T. Modic, MD, and Nancy A. Obuchowski, PhD

INTRODUCTION

Traditional approaches to prevention (primary and secondary) have combined a set of services, offering them to individuals at intervals throughout their lives based on considerations such as age, sex, occupation, and family history. These services usually include a directed physical examination and history and various screening and diagnostic tests, depending on circumstances. Screening in this context is the systematic testing of asymptomatic individuals for preclinical disease in an effort to detect and treat before the critical point is reached. Imaging tests such as conventional radiography and mammography usually have been a part of this approach. Of late, however, engineering advances have resulted in relatively noninvasive imaging acquisition devices with expanded capabilities and the potential for greater sensitivity and specificity in the detection of disease.

The net result of these engineering advances is that examinations of larger anatomical regions, such as the chest and abdomen, can be obtained in a single breath hold (less than 20 seconds) with excellent spatial resolution. Alternatively, the larger regions of coverage can be traded off for increased spatial resolution and shorter examination times. For example, isotropic images of the heart can be obtained with breath holds and cardiac gating, which can capture anatomical images of the heart during diastole, minimizing cardiac motion and allowing for detection and quantification of coronary artery calcification. Coupling such an acquisition with intravenous iodinated contrast medium allows for intravascular visualization of the coronary artery tree or other circulations that enable depiction of vascular diseases such as stenosis and aneurysms.

Such advances in technology tend to fuel new applications, often leading to controversy. For example, multi-slice computed tomography (CT) can enable detection of certain malignancies at an earlier stage than by routine history and physical examinations. However, early detection in a few patients is almost always accompanied by negative consequences for others: false labeling and unnecessary workup due to false-positives, false reassurance and delayed treatment due to false-negatives, and unnecessary workup and treatment due to lifetime latent and nonprogressive forms of disease.

Early detection of disease cannot be assumed to translate into improved patient outcomes. Determining whether these services should be recommended to patients necessitates an understanding of how often patients benefit by screening and how often they are harmed by screening. In clinical trials, the success or failure of a treatment often is quantified by the number of patients needed to be treated to benefit 1 patient (NNT) and the number of patients needed to be treated before harming 1 patient (NNH).[1] Additionally, it is helpful in screening to know the number of patients needed to be screened to benefit 1 patient (NNS) and the number of patients screened before harming 1 patient (NSH).

For purposes of illustration, this chapter will consider the use of multislice detector CT and mammography as screening tools and review current imaging screening programs targeted at detecting early disease and, in the case of coronary artery calcification, a risk factor for a disease. Using previously published criteria,[2] this chapter will attempt to identify the strengths and weaknesses of these approaches, shortcomings in the literature, and directions for future research, and discuss how these criteria can be used to estimate NNS and NSH.

CRITERIA FOR EFFECTIVE SCREENING

The basic logic behind screening asymptomatic individuals for disease is that earlier detection may lead to earlier intervention, when a disease process is more amenable to therapy. Ten criteria have been formulated for evaluating screening programs and are summarized in Table 5-1.[3] These criteria encompass the characteristics of the disease, the screening test, and the treatment. In the case of lung, breast, and colon cancers, screening is undertaken for the disease itself in an effort to prevent serious consequences by instituting treatment at an earlier time (ie, secondary prevention). These criteria must be modified (Table 5-2) in the case of calcium scoring, as it is a test that screens for a risk factor, rather than the actual disease (M.T.M., N.A.O., unpublished data, 2003) in an effort to prevent disease (ie, primary prevention).

Characteristics of the Disease

Earlier detection of disease does not always translate into improved patient outcomes. In fact, early detection of disease can lead to higher morbidity and mortality rates, which is especially true when the prevalence of the disease studied is low, prevalence of pseudodisease or false-positives is high, and potential follow-up diagnostic studies are encumbered with substantial morbidity. For the disease entities under discussion, there can be no doubt that there are potential serious consequences. Lung, colon, and breast cancers are the leading causes of death due to cancer in adults. Coronary artery disease is the leading cause of death in adults. Screening is more cost-effective if the disease screened for has a long and predictable detectable preclinical phase and a high prevalence among people who are screened (Fig 5-1[3]).

For screening lung cancer in a target population of men and women older than 40 years who have a history of smoking at least 10 packs of cigarettes a year, the prevalence of a detectable pulmonary cancer is 2% to 4%.[4-6] For colorectal cancer, the target population is asymptomatic individuals older than 50 years without risk factors. In this population, the prevalence of 1 cm or larger adenomatous polyps is 3%, increasing to 5% to 6%

by 80 years of age.[7] Both of these target populations have a significantly higher prevalence than that of breast cancer, for which the prevalence in the general population screened is only 0.6% to 1%.[8-10]

Unlike lung, colon, and breast cancer screening, in which the test detects the presence of disease, CT scanning for calcium scoring does not detect coronary artery disease. The detection and quantification of coronary artery calcium represents an approach based on the assumption that there is an association between coronary calcium scores and the risk of coronary events, and that primary prevention measures can lower the risk in the affected population.[11-15] The test then is employed to detect a marker for disease, the coronary calcium score. Ideally, a risk factor will be present only in patients in whom the disease will develop and will be absent in patients in whom the disease will not develop. However, coronary artery calcium, like most risk factors, is not nearly an ideal risk factor, as the noncalcified burden of atherosclerosis has been shown to be significantly greater than the calcified burden. In fact, the calcified portion of the atherosclerosis is likely to be more stable than the uncalcified portion, which may be at greater risk of a major symptom-producing event. Using the assumption that the amount of calcified plaque tracks the total amount of plaque, levels of probability of major coronary artery disease have been projected based on Agatston scores obtained with electron beam CT. It has been shown that these scores have a significant association with the risk of "hard" coronary events, but the reported associations were unadjusted for other cardiac risk factors.[16,17] A pooled analysis of the predictive values from these studies showed an increase in positive predictive value and a

---

TABLE 5-1

Criteria for Evaluating Effectiveness of Screening for Disease*

Characteristics of the disease
1. Disease has serious consequences.
2. Screening population has a high prevalence of the disease in a detectable preclinical phase.

Characteristics of the test
3. Screening test detects little pseudodisease.
4. Screening test has a high accuracy for detecting the detectable preclinical phase.
5. Screening test enables detection of the disease before the critical point.
6. Screening test causes little morbidity.
7. Screening test is affordable and available.

Characteristics of treatment
8. Treatment exists.
9. Treatment is more effective when applied before symptoms begin.
10. Prevention is not too risky or toxic.

*Adapted from *Am J Roentgenol.* 1997;168:3–11.[3]

TABLE 5-2

Criteria for Evaluating Effectiveness of Screening for Risk Factors

Characteristics of the disease
1. Disease has serious consequences.
2. Screening population has a high incidence* of disease.
3. Risk factor is a good predictor of disease.

Characteristics of the test
4. Screening test has a high accuracy for detecting the risk factor.
5. Screening test detects the risk factor before the critical point.
6. Screening test causes little morbidity.
7. Screening test is affordable and available.

Characteristics of prevention
8. Prevention exists.
9. Prevention is more effective than treatment of the disease.
10. Prevention is not too risky or toxic.

*Incidence is the rate of new occurrence of disease in a previously disease-free population over a particular period.

corresponding decrease in negative predictive value with increasing calcium scores.[18]

The currently used interpretation of these scores is as follows. An absent or low (less than 10) Agatston score indicates a very low risk of development of coronary heart disease.[18,19] A high score may be of value in patients considered to be at intermediate risk of coronary heart disease in elevating them to a higher risk category, a finding that may benefit an asymptomatic patient in whom other risk factors can be modified.[18,19] However, to date, published data have not defined which asymptomatic patients would benefit from calcium scoring.

Characteristics of the Test

Sensitivity and specificity

A screening test that detects a high frequency of pseudodisease will not be cost-effective. Two types of pseudodisease have been described:[3,20] type 1 disease, which never progresses and may regress naturally, and type 2 disease, which progresses so slowly that symptoms never develop. In the case of lung cancer, given that 80% to 100% of untreated cases die within 10 years,[21,22] the frequency of pseudodisease must be very small. In the case of colon cancer, there is evidence that many polyps smaller than 1 cm may regress (pseudodisease type 1).[23] The rate of progression from adenomatous polyps to cancer has been estimated at approximately 2.5 polyps per 1000 individuals per year.[24] The frequency of type 2 pseudodisease has been evaluated in a large autopsy series.[25] In that series, colorectal cancer unrelated to the cause of death was detected in 0.5% of 50- to 60-year-

olds, 1% of 60- to 70-year-olds, and 1.5% of 70- to 80-year-olds. These rates are lower than in breast cancer; the prevalence of ductal breast cancer in situ in women who died of other causes is 6% to 14%.[26-28]

To detect more true-positives than false-positives when the prevalence of a disease is less than 5%, which is the case for most disease, the screening test must have a sensitivity greater than 95% if the specificity is less than or equal to 95% and vice versa. Most tests, even diagnostic ones, do not meet these standards. An increase in specificity will increase cost-effectiveness of a screening test, but an increase in sensitivity may not.

To date, no good studies exist regarding the accuracy of slice CT for detecting pulmonary cancer. Recent studies compare CT to conventional chest radiographs,[6,29,30] but chest radiography is not an acceptable gold standard, nor does a gold standard exist. This absence of accuracy data is not unexpected at the introductory stage of a new screening technique. Tests that lack specificity may not be in the best interest of patients. In an asymptomatic population with a low prevalence rate of disease, a low specificity leads to unnecessary and sometimes invasive testing, adds monetary costs, and also adds patient costs in terms of false labeling and unnecessary worrying.

Criticism has been leveled against CT screening for lung cancer in that there may be a high frequency of detection of benign lung nodules, creating a high false-positive rate. However, the current approach is to view these indeterminate nodules over time rather than at a single testing. If an indeterminate nodule is identified, for instance, a noncalcified nodule less than 1 cm, follow-up

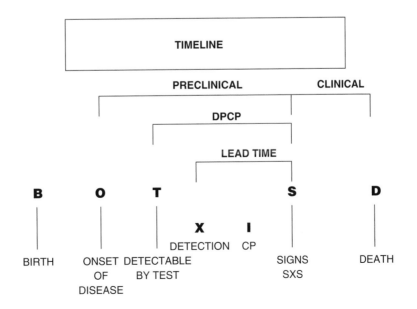

F I G U R E   5-1

Timeline from birth to death. Preclinical phase begins with onset of disease and ends when signs and symptoms appear. Clinical phase begins with onset of signs and symptoms. Detectable preclinical phase (DPCP) is interval during preclinical phase when disease is detectable by the test. Lead time is interval from disease detection to appearance of signs and symptoms. For screening to be effective, critical point (CP) must occur during DPCP. Reprinted with permission from *Am J Roentgenol.* 1997;168:3–11.[3]

intervals of 3, 6, 12, and 24 months are recommended to assess stability. The process of screening for lung cancer, then, should be viewed as dynamic with temporal factors rather than a single event.

In the case of colon cancer, recent studies have shown a sensitivity and specificity in excess of 90% for polyps measuring greater than 1 cm.[31-37] The argument for using a cutoff for polyp size in the analysis relates to the low prevalence of invasive cancer in polyps smaller than 1 cm vs a 10% prevalence in polyps between 1 and 2 cm.[38] The sensitivity for polyps smaller than 6 mm is less than 60%. For both lung and colon cancer screening, the acquisition and postprocessing techniques are important to consider. Studies have shown increasing sensitivity for thicknesses decreasing from 5 to 1 mm. Postprocessing techniques that include volumetric analysis are likely to improve the reproducibility and accuracy of lesion behavior over time. Mammography screening is an older test, and a number of studies have looked at accuracy. A meta-analysis published in 1998 reported a sensitivity range of 83% to 95% and false-positive rates ranging from 0.9% to 6.5%.[39]

The sensitivity and specificity of calcium scoring with mechanical scanners is based on data from electron beam CT. While both techniques are very sensitive and specific for the presence of calcification based on attenuation values, they are insensitive to the total atherosclerotic burden that is uncalcified. The current scoring methodology based on Agatston scores is further plagued by poor reproducibility. Efforts are under way to develop techniques that rely on volume or mass scores, which are more user independent and reproducible.

Critical point

Another important consideration relates to the ability of the screening test to detect disease, or the risk factor, before the critical point, the time in a disease process when treatment or prevention is no longer effective or is much less effective. To be effective, screening must occur (1) after the onset of the disease, (2) while the disease is detectable by the imaging test, and (3) before the critical point. For most cancers, the critical point occurs when the primary tumor metastasizes. Multiple models exist for determining the optimal timing if there are good natural history data.[40-44] Although recent studies have suggested that CT can help detect stage I lung cancer more effectively than any other method can, the critical point in the natural history may already have passed.[6,29,30] In these studies, 71% to 93% of people with detected pulmonary cancer had stage I disease. Yet the 5-year survival for stage I lung cancer is estimated at between 49% and 75% (dependent on cell type). For colorectal and breast cancers, the survival rates of patients with stage I disease are much higher, 92% and 97%, respectively.[45] The critical point for colon cancer is considered to be an adenomatous polyp greater than 1 cm, as metastasis from polyps smaller than 1 cm is considered very rare.[23] For

some patients with coronary artery disease, the critical point is when symptoms first appear. Unfortunately, for other patients, the first symptom can be sudden death secondary to a coronary event, and thus the critical point is earlier, during the development of ischemic disease before the onset of symptoms.

The morbidity of a screening test itself merits evaluation. In screening tests that employ ionizing radiation, no short-term morbidity occurs, and long-term morbidity relates to radiation exposure. Because CT screening subjects the individual screened to low levels of radiation exposure from X-rays, the theoretical possibility exists of him or her developing a radiation-induced cancer some time later in that person's life. Unfortunately, there is considerable confusion and speculation in the lay press and often uncertainty and imprecision from health care professionals when consulted about the risk of induced cancer. The risk due to exposure to ionizing radiation has been extrapolated backward from studies of survivors of the atomic bombs dropped on Hiroshima and Nagasaki, Japan, where high doses of ionizing radiation led to an increased incidence of cancer-related deaths. All available sources indicate that extrapolation downward is not justified. Cancer-inducing effects are not observed for exposure to dose levels below 200 mSv. In fact, radiation biology studies have demonstrated that in the low-dose region there may be positive effects from exposure to radiation.[46,47] Whole-body CT doses fall within the "low dose" (well below 100 mSv) and not the high-dose region (gt200 mSv), as some have suggested.[48] Within this low-dose region, it is not possible to make any definite predictions relative to any deleterious effect. Reference to the natural human environment appears to be more suitable and easiest to communicate. For this reason, dose values may be expressed as multiples of the natural background radiation, as suggested by Cameron.[49] The average yearly exposure to natural background radiation in the United States is 3.0 mSv, in contrast to the value of 200 mSv, which is the value below which the natural resistance and repair mechanisms of the human body are able to reduce the probability of damage. Conventional CT of the chest and abdomen has an effective dose of approximately 6.4 and 6.8 mSv, respectively, and if performed together has a total effective dose of 13.2 mSv. With the lower dose techniques employed in screening and technical improvements to reduce dose, the total dose from a screening examination is probably reduced by at least 50%. Portrayed in another way, the effective whole-body dose is probably equivalent to the radiation exposure of 2 years due to natural background radiation.

The affordability of a screening test is also important. At present, the cost of mammography, and in some cases conventional chest radiography, is covered by health care insurance providers. Screening with multisection detector CT currently is not covered. A recent survey in the United States revealed an average charge of $350 for each of the individual regions screened and an average charge of $900 for the chest, heart, and abdomen done as a single examination. The charges for virtual colonography in 2003 ranged from $700 to $900. Charges for screening mammography, covered by almost all payers, average about $200.

Characteristics of Treatment and Prevention

For lung, pulmonary, and breast cancers, treatment exists in the form of resection and often radiation or chemotherapy. For cardiovascular disease, prevention includes modification of risk factors, and treatment involves vascular, surgical, and drug interventions. For screening to be cost-effective, treatment must be more effective or less toxic when applied during the detectable preclinical phase compared with treatment applied after symptoms begin.[50] Demonstration of the benefits of early treatment may be difficult, even when treatment is known to be effective once symptoms occur. Four main problems plague comparisons of the outcomes of patients who are screened vs patients who are not screened (Table 5-3[19,51-56]). Because of these problems, researchers do not use length of survival when studying the effectiveness of early treatment. Currently, most researchers use disease-specific mortality,[20] computed as the number of deaths resulting from the specific disease divided by the number of people at risk. Two studies have shown promising increased lengths of survival from pulmonary cancer as the size of the detected tumor decreases,[57,58] but these studies are potentially flawed because of the biases listed in Table 5-3. In breast cancer screening, early detection and treatment may result in as much as a 50% reduction in mortality.

Treatment or prevention should also not be too risky or toxic, to offset long-term benefits. The 30-day mortality rate after pulmonary resection is high, 3.7%,[59] compared with endoscopic polypectomy and lumpectomy or mastectomy, which are effectively zero. There are also minor and major complications with lung resection, such as atelectasis, pneumothorax, pulmonary embolism, and infection.

ESTIMATION OF NNS AND NSH

The best estimate of the number of patients needed to be screened to benefit 1 patient (NNS) is a well-designed, controlled trial comparing outcomes of patients who underwent screening with those of patients who underwent usual care. This was done in the Swedish National Board of Health and Welfare Study, in which it was estimated that 1592 women aged 50 to 74 years had to be screened with mammography to prevent 1 death of breast cancer 7 years after the screening was instituted (ie, NNS = 1592).[23] Such data is available for mammography, being a mature screening test, but are not yet available for screening of colon and pulmonary cancers.

The estimate of the number of patients screened before harming 1 patient (NSH) can be calculated from published estimates of the prevalence of disease, the accuracy of the screening test, and the prevalence of pseudodisease. For breast cancer screening with mammography, this may be calculated to be 281.[2] To get even a crude estimate of NNS and NSH for calcium scoring, information needed includes the incidence of the disease in the relevant screening population, the probability of a high calcium score in patients destined for a coronary event, the probability of a low calcium score in patients who will not undergo a coronary event, the accuracy of CT, and the benefit of prevention vs treatment of disease. These parameters are currently unknown.

TABLE 5-3
Problems With Comparing Survival Times in Screened and Unscreened Patients

Bias Type	Definition
Lead time[51-54]	Length of time between disease detection and first appearance of signs or symptoms. Even if early treatment has no benefit, survival of screened patients may be greater than that of unscreened patients by addition of length of lead time.
Length[54,55]	Occurs because not all patients' disease progresses at the same rate. Slower progressing disease may be easier to detect in screening program and thus may be overrepresented in screening cohort.
Overdiagnosis[19]	Occurs when one does not adjust for occurrence of pseudodisease in screened cohort. Patients with pseudodisease do not die of specific disease under study, yet their survival is often falsely attributed to early treatment.
Stage migration[56]	Can occur when disease-specific survival rates of screened and unscreened patients are compared according to stage at which disease is detected. When malignant metastases are detected before any symptoms of metastasis appear, TNM stage is shifted from stage I or II to stage II or III. Then, survival in lower stages of screened patients appears greater than that of unscreened patients because patients with silent metastases have been removed from lower stages. Also, survival in higher stages appears better for screened patients because patients with early metastases tend to survive longer.

SUMMARY

Imaging screening tests enable detection of certain asymptomatic diseases at an earlier stage than by routine history and physical examinations. Most clinicians would agree that rather than competing, the 2 should be complementary. Evidence is mounting for the effectiveness of CT screening for lung and colon cancers. In the case of lung cancer, this screening test is clearly superior to anything else that exists, and early cancers are detected much more frequently using this tool. Recent trials have proved that screening for lung cancer in high-risk groups can be as effective and more cost-effective than similar programs, such as breast cancer screening with mammography, and that false-positives can be eliminated with simple follow-up, as part of the screening program.[60-62] Whether disease-specific mortality is affected by screening is unclear, but given the dismal 14% 5-year survival rate for lung cancer and the lack of other options for early detection, many view screening via this method as a practical approach.

On the other hand, a recent decision and cost-effectiveness analysis evaluated whether lung cancer screening using CT might be considered an appropriate strategy for adult smokers and those who have recently quit smoking. The authors predict a 13% lung cancer-specific mortality reduction but a 12% incidence of false-positive invasive procedures per 100,000 persons. This analysis found that such an approach is very expensive from both a health policy and societal perspective.[63] Unfortunately, cost-effectiveness analyses are highly dependent on a large number of assumptions and are only as good as those assumptions. In addition, with improvements in technology and interpretation, including computer-aided diagnosis, this type of analysis will have to undergo frequent revision and reassessment.[64]

Recently, the case has been made that all persons over the age of 50 years should undergo comprehensive evaluation of the entire large bowel.[65] While fiber-optic colonoscopy remains the gold standard, other options, such as barium enema, fecal occult blood testing, sigmoidoscopy, and CT colonoscopy, have been employed. In terms of its impact, any screening procedure requires patient acceptance and compliance to be effective. In this regard, studies suggest that CT colonography is considered less painful and less difficult for the patient overall than is fiber-optic colonoscopy.[66] Currently recommended American Cancer Society screening guidelines include fiber-optic and flexible sigmoidoscopy, which have low compliance.[67,68] Also, there is the advantage of optional abdominal screening at the same time; while infrequent, the identification of extracolonic CT findings, such as the detection of abdominal aneurysms, may be important.[69] Nevertheless, the required time and skills needed for CT colonography are not trivial, and whereas CT colonography may cost less, it is not clear what its accuracy is with flat lesions. The optimal practice of CT colonography is that suspicious lesions identified by this method also should be evaluated by fiber-optic colonoscopy and perhaps even should undergo biopsy on the same day with the same preparation.

Studies that included risk-adjusted outcomes that control for established cardiac risk factors have failed to consistently show the incremental value of coronary calcium scores over traditional multivariate risk assessment models, such as the Framingham risk model.[70,71] However, still other studies have suggested that there is a complementary role for these methods in identifying patients at high risk.[72] For instance, Taylor et al[73] suggested that the Framingham risk model significantly underestimates the presence of premature, subclinical calcified coronary atherosclerosis in a cohort of low-risk subjects and have recommended the use of calcium scoring as a means of identifying persons needing to be promoted to a higher risk category. Additional information for risk stratification can be gained from referencing a patient's calcium scores with asymptomatic individuals of the same sex and age to determine a percentile ranking.[74] Thus, the value of calcium scoring appears to be in providing a "biologic age" of the coronary artery to complement the chronological age employed in the Framingham risk model.

Controlled studies are needed that look at specific disease states and consolidate a database of these applied technologies from large multi-institutional experiences, to accumulate meaningful data. These data represent a longitudinal process, which can then assist high-risk populations and health care providers in making screening choices.

REFERENCES

1. Laupacis A, Sackett DL, Roberts RS. An assessment of clinically useful measures of the consequences of treatment. *N Engl J Med.* 1988;318:1728–1733.

2. Obuchowski NA, Graham RJ, Baker ME, Powell KA. Ten criteria for effective screening: their application to multi-slice CT screening for pulmonary and colorectal cancers. *Am J Roentgenol.* 2001;176:1357–1362.

3. Black WC, Welch HG. Screening for disease. *Am J Roentgenol.* 1997;168:3–11.

4. Eddy DM. Screening for lung cancer. *Ann Intern Med.* 1989;111:232–237.

5. Nesbitt JC, Putnam JB Jr., Walsh GL, Roth JA, Mountain CF. Survival in early stage non-small cell lung cancer. *Ann Thorac Surg.* 1995;60:466–472.

6. Henschke CI, McCauley DI, Yankelevitz DF, et al. Early Lung Cancer Action Project: overall design and findings from baseline screening. *Lancet.* 1999;354:99–105.

7. Neugut AI, Jacobsen JS, Rella VA. Prevalence and incidence of colorectal adenomas in asymptomatic persons. *Gastrointest Endosc Clin North Am.* 1997;7:387–399.

8. Braman DM, Williams HD. ACR accredited suburban mammography center: Three-year results. *J Fla Med Assoc.* 1989;76:1031–1034.

9. Burhenne LJW, Hislop TG, Burhenne HJ. The British Columbia Mammography Screening Program: evaluation of the first 15 months. *Am J Roentgenol.* 1992;158:45–49.

10. Linver MN, Paster S, Rosenberg RD, et al. Improvement in mammography interpretation skills in a community radiology practice after dedicated teaching courses: 2-year medical audit of 38,633 cases. *Radiology.* 1992;184:39–43.

11. Rumberger JA, Simmons DD, Fitzpatrick LA, et al. Coronary artery calcium area by electron beam computed tomography in coronary atherosclerotic plaque area: a histopathologic correlative study. *Circ J Am Heart Assoc.* 1995;92:2157–2162.

12. Mautner GC, Mautner SL, Froehlich J, et al. Coronary artery calcification: assessment with electron beam CT and histomorphometric correlation. *Radiology.* 1994;192:619–623.

13. Detrano R. Predictive value of electron beam computed tomography. *Circ J Am Heart Assoc.* 1997;95:534–536.

14. Carr JJ, Crouse JR, Joff DC Jr, et al. Evaluation of sub-second gated helical CT for quantification of coronary artery calcium and comparison with electron beam CT. *Am J Roentgenol.* 2000;174:915–921.

15. Shepherd J. Economics of lipid lowering in primary prevention: lessons from the West of Scotland Coronary Prevention Study. *Am J Cardiol.* 2001;87(5A):19B–22B.

16. Arad Y, Spadaro M, Goodman KG, et al. Prediction of coronary events with electron beam computed tomography: 19-month follow up of 1173 asymptomatic subjects. *Circ J Am Heart Assoc.* 1996;93:1951–1953.

17. Secci A, Wong N, Tang W, et al. Electron beam computed tomographic coronary calcium as a predictor of coronary events: comparison of two protocols. *Circ J Am Heart Assoc.* 1997;96:1122–1129.

18. O'Rourke R, Brundage B, Froelicher V, et al. American College of Cardiology/American Heart Association expert consensus document on electron beam computed tomography for the diagnosis and prognosis of coronary artery disease. *J Am Coll Cardiol.* 2000;36:326–340.

19. Wexler L, Brundage B, Crouse J, et al. Coronary artery calcification: pathophysiology, epidemiology, imaging methods and clinical implications: a statement for health professionals from the American Heart Association Writing Group. *Circ J Am Heart Assoc.* 1996;94:1175–1192.

20. Morrison AS. *Screening in Chronic Disease.* New York, NY: Oxford University Press Inc; 1992.

21. Sobue T, Suzuki R, Madsuda M, et al. Survival for clinical stage I lung cancer not surgically treated. *Cancer.* 1992;69:685–692.

22. Flehinger BJ, Kimmel M, Melamed MR. The effect of surgical treatment on survival from early lung cancer: Implications for screening. *Chest.* 1992;101:1013–1018.

23. Winawer SJ, Fletcher RH, Miller L, et al. Colorectal cancer screening: clinical guidelines and rationale. *Gastroenterology.* 1997;112:594–642.

24. Anderson LM, May DS. Has the use of cervical, breast, and colorectal cancer screening increased in the United States? *Am J Public Health.* 1995;85:840–842.

25. Berg JW, Downing A, Lukes RJ. Prevalence of undiagnosed cancer of the large bowel found at autopsy in different races. *Cancer.* 1970;25:1076–1080.

26. Kramer WM, Rush BF Jr. Mammary duct proliferation in the elderly. *Cancer.* 1973;31:130–137.

27. Alpers CE, Wellings SR. The prevalence of carcinoma in situ in normal and cancer-associated breasts. *Hum Pathol.* 1985;16:796–807.

28. Nielsen M, Thomsen JL, Primdahl S, et al. Breast cancer and atypia among young and middle-aged women: a study of 110 medicolegal autopsies. *Br J Cancer* 1987;56:814–819.

29. Kaneko M, Eguchi K, Ohmatsu H, et al. Peripheral lung cancer: screening and detection with low-dose spiral CT versus radiography. *Radiology.* 1996;201:798–802.

30. Mori K, Tominago K, Hirose T, Sasayawa M, et al. Utility of low-dose helical CT as a second step after plain chest radiography for mass screening for lung cancer. *J Thorac Imaging.* 1997;12:173–180.

31. Schreiber JP II. Assessment of techniques and efficacy of computed tomography colonography. *Appl Radiol.* 2003;(suppl) 31, no. 6:48–53.

32. Yee J, Akerkar GA, Hung RK, et al. Colorectal neoplasia: performance characteristics of CT colonography for detection in 300 patients. *Radiology.* 2001;219:685–692.

33. Fenlon HM, Nunes DP, Schroy PC III, Barish MA, Clarke PD, Ferrucci JT. A comparison of virtual and conventional colonoscopy for the detection of colorectal polyps. *N Engl J Med.* 1999;341:1496–1503.

34. Lees WR, Gillams AR. Is CT colography a reliable method for detecting colorectal cancer in symptomatic patients? *Radiology.* 2001;221(P):307.

35. Saito K, Mori M. Rate of progression to advanced stage in depressed-type colorectal adenoma. *Oncol Rep.* 2000;7:615–619.

36. Laghi A, Iannaccone R, Carbone I, et al. Multislice spiral CT colonography for the detection of colorectal polyps and neoplasms [abstract]. *Radiology.* 2001;221(P):307.

37. Johnson CD, Toledano A, Herman B, et al. CT colonography: performance evaluation in a multicenter setting (American College of Radiology Imaging Network Study 6653 [abstract]. *Radiology.* 2001;221(P):308.

38. Glick S. The significant polyp. Presented at the Second International Symposium on Virtual Colonoscopy, Boston, Mass, October 16–17, 2000.

39. Mushlin AI, Kouides RW, Shapiro DE. Estimating the accuracy of screening mammography: a meta-analysis. *Am J Prev Med.* 1998;14:143–153.

40. Parmigiani G. On optimal screening ages. *J Am Stat Assoc.* 1993;88:622–628.

41. Eddy DM. A mathematical model for timing repeated medical tests. *Med Decis Making.* 1983;3:34–62.

42. Kirch RLA, Klein M. Surveillance schedules for medical examinations. *Manage Sci.* 1974;20:1403–1409.

43. Shahani AK, Crease DM. Towards models of screening for early detection of disease. *Adv Appl Probl.* 1977;9:665–680.

44. Zelen M. Optimal scheduling of examinations for the early detection of disease. *Biometrika.* 1993;80:279–293.

45. Landis SH, Murray T, Bolden S, Wingo PA. Cancer statistics. *CA Cancer J Clin.* 1998;48:6–29.

46. Luckey TD. Physiological benefits from low levels of ionization radiation. *Health Phys.* 1982;43(6):771–789.

47. Cohen BL. Cancer risk from low level radiation. *Am J Roentgenol.* 2002;179:1137–1143.

48. Kalender WA. Dose. In: *Computed Tomography: Fundamentals, System Technology, Image Quality, Applications.* Munich, Germany: Publicis MCD Verlag; 2000:148.

49. Cameron JR. A radiation unit for the public. *Phys Soc.* 1991;20(2).

50. Cole P, Morrison AS. Basic issues in population screening for cancer. *J Natl Cancer Inst.* 1980;64:1263–1272.

51. Hutchinson GB, Shapiro S. Lead time gained by diagnostic screening for breast cancer. *J Natl Cancer Inst.* 1968;41:665–681.

52. Prorok PC. The theory of periodic screening: I. Lead time and proportion detected. *Adv Appl Probl.* 1976;8:127–143.

53. Prorok PC. The theory of periodic screening: II. Doubly bounded recurrence times and mean lead time and detection probability estimation. *Adv Appl Probl.* 1976;8:460–476.

54. Black WC, Welch HG. Advances in diagnostic imaging and overestimation of disease prevalence and the benefits of therapy. *N Engl J Med.* 1993;328:1237–1243.

55. Zelen M. Theory of early detection of breast cancer in the general population. In: Henson JC, Mattheiem WH, Rozencweig M, eds. *Breast cancer: trends in research and treatment.* New York, NY: Raven Press; 1976:287–300.

56. Feinstein AR, Sosin DM, Wells CK. The Will Rogers phenomenon: stage migration and new diagnostic techniques as a source of misleading statistics for survival in cancer. *N Engl J Med.* 1985;312:1604–1608.

57. Steele JD, Kleitsch WP, Dunn JE, Buell P. Survival in males with bronchogenic carcinomas resected as symptomatic solitary pulmonary nodules. *Ann Thorac Surg.* 1966;2:368–376.

58. Jackman R, Good CA, Clagett OT, Woolner LB. Survival rates in peripheral bronchogenic carcinoma up to four centimeters in diameter presenting as solitary pulmonary nodules. *J Thorac Cardiovasc Surg.* 1969;57:1–8.

59. Ginsberg RJ, Hill LD, Eagan RT, et al. Modern thirty-day operative mortality for surgical resection in lung cancer. *J Thorac Cardiovasc Surg.* 1983;86:654–658.

60. Sobue T, Suzuki T, Matsuda M, et al, for the Japanese Lung Cancer Screening Research Group. Survival for clinical Stage I lung cancer not surgically treated: comparison between screen detected and symptom detected cases. *Cancer.* 1992;69:685–692.

61. Henschke CI, McCauley DI, Yankelevitz DF, et al. Early lung cancer action project: overall design and findings from baseline screening. *Lancet.* 1999;354:99–105.

62. Henschke CI, Naidich DP, Yankelevitz DF, et al. Early lung cancer action project: initial findings on repeat screenings. *Cancer.* 2001;92:153–159.

63. Mahadevia PJ, Fleisher LA, Frick KD, et al. Lung cancer screening with helical computed tomography in older adult smokers. *JAMA.* 2003;289:313–322.

64. Grann VR, Neugut AI. Lung cancer screening at any price? *JAMA.* 2003;289:357–358.

65. Podolsky DK. Going the distance: the case for true colorectal cancer screening. *N Engl J Med.* 2000;343:207–208.

66. Svensson MH, Svensson E, Lasson A, Hellstrom M. Patient acceptance of CT colonography and conventional colonoscopy: prospective comparative study in patients with or suspected of having colorectal disease. *Radiology.* 2002;222:337–345.

67. Ferrucci JT. Colon cancer screening with virtual colonoscopy: promise, polyps, politics. *Am J Roentgenol.* 2001;177:975–988.

68. McMahon PM, Gazelle GS. The case for colorectal screening. *Semin Roentgenol.* 2000;35:325–332.

69. Hara AK, Johnson CD, MacCarty RL, Welch TJ. Incidental extracolonic findings at CT colonography. *Radiology.* 2000;215:353–357.

70. Wilson PWF, D'Agostino RB, Levy D, et al. Prediction of coronary heart disease using risk factor categories. *Circ J Am Heart Assoc.* 1998;97:1837–1847.

71. Detrano RC, Wong ND, Doherty TM, et al. Coronary calcium does not accurately predict near-term future coronary events in high-risk adults. *Circ J Am Heart Assoc.* 1999;99:2633–2638.

72. Taylor AJ, Burke AP, O'Malley PG, et al. A comparison of the Framingham risk index, coronary artery calcification, and culprit plaque morphology in sudden cardiac death. *Circ J Am Heart Assoc.* 2000;101:1243–1248.

73. Taylor AJ, Feuerstein I, Wong H, et al. Do conventional risk factors predict subclinical coronary artery disease? Results from the Prospective Army Coronary Calcium Project. *Am Heart J.* 2001;141:463–468.

74. Raggi P, Callister TQ, Cooil B, et al. Identification of patients at increased risk of first unheralded acute myocardial infarction by electron-beam computed tomography. *Circ J Am Heart Assoc.* 2000;101:850–855.

Behavioral and Psychological Influences in Health and Disease

chapter 6

Counseling for Health Behavior Change

Matthew M. Clark, PhD, and Kristin S. Vickers, PhD

INTRODUCTION

It has been well documented that the relationship between health care providers and their patients is a critical component of quality medical care. A positive relationship between the health care provider and patient is associated with increased patient satisfaction,[1] trust in the physician,[2] understanding of and adherence to physician instructions,[3] reduced litigation for malpractice,[4] and improved patient health status.[5] A recent systematic review evaluated the impact of various physician behaviors during the medical encounter on patient outcomes (eg, health status, quality of life, patient satisfaction, trust, and symptom resolution).[5]

Table 6-1 presents examples of the verbal and nonverbal behaviors found to be significantly associated with patient outcomes. A patient-centered approach that includes empathizing with the patient, reflective listening, and offering support and encouragement is not only associated with greater patient satisfaction, but also with improved patient behavior change.[5] In this chapter, we will review 2 models of health behavior that emphasize the use of these techniques.

Health behaviors are an important public health issue. A substantial number of adults in the United States would benefit from health behavior change in the areas of physical inactivity, tobacco use, or excess body weight. This chapter will focus on these 3 lifestyle factors as targets for health behavior change because these behaviors often coexist,[6] and each is associated with increased risk of chronic disease and related morbidity and mortality.[7-10] Furthermore, these are highly prevalent, high-risk health behaviors in US adults (approximately 23% smoke cigarettes, 65% are overweight or obese, and 70% are

TABLE 6-1

Examples of Physician Behaviors That Affect Patient Outcomes

Physician Verbal Behaviors Associated With Positive Patient Outcomes	Physician Verbal Behaviors Associated With Negative Patient Outcomes
Expressing empathy	Using mostly biomedical questioning style
Making statements of reassurance and support	Frequently interrupting patient
Being friendly and courteous	Behaving too formally
Using patient-centered questioning techniques	Collecting information without giving feedback to patient
Longer clinical encounter, with more time spent on health education	Antagonism
Expressing positive reinforcement in response to patient	Demonstrating irritation, anger, or nervousness
Appropriately using humor	Exerting dominance
Addressing patient's feelings, emotions, and social relations	**Physician Nonverbal Behaviors Associated With Positive Patient Outcomes**
Sharing medical data with patient	Nodding head
Discussing effects of treatment	Leaning forward toward patient
Listening to patient questions and statements	Uncrossed legs and arms
Summarizing information from patient	**Physician Nonverbal Behaviors Associated With Negative Patient Outcomes**
Giving explanations	Crossed arms
	Frequently touching patient during interview
	Orienting body away from patient

Adapted from *J Am Board Fam Pract.* 2002;15:25–38.[5]

physically inactive).[8,11] Although physician counseling is effective in modifying patient behavior[12,13] and is considered by physicians to be a valuable component of patient care, physicians counsel patients to change their health behaviors at a relatively low frequency.[14-18] However, many physicians do recognize and appreciate the importance of health behavior counseling.[19,20] The low frequency of physician counseling has given rise to a growing literature in the area of missed opportunities for physician counseling.[12,16] Given that most physicians believe that counseling is important but report a low frequency of providing counseling, there must be barriers to physician-delivered counseling that can help explain the low frequency of its delivery.

Previously identified barriers to counseling patients on lifestyle factors such as physical activity, diet, and smoking include the following:[17,21,22] lack of reimbursement for counseling-related activities, competing demands for the increasingly limited direct patient contact time, a perceived lack of counseling skills to help patients effectively make change, low confidence in counseling skills, and patient noncompliance with counseling recommendations.

In this chapter, we describe the prevalence of patient nonadherence and provide a case example of a patient in need of health behavior counseling. Two models of health behavior change are described along with their specific techniques, which have been found to be both useful in changing patient health behavior and appropriate for use in a medical setting. After presentation of the counseling strategies, we discuss the practical application of these techniques to the presented case.

PREVALENCE OF NONADHERENCE

Nonadherence to health care recommendations is a frequently experienced problem. Types of nonadherence can range from improper medication usage to not following a recommended low-calorie diet, not increasing the level of physical activity, not coming to follow-up appointments, or substance abuse. It has been estimated that nonadherence to health recommendations ranges from 20% to 95%.[23] For example, approximately 12% of those receiving a liver transplant to treat alcoholic liver disease will relapse to drinking alcohol the first year post-transplantation.[24] Despite the importance of continued exercise for patients enrolled in a cardiac rehabilitation program, almost 50% will demonstrate a reduction in their exercise level in the 3 months after their participation in a 12-week on-site cardiac rehabilitation program.[25] Finally, 78% of patients with lung cancer continue to smoke, despite having received counseling about nicotine dependence.[26] Thus, nonadherence to health behavior change is experienced by all patient populations and across all health behaviors.

CASE EXAMPLE

Ms Smith is a 55-year-old, successful, corporate attorney who has a range of health concerns. She experiences fatigue, insomnia, hip and knee pain, shortness of breath when walking up stairs, and some gastrointestinal distress. She is worried about her heart, because she has a family history of heart disease (her father died of a myocardial infarction at age 58 years and her brother had coronary artery bypass grafting at age 60 years). Her physical examination and full exercise stress test do not show any evidence of cardiac disease. However, she smokes 1 pack of cigarettes per day, is overweight with a body mass index (BMI) of 31 kg/m², and has a sedentary lifestyle. She has been informed that she has borderline hypertension and high cholesterol. When given this feedback, Ms. Smith says she is greatly relieved and that she is glad to know she has "nothing to worry about." You inquire about her smoking, eating, and exercise habits, and she responds, "Look, you just told me I'm healthy. I work 80 to 90 hours per week and don't have time to exercise or quit smoking, and why would I need to?" How would you respond?

MODELS OF BEHAVIOR CHANGE

Given the high frequency of nonadherence, several theoretical models have been proposed to promote health behavior change. Many counseling models assume that the individual patient is ready to implement behavior change. However, this assumption is not always true. For example, in a community sample of 756 smokers, only 30% of the smokers were considering quitting smoking in the next 30 days.[27] Among participants in cardiac rehabilitation programs, up to 30% may only be "considering adopting exercise."[25] Thus, many patients may have low levels of motivational readiness for change. The 2 models of health behavior change that we will review, the Transtheoretical Model and Motivational Interviewing, have the theoretical premise that motivation for health behavior change fluctuates not only among individuals but also within an individual over time. Both theories conceptualize motivational readiness as a state that will change, rather than conceptualizing motivation as a trait. Conceptualizing motivation as a trait would rely on the premises that an individual is either motivated to change or not motivated to change, this motivational level is fixed, and there is little the practitioner can do to intervene.

Our interest in these models originated in our clinical experience of working with obese, sedentary, and/or smoking patients. Frequently, these individuals have reported to us that although health care providers often have admonished them about their obesity or smoking, they, the patients, have not received the support, empathy, and guidance necessary for change. Although as health care providers we may be most inclined and perhaps best prepared to deliver action-oriented interventions (eg, pre-scribing nicotine replacement, recommending immediate adoption of regular physical activity), this approach may not match the patient's current readiness for change. At times, the goal of counseling for health behavior change may be to merely increase patient awareness of the problem or to offer support. Yet too often we have found ourselves wanting to instruct patients to immediately begin recording food intake, set a quit date for tobacco use, or start recording daily physical activity when these patients have clearly told us they are not ready to change. Conse-quently, health care providers may experience frustration with patient resistance to an action-oriented approach, while patients may feel overwhelmed and pessimistic about their ability to successfully make change. The goal then is to align practitioner and patient so that both are using the best methods to facilitate patient change.

TRANSTHEORETICAL MODEL

Stages of Change

The Transtheoretical Model of Behavior Change is founded on the conceptualization that motivational readiness is a changing state, rather than a "given" or a fixed personality trait.[28] According to this model, individuals can move across 5 levels of motivational readiness, or 5 stages of change. The stages of change are:

1. precontemplation: no consideration of change
2. contemplation: some limited motivation to change
3. preparation: making small changes
4. action: the first 6 months of change
5. maintenance: the period after the first 6 months of change

To clarify the stages, we will provide specific examples of how the stages of change are applied to smoking, inactivity, and obesity. The stages of change for tobacco use are as follows. In precontemplation, the individual is not considering stopping tobacco use, and in contemplation the person is seriously considering stopping in the next 6 months. Preparation involves the intention to stop smoking in the next 30 days and having made an attempt at quitting in the past year. The action stage is the first 6 months of stopping smoking, and maintenance is after the first 6 months of stopping tobacco use.[29] There is empirical support for the stages of change. Research examining patients with head and neck cancer found that those in the precontemplation stage for stopping smoking at the time of their cancer diagnosis were most likely to relapse to smoking after completion of their oncology treatment (surgery or radiation).[30]

For physical activity, those in precontemplation are not physically active and do not intend to become physically active in the next 6 months. Those in contemplation are not currently active but intend to become more physically active in the next 6 months. Those in preparation engage in some physical activity or exercise, but not at a total of 30 minutes per day, at least 5 days per week. Those in action participate in physical activity at least 30 minutes per day, at least 5 days per week, but have done so for less than 6 months. Those in maintenance have been physically active for more than 6 months.[31] Cross-sectional surveys have provided support for classifying people in these stages of change for physical activity. In a sample of 1172 partici-pants of work site health promotion programs, 24% were in precontemplation, 33% in contemplation, 10% in prepa-ration, 11% in action, and 22% in maintenance.[31]

For weight management, individuals in the precontemplation stage of change have no intention of losing weight in the next 6 months, even though it may be beneficial for them to lose weight. They may either deny the complications associated with their obesity or have low self-confidence from multiple cycles of weight loss followed by weight regain. Individuals in the contem-plation stage are considering change within the next 6 months but are not currently prepared to lose weight. Individuals in the preparation stage plan to lose weight in the next 30 days but may not know which weight-loss program to enroll in. The action stage is the period of changing behaviors, the time for dietary and exercise interventions. After 6 months of continuous successful action, individuals enter the maintenance stage, in which individuals continue to work on preventing relapse to inactivity and consolidating gains from the action stage.[32] Many obese patients seen in the medical setting will probably be in the precontemplation and contemplation stages and not ready to change. In a recent survey, 50% of overweight men and 30% of overweight women were not trying to lose weight.[33]

Although we have just presented the 5 stages of change in a linear fashion, the model proposes that individuals do not systematically progress from one stage to the next. Rather, the model proposes that the change is cyclic. Thus, although some individuals will advance in their stage of change, some will remain stationary, and some will relapse or slip back to a lower level of stage of change. Thus, the practitioner must anticipate setbacks, mistakes, and fluctuating performance from the individual they are counseling. This acceptance and anticipation of movement forward and backward is a hallmark of the model.

Processes of Change

Once a practitioner assesses an individual's stage of change, the model provides guidance on the selection of appropriate counseling strategies. It has been shown that individuals in different stages of change use different strategies and techniques to change. These strategies for change are called the processes of change and are related to the individual's stage of change. The processes of change include both the behavioral and cognitive strategies that an individual uses to implement change. Usually, the cognitive strategies (eg, learning more about a health problem, thinking about how a health problem impacts self-image) are used in the precontemplation and contemplation stages. The behavioral processes (keeping records; removing items from the environment, such as cigarettes, ashtrays, or junk food) are used in the action stage. Because individuals use different processes at different stages, the practitioner can match the strategy for change to the patient's stage of change.[34]

Decisional Balance

Also related to stage of change is decisional balance. Decisional balance is the perceived gains and perceived losses of a behavior change.[35] An individual may be perceiving that if he quits smoking his health will improve and he will save money, but he also anticipates experiencing very unpleasant withdrawal symptoms. These 2 major categories—the perceived positive aspects (pros) and the perceived negative aspects (cons) of a behavior—have been found to represent decisional categories for making behavior changes across the stages of change. For example, when individuals focus on the advantages, benefits, or pros of weight management, their motivation may increase. In contrast, when individuals focus on barriers, problems, or costs of weight management, their motivation for weight loss may diminish. Pros for weight management can include feeling healthier, being more energetic, or having an improved body image after weight loss. Cons for weight management include needing to consume unappetizing diet foods, believing that exercise is painful and boring, and anticipating hassles from family members about changes in meal planning. It has been demonstrated across 12 different behaviors that as individuals advance in their readiness to change, the pros of change become more important and the cons of change become less important.[36]

Self-efficacy

Another component of the Transtheoretical Model is self-efficacy. Self-efficacy, or self-confidence, is the individual's perceived ability to perform a specific behavior or task. An individual's self-efficacy for stopping smoking may be very different from his or her self-efficacy for weight-loss. Confidence level is very important in terms of initiating and maintaining motivational readiness. For example, baseline self-efficacy for stopping smoking has been found to be

predictive of smoking status at 7 weeks,[37] 3 months,[38] and 5 months[39] after treatment. In these studies, individuals with greater baseline self-reported confidence in making, following, and sustaining behavioral change regarding smoking cessation had greater success in treatment. Similarly, individuals who have experienced multiple cycles of weight loss followed by weight gain may doubt their ability to lose weight and, therefore, are in the precontemplation stage of change. In contrast, individuals who are managing their weight successfully (maintenance stage) are likely confident of their ability to manage their weight in the future. Assessing an individual's self-efficacy may provide information about his or her readiness to change and help identify specific strengths and weaknesses. Our research has shown that low self-efficacy for exercise is predictive of reduction in physical activity level in participants of cardiac rehabilitation programs[24] and is predictive of exercise relapse in college students.[40] We also have found that cognitive-behavioral treatment of binge eating disorder improves a participant's eating self-efficacy.[41] Thus, self-efficacy, the individual's confidence level, is important to assess and foster.

Application of Transtheoretical Model

As stated earlier, the Transtheoretical Model proposes that interventions tailored to the motivational readiness of the individual will enhance the effectiveness of the intervention. An outline of how to potentially match the individual's level of motivational readiness to the practitioner's counseling strategy is outlined in Table 6-2. It should be noted that most of the support for the Transtheoretical Model is from cross-sectional surveys or quasi-experimental design projects. However, several randomized, controlled trials have provided support for the effectiveness of tailoring interventions based on the stage-of-change model. For example, a controlled trial randomly assigned, stratified by stage of change for smoking, 756 cigarette smokers to receive one of the following: (1) standard self-help material; (2) self-help material matched to stage of change; (3) an interactive, expert-system computer that provided written, individualized, stage-matched feedback; or (4) individual counseling, stage manuals, and computer reports.[27] The expert-system computer provided participants with written individualized feedback on their stage of change, their use of the processes of change, their decisional balance, and their self-efficacy. The written feedback also provided tailored instructions on strategies for change. Researchers found at the 18-month follow-up that usage of the expert-system computer yielded the highest 24-hour point prevalence of smoking abstinence rate, 25.2%. In a follow-up study of 3967 smokers randomly assigned to an interactive expert system based on the

Transtheoretical Model or to stage-matched manuals, 21.6% of the expert-system participants, compared with 16.5% of those who received stage-matched manuals, demonstrated 24-hour point prevalence of abstinence at the 18-month follow-up.[42]

In a similar project involving exercise, 194 sedentary adults were randomized to receive either written feedback from a stage-matched computerized expert system or standard self-help booklets developed by the American Heart Association. At the 6-month follow-up, 43% of those in the expert-system group, vs 18% in the group receiving standard self-help materials, achieved the recommendation of the Centers for Disease Control and Prevention and the American College of Sports Medicine recommendation of participating in at least 30 minutes of moderately vigorous physical activity on most days of the week (defined in the project as 5 days).[43] Thus, several randomized controlled trials have demonstrated that individualized, motivationally tailored intervention can enhance the adoption of, and adherence to, health behavior change.

TABLE **6-2**

Stage-Matched Counseling Strategies

Stage of Change	Counseling Strategies
Precontemplation	Inquiry of past attempts Building of empathy Discussion of health problem Exploration of cons to change

Contemplation	Discussion of history of the
	  problem behavior
	Discussion of health consequences
	  of the behavior
	Discussion of benefits of change
	Building of self-confidence
	  for change

Preparation	Patient-treatment matching models Referral to appropriate providers Goals for small behavior change
Action	Standardized self-help materials Goal-setting strategies Support for health behavior change Problem-solving for barriers Relapse-prevention training

Maintenance	Ongoing support for lifestyle
	  changes
	Health feedback, with a focus
	  on improvements
	Pros of behavior change
	Addressing other issues
	  (eg, weight gain from
	  quitting smoking)

Adapted from *Am Psychol.* 1992;1102–1114.[34]

MOTIVATIONAL INTERVIEWING

As reviewed earlier, practitioner behaviors and the practitioner-patient relationship have been shown to have a substantial impact on patient outcomes and health behaviors.[5] In particular, Miller and Rollnick[44] have described the importance of practitioner behaviors in affecting patient motivation for and involvement in health behavior change. Motivational interviewing was developed from within the addiction treatment field and was based in part on the recognition that directly confronting patients about their need to quit drinking was an unhelpful strategy. It was found that confrontation frequently led to patient resistance rather than progress toward change.[45] Miller suggested that practitioners could be more effective in helping patients change by their facilitating a discussion in which the patients argue for changing their own behavior.[45] This is contrasted with a traditional approach in which the patient argues against change, while responding to the advice and pressure from the practitioner to change. However, motivational interviewing is not a passive approach either. Motivational interviewing is described as a directive, client-centered counseling style that facilitates behavior change by encouraging patients to think about and work toward resolving their ambivalence toward change.[44] Because motivational interviewing emphasizes preparing individuals to make change, this counseling style has an important role in health behavior interventions.[46]

Clinical Principles

Motivational interviewing incorporates the use of patient-centered counseling techniques and includes 4 guiding clinical principles: (1) express empathy, (2) develop discrepancy, (3) roll with resistance, and (4) support self-efficacy.[47]

The first principle suggests that accepting a patient can facilitate that patient making change. Acceptance of the patient does not mean that the clinician approves of the patient's behavior, but rather accepts the patient's perspectives and feelings. Reflective listening, which involves listening without judging, blaming, or criticizing, is a key strategy for expressing empathy.[44] To have accurate empathy for the patient, practitioners must understand that ambivalence toward change is normal.

Developing a discrepancy between current patient behavior and the broader goals and values of the patient is the second principle. This discrepancy is thought to underlie motivation toward change, and it is the patient, rather than the practitioner that should argue toward change. As previously mentioned, an unproductive approach to patient change involves having a clinician strongly advocate for change while the patient argues against such change.[45]

The third principle of rolling with resistance emphasizes the need to avoid arguing with patients or trying to force a change. When faced with resistance, a clinician using the motivational interviewing approach would see the resistance as a sign to respond differently and to try a different approach.

The fourth principle involves supporting patient self-efficacy, which reflects the confidence of patients in their own ability to successfully make and maintain a change. By supporting patient self-efficacy, the practitioner demonstrates that the patient is responsible for selecting the behavior for change and carrying out that change.[47] These 4 principles help emphasize the difference between motivational interviewing and more traditional approaches to the physician-patient relationship, in which the physician is seen as the expert whose role it is to give advice and advocate change.

Motivational interviewing often includes providing the patient with objective feedback (eg, laboratory and physical examination results) to enhance patient motivation to change.[46] The physician's role is to provide the facts about the test results, without interpreting the personal implications of the facts for the patient. The implications of the results are instead decided by the patient, and this approach may assist patients in evaluating their own behavior and recognizing the discrepancy between this and their broader goals and values. Feedback from tests has been shown to be an important motivator to patients.[48,49]

Motivational interviewing is more a style of interacting with patients than a narrow set of clinical techniques to be applied to patients.[47] Consequently, some consider motivational interviewing to be complex and difficult to distinguish from other patient-centered approaches.[50] Emmons and Rollnick[46] provide a concise overview of motivational interviewing as well as detail the opportunities and limitations of this health behavior change approach for health care settings. Furthermore, these authors provide a description of a brief motivational interviewing intervention appropriate for a health care setting (ie, time-limited and focused on 1 health behavior).

Application of Motivational Interviewing Model

A brief motivational interviewing intervention has been developed for primary care clinicians to use with their patients who smoke cigarettes.[51] The intervention requires approximately 10 minutes of clinical time, and it was rated as acceptable and satisfying by the health care providers trained to deliver the brief intervention. Key components of the intervention for smokers included first establishing rapport with the patient, assessing motivation and confidence to quit smoking, and assessing the patient's perception of the pros and cons of smoking. Then the clinician shared nonjudgmental information with the patient about tobacco use, collaborated with the patient in brainstorming possible solutions, supported the patient in setting a patient-centered and achievable goal, and arranged for follow-up. The following section provides an overview of the intervention components as well as examples of questions and strategies that are useful in motivating a patient to think about change and take steps toward quitting smoking.

The "teachable moments" that occur in medical settings provide health care providers with important opportunities for delivering motivational interviewing in support of patients' health behavior change.[52] Researchers reviewing the literature on motivational-interviewing interventions applied to patient health behaviors (eg, smoking, diet, physical activity) suggest that although the literature in this area is still emerging, motivational interviewing holds substantial promise as an approach to behavioral change in medical settings.[46,50,52,53]

Applying Motivational Interviewing Techniques: Tobacco Use Intervention

The following example is adapted from references 47 and 51.

Introduce topic and assess readiness for change

Introduce topic.   Use an open-ended, nonjudgmental question or comment to invite the patient to discuss smoking:

> "I'm interested in hearing you talk a little bit about your smoking."
>
> "I want to understand what it is like for you to be a smoker; please tell me about it."
>
> "How do you really feel about your smoking these days?"

Rate motivation.   Ask the patient to rate motivation to quit smoking:

> "I'd like to have you rate for me, on a scale from 1 to 10, your current motivation to quit smoking. If 1 is not at all motivated to quit smoking and 10 is completely ready to quit smoking, what number are you right now?"

Rate confidence.   Ask patient to rate confidence to quit smoking:

> "Again on a scale from 1 to 10, how confident are you that you could be successful at quitting smoking if you decided you wanted to quit right now? If 1 is not at all confident that you could quit and stay quit, and 10 is absolutely confident that you could be successful, what number are you right now?"

Address motivation and confidence

Discuss motivation. Elicit patient self-statements about change by having them explain their motivation rating:

"Why are you a _____ and not a 1 on the scale?"
"What would it take for you to move from a _____ to a (higher number)?"

Note that anchoring the question in the other direction (Why are you a _____ and not a 10?) is unhelpful because it encourages the patient to argue against change:

Weigh the pros and cons. Explore with the patient both the benefits of change and the barriers to change:

"What do you like about smoking?"
"What concerns you about smoking?"
"What are the roadblocks to quitting?"
"What would you like about being a nonsmoker?"

Summarize both the pros and the cons, then ask:

"Where does that leave you now?"

Provide personal risk information. Share nonjudgmental information about risk and/or objective data from medical evaluation, then ask the patient's opinion of this information (Avoid giving advice or attempting to shock or frighten the patient into change.):

"What do you make of these results?"
"Would current information about the risks of smoking be helpful to you now?"
"What do you need to hear from me about this?"

Discuss confidence. Elicit patient self-statements about confidence to quit smoking by discussing how confidence was rated:

"Why are you a _____ and not a 1?"
"What would help you move from a _____ to a (higher number)?"
"What can I do to support you in moving up to a (higher number)?"

Offer support and make patient-centered plan

- Work together to create a patient-centered plan that matches the patient's readiness to quit.
- Encourage the patient to consider what could work, rather than focus on what could not.
- Provide options (referral, nicotine replacement, patient education materials), but not direct advice.
- Ask the patient to select the next step.
- Reinforce any movement toward making a change.
- Follow-up on subsequent visits.

PSYCHIATRIC COMORBIDITY

In this chapter, the 2 models of health behavior change we have reviewed operate under the assumption that psychiatric comorbidity has been addressed. It has been well documented that psychiatric comorbidity can have an impact on adherence. For example, the presence of a major depressive episode has been shown to reduce medication adherence in elderly patients with coronary artery disease from 69% (nondepressed patients) to 45% (depressed patients).[54] Our own research has demonstrated that depression is predictive of attrition from a multidisciplinary weight management program[55] and that a history of being the victim of sexual abuse is related to nonadherence in a weight management program.[56] Thus, the practitioner should assess and evaluate for the presence of psychiatric comorbidity when addressing adherence. Appropriate treatment or referral may then be warranted for the psychiatric comorbidity.

CASE EXAMPLE CONTINUED

Ms Smith is expressing reluctance to even discuss her smoking, weight status, and sedentary lifestyle. She has minimal motivational readiness for change. Direct confrontation of her denial will probably lead to further resistance to change. In contrast, rapport building, expression of empathy, and support for what she has accomplished may build the groundwork for change. Open-ended questions, such as "Tell me more about your work responsibilities," "Let's briefly discuss what you have done in the past about your smoking," and "What are your beliefs about your current weight?" might provide important clinical guidance. Answers to these questions may provide information about past failures and insight into her confidence level, and identify her pros and cons for change. The counseling goal for the session could be to just have Ms Smith think more about her problem behaviors and to begin to identify what would be necessary for her to change. At a follow-up appointment, more direct information and advice about strategies for change may then be effective in helping Ms Smith change at least one of her problem behaviors.

SUMMARY

Many individuals will experience difficulty initiating and maintaining health behavior change. The health care provider is in an optimal position to provide counseling for health behavior change. We have reviewed 2 models of counseling, the Transtheoretical Model and Motivational Interviewing, both of which seek to tailor the counseling strategy to the individual's level of motivational readiness. Initial support for these models has been demonstrated, and numerous investigations are ongoing. Adoption of these counseling strategies will likely improve patients' health behavior change as well as enhance the practitioner's satisfaction with providing counseling in the health care setting.

REFERENCES

1. Flocke S, Miller W, Crabtree B. Relationships between physician practice style, patient satisfaction, and attributes of primary care. *J Fam Pract.* 2002;51:835–840.

2. Thom D, for Stanford Trust Study Physicians. Physician behaviors that predict patient trust. *J Fam Pract.* 2001;50:323–328.

3. Stewart M. What is a successful doctor-patient interview? A study of interactions and outcomes. *Soc Sci Med.* 1984;19:167–175.

4. Levinson W, Roter D, Mullooly J, Dull V, Frankel R. Physician-patient communication: the relationship with malpractice claims among primary care physicians and surgeons. *JAMA.* 1997;277:553–559.

5. Beck R, Daughtridge R, Sloane P. Physician-patient communication in the primary care office: a systematic review. *J Am Board Fam Pract.* 2002;15:25–38.

6. Emmons K, Marcus B, Linnan L, Rossi J, Abrams D. Mechanisms in multiple risk factor interventions: smoking, physical activity, and dietary fat intake among manufacturing workers. *Prev Med.* 1994;23:481–489.

7. Allison D, Fontaine K, Manson J, Stevens J, VanItallie T. Annual deaths attributable to obesity in the United States. *JAMA.* 1999;282:1530–1538.

8. Centers for Disease Control and Prevention. *The Burden of Chronic Diseases and Their Risk Factors.* Rockville, Md: US Department of Health and Human Services; 2002

9. Pastor P, Makuc D, Reuben C, Xia H. *Chartbook on Trends in the Health of Americans.* Hyattsville, Md: National Center for Health Statistics; 2002.

10. Russell L, Teutsch S, Kumar R, Dey A, Milan E. Preventable smoking and exercise-related hospital admissions: a model based on the NHEFS. *Am J Prev Med.* 2001;20:26–34.

11. Flegal KM, Carroll MD, Ogden CL, Johnson CL. Prevalence and trends in obesity among US adults, 1999–2000. *JAMA.* 2002;288:1723–1727.

12. Egede L, Zheng D. Modifiable cardiovascular risk factors in adults with diabetes. *Arch Intern Med.* 2002;162:427–433.

13. The Writing Group for the Activity Counseling Trial Research Group. Effects of physical activity counseling in primary care: The Activity Counseling Trial—A randomized controlled trial. *JAMA.* 2001;286:677–687.

14. Galuska D, Will J, Serdula M, Ford E. Are health care professionals advising obese patients to lose weight? *JAMA.* 1999;282:1576–1578.

15. Glasgow R, Eakin E, Fisher E, Bacak S, Brownson R. Physician advice and support for physical activity: results from a national survey. *Am J Prev Med.* 2001;21:189–196.

16. Centers for Disease Control and Prevention. Missed opportunities in preventive counseling for cardiovascular disease: United States, 1995. *MMWR Morb Mortal Wkly Rep.* 1998;47:91–95.

17. Stafford R, Farhat J, Misra B, Schoenfeld D. National patterns of physician activities related to obesity management. *Arch Fam Med.* 2000;9:631–638.

18. Wee C, McCarthy E, Davis R, Phillips R. Physician counseling about exercise. *JAMA.* 1999;282:1583–1588.

19. McIlvain H, Crabtree B, Backer E, Turner P. Use of office-based smoking cessation activities in family practices. *J Fam Pract.* 2000;49:1025–1029.

20. Wechsler H, Levine S, Idelson R, Schor E, Coakley E. The physician's role in health promotion revisited: a survey of primary care practitioners. *N Engl J Med.* 1996;334:996–998.

21. McIlvain H, Backer E, Crabtree B, Lacy N. Physician attitudes and the use of office-based activities for tobacco control. *Fam Med.* 2002;34:114–119.

22. Kushner R. Barriers to providing nutrition counseling by physicians: a survey of primary care practitioners. *Prev Med.* 1995;24:546–552.

23. Meichenbaum D, Turk D. *Facilitating Treatment Adherence: A Practitioner's Guidebook.* New York, NY: Plenum Press; 1987.

24. Jowsey S, Taylor M, Schneekloth T, Clark M. Psychosocial challenges in transplantation. *J Psychiatr Pract.* November 2001;404–414.

25. Bock BC, Albrecht AE, Traficante RM, Clark MM, Pinto BM, Tilkemeier P, Marcus BH. Predictors of exercise adherence following participation in a cardiac rehabilitation program. *Int J Behav Med.* 1997;4:60–75.

26. Sanderson Cox L, Patten CA, Ebbert JO, et al. Tobacco use outcomes among patients with lung cancer treated for nicotine dependence. *J Clin Oncol.* 2002;20:3461–3469.

27. Prochaska J, DiClemente C, Velicer W, Rossi J. Standardized, individualized, interactive, and personalized self-help programs for smoking cessation. *Health Psychol.* 1993;12:399–405.

28. Prochaska J, DiClemente C. Stages and processes of self-change of smoking: toward an integrative model of change. *J Consult Clin Psychol.* 1983;51:390–395.

29. Guise B, Goldstein M, Clark M, Thebarge R. Behavior change: the example of smoking cessation. In: Noble J, Greene H, Levinson W, Modest G, Young M, eds. *Textbook of Primary Care,* St Louis, Mo: Mosby; 1996:1650–1656.

30. Gritz E, Schacherer C, Koehly L, Nielsen I, Abemayor A. Smoking withdrawal and relapse in head and neck cancer patients. *Head Neck.* 1999;21:420–427.

31. Marcus B, Rossi J, Selby V, Niaura R, Abrams D. The stages and processes of exercise adoption and maintenance in a worksite sample. *Health Psychol.* 1992;11:386–395.

32. Clark M, Pera V, Goldstein M, Thebarge R, Guise B. Counseling strategies for obese patients. *Am J Prev Med.* 1996;12:266–270.

33. Kottke T, Clark M, Aase L, et al. Self-reported weight, weight goals, and weight control strategies of a midwestern population. *Mayo Clin Proc.* 2002;77:114–121.

34. Prochaska J, DiClemente C, Norcross J. In search of how people change: applications to addictive behaviors. *Am Psychol.* 1992;47:1102–1114.

35. Prochaska JO, Velicer WF, Rossi JS, et al. Stages of change and decisional balance for 12 problem behaviors. *Health Psychol.* 1994;13:39–46.

36. Velicer W, DiClemente C, Prochaska J, Bradenburg N. Decisional balance measure for assessing and predicting smoking status. *J Pers Soc Psychol.* 1985;48:1279–1289.

37. Borrelli B, Mermelstein R. The role of weight concern and self-efficacy in smoking cessation and weight gain among smokers in a clinic-based cessation program. *Addict Behav.* 1998;23:609–622.

38. Condiotte M, Lichtenstein E. Self-efficacy and relapse in smoking cessation programs. *J Consult Clin Psychol.* 1981;49:648–658.

39. DiClemente C, Prochaska J, Gibertine M. Self-efficacy and the stages of self-change of smoking. *Cogn Ther Res.* 1985;9:181–200.

40. Sullum J, Clark M, King T. Predictors of exercise relapse in a college population. *J Am Coll Health.* 2000;48:175–180.

41. Wolff G, Clark M. Changes in eating self-efficacy and body image following cognitive-behavioral group therapy for binge eating disorder: a clinical study. *Eating Behav.* 2001;2:97–104.

42 Velicer W, Prochaska J, Fava J, Laforge R, Rossi J. Interactive versus noninteractive interventions and dose-response relationships for stage-matched smoking cessation programs in a managed care setting. *Health Psychol.* 1999;18:21–28.

43. Marcus B, Bock B, Pinto B, Forsyth L, Roberts M, Traficante R. Efficacy of an individualized, motivationally-tailored physical activity intervention. *Ann Behav Med.* 1998;20:174–180.

44. Miller W, Rollnick S. *Motivational Interviewing: Preparing People to Change Addictive Behavior.* New York, NY: Guilford Press; 1991.

45. Miller W. Motivational interviewing with problem drinkers. *Behav Psychother.* 1983;1:147–172.

46. Emmons K, Rollnick S. Motivational interviewing in health care settings. *Am J Prev Med.* 2001;20:68–74.

47. Miller W, Rollnick S. *Motivational Interviewing: Preparing People for Change.* New York, NY: Guilford Press; 2002.

48. Miller W, Sovereign G, Krege B. Motivational interviewing with problem drinkers: II. The drinker's check-up as a preventative intervention. *Behav Psychother.* 1988;16:251–268.

49. Risser N, Belcher D. Adding spirometry, carbon monoxide, and pulmonary symptom results to smoking cessation counseling: a randomized trial. *J Gen Intern Med.* 1990;5:16–22.

50. Dunn C, Deroo L, Rivara F. The use of brief interventions adapted from motivational interviewing across behavioral domains: a systematic review. *Addiction.* 2001;96:1725–1742.

51. Rollnick S, Butler C, Stott N. Helping smokers make decisions: the enhancement of brief intervention for general medical practice. *Patient Education Counseling.* 1997;31:191–203.

52. Resnicow K, DiIorio C, Soet J, et al. Motivational interviewing in medical and public health settings. In: Miller W, Rollnick S, eds. *Motivational Interviewing: Preparing People for Change.* New York, NY: Guilford Press; 2002:251–269.

53. Burke B, Arkowitz H, Dunn C. The efficacy of motivational interviewing and its adaptations: what we know so far. In: Miller W, Rollnick S, eds. *Motivational Interviewing: Preparing People for Change.* New York, NY: Guilford Press; 2002:217–250.

54. Carney R, Freedland K, Eisen S, Rich M, Jaffe A. Major depression and medication adherence in elderly patients with coronary artery disease. *Health Psychol.* 1995;14:88–90.

55. Clark M, Niaura R, King T, Pera V. Depression, smoking, activity level and health status: pretreatment predictors of attrition in obesity treatment. *Addict Behav.* 1996;21:509–513.

56. King T, Clark M, Pera V. History of sexual abuse and obesity treatment outcome. *Addict Behav.* 1996;21:283–290.

RESOURCES

Hensrud D. *Mayo Clinic on Healthy Weight.* Mayo Foundation for Medical Education and Research. Rochester, MN; 2000.

Marcus B, Forsyth L. *Motivating People to be Physically Active.* Human Kinetics Publishers. 2003.

Miller W & Rollnick S. *Motivational Interviewing: Preparing People for Change.* New York, NY: Guilford Press; 2002.

Rollnick S, Mason P, Butler C. *Health Behavior Change: A Guide for Practitioners.* New York, NY: Churchill Livingstone; 1999.

chapter 7

Depression and Suicide: Recognition and Early Intervention

Donald A. Malone, MD, and Philip Lartey, MD

DEPRESSION

Introduction and Epidemiology

Depressive (mood) disorders are extremely common illnesses, probably affecting almost 10 million Americans at any one time. All ages, races, cultures, and socioeconomic classes are affected.[1] Fortunately, these disorders also represent the most treatable of psychiatric conditions, 80% to 90% of those affected respond to currently available treatments. Few people afflicted with these conditions, however, seek professional help. The rate of failure to seek help is estimated to be as high as 65% to 75%. Many who visit primary care physicians because of an array of somatic complaints may not be recognized as having an underlying or masked depression.

Too often depression is underrecognized, undertreated, or inappropriately treated.[2,3] Everyone experiences transient sad feelings, which usually accompany loss, perceived failure, unhappy incidents or events, emotional letdowns, or occupational and relationship difficulties. Grief is a special form of natural temporary reaction to the loss of a loved person, pet, or prized possession. With time, healing occurs. Despite these natural sad reactions, people continue to function occupationally and socially. In contrast, people with true depressive disorder have persistent difficulties with affective symptoms and signs for weeks, months, or even years. Depressive disorders pervasively affect feelings, thoughts, and actions, with *increasing inability to function in all meaningful areas of life.*

Depression is one of the most common problems that primary care physicians encounter. The prevalence of major depression in the general population is variously reported as 3% in a 6-month period, or 5% to 8% over a lifetime. Up to 30% of the population may develop depression at some point in their life.[4] Spontaneous remission occurs in up to 50% of those who experience depression;[5] in 50%, depression becomes chronic.[6] The incidence of depression is greatest among young, single, separated, or divorced women.[7] Separated or divorced individuals have 2.5 times more depression than those who are married, although marital discord increases risk, too.[8] Women are depressed twice as frequently as men.[9] Elderly adults are particularly vulnerable to depression.[1] Depression is present in 2% to 4% of elderly individuals in the community, 12% who are medically hospitalized, and 16% of those in long-term care. The estimated costs resulting from depression are approximately $30 to $44 billion a year in the United States.[3]

Diagnosis

Depression, as a transient feeling or symptom, is a universal experience. As a syndromal mental illness, it is probably experienced by 17% of the population at some point during their lifetime.[3,4] Depression may be seen as a continuum ranging from a symptom of sadness or the blues through normal grief to the full expression in the form of major depressive and psychotic syndromes. At one end of the spectrum are normal functioning and short-lasting symptoms; at the other end is total inability to function and prolonged illness. The best screening technique for depression is a psychiatric history and examination of mental status.

Clinical depression is best epitomized in the criteria for major depression found in the *Diagnostic and Statistical Manual of Mental Disorders, Fourth Edition Text Revision (DSM-IV-TR)*[10] (Table 7-1). These criteria can be remembered more easily using the helpful mnemonic: SIG E CAPS (Table 7-2).[11]

Signs and Symptoms

Mood may be described as depressed, sad, unhappy, discouraged, demoralized, irritable, nonspontaneous, or empty. Diurnal variations of mood may be present, with patients feeling worse in the morning and slightly better later in the day. Common warning signs are changes in appetite, sleep, and energy. Appetite usually is decreased, with attendant weight loss. Food becomes tasteless, and there is little pleasure in eating. A minority of depressed individuals have hyperphagia, with associated weight gain. Sleep usually shows middle insomnia, terminal

TABLE 7-1

DSM-IV-TR Diagnostic Criteria for Major Depressive Episode*

A. Five (or more) of the following symptoms have been present during the same 2-week period and represent a change from previous functioning; at least one of the symptoms is either (1) depressed mood or (2) loss of interest or pleasure. *Note:* Do not include symptoms that are clearly due to a general medical condition, or mood-incongruent delusions or hallucinations.

1. Depressed mood most of the day, nearly every day, as indicated by either subjective report (eg, feels sad or empty) or observation made by others (eg, appears tearful). *Note:* In children and adolescents, can be irritable mood.
2. Markedly diminished interest or pleasure in all, or almost all, activities most of the day, nearly every day (as indicated by either subjective account or observation made by others).
3. Significant weight loss when not dieting or weight gain (eg, a change of more than 5% of body weight in a month), or a decrease or increase in appetite nearly every day. *Note:* In children, consider failure to make expected weight gains.
4. Insomnia or hypersomnia nearly every day.
5. Psychomotor agitation or retardation nearly every day (observable by others, not merely subjective feelings of restlessness or being slowed down).
6. Fatigue or loss of energy nearly every day.
7. Feelings of worthlessness or excessive or inappropriate guilt (which may be delusional) nearly every day (not merely self-reproach or guilt about being sick).
8. Diminished ability to think or concentrate, or indecisiveness, nearly every day (either by subjective account or as observed by others).
9. Recurrent thoughts of death (not just fear of dying), recurrent suicidal ideation without specific plan, or suicide attempt or a specific plan for committing suicide.

B. The symptoms do not meet criteria for Mixed Episode.
C. The symptoms cause clinically significant distress or impairment in social, occupational, or other important areas of functioning.
D. The symptoms are not due to the direct physiological effects of a substance (eg, a drug of abuse, medication) or a general medical condition (hypothyroidism).
E. The symptoms are not better accounted for by bereavement, ie, after the loss of a loved one; the symptoms persist for longer than 2 months or are characterized by marked functional impairment, morbid preoccupation with worthlessness, suicidal ideation, psychotic symptoms, or psychomotor retardation.

*From *American Psychiatric Association: Diagnostic and Statistical Manual of Mental Disorders, Fourth Edition Text Revision.*[10]

insomnia (typical early morning awakening), or paninsomnia. Some show hypersomnia, sleeping 12 or more hours each day. The patient's energy may be decreased substantially to the point of lack of motivation, apathy, and chronic fatigue. Agitation shows itself in pacing, hand wringing, fidgeting, and nervous smoking. Psychomotor retardation may manifest by extremely slow movement and speech and delayed response to questioning. Anxiety often is associated with mood disorders,[12] particularly in the agitated depressive subtype. Other anxious symptoms may include phobias, obsessions, and panic attacks.[12,13] Loss of interest occurs in hobbies, work, personal relationships, and sexual activity. Cognitive difficulties include decreased attention span, difficulties with concentration, slowed thinking, poverty of content of thought, indecisiveness, inability to complete tasks, impaired abstract thinking, decreased memory, and disorientation. These symptoms may be confused with dementia.

Negative thinking, generalizations, and global negative conclusions are hallmarks of depression. Guilt can become so excessive as to reach the level of a full delusion for only minor previous transgressions. There may be extreme self-blame or shame, helplessness, hopelessness, crying spells, loss of capacity for pleasure,

and poor insight and judgment due to feelings of personal worthlessness. Obsessive negative ruminations and hypochondriacal preoccupation with bodily functions are frequent, including multiple somatic complaints: cardiac, gastrointestinal, genitourinary, and orthopedic. Patients with depressive symptoms experience poorer physical functioning than patients with many chronic medical conditions, including hypertension, diabetes, arthritis, and gastrointestinal and lung disorders.[14] In other words, depressed patients are as severely disabled as are those with chronic conditions.[15,16] Preoccupation with death, reuniting with loved ones after death, or thoughts of the survivors' responses to their deaths are common. Delusions may occur, which tend to have mood-congruent themes of guilt, poverty, nihilism, deserved persecutions, and somatic disturbances. Because of a belief that nothing will change, no attempts are made to improve things, thus reinforcing the belief that the situation is hopeless.[9] Depressed persons tend to blame themselves for everything bad. Psychotic features are present in 16% to 54% of those experiencing depression. Depressed individuals tend to become dependent, passive, helpless, insecure, needy, and rejection-sensitive and avoid interactions, leading to withdrawal, loneliness, and alienation.[9] Accident-proneness, frequent job changes,

TABLE 7-2
SIG E CAPS (Prescribe Energy Capsules)*

S	**Sleep** disturbance—insomnia or hypersomnia
I	Loss of **Interest** or pleasure in activities
G	Excessive **Guilt**, worthlessness, hopelessness
E	Loss of **Energy** or fatigue
C	Diminished **Concentration** ability, indecisive
A	Decreased **Appetite**, 5% weight loss or gain
P	**Psychomotor** retardation or agitation
S	**Suicidal** ideation, plan, or attempt

*From Rundell JR, Wise MG.[11]

marital discord, cynicism, loss of sense of humor, and all-or-nothing thinking may point to covert depression. Inappropriate self-medication with, for example, alcohol, can be a clue to the diagnosis.

Adolescents tend to present with acting-out behavior, covering their depression by acting angry, negative, or aggressive; running away; truancy; school difficulties; delinquency; promiscuity; pregnancy; sensitivity to rejection; poor peer relations; or poor hygiene.[1] Their tendency toward substance abuse also can complicate both the diagnosis and treatment of depression.

The elderly tend to present with cognitive deficits, such as disorientation and memory loss, distractibility, and confusion to the point of an affective "pseudodementia." Typically, these affective symptoms of pseudodementia can be misdiagnosed as Alzheimer's dementia, and the depression goes untreated. Issues of aging, declining health, loneliness through loss of friends and family, and financial difficulties are factors predisposing to the development of depression. Only occasionally do the elderly admit to feelings of depression. Instead, they tend to focus more on multiple somatic symptoms, such as various aches, pains, fatigue, insomnia, or constipation, particularly in individuals who are alexithymic (unable to express feelings in words, found particularly in men). These individuals tend to ascribe their symptoms to physical ailments and seek primary care rather than deal with the emotional issues. Many physical illnesses tend to affect older persons and are associated more commonly with depression, such as Parkinson's disease, cancer, arthritis, and Alzheimer's disease.[1] In addition, elderly individuals often take many medications, which may cause drug interactions.

Forms of Depression

Depressive disorders manifest in different forms.

Dysthymic disorder
Dysthymia is a chronic condition usually beginning early in life, in adolescence or young adulthood, lasting at least 2 years (1 year for children and adolescents) with symptoms similar to those of major depression but not of sufficient severity to warrant a diagnosis.[10,17] These individuals tend to say they have been depressed their whole lives and have a very negative view of their past, present, and future.

Bipolar disorder
Bipolar disorder depressed is very similar to major depression but characterized by a previous history of manic episodes. Bipolar II disorder shows similar depressive episodes but a previous history of only episodes of hypomania (less severe with reality contact maintained). Ten percent of unipolar depressions eventually proved to be bipolar in a 40-year follow-up study.[18]

Cyclothymic disorder is a much less severe form of bipolar disorder, with individuals showing depressive insecurity alternating with hyperactive aggressiveness.[9]

Seasonal affective disorder and organic mood disorder
Seasonal affective disorder (SAD) is depression that comes with decreased daylight in the fall and winter and disappears as the day lengthens in spring and summer. This condition is more common in latitudes farther from the equator with very low sunshine in winter (eg, Alaska).[17]

Organic mood disorders are secondary to an organic cause, such as medical illness or drugs.

Major depression
Major depression is characterized by the occurrence of 1 or more major depressive episodes (see Table 7-1) in the absence of any history of manic, mixed, or hypomanic episodes.

Forty percent of patients with major depression also have an Axis II (personality disorder) diagnosis, most commonly dependent, avoidant, narcissistic, or borderline personality disorders.[19] Unstable characterologic traits are the strongest predictor of poor social outcome.[20] Premorbid personality traits, such as introversion, may predispose to depression or affect the course of depression. Certain personality traits may represent attenuated forms of depression, and postmorbid personality changes may occur after depression.[19]

Secondary depression refers to depression occurring after other psychiatric conditions, such as alcoholism or schizophrenia. *Comorbid depression* exists alongside other psychiatric conditions and is often seen with alcoholism (33% to 59% of alcoholic persons have clinical depression), eating disorders (33% to 62% of anorexic and bulimic individuals are depressed), and anxiety.[19] Grief, especially when unresolved, may be complicated and culminate in a major depressive syndrome.

Etiology/Risk Factors

Genetic factors

Depressive disorders tend to run in families, and gradually accumulating evidence implicates a genetic factor, particularly in recurrent depressive disorders. Further evidence of a genetic factor has been demonstrated in the field of bipolar disorders. If 1 identical twin is affected, the other twin has a 70% likelihood of the illness developing. A nonidentical twin has a similar chance of the illness developing as do other first-degree relatives, such as parents, siblings, or children of the proband; the incidence is approximately 15%, about twice as high as that in the general population. In second-degree relatives, the relative risk drops to about 7%. Adoption studies have shown much higher correlations between depressed adoptees (particularly bipolar depressive persons) and their biologic parents rather than their adoptive parents. Response of family members to biologic treatments tends to be similar (eg, inherited patterns of metabolism of antidepressant medication). Children of depressed parents also may learn maladaptive ways of handling life stressors because of the distorted family environment, thereby developing increased vulnerability to depression.

Biochemical factors

Neurotransmitters have been shown to regulate mood in the limbic system. For instance, norepinephrine and serotonin are closely linked to areas of the brain that control the drives of hunger, sex, and thirst. Improper balance of neurotransmitters may be influential in the development of depressive symptoms. Norepinephrine is involved in the maintenance of arousal, alertness, and euphoria; disturbances in its availability might lead to lack of energy and depressed mood. Serotonin, an inhibitory neurotransmitter, when disturbed, may give rise to irritability, anxiety, and the sleep disturbance of depression.[1] Biochemical imbalance may represent a genetic vulnerability triggered by prolonged stress, trauma, physical illness, or environmental conditions.[1] There have been reports on the relationship between chronically low cholesterol levels and death due to violent behaviors, including suicide. It has also been suggested that low levels of cholesterol could lead to depression or increased risk of suicide due to changes in serotonin metabolism.[21,22]

Psychosocial factors

Any major change, loss, or stress, such as divorce, death, unemployment, moving, promotion, financial problems, midlife crisis, and sex-role expectations, may trigger depression. Premorbid personality, upbringing, and negative thinking contribute to its development. The loss may be of a person, attention from others, health, financial status, or control; may be real or only threatened or imagined; and may be seen as devastating by a patient but only trivial by others.[9] Losses are worse when they are unexpected, are related to ambivalently perceived objects, or occur after losses in very dependent persons. Retirement contributes to depression in older men who see their self-worth in terms of work and productivity. The highest rates of depression among women are found among single, young, poor mothers of young children who have little emotional or financial support.[23] Marital strains or disputes and parenting stresses often contribute to depression. Depressed patients tend to function poorly as parents by withdrawing from or acting hostile to their children, who, in turn, develop emotional problems themselves, including depression. Patients in an environment with high levels of expressed emotion (ie, the expression of criticism and hostility with overinvolvement of family members) are more likely to relapse.[24] Other issues that may contribute to depression include unexpressed anger, unresolved grief, all-or-nothing assumptions, negative self-fulfilling prophecies, and learned helplessness.[9]

Screening/Assessment

Early detection and treatment of depression alleviates symptoms sooner and speeds recovery, reducing morbidity and duration. The DART Program (Depression, Awareness, Recognition, and Treatment, since May 1988) is a major public health secondary prevention program sponsored by the National Institute of Mental Health to enhance professional (primary care and mental health specialist) and public awareness of depressive disorders as common illnesses requiring prompt diagnosis and treatment. Prospective studies of validated depression screening instruments suggest that they may help increase physicians' awareness and detection of depression.[25-27] Concern has been raised about possible harmful false-positive labeling[25] and the stigma still associated with psychiatric referral. Greater public acceptance of depression as a disorder, rather than a weakness, may help acceptance.[8]

Screening for depression in asymptomatic persons is not recommended by the US Preventive Services Task Force; rather, screening should be focused on those with risk factors for depression.[28] These risk factors include recent loss (real or perceived); previous history of depression; family history of depression (mania, suicide, alcoholism, or psychiatric treatment); symptoms of altered eating, sleep, or energy; chronic medical illness or pain; multiple unexplained somatic complaints; and history of substance abuse.

The prevailing standard for the diagnosis of clinical depression is the opinion of an examining physician that a patient's symptoms meet *DSM-IV-TR* criteria.[10] In other words, a detailed psychiatric history and mental-status examination is considered to be the essential diagnostic assessment.[29]

Several validated screening questionnaires are available to screen for depression. Subjective questionnaires are performed by the patients and include the following: Beck Depression Inventory (BDI), Zung Self-Rating Depression Scale (SDS), Center for Epidemiology Studies Depression Scale, General Health Questionnaire, The Hopkins Symptom Checklist, Mental Health Inventory, and Hospital Anxiety and Depression Scale.[2] Of these, the most widely used is the Zung Self-Rating Depression Scale. Among the objective questionnaires (those administered by a physician) is the Hamilton Psychiatric Rating Scale, which assesses depressive signs and symptoms. Other more complex psychologic tests that are helpful in diagnosis are the Minnesota Multiphasic Personality Inventory (MMPI) and projective tests, such as the Rorschach test and the Thematic Apperception Test (TAT).

The dexamethasone suppression test (DST) is the most widely used and studied biologic test in psychiatry. The DST is a research tool not found to be sufficiently accurate to warrant use as a screening tool.[30]

Sleep electroencephalographic recordings to look for or demonstrate characteristic disordered sleep patterns in depression also are not appropriate for routine screening because of poor sensitivity, large numbers of false-positive and false-negative results, invasiveness, and high cost. Functional brain techniques have been used to assess neuropathology of the depressive disorders, but findings have not been consistent enough to be of diagnostic value.

Primary Prevention

Insufficient epidemiologic data exist to support a risk factor intervention or primary prevention program for depression.[8] Primary prevention involves helping individuals to feel good about themselves by enhancing self-esteem and teaching problem solving, stress management, and appropriate coping skills to decrease vulnerability to depression.[31] Education offers the best hope for primary prevention.

Secondary Prevention/Treatment

In a high proportion of cases, depressive disorders respond well to treatment (secondary prevention)—some completely, others with some remaining morbidity. The type of treatment chosen depends on the particular presentation of the illness, its severity, and whether it is a single or recurrent episode (treatments that were successful in the past are likely to be effective again) as well as the patient's age, premorbid personality, and coping style.

Treatment tends to include somatic therapies in major depression with treatment of the underlying condition, removal of the offending medication, and/or biologic treatment of the underlying depression with antidepressant medications or electroconvulsive therapy (ECT), as appropriate. The more minor and reactive levels of depression usually respond well to psychotherapeutic interventions and counseling. Unfortunately, many people avoid treatment, believing they should get better through their own effort or simply live with depression until it passes. Many do not seek treatment because of feared effects on employment or perceived costs of treatment.[8] Depression frequently is treated inadequately.

Antidepressant medication

About 70% to 80% of depressed patients respond to antidepressants[8,32] or augmentation strategies. Approximately 10% to 30% of depressed patients do not respond to treatment.[33] Antidepressants tend to relieve neurovegetative symptoms most effectively. The ultimate mechanism of action of these medications remains unknown. The choice of a particular antidepressant, all of which are efficacious, depends primarily on side-effect profiles, previous responses to treatment or family members' responses, and the physician's familiarity with the chosen medication. Blood levels can be helpful and tend to correlate with clinical response with nortriptyline hydrochloride.[34] Blood levels for other antidepressants are helpful in terms of compliance, rapid metabolism, and tolerance but do not correlate as well with clinical response.

Side effects from antidepressants tend to occur early, and the patient often develops tolerance to them early. In other words, as long as the patient stays at the same dose, the side effect complained of will often improve within days. Exceptions to this general rule occur, such as dry mouth due to anticholinergic effects of antidepressants. It is often beneficial to teach patients to tolerate side effects in the initial phase so that they can receive the eventual rewards. Antidepressants take several weeks to become effective. Thus, it is important for the physician to maintain frequent early contact with the patient in the initial phases after a course of medication is begun. Education and support by the physician leads to improved compliance and improved prognosis. Antidepressants tend to improve appetite, weight, interest, pleasure, energy, psychomotor function, hopelessness, helplessness, and guilt, and to avert suicidal thoughts between 2 and 6 weeks after onset of therapy. Sleep pattern may improve first, during the first week (a hopeful sign). It is essential to treat adequately, that is, allow sufficient time (up to 6 weeks) and prescribe sufficient dosages, before trying an alternate strategy.

Selective serotonin reuptake inhibitors (SSRIs) have been shown to be safe and effective. Frequently, SSRIs are better tolerated than conventional tricyclic antidepressants and have a superior safety profile in overdosage. Potential drug interactions exist with these medications related to effects on the cytochrome P-450 system. Considerable evidence suggests that these drugs are indicated for a broad spectrum of psychopathology,[18] including panic disorder, post-traumatic stress disorder, obsessive-compulsive disorder, and bulimia.

Monoamine oxidase inhibitors (MAOIs) tend to have special effectiveness in atypical depressions characterized by marked anxiety; increased appetite; carbohydrate craving; hyperphagia; weight gain; excessive sleepiness (hypersomnolence); fatigue; self-pity; hypochondriacal, phobic, and obsessive-compulsive features; and reverse diurnal variation of mood (worse in evening).[35] Generally, MAOIs are used as the second or third choice in the treatment of depression.

Lithium revolutionized the treatment of bipolar (manic-depressive) disorder, both acutely and prophylactically, by decreasing the frequency and severity of manic and depressive episodes. Stimulants, such as amphetamine, methylphenidate, or pemoline, may be helpful in elderly, medically ill patients.

Maintenance of antidepressant treatment is extremely important after the acute episode. Many patients respond to the antidepressants initially and prematurely discontinue them. Within a few weeks thereafter, these patients often relapse. When the drug therapy is continued long enough, relapse of the underlying depression is prevented. It is wiser to continue treatment for at least for 4 to 6 months after resolution of multiple depressive symptoms and return to usual functioning to ensure that the episode has run its course. Length of time has been variously recommended from 4 to 12 months[36] before discontinuation by gradual taper of the dosage. If the dosage is discontinued too rapidly, there can be a brief period of discomfort with gastrointestinal complaints, listlessness, anxiety, and rapid eye movement rebound with nightmares.[37] Initially, maintenance was recommended at a reduced dose, but increasing evidence suggests that it is better to use the full acute therapeutic dosage, even for prevention. In patients with 2 or more depressive episodes, indefinite maintenance medication is probably appropriate.

Noncompliance with treatment occurs frequently (probably in 25% to 50% of patients),[32] particularly in individuals who do not believe anything will help them or that they do not deserve to get better. Noncompliance also can occur when patients feel threatened by or cannot handle the responsibility of becoming well, preferring their dependent depressive lifestyles.[9]

Phototherapy

In patients with seasonal affective disorder (SAD), phototherapy—exposure to bright (>10,000 lux) full-spectrum lights for various periods each day—often alleviates and, in certain cases, totally resolves these depressions.[38] If a major geographic factor is contributing to the depression, for example, the Alaskan latitudes, a move toward the equator may increase exposure to daily sunlight and thus improve the disorder.

Changes in sleep patterns

Sleep deprivation may be an effective technique to relieve depression temporarily.[20] Unfortunately, it lasts only a day or 2 in most people, and the person may feel worse after recovery sleep. Depriving people of the latter part of their sleep (partial sleep deprivation) may be more effective.[39] Phase shifting, in which the time that people go to sleep is progressively advanced, can be helpful.[40] This approach resets the biological clock involved in controlling normal life rhythms, such as eating and sleeping cycles, which are disrupted during depression.

Psychotherapy

Psychological therapies have been developed or modified specifically for the treatment of depression over the past 15 years, and their effectiveness has been supported through controlled studies. Combined treatments, blending psychotherapy and pharmacotherapy, often are more effective than a single-treatment approach.

Psychotherapy alone is useful in persons who do not respond well to medications, persons who are intolerant to drug side effects, or those with medical contraindications to antidepressants.[39] Some patients prefer psychotherapy, wanting to avoid drugs. Psychotherapy may increase compliance with treatment and improve social and occupational functioning and coping capacity. Many studies have shown psychotherapy to be the equal of medications in mild- to moderate-severity depressions.

The physician-patient relationship is extremely important for treatment success. Empathy and establishing a trusting relationship in a supportive holding environment, characterized by positive expectations and the reversal of demoralization, may be the most important basis for all other therapies to work.

Insight-oriented (psychodynamic, psychoanalytic) therapies deal with internal conflicts, such as dependence-independence struggles or ambivalence about relationships, which are thought to cause the patient's disorder. Therapy is directed toward resolving these conflicts, many of which are rooted in early childhood from child-parent relationships. These conflicts are subsequently played out in transferential reactions in therapy. In the past, psychoanalysis typically took several years and required several treatments per week with the goal of changing personality structure and not merely alleviating symptoms. Today, weekly short-term versions are increasingly used, such as those proposed by Malan[41] and Sifneos,[42] which tend to focus on a single dynamic issue. Other short-term psychotherapies, such as cognitive, behavioral, and interpersonal therapies, tend to have standardized treatment manuals and explicit training procedures and seem to be supplanting or augmenting purely psychodynamic approaches. These approaches also have undergone the greatest empirical research.[39]

Cognitive therapy is based on the premise that people's thoughts, attitudes, and views of the world and their experiences determine their emotions and subsequent behaviors. Because depressed people tend to think negatively about themselves, their environment (the world), and their future (the negative cognitive triad), they expect to fail and make faulty conclusions (inferences) about the behaviors and thoughts of others. Treatment is devoted to correcting maladaptive beliefs and negative thought patterns and habits. Eventual acceptance of reality and logical thinking leads to enhanced functioning and improved self-esteem, thereby improving mood. The preventive aspect of the therapy is presumed to be the alteration of dysfunctional attitudes, such as associating self-worth with the approval of specific others or excessively high standards, dependency, or self-criticism. Cognitive therapy lowers relapse and recurrence rates of unipolar nonpsychotic depressions and has been demonstrated to be as efficacious as antidepressant drugs in treating outpatient depression.[24]

Behavior therapy focuses on action and homework involving specific behaviors (eg, positive activities and developing social skills), thereby giving patients a sense of accomplishment by setting realistic goals in a stepwise fashion. Because depressed individuals give themselves too little self-reinforcement and too much self-punishment, behavioral strategies and techniques are designed to increase positive and decrease negative interactions and activities.[39]

Interpersonal therapy focuses on disturbed relationships rather than intrapsychic functions. These disturbed relationships are thought to cause depressive symptoms. By focusing on current interpersonal issues, patients are encouraged to become more aware of their patterns and develop better methods of relating and improved social functioning. Improved communication skills and the appropriate expression of suppressed emotions, including anger and grief, are encouraged.[39]

Depressed individuals tend to marry similar souls (assortative mating) who also need treatment. Marital maladjustment is common, often leading to separation or divorce. Some depressed individuals even provoke their partners to leave, thereby avoiding having to wait passively for abandonment.[9] Marital therapy may be essential.

Support from others

Family and friends can be helpful by encouraging the depressed person to seek appropriate treatment, providing support and encouragement while the patient is depressed, and making the patient feel worthwhile by maintaining the relationship with kindness, affection, respect, and caring.[1] Accepting that the person is suffering and in pain without being critical or disapproving is very supportive. Encouraging patients to "pull themselves up by their bootstraps" is not helpful. Helping the patient be busy and active breaks the cycle of withdrawal. It is important for family members to show patience and indicate that depression is not a sign of weakness. During times when suicide is a major risk, family also can be invaluable by providing containment and support.

Grief interventions

Not all people who are in a state of grief need formal intervention. Some grieving persons tend to respond to moral support and reassurance from family, friends, or religious support. Others are helped by physicians, psychiatrists, and other health professionals who review the history of the relationship with the departed person and use individual psychotherapy for persons who are overwhelmed. Self-help support groups, avoidance of alcohol and drug use, and specific antidepressants if grief gives way to major depression are indicated. Treatment-resistant cases should be referred to psychiatrists with special interest in the treatment of mood disorders or to tertiary care hospitals and universities.

SUICIDE

Epidemiology

Suicide is defined as intentional, self-inflicted death. Suicidal behavior is an extreme expression of underlying psychopathology, not a diagnosis in itself.[43] Suicide exists as a spectrum, from ideation to threat to intent and then attempt and finally completion. Suicide is the ultimate complication of depression in approximately 15% of cases. Identifiable depression may be causally related to 60% of suicides.[44] More than 90% of suicide victims have a diagnosable psychiatric illness.[45,46] Suicide attempts occur in 1% of the population without a lifetime mental disorder, 17% of dysthymic persons, 18% of those with major depression, and 24% of those with bipolar disorders.[8] Suicide is the eighth leading cause of death for all Americans, accounting for more than 30,000 deaths per year in the United States,[31,45,47] although suicide is thought to be underreported.

Despite extensive efforts of prevention over the last 3 decades, the incidence of suicide in the United States has not been reduced.[48] Higher rates are consistently found in the West and South than in the Midwest and Northeast.[49] American teenagers have the highest suicide rate in the world.[50] This rate increased dramatically in recent years,[51,52] rises with each teenage year, and peaks for youth at age 23.[53,54] A particularly disturbing trend in adolescents has been suicide clusters, where several adolescents in the same community commit suicide in rapid copycat succession.[55] People over 65 years of age account for 25% of all suicides. Female suicides peak at age 50 years, males at 75 years. Women attempt suicide 3 times more often than men do, but men commit suicide 3 times more often than women.[53,56]

Risk Factors

Although those at risk of suicide can be identified, those who will actually commit suicide are less easily determined because suicide is a rate event.[48] Most people who engage in suicidal behavior are mentally ill.[57] Most people who commit or attempt suicide have mood disorders (65% to 75%),[45,58] substance abuse (alcoholism in 25%),[58] or schizophrenia (depression rather than delusions increase the risk).[50,59] Three fourths of alcoholic persons who commit suicide concurrently have depression.[60] The risk of suicide is 5 to 6 times higher in psychotic depression. Some suicides are covertly encouraged by hostile or depressed significant others who also may need to be treated to reduce suicidal risk.[9,59,61]

All suicide attempts or threats should be taken seriously, even though 85% to 95% of attempters do not commit suicide. The apparent triviality of a suicide attempt may not be proportional to the seriousness of the risk and may be a rehearsal for a lethal attempt. Of those who attempt suicide, 1% to 2% of attempters do commit suicide each year, and a significant percentage (10% to 40%) of eventual suicide victims have made previous attempts.[49,62]

In a prospective study of patients with major affective disorders, suicide was found to occur relatively early in the course of affective illness.[63] Predictors of these early suicides were severe hopelessness, near total anhedonia, severe anxiety, recent state-dependent panic attacks, rapid switching from depression to anxiety to anger, and moderate alcohol abuse. Suicides occurring after 1 year from presentation were associated with suicidal ideation, history of previous attempts, and suicidal intent.[64]

Dependence increases risk of suicide, particularly in those who require constant reassurance and attention or who have unrealistic, frequently unmet expectations. People with small social networks or with few ties to the community have a much greater risk of death than those with larger networks.[45,65] Marital status affects suicide risk with increasing order of risk being single, widowed, divorced, separated.[66] Recent life changes and bereavement increase risk.[50] The elderly widower may be particularly vulnerable to fantasies of reunion with his spouse, particularly around anniversaries.[57] Intractable relationship problems, living alone, unemployment, poverty, and dropping out of school can contribute to risk. Terminal illness, recent surgery, and facial disfigurement are particularly important risk factors. Similarly, a history of physical violence or previous child, animal, or spouse abuse predicts a greater likelihood of suicide. Settings and professions that portend a higher rate of suicide are rural areas because of high rates of gun ownership and social isolation;[45,65] dentists, physicians, pharmacists, lawyers, musicians, police officers, and unskilled workers;[58] and prison inmates.[2] Alienated or stigmatized groups, such as homosexual adolescents, also have a higher suicide rate.[12]

A concrete suicidal plan, particularly if there has been rehearsal, is ominous. The most lethal method, firearms, is used by 60% of men and more than 33% of women.[53] Drug overdose was preferred during the 1970s and today is the second most common means. Women tend to take drug overdoses, particularly psychotropic drugs mixed with alcohol or poisons, or to slash their wrists.[58] Alcohol intoxication is associated with 25% to 50% of all suicides[50] and is especially common in suicides involving firearms.

Clinical Intervention

Although the US Preventive Services Task Force does not recommend routine screening of asymptomatic adult persons for suicidal intent,[28] the American Academy of Pediatrics advises questioning all adolescents about suicidal thoughts during the routine medical history.[67] In the course of standard practice, a primary care practitioner should assess risk factors for suicide and extent of preparatory actions as well as evaluate for depression, psychosis, intoxication, chronic alcohol abuse, recent loss, and social support. Seventy-five percent of patients who subsequently commit suicide see a physician (usually not a psychiatrist) within 6 months of their death, and more than 50% see a physician within 1 month of their death. Their complaints, mainly about somatic symptoms associated with depression, give the physician an opportunity to anticipate the possibility of suicide and refer the patient for psychiatric help. Even though two thirds communicate intent to commit suicide to a friend, family, or physician, the communications are often difficult to interpret.[9] Current suicidal intent scales lack sufficient sensitivity or specificity to be useful.[48] When the cutoff point on the Beck Hopelessness Scale is set to correctly identify 90% of suicides, it also yields 88% false-positive results.[68] The single greatest contributor to suicide prevention is an early diagnosis of mood disorder.[60] Patients with mood disorders who receive comprehensive psychiatric care have lower suicide rates than do patients with other psychiatric illnesses.[69,70]

Patients with serious suicidal intent should be referred for psychiatric consultation and intervention. A policy of routine psychiatric consultation after attempted suicide reduces the risk of suicide.[2] Hospitalization is mandatory for patients with overt suicidal ideation complicated by injurious behavior, encephalopathy, substance abuse, or intoxication.[57] Previous attempters are less likely to seek help or share their feelings with others and are more likely to react negatively to suicide prevention programs.[71] The family should be contacted despite the patient's objections if suicidal risk is judged to be high.[57] The closest available family member should be called to gain information and increase support. Patients and their families or friends should be aware of available community resources, such as local community mental health centers. Significant others, including parents, should be counseled to remove potentially lethal prescription drugs and firearms from the home. Other family members may also be suicidal and merit assessment.[66]

Suicide hotlines and suicide prevention centers can provide crisis intervention and triage. Evidence for the effectiveness of suicide hotlines in decreasing suicide rates has not been conclusive,[2] although a small reduction was found in one study.[72] In the United States, more than 200 centers offer educational, outreach, and supportive programs. Only 2% of suicide victims have contacted a center before taking their lives.[48] The Canadian Task Force on the Periodic Health Examination found little evidence to support the effectiveness of crisis intervention in preventing suicide.[2] Crisis intervention appears to postpone rather than prevent suicide in the chronically suicidal person.[48]

Hospitalization is indicated if risk is sufficiently high and evidence suggests that a person is actively suicidal. Assessment of intent is an important distinguishing factor. Overtly suicidal patients who refuse treatment should be hospitalized involuntarily, following state guidelines. Hospitalization, however, does not assure resolution of the problem, as many patients commit suicide in the hospital. The immediate post-hospital discharge period of these patients also is characterized by a particularly high rate of suicide.[63]

Outpatient treatment may be a valid alternative to hospitalization for patients who have suicidal ideation without a plan, no severe psychiatric disturbance, low levels of anxiety and perturbation, supportive and responsible family members to watch over them, and willingness and commitment to complete outpatient treatment. Preventing suicide is a family concern and families need family therapy to understand, cope with, and monitor their own feelings evoked by self-destructive behavior in their loved one.[69]

Contracts against suicide are a frequently used preventive therapeutic strategy.[57] The patient contracts, orally and in writing, to refrain from attempting suicide and to communicate with the physician if his or her resolve weakens. Contact with the patient by telephone and in person should initially be made daily and frequently thereafter.

Pharmacotherapy

The risk of suicide decreases with appropriate pharmacotherapy. Patients with major depression should be treated with antidepressant medications or ECT. The choice of antidepressants in the suicidal patient should be based on safety for risk of overdose. Newer antidepressants such as SSRIs, trazodone hydrochloride, nefazodone hydrochloride, mirtazapine, and bupropion hydrochloride tend to be safer than tricyclic antidepressants.[18,73] Psychotic symptoms merit antipsychotic medication. Severe agitation may require antipsychotics or parenteral benzodiazepines. Drugs prescribed by the physician are often used as a means of suicide, and in more than 50% of suicides the drugs were prescribed by a physician within the preceding week or as a refillable prescription.[74] Therefore, nonlethal quantities of prescription should be prescribed, (eg, less than 1500 or 2000 mg of standard tricyclic antidepressant at any one time). Because an overdose of 2 g of many antidepressants is potentially lethal, the prescription amount should be limited and nonrefillable.

Psychotherapy

The suicidal patient benefits from a therapeutic alliance and communication of hope. To relieve a sense of hopelessness, the patient should be encouraged to explore available options and alternative solutions and to focus on the temporary nature of suicidal feelings and intent. Psychotherapy helps to keep self-destructive dynamics in perspective. Involving family, friends, and significant others, considering family therapy, and restructuring of the patient's environment by attending to worrisome matters that can be changed (eg, contact with employer or significant other) help reduce anxiety. Continued reassessment is essential, particularly in the first phase of improvement from depression, when the patient develops sufficient energy to carry out a plan. Abrupt cessation of physician contact may be interpreted by the patient as rejection.[60] Suicide "completers" are less likely to be in or stay in psychiatric treatment.[63]

Valente[12] notes that suicidal risk decreases as adolescents learn to clarify problems; expand resources; use safer, more appropriate coping strategies; and rally significant others. These same principles are applicable to other age groups in applied prevention.

SUMMARY

No community has the resources to provide comprehensive care to all suicidal individuals,[48] and caring for these patients can be stressful. Many physicians who have a patient who committed suicide have many unresolved feelings and should be encouraged to discuss them with colleagues or supervisors. Suicide has been described as the ultimate hostility against the survivors. This sometimes includes the physician, giving rise to marked countertransference feelings, guilt, and grief. Physicians never know how many suicides they prevent and never forget the ones that are completed despite their best efforts. Psychiatrists need to limit the number of acutely suicidal patients they are treating, as these patients produce considerable emotional drain and stress.[58]

REFERENCES

1. Sargent M. *Depressive Disorders: Treatments Bring New Hope.* Rockville, Md: Dept of Health and Human Services; 1985. DHHS Publication No. (ADM) 86–1491.

2. Canadian Task Force on the Periodic Health Examination. 1990 update: early detection of depression and prevention of suicide. *Can Med Assoc J.* 1990;142:1233–1238.

3. Louise BA. Depression and suicide. *emedicine.* Available at: www.emedicine.com/. Accessed January 2003.

4. Rosenthal MP, Goldfarb NI, Carlson BL, et al. Assessment of depression in a family practice center. *J Fam Pract.* 1987;25:143–149.

5. Hankin JR, Locke BZ. The persistence of depressive symptomatology among prepared group practice enrollees: an exploratory study. *Am J Public Health.* 1982;72:1000–1007.

6. Caribbean Epidemiology Centre/Pan American Health Organization (CAREC/PAHO). *Paraquat Poisoning in Two Caribbean Countries.* Trinidad, West Indies: CAREC/PAHO; 1986:1–9. CAREC Surveillance Report No. 12.

7. Weissman MM. Advances in psychiatric epidemiology: rates and risks for depression. *Am J Public Health.* 1987;77:445–451.

8. Regier DA, Hirschfeld RMA, Goodwin FK, et al. The NIMH depression awareness, recognition and treatment program: structure, aims and scientific basis. *Am J Psychiatry.* 1988;145:1351–1357.

9. Dubovsky SL, Dubovsky AN. *Concise Guide to Mood Disorders.* Washington, DC: American Psychiatric Publishing Inc; 2002.

10. American Psychiatric Association. *Diagnostic and Statistical Manual of Mental Disorders, Fourth Edition Text Revision.* Washington, DC: American Psychiatric Association; 2000.

11. Rundell JR, Wise MG. *Concise Guide to Consultation Psychiatry.* Washington, DC: American Psychiatric Association; 2000: 61–80.

12. Valente SM. Adolescent suicide: assessment and intervention. *J Child Adolesc Psychiatr Ment Health Nurs.* 1989;2:34–39.

13. Roy-Byrne PP, Stang P, Wittchen H, Ustun B, Walters EE, Kessler RC. Lifetime panic depression comorbidity in the National Comorbidity Survey: association with symptoms, impairment, course and help-seeking. *Br J Psychiatry.* 2000;176:229–235.

14. Keller MB. Depression: underrecognition and undertreatment by psychiatrists and other health care professionals. *Arch Intern Med.* 1990;150:946–948.

15. Roose SP, Glassman AH, Seidman SN. Relationship between depression and other medical illnesses. *JAMA.* 2001;286:1687–1690.

16. Wells KB, Stewart A, Hays RD, et al. The functioning and well-being of depressed patients: results from the Medical Outcomes Study. *JAMA.* 1989;262:914–919.

17. Dubovsky SL, Randall B. Mood disorders. In: Hales RE, Yudofsky SC, eds. *Essentials of Clinical Psychiatry.* Washington, DC: American Psychiatric Association; 1999:277–344.

18. Winokur G, Tsuang MT, Crowe RR. The Iowa 500: affective disorder in the relatives of manic and depressed patients. *Am J Psychiatry.* 1982;139:209–212.

19. Keller MB. Diagnostic issues and clinical course of unipolar illness. In: Frances AJ, Hales RE, eds. *Review of Psychiatry.* Vol 7. Washington, DC: American Psychiatric Association; 1988.

20. Pflug B, Tolle R. Disturbance of the 24-hour rhythm in endogenous depression and the treatment of endogenous depression by sleep deprivation. *Int Pharmacopsychiatry.* 1971;6:187–196.

21. Steegmans PH, Hoes AW, Bak AAA, et al. Higher prevalence of depressive symptoms in middle-aged men with low serum cholesterol levels. *Psychosom Med.* 2000;62:205–211.

22. Davey SG, Shipley MJ, Marmot MG, et al: Plasma cholesterol concentration and mortality: the Whitehall Study. *JAMA.* 1992;267:70–76.

23. Schligen B, Tolle R. Partial sleep deprivation as therapy for depression. *Arch Gen Psychiatry.* 1980;37:267–271.

24. Shaw BF. Cognitive-behavior therapies for major depression: current status with an emphasis on prophylaxis. *Psychiatr J Univ Ottawa.* 1989;14:403–408.

25. Campbell TL. Controversies in family medicine: why screening for mental health problems is not worthwhile in family practice. *J Fam Pract.* 1987;25:184–187.

26. Prestidge BR, Lake CR. Prevalence and recognition of depression among primary care outpatients. *J Fam Pract.* 1987;25:67–72.

27. Rucker L, Frye EB, Cygan RW. Feasibility and usefulness of depression screening in medical outpatients. *Arch Intern Med.* 1986;146:729–731.

28. US Preventive Services Task Force. *Guide to Clinical Preventive Services: Screening for Depression.* Rockville, Md: Agency for Health Care Policy and Research, US Dept of Health and Human Services; 1989:173–178.

29. Gaviria FM, Flaherty JA. Depression: In: Flaherty JA, Shannon RA, Daviss JM, eds. *Psychiatry: Diagnosis and Therapy.* East Norwalk, Conn: Appleton & Lange; 1988.

30. Ballenger JC. Biological aspects of depression: implications for clinical practice. In: Frances AJ, Hales RE, eds. *Review of Psychiatry.* Vol 7. Washington, DC: American Psychiatric Association; 1988.

31. Public Health Service, US Department of Health and Human Services. *Promoting Health/Preventing Disease: Year 2000 Objectives for the Nation; Mental and Behavioral Disorders (Draft).* Philadelphia, Pa: WB Saunders Co; 1989. Publication PHS 19-1-19-19.

32. Prien RE. Somatic treatment of unipolar depression disorder. In: Frances AJ, Hales RE, eds. *Review of Psychiatry.* Vol 7. Washington, DC: American Psychiatric Association; 1988.

33. Charney DS, Berman RM, Miller HL. Treatment of depression. In: Schatzberg AF, Nemeroff CB, eds. *Essentials of Clinical Psychopharmacology.* Washington, DC: American Psychiatric Association; 2001:353–386.

34. Task Force on the Use of Laboratory Tests in Psychiatry. Tricyclic antidepressants, blood level measurements and clinical outcome. *Am J Psychiatry.* 1985;142:155–162.

35. Davidson JT, Miller RD, Turnbull CD, et al. Atypical depression. *Arch Gen Psychiatry.* 1982;39:527–534.

36. Prien RF, Kupfer DJ. Continuation drug therapy for major depressive disorder: how long should it be maintained? *Am J Psychiatry.* 1986;143:18–23.

37. Lawrence JM. Reactions to withdrawal of antidepressants, antiparkinsonian drugs and lithium. *Psychosomatics.* 1985;11:869–877.

38. Rosenthal NE, Sack DA, Carpenter CJ, et al. Antidepressant effects of light in seasonal affective disorder. *Am J Psychiatry.* 1985;142:163–170.

39. Shea MT, Elkin I, Hirchfeld RMA. Psychotherapeutic treatment of depression. In: Frances AJ, Hales RE, eds. *Review of Psychiatry.* Vol 7. Washington, DC: American Psychiatric Association; 1988.

40. Sack DA, Nurnberger J, Rosenthal NE, et al. The potentiation of antidepressant medications by phase advance of the sleep-wake cycle. *Am J Psychiatry.* 1985;142:606–608.

41. Malan DH. *The Frontier of Brief Psychotherapy.* New York, NY: Plenum Publishing; 1976.

42. Sifneos PE. Short-term anxiety- provoking psychotherapy: its history, technique, outcome and instruction. In: Budman S, ed. *Forms of Brief Therapy.* New York, NY: Guilford Press; 1981.

43. Davidson L. Assessment and management of suicidal patients. *J Med Assoc Ga.* 1988;77:834–835.

44. Stoudemire A, Frank R, Hedermark N. The economic burden of depression. *Gen Hosp Psychiatry.* 1986;8:387–394.

45. Mann JJ. A current perspective of suicide and attempted suicide. *Ann Intern Med.* 2002;136:302–311.

46. Shaffer D, Gould MS, Fisher P, et al. Psychiatric diagnosis in child and adolescent suicide. *Arch Gen Psychiatry.* 1996;53:339–348.

47. National Center for Health Statistics. *Advance Report of Final Mortality Statistics, 1986.* Monthly Vital Statistics Report, Vol 37, No 6. Hyattsville, Md: US Department of Health and Human Services; 1988.

48. Greenberg SI. Suicide prevention update: thirty years later. *J Fla Med Assoc.* 1988;75:610–613.

49. Prevention: the endpoint of suicidology [editorial]. *Mayo Clin Proc.* 1990;65:115–118.

50. Blumenthal SJ. Suicide: a guide to risk factors, assessment, and treatment of suicidal patients. *Med Clin North Am.* 1988;72:937–971.

51. Centers for Disease Control. *Youth Suicide in the United States, 1970–1980.* Atlanta, Ga: Centers for Disease Control; 1986.

52. Fingerhut LA, Kleinman JC. Suicide rates for young people. *JAMA.* 1988;259:356.

53. National Center for Injury Prevention and Control. *Suicide in the United States.* Atlanta, Ga: Centers for Disease Control and Prevention; November 2002.

54. Shaffer D, Garland A, Gould M, et al. Preventing teenage suicide. *J Am Acad Child Adolesc Psychiatry.* 1988;27:675–687.

55. Anonymous Leads from the MMWRCluster of suicides and suicide attempts: New Jersey. *JAMA.* 1988;259:2666–2668.

56. Jamison KR. Suicide prevention in depressed women. *J Clin Psychiatry.* 1988;49(suppl 9):42–45.

57. Pary R, Lippman S, Tobias CR. A preventive approach to the suicide patient. *J Fam Pract.* 1988;26:185–189.

58. Fawcett J, Shaugnessy R. The suicide patient. In: Flaherty JA, Channon RA, Davis JM, eds. *Psychiatry: Diagnosis and Therapy.* East Norwalk, Conn: Appleton & Lange; 1988.

59. Drake RE, Gates C, Cotton PG, et al. Suicide among schizophrenics: who is at risk? *J Nerv Ment Dis.* 1984;172:613–617.

60. Murphy GE. Prevention of suicide. In: Frances AJ, Hales RE, eds. *Review of Psychiatry.* Vol 7. Washington, DC: American Psychiatric Association; 1988.

61. Roose SP, Glassman AH, Walsh BT, et al. Depression, delusions and suicide. *Am J Psychiatry.* 1983;140:1159–1162.

62. Robins PV, Harvic K, Koven S. High fatality rates of late-life depression associated with cardiovascular disease. *J Affective Disord.* 1985;9:165–167.

63. Brent DA, Kupfer DJ, Brochet EJ, et al. The assessment and treatment of patients at risk for suicide. In: Frances AJ, Hales RE, eds. *Review of Psychiatry.* Vol 7. Washington, DC: American Psychiatric Association; 1988.

64. Fawcett J. Predictors of early suicide: identification and appropriate intervention. *J Clin Psychiatry.* 1988;49(suppl 10):7–8.

65. Beautrais AL, Joyce PR, Conn JM. Access to firearms and the risk of suicide: case control study. *Aust N Z J Psychiatry.* 1996;30:741–748.

66. Morgan HG, Vassilas CA, Owen JH. Managing suicide risk in the general ward. *Br J Hosp Med.* 1990;44:56–59.

67. American Academy of Pediatrics Committee on Adolescence: suicide and suicide attempts in adolescents and young adults. *Pediatrics.* 1988;81:322–324.

68. Beck AT, Steer RA, Kovacs M. Hopelessness and eventual suicide: a ten year prospective study of patients hospitalized with suicidal ideation. *Am J Psychiatry.* 1985;142:559–563.

69. Jamison KR. Suicide and bipolar disorders. *Ann N Y Acad Sci.* 1986;487:301–315.

70. Martin RL, Cloninger R, Guze SB, et al. Mortality in a follow-up of 500 psychiatric outpatients. *Arch Gen Psychiatry.* 1985;42:58–66.

71. Shaffer D, Vieland V, Garland A, Rojas M, Underwood M, Busner C. Adolescent suicide attempters: response to suicide-prevention programs. *JAMA.* 1990;264:3151–3155.

72. Miller HL, Coombs DW, Leeper JD. An analysis of the effects of suicide prevention facilities on suicide rates in the United States. *Am J Public Health.* 1984;74:340–343.

73. Mann JJ, Sanley M. Afterward: suicide. In: Frances AJ, Hales RE, eds. *Review of Psychiatry.* Vol 7. Washington, DC: American Psychiatric Association; 1988.

74. Murphy GE. The physician's responsibility for suicide. I. An error of omission. *Ann Intern Med.* 1975;82:301–314.

RESOURCES

American Association of Suicidology, 4201 Connecticut Ave NW, Suite 408, Washington, DC 20008; 202 237-2280.
Web site: www.suicidology.org.

Centers for Disease Control and Prevention, 1600 Clifton Rd, Atlanta, GA 30333; 800 311-3435.
Web site: www.cdc.gov.

Depression and Bipolar Support Alliance (formerly National Depressive and Manic-Depressive Association), 730 N Franklin St, Suite 501, Chicago, IL 60610; 800 826-3632.
Web site: www.dbsalliance.org.

Depression Awareness, Recognition and Treatment (DART) Program, National Institute of Mental Health, 6001 Executive Boulevard, Room 8184, MSC 9663, Bethesda, MD 20892-9663; 301 443-4513.
Web site: www.nimh.nih.gov.

National Alliance for the Mentally Ill, Colonial Place Three, 2107 Wilson Blvd, Suite 300, Arlington, WV 22201; help line 800 950-NAMI (6224).
Web site: www.nami.org.

National Foundation for Depressive Illness, PO Box 2257, New York City, NY 10116; 800 239-1265.
Web site: www.depression.org.

National Mental Health Association, 2001 N Beauregard St, 12th Floor, Alexandria, VA 22311; 703 684-7722.
Web site: www.nmha.org.

Substance Abuse and Mental Health Administration (SAMHSA), Room 12-105 Parklawn Building, 5600 Fishers Ln, Rockville, MD 20857.
Web site: www.samhsa.gov.

World Health Organization.
Web site: www.who.int/en.

chapter 8

Stresses of Daily Life

Michael G. McKee, PhD, and Kathleen Ashton, PhD

INTRODUCTION

Frequency, Nature, and Cost of Stress Problems

The pervasiveness of stress as a cause of illness affecting mental health as well as physical health is well recognized. According to the *Healthy People 2010* report of the US Department of Health and Human Services, "There is increasing awareness and concern in the public health sector regarding the impact of stress, its prevention and treatment, and the need for enhanced coping skills. Stress may be experienced by any person and provides a clear demonstration of the mind-body interaction."[1] Mental health problems such as anxiety and depression are clearly affected by stress. The effects of stress have been determined through research to be significant contributors to many clinically defined illnesses, including hypertension, head and back pain, cardiovascular disease, immune disorders, gastrointestinal disorders, anxiety and depressive disorders, and eating disorders, as well as to injuries, violence, and suicide.[2] Health care expenses are nearly 50% greater for workers who report high levels of stress.[3]

The majority of adults in the United States report that they have emotional problems during a given year, yet only a minority of them seeks professional help. When they do reach out to a professional, physicians are frequently consulted. In fact, persons with emotional problems are more likely to use a medical problem as a reason to visit physicians.[1] Stress-related symptoms may be presented without a description or even awareness of the stress. Physicians are increasingly called on to learn how to decode messages about stress and to recognize stress-related symptoms however they are presented. Almost none of the physicians has received formal education in stress,[4] and some researchers suggest that 58% of physicians themselves may experience enough stress to feel "emotionally exhausted."[5]

Because of data such as these, the *Healthy People 2000* report set objectives to prevent and treat mental and behavioral disorders related to stress by: reducing adverse health effects from stress, increasing the number of people who seek help for emotional problems, decreasing the number of people who have high stress levels and do not take steps to control it, increasing the number of employers who provide stress reduction programs for their workers, and increasing how often primary care providers review emotional, cognitive, and behavioral functioning of their patients. Data from the *Healthy People 2000 Final Review* indicated that stress continues to be a major concern for the health care field.[6]

Healthy People 2010 continues to emphasize that the public and the health care community need to recognize the importance of stress and dealing with it effectively. "Coping skills, acquired through the lifespan, are positive adaptations that affect the ability to manage stressful events," the report says. "Additional research can help to quantify the public health burden of stress and identify ways to prevent or alleviate it through environmental or individual strategies."[1]

Healthy People 2010 also continues to point out that health problems related to stress are among the most pressing concerns in public health. For example, 5 of the 10 Leading Health Indicators (high-priority public issues) identified by the Office of Disease Prevention and Health Promotion are significantly interrelated with stress. These include mental health, obesity, smoking, physical activity, and substance abuse.

DEFINITION OF STRESS

The term stress is used popularly in at least 3 major senses: (1) stressors, events experienced as stressful; (2) stress reactions, with particular emphasis on the physiological responses detailed by Cannon[7] and Selye;[8] and (3) further consequences of stress reactions, with impairment of mental or physical well-being or functioning. The commonsense view of stress implies that stressful events rather inevitably lead to stress reactions and further consequences (ie, that the relationship is linear); however, data suggest that the stress system is more complex than this. Much of stress is transactional in nature, with perception and cognition playing major roles in the definition of an event as stressful. A given event becomes a stressor when it is perceived and defined as a threat, and except for a few universal stressors such as starvation or exposure to extreme cold, most stressors appear to exist in the eye of the beholder. Lazarus and Folkman[9] define psychological stress as "a particular relationship between the person and the environment that is appraised by the person as taxing or exceeding his or her resources and endangering his or her well-being." Once an event is defined as stressful and reacted to as such, the sequence is not linear but a homeostatic network with reverberating feedback loops involving the central nervous system, autonomic nervous system, endocrine system, and immune system.

STRESS DISORDERS

Stress disorders can be grouped into 6 main categories: (1) psychophysiologic disorders, (2) emotional disorders, (3) interpersonal disorders, (4) performance problems, (5) bad habits and addictive behaviors related to stress, and (6) burnout.

Commonly, medical departments refer patients who are thought to have physical symptoms primarily related to stress or secondarily exacerbated by stress. Similarly, surgical departments refer patients for assistance in managing stress before surgery and reducing stress during the recovery.

Emotional symptoms of stress include various dimensions of fear and anger, such as panic and anxiety, irritability, hostility, and rage. Acute stress and hyperarousal often cause motoric restlessness, hypervigilance, apprehensive expectation that something bad is about to happen, autonomic overarousal in the sympathetic nervous system, and feelings of pressure. With prolonged stress, there often is lowered self-esteem and symptoms of depression, including disturbed sleep and changes in eating patterns, loss of initiative and interest in involvement with others, tearfulness, and feelings of being blue or sad.

In interpersonal disorders, disruption of social and family relationships occurs with tendencies to be either sad and withdrawn or irritable and difficult to get along with. Often a whole family is stressed by the anger, anxiety, and depression of 1 stressed member.

Performance problems develop because chronic stress may impair both mental and physical functioning, as does extreme acute stress. Increased difficulty focusing and concentrating, impairment of memory, and increased confusion are all characteristic mental symptoms. Physical symptoms include increased difficulty with coordination and loss of stamina. In general, the relationship between arousal and performance can be charted by an inverted U, with too little arousal leading to low performance, and too high arousal leading to poor performance. The acute stress response often initiates hyperarousal and the chronic stress response hypoarousal.

Smoking, drinking alcohol, overusing caffeine or tranquilizing medication, using illicit drugs, overeating, and sexual addictions are among the common habit problems that frequently develop in part as an effort to alleviate other stress symptoms. Stress usually becomes greater as the problems contributing to the original stress responses are not dealt with and as the habits themselves constitute additional problems.

One of the ironies of stress is that stress reactions themselves constitute a major source of stress, so that people in stress tend to spiral downward, often resulting in burnout. Freudenberger[10] describes burnout as starting with an intense commitment to prove oneself, with the need to be of service, leading to a denial and dismissal of one's own needs, followed by increased disengagement from others, and finally feelings of emptiness and depression. In the middle stages of burnout, one often is fatigued and forgetful, works harder than ever, worries more, sleeps badly, loses interest in sex, has vague physical complaints, is increasingly cynical and isolated from others, and is irritable and tense. Burnout tends to happen to the best and the brightest. If one does not care to begin with, the personal commitment, dedication, caring, and giving that ultimately lead to burnout is unlikely.

Individual, work group, and organization factors all contribute to burnout. Individuals who are perfectionistic, relate self-worth to achievement, have difficulty saying no, tend to keep all feelings inside, and isolate themselves from others are at higher risk of burnout. So, too, is the worker whose workplace is characterized by excessive demands, competitiveness rather than cooperativeness, and punishment rather than reward. An organization that does not provide an opportunity for self-assessment and self-expression, and for stress reduction and problem-solving groups contributes to the development of burnout.[11]

STRESSORS

Some stressors seem to be primarily external (ie, encountered), while others seem mainly internal (ie, self-imposed).

External Stressors

External stressors include change, work environment, family, difficult people, daily hassles, discrimination, trauma, and medical illness. Many studies have documented that major life changes are stressful for the average person.[12] Holmes and Rahe[13] constructed a scale that assigns a value which can be interpreted as representing the amount of energy it takes to cope with any given change that one has experienced during the past year. The most severe stressor on the scale is the death of a spouse. Because both positive events and negative events are stressful, getting married was set arbitrarily as the scale's midpoint. A life crisis can be defined as any change that requires one to modify important living patterns. Even going on a vacation temporarily disrupts normal patterns of living and in this sense constitutes a stressful demand. The more stress units accumulated during a given year, the greater the likelihood of illness or injury in the following year.

We live in a time of major change. Toffler,[14] in *Future Shock,* described the J curve of change, which characterizes much of life. In the last 10 years, an explosion of changes has affected not only our culture but also how each of us copes with his or her life. Examples include widespread use of the Internet and cellular telephones, the economic boom and recession, and increased domestic and foreign terrorism. As each decade produces a similarly accelerated number of changes, our ability to adapt becomes more and more challenged.

According to the National Institute for Occupational Safety and Health, job stress has become "a costly problem in the American workplace, leaving few workers untouched."[15] Three fourths of employees believe that today's worker has more job stress than workers did a generation ago.[16] In addition, problems at work account for more health complaints than stressors in other areas, including financial problems or family problems.[17] In a national survey using a representative sample of people at all levels of the workplace hierarchy in all geographic areas, 70% of people said that work stress alone resulted in frequent health and performance problems. One third said that they had seriously considered quitting their jobs in the previous year because of stress, and another third said they expected to burn out in the near future. Forty-six percent found their jobs to be highly stressful.[18]

The most stressed employees were those who had too much work or too little control over their job. The combination of too much responsibility and too little authority appears to be almost a prescription for job stress. Erratic work schedules and too little work can also be stressful. Role ambiguity is an additional source of job stress, in which there is uncertainty where responsibilities begin and end. A corporate culture in which loyalty is expected from the employee but not extended in return is also a significant source of stress. Uncertainty and insecurity in the workplace are added sources of stress, with rumors of takeovers increasing stress reactions and stress-related illnesses in the workplace. Deadlines and the need to work fast, inadequate information, vague objectives, and inadequate or vague feedback about performance increase stress reactions among workers. Social isolation in the workplace is stressful for most people,[19] as are people and politics in the workplace. Nonsupportive supervisors, the working environment, physical conditions, and ambiance are major sources of stress for employees. Additionally, lack of opportunity for professional or personal advance-

ment is stultifying and stressful. American society is increasingly becoming an around-the-clock society, and shift work and on-call duty are a separate major category of job stress.[20] Table 8-1 provides a tool to help identify sources of stress on the job.

Lack of work, or unemployment, is also a significant stressor for our society, especially in light of the volatile economy in recent years. Major job cuts, which were largely confined to blue collar workers in the 1980s, have increasingly threatened middle-class and white collar professionals. According to Broman et al,[21] downsizing can lead to major emotional difficulties, including depression, low self-worth, and interpersonal difficulties in additional to obvious financial stress. Unemployment and the fear of unemployment can negatively affect family harmony and damage family life, resulting in arguments, physical aggression, and breaking family ties.

People with stress-related disorders commonly identify conflict with 1 or more family members as a major source of stress. Family stressors relate to change, birth, death, members leaving for school, jobs, and marriage. Divorce is a major stressor for the American family. Additionally, conflict with a loved one is stressful.[22] Families have become more and more difficult to maintain. Demographers project that half of all first marriages will end in divorce and that about 60% of second marriages will end in divorce. Data from the US Census Bureau indicate that, in 1998, 27.4% of all children lived in single-parent homes, with most of them being mother-child families.[23] Of these families, 42.2% of the mothers had never been married.

In addition, family roles are changing, constituting a source of stress for many. With women becoming increasingly active members of the workforce during the childbearing years, 75% of all children under age 5 years participate in day care outside of their parents.[24] Fathers are playing a major role in child care as well. Fathers are the primary caregivers for 18.5% of children under 5 years of age, with an additional 25% providing some care for their young children. However, in general the percentage of men sharing home responsibilities has lagged behind the number of women sharing the pressure of providing income; studies suggest that less than 25% of men help equally at home.

Difficult people may be stressors. They are angry or meek, blunt or indirect, too talkative or silent, blaming others or blaming themselves, hyperemotional or hyperrational. Difficult people tend to exceed the normal boundaries of behavior.[22]

Daily hassles are the other side of the stress picture, the opposite of enduring patterns or major life changes. Daily hassles are the small things that cause frustration in our daily lives: the traffic light stuck on red, the driver who cuts in front of us or who drives too slowly, a child who is not ready for school in the morning, the shoelace that breaks, the inopportune phone call. When physiological

T A B L E   8-1

Sources of Stress

Rate the following in terms of how much stress they cause you.

	Very Much				Very Little
Too much work	1	2	3	4	5
Too little authority	1	2	3	4	5
Politics	1	2	3	4	5
Difficult customers	1	2	3	4	5
Difficult supervisors	1	2	3	4	5
Difficult coworkers	1	2	3	4	5
Lack of clarity in job description	1	2	3	4	5
Lack of feedback	1	2	3	4	5
Excessive need for approval	1	2	3	4	5
Perfectionistic tendencies/unrealistic idealism	1	2	3	4	5
Too frequent interruptions	1	2	3	4	5
Juggling job and family demands	1	2	3	4	5
Sexual harassment	1	2	3	4	5
Erratic work schedule and take-home work	1	2	3	4	5
Disparity between what I have to do on the job and what I would like to accomplish	1	2	3	4	5
Ambiguity of work tasks, territory, and role	1	2	3	4	5
Expecting too much of myself	1	2	3	4	5
Financial problems	1	2	3	4	5
Sexual problems	1	2	3	4	5
Marital or significant-other problems	1	2	3	4	5
Problems with parents	1	2	3	4	5
Problems with children	1	2	3	4	5
Problems with other relations	1	2	3	4	5
Chronic illness in family member	1	2	3	4	5
Trouble speaking up for myself	1	2	3	4	5
Poor time management	1	2	3	4	5
Loneliness	1	2	3	4	5
Lack of confidence	1	2	3	4	5
Feeling of powerlessness	1	2	3	4	5
Effects of childhood abuse	1	2	3	4	5
Death of someone close	1	2	3	4	5
Divorce or separation	1	2	3	4	5
Spiritual alienation	1	2	3	4	5
Change in job	1	2	3	4	5
Change in residence	1	2	3	4	5
Health problems	1	2	3	4	5
Poor exercise and diet habits	1	2	3	4	5
Smoking	1	2	3	4	5
Drinking too much	1	2	3	4	5
Type A personality	1	2	3	4	5
Other	1	2	3	4	5

reactivity is monitored during the day, daily hassles tend to produce fight or flight reactions on a recurring basis.

Discrimination based on race, sex, age, religion, or social class constitutes a heightened risk of vulnerability.[25] An example by Miller et al[26] of the stressors experienced by urban African American adolescents helps to capture the impact of poverty, urban living, and discrimination. More than half the adolescents whom these authors surveyed said that they experienced any of the following:

- being asked for money by drug addicts
- pressure by friends to join a gang
- being made fun of because of grades
- worry that someone would try to take their clothes, shoes, or money
- pressure to carry weapons for protection
- pressure for sex by boyfriend or girlfriend
- must work to help pay bills at home
- nervous about gunshots and sirens at night
- keeping fear about safety secret from friends
- being offered sex by drug addicts for money

Traumatic stresses can lead to post-traumatic stress disorder (PTSD). Children have been shown to be particularly vulnerable to PTSD. According to the American Psychiatric Association's *Diagnostic and Statistical Manual of Mental Disorders, Fourth Edition (DSM-IV)*, PTSD involves characteristic symptoms that occur "following exposure to an extreme traumatic stressor involving direct personal experience of an event that involves actual or threatened death or serious injury, or other threat to one's physical integrity; or witnessing an event that involves death, injury, or a threat to the physical integrity of another person; or learning about unexpected or violent death, serious harm, or threat of death or injury experienced by a family member or other close associate."[27] Traumatic events may include life-threatening situations, such as encountering a sexual assault; sustaining a serious car accident; being caught in a hurricane; witnessing a murder; or dealing with national traumas, including the Oklahoma City bombing, the Columbine (Colo) school massacre, and the World Trade Center and US Pentagon terrorist attacks.

The psychological effects of such traumas may not be limited to those persons who experienced the events directly. For example, researchers using a nationwide survey of US residents outside of New York City reported that 17% of those surveyed reported post-traumatic stress symptoms 2 months after the attacks on September 11, 2001, and 5.8% continued to report symptoms 6 months after September 11.[28]

Medical illness is a major source of stress for many individuals. The emotional stress triggered by a medical illness may be more problematic than the illness itself, especially if the illness is chronic.[29] If the medical illness

requires hospitalization, the degree of emotional distress is amplified.[30] Estimates of medical patients who experience emotional distress leading to depression or anxiety range from 24% to 50%.[29] Several factors contribute to the stress of medical illness and hospitalization.[31] Patients may feel a reduced sense of independence and autonomy as they are expected to follow orders from medical professionals. They are exposed to a strange environment, without the comforting routines of their everyday life. Medical patients must negotiate a host of new relationships with their medical providers and other patients. They may fear potential losses of income, employment, or physical functioning. Invasive procedures require individuals to adapt to their intrinsic fear of pain. Patients may struggle with widely held beliefs that "bad things happen to bad people" and feel a sense of guilt or punishment. The additional pragmatic stresses of coping with a medical illness include extended travel, large and confusing hospital environments, multiple appointments to schedule and remember, and dealing with several medications that may need to be taken with specific instructions. Dealing with medical bills and insurance issues can add to the stress of coping with a medical illness. Many people have phobias of medical procedures such as injections and scans.[32] Some medical illnesses or injuries and their treatments have even been postulated to be so stressful as to cause a post-traumatic stress reaction. These include heart attacks, delirium, cancer, childbirth, burns, and major injuries.[32]

The impact of stress due to medical illness can be illustrated by the experience of the cardiology patient. Patients may take several weeks to recover after a myocardial infarction. They recently have experienced a life-threatening event and possibly have undergone invasive procedures to treat their illness. After a hospital stay, lifestyle changes may be stressful such as losing weight, exercising, quitting smoking, or needing to retire from a job for medical reasons.

Although much research has focused on how stress may exacerbate medical illness, the importance of medical illness producing stress is being recognized and is being better managed to produce better health outcomes. As new advances in health care lower mortality and lengthen the lifespan, chronic medical illnesses increasingly become stressors with which people must cope.

Internal Stressors

Internal stressors include behavior type, thought patterns, and life stages. In 1974, Friedman and Rosenman's[33] *Type 'A' Behavior and Your Heart* had a profound impact on the public. In 1984, Friedman and Ulmer[34] reported a study indicating that individuals with type A behavior who receive special counseling cut their heart attack rate by half, presumably as a result of changing their behavior patterns. Individual components of type A behavior have been identified in subsequent research as (1) emotional, including anger, contempt, and scorn; (2) behavioral, including verbal and physical aggression; and (3) cognitive, including hostility toward others.[35]

Recent studies have indicated that hostility and anger were predictive of new coronary events in previously healthy people.[36,37] In addition, hostility has been related to heightened cardiovascular and neuroendocrine reactivity to stressful social situations.[38] Fredrickson et al[39] found that hostile persons show a prolonged period of increased blood pressure when recalling events that made them angry.

People tend to live by rules. Common rules that increase stress and lead to perfectionistic striving and excessive work are "anything worth doing is worth doing well" and "anything worth starting is worth finishing." As Ellis and Harper[40] pointed out, stress does not go from action A to consequence C in the individual. Rather, it goes from A to B to C, where B indicates a person's belief about a situation. This is a philosophy espoused eloquently by Epictetus, who developed the philosophy of stoicism. Fundamental among his dicta was "It is not events which disturb our lives, it is our judgement of events." Thus, never say, "That man's words make me angry"; always say, "I react with anger to that man's words." The notion that one reacts to anger, rather than someone else making you angry, is contrary to daily parlance. "He really tics me off" and "She makes me furious" are examples of ways of talking that imply that somebody else has control over one's feelings and one's stress.

Externalization of causality contributes to stress. So, too, does permanence, in which stressors are seen as never changing—"It will always be that way." A third stress-producing attitude is global attribution in which one does not focus on the effects of the immediate specific stress but instead says, "Everything's going down the drain."

Phases of the life cycle are developmental internal stressors. The *DSM-IV* states: "In addition to the above, for children and adolescents the following stressors may be considered: cold or distant relationship between parents; overtly hostile relationship between parents; physical or mental disturbance in family members; cold or distant parental behavior toward child; overtly hostile parental behavior toward child; parental intrusiveness; inconsistent parental control; insufficient social or cognitive stimulation; anomalous family situation, eg, single parent, foster family; institutional rearing; loss of nuclear family members."[27]

Karraker and Lake[41] note that infants are subject to stressors that William James has described as "the blooming, buzzing confusion" of the world. Psychologically, separation is probably the major stressor for infants, starting around 7 or 8 months. Distressing interactions,

such as with a depressed mother, are also major stressors for infants. The events that infants experience as stressful might not appear to be stressful to adults, but they are categories of events that adults do find stressful: unpredictability, feeling out of control, uncertainty, and events inconsistent with our expectations and understandings.

Humphrey[42] has summarized sources of stress in children as including self-concerns, home conditions, and school conditions. In the latter, it is noted that school tends to be more stressful for boys than for girls. Test anxiety and subject anxiety are prevalent and manifest in increased muscle tension, difficulty concentrating, and restlessness. The one thing that seems to worry children most in school is pressure from teachers for competitiveness. At home, pressure to do things the parents' way, lack of concern, and lack of support are major stressors. Self-imposed stressors may relate to personal goals, self-esteem, values, social standards, ability, and personal characteristics.

Each stage of life embodies certain tasks.[43,44] In adolescence these tasks center on establishing an identity—learning to answer "Who am I?" In their search, teenagers must learn to accept new physical and sexual roles, establish new friendships, strive toward emotional independence from their parents, and take steps toward economic independence. They must develop a greater capacity for abstract thinking, deal with social issues and personal values, develop socially responsible behavior, and start to prepare for marriage and family life.

After adolescence, young adults typically are oriented toward moving out of the house and developing families and careers of their own. In this stage, there is the continued task of trying to define identity, followed by the task of becoming able to establish intimacy.

Many adults experience a midlife crisis near age 40.[43] This occurs at a time when one perceives that one's life has reached the halfway point and is no longer going uphill but is sliding downhill toward retirement, old age, and death. This perception leads many people to go through an agonizing appraisal of their personal and work lives. This philosophical crisis coincides with the reality that many parents are coping with adolescent children for the first time, often simultaneously having to deal with ill or dying parents. In addition, they may be coping with major job responsibilities that have accrued by midlife. Heavy work demands and multiple roles often overload one's coping abilities.

With the dramatic increase in the US elderly population, attention to the impact of stress on older adults is more important than ever before. Currently, 32 million Americans are age 65 or older, and by the year 2030 the figure is expected to more than double to nearly 65 million.[45] Whereas the average American born in the year 1900 had a life expectancy of 49 years, 4 out of 5 Americans can expect to live to at least 65 years of age today.

Thus, stressors affecting the elderly are likely to gain in prominence and public awareness in the coming years.

Retirement, financial responsibilities, increased medical problems, and changes in social relationships are a few of the most common stressors for older adults. Often, the elderly are forced to deal with a lower standard of living due to reduced income.[46] Long-term care of older adults with progressive dementia may be a particular economic hardship for the elderly and their families. Beyond the financial burden of health care, coping with medical illness is a significant stressor for older adults. More than 80% of Americans over the age of 65 years report at least one chronic medical problem, and most have multiple medical conditions.

Research suggests that older adults may be more vulnerable to stressors due to the physiological changes that occur with aging.[47] More than half of older adults surveyed in an epidemiologic study reported severe sleep problems, putting them at higher risk of depression and anxiety.[48] Stress hormones, such as epinephrine and norepinephrine, tend to be elevated in the elderly compared with younger adults.[49] The increased physical vulnerability to stress along with multiple new stressors puts the elderly at a high risk of emotional problems such as depression, anxiety, and suicidal thoughts or impulses.

Death of a family member is a major stressor whenever it occurs. On the life crisis scale, the most stressful item is death of a spouse. This is an event more likely to be faced in late adulthood than at other times of life, with women 4 times as likely as men to have a spouse die.[50] The stages of reaction to death have been described as denial, bargaining, anger, sadness and loss, and finally acceptance. Developing a new life at this stage parallels developing a life in young adulthood, leaving home but without all the excitement of looking forward to a new life. The majority of persons over age 65 have grandchildren as well as children, and often the grandchildren offer a relationship that is extremely satisfying and can help rebuild the will to live after a spouse's death. Group support can be particularly helpful during the grieving period.[51] (See "Resources" at the end of the chapter.)

ASSESSING STRESS

In the clinical setting, when stress is thought to be an important issue, helpful questions include:

- How do I know how stressed this person is?
- What are his or her symptoms of stress?
- What are the causes of the symptoms?
- What can I do to help keep the person physically and mentally healthy?

Asking a patient to complete an assessment tool of stress symptoms and sources of stress may help to establish effective communication (Tables 8-1 and 8-2).

TABLE 8-2

Symptoms of Stress

Rate how much you experience these symptoms.	Very Much				Very Little
Physical symptoms (eg, headaches, gastrointestinal upset, hypertension)	1	2	3	4	5
Deterioration in work performance (difficulty concentrating, increased errors, decreased efficiency)	1	2	3	4	5
Unhealthy habits (eg, smoking, alcohol and substance abuse, overeating)	1	2	3	4	5
Deterioration in interpersonal relationships (eg, increased conflict, decreased satisfaction, social withdrawal)	1	2	3	4	5
Subjective distress that interferes with well-being (eg, tension, pressure, anxiety, depression)	1	2	3	4	5
Attitude change (eg, decreased motivation, cynicism)	1	2	3	4	5
Fatigue, chronic tiredness	1	2	3	4	5
Insomnia (difficulty falling asleep and/or awakening frequently or early)	1	2	3	4	5
Anger and irritability	1	2	3	4	5
Other (List)	1	2	3	4	5

All persons are under stress, so people generally respond positively to a request to identify which stressors are present in their life and which stress reactions are bothersome. In assessing stress, there are formal instruments such as the Minnesota Multiphasic Personal Inventory (MMPI-2), which measures psychological pathology along various dimensions. The Symptom Checklist-90 is a briefer measure that has scales for symptoms in various systems. Computerized self-assessment questionnaires can be taken online at the office, such that assessment of stress can become a routine part of examinations. The simplest self-report methods are visual analog scales and ratings of magnitude. Such a scale can be constructed by drawing a line from 1 to 10 and making a self-anchoring scale, in which one end is defined as no stress and the other end is the worse stress imaginable. The person then assesses where he or she falls on the scale according to no stress and worst stress.

Typically, one recognizes times of stress because the body develops various symptoms, including aches and pains; the mind sends apprehensive thoughts and feelings of being pressured and harassed; bad habits begin to escalate to try to reduce stress; and performance declines noticeably. Often family members can help to assess stress. Spouses of type A personalities are always acutely aware of the type A behavior with which they live, even though the type A person may deny it. Anyone living with someone else who is irritable and/or withdrawn because of stress will be able to report the situation clearly. Often, it is a family member who sees the relationship between excessive drinking and stress or between school or work worries and physical symptoms. Asking a relevant family member to fill out the forms in this section, as they relate to the designated patient, can provide important information.

The *Healthy People 2010* report states, "Attention to mental state in primary care can promote early detection and intervention for mental health problems."[1] In particular, it is worthwhile to give attention to major life stressors, including recent divorce or separation, death of a family member, legal problems, unemployment, or serious medical illness, as well as symptoms of emotional and behavioral problems, including depression and substance abuse.

Normalizing stress is a key technique to obtain information from people who feel stigmatized by reporting stress or who feel that being stressed is a sign of personal weakness. A comment such as "I know we are all under a lot of stress in the world we live in today; tell me about yours" can be a good starting point. An acknowledgment that stress happens to people who care and who try is another way to offset possible feelings of stigma. Once the door is opened, using forms such as those in Tables 8-1 and 8-2 can constitute a guided interview. Patients will also communicate a great deal

about themselves in nonverbal ways. The anxious patient will have motoric restlessness, autonomic hyperarousal, vigilant scanning behavior, and apprehensive expectations. Posture, movement, intonation, inflection, volume of voice, eye contact, expression, and grooming all make powerful statements about one's self-esteem and about how effectively one is coping with the multiple pressures in life.

MANAGING STRESS

Patients who need to reduce stress in their lives can be helped in many ways. Psychotherapy, biofeedback, and psychopharmacologic interventions all have documented effectiveness.

Social support protects one in stressful situations. Loving and caring friends and family help reduce stress reactivity. Self-help groups offer social support and acceptance along with a shared focus on a particular problem area. The *Healthy People 2000* report says[52]

> During the past decade, autonomous mutual help groups have gained increasing recognition as complementary to clinical practice. Often referred to as self-help organizations, their members include people who share or have shared specific physical, mental, or emotional problems. These groups make significant contributions to positive outcomes for persons affected by mental and behavioral disorders, including the family members and formal and informal caregivers of individuals with chronic conditions. An estimated 10 million to 15 million people are members of mutual help groups in the United States, with some 1.9 million adults turning to nonprofessional mutual help resources for personal or emotional problems in the course of a year.

To locate a group that fits a particular situation, national self-help clearinghouses can point the way (see "Resources" at the end of the chapter). Techniques to minimize stress symptoms and impairments are, in part, age-old and commonsense: eat a healthy diet, exercise regularly, avoid alcohol or caffeine, and don't smoke. Additional strategies reflecting psychological input include mastering and practicing a relaxation technique, setting realistic expectations, developing a support network, identifying and eliminating distorted cognitions, setting realistic goals, and taking responsibility for one's own feelings and behavior.

SUMMARY

The research describing the relationship between life stress and disease can be summarized briefly. The results are equivocal and contradictory but overall strongly suggestive that stress is one of the factors in the cause-and-effect chain in the etiology of many diseases. The research is nomothetic, looking for statistical relationships that hold across groups in which general principles of relationship exist. Clinical work is idiographic, dealing with individuals. The challenge to the clinician is to define the way in which stress is relevant for each individual patient.

Excessive stress impairs mental health as well as physical health, reduces effectiveness at many tasks, and often contributes to bad habits that are intended to relieve tension. A physician's assessment of a patient's stress reactions and stressors can help patients change both themselves and their environments to reduce the negative effects of stress. In time, this approach will contribute to improving the health, happiness, and effectiveness of the population and reduce mental health costs.

REFERENCES

1. US Dept of Health and Human Services. *Healthy People 2010.* 2nd ed. *With Understanding and Improving Health and Objectives for Improving Health.* Vols 1 and 2. Washington, DC: US Dept of Health and Human Services; November 2000.

2. Pelletier K, Herzing D. Psychoneuroimmunology: toward a mind and body model—critical review. Advances. *J Inst Adv Health.* 1988;5:27–56.

3. Goetzel RZ, Anderson DR, Whitmer RW, Ozminkowski RJ, Dunn RL, Wasserman J, for Health Enhancement Research Organization (HERO) Research Committee. The relationship between modifiable health risks and health care expenditures: an analysis of the multi-employer HERO health risk and cost database. *J Occup Environ Med.* 1988;40:843–854.

4. Shapiro S, Shapiro DE, Schwartz GER. Stress management in medical education. *Acad Med.* 2000;75:748–759.

5. Deckard G, Meterko M, Field D. Physician burnout: an examination of personal, professional, and organizational relationships. *Med Care.* 1994;32:745–754.

6. National Center for Health Statistics. *Healthy People 2000 Final Review.* Hyattsville, Md: US Public Health Service; 2001.

7. Cannon WB. *Bodily Changes in Pain, Hunger, Fear and Rage.* Boston, Mass: CT Branford Co; 1929.

8. Selye H. *Stress in Health and Disease.* Boston, Mass: Butterworths; 1976.

9. Lazarus RS, Folkman S. *Stress Appraisal, and Coping.* New York, NY: Springer-Verlag; 1991.

10. Freudenberger H. *Burnout: How to Beat the High Cost of Success.* New York, NY: Bantam Books; 1981.

11. Maslach C, Leiter M. *The Truth About Burnout: How Organizations Cause Personal Stress and What to Do About It.* San Francisco, Calif: Jossey-Bass; 1997.

12. Miller T, ed. *Stressful Life Events.* Madison, Wis: International Universities Press; 1989. *Stress and Health Series.* Monograph 4.

13. Holmes TH, Rahe RH. The social readjustment rating scale. *J Psychosom Res.* 1967;11:213–218.

14. Toffler A. *Future Shock.* New York, NY: Random House Inc; 1970.

15. National Institute for Occupational Safety and Health. *Stress at Work.* Washington, DC: US Dept of Health and Human Services. Publication No. 99–101.

16. Princeton Survey Research Associates. *Labor Day Survey: State of Workers.* Princeton, NJ: Princeton Survey Research Associates; 1997.

17. St Paul Fire and Marine Insurance Co. *American Workers Under Pressure.* St Paul, Minn: St Paul Fire and Marine Insurance Co; 1992. Technical report.

18. Northwestern National Life Insurance Co. *Employee Burnout: America's Newest Epidemic,* 1991.

19. Cummings ME, Greene AL, Karraker KH, eds. *Life-span Developmental Psychology: Perspectives on Stress and Coping* (West Virginia Univ Conference on Life-Span Development, No. 11). Hillsdale, NJ: Lawrence Erlbaum Associates Inc; 1991.

20. Coleman RM. *Wide Awake by 3 AM: By Choice or by Chance.* New York, NY: WH Freeman & Co; 1986.

21. Broman CL, Hamilton VL, Hoffman WS. *Stress and Distress Among the Unemployed.* New York, NY: Kluwer/Plenum Publishers; 2001:226.

22. Davis M, Eshelman ER, McKay M. *The Relaxation and Stress Reduction Workbook.* 5th ed. Oakland, Calif: New Harbinger Publications; 2000.

23. Caspar LM, Bryson K. Population characteristics. Washington, DC: US Census Bureau 1998:20–515.

24. Smith K. *Who's Minding the Kids?* Washington, DC: US Census Bureau; 2000:70–75.

25. Adams P. Prejudice and exclusion in social traumata. In: Noshpitz JD, Coddington RD, eds. *Stressors and the Adjustment Disorders.* New York, NY: John Wiley & Sons Inc; 1990:363–391.

26. Miller DB, Webster SE, MacIntosh R. What's there and what's not: measuring daily hassles in urban African American adolescents. *Res Soc Work Pract.* 2002:12:375–388.

27. American Psychiatric Association. *Diagnostic and Statistical Manual of Mental Disorders, Fourth Edition.* Washington DC: American Psychiatric Association; 1994.

28. Silver RC, Holman EA, McIntosh DN, Poulin M, Gil-Rivas V. Nationwide longitudinal study of psychological responses to September 11. *JAMA.* 2002;288:1235–1244.

29. Gibson RL, Burch EA. Emotional disorders and medical illness. In: Sutker PB, Adams HE, eds. *Comprehensive Handbook of Psychopathology.* 3rd ed. New York, NY: Kluwer/Plenum Publishers; 2001:797–811.

30. Burch EA.. Emotional disorders in chronic medical illness. In: Sutker P, Adams HE, eds. *Comprehensive Handbook of Psychopathology.* 2nd ed. New York, NY: Plenum Press; 1993:671–688.

31. Strain JJ, Grossman S. *Psychological Care of the Medically Ill: A Primer in Liaison Psychiatry.* New York, NY: Appleton-Century-Crofts; 1975.

32. Mayou RA, Smith KA. Post-traumatic symptoms following medical illness and treatment. *J Psychosom Res.* 1997;43:121–123.

33. Friedman M, Rosenman R. *Type 'A' Behavior and Your Heart.* New York, NY: Alfred Knopf; 1974.

34. Friedman M, Ulmer D. *Treating Type A Behavior and Your Heart.* New York, NY: Alfred A. Knopf; 1984.

35. Smith TW, Ruiz JM. Psychosocial influences on the development and course of coronary heart disease: current status and implications for research and practice. *J Consult Clin Psychol.* 2002;70:548–568.

36. Chang PP, Ford DE, Meoni LA, Wang N, Klag MJ. Anger in young men and subsequent premature cardiovascular disease. *Arch Intern Med.* 2002;162:901–906.

37. Williams JE, Paton CC, Siegler IC, Eigenbrodt ML, Nieto FJ, Tyroler HA. Anger proneness predicts coronary heart disease risk: prospective analysis from the Atherosclerosis Risk in Communities (ARIC) study. *Circulation.* 2002;101:2034–2039.

38. Suarez EC, Kuhn CM, Schanberg SM, Williams RB, Zimmerman EA. Neuroendocrine, cardiovascular, and emotional responses of hostile men: the role of interpersonal challenge. *Psychosom Med.* 1998;60:78–88.

39. Fredrickson BL, Maynard KE, Helms JJ, Haney TL, Siegler IC, Barefoot JC. Hostility predicts magnitude and duration of blood pressure response to anger. *J Behav Med.* 2000;23 :229–243.

40. Ellis A, Harper RA. *A New Guide to Rational Living.* New York, NY: Institute for Advanced Study in Rational Psychotherapy; 1975.

41. Karraker KA, Lake M. *Normative Stress and Coping Processes in Life-span Developmental Psychology: Perspectives on Stress and Coping.* Hillsdale, NJ: Lawrence Erlbaum Associates Inc; 1991.

42. Humphrey JH. *Stress in Childhood.* New York, NY: AMS Press; 1984.

43. Berger KS. *The Developing Person Through the Life Span.* New York, NY: Worth Publishers; 1983.

44. Duvall EM. *Family Development.* 4th ed. New York, NY: JB Lippincott; 1971.

45. MacNeil RD. Bob Dylan and the Baby Boom Generation: "the times they are a-changin'"—again. *Activities Adaptation Aging.* 2001;25:45–58.

46. Koenig HG, George LK, Schneider R. Mental health care for older adults in the year 2020: a dangerous and avoided topic. *Gerontologist.* 1994;34:674–679.

47. Nguyen CTMH, Goldberg JH, Sheikh JI. The geriatric patient. In: Motofsky DI, Barlow DH, eds. *The Management of Stress and Anxiety in Medical Disorders.* Needham Heights, Mass: Allyn & Bacon; 2000:180–193.

48. Foley DJ, Monjan AA, Brown SL, Wimonsick EM, Wallace RB, Blazer DG. Sleep complaints among elderly persons: an epidemiologic study of three communities. *Sleep.* 1995;18:425–432.

49. Sapolsky RM. *Why Zebras Don't Get Ulcers.* New York, NY: Freeman; 1994.

50. Caine L. *Being a Widow.* New York, NY: Penguin Books; 1988.

51. Einstein E. *The Step-family: Living, Loving and Learning.* Boston, Mass: Shambhala; 1985.

52. Louis Harris Associates Inc. *A Study of the Sources,Correlates and Manifestations of Perceived and Experienced Stress in the United States.* Report submitted to the Office of Disease Prevention and Health Promotion, US Dept of Health and Human Services; 1985. DHHS Contract No. 282-85-0063.

RESOURCES

Alcoholics Anonymous, PO Box 459, Grand Central Station, New York, NY 10163; 212 870-3400.
Web site: www.alcoholics-anonymous.org.

American Association of Retired Persons, 601 E St NW, Washington, DC 20049; 800 424-3410.
Web site: www.aarp.org.

American Association of Suicidology, 4201 Connecticut Ave NW Suite 408, Washington, DC 20008; 202 237-2280.
Web site: www.suicidology.org.

American Psychiatric Association, 1000 Wilson Blvd, Suite 1825, Arlington, VA 22209-3901; 888 35-PSYCH.
Web site: www.psych.org.

American Psychological Association, 750 First St NE, Washington, DC 20002-4242; 800 374-2721.
Web site: www.apa.org.

American Self-Help Clearinghouse. St Clare Health Services. Denville, NJ 07834; 973 625-3037.
Web site: www.mentalhelp.net.

Association for Applied Psychophysiology and Biofeedback, 10200 W 44th Ave, Suite 304, Wheat Ridge, CO 80033-2840; 303 422-8436.
Web site: www.aapb.org.

Children of Aging Parents, 1609 Woodbourne Rd, Suite 302A, Levittown, PA 19057; 800 227-7294.
Web site: www.caps4caregivers.org.

Communities Against Violence Network (domestic violence resources). Web site: www.cavnet2.org.

Corporation for National and Community Service, 1201 New York Ave NW, Washington, DC 20525; 202 606-5000.
Web site: www.nationalservice.org.

Emotions Anonymous International, PO Box 4245, St Paul, MN 55204-0245; 651 647-9712.

Web site: www.emotionsanonymous.org.

God Grant Me the Serenity: Self-Help and Recovery (addiction resources).

Web site: www.open-mind.org.

National Council of Senior Citizens, 8403 Colesville Rd, Suite 1200, Silver Spring, MD 20910-3314; 301 578-8800.

Web site: www.ncscinc.org.

National Council on Aging, PO Box 75556, Baltimore, MD 21275-5556; 202 479-6606.

Web site: www.ncoa.org.

National Mental Health Consumers Clearinghouse, 1211 Chestnut St, Suite 1207, Philadelphia, PA 19107; 800 553-4539.

Web site: www.mhselfhelp.org.

National Self-Help Clearinghouse. Graduate School and University Center of the City University of New York, 365 Fifth Ave, Suite 3300, New York, NY 10016; 212 817-1822.

Web site: www.selfhelpweb.org.

Older Women's League, 666 11th St NW, Suite 700, Washington, DC 20001; 800 825-3695.

Web site: www.owl-national.org.

Parents Without Partners Inc, 1650 South Dixie Hwy, Suite 510, Boca Raton, FL 33432; 561 391-8833.

Web site: www.parentswithoutpartners.org.

US Administration on Aging, 200 Independence Ave SW, Washington, DC 20201; 202 619-0724.

Web site: www.aoa.gov.

Benson H. *Beyond the Relaxation Response.* New York, NY: Berkley; 1984.

Benson H. *The Relaxation Response.* New York, NY: Avon Books; 1976.

Cummings N, VandenBos G. The 20 years Kaiser-Permanente experience with psychotherapy and medical utilization: implications for national health policy and national health insurance. *Healthcare Policy Q.* 1981;1:159–175.

Everly G. *A Clinical Guide to the Treatment of the Human Stress Response.* New York, NY: Plenum Press; 1989.

Field TM, McCabe PM, Schneiderman N. *Stress and Coping Across Development.* Hillsdale, NJ. Lawrence Erlbaum Associates Inc; 1988.

Hanson RW, Gerber KE. *Coping With Chronic Pain: A Guide to Patient Self-management.* New York, NY: Guilford Press; 1990.

Karasek R, Theoreil T. *Healthy Work: Stress, Productivity, and the Reconstruction of Working Life.* New York, NY: Basic Books; 1990.

McCabe PM, Schneiderman N, Field TM, et al, eds. *Stress, Coping and Disease.* Hillsdale, NJ: Lawrence Erlbaum Associates Inc; 1991.

McGuigan FJ, Sime WE, Wallace JM, eds. *Stress and Tension Control: 1.* New York, NY: Plenum Press; 1980.

McGuigan FJ, Sime WE, Wallace JM, eds. *Stress and Tension Control: 2.* New York, NY: Plenum Press; 1984.

McGuigan FJ, Sime WE, Wallace JM, eds. *Stress and Tension Control: 3.* New York, NY: Plenum Press; 1990.

McKee MG. Mixed messages and missed messages: communications gone awry. In: Eisenberg MG, Falconer J, Sutkin LC, eds. *Communications in a Health Care Setting.* Springfield, Ill: Charles C Thomas Publishers; 1980:17–34.

Michelson L, Ascher L, eds. *Anxiety and Stress Disorders: Cognitive-Behavioral Assessment and Treatment.* New York, NY: Guilford Press; 1987.

Pelletier K. *Mind as Healer, Mind as Slayer.* New York, NY: Dell Publishing Co; 1977.

Pelletier KB, Lutz RW. Healthy people-healthy business: a critical review of stress management programs in the workplace. In: Weiss SM, Fielding JE, Baum A, eds. *Perspectives in Behavioral Medicine: Health at Work.* Hillsdale, NJ: Lawrence Erlbaum Associates Inc; 1991:189–204.

Peterson C, Prout MF, Schwarz RA. *Post-traumatic Stress Disorder: A Clinician's Guide.* New York, NY: Plenum Press; 1991.

Roskies E. *Stress Management for the Healthy Type A.* New York, NY: Guilford Press; 1987.

Sedlacek K. *The Sedlacek Technique: Finding the Calm Within You.* New York, NY: McGraw-Hill; 1989.

Selye H. *The Stress of Life.* New York, NY: McGraw-Hill; 1978.

Selye H. *Stress Without Distress.* New York, NY: McGraw-Hill; 1974.

Speilberger CD, Sarason IG. *Stress and Anxiety.* Washington, DC: Hemisphere Publications Corp; 1986.

US Dept of Health and Human Services. *Healthy People 2000: National Health Promotion and Disease Prevention Objectives.* Washington, DC: US Dept of Health and Human Services; 1990.

Willing JZ. *The Reality of Retirement: The Inner Experience of Becoming a Retired Person.* New York, NY: William Morrow & Co; 1981.

Woolfolk RL, Lehrer PM. *Principles and Practice of Stress Management.* New York, NY: Guilford Press; 1984.

chapter 9

Alcohol and Drug Abuse

Gregory B. Collins, MD

INTRODUCTION

Substance abuse disorders and dependence are large-scale public health problems that cause morbidity and mortality and are seen in nearly every type of medical practice. Abuse of alcohol and drugs affects nearly every American family in some way, as the lifetime expected prevalence rate of substance abuse is 17%.[1] A recent government estimate of the cost of these disorders to our society exceeded $245 billion annually (study prepared by the Lewin Group for the National Institute on Drug Abuse and the National Institute on Alcohol Abuse and Alcoholism), and the human cost in suffering and waste of lives is beyond measure. Because alcoholic individuals and drug abusers use medical services excessively in proportion to their numbers, they are overrepresented in hospitals and clinics, where the medical, surgical, and psychologic sequelae of their disorders are treated. Although the physician is generally called on to diagnose and treat only the medical consequences of substance abuse, the physician also needs to recognize the opportunity to intervene in the underlying, often hidden, self-destructive, relentless, and perhaps fatal addictive process.[2]

Effective prevention for the office-based physician begins with an appreciation of the fact that abuse can easily become dependence, which is synonymous with addiction. People who are chemically dependent are addicted to the substance that is destroying their lives. Not all users of potentially addicting substances will go into a cycle of abuse and dependence, but, for reasons not completely understood, some people slowly or quickly succumb to the allure of these substances. Some individuals start with light social drinking of the legal drug alcohol or with a drug legitimately prescribed for a medical condition. In susceptible people, the pattern of use becomes one of misuse, overuse, problematic use, and, eventually, uncontrollable use. This progressive and destructive pattern has long been recognized as a disease process by the American Medical Association and the World Health Organization.

Primary prevention involves cautious prescribing on the part of the doctor, limiting access to large quantities of addictive medications, and controlling and carefully documenting all such prescriptions. The physician should transmit a message of caution and healthy respect for the potentially destructive power of all abusable substances, emphasizing that anyone, regardless of sex, race, religion, education, or age, can have this disease. A corollary message is that help is available and effective, and that one should discuss substance use with the physician, and should not postpone treatment or a lifestyle change if substances are becoming a problem.

Recognition of individuals at risk or of those who have early signs is key to an effective prevention strategy. The physician should ask and pay close attention to family history as a clue to substance abuse, particularly alcoholism. Alcoholism often "runs in families" for reasons that are probably both genetic and environmental. Males with alcoholic fathers have a threefold increase in alcoholism compared with controls.[3] Studies done of adopted infants demonstrate that infants of alcoholic parents are more likely to develop alcoholism later in life, even if raised by nonalcoholic adoptive parents.[4] Identical twins (with identical genetic material) have a higher incidence of concordance of alcoholism than do fraternal twins, who share only half of the same genes.[5] These studies and many more confirm that the tendency for alcoholism is strongly influenced by heredity, but the exact nature of the inherited genetic substrate is unknown. For the office-based physician, these studies indicate a need to be alert to a strong family history of alcoholism, as such individuals are at particular risk. Premorbid education of such at-risk individuals may alter their pattern of drinking while still in the volitional stage, before loss of control over the alcohol sets in.

Secondary prevention involves early recognition and treatment of developing cases. Recognition of alcohol-related medical conditions is such a secondary prevention paradigm. Alcohol causes numerous medical complications, such as tremor, diaphoresis, hypertension, gastritis, esophagitis, pancreatitis, and hepatitis. Elevated levels of liver function tests, especially (gamma-glutamyltransferase (GGT), aspartate aminotransferase (AST), and alanine aminotransferase (ALT), will provide early sensitive clues to diagnosis. Because erythrocyte formation is inhibited, blood cells are large, and thus mean corpuscular volume (MCV) and mean corpuscular hemoglobin (MCH) levels are frequently elevated. The platelet count is often low. These conditions are generally seen early in the course of the disease.

In more advanced cases, flushed facies, enlargement of the nose, and signs of advanced disease of the liver and nervous system are more readily apparent. Gross derangement of results of liver function tests may indicate progression to cirrhosis with icterus, ascites, esophageal varices, and death. Chronic poisoning of the nervous system with ethanol, with or without malnutrition, often leads to ataxia, a sign that may indicate long nerve tract degeneration, cerebellar degeneration, or both. Cerebral tissue loss with enlargement of the ventricles is an ominous sign that alcohol-induced dementia is progressing. Alcohol withdrawal is the most common etiology for a first seizure in a patient over 40 years of age. Severe cases of alcohol withdrawal can cause a gross delirium with life-threatening derangement of the sympathetic nervous system, leading to marked tachycardia, hypertension, hyperthermia, uncontrollable agitation, profound mental confusion, and electrolyte derangement. Accidents, falls, violent altercations, and suicide also account for much of the high level of morbidity and mortality associated with this disease. Women are prone to develop more severe complications of alcoholism than men at an earlier age.

Some physicians use simple screening devices such as the CAGE test.[6] In this test, the patient is asked if he or she has tried to **C**ut down on drinking, or has gotten **A**nnoyed when confronted about drinking, or has experienced **G**uilt over drinking, or has resorted to a morning **E**ye-opener drink to settle tremors and reduce sweating and cravings. Even 1 or 2 positive responses should trigger concern by the physician and should lead to a more probing discussion with the patient or the patient's spouse about the drinking pattern and related problems.

Early diagnosis and prevention intervention for drug abuse is usually a more subtle challenge to the physician than for alcohol abuse. Medication abuse is often difficult to detect because the addicted person offers plausible medical or psychosomatic reasons for needing the medications. Often such individuals can seem very ingratiating and trustworthy, and the physician can easily be taken in. Soon the signs of addiction begin to appear: "lost" prescriptions, which need early replacement, or worsening complaints that "require" stronger medications or more direct routes of administration, even indwelling intravenous (IV) lines or subarachnoid pumps. Even then,

with massive amounts of medication being offered through high-potency access ports to the nervous system, the patient is not satisfied. Soon the doctor gets a call from the pharmacy indicating that other doctors are prescribing for the same patient, or the astute doctor requests a toxicology screen, which indicates other nonprescribed addictive drugs. The clinician should watch closely for such signs and always obtain a substance abuse history before prescribing scheduled drugs. A few simple questions can serve as a good screen: "Have you ever been treated for a substance abuse problem (including alcohol)? Has anyone complained or expressed concern about your use of drugs or alcohol? Have you ever been to a meeting of Alcoholics Anonymous (AA) or a similar self-help organization? Have you ever been arrested for any offense involving drugs or alcohol?" It is best to remember that dependence is chronic and life-long, and that persons with a history of past drug or alcohol abuse or dependence are always at high risk of addictive relapse if scheduled drugs or street drugs are reintroduced to them.

In addition to asking the above screening questions, the physician should be wary of prescribing controlled or scheduled substances in patients who:

- present with a subjective or psychosomatic disorder, with complaints out of proportion to an anatomic cause, or with symptoms that fit no consistent anatomic or pathophysiologic cause
- insist on a particular controlled substance for treatment, to the exclusion of all other drugs or modalities
- refuse consultations or second opinions from experts on the presenting problem
- call for emergency refills of a controlled substance, especially at night to cross-covering physicians
- return very frequently to the doctor, with an endlessly growing list of complaints requiring 1 or more scheduled drugs
- alter a prescription or call in their own refills
- see more than 1 physician at a time
- visit emergency rooms often for acute crises requiring "emergency" scheduled drugs

Prevention, then, very often depends on the physician's awareness of the enormous prevalence of substance abuse in any patient population, recognition of classic behavioral signs and patterns suggesting addiction, and discretion and judgment in refusing to prescribe addictive medications and offering alternative treatments when deemed necessary. The phenomenon of substance abuse can present a frustrating and puzzling challenge to the physician. The physician may perceive clear-cut evidence of drug-induced medical complications, trauma, or psychosocial consequences, but the patient may meet these findings with denial and resistance. The patient's attitude and behavior are made more problematic at times by concealment of drug history, noncompliance, or even hostility. These substance-related behaviors place formidable obstacles in the path of the treating physician and challenge even the most experienced clinicians.

Intervention with the substance-involved patient concerns 4 major areas: diagnosis, intervention that often may be confrontation, detoxification and treatment, and follow-up. Diagnosis of any medical condition, including substance abuse, is predicated on understanding and recognizing the disorder. However, there is something elusive and problematic about defining drug abuse. When does prudent, recreational use become abuse? At what point does abuse become dependency, and is dependency the same as addiction? It is easy for the treating physician to be caught up in these issues, especially if the involved patient wishes to impress the physician that his use is occasional, recreational, or medically necessary. If the drug use has created any problem serious enough to come to the attention of a physician, the problem is probably serious. As a general rule, minor problems of occasional misuse do not come to the attention of a physician. It is best to maintain a high index of suspicion, assuming that a serious problem is present, in the hope that additional information will clarify the diagnostic picture.

All the drugs of abuse, including the drug alcohol, afford the user a measure of temporary chemical pleasure. These drugs, regardless of their class or pharmacologic effect, produce a type of chemical experience perceived by the user as positive. Although the initial use of these substances may be experimental or even medically necessary, the user soon learns that they afford a chemically pleasurable experience and soon begins to take them for their own sake. This process may happen fully outside the user's conscious awareness, but the net effect is the same: the drugs induce their own taking. Use progresses to abuse and to loss of control. Generally, patients deny any loss of control. They feel they are in complete volitional control of their actions, including drug taking or avoidance. Although the drug use itself may be heavy and frequent, this fact may seem only dimly apparent to the users, who seem instead preoccupied with reasons and excuses for drug use. These "causes" may be situational, medical, or psychological, but users become convinced of the reasonableness of continued heavy involvement with mood-altering drugs. Thus, the loss of control is apparent to everyone but the users themselves. It is the loss of control that marks the phenomenon as the self-perpetuating malignant disease process called chemical dependency or drug addiction. Bearing in mind that substance abusers may have an addiction or sick compulsion may help you as the physician to understand better the abusers' behavior, relapses, mood swings, manipulations, and physical complications.

PATHOPHYSIOLOGY AND CHEMICAL DEPENDENCY

Addictions can be regarded as having both psychological and physical components, but their pathophysiology has not yet been entirely elucidated. For now, the only practical way to diagnose addictions is to observe their consequences or symptoms. Usually, these symptoms are reflected in the deterioration of marital, occupational, emotional, spiritual, legal, financial, or physical well-being. If the substance use repeatedly causes problems in 1 or more of these areas, the diagnosis of chemical dependency or addiction can be made, even though the patient may believe that he or she can stop using drugs or alcohol.

Current thinking favors the view that chemical dependency is a result of complex genetic, environmental, psychological, physical, and social factors. Because of these complexities, most professionals pay little attention to how the chemically dependent person came to be addicted. Looking for underlying problems or causes before a period of stable abstinence has been achieved may at times be fruitless and even detrimental. Often, a better approach is to direct treatment at eliminating the use of psychoactive substances, while recognizing that the patient is suffering from a compulsion to return to active substance use. Chemical dependency is a great masquerader, often disguising itself as a medical or psychiatric complaint. Patients rarely seek treatment of substance problems. Usually they are in the physician's office for 1 or more secondary disorders, such as seizures, systemic or local infections, accidents, trauma, burns, gastritis, pancreatitis, or hepatitis. The presenting complaint also may be psychiatric with the appearance of anxiety, depression, personality disorder, or paranoid ideation. Complaints of chronic pain may present, such as fibromyalgia, arthritis, disk disease, or other painful conditions "requiring" opiate medication. The role of the physician is to see through the presenting symptoms and diagnose the chemical problem. If alcohol, drugs, or both have anything to do with the problem, the possibility of chemical abuse should be investigated further.

Problems often arise because physicians tend to recognize only late-stage physical complications and withdrawal symptoms as indicative of chemical dependency. They should, however, cultivate the skill of diagnosing substance dependency at a much earlier point in this progressive disability, when manifestations are subtle. The earliest symptoms are generally adverse effects on marriage and job, which often antedate by many years any detectable physical consequences. It is therefore a good idea to ask, "Did this problem have anything to do with your drug use or alcohol?" or "Were you using a drug or alcohol when the problem occurred?" If the answer is yes, the physician should explore the possibility of a chronic, serious, or incipient problem with substance abuse.[2]

SCREENING AND DIAGNOSIS

The diagnosis of chemical dependence is usually made on the basis of information obtained from the medical history, physical examination, psychological assessment, laboratory tests, and reports of concerned others.

The medical history should survey recent drug use, including alcohol, cigarettes, analgesics, sedatives, tranquilizers, cocaine, marijuana, and any others. Has there been a pattern of increasing the dosage or frequency of these drugs? Has the patient received treatment from numerous doctors or hospitals? Is the patient unwilling to reveal the names or places of the previous treatment? Does the individual have a vague physical problem such as back pain without radiologic changes, or conversely, does he or she report an exotic chronic disease that causes intermittent bouts of pain? Is there any deception or major omission in the medical or psychiatric history? Does the patient acknowledge an earlier alcohol problem or previous drug treatment? Are other risk factors present, such as easy access to drugs (in the case of health care professionals) or peer pressure (eg, in sports or entertainment figures)? Has the patient been arrested for driving while intoxicated? Have there been any other drug- or alcohol-related arrests? Is there a history of drug-involved marital discord or job trouble? Has there been any drug-related trauma, violence, explosion, or burns? Is there a history of any drug withdrawal symptoms, such as sweating, nausea, vomiting, or seizures?

The physical examination should be comprehensive, since chronic substance misuse can adversely affect virtually any organ system. The physician should look for signs of drug use, such as residual white powdery substance (cocaine or heroin) around the nares or alcohol on the breath. Complications of chronic drug administration may be present. These may include any of the following:

- needle marks, injection "tracks" over veins, scars, ulcerations, cellulitis, or necrotic areas of skin
- "no veins," making it difficult to obtain blood for laboratory sampling
- aseptic necrosis of large muscle masses, often with scarring and fibrosis, and muscles taking on a boardlike consistency
- elevated blood pressure, decreased or increased pulse rate, tremors, and diaphoresis
- brisk reflexes
- pupillary constriction (opiates) or dilation (stimulants or opiate withdrawal)
- jaundice of skin and icteric sclerae
- heart murmurs (possible subacute bacterial endocarditis with valvular vegetations)
- liver tenderness or enlargement
- nasal mucosal inflammation or septal perforation
- coarsened voice or chronic bronchitis from cocaine freebasing or marijuana smoking

Psychological manifestations may include a recent drug-related personality change of any type. There may be evidence of intoxication: staggering gait, slurred speech, "nodding off," not making sense, or forgetfulness. Clothing and personal effects may reveal an interest in drugs or the drug culture or shown by the presence of medications or drugs, as well as administering paraphernalia including syringes, needles, cellophane "bags," paper wrappers, crack pipe, volatile ether, sodium bicarbonate, quinine, razor blades, and tiny spoons. The patient may wear drug-related insignias on belts, shirts, and rings. Anxiety and nervousness may be present with anger, irritability, and impatience. Agitation or even assaultiveness may require emergency protective precautions. The patient may be confused or disoriented and may have evidence of hallucinosis or paranoid delusions. Conversely, behavior may be dull, apathetic, and listless. Drug seeking may be in evidence.

Laboratory testing may help to confirm the presence of alcohol or drugs, may establish evidence of organ damage, or may suggest the presence of a drug or alcohol problem. Negative or normal results of laboratory studies do not rule out a substantial drug problem. A toxicology screen for substance abuse is warranted in any suspicious circumstance. A supervised urine collection is best for drugs. Alcohol requires testing of the blood or breath. Blood studies may indicate effects on internal organs, toxicity, or related infections.

It is always helpful for a physician to receive confirmation about a patient's substance abuse from concerned others, such as the spouse or persons close to the patient. In this regard, physicians must be discreet in their inquiries so as not to reveal privileged information or jeopardize the patient's reputation. Generally, eliciting information from the family is the best way to proceed. If family members reveal serious concerns because of substance use, the physician can support these concerns and assist the family to motivate the patient to accept help.

SPECIFIC DRUGS

Alcohol

Alcohol is a depressant drug, is marketed aggressively in beverage form, and is legal in the Western world. Alcohol tends to exert its soporific effects starting from the newer, frontal cortical lobes and progressing later to the older basilar brain structures. As a result, judgment is affected first, and life-sustaining functions are affected last. Alcohol is an addictive drug, but not everyone is susceptible to this addiction. There appears to be genetic, metabolic, emotional, social, and cultural differences that predispose or protect certain individuals or groups. Those at risk often have a strong family history of alcoholism and, when young, appear less intoxicated than others after equivalent doses of alcohol. Often the signs of excessive drinking and significant consequences begin early in life as problem drinking becomes evident in high school, college, or military. The progression to compulsive, daily, excessive drinking can be rapid or slow, but serious consequences to marriage, job, health, finances, and legal status are typical. Dramatic deterioration of personality is commonly seen, with loss of interest in nondrinking people and activities. Morbid depressive self-absorption, emotional outbursts of temper, paranoia, violence, and suicide are not uncommon.

For heavy drinkers, alcohol withdrawal begins within 24 hours. Early signs comprising the minor phase of alcohol withdrawal include tremor, diaphoresis, hallucinosis, and seizures, with moderate elevations of pulse and blood pressure. Prevention of withdrawal depends on the clinician obtaining from the patient a history of continuous heavy drinking, followed by abrupt cessation or reduction in amount. The presence of the early signs listed above should hasten the prevention efforts, which should include the following: replacement of alcohol with chlordiazepoxide hydrochloride, 25 to 50 mg by mouth 4 times a day or another equivalent benzodiazepine, then tapering the dosage over 3 to 7 days. The major phase, or classical delirium tremens (alcohol withdrawal delirium), occurs 2 to 4 days after drinking cessation and is characterized by gross confusion, agitation, and severe dysregulation of autonomic functions such as temperature, pulse, and blood pressure. Electrolyte derangement is seen, especially low levels of potassium and magnesium. Detoxification from alcohol must be guided by the intensity and duration of drinking, the clinical presentation, and past history of withdrawal patterns and effective treatment. Benzodiazepines are prescribed, such as chlordiazepoxide (Librium), 25 to 50 mg by mouth 4 times a day, or lorazepam (Ativan), 1 to 4 mg orally 4 times a day, titrated up or down for severity. Less medication is used in the event of liver disease. If seizure history is present, phenytoin (Dilantin), 100 mg orally 3 times a day for women or 4 times a day for men, will usually prevent withdrawal seizures. Serum electrolytes, especially potassium, should be normalized. Multivitamins, plus thiamine, 100 mg orally or intramuscularly, and folic acid, 1 mg orally, should be given for 3 days. Hydration should be optimized, avoiding overhydration or underhydration. Once the patient is stabilized on a regimen of benzodiazepines, tapering the dosage can proceed as tolerated by the patient. Most patients will tolerate a 20% to 25% reduction per day, but some patients cannot have the dosage tapered this quickly. After detoxification, transition is necessary to rehabilitation programs, AA, and aftercare.

Barbiturates

Barbiturate addicts are becoming rare. Their recognition comes about by observing a pattern of increasingly heavy use of barbiturate sedatives or, more commonly, barbiturate analgesics, such as butalbital (Fiorinal). The problem becomes more severe in conjunction with alcohol intake or use of other sedative-hypnotic drugs. Initially used as sedatives, calmatives, or analgesics, barbiturates produce rapid tolerance and sedation. These drugs can cause respiratory suppression at high doses and withdrawal convulsions if the dosage is reduced too rapidly. These problems make preventive reduction and detoxification difficult outside a hospital. For barbiturate detoxification, an initial challenge dose of 200 mg of pentobarbital sodium (Nembutal) is used to see if the person can tolerate it. If the patient becomes sleepy or ataxic or shows nystagmus, tolerance is mild, and a modest dosage schedule is indicated, such as 100 to 200 mg of pentobarbital by mouth 4 times a day. If no effect is seen 2 hours after the initial 200-mg challenge dose, a stronger regimen may be required, such as 300 to 400 mg by mouth 4 times a day. A slow taper of the dosage from these starting levels, supplementing with anticonvulsants such as phenytoin, should then be undertaken.

Amphetamines

Medical uses of amphetamine compounds generally are limited to treatment of narcolepsy and attention deficit disorders, certain types of depression (particularly in older patients with medical illnesses), and certain atypical depressions[7] or as adjuncts to tricyclic or selective serotonin reuptake inhibitor (SSRI) antidepressant therapy. Although amphetamine has been used for weight loss, many doubts have been raised about the long-term efficacy and safety of such treatments.[8] The anorectic effect of amphetamines is not long-lasting, and the risk of abuse or addiction exceeds the short-term benefit of weight loss. Today, amphetamines are abused by sophisticated addicts, and the newer amphetamine-like drugs, such as "ice" or "crystal" (crystal methamphetamine) are fashionable among stimulant abusers.

The acute effects of intoxication usually begin within 20 to 60 minutes after oral ingestion and immediately after IV administration of amphetamines. In high doses, they can produce euphoria or a rush (a burst of energy accompanied by a physical sensation in the head and neck). Other symptoms of the amphetamines' sympathomimetic effects during intoxication include increased confidence, elation, grandiosity, hyperarousal, hypervigilance, irritability, aggressiveness, hostility, hyperactivity, loquacity, emotional lability, anorexia, anxiety, panic, resistance to fatigue, decreased need for sleep, and impaired judgment. Amphetamines can also cause abdominal pain that can mimic acute abdomen and may cause chest pain. Clinical signs of amphetamine use include dilated but reactive pupils, tachycardia, elevated temperature, elevated blood pressure, dry mouth, flushed skin, perspiration, chills, nausea, vomiting, psychomotor excitement, tremulousness, and hyperactive reflexes; with prolonged use, signs include repetitious compulsive behavior and body movements, such as bruxism, biting, and facial grimacing.[2]

Prolonged use of high-dose amphetamines can result in a delusional state characterized by paranoid ideations that strongly resemble paranoid schizophrenia or bipolar mania.[8,9] The drug-induced state may be characterized by restlessness, irritability, and heightened perceptual sensitivity. Delusions of persecution or bizarre visual and auditory hallucinations may develop. Tactile hallucinations are distinct features in advanced cases and may range from vague skin discomfort to delusions and hallucinations of bugs crawling under the skin, much like Magnan sign, or the "cocaine bugs" seen with cocaine use.[10] Disorientation and memory impairment, however, are not part of the syndrome. Amphetamine psychosis is frequently dose-related, is often associated with sleep deprivation, and generally resolves as amphetamines are excreted. Acute psychotic symptoms usually disappear within days or at most weeks after the drug is withdrawn, but fixed delusions and the tendency toward suspiciousness, misinterpretation, and mild paranoia may persist for months after the overt psychosis has ceased. Amphetamines also can precipitate latent psychotic reactions, which do not subside when the drug use ends.[11]

After prolonged heavy use of amphetamines, a withdrawal syndrome may occur. Often referred to as "crashing," this phenomenon is characterized by depressed mood, fatigue, disturbed sleep, and increased dreaming. Amphetamines suppress rapid eye movement (REM) sleep and cause a rebound increase in REM sleep after the drug is withdrawn.[12] Beginning within 24 hours after the last dose, the patient may sleep for increasing periods, up to 18 to 20 hours per day for the next 72 hours. Other symptoms include irritability, impulsivity, insatiable hunger, headaches, profuse sweating, muscle cramps, and stomach cramps. The depression generally peaks 48 to 72 hours after the last dose and persists for several weeks. Suicidal ideation occasionally occurs during this period. If depression persists longer, an underlying disorder should be considered and antidepressant therapy should be instituted.

Treatment of patients presenting with amphetamine-induced psychosis, with an acutely intoxicated, agitated, or delusional state requires inpatient supervision. These patients should be placed in a quiet room and given reassurance. Intramuscular treatment with haloperidol (1 to 5 mg 3 times a day for the first day, and as needed thereafter) should be started, if necessary, for control of agitation. Diazepam (10 to 20 mg orally or intra-muscularly) may be substituted. Diazepam may also be the drug of choice if the patient has had seizures in the past. Later, if episodes of depression become notable during the withdrawal period, an antidepressant (not a monoamine oxidase inhibitor) may be added to the regimen. It is also vitally important to establish a follow-up relationship with the patient, explaining that episodes of depression, apathy, and lack of initiative may occur over the next 2 to 4 months and that this may tempt the patient to resume amphetamine use.[2]

Cocaine

Cocaine is one of the most potent addictive substances known. Pharmacologically, cocaine is an alkaloid, similar to atropine and belladonna; it is a potent vasoconstrictor and nerve-conduction blocker when administered locally. Recreational users generally begin by snorting powdered cocaine or by smoking crack cocaine. Taken by these routes, the drug is rapidly absorbed and quickly enters the bloodstream. Once hooked, heavy users and addicts rely on the more efficient methods, such as crack smoking, freebase smoking, or IV administration. These methods allow the cocaine to reach the brain very rapidly, with the attainment of a nearly instantaneous high.

Cocaine stimulates the central nervous system (CNS) "from above downward," affecting cognitive and mood centers first. Small amounts of the drug produce talkativeness, elation, euphoria, motor restlessness, diminished fatigue and depression, and a sense of increased mental, physical, and sexual ability. However, severely depressed individuals who use the drug do not experience mood elevation.[13] Depending on the individual's predisposition, other effects can include extreme hyperactivity, grandiose or paranoid delusions, and violence. The period of intense pleasure—30 to 60 minutes—is followed by depression and profound dysphoria; thus, users want to repeat the experience to relieve "let-down" depression. At higher doses, users may become anxious and suspicious. They may resort to simultaneous use of IV opiates with cocaine (speedballing) to reduce the dysphoric letdown effect. In the letdown phase, marked depression is common, with crying and suicidal thoughts. Some users may acutely experience seizures, respiratory arrest, or sudden death.

Cocaine potentiates sympathetic neurons with both excitatory and inhibiting functions. The drug prevents reuptake of catecholamines in the neuronal synapse and may sensitize neurons to sympathomimetic amines. Taken short term, cocaine acts as a powerful, pleasurable stimulant but chronic cocaine use results in insomnia, depression, delusions, diminished appetite, and preoccupation with the drug.[2] Severe cocaine addictions can be difficult to treat and often require inpatient or residential sequestering of the patient. Psychosis, suicidality, or cocaine-induced angina will also require initial inpatient care. Once the patient's condition is stable, progression to outpatient modalities can proceed, including group or individual supervision, toxicology monitoring, family therapy, and self-help groups, such as Cocaine Anonymous, Narcotics Anonymous, or AA. Residual dysphoria may be medicated with an activating antidepressant such as imipramine hydrochloride, fluoxetine hydrochloride, or bupropion hydrochloride.

Marijuana (Cannabis)

Although the use of marijuana has declined moderately over the last decade, it is still the most commonly used illicit substance in the United States. It is estimated that 10 to 12 million people use cannabis on a regular basis, down from a peak of 20 million users in the late 1970s.[14] It is also estimated that up to 40 million people in the United States have tried marijuana at least 1 time.[15] Occasional use of marijuana is far more common than daily use. Peer and sibling influence appears to be the strongest predictor of the initiation of cannabis use.[15] Children whose parents actively use cannabis are far more likely to initiate and continue its use. Some evidence suggests that children from homes where alcohol is consumed regularly are more likely to begin experimentation with marijuana.

Marijuana consists of the leaves, flowers, stems, and seeds of the plant *Cannabis sativa.* This fibrous plant grows wild throughout most tropical regions of the world and has been used medicinally and recreationally for thousands of years. It was banned in the United States by the 1937 Marijuana Tax Act, as marijuana became recognized as a drug of abuse, used mainly by counterculture groups of musicians and intellectuals. Marijuana again became popular with the youth of the 1960s generation, continuing in popularity throughout the 1970s and 1980s. Only recently has a slight decrease in numbers of marijuana users been observed.

The term *cannabis* is used to describe the bioactive substances of the marijuana plant.[14] The most common method of using cannabis is to smoke or to ingest the dried plant parts. Other preparations of cannabis can be obtained by collecting the resin from the flowering tops of the plant, commonly referred to as hash or hashish. Plant material also can be processed into a dark concentrated liquid called hash oil. In recent years more marijuana has been grown domestically by growers who develop potent, seedless strains called sinsemilla, sometimes doubling the percentage of bioactive substance within the plant.

Delta-9-tetrahydrocannabinol (Δ-9-THC) is the substance primarily responsible for the mood-altering euphoria associated with cannabis use. The drug Δ-9-THC has a high lipid solubility and is quickly absorbed into fatty tissue, resulting in a slow elimination time, up to 4 to 10 weeks in heavy cannabis users.[14] This slow elimination time becomes important in the treatment of cannabis abusers because measurable levels of marijuana metabolites can be obtained in urine samples long after smoking has stopped and long after the mood-altering effects have passed. These acute effects in humans usually last only 3 to 5 hours when cannabis is smoked. The liver is responsible for almost complete metabolism of Δ-9-THC, which is then excreted in urine.[14] Marijuana is one of the drugs forbidden under US Department of Transportation rules for safety-sensitive jobs.

Due to a low level of toxicity, marijuana poses few acute medical problems. Emergency room visits are rare for exclusive use of cannabis, and a lethal dose of cannabis has yet to be determined in humans. The physician will be more likely to encounter medical complications associated with long-term chronic abuse of cannabis, rather than acute medical crises. For the primary care physician, the diagnosis may be obvious, as the person has been found to possess the drug or drug paraphernalia or to have a positive drug screen; or diagnosis may be difficult, with few definitive signs present. Suspicion should arise when there is any symbol of the drug on the person, such as a marijuana leaf tattoo or emblem, or in a dazed, inattentive individual. The age group most affected is the college age group. A urine toxicology test, collected under carefully controlled circumstances, is the only sure way to confirm the presence of the drug. Often adulterants or "clean" (drug-free) substituted urine (both commercially available) are used to frustrate testing.

The CNS is the most affected system in cannabis intoxication, with most users experiencing a change in mood, described as a feeling of well-being or euphoria.[14] There is also a decrease in attention span, short-term memory, and the ability to perform memory-dependent tasks. Most users also experience an increase in appetite and lethargy. Simple reaction time appears to be unchanged, but complex reactions, in which information must be quickly processed by the brain, are impaired.[14] This effect may have serious consequences in the operation of automobiles or other equipment, during which information must be processed before a proper reaction is made. Learning is clearly made more difficult while intoxicated with cannabis due to decreased attention span and short-term memory and increased lethargy. Chronic use of cannabis among adolescents is said to produce an amotivational syndrome, but current research is controversial.[14]

Cannabis has an extremely dysphoric effect on some users, causing an increase in anxiety, severe panic reactions, hallucinations, and confused thinking[16] in a marijuana-induced "psychosis." Usually hospitalization in a secure setting with low-dose benzodiazepines or neuroleptics will allow the psychosis to clear in a few days.

The most medically significant effects of cannabis appear to be on lung tissue. Cannabis smoke is usually drawn deeply into the lungs and is held for the longest possible time to potentiate the absorption of cannabinoids into the bloodstream. By weight, cannabis contains approximately 10 times the respiratory irritants and has more carcinogens than tobacco. Evidence shows that chronic cannabis smokers face the same risks of developing lung cancer as do tobacco smokers.[14]

Effects of cannabis on the cardiovascular system are usually minimal but can be detrimental to persons with known arteriosclerotic heart disease. After using cannabis, most people experience mild tachycardia and orthostatic hypotension. People with known angina have reduced tolerance for exercise and increased complaints of chest pain.[14] Patients with known heart disease should avoid the use of cannabis.

Effects on the endocrine system are controversial. Serum testosterone levels and sperm production are slightly decreased, with a slight decrease in fertility.[15] In women, some research has shown inhibition of ovulation, with more anovulatory menstrual cycles in women who are heavy marijuana users. The levels of luteinizing hormones are also slightly decreased with heavy marijuana use.[15] The physician should advise all women planning pregnancy to avoid the use of cannabis products.

The therapeutic potential of cannabis has been controversial for years. Recent research has shown antiemetic effects of cannabis products in patients with chronic nausea due to chemotherapy treatments. Although therapeutic effects are measurable with the use of THC, adverse effects are also frequently reported.[15] In light of the frequency of adverse reactions, other pharmacologic treatments are more effective at this time. Cannabis has also been shown to lower intraocular pressure, with possible therapeutic effects in treating glaucoma. Studies have shown 30% to 50% decreases in intraocular pressure in patients with ocular hypertension.[15] However, more research is needed in this area to understand better the long-term benefits of cannabis in the treatment of glaucoma.

Although marijuana does not show the severe physical withdrawal or acute medical problems associated with other substances of abuse, such as alcohol, opiates, and cocaine, signs of addiction are common in heavy cannabis abusers. The American Medical Association defines the characteristics of marijuana addiction as a preoccupation and compulsivity with the drug and potential for relapse.[17] The person compulsively using cannabis will show a preoccupation with all aspects of this drug. Obtaining and using cannabis will become the driving forces in the daily life of the addicted person, who will often risk loss of employment or relationships to use it.[17]

When cannabis addiction is present, outpatient treatment usually is recommended to disrupt the cycle of addiction and to confront denial and rationalization. The marijuana-addicted person should be followed up closely, with referral to individual counseling and a Twelve-Step program of recovery through AA or Narcotics Anonymous or both. Compliance with the program increases with random urine toxicology screens.

Opiates

Opiates refer to a class of powerful analgesics derived from the poppy plant, *Papaver somniferum,* which contains more than 20 alkaloids, including morphine and codeine. The major medical uses of opiates are for the relief of pain, treatment of diarrhea, and the suppression of cough. Opioids are opiumlike drugs that occur naturally or are synthetically produced and are used for analgesia and anesthesia.

Opiates can be classified into groups according to their functions: morphine-like agonists, mixed agonist-antagonists, and pure antagonists. Agonists such as morphine, heroin, codeine, and methadone produce their principal pharmacologic effects on the CNS and gastrointestinal tract by activation at the opioid receptor site on neurons throughout the brain and body. These agonists typically have the strongest effects in producing analgesia and euphoria and have the highest addictive potential among opiates. Mixed agonists-antagonists have properties similar to opiates and have the ability to block the effects of the drug at the opioid receptor sites. Butorphanol tartrate (Stadol), pentazocine hydrochloride (Talwin), and buprenorphine hydrochloride (Subutex) are representatives of the agonist-antagonist class of opiates. Antagonists, such as naloxone hydrochloride and naltrexone hydrochloride, block the effects of opioids at the opioid receptor site and have no potential for abuse. Naloxone (Narcan) produces rapid withdrawal symptoms in opioid-dependent addicts. It is also the drug of choice to treat respiratory distress after acute opioid intoxication or overdose. Naltrexone (Revia) has been found useful in the treatment of chronic opioid abusers. It may be taken orally and is effective in blocking the euphoric state that results from illicit opioid use.[18]

Psychologically, opioids usually cause a pleasant euphoria. Occasionally, and especially with the first use, some individuals experience a dysphoria, consisting of anxiety and fear, lethargy, apathy, sedation, mental clouding, lack of concern, inability to concentrate, nausea, and vomiting.[19] Frequent users describe either a euphoric state marked by feelings of peacefulness and increased energy, or a feeling of sedation with a dreamlike quality.

Clinicians use several criteria to diagnose an addiction to opiates: a preoccupation with the acquisition of the drug, compulsive use despite adverse consequences, an inability to reduce the amount of use consistently to avoid adverse consequences, and a pattern of relapse after a period of abstinence.[20] Tolerance to opioids may develop at different rates among users. Dose, frequency of administration, and particular physiologic and psychologic responses are the influencing factors. Drug tolerance can be extreme; if a pattern of repeated administration occurs, the clinician may find that the patient may need a phenomenal increase in dose to prevent withdrawal discomfort or to induce the euphoric state. Physiologically, tolerance appears to be due to both the induction of drug-metabolizing enzymes in the liver and the adaptation of neurons in the brain to the presence of the drug.[19] Clinicians also must be aware of the phenomenon of cross-tolerance with opioid addiction; that is, as a patient develops a tolerance to one particular opioid, he or she will have the same level of tolerance for all other natural or synthetically manufactured opioids. Cross-tolerance to other drugs, namely barbiturates and benzodiazepines, and alcohol, does not occur with opiates.

Withdrawal from opioids is rarely life threatening, although the user is extremely uncomfortable and anxious and seeks drugs. Symptoms of withdrawal from opioids are restlessness, craving for the drug, sweating, extreme anxiety, fever, chills, violent retching and vomiting, increased respiratory rate (panting), cramping, insomnia, explosive diarrhea, and unbearable aches and pains. The magnitude of these withdrawal symptoms depends on the dose, frequency of drug administration, and individual host factors.

One group of abusers of opioids is the nonmedical, or "street," user, estimated to number well over 500,000 in the United States. These individuals use multiple daily IV injections of various street opioids, often impure and unsterile. If intermittent IV abuse is considered, the number of abusers may be well over 2 million.[18] The most often abused drug in this category is heroin, and, because it is illegal, procurement and use often lead to criminal activities. A heroin addict may use more than $500 worth of heroin in a day. Those most likely to use heroin are males living in urban settings, although use by females and persons in rural settings is increasing. An antisocial disorder often predates heroin use, but, if not, such a disorder frequently develops because of the pharmacologic effects of heroin addiction combined with the high cost of obtaining it.[20]

Drug dependence also may occur in the context of medical treatment of acute or chronic illnesses for which pain control is a factor. According to Ford et al,[21] this type of opioid-dependent patient often will try to obtain prescriptions from more than 1 physician and also will be resistant to any other methods of pain control. As the dependence develops, patients may become involved in criminal activities, such as altering prescriptions and purchasing street supplies of drugs.

Dole and Nyswander,[22] in studies performed in the mid-1960s, found that methadone would block the effects of heroin and thus negate the euphoric properties of heroin use.[22] The goal of maintenance therapy is to give the abuser enough methadone to prevent the opioid withdrawal syndrome and also to block the euphoria produced by further opioid abuse. Studies have shown that, with methadone maintenance, as the overall health status of users improves, a decrease of criminal activities is seen, and the controlled addict may hold stable employment for the first time in many years.[23]

Opiate detoxification is usually accomplished by discontinuing the abused drug (agonist) and substituting a noneuphoric drug. Typically, this substitute is methadone or buprenorphine. The dosage of the substitute drug is then tapered to a maintenance level or is discontinued altogether. For cases of street opiate (heroin) use, usually

20 to 30 mg/day of methadone hydrochloride in divided doses of 4 times a day will suffice to start. For recently acquired addictions or for patients abusing milder opiates (codeine, propoxyphene), 2 to 10 mg of methadone in divided doses will often be adequate. Clonidine hydrochloride, by mouth, can be used 2 to 3 times a day for milder addictions, perhaps with as-needed supplementation of 100 mg of oral propoxyphene napsylate (Darvon) or tramadol hydrochloride (Ultram) every 6 hours to reduce craving if this is a problem. Hypotension may occur with both methadone and clonidine detoxification; if blood pressure falls, this should lead to withholding doses or to changing the detoxification regimen. Addicts tolerant to daily large doses of high-grade pharmaceutical opiates may need 60 to 100 mg/day or more of methadone, usually given in 4 divided doses, with respirations closely monitored. Smaller test doses of 10 to 15 mg orally are usually given first to ensure that the patient is telling the truth and is not exaggerating drug use, as sudden administration of high doses to a nontolerant person could be fatal. Naloxone (Narcan) injections of 0.4 mg are kept handy in case of overdose. Somnolence and slowed respirations are the best indicators of overtitration, and, when present, medication should be held back. If overdosed on heroin or methadone, the patient should be given frequent intramuscular or IV injections of naloxone, approximately every 30 minutes while being monitored closely, as the duration of action of Narcan is short. As soon as the patient no longer lapses into narcotic sedation, naloxone can be discontinued. Once the patient's condition is stabilized using the detoxification dosage, the dosage can be tapered.

Hallucinogens

When ingested, hallucinogenic substances have the potential to cause perceptual distortions or hallucinations. Although tolerance occurs quickly with most hallucinogenic substances, withdrawal symptoms have not been observed.[24] Because of the sensory distortion and intensity of the intoxication, these drugs rarely are used on a continuous, daily basis. More often, it is the episodic experimentation by novice users who do not understand or expect the drastic mind-altering effect that comes to the attention of the physician. Education on the unpredictable and potentially violent effects of the hallucinogenic drugs is probably the best method of reducing the incidence of experimentation with these substances.

Lysergic acid diethylamide
Although lysergic acid diethylamide (LSD) was first synthesized in the laboratory in 1938, it was not until the mid-1960s that it became a recreational drug. The rise in popularity followed the experimental use of LSD and publication of the findings by 3 Harvard University professors, T. Leary, R. Alpert, and R. Metzner.[25] The

popularity of LSD peaked in the late 1970s and declined throughout the early 1980s, with an estimated 6% of high school students and young adults now reporting experimentation with this drug.[26]

The most common method of administering LSD is oral ingestion, usually in small pills (microdots) or liquid LSD, often dropped on small pieces of blotter paper and sugar cubes. LSD also can be added to gelatin with the street name of "window pane." Other routes of administration include inhalation, IV and subcutaneous injection, smoking, and conjunctival instillation of liquid LSD.[24] This hallucinogen is quickly absorbed from the gastrointestinal tract, with effects perceived in 30 minutes or less. The user first may feel a sense of being more alert and connected with the environment, followed by time distortion, visual illusions, and sound misperception. There may be a feeling of euphoria and peace, often described as a mystical or religious experience. Physiological changes include tachycardia, hypertension, nausea, dilated pupils, and tremors.[24]

The experience may last from 6 to 18 hours, depending on the dose. The extended duration of the intoxication along with the sensory distortions may become very frightening and anxiety provoking in individuals not expecting this experience or reaction. Fear and anxiety, combined with the intense high, can trigger a bad trip, characterized by panic and feelings of breaking with reality. Long-term LSD psychosis has been disputed by many professionals, but similarities to schizophrenia have been observed.[24] Flashbacks are another controversial aspect of the LSD experience. It is unclear why some individuals experience flashbacks, but predisposing personality characteristics may be an important factor. Although withdrawal symptoms have not been observed with LSD, tolerance can develop quickly.[24]

Psilocybin, mescaline, and other substances

Psilocybin and mescaline are 2 naturally occurring substances with hallucinogenic effects when ingested. Psilocybin is produced by a species of mushroom that grows wild in many regions of the world. Often these mushrooms are ingested whole or are boiled in tea. The intoxication is very similar to that of LSD, and the duration of the effects may be slightly shorter, but management of symptoms is the same as for LSD. Mescaline is a substance derived from the peyote cactus, often introduced into the body by ingestion of cactus buds, or "buttons." Mescaline intoxication is similar to LSD, with adverse reactions much the same. Psilocybin and mescaline both have potential for causing bad trips, which are best treated by supportive measures.

Throughout the 1980s, other substances with hallucinogenic effects have appeared on the illicit market. These mostly synthetic drugs are produced in clandestine laboratories. The most common synthetic drugs are the amphetamine derivatives, methylenedioxyamphetamine (MDA) and 3,4-methylenedioxymethamphetamine (MDMA), or "Ecstasy," as it is commonly known. These substances produce a sympathomimetic response, visual illusions, and sound distortions, much the same as LSD, but with far more serious toxic effects. Overdose of these substances can produce lasting psychosis, anxiety, and panic. Physiologic symptoms may include tachycardia, hypertension, hyperthermia, and possible death.[27] Toxic doses of these drugs have not been determined because little human research has been performed.

Phencyclidine

Phencyclidine (PCP) was developed and used as an anesthetic agent but was discontinued for human use because of the high incidence of adverse postanesthetic reactions. These reactions included hallucinations, agitation, violence, and prolonged depression of consciousness.[28] These same symptoms pushed PCP into the illicit market as a recreational drug. The drug is commonly referred to as "angel dust" and may be sold mislabeled as THC or LSD. Its popularity began in the 1960s, reached a peak in the late 1970s, and gradually decreased in popularity to a relatively stable level throughout the 1980s, with 5% of high school students and young adults reporting use of PCP.[26]

The most common method of using PCP is smoking, usually by mixing the powdered drug with tobacco or marijuana and rolling it into a cigarette. Another means of PCP use is the smoking of "wet" marijuana dipped in formaldehyde, which when burned, produces PCP. Phencyclidine also can be injected intravenously, ingested orally, or taken intranasally.

The effects of the drug usually are recognized within a few minutes after administration and last from 12 to 15 hours, depending on the dose. The most common effects are feelings of euphoria and distortions of reality perception, time, space, and body image.[26] To the user, arms and legs may appear longer or shorter, and physical environments may seem larger or smaller than they actually are. These effects can produce extreme fear and panic in the user, causing bizarre behavioral changes, agitation, and violence.

Medical complications may include hypertension, hyperthermia, seizures, rhabdomyolysis, acute renal failure, apnea, cardiac arrest, and trauma. Medical management of PCP intoxication is mostly supportive, with symptomatic treatment of specific complications. Tranquilizing agents such as benzodiazepines and haloperidol may be used with the extremely agitated patient, and physical restraints are indicated for the combative patient.[26,28] Since the drug PCP is a strong base, it is attracted to acidic areas of the body; thus, nasogastric suction is employed as well as urinary acidification with ammonium chloride, 1 g 4 times a day, and with water or cranberry juice, at least 504 g/day (18 oz/day) by mouth or nasogastric tube.[29] Symptoms usually diminish within a few hours with supportive treatment but can last days or weeks.[28] Phencyclidine can accumulate in adipose tissue with delayed release, causing a flashback or a recurrence of symptoms, making it an unpredictable and dangerous substance for recreational use.

GENERAL MANAGEMENT CONSIDERATIONS

Detoxification

In general, great care must be exercised in establishing the initial detoxification dosage. After receiving the first dose, patients must be observed carefully for the next 2 to 6 hours to determine if the medication is adequate to "hold" them, that is, to replace their usual drug but also to determine that the dose is not excessively high, which could produce somnolence, lethargy, intoxication, or even respiratory suppression and death. One can be a little more generous with the "safe" drugs such as benzodiazepines, but one should be more cautious with drugs that have the capability to suppress respiration, such as barbiturates or opiates. Concern about the possibility of respiratory suppression is the reason for test doses and divided dosage schedules so that patients do not receive large quantities of drug at any one time. It should also be remembered that most of these drugs are metabolized in the liver and excreted by the kidney. Thus, liver disease, often present in addicts, may impair the conjugation and excretion of these drugs and their metabolites, and may cause a corresponding accumulation of drug in the bloodstream. Lethargy and somnolence usually indicate this phenomenon, which calls for discontinuation or sharp curtailment of the detoxification drug. Lorazepam (Ativan) may work better with patients with liver disease.

Once the comfortable start-up dosage is established, one can generally proceed to reduce the amount of detoxification drug by approximately 10% to 25% per day. Periodic toxicology checks of the urine are advisable during the detoxification period to determine whether the patient is obtaining any additional medication surreptitiously. The patient should be medicated to a level of mild irritability and tremor. Violent withdrawal reactions, including nausea, vomiting, abdominal spasms, or seizures, are to be avoided. These symptoms generally indicate that more detoxification medicine is needed. Usually the first signs of undermedication are irritability, anger, noncooperation, and a desire to leave the hospital. It is remarkable how many discharges against medical advice can be avoided by prompt supplements to medication.

Symptoms and reactions to the medications are scrutinized closely and discussed freely. Dosing schedules on a basis of 4 times a day reduce the operant conditioning of patients who seek drugs by complaining. Insomnia is often present during the first few days of detoxification. For this reason, one occasionally should allow a sedative to be administered at bedtime. One can use trazodone hydrochloride, 25 to 100 mg orally, or zolpidem tartrate (Ambien), 5 to 10 mg at bedtime, for 1 to 3 days. In almost all cases, however, no bedtime sedatives are given.

Nursing Care

There is much to be said for good nursing care during the detoxification process. Verbal and emotional reassurance, patience, and encouragement help patients endure difficult and uncomfortable days and nights. Heating pads, hot baths, and relaxation therapies presented in a calm and dignified milieu do much to relieve tension and anxiety. If complaints of localized pain emerge as detoxification progresses, dosage reduction can be slowed, or ibuprofen can be allowed for minor discomforts. Acetaminophen should be avoided in alcoholic patients. Most patients addicted to analgesics experience recurrences of localized pain as withdrawal progresses. Interestingly, this pain is generally experienced in the region that was originally painful, triggering the dependence on narcotics, perhaps years earlier. Pain is once again "felt" in that area even though the "painful" organ or limb may be normal or may have been removed. Nonsteroidal anti-inflammatory drugs, physical therapy, exercise, or heat may help these discomforts. Since many addicts are malnourished, aggressive nutritional support is advised, generally with vitamin supplementation. Multivitamin preparations with additional vitamin C and thiamine should be encouraged.

FOLLOW-UP

During hospitalization, the patient and physician must lay the groundwork for a long-term follow-up program and other specialized treatments. It must be decided whether a residential chemical dependency rehabilitation program might be beneficial. There is much to recommend these programs in most cases; they generally provide an intense educational-motivational experience, overcoming denial and resistance in a supportive milieu. If the patient has been through one or more of these programs recently, it may not be beneficial to repeat the experience if it appears that he or she is adequately motivated and insightful. Outpatient aftercare programs are appropriate once reasonable abstinence and emotional and physical stability are achieved.

Urine Monitoring

Urine monitoring is an indispensable tool in dealing with drug-involved patients. Frequent, randomized urine tests are recommended for a minimum of 1 to 2 years for most such patients. Most of these urine checks are obtained randomly, approximately once a week, and are collected under direct supervision.

Self-Help Groups

Addiction self-help groups should also be considered part of the recovery program. Such groups, including AA, Narcotics Anonymous, Cocaine Anonymous, and others affiliated with treatment centers, provide frequent, powerful, therapeutic reinforcement for recovering patients. As a rule, patients must go to these self-help groups to maintain sobriety. Your task as a physician should be to endorse these organizations strongly and facilitate patients' participation. Avoid offering treatment alternatives to the self-help groups. Many physicians who are successful with chemical dependents will not even see them unless they are willing to be involved in the self-help groups. Knowledgeable physicians develop familiarity with local groups and cultivate friendships within them. Patients should become involved with the self-help groups while in the hospital. They should call the local representatives, who will visit them in the hospital or shortly after discharge.

Aftercare

As the treatment physician, the physician's role in aftercare is to ask about abstinence and participation in the other treatment modalities. Continued sobriety usually hinges on regular and frequent attendance at self-help groups and professional counseling. Try to continue a physician-patient relationship after the detoxification phase. Encourage patients to bring all requests for medication and other medical consultations to you first for your opinion. Generally, prohibit the taking of any medicine other than ibuprofen without expressed approval. Periodically check needle-using addicts for physical evidence of injection; examine the entire body surface carefully. Maintain contact with the toxicology laboratory to ascertain results of urine checks. If patients become lax in participating in any of these modalities, encourage reactivation. After detoxification, avoid the use of psychoactive drugs, especially sedatives, analgesics, and tranquilizers. These medications, even when taken under the supervision of a well-meaning physician, are poorly tolerated by such patients; they carry substantial risk of reinducing medication dependency. Strongly recommend to medication-dependent patients that they abstain from drinking alcohol. In many such patients, drinking escalates rapidly to full-blown alcoholism, whereas in other people, drinking leads to relapse of drug abuse. Regard alcohol as another mood-altering drug and insist on rigorous abstinence from it.

Maintain close contact with both the patient and the patient's spouse or other close family member for at least 1 to 2 years. It is best to regard addiction as a chronic, relapsing condition that is never cured, only held in remission. Follow-up visits may be scheduled to conform to a pattern of weekly, then biweekly, then monthly office visits, generally with the spouse attending or at least telephoned to ascertain compliance. As solid drug-free stability is achieved, visits can be spread out to quarterly or even yearly intervals. Give recovering patients respect and praise for maintaining an abstinence program and for participating in the treatment modalities. They have to sacrifice much in time, energy, and expense to conquer this potentially fatal illness. Understanding, praise, and firm support for adhering to the treatment program are the physician's most valuable psychotherapeutic tools.

REFERENCES

1. Robins LN, Helzer JE, Weissman MM, et al. Lifetime prevalence of specific psychiatric disorders in three sites. *Arch Gen Psychiatry.* 1984;41:949–958.

2. Collins GB, Carlson K, Conroy T, Frankel O, Golden D, Moliff H. Drug dependence and substance abuse. In: Matzen R, Lang R, eds. *Clinical Preventive Medicine.* St Louis, Mo: Mosby Yearbook Inc; 1993:239–255.

3. Schuckit MA, Smith TL. An 8-year follow-up of 450 sons of alcoholic and control subjects. *Arch Gen Psychiatry.* 1996;53:202–210.

4. Goodwin DW, Schulsinger F, Hermansen L, Guze S, Winokur G. Alcohol problems in adoptees raised apart from biological parents. *Arch Gen Psychiatry.* 1973;28:238–243.

5. Kaij L. Studies on the etiology and sequels of abuse of alcohol dissertation. Lund, Sweden: University of Lund, Department of Psychiatry; 1960.

6. Ewing JA. Detecting alcoholism: the CAGE questionnaire. *JAMA.* 1984;252:1905–1907.

7. Raskin DE. Amphet use [letter]. *J Clin Pharmacol.* 1983;3:262.

8. Grinspoon L, Bakalar JB. Drug dependence: non-narcotic agents. In: Kaplan HI, Sadock BJ, eds. *Comprehensive Textbook of Psychiatry.* Vol 4. Baltimore, Md: Williams & Wilkins; 1985.

9. Griffith JD, Cavanaugh J, Held J, et al. Dextroamphetamine: evaluation of psychomimetic properties in man. *Arch Gen Psychiatry.* 1972;26:97–100.

10. Magnan V, Saury. Trois cas de cocainisme chronique. *C R Soc Biol Paris.* 1889;1:series 9.

11. Slaby AE, Martin SD. Drug and alcohol emergencies. In: Miller N, ed. *Comprehensive Handbook of Drug and Alcohol Addiction.* New York, NY: Marcel Dekker; 1991.

12. Gossop MR, Bradley BP, Brewis RK. Amphetamine withdrawal and sleep disturbance. *Drug Alcohol Depend.* 1982;10:177–183.

13. Post RM, Kotin J, Goodwin FK. Effects of cocaine on depressed patients. *Am J Psychiatry.* 1974;131:511–517.

14. Clark RF, Curry SC, Selorn BS. Marijuana. *Emerg Med Clin North Am.* 1990;8:527–539.

15. Hollister LE. Cannabis. *Acta Psychiatr Scand Suppl.* 1988;345:108–118.

16. Tunving K. Psychiatric effects of cannabis use. *Acta Psychiatr Scand Suppl.* 1985;72:209–217.

17. Miller NS, Gold MS, Pottash AC. A 12-step treatment approach for marijuana (Cannabis) dependence. *J Subst Abuse Treat.* 1989;6:241–250.

18. Kreek MJ. Tolerance and dependence: implications for the pharmacological treatment of addiction. *Natl Inst Drug Abuse Res Monogr Ser.* 1987;76:53–62.

19. Julien R. *A Primer of Drug Action.* 5th ed. New York, NY: WH Freeman & Co; 1988.

20. Belkin BM, Gold MS. Opioids. In: Miller N, ed. *Comprehensive Handbook of Drug and Alcohol Addiction.* New York, NY: Marcel Dekker; 1991.

21. Ford M, Hoffman RS, Goldfrank LR. Opioids and designer drugs. *Emerg Med Clin North Am.* 1990;8:495–511.

22. Dole VP, Nyswander ME. The use of methadone for narcotic blockade. *Br J Addict.* 1968;63:55–57.

23. Senay E. Methadone maintenance treatment. *Int J Addict.* 1985;20:803–821.

24. Kulig K. LSD. *Emerg Med Clin North Am.* 1990;8:551–559.

25. Smith DE, Seymour RB. Dreams become nightmares: adverse reactions to LSD. *J Psychoactive Drugs.* 1985;17:297–303.

26. Carroll ME. PCP and hallucinogens. *Adv Alcohol Subst Abuse.* 1990;9:167–190.

27. Hayner GN, McKinney H. MDMA: the dark side of ecstasy. *J Psychoactive Drugs.* 1986;18:341–347.

28. Baldridge EB, Bessen HA. Phencyclidine. *Emerg Med Clin North Am.* 1990;8:541–550.

29. Simpson GM, Khajawall AM. Urinary acidifiers in phencyclidine detoxification. *Hillside J Clin Psychiatry.* 1983;5:161–168.

RESOURCES

Alcoholics Anonymous.
Web site: www.alcoholics-anonymous.org.

American Society of Addiction Medicine.
Web site: www.asam.org.

Betty Ford Center. Web site: www.bettyfordcenter.org.

The Cleveland Clinic Foundation Alcohol and Drug Recovery Center.
Web site: www.clevelandclinic.org/psychiatry/services/drugrecovery.htm.

Hazelden Foundation. Web site: www.hazelden.org.

National Council on Alcoholism and Drug Dependence Inc.
Web site: www.ncadd.org.

National Institute on Alcohol Abuse and Alcoholism.
Web site: www.niaaa.nih.gov.

National Institute on Drug Abuse.
Web site: www.nida.nih.gov.

chapter 10

Intimate-Partner Violence

Patricia A. Barrier, MD, MPH

INTRODUCTION

Physical, psychological, or sexual abuse is often inflicted by a family member. Family violence is increasingly recognized to be an important issue in the United States and internationally with significant medical, social, economic, and public health implications. In the broadest sense, family violence includes child abuse, intimate-partner violence (IPV), sibling abuse, elder abuse, and abuse of vulnerable adults. This chapter will focus on the magnitude and consequences of IPV in the United States as well as recognition and prevention strategies in the clinical setting. Violence from guns also will be discussed.

Intimate-partner violence is defined as physical, sexual, and/or psychological abuse perpetrated by a current or former intimate partner. An intimate partner is defined as a current or former spouse, partner, or dating partner without regard to cohabitation or genetic sex.[1]

Intimate-partner violence is a cyclic pattern of violence grounded in a dynamic of unequal power and control. In a particular relationship, one form of violence may predominate, but the partner usually experiences physical, psychological, and sexual abuse at some time in the escalating process. The cycle of violence may begin with psychological abuse designed to erode the partner's self-esteem, to intimidate, and to exert control. This may take the form of demeaning remarks about the partner's appearance, intelligence, abilities, family, and friends as well as threats of harm to the partner or the partner's children, pets, or possessions. Isolation is an important aspect of IPV. The perpetrator will isolate the partner from family and friends by various means, such as restricting transportation, money, and phone access. This psychological abuse can escalate to a physical act such as a push, shove, or slap triggered by a mild infraction, for instance, a burned steak. After this physical event, there is usually a period of remorse when the perpetrator apologizes for the act and attempts to make amends with some gift or special act. The partner usually believes in the remorse of the perpetrator. After a period of congenial behaviors, the cycle

renews and escalates. The perpetrator again engages in increasing psychological abuse, which leads to another physical episode that may be more severe. Abusive, forced sexual activities may be occurring simultaneously. Rarely does IPV resolve without intervention.[2]

DEMOGRAPHICS AND EPIDEMIOLOGY

Most victims of IPV in the United States are women with male perpetrators. Between November 1995 and May 1996, the National Institute of Justice and the Centers for Disease Control and Prevention (CDC) conducted the National Violence Against Women Survey (NVAWS). This survey consisted of telephone interviews with a nationally representative sample of 8000 women and 8000 men. Estimates from the NVAWS indicate that annually about 1.5 million women and 840,000 men are victims of physical or sexual assault by a current or former intimate partner.[3] Data from federal law enforcement agencies indicate that 30% to 40% of female homicides and 4% of male homicides are committed by past or present intimate partners. Intimate-partner violence is the leading cause of injuries to US women in the 15- to 44-year-old age group and the second leading cause of injury to all women. Data from the US Department of Justice indicate that a woman in the United States is more likely to be physically or sexually assaulted or murdered by a current or former intimate partner than by any other assailant. Approximately 25% to 45% of abused women are abused during pregnancy. Children often are abused along with the female victim.[2]

There are no demographic, racial, ethnic, socioeconomic, religious, geographic, educational, or gender preference boundaries to IPV. Rates differ in various racial and socioeconomic groups, but no factor or combination of factors emerges as a significant predictor of IPV risk. Violence between intimate partners occurs in both heterosexual and same-sex relationships. Studies on

IPV in gay and lesbian relationships are limited. However, the NVAWS indicated that it was slightly less common in lesbian relationships, with approximately 11% of same-sex female partners reporting physical or sexual assault by an intimate partner vs 30.4% of women in heterosexual relationships. Fifteen percent of men with male partners report physical or sexual abuse by an intimate partner vs 7.7% of men with female partners. According to the NVAWS, most IPV incidents are not reported to law enforcement agencies.[3]

A recent population-based survey in Montana sampled 1804 individuals (56% women, 44% men) using the Behavioral Risk Factor Surveillance System, a telephone survey from the CDC. This survey reported that 5% of men and 3% of women surveyed had experienced physical violence in the past year. Additionally, this study found that women more frequently reported that the perpetrator was a current or former partner and that the violence occurred in their home.[4]

Estimates of the incidence and prevalence of IPV nationally and by individual states vary depending on the data source and the definition of IPV used. As noted above, law enforcement data may yield an underestimate because IPV incidents are not often reported. Data from emergency departments, hospitals, clinics, and health plans may yield a different estimate. A narrow definition confined to physical or sexual assault will yield a lower estimate than a wider definition that includes psychological abuse. Therefore, use of multiple data sources is necessary to get an accurate picture in any community or in the United States as a whole.[5] The CDC, through the programs of the National Center for Injury Prevention and Control, Division of Violence Prevention, has developed a number of surveillance strategies, including the state-implemented Behavioral Risk Factor Surveillance System.[1]

HEALTH EFFECTS OF IPV

A woman who is experiencing IPV may present with physical injuries such as broken bones, burns, cuts, whip marks, or bruises. Trauma to the head, neck, abdomen, and breasts; multiples injuries in different stages of healing; or injuries during pregnancy can be indicative of IPV. Trauma from IPV-related physical assault (excluding sexual assault) is estimated to result in about 460,000 emergency department visits, 400,000 hospital admissions, and 860,000 physician visits per year.[3]

Often the presentation can be subtle and nonspecific. Resnick and colleagues[6] suggest 1 model of the health effects of violence with 3 outcome mechanisms. Acute injuries can lead to chronic problems. Increased stress can impair immune and endocrine function and lead to increased infections and stress-related diseases. Psychological trauma can lead to psychiatric conditions and multiple unhealthy behaviors, such as smoking and alcohol and drug abuse, with the related negative health consequences.[6]

Besides direct trauma, multiple studies show that women experiencing IPV report poorer physical and mental health and increased use of medical services compared with women who have never been abused. This appears evident whether the abuse is current or past. Presenting signs and symptoms may include headache, backache, gastrointestinal (GI) problems, pelvic pain, vaginal complaints, fatigue, chest pain, and other nonspecific somatic complaints. Psychiatric problems such as depression, anxiety, dissociative reactions, suicide attempts, eating disorders, and drug and alcohol abuse can be common mental health problems for women experiencing IPV. Many stress-related problems manifest, such as chronic pain, hypertension, irritable bowel syndrome, and upper respiratory tract infections. Gynecologic problems can include sexually transmitted diseases (STDs) and infection with human immunodeficiency virus (HIV) from unprotected sex after the abusing partner has engaged in sexual activity with multiple partners. Unwanted pregnancy can occur when the abusing partner controls the use of contraception.

There are also issues of poor compliance with medication regimens and follow-up visits if the controlling partner interferes with the woman's attendance at appointments or limits money for prescriptions. A number of studies indicate that abused women seek routine health services such as Papanicolaou tests and breast examinations at the same rate as do women who have never been abused. This increased use of health services has implications for screening in multiple health care settings.[7-14] One study has shown a dose-response relationship between the severity of IPV and the increase in physical and psychological health effects. The authors assessed the health outcomes of exposure to "low-severity violence" encompassing pushing, grabbing, or threats of harm compared with exposure to "high-severity violence." The latter included more serious physical contact, such as slapping, kicking, burning, choking, forcing sexual acts, or threatening or injuring with a weapon. The study showed that low-severity violence was associated with poor health and that the effects on health intensified with high-severity violence.[15]

The relationship to poor health appears to exist whether the abuse is physical or psychological. One study of 1152 women aged 18 to 65 years from a family medicine practice showed that women experiencing psychological abuse alone experienced poorer health compared with women who had never been abused. The abused women in this study had an increase in chronic neck and back pain, migraines or other frequent headaches, work disabilities, arthritis, STDs, chronic pelvic pain, and GI symptoms. This highlights the need to screen for psychological abuse as well as physical and sexual abuse.[16]

Studies of the effects of IPV on pregnancy outcomes have yielded mixed results. Obviously, severe physical trauma may lead to adverse outcomes or complications. There is some indication that the stress associated with IPV of a physical, psychological, or sexual nature may be associated with low birth weight or lower mean birth weight.[17] The increased risk of infection, possible inadequate prenatal care, and the impact of negative health habits can lead to indirect adverse pregnancy effects due to IPV.

Children often experience physical and psychological abuse in IPV. They may experience physical abuse from the abuser or the victim. They are subject to the psychological trauma of witnessing abuse, which may be predictive of engaging in future abusive relationships. The dysfunction in the abusive family unit may also adversely affect many developmental parameters, such as school performance.[13,18]

Intimate-partner violence is associated not only with direct trauma and all its consequences but also with many other physical and mental health problems, poorer overall health, and increased use and cost of health services for the victim and victim's children. Women experiencing IPV interact with health care providers frequently and in many health care venues. Health care providers are very important in the early detection of and intervention in IPV.

CHARACTERISTICS OF PERPETRATORS

Just as it is difficult to define a profile of a person at high risk of IPV, so it is difficult to define a profile of someone likely to be a perpetrator of IPV in terms of socio-economic, racial, ethnic, religious, geographic, or educational factors. What seems to be most correlated with becoming a perpetrator is witnessing IPV as a child. The next most predictive factor seems to be experiencing abuse as a child. Some data suggest an increased use of drugs or alcohol among IPV perpetrators.[19]

In the clinical environment, there may be behaviors that raise suspicion of IPV. The perpetrator may accompany the victim of IPV to an emergency department visit or routine medical visits and be overly attentive, answer for the victim, and be unwilling to leave her alone with the health care provider. Although women experiencing IPV frequently interact with the health care system as noted above, perpetrators seem to be less frequent users of health services. However, one small study showed that 42% of men in a treatment program for batterers (perpetrators) had visited a health care provider within the 6 months before the battering episode for an injury, medical illness, or checkup. Twenty-nine percent of those men had been seen by a primary care provider. This suggests the potential to identify perpetrators in the medical setting, but the full implications and ramifications of this are very clouded at best. Routine screening for perpetrators of IPV is not yet recommended.[20]

Estimates of how often women are the perpetrators of IPV are unclear. In a recent study with 225 military and civilian domestic violence professionals, 80% indicated that they encountered women who initiated the IPV and 69% indicated that the violence was unprovoked by partner violence. Fifty-nine percent reported that the violence inflicted by women was just as serious as that by men.[21]

PRIMARY PREVENTION

Intimate-partner violence is a community and society issue as well as an individual issue. Interventions with individual victims, although extremely important, will not influence the overall incidence and prevalence of IPV. Primary prevention is a much more complex process involving social and behavioral norms, attitudes about violence in society, and attitudes about women and relationships with women.

As previously noted, one predictive factor for future intimate-partner abusive behavior has been identified as exposure to IPV in childhood. To break this cycle of violence, primary prevention must start at the earliest age possible. The environment and attitudes that promote violence and victimization must be modified. It may be critical to begin school programs very early that raise awareness about violence and focus on alternate ways to manage anger and conflict. In adolescence, the emphasis can expand to dating violence.[22]

Intimate-partner violence is also a problem that involves far more than law enforcement, schools, and medical and mental health communities. Religious communities, workplaces, community and service organizations, and media must all be involved in public education and primary prevention of IPV and other forms of violence.[23] Primary prevention must focus on the overall reduction of violence as a pervasive aspect of our society.[1,24-26]

SECONDARY PREVENTION: DETECTION OF IPV IN THE CLINICAL ENVIRONMENT

Secondary prevention must focus on early detection and intervention to decrease the morbidity and mortality associated with IPV. The costs of IPV in terms of personal and medical costs, lost workdays, years of potential life lost, and effects on children are staggering. As previously stated, women experiencing IPV frequently interact with health care providers in a number of acute- and chronic care settings. A health care setting can be the one place where the victim escapes the calculated isolation of IPV. It behooves health care providers to be involved in the secondary prevention of IPV through early detection and mitigation of the effects of future violence by routinely screening for victims of IPV. Most victims of IPV will not spontaneously disclose this to a health care provider because of shame, self-blame, fear, isolation, belief in the remorse of the perpetrator, or economic or social dependence on the perpetrator. Even when screened, women may decline to disclose IPV because of fear of the partner and escalating violence to themselves or their children. However, overall, a number of studies show that many women will disclose if asked directly by a health care provider.

The Council on Ethical and Judicial Affairs of the American Medical Association has indicated that physicians should routinely screen for domestic violence.[27] Several other professional organizations (the American College of Obstetricians and Gynecologists, the American College of Physicians, the American Academy of Family Physicians, and the Joint Commission on Accreditation of Healthcare Organizations) have also recommended either screening or increased awareness. The US Preventive Services Task Force indicates that there is insufficient evidence to recommend for or against screening for IPV but concludes that inclusion of questions on physical abuse of adults is indicated on other grounds. As stated in their document, "These other grounds include the substantial prevalence of undetected abuse among adult female patients, the potential value of this information in the care of the patient, and the low cost and low risk of harm from such screening."[28]

Despite the above recommendations for IPV screening by health care providers, few providers screen on a regular basis. One recent study of 610 primary care physicians indicated that 86% thought that IPV screening was an essential part of their role, but only 19% of the physicians sampled screened new patients for IPV. Indeed, screening rates for IPV were significantly less than their rates of screening for tobacco use, alcohol abuse, or HIV/STD risk.[29] Another study sampled 2400 physicians (600 each in general internal medicine, family practice, obstetrics and gynecology, and emergency medicine). Of these physicians, 46% to 50% screened less than 10% of their female adult patients for IPV despite the fact that most believed it was their responsibility to screen and most knew women in their practices who had experienced IPV.[30]

Multiple factors have been cited as reasons for lack of provider screening. These include lack of education about IPV and how to screen, lack of time to screen, lack of effective interventions, concerns about what to do if a patient indicates she is a victim of IPV, and fear of offending patients. Physicians have also expressed the belief that IPV is not a medical problem or does not occur in their particular practice.[31]

One reason that health care providers cite for not screening all female patients for IPV is that they may offend their patients. However, there is evidence to suggest that screening is acceptable and effective in prompting women to disclose IPV. In a recent study of 375 racially and ethnically diverse women, Rodriguez and colleagues[32] found that only 28% of the sample were directly questioned about IPV. Of those who were directly questioned, 85% disclosed information in response to the question; only 25% disclosed IPV without direct

questioning. Issues involved in nondisclosure were concerns about confidentiality, beliefs that physicians lacked time and interest in IPV issues, fear of police and courts, and immigrant status. In this study, the strongest determinant of IPV disclosure was a care provider's inquiry.[32] In a case-control study of 202 abused women, 48% of women agreed that providers should routinely screen all women, and positive responses were 1.5 times more likely from abused women. Eighty-six percent of those interviewed agreed that screening would help abused women get assistance.[33]

The goal of IPV screening is secondary prevention—preventing further abuse and the sequelae of abuse by early detection. One must then examine the validity of screening as a predictor of further abuse. To accomplish this, a valid screening tool must be in place. A recent study examined the validity of a brief IPV screen as a predictor of future violence. In this prospective cohort study, 679 adult women in Colorado were screened by telephone survey using the CDC Behavioral Risk Factor Surveillance System. Of the initially screened women, 409 were followed up in 3 to 6 months and interviewed again with questions regarding IPV occurrences since the initial interview. Of the respondents, 8.4% had an initial screen that was positive for IPV. When interviewed during follow-up, these women were 46.6 times more likely to experience severe physical violence, 11.7 times more likely to experience any physical violence, 3.6 times more likely to experience verbal abuse, and 2.5 times more likely to experience sexual abuse than those who had responded negatively to the initial screening questions. Thus, a positive screen for IPV seems to be a good predictor of future violence and harm.[34]

Health care providers can screen routinely for IPV by a number of means. Because women who are victims of IPV seem to access routine medical services at the same rate as women who are not abused and also access acute- and chronic-care medical services more often, screening in a variety of clinical settings is indicated. Physicians can make screening for IPV a routine part of their interaction with new and follow-up patients. Questions such as "Have you ever been physically, emotionally, or sexually abused? Is this a past or a current problem?" can be either included on history forms that patients complete or asked directly as part of the medical interview. Physicians may want to tell patients that screening for IPV is included in good preventive screening in the same way that screening for tobacco, alcohol, and drug use, or diet and exercise is included. This may decrease any physician or patient discomfort about IPV-related questions.

Many screening tools have been developed to help providers screen for IPV. Fogarty et al[35] provide a concise summary of short screening instruments that have validity and reliability determinations. These include the Woman Abuse Screening Tool, to detect current IPV; Women's Experience With Battering Scale, to measure both physical and psychological abuse; Hurt, Insult, Threaten, and Scream (HITS), which is a 4-question tool for the outpatient setting; Abuse and Assessment Screen to detect abuse during pregnancy; and Partner Violence Screens for use in emergency departments.

Once the health care provider screens for IPV and receives a positive response, the degree and duration of violence should be ascertained. Patients should be questioned regarding the types of violence they experience (physical, sexual, psychological), injuries they have sustained, how long this has been occurring, if children have been involved in the violence, and if there are weapons in the home or in the possession of either the victim or the perpetrator. It is also important to assess the level of the victim's isolation by asking whether family or friends know what is going on. Finally, the physician should inquire if the victim has an escape plan for herself and her children if violence escalates to a serious level.

A good mnemonic for assessing for IPV and the level of threat is **SAFE**[36,37]:

Stress/safety

Afraid/abused

Friends/family

Emergency plan

It appears that education of physicians about IPV and IPV screening is not sufficient to implement this in practice. Salber and McCaw[38] suggest that the emphasis should shift from identifying the barriers to screening to what can be done to help physicians to screen. They advocate a systems approach to IPV screening and awareness that involves all aspects of a health care setting. They describe the Family Violence Prevention Project that was implemented at the Kaiser Permanente-Richmond (Calif) Medical Center from 1998 to 1999. The program involved the whole medical center and included physician and health care provider training; visual information throughout the medical center, such as posters and information in examination rooms; patient materials; onsite domestic violence evaluators to assist when a provider identified a patient with IPV issues; and feedback to providers regarding IPV interventions via a confidential database. The results of this project included increased clinician detection of IPV and referrals for IPV-related services as well as greater self-reporting by victims.[38]

To summarize, the goal of screening for IPV is secondary prevention. We have evidence that screening is predictive of future violence and, thus, has important implications for both health care providers and victims. There seems to be acceptance of screening by women, and, indeed, direct physician questioning may be the most important factor in disclosure. With screening, it is most important to ask the question in a nonjudgmental fashion, convey the message that no one deserves to be treated this way, offer information regarding resources for help, and offer follow-up care. Provider screening is one aspect of a continuum to prevent and intervene in IPV but is a very critical one because of the frequent interface between the health care system and IPV victims. Through asking questions about IPV, the health care provider may be providing the first intervention, even if the patients do not respond or respond but do not take any action to extricate themselves from the IPV situation after the initial discussion.

INTERVENTIONS

Once IPV occurs and a person presents with acute injuries, the first obligation is to appropriately treat those injuries and carefully document the history and description of the injuries in the medical record. This careful documentation, including photographs with the victim's consent, is essential for any legal action that the victim may wish to pursue. Whether the IPV has been identified acutely and directly or through health care provider screening, the next step is to decrease future exposure to violence by providing the victim with information about IPV intervention services. Services available in most communities include social services, victim services, rape and assault crisis hotlines, legal services, law enforcement, battered women's shelters, national and local domestic violence hotlines, and victim advocacy groups. Health care providers can access many excellent resources on the Internet[39] (see "Resources" at the end of the chapter). Developing a list of resources in the provider's own community is a good starting point. Providers must be careful about giving IPV victims printed material, which may trigger more violence if found by the perpetrator.

Mandatory reporting of IPV by health care providers has been implemented in some states for prevention, intervention, and data collection. Providers should become familiar with the laws in their states. Houry et al[40] recently surveyed state legislatures and state domestic violence coalitions in all 50 states and the District of Columbia between July 1999 and April 2000. They found that domestic violence is a crime in all states. Twenty-three states had laws requiring reporting injuries from crimes. Seven states (California, Colorado, Kentucky, Mississippi, Ohio, Rhode Island, and Texas) had specific laws requiring reporting of injuries resulting from domestic violence. All states mandating reports grant immunity to the reporter. The outcome of reports varies from data collection only (Rhode Island) to a requirement to document domestic violence in the medical record, refer victims to shelters, and inform the victim that domestic violence is a crime (Texas). Some states have specific consequences for failure to report domestic violence, ranging from fines to imprisonment.[40]

Mandatory reporting is controversial. Questions exist as to whether mandatory reporting would deter both physician screening and patient reporting and cause more endangerment of the victim. Attitudes of patients have been assessed. One study assessed attitudes of patients in emergency departments in California, which has a mandatory reporting law, and in Pennsylvania, which does not have mandatory reporting. Of the 1218 women studied, 12% reported physical or sexual IPV within the past year. Of the abused women, 56% supported mandatory reporting. Of the 43% who opposed mandatory reporting, 8% favored no reporting and 36% favored reporting only with the woman's consent. Of women who reported no experience of abuse, 71% supported mandatory reporting. Those who supported reporting felt that it would improve data collection, encourage provider identification, and lead to increased prosecution of perpetrators. Those who opposed mandatory reporting felt it may increase violence, decrease patient autonomy, and compromise patient-provider confidentiality. Factors that predicted opposition included currently living with or seeing the abusing partner, not speaking English at home, and physical abuse within the past year. There was no difference in attitudes between women in California and in Pennsylvania.[41]

In another study involving women in an urban health maintenance organization, 48% favored mandatory reporting only with the woman's consent and 66% thought they would be less likely to disclose because of fear of more abuse.[33] These surveyed women preferred referral to counseling services, shelters, and confidential hotlines over mandatory reporting. Clearly, the physician must be cognizant of the laws in his or her state. However, the issue of mandatory reporting needs much more study before it is universally implemented in all states.

Civil protection orders (restraining orders) are another intervention for IPV. It is estimated that 20% of women experiencing IPV obtain civil protection orders, and evidence suggests that civil protection orders do reduce further IPV. Holt et al[42] studied a retrospective cohort of women who had reported IPV to law enforcement and had obtained a 12-month permanent protection order. This study showed an 80% reduction in police-reported IPV with an order in place. This may be an important intervention for physicians to inform and counsel patients about when screening or patient disclosure reveals IPV.

Interventions with perpetrators have yielded limited success. Most intervention programs are court-mandated group interactions and focus on anger management. Few programs address the deeper issues stemming from childhood exposure to violence, attitudes about women, relationships with women, and concomitant substance abuse problems. Clearly, more research is needed to develop the most effective interventions for perpetrators. Counseling of couples can lead to major escalation of the violence and should not be attempted.[19]

GUNS AND IPV

Another important aspect of prevention and intervention in IPV is to ascertain the presence of guns in the home or in the possession of the perpetrator or victim. The pres-

ence of a firearm in the milieu of IPV greatly increases the mortality and morbidity. The perpetrator may possess the weapon, or the victim may have been advised to obtain a weapon for her protection from the perpetrator. Both situations escalate the risk of serious IPV.

Firearms are a pervasive aspect of life in the United States. In their review, Kellerman and Heron[44] indicate that about 40% of US homes have firearms and that 33% of all privately owned firearms are handguns. They cite data from the Federal Bureau of Investigation's Uniform Crime Reports that indicate that guns are used in 61% of domestic homicides and that handguns are more frequently used than rifles or shotguns. Women are more likely to be shot and killed by an IPV perpetrator than by a stranger. When women kill with a firearm, they are more likely to kill an intimate partner or family member than a stranger.[43]

Self-defense is frequently cited as the reason for ownership of a firearm, especially a handgun. Self-defense is also the reason used to advocate for gun possession by victims of IPV. However, numerous studies indicate that handguns are used infrequently for self-defense and that their use more frequently results in suicide or homicide. The National Crime Victimization Survey estimated that guns were used defensively only 1% to 3% of the time. Also, if a weapon is kept for self-defense, it is more likely to be loaded and easily accessible, increasing not only the suicide and homicide risk but the risk of childhood injury or death by the firearm.[43]

The increase in suicide rate from handgun possession was studied in a population-based cohort study by Wintemute and colleagues.[44] They compared the mortality of 238,292 persons in California who purchased handguns from licensed dealers in 1991 vs the general adult population of California. They found that suicide was the leading cause of death among the purchaser group within the first year of handgun purchase, accounting for 24.5% of all deaths in this group and 51.9% were women ages 21 to 44 years. The rate of suicide within the first week after purchase was 57 times higher than that in the general population and may reflect purchase with suicidal intent. However, the increased risk of suicide persisted up to 6 years after handgun purchase, and the female dominance was also sustained.[45] In another study comparing gun mortality in rural and urban settings, it was found that in rural settings a higher percentage of gun-related deaths were from shotguns and rifles and a higher percentage were from suicides and accidents compared with urban settings. However, in both settings, more than 50% of the deaths due to gunfire were from handguns, and suicides accounted for 70% of the gun deaths.[45]

The morbidity and cost of nonfatal gunshot wounds are very high. Cook et al[46] examined data from multiple sources, including hospital discharges from Maryland and New York in 1994, emergency department discharges in South Carolina in 1997, the 1994 National Electronic

Injury Surveillance System, the National Spinal Cord Injury Statistical Center, and 1994 vital statistics. In their analysis, they estimated that the lifetime cost of gunshot wounds (in 1994 dollars) was $2.3 billion, with about $1.1 billion being covered by government programs.[46]

Primary prevention can occur at the legislative level either nationally or in individual states. A classic study suggests that legislative approaches can be very effective. Sloan et al[47] compared homicide and other crime and violence rates between a community with restriction of handgun access (Vancouver, British Columbia) and a comparable neighboring community with easier access to handguns (Seattle, Wash). The authors found a 63% increase in homicide rate in Seattle compared with Vancouver during the 7-year period of study. Most of the increase in homicide was due to handgun deaths.[47] The Violent Crime Control and Law Enforcement Act of 1994 (Brady Act) includes a provision that prohibits anyone under a restraining order to possess a firearm. This was further strengthened by the 1996 amendment to the Brady Act, the Domestic Violence Offenders Gun Ban. This amendment prohibits gun possession or purchase by anyone convicted of a domestic violence offense.[44]

Physicians can engage in lobbying at the legislative level to reduce the number of firearms in possession. In terms of secondary prevention in clinical practice, it is important to begin to screen for firearm possession and to counsel patients regarding firearms as part of overall preventive screening. Discouraging firearm possession, especially handguns, and countering the self-defense argument may be very appropriate to promote safety among adults and children in the household. Next to deterring ownership, physicians should promote firearm safety, such as keeping a gun in locked storage, separate storage of ammunition, trigger locks, and careful education of children regarding firearm safety.[45]

Because of the increased potential for homicide or suicide in IPV if there is a weapon involved, especially a handgun, it is extremely important for health care providers to inquire about weapons in the IPV setting. It is also important to warn IPV victims of these increased risks, even if they keep a gun for self-defense, since they are more likely to be killed or injured by their own weapon in these circumstances.

SUMMARY

Intimate-partner violence is a major public health problem in the United States, causing substantial morbidity and mortality. Most victims are female with male perpetrators. Intimate-partner violence can occur in any population group and between same-sex as well as heterosexual partners. Victims of IPV have increased visits to health care providers for both acute and chronic problems. Thus, health care providers can provide the first intervention to break the cycle of violence by universal screening and being familiar with community resources to assist victims of IPV.

REFERENCES

1. Saltzman LE, Green YT, Marks JS, Thacker SB. Violence against women as a public health issue: comments from the CDC. *Am J Prev Med.* 2000;19:325–329.

2. Barrier PA. Domestic violence. *Mayo Clin Proc.* 1998;73:271–274.

3. Tjaden P, Thoenes N. *Extent, Nature and Consequences of Intimate Partner Violence: Findings From the National Violence Against Women Survey.* Washington, DC: US Department of Justice, NCJ 181867. National Institute of Justice and Centers for Disease Control and Prevention; 2000.

4. Harwell TS, Spence MR. Population surveillance for physical violence among adult men and women, Montana 1998. *Am J Prev Med.* 2000;19:321–324.

5. Verhoek-Oftedahl W, Pearlman DN, Babcock JC. Improving surveillance of intimate partner violence by use of multiple data sources. *Am J Prev Med.* 2000;19:308–315.

6. Resnick HS, Acierno R, Kilpatrick DG. Health impact of interpersonal violence: II. Medical and mental health outcomes. *Behav Med.* 1997;23:65–78.

7. Mcnutt LA, Carlson BE, Persaud M, Postmus J. Cumulative abuse experience, physical health and health behaviors. *Ann Epidemiol.* 2002;12:123–130.

8. Cambell JC. Health consequences of intimate partner violence. *Lancet.* 2002;359:1331–1336.

9. Campbell J, Jones AS, Dienemann J, et al. Intimate partner violence and physical health consequences. *Arch Intern Med.* 2002;162:1157–1163.

10. Hathaway JE, Mucci LA, Silverman JG, Brooks DR, Mathews R, Pavlos CA. Health status and health care use of Massachusetts women reporting partner abuse. *Am J Prev Med.* 2000;19:302–307.

11. Yeager K, Seid A. Primary care and victims of domestic violence. *Primary Care.* 2002;29:125–150.

12. Plichta SB, Falik M. Prevalence of violence and its implications for women's health. *Women's Health Issues.* 2001;11:244–258.

13. Campbell JC, Lewandowski LA. Mental and physical health effects of intimate partner violence on women and children. *Psychiatr Clin North Am.* 1997;20:353–374.

14. Kernic MA, Wolf ME, Holt VL. Rates and relative risk of hospital admission among women in violent intimate partner relationships. *Am J Public Health.* 2000;90:1416–1420.

15. McCauley J, Kern DE, Kolodner K, Derogatis LR, Bass EB. Relation of low-severity violence to women's health. *J Gen Intern Med.* 1998;13:687–691.

16. Coker AL, Smith PH, King BL, McKeown RE. Physical health consequences of physical and psychological intimate partner violence. *Arch Fam Med.* 2000;9:451–457.

17. Altarac M, Strobino D. Abuse during pregnancy and stress because of abuse during pregnancy and birth. *J Am Med Womens Assoc.* 2002;57: 208–214.

18. Stiles MM. Witnessing domestic violence: the effect on children. *Am Fam Physician.* 2002;66:2052–2066.

19. Lee WV, Weinstein SP. How far have we come? A critical review of the research on men who batter. In: Galanter M ed. *Recent Developments in Alcoholism, Volume 13: Alcoholism and Violence.* New York, NY: Plenum Press; 1997;13:337–355.

20. Coben JH, Friedman DI. Health care use by perpetrators of domestic violence. *J Emerg Med.* 2002;22:313–317.

21. Adams SR, Freeman DR. Women who are violent: attitudes and beliefs of Wolfe professionals working in the field of domestic violence. *Mil Med.* 2002;167:445–450.

22. DA, Jaffe. Emerging strategies in the prevention of domestic violence. *The Future of Children.* 1999;9(3):133–144.

23. Petersen R, Gazmararian J, Andersen Clark K. Partner violence: implications for health and community. *Womens Health Issues.* 2001;11:116–125.

24. Hyman I, Guruge S, Stewart DE, Ahmad F. Primary prevention of violence against women. *Womens Health Issues.* 2000;10:288–293.

25. Gundersen L. Intimate-partner violence: the need for primary prevention in the community. *Ann Intern Med.* 2002;136:637–640.

26. Weinbaum Z, Stratton TL, Chavez G, et al. Female victims of intimate partner physical domestic violence (IPP-DV), California 1998. *Am J Prev Med.* 2001;21:313–319.

27. Council on Ethical and Judicial Affairs, American Medical Association. Physicians and domestic violence: ethical considerations. *JAMA.* 1992;267:3190–3193.

28. US Preventive Services Task Force. Screening for family violence. In: *Guide to Clinical Preventive Services.* 2nd ed. Alexandria, VA: International Medical Publishing; 1996:555–565.

29. Gerbert B, Gansky SA, Tang JW, et al. Domestic violence compared to other health risks: a survey of physicians' beliefs and behaviors. *Am J Prev Med.* 2002:23:82–90.

30. Elliiot L, Nerney M, Jones T, Friedmann PD. Barriers to screening for domestic violence. *J Gen Intern Med.* 2002;17:112–116.

31. Waalen J, Goodwin MM, Spitz AM, Petersen R, Saltzman LE. Screening for intimate partner violence by health care providers. *Am J Prev Med.* 2000;19:230–237.

32. Rodriguez MA, Sheldon WR, Bauer HM, Perez-Stable EJ. The factors associated with disclosure of intimate partner abuse to clinicians. *J Fam Pract.* 2001;50:338–344.

33. Gielen AC, O'Campo PJ, Campbell JC, et al. Women's opinions about domestic violence screening and mandatory reporting. *Am J Prev Med.* 2000;19:279–285.

34. Koziol-McLain J, Coates CJ, Lowenstein SR. Predictive validity of a screen for partner violence against women. *Am J Prev Med.* 2001;21:93–100.

35. Fogarty CT, Burge S, McCord EC. Communication with patients about intimate partner violence: screening and interviewing approaches. *Fam Med.* 2002;34:369–375.

36. Ashur MLC. Asking about domestic violence: SAFE questions. *JAMA.* 1993;269:2367.

37. Neufeld B. SAFE questions: overcoming barriers to the detection of domestic violence. *Am Fam Physician.* 1996;53: 2575–2580, 2582.

38. Salber PR, McCaw B. Barriers to screening for intimate partner violence: time to reframe the question. *Am J Prev Med.* 2000;19:276–278.

39. Goodman P. Domestic violence resources on the Internet. *JAMA.* 1998;280:477–478.

40. Houry D, Sachs CJ, Felhaus KM, Linden J. Violence-inflicted injuries: reporting laws in the fifty states. *Ann Emerg Med.* 2002;39:56–60.

41. Rodriguez MA, McLoughlin E, Nah G, Campbell JC. Mandatory reporting of domestic violence injuries to the police: what do emergency department patients think? *JAMA.* 2001;286:580–583.

42. Holt VL, Kernic MA, Lumley T, Wolf ME, Rivara FP. Civil protection orders and risk of subsequent police-reported violence. *JAMA.* 2002;288:589–594.

43. Kellermann A, Heron S. Firearms and family violence. *Emerg Med Clin North Am.* 1999;17:699–716.

44. Wintemute GJ, Parham CA, Beaumont JJ, Wright M, Drake C. Mortality among recent purchasers of handguns. *N Engl J Med.* 1999;341:1583–1589.

45. Dresang LT. Gun deaths in rural and urban settings: recommendations for prevention. *J Am Board Fam Pract.* 2001;14:107–115.

46. Cook PJ, Lawrence BA, Ludwig J, Miller TR. The medical costs of gunshot injuries in the United States. *JAMA.* 1999;282:447–454.

47. Sloan JH, Kellermann AL, Reay DT, et al. Handgun regulations, crime, assaults, and homicide: a tale of two cities. *N Engl J Med.* 1988;319:1256–1262.

RESOURCES

Family Violence Prevention Fund.
 Web site: www.endabuse.org

Institute for Law and Justice.
 Web site: www.ilj.org/dv/

National Domestic Violence Hotline: 800 799-SAFE.
 Web site: www.ndvh.org

US Department of Justice, Office on Violence Against Women.
 Web site: www.usdoj.gov/vawo/

chapter 11

Tobacco and Smoking Cessation

J. Taylor Hays, MD

INTRODUCTION

Tobacco use continues to be one of the most common preventable causes of death in the United States, accounting for about 20% of all cause-specific mortality.[1] Current surveys indicate that approximately 23% of adult Americans, or 47 million people, smoke cigarettes.[2] Despite the known serious health consequences of smoking, clinicians often fail to assess smoking status or offer intervention for tobacco use.[3] Among the barriers to intervention are inadequate knowledge of effective treatment strategies that can be applied in the office and uncertainty about the relative efficacy of treatments that are currently available.

This chapter will present office-based strategies for effective tobacco-use intervention and discuss the relative efficacy of the various treatments. Although tobacco use of all types presents a health risk, the population attributable risk is greatest for cigarette smoking. The assessments and treatments recommended in this review refer to treatment of cigarette smoking in particular, but many principles can be generalized to the treatment of other tobacco use disorders as well.

CHRONIC DISEASE MODEL

Tobacco use and dependence is a chronic, remitting, and relapsing condition. Approximately 46% of smokers try to quit each year although few remain abstinent after 1 year.[3] In addition, treatment advances may falsely suggest that simply applying the most recent treatment will result in permanent abstinence. However, the true nature of tobacco use is that of a chronic disorder. For the clinician, this means that relapse is expected and that an acute treatment approach alone is bound to fail to meet the needs of patients. Successful treatment will incorporate counseling and advice and a long view of the therapeutic relationship between clinician and patient.

ADDICTION MODEL

Nicotine is the addictive substance in tobacco.[4] The continued use of tobacco is due, in large part, to addiction to nicotine. All drug addictions have in common a complex interplay of stereotypical behavior surrounding drug use and the positive and negative reinforcing effects of the particular drug. The major effect of nicotine is an increase in midbrain dopamine levels,[5] an effect believed to be at the heart of the positive reinforcing effects of nicotine as well as cocaine, amphetamines, and opiates.[6] The positive reinforcing effects on the smoker include relaxation, reduced stress, enhanced cognitive performance, and enhanced vigilance.[4] The nicotine withdrawal syndrome provides strong negative reinforcement for continued smoking.[7] Because smoking provides immediate relief of abstinence-induced symptoms, relapse to smoking is common over the first days and weeks of an attempt at smoking cessation. In addition, because of the strong positive and negative reinforcement for continued tobacco use, relapse typically occurs many times before permanent abstinence is achieved. Finally, each smoker associates certain behaviors, situations, emotions, and activities with the reinforcing effects of nicotine. The more closely these stimuli are linked to smoking, the more powerful is the conditioned response (smoking) to these "cues." The addiction model, in keeping with the chronic disease model, indicates that combined behavioral and pharmacologic treatment will be the most effective approach. Relapse is expected and should be viewed as part of the process of achieving long-term abstinence.

BEHAVIORAL SUPPORT FOR SMOKING CESSATION

Assessing Tobacco Use

Although nearly 70% of smokers report a desire to quit, few are offered assistance when visiting a clinician.[3]

To reverse this trend, the first step will be proper assessment of smoking status for every individual who is seen for care in the office. The office-based assessment of tobacco use should include assessment of both current and past use. Evidence suggests that the systematic assessment of tobacco use as "the new vital sign" will improve identification and intervention with smokers.[8] Current smokers will require further intervention to encourage an attempt to quit. The intervention in the office does not need to be excessively time-consuming but does require the active involvement of the clinician. The steps involved in the intervention are:

- Assess readiness to stop smoking
- Provide brief counseling
- Provide appropriate pharmacologic intervention
- Follow up for relapse prevention

Assessing Readiness to Stop Smoking

The transtheoretical model of change has become a commonly used tool for assessing readiness to change health behavior.[9] Many of the details of this model are presented in Chapter 6. For the clinician, the model serves as a valuable staging tool that can be used to guide and tailor the intervention to the particular needs of the patient. The stages of change represent a continuum of motivation for initiating and maintaining abstinence from tobacco (Table 11-1). Proper staging will allow the clinician to limit the time required to provide appropriate "stage-matched" interventions. The staging assessment for current smokers requires 2 simple questions:

1. Are you planning to quit smoking in the next 6 months?
2. If yes, are you planning to quit smoking in the next month?

The interventions appropriate for each stage range from providing a brief personalized message to quit to a more detailed discussion of a plan to quit and a discussion about the use of medications to aid in the attempt.

For those individuals in earlier stages of change (precontemplation and contemplation), the role of the clinician is to promote motivation and movement along the stages of change. Motivation can be stimulated by providing a consistent message such as the "5 Rs."[3]

1. *Relevance:* The message must be personalized to have the greatest impact.
2. *Risk:* Identify some immediate and longer-term risks of continuing to smoke (eg, immediate—bad breath; long-term—lung disease).
3. *Rewards:* Identify potential benefits of stopping tobacco use.
4. *Roadblocks:* What are the barriers to quitting now? Identify ways these might be overcome.
5. *Repetition:* Repeat the message with every unmotivated smoker at every visit. Encourage repeated attempts to quit for those who have relapsed.

More intense counseling efforts will be required and should be reserved for smokers who are in the preparation and action stages. By assessing the stage of change and providing only the intervention indicated, clinicians will find that time is used more efficiently. For example, a smoker who is in the "contemplation" stage usually will respond best to a brief message that increases awareness of the problems that smoking may cause, rather than a more lengthy discussion of behavioral strategies for coping with abstinence-induced symptoms. The stage-matched approach will also reduce a clinician's frustration over patients who fail to take action, since unrealistic expectations will be tempered by recognition of a "precontemplation" or "contemplation" stage of change.

T A B L E   11-1

Stages of Change and Appropriate Interventions

Stage of Change	Definition	Intervention
Precontemplation	Not seriously thinking of quitting in next 6 mo	Advise patient to quit; give brief motivational message
Contemplation	Seriously thinking of quitting in next 6 mo	Advise patient to quit; give brief motivational message; discuss pharmacotherapy
Preparation	Desire to quit tobacco use in next 30 d and made a quit-attempt of at least 24 h within the last year	Set quit date; develop a quit plan; prescribe pharmacotherapy; provide behavioral therapy
Action	Currently not smoking and abstinent <6 mo	Review pharmacotherapy; provide support; discuss relapse prevention
Maintenance	Currently not smoking and abstinent ≥6 mo or more	Discuss relapse prevention; provide encouragement

Brief Office Counseling for Smoking Cessation

Every smoker should receive a clear, personalized message to quit and a motivational message to encourage an attempt to quit. For those smokers who are motivated to change, brief office counseling may be employed to aid in developing specific plans for quitting.

Brief office counseling is an effective tool to facilitate increased quitting activity and abstinence from tobacco in smokers who are motivated to change.[10] Counseling by a physician lasting 3 minutes or less results in a 30% increase in abstinence compared with no intervention.[3] For a brief intervention to be most effective, it should be practical in approach and patient-centered. Practical counseling includes problem solving and a review of coping skills that the patient can readily learn to employ. Problem-solving strategies may be as simple as advising removal of all tobacco products from home and work before quitting and planning for high-risk relapse situations. Coping strategies are key to learning successful self-management and maintaining abstinence.[11] Examples are suggesting deep breathing for relaxation or changing a routine in which smoking is often involved. A patient-centered approach to office counseling calls for the clinician to determine the resources a patient possesses for smoking cessation. Questions about past attempts to quit and previous successes or failures provide information for developing the quitting plan.

Beyond simple advice and encouragement to quit, a brief counseling intervention may include a number of components:

- Give clear and personalized advice to quit.
- Encourage a quit date.
- Develop a quit plan.
- Provide support for the quit attempt.
- Prescribe appropriate pharmacotherapy.
- Discuss a plan for relapse prevention.
- Set a follow-up date.

At minimum, the clinician should assist the patient in setting a stop date and developing a plan for quitting. Using the patient-centered approach, these minimal goals can be accomplished in 3 minutes or less. More extensive office-based counseling may be employed to develop detailed plans for quitting and relapse prevention.

There is a dose-response relationship between time spent in counseling for smoking cessation and abstinence rates; higher intensity counseling lasting more than 10 minutes results in near doubling of abstinence rates compared with minimal (less than 3 minutes) counseling.[3] Because clinician time is limited, higher intensity counseling is reserved for patients who are motivated to quit and develop a detailed plan for smoking cessation (patients who are in the "preparation" or "action" stage of change).

Quit plan

Clinicians can effectively guide the plan for quitting using a patient-centered approach to counseling. The stop date should occur within 2 weeks of the office visit and the patient should be advised to stop all tobacco use on that date. Complete abstinence from tobacco is the clearly stated goal. It is unclear whether reduced tobacco consumption without complete abstinence is sustainable or results in substantially reduced harm from smoking.[12] Appropriate pharmacologic treatment should commence on or before the planned stop date. Follow-up with brief office visits or by telephone improves abstinence rates.[13] Follow-up contacts are used to reinforce the importance of maintaining abstinence, to review medication recommendations, and to promote relapse prevention.

Relapse prevention

The goal of treatment of tobacco use and dependence is permanent abstinence. However, relapse occurs in approximately 80% of smokers within 1 year of an attempt to quit.[14] Most relapse episodes occur within the first 3 months of quitting tobacco use, whether or not nicotine replacement medication is used.[15] Risk factors for relapse provide the clinician with an indication about which smokers will need the most intense support and follow-up. The risk factors for relapse are:

- High nicotine dependence (smokes more than 25 cigarettes per day or within 30 minutes of waking)
- No previous abstinence of 30 days or more
- History of major depression
- Current or past alcohol abuse or dependence
- Other smokers in the household

Relapse occurs in a vulnerable individual who is in a triggering situation and has inadequate coping responses. Office counseling for relapse prevention should include planning for high-risk situations, avoidance of strong triggers (eg, alcohol), encouragement for successes, continued troubleshooting of problem areas, and offering continued support and follow-up. The support required for some smokers may be extensive and beyond the reach of clinicians with busy office practices. In these cases, referral to a trained tobacco counselor or treatment center for higher intensity treatment is appropriate.[16]

Alternatives for providing physician office-based support include training a member of the office staff to provide supportive counseling or referral to a telephone counseling service.

Referral to Telephone Counseling

Telephone counseling is an effective way to deliver smoking-cessation counseling.[17] Proactive telephone counseling results in abstinence rates comparable to individual counseling by a physician. Telephone counseling services are supported by more than 30 states for their residents and are provided to enrollees of many large health plans. This type of counseling may serve as a valuable adjunct to low-intensity, clinician-provided office counseling by providing important follow-up contact. Clinicians should become familiar with telephone counseling resources for their patients.

PHARMACOTHERAPY FOR SMOKING CESSATION

Pharmacotherapy has dramatically changed the treatment of tobacco use and dependence over the past decade and may become increasingly important for successful treatment in the future. Because of the declining prevalence of smoking, the remaining population of smokers may become more difficult to treat—the so-called "hardening hypothesis." There is evidence to suggest that this hardening has taken place.[18] The hardening of smokers is likely due to higher levels of nicotine dependence and will require adequate pharmacotherapy to achieve abstinence.

A number of different pharmacotherapy options are available to clinicians, and many are being developed (Table 11-2). Systematic reviews and meta-analyses of pharmacotherapy indicate that the odds of prolonged abstinence increase by 1.5 to 2.0 times for active pharmacotherapy compared with placebo.[3,19,20] No evidence has shown that any one of the approved medications for smoking cessation is superior to the others. For this reason, the patient's preference, confidence in the treatment, and past experience with a particular medication are important considerations in recommending pharmacotherapy.[21] Clinicians should be familiar with all the available pharmacotherapy options to optimize abstinence outcomes.

A brief discussion of available pharmacotherapy should be presented to every smoker as part of a motivational message. Every patient who is motivated to make a stop attempt will require a review of the pros and cons of the pharmacotherapy choices as part of the office intervention. The evidence is clear that the combined approach of behavioral treatment provided by a clinician and effective pharmacotherapy results in superior abstinence outcomes.[3]

Nicotine Replacement Therapy

Rationale

The rationale for the use of nicotine replacement therapy (NRT) for smoking cessation is twofold. First, therapeutic use of nicotine reduces withdrawal symptoms precipitated by tobacco abstinence. Blocking the negative reinforcement of smoking is thought to promote abstinence. Second, NRT is believed to reduce satisfaction derived from smoking by desensitizing nicotinic receptors in the brain. Reduction in the positive reinforcing effects of smoking results in fewer urges to smoke and less satisfaction if tobacco is used.[22] Regardless of the mechanism of action, the efficacy of NRT has been supported empirically over many years of observation.

In a recent systematic review of all NRT studies, the odds ratio of abstinence with active therapy at 6 to 12 months was 1.74 (95% confidence interval of 1.64 to 1.86).[20] The efficacy of NRT appears to be independent of the intensity of adjunctive behavioral treatment and support. As previously noted, higher intensity behavioral support facilitates quitting in a dose-response fashion. Thus, behavioral support does not appear to be essential for the success of NRT, but the absolute rates of abstinence will be positively influenced by the degree of behavioral support provided.[21] A number of NRT products are approved for use in the United States both by prescription and for over-the-counter sale. Specific recommendations for treatment are provided, but dose and

T A B L E   11-2

Pharmacotherapy for Smoking Cessation*

First-line Medications	Second-line Medications	Combination Regimens	Not Recommended
Nicotine replacement	Nortriptyline	Bupropion + nicotine patch	Anxiolytics
Nicotine patch	Clonidine	Nicotine gum + nicotine patch	Mecamylamine
Nicotine gum		Nicotine nasal spray + nicotine patch	SSRI antidepressants
Nicotine nasal spray			Silver acetate
Nicotine inhaler			Naltrexone
Nicotine lozenge			Lobeline
Nonnicotine medication			
Bupropion SR			

*SSRI indicates selective serotonin reuptake inhibitor; SR, sustained release.

duration of treatment should be individualized to meet the needs of each patient for relief of withdrawal symptoms and support of abstinence.

Nicotine replacement products

Nicotine patch.   Although some brands of nicotine patches still require a prescription, most are available over-the-counter as either a 16-hour or 24-hour preparation. There is no evidence that any brand has better efficacy compared with the others. A nicotine patch is applied once daily and requires no other intervention on the part of the smoker. Steady-state blood levels of nicotine are achieved in 4 to 6 hours from application and are maintained for the life (16 or 24 hours) of the patch.

Studies have shown that a standard dose of a nicotine patch (15 mg per 16 hours or 21 mg per 24 hours) achieves only approximately a 50% replacement dose compared with baseline levels of smoking.[23,24] This suggests that heavier smokers may need higher doses of replacement for the best outcomes. Studies of higher dose nicotine patch therapy (requiring more than one patch as the initial dose) have shown an early dose-response effect in favor of higher doses.[25] However, to date no studies have shown that higher dose nicotine patch therapy provides greater efficacy with regard to long-term abstinence over standard-dose treatment.[26]

Nicotine patch treatment should be initiated on the stop date with a 15-mg or 21-mg patch. Higher dose therapy may be needed for smokers who have previously relapsed or who have experienced withdrawal symptoms that were unrelieved using standard-dose treatment. If higher dose treatment is used, the dose should be matched to the baseline smoking rate or to a blood cotinine level (Table 11-3). Cotinine, a major metabolite of nicotine, can be used to quantify nicotine exposure and guide nicotine replacement.[27] The appropriate starting dose for light smokers (fewer than 10 to 15 cigarettes per day) is uncertain, although toxicity from a nicotine patch among light smokers is uncommon.[28] The recommended duration of treatment is 6 to 8 weeks, since there is no evidence that longer treatment provides greater efficacy. The 24-hour patch is available in 3 dose sizes (21 mg, 14 mg, and 7 mg) to allow for a tapering dosage schedule. Most smokers find that tapering is more acceptable than stopping treatment, although no studies have shown that tapering is more effective than simply stopping treatment after 6 to 8 weeks of standard-dose therapy.[20] A typical course involving tapering would include 4 weeks at 21 mg/day, followed by 2 weeks each at 14 mg/day and 7 mg/day. The most troublesome adverse effect of a nicotine patch is a rash at the patch application site, which may occur in up to 50% of individuals.[29] Rotation of patch sites to a different area of skin each day will minimize this problem. Topical corticosteroids may be used to treat the rash. The course

of therapy may need to be shortened depending on the severity of the skin reaction.

Nicotine gum.   Nicotine gum has been available over-the-counter in the United States since 1996 in both a 2-mg and 4-mg form. Systemic absorption through the buccal mucosa from a dose of nicotine gum occurs in 20 to 30 minutes, causing only mild subjective effects. It is important to individually instruct patients to begin using nicotine gum on their stop date and to instruct them in the proper use of nicotine gum to enhance effectiveness. The gum should be chewed slowly until a distinctive taste or tingling sensation occurs, indicating release of nicotine from the gum. At that point, the gum should be placed against the buccal mucosa between the gum and cheek and left there for 30 to 60 seconds. The gum should then be removed and chewed again slowly a few times until a similar sensation occurs, and the gum then should be "parked" again. This cycle of "chew-and-park" should be repeated for approximately 30 minutes for each piece of gum. Because the absorption of the nicotine from the gum is dependent on pH, the patient should drink no beverages, with the exception of water, while chewing the gum. The consumption of beverages other than water will lower pH and will significantly reduce the absorption of nicotine from each piece of gum.[30]

Smokers may be instructed to use the gum ad lib in response to urges to smoke or on a schedule of 1 piece every 1 or 2 hours. Most patients find that approximately 10 to 15 pieces per day will substantially suppress withdrawal symptoms. The usual starting dose is 2 mg, but smokers who smoke more than 25 cigarettes a day should receive the 4-mg gum. The usual recommended duration of therapy is about 12 weeks of ad lib use followed by 6 to 12 weeks of tapering. The most common adverse effects are nausea, hiccups, and oral or jaw pain. These effects are generally mild and may be managed with a proper chewing technique.

Nicotine nasal spray.   Nicotine nasal spray requires the smoker to intermittently use the medication to relieve symptoms of withdrawal as needed. Systemic absorption

T A B L E   11-3

Nicotine Patch Dose Based on Smoking Rate or Blood Cotinine Level

Cigarettes per Day	Cotinine (nmol/L)*	Patch Dose (mg/d)
<10	<568	7–14
10–20	568–1136	14–22
21–40	1137–1704	22–44
>40	>1704	>44+/–

*Conversion factor from nanomoles per liter to nanograms per milliliter is to divide by 5.68.

is achieved within minutes of application and is accompanied by mild subjective effects. The spray is delivered via a metered-dose dispenser that dispenses 0.5 mg of nicotine with each spray. Each 1-mg dose is obtained by spraying once in each nostril. It is recommended that patients start the medication on their stop date and begin by using 1 to 2 doses per hour on a regular basis in addition to as needed when urges to smoke occur, up to a maximum dose of 5 per hour. Most patients will achieve adequate relief of symptoms with 1 to 2 doses per hour or approximately 15 doses per day. The maximum recommended daily dose is 40 per day. Typical side effects include nasal and throat irritation, both of which tend to ameliorate over the first week of use.[31]

There is little evidence to guide the appropriate duration of therapy for nicotine nasal spray. However, a standard approach is to have individuals use the nasal spray as needed for up to 12 weeks. After 12 weeks of ad lib use, attempts should be made to taper the dosage by gradually reducing the number of doses per day. By 6 months, most individuals should complete tapering. In clinical trials, a minority of subjects continued to use nasal spray for as long as 1 year.[32-34] There was no indication that longer use promoted greater abstinence, nor were there any significant long-term adverse effects on the nasal mucosa or sinuses.[33]

Nicotine inhaler.   The nicotine inhaler became available as a prescription drug in 1998. The inhaler is a plastic cylinder in which a small capsule containing nicotine-impregnated cotton is inserted. One end of the plastic cylinder has a tapered tip and is placed in the mouth for puffing nicotine vapor that is absorbed through the buccal mucosa in a fashion similar to nicotine gum. Absorption through the buccal mucosa (and not pulmonary alveoli) occurs regardless of the inhalation technique.[35] A nicotine inhaler may substitute for some of the behavioral features of smoking by simulating the tactile and sensory stimulation of cigarette puffing.

Each capsule of nicotine-impregnated cotton contains 10 mg of nicotine, of which approximately 4 mg may be deliverable through the device. The product is used by continuously puffing on the plastic cylinder for several minutes. About 80 puffs over 20 minutes are needed to obtain 2 mg of nicotine (half of the maximum deliverable dose). Treatment should be started on the stop date and used intermittently throughout the day to suppress urges to smoke and withdrawal symptoms. The recommended initial daily dose is approximately 6 capsules per day up to a maximum of about 16 capsules per day. Adverse effects with a nicotine inhaler are mild, but some individuals may report slight mouth and throat irritation. Similar to other NRT products, the appropriate duration of therapy is uncertain. Most individuals should be instructed to use the nicotine inhaler ad lib for up to 12 weeks and then taper and discontinue use of the inhaler over the subsequent 12 weeks.

Nicotine lozenge and sublingual nicotine.   Other forms of oral, self-administered NRT have been found to be efficacious for smoking cessation. The nicotine lozenge was released for over-the-counter sale in the United States in 2002. It is available in both 2-mg and 4-mg tablet sizes. The lozenge is allowed to dissolve in the mouth without biting or chewing. Because the lozenge completely dissolves without the chewing required for nicotine gum, it is simpler to use and delivers about 25% more nicotine than comparable doses of nicotine gum. In the only clinical trial describing its use, abstinence rates were significantly greater for both the 2-mg and 4-mg treatment groups compared with placebo.[36] Recommendations for use, duration of use, and common adverse effects are similar to nicotine gum. A sublingual nicotine tablet has been tested in a small, randomized, clinical trial and found to be efficacious for smoking cessation.[37] It has been released in a limited number of countries in Europe but not in the United States.

Combination NRT.   Combinations of slow-release NRT (nicotine patch) plus an immediate-release form of NRT (nicotine-containing gum, nasal spray, inhaler, or lozenge) are attractive. These combinations provide both a constant nicotine replacement dose along with the opportunity for intermittent dosing under the control of the individual in response to urges to smoke. A limited number of clinical trials investigating combination therapy have been published. Many show combination therapy to be superior to single-agent treatment at short-term follow-up but little or no difference in abstinence rates at 12 months.[38-41] Combinations of the nicotine patch plus nicotine gum, nasal spray, or inhaler may be recommended in smokers who are unable to quit using single-agent NRT.[3]

Nonnicotine Pharmacotherapy

First-line therapy

Only one medication that does not contain nicotine has a labeled indication for smoking cessation, although second-line options also contain no nicotine.

Bupropion hydrochloride is an atypical antidepressant that is the only nonnicotine medication approved for the treatment of tobacco dependence. It is available as sustained-release tablets of 100 mg and 150 mg. Bupropion inhibits the reuptake of dopamine and norepinephrine in the central nervous system. It appears that increasing levels of dopamine in the so-called "pleasure and reward centers" of the brain may be important for the efficacy of bupropion in smoking cessation.[6] Published studies report abstinence rates with bupropion treatment that are double that of placebo treatment.[42,43] Additional clinical trials have demonstrated the efficacy of bupropion for smoking cessation in smokers with chronic lung disease, as treatment of relapsed smokers, and in African Americans.[44-46]

Bupropion is appropriate as first-line therapy for any smoker who is motivated to make a stop attempt. There are no specific indications for choosing bupropion over NRT products. Past failed attempts to stop smoking with NRT or a desire to use a nonnicotine medication may be motivating factors in choosing bupropion. Although bupropion is an antidepressant, it does not appear to have greater efficacy in individuals with past major depression over those without a history of major depression.[47] Unlike NRT, bupropion treatment should be started approximately 1 week before the target quit date. The initial dose of sustained-release bupropion (bupropion SR) is 150 mg daily for 3 days followed by 150 mg twice a day. The recommended duration of therapy after the target quit date is 7 to 12 weeks, although longer durations of treatment may be useful in some patients. A long-term study of bupropion found that it delayed relapse to smoking and was safe for use up to 1 year.[48] Combination therapy of nicotine patch with bupropion SR appears to boost abstinence rates over nicotine patch therapy alone.[43] Bupropion may have an effect on attenuating postcessation weight gain, which may make this treatment option more attractive to smokers who have a concern about weight gain.[42,48]

Side effects with bupropion are generally mild and well tolerated. The most commonly reported side effects of dry mouth, sleep disturbance, and nausea tend to ameliorate over time.[49,50] The sleep disturbance may be decreased by advising individuals to take the evening dose of bupropion before 6 pm. Seizures have also been reported with bupropion treatment but are not common.[51] There are no reported seizures in any of the published trials evaluating smoking cessation using bupropion. Both a history of a seizure disorder or any predisposition to seizures are contraindications for the use of bupropion (Table 11-4).

Other nonnicotine medications have been used in the treatment of tobacco dependence, but few investigators have evaluated these medications for their effects on long-term (6- and 12-month) efficacy. Alternatives to NRT and bupropion that have been studied for their long-term efficacy include nortriptyline hydrochloride and clonidine hydrochloride. Because of more limited data on efficacy or an unfavorable side-effect profile, these drugs should be considered only when clear contraindications for using first-line pharmacotherapy exist.

Nortriptyline.   Three randomized clinical trials have shown that the tricyclic antidepressant nortriptyline has significant effects on smoking cessation compared with placebo.[52-54] Nortriptyline does not appear to be more effective among patients with past major depression than in those without past major depression.[53] The positive effects of nortriptyline for smoking cessation do not generalize to other tricyclic antidepressants or to other classes of antidepressants.[19] Nortriptyline may be a more useful second-line agent than clonidine for smokers who are unable to tolerate first-line therapy.

T A B L E 11-4

Contraindications for Use of Sustained-release Bupropion Due to Risk of Seizures

Known seizure disorder
 Idiopathic epilepsy
 Febrile childhood seizures
 Other seizure disorder (eg, alcohol withdrawal seizure)
History of serious brain injury
 Closed head trauma
 Stroke
 Brain surgery
Drugs that lower seizure threshold (relative contraindication)
 Phenothiazines
 Alcohol (in patients clinically thought to be at increased risk of withdrawal seizures)
 Benzodiazepines (in patients clinically thought to be at increased risk of withdrawal seizures)
Eating disorders
 Anorexia
 Bulimia

Clonidine.   Clonidine is a centrally acting antihypertensive agent that has been used in the treatment of other drug addictions to reduce withdrawal. An early efficacy trial of clonidine treatment suggested an increased benefit for clonidine over placebo therapy.[55] However, later studies using clonidine in a primary care setting or using transdermal clonidine did not confirm any efficacy for clonidine treatment over placebo.[56, 57] Clonidine appears to have limited efficacy and is associated with major side effects such as dry mouth, constipation, and drowsiness. The use of clonidine should be limited to those smokers who cannot tolerate or who have a definite contraindication to the use of NRT, bupropion, or nortriptyline.

SUMMARY

Clinicians should assess the level of tobacco use of every patient at every visit. Patients who have sustained abstinence for longer than 6 months need only continued encouragement and support. Smokers who are recently abstinent may need more frequent support through office or telephone follow-up and may need continued pharmacotherapy until they feel stable in their recovery. Current smokers require an assessment of motivation for change. For smokers who are in early stages of change (so-called precontemplation and contemplation), brief advice to quit and a motivational message are needed. Smokers who are motivated to change will benefit from more extensive office counseling, including assistance with a quit plan, prescription for pharmacotherapy, and follow-up contact for relapse prevention. Counseling through a proactive telephone counseling service may be as effective as individual office counseling. If relapse occurs, reassessment of stage of change and reinstitution of higher intensity treatment or referral to a treatment center for specialized tobacco dependence treatment is appropriate. Consistent application of these principles will result in the best outcomes and is a cost-effective approach for patients.[58]

REFERENCES

1. McGinnis JM, Foege WH. Actual causes of death in the United States. *JAMA*. 1993;270:2207–2212.

2. Giovino GA. Epidemiology of tobacco use in the United States. *Oncogene*. 2002;21:7326–7340.

3. Fiore MC, Bailey WC, Cohen SJ, et al. *Treating Tobacco Use and Dependence: Clinical Practice Guideline*. Rockville, Md: US Dept of Health and Human Services, Public Health Service; 2000.

4. US Dept of Health and Human Services. *The Health Consequences of Smoking: Nicotine Addiction—A Report of the Surgeon General*. Washington, DC: US Dept of Health and Human Services; 1988.

5. Watkins SS, Koob GF, Markou A. Neural mechanisms underlying nicotine addiction: acute positive reinforcement and withdrawal. *Nicotine Tobacco Res*. 2000;2:19–37.

6. Pontieri FE, Tanda G, Orzi F, et al. Effects of nicotine on the nucleus accumbens and similarity to those of addictive drugs. *Nature*. 1996;382:255–257.

7. Hughes JR, Hatsukami D. Signs and symptoms of tobacco withdrawal. *Arch Gen Psychiatry*. 1986;43:289–294.

8. Fiore MC, Jorenby DE, Schensky AE, et al. Smoking status as the new vital sign: effect on assessment and intervention in patients who smoke. *Mayo Clin Proc*. 1995;70:209–213.

9. Prochaska JO, Goldstein MG. Process of smoking cessation: implications for clinicians. *Clin Chest Med*. 1991;12:727–735.

10. Ockene JK. Physician-delivered interventions for smoking cessation: strategies for increasing effectiveness. *Prev Med*. 1987;16:723–737.

11. Shiffman S, Read L, Maltese J, et al. Preventing relapse in ex-smokers: a self-management approach. In: Marlatt GA and Gordon JR, eds. *Relapse Prevention: Maintenance Strategies in the Treatment of Addictive Behaviors*. New York, NY: Guilford Press; 1985:472–520.

12. Hurt RD, Croghan GA, Wolter T, et al. Does smoking reduction result in reduction of biomarkers associated with harm? A pilot study using nicotine inhaler. *Nicotine Tobacco Res*. 2000;2:327–336.

13. Wilson DM, Taylor DW, Gilbert JR, et al. A randomized trial of a family physician intervention for smoking cessation. *JAMA*. 1988;260:1570–1574.

14. Brigham J, Henningfield JE, Stitzer ML. Smoking relapse: a review. *Int J Addict*. 1991;9A–10A:1239–1255.

15. Stapleton J. Cigarette smoking prevalence, cessation and relapse. *Stat Methods Med Res*. 1998;7:187–203.

16. Hays JT, Wolter TD, Eberman KM, et al. Residential (inpatient) treatment compared with outpatient treatment for nicotine dependence. *Mayo Clin Proc*. 2001;76:124–133.

17. Zhu SH, Anderson CM, Tedeschi GJ, et al. Evidence of real-world effectiveness of a telephone quitline for smokers. *N Engl J Med*. 2002;347:1087–1093.

18. Irvin JE, Brandon TH. The increasing recalcitrance of smokers in clinical trials. *Nicotine Tobacco Res*. 2000;2:79–84.

19. Hughes JR, Stead LF, Lancaster T. *Antidepressants for Smoking Cessation (Cochrane Review)* [software]. Vol 1. Oxford, England: Cochrane Library; 2002.

20. Silagy C, Lancaster T, Stead L, et al. *Nicotine Replacement Therapy for Smoking Cessation (Cochrane Review)* [software]. Vol 4. Oxford, England: Cochrane Library; 2002.

21. Hughes JR, Goldstein MG, Shiffman S. Recent advances in the pharmacotherapy of smoking. *JAMA*. 1999;281:72–76.

22. Benowitz NL. Pharmacology of nicotine: addiction and therapeutics. *Annu Rev Pharmacol Toxicol*. 1996;36:597–613.

23. Hurt RD, Dale LC, Offord KP, et al. Serum nicotine and cotinine levels during nicotine patch therapy. *Clin Pharmacol Ther*. 1993;54:98–106.

24. Hurt RD, Dale LC, Frederickson PA. Nicotine patch therapy for smoking cessation combined with physician advice and nurse follow-up: one-year outcome and percentage of nicotine replacement. *JAMA*. 1994;271:595–600.

25. Hughes JR, Lesmes GR, Hatsukami DK, et al. Are higher doses of nicotine replacement more effective for smoking cessation? *Nicotine Tobacco Res*. 1999;1:169–174.

26. Jorenby DE, Smith SS, Miore MC, et al. Varying nicotine patch dose and type of smoking cessation counseling. *JAMA*. 1995;274:1347–1352.

27. Lawson GM, Hurt RD, Dale LC, et al. Application of serum nicotine and plasma cotinine concentrations to assessment of nicotine replacement in light, moderate, and heavy smokers undergoing transdermal therapy. *J Clin Pharmacol*. 1998;38:502–509.

28. Dale LC, Hurt RD, Offord KP, et al. High dose nicotine patch therapy: percent replacement and smoking cessation with placebo 11, 22 and 44 mg/24 hour doses. *JAMA*. 1995;274:1353–1358.

29. Fiore MC, Smith SS, Jorenby DE, et al. The effectiveness of the nicotine patch for smoking cessation: a meta-analysis. *JAMA*. 1994;271:1940–1947.

30. Henningfield JE, Aleksandras R, Cooper TM, et al. Drinking coffee and carbonated beverages blocks absorption of nicotine from nicotine polacrilex gum. *JAMA*. 1990;264:1560–1564.

31. Hurt RD, Dale LC, Croghan GA, et al. Nicotine nasal spray for smoking cessation: pattern of use, side effects, relief of withdrawal symptoms and cotinine levels. *Mayo Clin Proc*. 1998;73:118–125.

32. Sutherland G, Stapleton JA, Russell MAH, et al. Randomized controlled trial of nasal nicotine spray in smoking cessation. *Lancet*. 1992;340:324–329.

33. Hjalmarson A, Franzon M, Westin A, et al. Effect of nicotine nasal spray on smoking cessation. A randomized, placebo-controlled, double-blind study. *Arch Intern Med*. 1994;154:2567–2572.

34. Schneider NG, Olmstead R, Mody FV, et al. Efficacy of a nicotine nasal spray in smoking cessation: a placebo-controlled, double-blind trial. *Addiction*. 1995;90:1671–1682.

35. Bergstrom M, Nordbert A, Lunell E, et al. Regional deposition of inhaled 11C-nicotine vapor in the human airways as visualized by positron emission tomography. *Clin Pharmacol Ther*. 1995;57:309–317.

36. Shiffman S, Dresler CM, Hajek P, et al. Efficacy of a nicotine lozenge for smoking cessation. *Arch Intern Med*. 2002;162:1267–1276.

37. Glover ED, Glover PN, Franzon M, et al. A comparison of nicotine sublingual tablet and placebo for smoking cessation. *Nicotine Tobacco Res*. 2002;4:441–450.

38. Kornitzer M, Boutsen M, Dramaix M, et al. Combined use of nicotine patch and gum in smoking cessation: A placebo-controlled clinical trial. *Prev Med*. 1995;24:41–47.

39. Puska P, Korhonen HJ, Vartiaaninen, et al. Combined use of nicotine patch and gum compared with gum alone in smoking cessation. *Tobacco Control*. 1995;4:231–235.

40. Blondal T, Gudmundsson LJ, Olafsdottir I, et al. Nicotine nasal spray with nicotine patch for smoking cessation: randomized trial with six year follow up. *Br Med J*. 1999;318:285–289.

41. Bohadana A, Nilsson F, Rasmussen T, et al. Nicotine inhaler and nicotine patch as a combination therapy for smoking cessation: a randomized, double-blind, placebo-controlled trial. *Arch Intern Med*. 2000;160:3128–3134.

42. Hurt RD, Sachs DP, Glover ED, et al. A comparison of sustained-release bupropion and placebo for smoking cessation. *N Engl J Med*. 1997;337:1195–1202.

43. Jorenby DE, Leischow SJ, Nides MA, et al. A controlled trial of sustained-release bupropion, a nicotine patch, or both for smoking cessation. *N Engl J Med*. 1999;340:685–691.

44. Tashkin DP, Kanner R, Bailey W, et al. Smoking cessation in patients with chronic obstructive pulmonary disease: a double-blind, placebo-controlled, randomised trial. *Lancet*. 2001;357:1571–1575.

45. Gonzales DH, Nides MA, Ferry LH, et al. Bupropion SR as an aid to smoking cessation in smokers treated previously with bupropion: a randomized placebo-controlled study. *Clin Pharmacol Ther*. 2001;69:438–444.

46. Ahluwalia JS, Harris KJ, Catley D, et al. Sustained-release bupropion for smoking cessation in African Americans: a randomized controlled trial. *JAMA*. 2002;288:468–474.

47. Hayford KE, Patten CA, Rummans TA, et al. Efficacy of bupropion for smoking cessation in smokers with a former history of major depression or alcoholism. *Br J Psychiatry*. 1999;174:173–178.

48. Hays JT, Hurt RD, Rigotti NA, et al. Sustained-release bupropion for pharmacologic relapse prevention after smoking cessation: a randomized, controlled trial. *Ann Intern Med*. 2001;135:423–433.

49. Settle EC, Stahl SM, Batey SR, et al. Safety profile of sustained-release bupropion in depression: results of three clinical trials. *Clin Ther*. 1999;21:454–463.

50. Hays JT, Ebbert JO. Bupropion for the treatment of tobacco dependence: guidelines for balancing risks and benefits. *CNS Drugs*. 2003;17:71–83.

51. Johnston JA, Lineberry CG, Ascher JA, et al. A 102-center prospective study of seizure in association with bupropion. *J Clin Psychiatry*. 1991;52:450–456.

52. Prochazka AV, Weaver MJ, Keller RT, et al. A randomized trial of nortriptyline for smoking cessation. *Arch Intern Med*. 1998;158:2035–2039.

53. Hall SM, Reus VI, Munoz RF, et al. Nortriptyline and cognitive-behavioral therapy in the treatment of cigarette smoking. *Arch Gen Psychiatry*. 1998;55:683–690.

54. da Costa CL, Younes RN, Cruz-Lourenco MT. A prospective, randomized, double-blind study comparing nortriptyline to placebo. *Chest*. 2002;122:403–408.

55. Glassman AH, Stetner F, Walsh BT, et al. Heavy smokers, smoking cessation and clonidine: results of a double-blind, randomized trial. *JAMA*. 1988;259:2863–2866.

56. Franks P, Hays J, Bell B. Randomized, controlled trial of clonidine for smoking cessation in a primary care setting. *JAMA*. 1989;262:3011–3013.

57. Prochazka AV, Petty TL, Nett L, et al. Transdermal clonidine reduces some withdrawal symptoms but did not increase smoking cessation. *Arch Intern Med*. 1992;152:2065–2069.

58. Croghan IT, Offord KP, Evans RW, et al. Cost-effectiveness of treating nicotine dependence: the Mayo Clinic experience. *Mayo Clin Proc*. 1997;72:917–924.

RESOURCES

All Surgeon Generals reports on smoking and health available online.

Web site: sgreports.nlm.nih.gov/NN/

The American Legacy Foundation was established with money from the tobacco litigation master settlement agreement and contains important information on tobacco treatment and advocacy issues.

Web site: www.AmericanLegacy.org

The Behavioral Risk Factor Surveillance System of the CDC contains the most useful health risk factor data including detailed tobacco use statistics.

Web site: www.cdc.gov/brfss

The CDC Office on Smoking and Health has useful up-to-date information on treatment and tobacco control issues.

Web site: www.cdc.gov/tobacco/

The Tobacco Use and Dependence Guideline Panel. *A clinical practice guideline for treating tobacco use and dependence.* JAMA 2000;238:3244–3254. [A summary of the practice guideline produced by the USPHS for tobacco dependence treatment.]

West R, McNeill A, Raw M. *Smoking cessation guideline for health professionals.* Thorax 2000;55:987–999. [The evidence-based practice guideline published by the Health Education Authority of the UK for smoking cessation.]

chapter 12

Sleep Disorders

Lois E. Krahn, MD

INTRODUCTION

The relatively new field of sleep medicine has not matured to the point where a great deal of research has been conducted regarding prevention strategies for sleep disorders. Most studies in sleep medicine to date have been designed to examine the diagnostic procedures, etiology, clinical course, and treatment options. This chapter will review the available data about the interventions that may help in the prevention of specific sleep disorders. In general, much of what is known about the prevention of sleep disorders relates to insomnia and shift work. Prevention strategies in sleep medicine depend on individuals taking responsibility to promote healthy sleep, in addition to workplace measures that facilitate adjustment to changing work schedules. Medical interventions such as medications should not play a major role.

The primary care physician has a special role in helping to improve the quality of sleep and prevent the development of specific sleep disorders. Sleep disorders are common, yet few patients specifically seek health care because of their sleep complaints.[1] If patients mention insomnia or other sleep concerns, they do so during an assessment of another medical issue. Accordingly, physicians should inquire about the quality and quantity of a patient's sleep.[2] Using a standardized form to collect patient-provided information about a variety of health matters may be most efficient. Follow-up questioning can identify specific factors and behaviors that may compromise sleep. Queries should be made into the patient's attempts to hasten or extend sleep and specifically look for practices, such as the habitual consumption of alcohol, that are actually detrimental. The primary care physician has a clear opportunity to provide patient education about the importance of getting adequate sleep, as well as the means to promote healthy sleep.

PHYSIOLOGY OF NORMAL SLEEP

A brief discussion about sleep physiology is included to help define the 2 major components of sleep. Sleep can be divided into rapid eye movement (REM) sleep, which is characterized by high levels of cortical activation in the presence of muscle atonia to prevent corresponding movements, and non-REM (NREM) sleep, which consists of 4 stages. Table 12-1 summarizes the characteristics and percentage of time spent in each sleep stage in healthy middle-aged adults.

As the sleep cycle progresses, the electroencephalogram (EEG) progresses to stage 3/4 sleep and gradually returns to the most common stage, stage 2 sleep. Stage 2 sleep evolves into the first REM sleep episode of the night. The first REM episode is often brief and typically begins 70 to

TABLE 12-1

Sleep Stages in Healthy Adults

Stage	Percentage	PSG Characteristics	Physiological Changes
Stage 1	2–5	Slow eye movements	Easy to arouse
Stage 2	45–55	Spindles, K complexes	More difficult to arouse
Stage 3/4	13–23	Slow EEG frequency	Difficult to arouse
REM	20–25	Rapid eye movements, muscle atonia, increased EEG frequency	Variable arousal threshold; penile engorgement

PSG indicates polysomnography; REM, rapid eye movement; and EEG, electroencephalographic.

100 minutes after the patient falls asleep. The sleep cycle repeats 4 to 5 times during the night, with the subsequent REM episodes lasting longer than the first (Fig 12-1). In general, slow wave (NREM) sleep is more common early in the night, and REM sleep periods become longer toward morning. Because the last REM episode occurs at the very end of the major sleep period, people recall their dreams and men experience morning erections.

The data in Table 12-1 are useful as normative data since sleep study reports typically describe the percentage of the night spent in each complete stage, allowing comparison between individuals without sleep disorders and patients with sleep disorders. In healthy elderly subjects, the relative percentage of time spent in slow wave (stages 3 and 4) sleep decreases, and sleep is generally more fragmented. Patients with disrupted sleep often spend most of the night in stages 1 and 2, with little slow wave or REM sleep. The exact role that slow wave sleep and REM sleep play in a refreshing night's sleep is not well understood, but substantial reductions in either state can lead to undesirable results, including daytime sleepiness, depressed mood, and cognitive impairment. In animal studies, prolonged total sleep deprivation has resulted in death attributed to sepsis due to suspected underlying autoimmune compromise.[3]

SOCIETAL CONSEQUENCES OF PARTIAL SLEEP DEPRIVATION

Inadequate sleep, otherwise known as partial sleep deprivation, is a major public health problem. Total sleep deprivation, where a person does not obtain any sleep whatsoever for more than 24 to 30 hours is uncommon under normal circumstances and does not warrant discussion in this chapter. Nevertheless, partial sleep deprivation is widespread. One difficulty in doing research in this area is that no consensus exists regarding

the minimum number of hours of sleep considered sufficient. Determining a minimum is difficult because of the variability in individual need for sleep, with a range as wide as 5 to 12 hours.

Sleep deprivation is a well-recognized cause of accidents on roadways and in industrial settings. Sleepy and inattentive drivers contribute to 30% of motor vehicle accidents and 83% of fatalities.[4] Drivers younger than 30 years are at highest risk and are responsible for 60% of all sleep-related crashes. In many circumstances, a synergistic combination of sleep deprivation and alcohol intoxication contributes to poor judgment, reckless behavior, and impaired response time. Other than getting adequate sleep, the recommended strategy for combating driver sleepiness is a 30-minute break with at least a 15-minute nap or 150 mg of coffee.[5] Exercise, cold air, and listening to the radio are ineffective. In industrial settings, sleep deprivation can lead to workplace accidents. Often, sleep deprivation is related to shift work, which will be discussed later in this chapter.

INSUFFICIENT SLEEP

In our society, with numerous 24-hour services and conveniences becoming more common, people do not make sleep as high a priority as other activities. This condition of voluntary sleep deprivation is called the insufficient sleep syndrome. Since the introduction of artificial lighting that permits people to pursue activities after dark, the amount of time spent asleep has steadily decreased. The scope of this problem is not well known. Few studies have been designed to investigate patients who are sleep-deprived without reporting difficulty attaining sleep. One study of 24,600 European subjects in the general population described a prevalence rate of 2.1%.[6] However, many experts believe this condition to be more common than this single study suggests. Nonetheless, persons choosing not to obtain sufficient

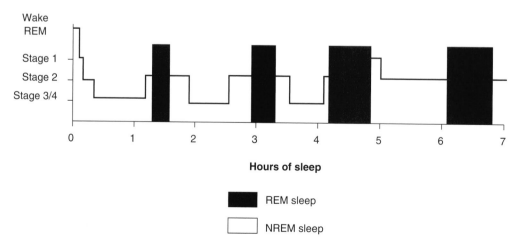

FIGURE 12-1

Hours of Sleep

sleep, unrelated to other problems such as shift work or insomnia, can be at higher risk of both motor vehicle accidents and workplace accidents. Affected persons generally do not present to physicians or sleep specialists because they are aware of the cause of their daytime sleepiness and fatigue. Patient education about the value of adequate sleep is of great importance relative to this condition.

INSOMNIA

Insomnia is another major cause of sleep deprivation. In contrast to the insufficient sleep syndrome in which people do not make an adequate effort to sleep, insomniacs try to sleep adequately but complain of insufficient sleep leading to adverse daytime circumstances. Insomnia is present when someone perceives obtaining inadequate sleep. Because objective data regarding the duration or continuity of sleep is not necessary, sleep studies are not required for the assessment of insomnia. Insomnia can take several forms. The 2 most common are initial insomnia (also referred to as delayed sleep onset or difficulties with initiating sleep) and sleep maintenance difficulties (awakenings in the middle of the night or prematurely in the morning).

According to a study reported by Mallon, Broman, and Hetta in *International Psychogeriatrics* in 2000, the incidence of insomnia increases with age with chronic insomnia affecting 36% of people over the age of 65 years. In the United States, approximately 30% of adults report occasional insomnia and 10% describe persistent insomnia. The consequences of untreated insomnia include impaired concentration, decreased memory, reduced ability to fulfill roles, and decreased enjoyment of interpersonal relationships.[7] Chronic insomnia frequently develops in conjunction with a psychiatric disorder, typically a depressive, anxiety, or substance abuse disorder.

Because the term *insomnia* refers to both a symptom and a diagnosis, a careful evaluation is required to understand the condition's significance for an individual patient. In addition to the psychiatric disorders that are associated with unsatisfactory sleep, a plethora of medical disorders also can have symptoms that compromise the quality or quantity of sleep. These include gastroesophageal reflux disease, chronic obstructive pulmonary disease, congestive heart failure, chronic pain, and endocrine conditions such as hyperthyroidism. In circumstances when a psychiatric or medical condition appears to interfere with the patient getting adequate sleep, stabilizing the primary disease should be the first step in trying to improve or prevent sleep difficulties. In rare cases after an extensive evaluation when no psychiatric or medical causes are identified, primary insomnia is considered a separate diagnosis rather than a symptom or complaint.

PRIMARY PREVENTION OF SLEEP DISORDERS

This section will review the factors that promote high-quality sleep. The term *sleep hygiene* frequently is used to describe optimal sleep conditions. Nonetheless, relatively few physicians or patients have a complete understanding of all the issues that fall into this area. Sleep is a sensitive and dynamic state that can be perturbed by a multitude of avoidable factors. For the purposes of this chapter, sleep hygiene will be divided into these categories: sleep environment, lifestyle choices while preparing to sleep, relaxation techniques, regular sleep-wake schedule, exercise, avoiding alcohol use close to bedtime, limiting caffeine intake, proper diet, avoiding weight gain, and prevention of anemia (Table 12-2).

Sleep Environment

Falling and staying asleep depend on a conducive environment. Many different environmental factors can interfere with falling asleep or staying asleep. These include loud noise (traffic, alarms, mechanical sounds, conversations, television), extreme temperature (cold or heat), body position (standing, seated), pillow choice (feather, synthetic, other), and bedding (mattress type and firmness). Surprisingly, some people consistently attempt to sleep in adverse circumstances, such as a night shift worker sleeping at home with his spouse's child care business in the same dwelling, without fully appreciating the impact on their sleep. When traveling, difficult circumstances may make it necessary to tolerate

TABLE 12-2

Means to Prevent Insomnia and Other Sleep Disorders

Sleep Disorder	Technique
Primary insomnia	Optimal sleep environment Appropriate bedtime activities Stress management skills Regular sleep-wake schedule Carefully timed exercise Limited alcohol use Limited caffeine use
Secondary insomnia	Treatment of depressive and anxiety disorders Stabilization of chronic pain, nausea, gastroesophageal reflux, and other conditions
Obstructive sleep apnea	Lean body weight Adequate nasal and oral airways Avoidance of alcohol close to bedtime
Restless legs syndrome	Prevention of anemia

suboptimal sleeping conditions for a short time. Despite getting inadequate sleep for several days, people can generally adapt and continue to function.

Lifestyle Choices While Preparing to Sleep

Lifestyle choices may compromise sleep quality. The 30 to 60 minutes before desired sleep onset should be treated as a transitional time from the stimulatory activities of the day to relaxed state of sleep. Many individuals with hectic schedules and multiple responsibilities continue engaging in mentally or physically demanding activities right up to bedtime.[8] Diverse activities such as preparing for the next day's work by answering e-mails or reading professional materials can contribute to heightened anxiety. Stressful nonprofessional activities, such as preparing taxes or planning a social event, can be equally invigorating. When a person pursues cognitively demanding tasks, muscle tension increases. This situation is a far cry from the generalized muscle relaxation that is the prerequisite for sleep onset. Some individuals take considerable time to cease thinking about these matters and relax their mind and body.[9] Although relaxation techniques may be helpful in many cases, the preferable approach is to refrain from these stimulating activities before bedtime. More suitable activities include routine hygiene practices, watching relaxing television, reading for pleasure, and romantic activities.[10]

Insomnia can develop when persons no longer associate their bed or bedroom with sleep. The prevalence of this phenomenon is unknown. If patients use their bed for other activities, for example, writing term papers or paying bills, they eventually may no longer view their bed as a place for sleep. Some patients with insomnia have developed conditioning because they have pursued activities associated with arousal in bed, and they no longer expect to fall asleep. Patients with this type of conditioned insomnia typically fall asleep more readily in an unfamiliar bed where these expectations do not apply. Prevention of this maladaptive conditioned state is more desirable than later attempting to regain the patient's confidence in their ability to fall asleep in their own bed.

Relaxation Techniques

All persons under stress can benefit if they are able to consciously relax the body and mind. Many individuals develop relaxation techniques intuitively. Supplemental instruction and practice of relaxation techniques are universally helpful. Given enough psychological stress, negative or positive, all persons have a threshold above which they may respond by feeling anxious and physically tense. For example, elite athletes vying to perform at a stellar level under extreme stress may seek the input of a

sports psychologist to enhance their relaxation techniques. Having a "toolbox" of cognitive and/or behavioral techniques allows a person to adapt to adversely stressful circumstances. An individual can employ these tools to avoid prolonged sleeplessness. The effectiveness of these practices has been repeatedly demonstrated in well-designed clinical trials of young and aging patients when insomnia interventions are overseen by expert sleep psychologists.[11,12] Their applicability, when recommended as prevention strategies for normal sleepers or when prescribed in routine clinical practice, has not been studied. Probable limitations of applying cognitive or behavioral techniques include the physician's lack of knowledge, having adequate time to teach the intervention, patient acceptance, and patient adherence to employing them when the need arises. For these reasons, when patients complain of insomnia, hypnotic medications are more routinely provided than is relaxation training.

Multiple relaxation techniques are known to be beneficial for hastening sleep onset, allowing the individual to select the ones with which he or she feels most comfortable. Some people are able to consciously relax by simply listening to music, watching television, or reading. Others need to start relaxing by using a relaxation tape with cues designed to encourage peaceful thoughts and release of muscle tension.[13] Other practices include a technique similar to yoga and progressive muscle relaxation, where the participant sequentially constricts and then slowly relaxes each muscle group.[14] This approach should be used cautiously with patients with preexisting chronic pain, since it may cause them to remain preoccupied with their physical state. An alternative relaxation exercise is diaphragmatic breathing, encouraging the patient to concentrate on slow, deep breathing.

Other relaxation practices focus more specifically on thoughts. In guided visual imagery, a person spends an extended time (eg, 15 minutes) imagining himself or herself to be in a serene setting. Depending on the person's life experience, he or she may conjure up images of an alpine lake, tropical beach, shady hammock, or other scene. The image is elaborated to encompass all the senses, including vision, hearing, touch, and smell.

Regular Sleep-Wake Schedule

Human beings have many bodily functions, including temperature and hormonal shifts, as well as sleep, that conform to a 24-hour circadian rhythm. In general, people have less difficulty falling asleep if they strive for the same bedtime day after day, which produces a predictable sleep-wake rhythm. A study examined the sleep habits of adolescents, looking at the relationship between an irregular sleep-wake schedule and unsatisfactory daytime functioning. They found that during the school week adolescents were staying up later but keeping their wake-up time consistent, with the result being 40 to 50 minutes less sleep than on the weekends.[15] Students getting less sleep (<6 hours, 45 minutes) had a later bedtime during the week as well as a more pronounced tendency to stay up later (>120 minutes) on weekends. They were likely to have poorer academic performance, depressed mood, and increased excessive daytime sleepiness. Adolescents may have more of a vulnerability to a delayed sleep phase (late bedtime and late wake-up time, but satisfactory daytime functioning as long as they get adequate sleep) than do adults. Young adults are likely at higher risk of an irregular sleep schedule that resolves as they mature and develop the sleep schedule of middle adulthood. Improving the consistency of sleep-wake schedules in college undergraduate students by recommending a minimum of 7.5 hours sleep a night on a regular schedule increased daytime alertness and decreased subjective daytime sleepiness.[16]

Exercise

Recent studies have demonstrated the positive impact of habitual moderate exercise on sleep initiation, duration, and quality.[17] A reduced risk of sleep problems was noted with regular physical activity at least once a week and at an intensity for men of walking briskly for at least 6 city blocks.[18] Extremely prolonged strenuous exercise, however, may be detrimental for sleep, possibly because of physical discomfort. The timing of exercise should be carefully considered. A vigorous physical workout within several hours of bedtime increases body temperature and muscle tension and can promote an excited stimulated mindset. These conditions take time to fade and, in the meantime, can interfere with sleep onset. Exercise is preferable at least 4 hours before the desired bedtime so as not to delay sleep onset.

Alcohol Use

Alcohol is a sedating agent and, for this reason, people sometimes deliberately consume alcohol to facilitate sleep. An estimated 28% of patients presenting with insomnia have substance abuse disorders. A recent study in people with insomnia found 10% used alcohol; 10%, over-the-counter medications; and 8%, prescription medication. Five percent of respondents used both alcohol and medications.[19] In this study, persons who exclusively used alcohol to facilitate sleep were more likely to be younger, male, and single and complained of excessive daytime sleepiness more than the other user groups. Sometimes, alcohol use becomes more habitual because of a mistaken belief that it prevents insomnia. In actuality, alcohol has several detrimental effects on sleep that outweigh the benefits. The initial sedation is short-lived and within hours alcohol is metabolized. Use of alcohol at bedtime contributes to difficulties with sleep maintenance, that is, increased awakenings later in the night.[20] The decreased quality of sleep in the second half of the night has been associated with excessive daytime sleepiness.[21] Long-term alcohol use, as well as long-term use of benzodiazepines, can lead to a reduction in the time spent in slow wave sleep. Although empirical data are limited, decreased slow wave sleep is viewed as incompatible with refreshing, high-quality sleep.

Since alcohol is a potent muscle relaxant, the musculature of the upper airway is more prone to collapse, leading to snoring. Patients with a tendency toward upper airway narrowing signified by preexisting snoring can experience more airway obstruction. Hypopneas and apneas, which in turn trigger arousals from sleep, can develop after alcohol ingestion, revealing the incremental decrease in airway patency until the alcohol is metabolized. Patients should be advised to refrain from drinking alcohol within 1 hour of bedtime.

Especially in younger patients, alcohol consumption can put them at risk of sleepwalking and other abnormal behaviors arising out of NREM sleep. The typical scenario is binge drinking, in conjunction with staying up later than usual. The abnormal behaviors, classed by sleep specialists as parasomnias, can range from mild sleep talking to life-threatening sleepwalking, in which the person may fall from a height or otherwise go in harm's way. The NREM parasomnias can develop for the first time under these fertile conditions. Not unexpectedly, if the patient has a history of sleep-walking or related behaviors during childhood, they are at higher risk of engaging in inappropriate behaviors when intoxicated.

Caffeine Use

Caffeine is one of the most widely used stimulants. Recently some brands of water and mints have added caffeine, promoting that these improve vigilance. Judicious use of small quantities of caffeine (no more than 300 mg or 3 cups of regular coffee and restricted to the morning) is tolerated by most people.[22] Many persons enjoy coffee with their breakfast and perceive coffee to be desirable to promote a bright mood and alertness. Daily caffeine use quickly leads to a physical dependence. If caffeine is abruptly discontinued, a headache of varying intensity can develop. Other, more serious withdrawal symptoms are absent. Patients with a history of cardiac arrhythmia, tachycardia, palpitations, or anxiety are typically advised to avoid caffeine use. If ingested after noon or in larger than 300-mg quantities, caffeine can lead to initial insomnia or sleep maintenance difficulties. Studies have shown increased arousals from sleep throughout the night even when 200 mg of caffeine is consumed in the morning.[23] Poor quality sleep at night can lead to daytime fatigue. Patients may increase their consumption of caffeine to self-medicate the fatigue, unaware that they are aggravating the situation.[24]

Patients can easily avoid this situation by partially or totally substituting decaffeinated products. A gradual taper of caffeine may be initially necessary for patients consuming excessive quantities.

Diet

The relationship between sleep and diet is of interest to many patients but has not been extensively studied. Each year around Thanksgiving, television talk shows discuss the possibility that tryptophan-rich turkey will promote sleep. Although tryptophan is thought to enhance sleep, few studies have been conducted of tryptophan-rich foods such as poultry and milk, resulting in a paucity of evidence demonstrating its benefits.[25]

More is known about foods that may be detrimental to sleep. Any dietary factor that enhances the dilation of the lower esophageal sphincter (eg, citrus juice) can contribute to gastroesophageal reflux disease. Reflux and dyspepsia are well known to delay sleep initiation and trigger arousals from sleep.[26]

Weight Gain

Obesity is a growing public health crisis in North America in unprecedented numbers of children, adolescents, and adults. In the absence of obstructive sleep apnea, obese adolescents obtained less sleep and were less physically active than were adolescents who were not obese.[27] Furthermore, the relationship between obesity and sleep-disordered breathing, specifically obstructive sleep apnea, is well accepted. Excessive adipose tissue, especially if distributed to the upper body and neck region, increases the resistance and collapsibility of the upper airway. A neck circumference in men of 16.5 cm or larger is accepted as a risk factor for obstructive sleep apnea.[28] A narrowed upper airway can lead to snoring (vibrations of the soft tissue) and partial airway closure. Obstruction of airflow during sleep leads to hypopneas and apneas. A large population-based study demonstrated that more than 11 apneas and hypopneas per hour leads to a 42% increase in the odds of cardiovascular disease vs fewer than 2 apneas and hypopneas per hour.[29]

The presence of obstructive sleep apnea increases the risk of several other preventable medical disorders, including hypertension, coronary artery disease, congestive heart failure, and stroke. Additional factors that are associated with an increased risk of obstructive sleep apnea, particularly when comorbid with obesity, are enlarged tonsils and adenoids, retrognathia or micrognathia, nasal septal deviation, seasonal allergies associated with nasal obstruction, severe hypothyroidism, neuromuscular weakness, and craniofacial abnormalities. These conditions create either an increased risk of upper airway obstruction or decreased neuromuscular tone that compromises airway patency.

Moderate weight loss of 5% to 10% of body weight usually decreases apneas and hypopneas and improves sleep quality in people with obstructive sleep apnea.

Anemia

Restless legs syndrome is a condition that affects 10% of the population.[30] Four cardinal symptoms are recognized:

- Symptoms worse in the evening or night
- Symptoms present during rest or inactivity
- Symptoms relieved by movement or stretching
- Unpleasant leg sensations accompanied by a need to move the legs

Iron deficiency is now established as a cause of restless legs syndrome. Iron is an essential cofactor for tyrosine hydroxylase, the rate-limiting step in the synthesis of dopamine. The severity of the symptoms is increased when serum ferritin levels are less than 50 mg/(g/L).[31] Patients should be asked about any anemia, gastrointestinal blood loss, menorrhagia, or frequent blood donation. Restless legs syndrome also has been associated with peripheral neuropathy, certain medications, chronic renal failure, and pregnancy. Familial cases have been described. Restless legs syndrome currently is treated with iron replacement as well as medications largely from the dopamine agonist category.

SHIFT WORK

An increasing number of people are employed in jobs that involve working shifts. The type of shift varies but can encompass early morning start times; on-call responsibilities; and evening, night, split, or 24-hour shifts. Shift workers have higher rates of both insomnia and excessive daytime sleepiness. Workers with rotating schedules, as opposed to working a straight second (evening) shift or third (night) shift, are at higher risk of complications because their sleep-wake circadian rhythm is constantly adapting to a new timetable.[32] Environmental factors, such as neighborhood noise or sunlight, make initiating or maintaining sleep during the day difficult. Many shift workers obtain insufficient sleep because they sacrifice daytime sleep due to a preference to spend time with family, perform leisure activities, or run errands. Shift work puts individuals at higher risk of several problems. A coexisting sleep disorder such as obstructive sleep apnea increases the probability of excessive daytime sleepiness.[33]

Working when not fully alert poses the risk of performance problems due to inadequate vigilance. Fatigue can predispose an individual to cognitive or motor impairment.[34] Many industrial or transportation incidents, including the Exxon Valdez oil spill in Prince William Sound, Alaska, and the Three Mile Island nuclear power accident near Harrisburg, Pa, have occurred at night or in the predawn hours, suggesting that worker fatigue may have been a contributing factor.

Missing opportunities to interact with family or friends due to shift work or recovery sleep can lead to social problems and family strain. Young children in particular may have difficulty understanding that a parent must be allowed to get adequate sleep after returning home from work. Recent work has found an increase in common respiratory infections and gastroenteritis in shift workers—the third shift more than the second—and it has been postulated that fatigue renders employees vulnerable to infection.[35]

Some individuals have an affinity for functioning well at certain times. For example, people with a tendency toward a delayed sleep phase may actually cope satisfactorily with an evening work schedule provided that they can sleep late the following morning. For others, several strategies have been identified to assist workers who must incorporate shift work into their lifestyle. In general, older persons find it harder to adapt to shift changes than younger individuals. Meals should be timed to promote sleep. Hunger or foods that cause dyspepsia may fragment sleep. The workplace environment should be carefully planned to take into account the worker's safety and sleep needs. Bright lights and a slightly cool air temperature may improve alertness. Ideally, attention should be given to the type of tasks undertaken by employees, especially on the night shift, with monotonous duties interspersed with more stimulating activities.

The sleeping environment at home may need to be more extensively modified for a shift worker. A quiet and dark bedroom can be arranged for a shift worker sleeping during the day. Special window coverings may be required. The telephone should be switched off and messages collected with an answering machine or voice mail. Family members should be urged not to awaken someone in the midst of their major sleep period. Sleep hygiene should be optimized.

Studies have shown that workers cope better when switching from one shift to another if they delay, rather than advance, their work and sleep time. For instance, if they move from evening to night shift, most individuals adjust more easily to the change. Preparing for an approaching shift change by gradually shifting the bedtime and wake-up time by 2 hours, starting several days before the switch, has been found to be beneficial. Family responsibilities often complicate careful sleep schedule adjustments of this type, however.

Other effective coping strategies include taking a break during work hours. Recent study has focused on the transportation industry, specifically airline personnel, for whom a 30-minute nap part way through the shift increases productivity, reduces fatigue, and improves employee satisfaction. Long-haul aircraft now have been designed to include bunks or reclining seats for scheduled naps.[36]

Some employers and employees prefer work schedules that use permanent shift assignments. Night shift workers should endeavor to keep to a consistent sleep-wake schedule even on days when they do not work. Reverting to nighttime sleep over a weekend or a single day off presents adjustment problems similar to those faced by workers assigned to rotating shifts. Once again, family responsibilities and the need to perform business and errands at institutions that operate exclusively during the day make it difficult for people to follow an exclusive night activity schedule.

On-call arrangements present another complication. These individuals cannot predict when they will be required to perform a task. Typically the time block for on-call workers is longer, for example, 24 hours, than for most other shift work. Workers cannot plan their sleep-wake schedule. Naps may be especially important under these circumstances. Although in general people are urged to have a major sleep period every 24 hours as opposed to several shorter stretches of sleep, naps are reasonable if that is the only means by which adequate sleep can be obtained.

Medications have been examined to help shift workers initiate sleep at the desired time. Regular use of long-acting benzodiazepines creates the risk of physical dependence as well as a hangover effect, especially with longer acting agents. Short-term use of a newer nonbenzodiazepine hypnotic such as zaleplon or zolpidem tartrate is preferable to a benzodiazepine. Caution must be taken even with these agents, since they have not been studied or approved for long-term use. Shift workers should first fully explore means to get adequate sleep by means of careful schedule changes, making sufficient sleep a priority, and taking naps if indicated. The hypnotics provide symptomatic relief without addressing the underlying circadian rhythm disturbance inherent in shift work.[37] In general, there is agreement that prescribed psychostimulant medications are not an appropriate means to treat shift work-related sleep disorders. As with the benzodiazepines, patients should be discouraged from what might become long-term use of a habituating medication and instead be encouraged to rely on scheduling issues and naps.

Alcohol should be avoided as a means of inducing sleep because of its detrimental effects on the patency of the upper airway and tendency to reduce the quality of NREM sleep. Caffeine may be useful to boost alertness but should be avoided close to bedtime in order not to interfere with sleep onset.[38] As in jet lag, bright light therapy delivered at precise times may be a useful option to treat shift work-related sleep disorders. Melatonin has been explored as a possible chronotherapy agent, although it is not currently in wide use. Very recently, melatonin agonists have been synthesized and show promise in pilot studies.[39]

REFERENCES

1. Ancoli-Isreal S, Roth T. Characteristics of insomnia in the United States: results of the 1991 National Sleep Foundation Survey. *Sleep.* 1999;229(suppl)2:S347–S353.

2. National Center on Sleep Disorders Working Group. Recognizing problem sleepiness in your patients. *Am Fam Physician.* 1999;59:937–944.

3. Bergmann B, Gilliland M, Feng P, et al. Are physiological effects of sleep deprivation in the rat mediated by bacterial invasion? *Sleep.* 1996;19:554–562.

4. McCall W, Rakel R. *A Practical Guide to Insomnia.* New York, NY: McGraw-Hill Healthcare Information Programs;1999:1–10.

5. Horne J, Reyner L. Vehicle accidents related to sleep: a review. *Occup Environ Med.* 1999;56:289–294.

6. Ohayon M, Roth T. What are contributing factors for insomnia in the general population? *J Psychosom Res.* 2001;51:745–755.

7. Roth T, Ancoli–Isreal S. Daytime consequences and correlates of insomnia in the United States: results of the 1991 National Sleep Foundation Survey. *Sleep.* 1999;22(suppl 2):S354–S358.

8. Hauri P, Linde S. *No More Sleepless Nights.* Rev ed. New York, NY: John Wiley & Sons Inc; 1996:33–42.

9. Nowell P, Buysse D, Reynolds C III, et al. Clinical factors contributing to the differential diagnosis of primary insomnia and insomnia related to mental disorders. *Am J Psychiatry.* 1997;154:1412–1416.

10. Ellis C, Lemmens G, Parkes D. Pre-sleep behaviour in normal subjects. *J Sleep Res.* 1995;4:199–201.

11. Rybarczyk B, Lopez M, Benson R, Alsten C, Stepanski E. Efficacy of two behavioral treatment programs for comorbid geriatric insomnia. *Psychol Aging.* 2002;17:288–298.

12. Morin C, Hauri P, Espie C, Spielman A, Buysse D, Bootzin R. Nonpharmacologic treatment of chronic insomnia: an American Academy of Sleep Medicine review. *Sleep.* 1995;18:1134–1156.

13. Pallesen S, Nordhus I, Kvale G, et al. Behavioral treatment of insomnia in older adults: an open clinical trial comparing two interventions. *Behav Res Ther.* 2003;41:31–48.

14. Viens M, De Konick J, Mercier P, St-Onge M, Lorrain D. Trait anxiety and sleep-onset insomnia: evaluation of treatment using anxiety management training. *J Psychosom Res.* 2003;54:31–37.

15. Wolfson A, Carskadon M. Sleep schedules and daytime functioning in adolescents. *Child Dev.* 1998;69:875–887.

16. Manber R, Bootzin R, Acebo C, Carskadon M. The effects of regularizing sleep-wake schedules on daytime sleepiness. *Sleep.* 1996;19:432–441.

17. Montgomery P, Dennis J. Physical exercise for sleep problems in adults aged 60+. *Cochrane Database Systematic Rev.* 2002;4:CD003404.

18. Sherrill D, Kotchou K, Quan S. Association of physical activity and human sleep disorders. *Arch Intern Med.* 1998;158:1894–1998.

19. Roehrs T, Hollebeek E, Drake C, Roth T. Substance use for insomnia in Metropolitan Detroit. *J Psychosom Res.* 2002;53:571–576.

20. Rosenthal L. The Sleep Wake Inventory: a self-report measure of daytime sleepiness. *Biol Psychiatry.* 1993;34:810–820.

21. Roehrs T, Roth T. Sleep, sleepiness, and alcohol use. *Alcohol Res Health.* 2001;25:101–109.

22. Smith A. Effects of caffeine on human behavior. *Food Chem Toxicol.* 2002;40:1243–1255.

23. Landolt H, Werth E, Borbely A, Dijk D. Caffeine intake (200 mg) in the morning affects human sleep and EEG power spectra at night. *Brain Res.* 1995;675:67–74.

24. Brown S, Salive M, Pahor M. Foley D, Corti M, Langolis J, Wallace R, Harris T. Occult caffeine as a source of sleep problems in an older population. *J Am Geriatr Soc.* 1995;43:860–864.

25. Regestein Q. Postprandial drowsiness. *JAMA.* 1972;221:601–602.

26. Suganuma N, Shigedo Y, Adachi H, et al. Association of gastroesophageal reflux disease with weight gain and apnea and their disturbance on sleep. *Psychiatry Clin Neurosci.* 2001;55:255–256.

27. Gupta N, Mueller W, Chan W, Meininger J. Is obesity associated with poor sleep quality in adolescents? *Am J Hum Biol.* 2002;14:762–768.

28. Young T, Peppard P, Gottlieb D. Epidemiology of obstructive sleep apnea: a population health perspective. *Am J Respir Crit Care Med.* 2002;165:1217–1239.

29. Shahar E, Whitney C, Redline S, et al. Sleep-disordered breathing and cardiovascular disease: cross-sectional results of the Sleep Heart Health Study. *Am J Respir Crit Care Med.* 2001;163:19–25.

30. Phillips B, Young T, Finn L, Asher K, Hening WA, Purvis C. Epidemiology of restless legs symptoms in adults. *Arch Intern Med.* 2000;160:2137–2141.

31. Milligan S, Chesson A. Restless legs syndrome in the older adult: diagnosis and management. *Drugs Aging.* 2002;19:741–751.

32. Folkhard S, Tucker P. Shift work, safety, and productivity. *Occup Med.* 2003;53:95–101.

33. Garbarino S, De Carli F, Nobili L, et al. Sleepiness and sleep disorders in shift workers: a study on a group of Italian police officers. *Sleep.* 2002;25:648–653.

34. Akerstedt T. Shift work and disturbed sleep/wakefulness. *Occup Med.* 2003;53:89–94.

35. Moran D, Jansen K, Kant I, Galana J, van der Brandt P, Sween G. Prevalence of common infections in employees on different work shifts. *J Occup Employee Med.* 2002;44:1003–1011.

36. Rosekind M, Smith R, Miller D, et al. Alertness management: strategic naps in operational settings. *J Sleep Res.* 1995;4(suppl 2):62–66.

37. Stone B, Turner C. Promoting sleep in shiftworkers and intercontinental travelers. *Chronobiology Int.* 1997;14:133–143.

38. Muehlbach M, Walsh J. The effects of caffeine on simulated night-shift work and subsequent daytime sleep. *Sleep.* 1995;18:22–29.

39. Nickelsen T, Samel A, Vejvoda M, Wenzel J, Smith B, Gerzer R. Chronobiotic effects of the melatonin agonist LY 156735 following a simulated 9h time shift: results of a placebo-controlled trial. *Chronobiology Int.* 2002;19:915–936.

PART 3

Physical Activities and Fitness

chapter 13

Physical Activity and Programs for Fitness

Donald T. Kirkendall, PhD

INTRODUCTION

Habitual physical conditioning is known to have many different health benefits. In addition, training can improve efficiency and overall physiological function. For patients with specific medical problems, training can be an important adjunct to therapy. Consistent physical training is recommended for patients with coronary heart disease. However, there is increasing evidence that exercise is justified in a wide array of applications in the primary and tertiary prevention of disease and in the treatment of conditions such as cancer, stroke, and obesity.

An old adage suggests that exercise does not necessarily help one live longer, but helps one live "younger longer." Blair et al[1] suggested that consistent physical activity may influence longevity. They observed that all-cause mortality, independent of one's sex, was reduced with increasing levels of fitness (Fig 13-1). The greatest reduction in death rates occurred between the sedentary group and those of low fitness. Further reductions in death rate were evident with increasing levels of fitness, but not to the degree seen between the 2 lowest categories. This indicates that even a moderate increase in physical activity has health benefits. It is important to recognize that any form of physical activity can benefit health, including exercise and activities performed throughout the day within an active lifestyle. However, this chapter will primarily focus on the basic components of exercise training and the application of exercise in the tertiary prevention of various clinical conditions.

In some illnesses (eg, coronary disease), the proper use of exercise coupled with other therapies can favorably modify the disease process. In other conditions, exercise can serve as a supplement to therapeutic regimens and improve function and outcome, although the effect on the underlying disease may be minor. At a minimum, training typically increases the patient's functional reserve, permitting a greater range of activities of daily living and improved quality of life.

Before placing a patient in an exercise program, a physician should conduct a complete history and physical examination, which often includes a stress test. Following this essential evaluation, the principles of an exercise prescription outlined here have broad application across numerous clinical populations. It is important to understand the adaptations that occur from physical training and how these adaptations improve the clinical status of

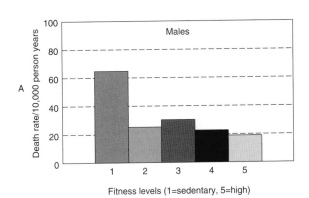

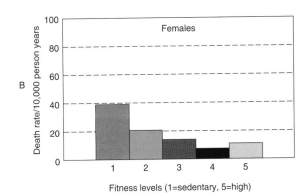

FIGURE 13-1

Age-adjusted all-cause death rates by fitness level and gender. **A**, Males; **B**, Females. Adapted from Blair SN, Kohl HW III, Paffenberger RS Jr, Clark DG, Cooper KH, Gibbons LW. Physical fitness and all-cause mortality: a prospective study of healthy men and women. *JAMA*. 1989; 262:2395–2401.

patients with specific health conditions, so exercise can best be used in patients with these conditions. The application of exercise in selected disease states should generally be supervised and directed by an appropriate specialist and his or her associates (eg, the cardiologist and exercise physiologist).

BASIC COMPONENTS OF TRAINING

Frequency

The number of days per week that lead to an adaptation can vary according to the muscle group being trained. The general consensus is that for training to be effective, at least 3 to 5 days per week of exercise is needed. Fewer days leads to less adaptation, which plateaus between 3 and 5 days of work. Six or 7 days of training per week may increase the risk of an overuse injury. There are a couple of exceptions to the 3- to 5-day guideline. For example, 1 day per week of extension training of the spine is as effective as 2 or 3 days of training per week. In general, strength training of trunk muscles needs 1 to 2 days per week, but strength training of the limbs needs the typical 3 to 5 days per week.

Duration

In each training session, the general goal is 20 to 60 minutes of work. This can be accomplished in one session or multiple 10-minute sessions. There is an inverse relationship between intensity and duration; the more intense the exercise, the less duration it can be maintained, and vice versa.

Intensity

The overall intensity of exercise can be determined in many ways—heart rate, heart rate reserve, oxygen consumption, rating of perceived exertion, and metabolic equivalents (METs), among others. The best method is the one the person will use during exercise. Oxygen consumption is an impractical tool, and METs assume some consistency of exercise energy expenditure. Therefore, heart rate and rating of perceived exertion are often used. Using heart rate, the desired intensity of exercise should be between 55% and 90% of maximum heart rate or between 45% and 85% of maximum heart rate reserve (the fraction of the difference between rest and maximal exercise pulse rate added to the resting pulse rate). In either case, it is best to use a known, measured maximal heart rate (usually from a stress test). Using rating of perceived exertion (Fig 13-2) the person answers the question, How hard is the exercise? The individual should strive to maintain an intensity of 3 (moderate), 4 (somewhat strong), or 5 (strong). After the initial period of time adjusting

to the program, most people end up exercising to some conscious perception of intensity.

Types of Exercise

Most people want to train the whole body, so use of a mode that incorporates many large muscle groups is advisable. Possible activities include walking (although it may be difficult to get into the target heart rate zone while walking), running, swimming, biking, cross-country skiing, "aerobic" dance programs, rope skipping, rowing, skating, or stair climbing.

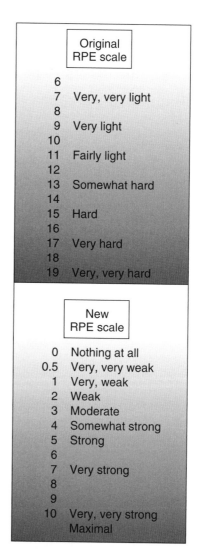

F I G U R E   13-2

Scales used for ratings of perceived exertion (RPE). Original scale (6–19) above and revised briefer scale (1–10) below. These scales are related to physiologic stress and can be used to establish exercise intensity for the purpose of training. From Borg GA. Psychological bases of perceived exertion. *Med Sci Sports Exerc.* 1982;14:377.

Rate of Progression

Recommendations vary on the order in which the 3 factors of training—frequency, duration, and intensity—should be increased. People must be counseled not to try to do too much too soon. If they do, the incidence of overuse injuries rises dramatically. Maintenance of fitness is simple; just remain at the level of work. Reduction of any of the 3 primary factors of training will decrease fitness. Studies have shown the fastest way to lose fitness is to decrease intensity. If frequency or duration must decrease, fitness can be maintained if the intensity is held constant.

Resistance Training

The goal of resistance training is local muscle strength, endurance, and maintenance or growth of lean muscle mass. This, too, should be progressive and should provide a stimulus to all the major muscle groups. Most people find doing compound lifts (those requiring multiple joints, not just one) are very effective and an efficient use of time. The general guideline for basic resistance training is one set of 8 to 10 repetitions of each exercise 2 to 3 times per week. The intensity is somewhat subjective, but each set should induce some fatigue in the final few repetitions. More sets can be used if the person has the time and if the goal is greater strength. For elderly persons, the weight should probably be less, with 10 to 15 repetitions of each exercise.

Flexibility Training

Most people stretch as a warm-up to exercise. Warm-up is preparing the body for work, and this may not be the optimal time to stretch. Flexibility training is real training designed to increase the range of motion of each joint and improve mechanical characteristics of muscle. The major muscle groups should all be trained 2 to 3 times per week. Flexibility training should be performed at the end of a workout when the muscles are very warm and most responsive to stretching. The American College of Sports Medicine offers a complete treatment of the exercise prescription in its position stand.[2]

ADAPTATIONS TO TRAINING

Nearly all clinical applications of exercise use aerobic training. This section will focus on aerobic training and discuss selected aspects of resistance training. Physical training influences the ability of the body to transport oxygen to the working muscles and the working muscle's ability to use the delivered oxygen. These central and peripheral adaptations to training are the foundation of the clinical application of exercise.

In addition, selected principles influence the responses to training. For example, training programs need to *overload* the person. The training should be *progressive;*

training volume or intensity should be increased systematically. Training is *specific.* Only those tissues that are stressed will adapt. *Individual differences* affect training responses, and if training is interrupted, the adaptations *reverse,* unfortunately quickly.

Adaptations Seen at Rest

Cross-sectional and longitudinal studies of cardiac mass point to an enlargement of the heart, mainly in left ventricular mass. In endurance training, the left ventricular internal dimension increases and the mass increases out of proportion to lean body mass, resulting in a true hypertrophy. Total hemoglobin levels may increase by nearly 25%, but plasma volume increases more, thus lowering hemoglobin concentration and resulting in occasional pseudoanemia, especially in females. The most recognized training adaptation is a decrease in resting heart rate secondary to an increase in vagal tone and a decrease in sympathetic influence and intrinsic atrial rate. Blood pressure at rest tends to mildly decrease. Other changes at rest include a more favorable lipoprotein profile. Training elevates high-density lipoprotein cholesterol (HDL-C) levels while lowering triglyceride levels, although the effect is variable.

Training, especially in concert with caloric (energy) restriction, can reduce fat mass with little or no change in fat-free mass. This makes the use of exercise and decreased caloric intake the methods of choice for weight reduction. Connective tissue changes are seen, as is an increase in trabecular bone thickness, resulting in increased bone density.

CORONARY DISEASE

Coronary disease represents probably the widest area of application of systematic exercise training in clinical medicine. Cardiac rehabilitation programs place the postinfarction or postsurgical patient into the treatment (ie, tertiary prevention) mainstream not many years after absolute bed rest for extended periods was the norm. Although exercise is used in many circumstances, some situations still require caution (Table 13-1).

Rehabilitation programs are well defined. Typically, soon after a coronary event, a phase 1 program of physical therapy and education begins. Phase 2 is usually initiated in the early outpatient period under medical monitoring. Activities are frequently of a light intensity and involve a variety of exercises. Phase 3 is a totally outpatient program but still includes some medical guidance. Monitoring is minimal (exercise intensity is monitored either by heart rate or rating of perceived exertion) and frequently is conducted at community centers. Activities include games and aerobic exercises and are consistent with the exercise prescription guidelines of the American College of Sports Medicine. Occasionally a phase 4 is

T A B L E   13-1

Contraindications to Exercise Training and Conditions
Requiring Special Precautions*

Absolute contraindications
  Acute myocardial infarction
  Manifest circulatory insufficiency (congestive
      heart failure)
  Rapidly increasing angina pectoris with effort
  Dissecting aneurysm
  Ventricular tachycardia at rest
  Severe aortic stenosis
  Active myocarditis
  Recent embolism, either systemic or pulmonary
  Thrombophlebitis
  Acute infectious disease
Relative contraindications
  Repetitive or frequent ventricular ectopic activity
  Uncontrolled or high-rate supraventricular dysrhythmia
  Ventricular aneurysm
  Moderate aortic stenosis
  Severe myocardial obstructive syndrome (subaortic
      stenosis)
  Untreated severe systemic or pulmonary hypertension
  Marked cardiac enlargement
  Severe anemia
  Uncontrolled metabolic disease (diabetes,
      thyrotoxicosis, or myxedema)
  Neuromuscular, musculoskeletal, or arthritic disorder
      that would prevent activity
  Overt psychoneurotic disturbance requiring therapy
Conditions requiring special consideration or precautions
  Controlled dysrhythmia
  Conduction disturbance (complete atrioventricular
      block, left bundle branch block, Wolff-Parkinson-
      White syndrome)
  Fixed-rate pacemaker
  Electrolyte disturbance
  Use of certain medications (digitalis, β-blockers, and
      drugs of related action)
  Angina pectoris and other manifestations of coronary
      insufficiency
  Cyanotic heart disease
  Intermittent or fixed right-to-left shunt
  Marked obesity
  Renal, hepatic, and other metabolic insufficiency

*From American College of Sports Medicine.[2]

included, which the patient conducts independently with
only periodic checks with a physician. Time since the
coronary event or selected performance variables are the
"graduation" criteria from phase 3.

When compliant with a prescribed exercise program,
physical work capacity will improve. The threshold for
angina or ST-segment depression occurs at a higher
absolute power output, which may lead to reductions
in antianginal medications. The improvement in work
capacity is primarily related to peripheral factors. If
the oxygen consumption needed for any task is slightly
reduced, then cardiac output is also reduced, thus lowering
the myocardial work requirement. The improvements in
aerobic metabolism that influence the increase in the
A-VO2 difference will also reduce the heart rate, blood
pressure, and muscle blood flow during submaximal
exercise, further reducing the myocardial demand.

The application of training after a coronary event is
one of the most widely used applications of exercise in
clinical practice. Improvements in work capacity, psychological well-being, productivity, and other social and
economic benefits, although sometimes difficult to document, are additional reasons to include training as a part
of a therapeutic regimen. More details on all aspects of
cardiac rehabilitation are provided in recent reviews.[3-5]

PERIPHERAL VASCULAR DISEASE

Foley[6] first demonstrated that daily physical training
(walking) was beneficial for patients with vascular disease. This contradicted standard treatment at the time,
which included a reduction in walking intensity and
smoking cessation in concert with medical or surgical
management. Patients feared the onset of ischemic pain.
However, it was demonstrated that, with training, time
(or distance) to the onset of pain could be increased.

Many studies have addressed the aspect of training
in patients with peripheral vascular disease. The most
common mode of training was walking. Training programs suggested in the literature were typically 2 to 3 days
per week, 30 to 60 minutes per day. In some cases, basic
calisthenics were performed (eg, toe raises, stair climbing,
leg raises, sit-stand, and "squats"). In nearly every study,
exercise to and beyond the onset of pain was a requirement. Training programs varied from 2 to 11 months, and
the average age of patients was more than 60 years.

In many studies, patients who adhered to the program,
including time (or distance) to the onset of pain and total
distance walked, often improved by up to 100% or more,
as estimated by the use of blood flow measurement during
exercise. However, a few studies showed no change in
blood flow as a result of the training program.

More efficient use of oxygen by muscles, in the
absence of blood flow changes, allows time to pain to be
increased as well as total walking distance. In this situation, exercise does little to the underlying disease process
of vascular narrowing. Rather, exercise allows the tissue
distal to the lesion to raise its function despite its blood
flow limitation.

The consistent requirement of walking to pain means that the exercise prescription needs to be modified to the patient's level of tolerance. A patient should walk to pain, then rest before continuing until a time (eg, 10 to 15 minutes to start with) or a distance requirement has been met. With training, the time or distance requirement will increase. Reviews are available that expand on this discussion.[3,7,8]

HYPERTENSION

The effect of exercise training on hypertension remains somewhat controversial. Methodological reasons make it challenging to determine the independent effect of exercise on blood pressure. Overall, however, most studies support a mild effect of decreased resting blood pressure from exercise, particularly aerobic exercise. During aerobic exercise, systolic pressure rises to a steady level while diastolic pressure changes little, with only slight changes in the mean arterial pressure. During resistance exercise, both systolic and diastolic pressures rise, sometimes to dramatic levels. Resistance training has only a slight effect or no effect on decreasing resting blood pressure. Patients with uncontrolled hypertension should first have their blood pressure brought under control before undertaking an exercise program.

STROKE

The goals for the patient who has had a stroke are to improve mobility and independence and to reduce the risk of future disease and impairment. Generally, there is major improvement in function during the first 6 months, whereas others may continue to see improvement for a year.

Because of the wide variability in age, severity, comorbidities, and disability, the stroke-affected patient should exercise under supervision. The general core of rehabilitation for patients after a stroke has been strength and gait training, but the inclusion of endurance work as tolerated has been gaining support. The main outcome of exercise is an improvement in the conduct of daily activities, with an improvement in overall capacity secondary to reduced cardiac demand.

CHRONIC OBSTRUCTIVE PULMONARY DISEASE

Obstructive pulmonary diseases (chronic airflow obstruction, asthma, or chronic bronchitis) present a central limitation to the performance of exercise. Normally, the lungs offer little limitation to exercise. However, when ventilatory function is compromised, physical work capacity and subsequent activities of daily living become difficult. With increasing disability, a reduction in exercise intensity is necessary.[9] For patients who undertake

an exercise program, the improvement in work capacity is unrelated to modification of the underlying disease. Rather, improvements are related to adaptations to exercise training.

DIABETES

Even before 1959, when Joslin described the interaction of diet, exercise, and insulin, exercise served as a basic therapy for patients with diabetes mellitus. Practical information for the diabetic individual is a result of the expanding knowledge base on the effects of physical training on metabolism.

Type 1 Diabetes Mellitus

Type 1 diabetes typically begins when physical activity is normally part of everyday life. However, the fear of precipitating hypoglycemia by exercise may cause some patients to severely limit their activities. This inactivity may lead to other complications associated with a sedentary life, which can add more medical problems to an already difficult condition. However, if diabetic persons are knowledgeable about the disease, they can avoid potential risks associated with activity. There are many instances of professional athletes who have successfully competed while managing type 1 diabetes.

The most important aspect of exercise in patients with type 1 diabetes is the timing of insulin administration, food, and exercise. Similar to food intake, regularity in exercise can help facilitate good control of blood glucose without wide fluctuations. Because patients with type 1 diabetes are at increased risk of cardiovascular disease, exercise is particularly important in helping to control other risk factors. The lipid profile of the diabetic patient is usually improved with training, resulting in a reduction in triglycerides and an increase in HDL-C levels. In addition, insulin sensitivity is improved by up to 20% with training. These metabolic changes quickly disappear with a return to inactivity, and the insulin-resistant condition can worsen with bed rest.

A series of complications associated with type 1 diabetes deserve special mention. Patients with *diabetic retinopathy* are discouraged from participating in activities of very high intensity or activities that require a Valsalva maneuver. This should not be interpreted to mean that exercise accelerates the progression of retinopathy.

Exercise-related *albuminuria* is a common finding in diabetics and seems to be related to the degree of elevation in systolic pressure. Thus, activities that elevate systolic pressure above 180 to 200 mm Hg are to be avoided, with activities such as walking or cycling encouraged.

Patients with *autonomic neuropathy* are predisposed to postexertional hypotension and should be counseled to avoid exercises that result in rapid changes in body position, heart rate, or blood pressure, such as ball games and weight training. These patients also seem to have problems exercising in heat, as it makes them more likely to become dehydrated. Patients with *peripheral neuropathy* need to pay particular attention to shoe selection and inspect their feet after each exercise session. Cycling and swimming, because of reduced stress on the feet, are the exercises of choice. In addition, the loss of sensation increases the risk of excessive stretching on muscles and connective tissues.

Myocardial ischemia is a common problem in diabetic persons. Thus, before starting an exercise program, diabetic patients should have a thorough cardiovascular examination and stress test.

Type 2 Diabetes Mellitus

Two phases of type 2 diabetes exist. In the first, there is an impaired sensitivity to insulin, and in the other, usually after long-term type 2 diabetes with exhaustion of the beta cells, there is an inability to secrete insulin.

Acute exercise decreases blood glucose levels well into the recovery period. This decrease appears to be related to exercise duration and is most common in patients being treated with sulfonylureas or insulin. After maximal, exhaustive exercise, a hyperglycemic condition can occur.

Physical training (again following standard prescription guidelines for exercise) has been shown to mildly improve metabolic control, especially in younger diabetic patients. If weight loss also occurs, substantially greater improvement in metabolic control is often achieved. Insulin sensitivity is improved most in skeletal muscle among patients with high insulin levels, whereas patients with low insulin levels appear to show increased levels of insulin secretion.

The association between obesity and type 2 diabetes clearly makes weight reduction a priority in any treatment plan. Most people are aware that the most efficient method of weight loss is the combination of diet and exercise, and this is true for the diabetic also. The preferred type of exercise is long-duration, low-intensity exercise that is most likely to lead to increased energy expenditure. The increased risk of coronary disease in diabetics makes the improvement of lipid profiles important, and exercise will decrease triglycerides and raise HDL-C levels.

In the care of the exercising patient with type 2 diabetes, it is usually not necessary to increase carbohydrate intake unless the activity is of extended duration. Patients under treatment with sulfonylureas may need some additional carbohydrate before and during the activity. The activity should be aerobic and chosen by the individual. Table 13-2 shows some potential benefits to the patient with type 2 diabetes. Further information on exercise and diabetes can be found elsewhere.[10-12]

OSTEOPOROSIS

Among the natural consequences of aging, the loss of bone density constitutes a major public health concern, especially in Western societies. The maintenance of bone health may reduce fractures, and the role of exercise in maintaining such health could be one of the most effective applications of exercise. The maintenance of bone health depends on the interaction of 3 variables: nutrition (calcium intake, vitamin D), functional stress (gravity and activity), and hormones (eg, parathyroid hormone, calcitonin, estrogen, and growth hormone). Reducing any of these may result in a reduction in bone density.

Elimination of gravity (space flight) results in a rapid decrease in bone density. Bed rest and immobilization can also reduce bone density, and excess weight can overload the bones and increase bone density. In female subjects who exercise heavily, particularly when associated with low body weight, the normal menstrual cycle can be disrupted. With the resulting loss of estrogen comes a reduction in bone density and increased risk of stress fractures, most often documented in female runners during stressful training.[13]

Dense cortical and spongy trabecular bone has been the subject of intense study. Bone mass is gained throughout adolescence. About 60% of the final bone mass is built up during the 2- to 3-year pubertal growth spurt, making nutrition in this period a critical factor. A plateau is reached in about the third to fourth decades, followed by a progressive thinning or even disappearance of the trabecular aspects of the tissue. The loss of mass during menopause proceeds at a rapid rate during the first 5 years (nearly 3.5% per year), followed by a small loss (<1% per year by the ninth year) in subsequent years.

According to the Wolff law, bone will adapt to the recurring demands placed on it. The load must be progressive. If one trains to jog a specific distance, the bone will adapt to some equilibrium by thickening trabecular bone.

The specific type of exercise is important when prescribing exercise for osteoporosis. Weight-bearing

TABLE 13-2

Long-term Possible Positive Effects of Regular Exercise in Type 2 Diabetes Mellitus*

1. Improved blood glucose control
2. Increased peripheral insulin sensitivity
3. Improved blood lipid profile
4. Decreased hypertension
5. Contributing factors (together with diet) to weight reduction
6. Increased physical work capacity
7. Increased sense of well-being and quality of life

*From Wallberg-Henricksson H. Exercise and diabetes mellitus. *Exerc Sports Sci Rev.* 1992;20:339.

exercise, such as walking or running, particularly when combined with calcium supplementation, show greater increases in bone density compared with controls or non–weight-bearing exercise. Weight-bearing exercise can be improved by supplementing specific sites (eg, arms, lumbar vertebrae) or by incorporating resistance exercise (weight lifting) and cross training, such as rowing. Specific loading (weight lifting) will increase bone density while non–weight-bearing aerobic exercise has little effect on bone density. To some extent, muscle strength predicts bone strength in adjacent bones. In general, although training can improve bone density, the degree of improvement is relatively small, requires months or years, and shows the greatest percentage of improvement in sedentary people rather than in those already trained.

Low-intensity work has been suggested for elderly individuals with osteoporosis. Recommended activities include supervised rhythmic activities, supported exercise (holding onto a chair), and low-intensity resistance training (sandbags, similar to what a physical therapist might use). These exercises need not be done to fatigue or exhaustion. Higher-intensity work should be primarily recommended for younger people still laying down bone. However, training studies in nonagenarians show that even this age group can tolerate weight training as well as show beneficial training effects. Further details can be found in reviews on this topic.[14,15]

PREGNANCY

The most obvious benefit of exercise during pregnancy is the maintenance of the fitness of the mother. Other possible outcomes include facilitation of labor, quicker recovery from birthing, improved emotional well-being, and improved lifestyle habits. Generally, if a woman is training and becomes pregnant, she can continue training with some modifications. However, pregnancy is not the time to begin a vigorous training program.

The American College of Sports Medicine offers recommendations regarding exercise and pregnancy. The frequency of exercise should be 3 to 5 days per week, with a duration of 15 to 30 minutes. Intensity should be monitored by the perceived exertion scale rather than by heart rate because the maternal heart rate is elevated during pregnancy. Activities of choice include walking or weight-supporting exercises such as cycling or water-based programs. Whether weight training should be advised is still unknown. Extremes of heat (especially during the first trimester because of fear that hyperthermia might affect neural closure), humidity, hypoxia, or exercise duration should be avoided. For the female in training, exercise in the first trimester should follow the routine exercise prescription, including the avoidance of excessive heat. During the time when the risks of exercise are low (second trimester), exercise can continue until discomfort requires a reduction in exercise duration or intensity. Third-trimester exercise is usually limited by fatigue.

Certain conditions require special consideration (Table 13-3). Certain signs and symptoms (Table 13-4) may also force cessation of an exercise program. Although musculoskeletal complaints are frequent in the pregnant female, some evidence suggests a reduction in musculoskeletal problems during training.

Risks of exercise include the concern of hyperthermia mentioned previously. In addition, there have been reports of variable fetal heart rates (absent medical intervention or birth abnormalities) in untrained women after exhaustive exercise. The application of exercise in pregnant women

TABLE 13-3

Contraindications for Exercise During Pregnancy*

Absolute Contraindication	Relative Contraindication
Heart disease	High blood pressure
Ruptured membranes	Anemia or other blood disorders
Premature labor	Thyroid disease
Multiple gestation	Diabetes
Bleeding	Palpitations or irregular heart rhythms
Placenta previa	Breech presentation in last trimester
Incompetent cervix	Excessive obesity
History of ≥3 spontaneous abortions or miscarriages	Extreme underweight
	History of precipitous labor
	History of intrauterine growth retardation
	History of bleeding during pregnancy
	Extremely sedentary lifestyle

*From American College of Obstetricians and Gynecologists (ACOG). *Exercise During Pregnancy and Postnatal Period: Home Exercise Programs.* Washington, DC: ACOG; 1985.

TABLE 13-4

Indications for Discontinuing Exercise During Pregnancy*

Pain or bleeding
Dizziness or faintness
Pubic pain
Palpitations
Rapid heart rate
Back pain
Shortness of breath
Difficulty walking

*From American College of Obstetricians and Gynecologists (ACOG). *Exercise During Pregnancy and Postnatal Period: Home Exercise Programs.* Washington, DC: ACOG; 1985.

with either coexisting disease or diseases particular to pregnancy has received little attention. In the absence of sound data, clinical judgment should influence the physician in such cases. Three good reviews are available to guide the physician in discussing exercise for pregnant women.[16-18]

CANCER

Epidemiologic reports point out that lifetime physical activity, whether occupational or recreational, can lower one's risk of colon or breast cancers.[19-21] Controlled studies are difficult because of the many factors associated with cancer. Many statements about the use of exercise in the prevention of cancer come from extensions of epidemiologic literature.

The American College of Sports Medicine offers suggestions regarding the use of exercise in patients with cancer. Before a patient begins an exercise program, functional capacity should be assessed through an exercise test. A low initial level of fitness is not uncommon in these patients. In addition, patients whose disease has metastasized to bone may need to be tested on a cycle for weight support.

Exercise intensity should start low (40% to 65% of heart rate reserve) and progress according to patient tolerance. The clinical status of the patient governs frequency. Treatment regimens may require a more flexible approach to training days. Patients may have poor blood cell counts, side effects from treatment, or other limitations that may require postponing a training session. Weight training has been suggested to counter the muscle wasting sometimes seen in patients with cancer. Low-intensity, high-repetition training using any of the commercial machines (for safety) is suggested. Serum enzyme levels are frequently used to follow the course of patients, and weight training elevates serum enzyme levels. Thus, weight training should be avoided for at least 36 hours before venipuncture. A concise discussion on the role of exercise for the patient with cancer is available elsewhere.[22]

EXERCISE AND EMOTIONAL WELL-BEING

Improvement in emotional health is widely believed to be a benefit of physical training. Anecdotal evidence can be easily found to support better mental health. Executives say their efficiency and decision-making capacity are greater during training. Mental health professionals believe that exercise helps to manage stress; decrease anxiety; and improve self-esteem, alertness, and attitudes toward work.

Stress management is frequently mentioned as a prime reason to pursue an exercise program. Whether stress reduction is in response to some biochemical alteration, such as a release of endorphins, or a sympathetic hormonal adaptation to physical or psychological stress has not been conclusively demonstrated. Some experts believe that stress relief is a response to a "time-out" from the stressful environment. Others suggest that the threshold for stress hormone release is raised such that stress levels previously perceived as grave would no longer be perceived as threatening. The influence of exercise on a variety of mental health dimensions seems to suggest that both short-term and long-term emotional well-being can be improved by training. More details on adding exercise in support of mental health can be found in recent reviews.[23,24]

SUMMARY

The role of exercise in the development and maintenance of fitness for the apparently healthy adult, the primary prevention of disease, and the tertiary prevention of a wide range of clinical conditions underscores its importance and wide applicability. The trained human operates at a much more efficient manner, reducing the overall load on the system. Virtually anyone can safely realize these benefits if he or she follows and adheres to a sound training program designed to meet personal needs.

REFERENCES

1. Blair SN, Kohl HW III, Paffenberger RS Jr, Clark DG, Cooper KH, Gibbons LW. Physical fitness and all-cause mortality: a prospective study of healthy men and women. *JAMA*. 1989;262:2395–2401.

2. American College of Sports Medicine. *Guidelines for Exercise Testing and Rehabilitation*. 6th ed. Philadelphia, Pa: Lippincott, Williams & Wilkins; 2000.

3. Armen J, Smith B. Exercise considerations in coronary artery disease, peripheral vascular disease and diabetes mellitus. *Clin in Sports Med*. 2003;22:123–133.

4. Batty G. Physical activity and coronary heart disease in older adults: a systematic review of epidemiological studies. *Eur J Public Health*. 2002;12:171–176.

5. Franklin B, Swain D, Shepard RJ. New insights in the prescription of exercise for coronary patients. *J Cardiovasc Nurs*. 2003;18:118–123.

6. Foley WT. Treatment of gangrene of the feet and legs by walking. *Circulation*. 1957;15:689.

7. Burns P, Gough S, Bradbury AW. Management of peripheral arterial disease in primary care. *BMJ*. 2003;326:584–588.

8. Treat-Jacobson D, Walsh M. Treating patients with peripheral arterial disease and claudication. *J Vascular Nursing*. 2003;21:5–14.

9. Jones N. Chronic obstructive respiratory disease. In: Skinner J, ed. *Exercise Testing and Exercise Prescription for Special Cases*. Philadelphia, Pa: Lea & Febiger; 1987.

10. Galbo H. *Hormonal and Metabolic Adaptations to Exercise*. Stuttgart, Germany: Georg Thieme Verlag; 1983.

11. Horton E. Role and management of exercise in diabetes mellitus. *Diabetes Care*. 1988;11:201–211.

12. Vitug A, Schneider SH, Ruderman NB. Exercise and type I diabetes mellitus. *Exerc Sport Sci Rev*. 1988;16:285–304.

13. Drinkwater BL, Nilson K, Chesnut CH III, Bremner WJ, Shainholtz S, Southworth MB. Bone mineral content of amenorrheic and eumenorrheic athletes. *N Engl J Med*. 1984;311:277–281.

14. Snow-Harter C. Exercise, bone mineral density and osteoporosis. *Exerc Sports Sci Rev*. 1991;19:351–388.

15. Bonaiuti D, Shea B, Iovine R, Negrini S, Robinson V, Kemper HC, Wells G, Tugwell P, Cranney A. Exercise for preventing and treating osteoporosis in postmenopausal women. *Cochrane Database Syst Rev*. 2002;3:CD000333.

16. Clapp J. Exercise during pregnancy: a clinical update. *Clin Sports Med*. 2000;19:273–286.

17. Brown W. The benefits of physical activity during pregnancy. *J Sci Med Sport*. 2002;5:37–45.

18. Kramer M. Aerobic exercise for women during pregnancy. *Cochrane Database Syst Rev*. 2002;2:CD000180.

19. Garabrant DH, Peters JM, Mack TM, Bernstein L. Job activity and colon cancer risk. *Am J Epidemiol*. 1984;119:1005–1114.

20. Vena JE, Graham S, Zielezny M, Swanson MK, Barnes RE, Nolan J. Lifetime occupational exercise and colon cancer. *Am J Epidemiol*. 1985;122:357–365.

21. Frisch R., Wyshak G, et al. Lower prevalence of breast cancer and cancers of the reproductive system among former college athletes compared to non-athletes. *Br J Cancer*. 1985;52:885–891.

22. Feiedenreich C, Orenstein M. Physical activity and colon cancer: etiologic evidence and biological mechanisms. *J Nutr*. 2002;132:3456S–3464S.

23. Dunn AL, Trivedi MH, O'Neal HA. Physical activity dose-response effects on the outcomes of depression and anxiety. *Med Sci Sports Exerc*. 2001;33:S587–S597.

24. Brosse AL, Sheets ES, Lett HS, Blumenthal JA. Exercise and the treatment of clinical depression in adults: recent findings and future directions. *Sports Med*. 2002;32:741–760.

RESOURCES

American College of Sports Medicine. *Exercise Management for Persons with Chronic Diseases and Disabilities*. Philadelphia, Pa: Lippincott, Williams & Wilkins; 1997.

American College of Sports Medicine. *Guidelines for Exercise Testing and Rehabilitation*. 6th ed. Philadelphia, Pa: Lippincott, Williams & Wilkins; 2000.

American College of Sports Medicine. *Resource Manual for Guidelines for Exercise Testing and Prescription*. 4th ed. Philadelphia, Pa: Lippincott, Williams & Wilkins; 2001.

American College of Sports Medicine. *Resources for Clinical Exercise Physiology: Musculoskeletal, Neuromuscular, Neoplastic, Immunologic and Hematologic Conditions*. Philadelphia, Pa: Lippincott, Williams & Wilkins; 2002.

Fox EL, Bowers RW, Foss ML. *Physiological Basis of Physical Education and Athletics*. 4th ed. Dubuque, Iowa: William C Brown Publishing; 1988.

Galbo H. *Hormonal and Metabolic Adaptations to Exercise*. Stuttgart, Germany: Georg Thieme Verlag; 1983.

McArdle WD, Katch FL, Katch VL. *Exercise Physiology: Energy, Nutrition and Human Performance*. 4th ed. Philadelphia, Pa: Lippincott, Williams & Wilkins; 1996.

Pollack ML, Wilmore JH, Fox SM. *Exercise in Health and Disease*. Philadelphia, Pa: WB Saunders Co; 1984.

Skinner JS. *Exercise Testing and Exercise Prescription for Special Cases: Theoretical Basis and Clinical Application*. Philadelphia, Pa: Lea & Febiger; 1987.

Wilson PK, Fardy PS, Froelicher VF. *Cardiac Rehabilitation, Adult Fitness and Exercise Testing*. Philadelphia, Pa: Lea & Febiger; 1981.

chapter 14

The Team Physician and the Preparticipation Physical Examination

Donald T. Kirkendall, PhD

INTRODUCTION

Being a team physician might be considered an ideal situation for the care and prevention of athletic injuries. However, it is also a position that demands good balance when working for both the team and the athlete. This balance can determine whether the position of team physician is a great or grim opportunity. The decisions made can have an impact on not only the player but also the team, coach, and entire sports organization as it pertains to health, career longevity, and income.

REQUIREMENTS OF THE TEAM DOCTOR

Any survey of suburban high schools for the specialty interests of the team doctor will show that the common requirement is an MD or DO degree. Cardiologists, orthopedists, internists, pediatricians, family medicine physicians, or members of any other medical specialty have spent time on the sidelines of scholastic sports. Regardless of specialty, the physician must have a comprehensive approach to this corner of medicine. This comprehensive approach must meet not only the physical needs of the athletes but also their emotional needs and possibly their spiritual needs. The physician's broad base in medicine must go beyond the musculoskeletal system to the cardiovascular, pulmonary, skin, reproductive, neurologic, and gastrointestinal systems, among others. For example, some physicians make international trips with teams and have to deal with traveler's diarrhea. In addition, the physician is frequently the professional who will hear an athlete's anxiety about playing time in relation to an injury or illness, motivation to train, or performance. An understanding of the athlete's psyche is almost as important as medical knowledge. The physician is usually the person asked about whether some new method of training is appropriate. Finally, the issues of prescribed medications, performance-enhancing drugs,

and recreational drugs get to the team doctor one way or another. A superior athlete may make an international trip that could include drug testing, and the issue could arise of whether any supplements, prescribed medications, or over-the-counter drugs might trigger a positive drug test result. All of these scenarios raise the possibility of extending physicians far beyond their personal medical training. The opportunity may present itself to save a spectator who has a heart attack, to answer honestly and knowledgeably whether a certain supplement is allowed, or to suggest a cold remedy when the next day the athlete has to give a urine sample prior to getting on the plane as part of a national team.

Orthopedists and family physicians often have the responsibility as team physicians. However, Lombardo[1] has referred to the team physician as the "captain of the ship, the director of the symphony and jack-of-all-trades." The physician considering serving as a team doctor needs to be aware of the differences between daily medical practice and this role. The front line of sports medicine is the athletic field, not the stands or the office. Although it is important for a physician to be available for all patients, the athlete has unique demands. Frequently, injuries are acute and require immediate attention so the physician needs to have a system in place to provide prompt evaluation in the office. However, the physician will usually have a better relationship with the team in the athlete's setting, which means seeing patients there, as opposed to the office. Being on the sidelines during competition is a necessity, as is traveling. When traveling with the team, it is important that the physician not bury his or her head in journals but instead function as part of the team. The team is not the only entity with which the physician needs to have a relationship. The coach, athletic trainer, or therapist, as well as management personnel at the college or professional level, must be comfortable with the team doctor. Informal banter can go a long way to help cement a good professional relationship.

DIFFERENT ROLES OF THE TEAM PHYSICIAN

The clinical role is the role that most physicians enjoy, but the team physician has added responsibilities.[2] These roles change with time but include the following.

Clinical Role

This role is obviously the foundation of the interaction between the physician and athlete. It requires the most current diagnostic and therapeutic regimens, from general medicine to specialty interests particular to the sport. The physician's knowledge base should include basic and advanced cardiac life support (BCLS and ACLS), advanced trauma life support (ATLS), and on-the-field sports medicine. One goal is to keep players in the game; therefore, prevention and proper safeguards are the primary aspects of the clinical responsibilities. Physicians performing this role should consider taking the Certificate of Added Qualification in Sports Medicine created by 4 medical specialty boards, including the American Board of Family Practice.

Educational Role

While the physician is forever a student, as new knowledge is produced so quickly, the role as educator is equally critical, because trainers, players, coaches, and parents cannot be expected to keep up with new medical information. It also must be emphasized that this role is a 2-way street, especially between the physician and other members of the health care team.

Medicolegal Role

In sports medicine, as in all aspects of medicine, it is critical to keep abreast of the current opinions regarding the legal ramifications of sports medicine and personal liability.

Research Role

Research could involve collecting, analyzing, and publishing new data. It also means continually reviewing the medical literature and other outlets for any new information that might pertain to sports and medicine. Research also involves determining best practices and the most current and evidence-based information applied to sports medicine.

Political Service Role

The team physician can provide valuable contributions to professional associations, athletic conferences, parent booster clubs, and more. The medical leader on the field, the team physician is best positioned to hold the same role off the field.

PREPARTICIPATION PHYSICAL EXAMINATION

The physician generally has 2 global responsibilities with any athletic team. The role the public sees is the treatment of athletic injuries. This also includes injury prevention and other responsibilities described above. The other role is in qualifying athletes for participation in sports. The level of competition determines the specific criteria for this evaluation. The foundation of any examination is the health and safety of every athlete. If participation in sports is likely to place the health of an athlete at risk, the athlete must be counseled about these risks. Additional goals of the examination are to:

1. Detect disabling or life-threatening conditions.
2. Detect any conditions that potentially could limit the athlete's ability to compete.
3. Detect any factors that may predispose an athlete to injury.
4. Meet insurance and legal guidelines.

Whereas these are the basic objectives, the evaluation can be expanded to include such aspects as counseling on fitness and determination of health status and maturity.

TIMING OF SCREENING

Practical considerations influence the timing of a screening evaluation. For example, most team screening sessions involve a station approach, meaning many people need to be involved. Thus, if the screening is done before each competitive season, multiple people must be available on more than one date. If the screening is done in the summer, the session must be coordinated with family and professional schedules. Usually, most screening sessions take place in the 1 or 2 months before the opening of a training camp so that any uncovered deficiencies can be corrected before the sport's season.

FREQUENCY OF EVALUATIONS

There is no consensus on the frequency that an athlete should undergo a preparticipation physical examination. The American Heart Association (AHA) previously recommended a screening history and physical examination looking for cardiovascular abnormalities before sports participation in high school and college, followed by repeated evaluations every 2 years with a brief history in the off years.[3] A year later, the Committee on Competitive Safeguards and Medical Aspects of Sports of the National Collegiate Athletic Association (NCAA) announced that there were little data to justify the second evaluation for cardiovascular problems in college athletes. This led the AHA to modify its stand to recommend an interim history and blood pressure measurement in the years after the initial evaluation.[4] Any changes detected would necessitate another complete evaluation. An evaluation should probably be performed upon entry to each new level of competition. Professional athletes usually undergo an extensive evaluation each year.

DAY OF THE EXAMINATION

The preparticipation physical examination is typically performed either individually in the physician's office or with the whole team in the athletes' environment.

Office Setting

The physician's office offers the setting where all the needs of the physician are located and there is a history of doctor-patient interaction. Full records are available and the setting is private and confidential. Unfortunately, the appointment slots for this may be limited, and there is a wide variety of expertise among primary care physicians with regard to sports participation. There are other limitations, such as the expense of the appointment. The alternative is to take the "office" to the athlete and examine as many athletes as possible of those that are available. To do this, a station approach is organized using a team of health care providers plus other assistants associated with the team.

Mass Screening

Using the station approach, multiple stations are set up and staffed by someone who is experienced in that specific area. The final station must be filled by the experienced sports physician, who will review the information collected, decide on medical clearance, and make whatever recommendations might be needed. Although this type of setting requires a good deal of organization, it does offer many practical advantages. A large number of athletes can be handled at one time in one location. Among the disadvantages of the station approach is that privacy may be compromised because the location typically does not have private examination rooms. Also, counseling is limited and follow-up is rare. Adequate staffing should be available to limit potential bottlenecks. The specific organization and order of the stations can be flexible based on each team's health care and athletic needs. Staff should be aware of confidentiality concerns and privacy regulations of the Health Insurance Portability and Accountability Act (HIPAA). In some settings, fitness evaluations have been added to the basic health and well-being of the athlete, which adds a layer of complexity to the examination. If this is done, someone must assume responsibility for making decisions on the fitness needs of the sport, then select the necessary tests to determine if the athlete has any weaknesses that can be corrected before the formal opening of training. It is difficult for physicians to assume these additional

responsibilities. An exercise physiologist is the obvious choice for organizing this aspect of the evaluation, yet people with this training may not be available and the responsibility can fall on a trainer or physical therapist. The advantage of including fitness in the evaluation is a more complete picture of the athlete's capability as well having a more objective assessment of that person's fitness. Disadvantages are the added time, space, and personnel needed. In addition, many coaches feel that the fitness evaluation is part of their domain.

The stations for the preparticipation physical examination are as follows:

Sign-in

The first station does not entail actually filling out the forms. Optimally, forms should be filled out ahead of time (with the help of parents or guardians for younger athletes), to obtain accurate information and save time. At the sign-in station, all forms are checked for completeness, and the paperwork for the full evaluation is dispensed to each athlete. The general setup of the screening is described. Anyone who knows the athletes, such as an assistant coach, can staff this station.

History review

It is important that someone who is comfortable asking for clarity of information based on the history forms carefully perform the history review (Table 14-1). This person may have to make recommendations on how the rest of the session will be handled. A physician, nurse,

TABLE 14-1

AHA Recommendations for Cardiovascular Screening in Preparticipation Examination[*]

History	Physical Examination
Sudden death in family member <50 y old	Blood pressure
Prior heart disease in family member	Heart murmur[†]
Exertional dyspnea or chest pain	Peripheral (femoral) pulses
Syncope	Marfan stigmata[‡]
Excessive fatigability	
Heart murmur	
Systemic hypertension	
Parental verification of history	

[*]Reprinted from American Heart Association (AHA).[3]

[†]Precordial auscultation is recommended in supine, sitting, and standing positions to identify heart murmurs reflecting hypertrophic cardiomyopathy.

[‡]Tall stature, arachnodactyly, kyphoscoliosis, anterior chest deformity, arm span greater than height, decreased upper body length-to-lower body length ratio, heart murmur or midsystolic click, ectopic lens, or family history of Marfan syndrome.

physician assistant, or experienced trainer or therapist should be chosen to staff this position.

Height and weight

To accurately establish body mass index, these factors must be measured. An assistant coach, trainer, or other volunteer such as a parent can handle this station.

Vision

The basic vision screening can be taught to be administered by a layperson, or a nurse or trainer can administer it.

Vital signs

A health care professional should staff this station to ensure accurate measurements.

Medical evaluation

The medical station or stations offer a comprehensive evaluation. A further review of history is followed by a physical examination (Fig 14-1). A physician, physician assistant, or nurse practitioner should staff this station. Time limits may affect this station and the orthopedic station. The potential for a bottleneck exists, so multiple stations and personnel might be needed.

Orthopedic evaluation

A detailed musculoskeletal examination requires sport and joint-specific screening. The asymptomatic athlete may not require the same extensive review as those with a history of an injury.

Fitness evaluation

Depending on the breadth of the physical examination, fitness tests may be conducted. These are usually field tests of fitness that require a minimum of equipment, yet give reasonable results. Examples include the 12-minute run or a paced shuttle test (endurance), 300-m sprint (anaerobic capacity), 10- to 30-m sprints (speed), skinfold calipers (body composition), sit-reach test (hamstring and low back flexibility), vertical jump (power), agility test, and 30 sit-ups or push-ups in 30 seconds (local muscle endurance). An overall profile can be developed of the team and sport. The examiner may determine individual weaknesses (in the team or in the sport overall) and offer training suggestions.

Review and clearance

The outcome of the preparticipation physical examination is 1 of 3 possibilities: medical clearance to participate in the sport, no clearance, or further evaluation is needed. This station is always the last in a mass screening setting and might be considered as a checkout in some circumstances.

CLEARANCE TO PARTICIPATE

The American Academy of Pediatrics Committee on Sports Medicine and Fitness has produced specific guidelines for medical clearance[5] (Fig 14-2). Findings are then checked against sports that are classified according to degree of physical contact and specific sport demands.

Highlights from the guidelines in Fig 14-2 include:

- Answers to questions on the history form and current medications can give valuable clues to current or underlying conditions. Particular attention is paid to any responses suggesting dizziness, passing out, shortness of breath, and family history of premature death.

- Elevated blood pressure is one of the most common findings in the preparticipation examination. If the blood pressure is mildly above acceptable age group norms, is not related to underlying heart disease, and is without evidence of target organ damage, the athlete usually can be cleared to play. The athlete should have his or her blood pressure checked regularly. Any athlete with severe hypertension needs to sit out until the blood pressure is controlled.

- Any cardiac rhythm disorder or nonphysiological murmur needs to be worked up before an athlete can be given clearance for competition. Specific recommendations for cardiovascular evaluation and clearance are published and are a valuable resource for all team physicians (Table 14-1).[6]

- Any athlete with a history of concussion presents unique challenges. First, there is no accepted, validated grading scale for concussion; many scales exist. Second, the return-to-play guidelines are also problematic. Third, there is the concern over the so-called second impact syndrome that some professionals believe exists. Special attention needs to be paid to high-risk sports, such as football, soccer, lacrosse, ice hockey, field hockey, wrestling, and gymnastics. The physician need not become an expert on all the various schemes of grading and clearing. However, the potential for handling a concussed athlete requires that the team physician be familiar and comfortable with one scale and set of clearance guidelines. The bottom line is: no play if there are any symptoms at all. The old line "when in doubt, hold them out" is an important guideline to follow. It is important to keep in mind that when an athlete has sustained a mild head injury and questions are asked regarding symptoms or memory, the urge to return to play can lead to outright lying by the player. Being skeptical of an athlete's answers to oral questions is a prudent stance to adopt.

- An athlete with a stinger or burner can play in the absence of symptoms and a normal physical examination.

- Any skin infection needs proper treatment before the athlete can be allowed to return to training and competition. Particular emphasis needs to be paid to wrestlers and their mats.

Preparticipation Physical Evaluation

PHYSICAL EXAMINATION

Name _____   Date of birth _____

Height _____ Weight _____ % Body fat (optional)_____ Pulse _____ BP ____/____ (____/____ , ____/____)

Vision R 20/_____   L 20/_____   Corrected: Y N   Pupils: Equal _____ Unequal _____

	NORMAL	ABNORMAL FINDINGS	INITIALS*
MEDICAL			
Appearance			
Eyes/Ears/Nose/Throat			
Lymph Nodes			
Heart			
Pulses			
Lungs			
Abdomen			
Genitalia (males only)			
Skin			
MUSCULOSKELETAL			
Neck			
Back			
Shoulder/arm			
Elbow/forearm			
Wrist/hand			
Hip/thigh			
Knee			
Leg/ankle			
Foot			

*Station-based examination only

CLEARANCE

❏ Cleared

❏ Cleared after completing evaluation / rehabilitation for: _____

_____

_____

_____

❏ Not cleared for: _____ Reason: _____

Recommendations: _____

_____

_____

_____

Name of physician (print / type): _____ Date: _____

Address: _____ Phone: _____

Signature of physician _____ MD, DO

© 1997 *American Academy of Family Physicians, American Academy of Pediatrics, American Medical Society for Sports Medicine, American Orthopaedic Society for Sports Medicine, and American Osteopathic Academy for Sports Medicine*

FIGURE 14-1

Preparticipation physical evaluation. Reprinted from *Physician Sportsmed.*

Preparticipation Physical Evaluation

HISTORY

DATE OF EXAM: _____

Name _____ Sex _____ Age _____ Date of Birth _____

Grade _____ School _____ Sport(s) _____

Address _____ Phone _____

Personal physician _____

In case of emergency, contact

Name _____ Relationship _____ Phone (H) _____ (W) _____

Explain "Yes" answers below.
Circle questions you don't know the answers to.

	Yes	No
1. Have you had a medical illness or injury since your last check up or sports physical?	❏	❏
Do you have an ongoing or chronic illness?	❏	❏
2. Have you ever been hospitalized overnight?	❏	❏
Have you ever had surgery?	❏	❏
3. Are you currently taking any prescription or nonprescription (over-the-counter) medications or pills or using an inhaler?	❏	❏
Have you ever taken any supplements or vitamins to help you gain or lose weight or improve your performance?	❏	❏
4. Do you have any allergies (for example, to pollen, medicine, food, or stinging insects)?	❏	❏
Have you ever had a rash or hives develop during or after exercise?	❏	❏
5. Have you ever passed out during or after exercise?	❏	❏
Have you ever been dizzy during or after exercise?	❏	❏
Have you ever had chest pain during or after exercise?	❏	❏
Do you get tired more quickly than your friends do during exercise?	❏	❏
Have you ever had racing of your heart or skipped heartbeats?	❏	❏
Have you ever had high blood pressure or high cholesterol?	❏	❏
Have you ever been told you have a heart murmur?	❏	❏
Has any family member or relative died of heart problems or of sudden death before age 50?	❏	❏
Have you had a severe viral infection (for example, myocarditis or mononucleosis) within the last month?	❏	❏
Has a physician ever denied or restricted your participation in sports for any heart problems?	❏	❏
6. Do you have any current skin problems (for example, itching, rashes, acne, warts, fungus, or blisters)?	❏	❏
7. Have you ever had a head injury or concussion?	❏	❏
Have you ever been knocked out, become unconscious, or lost your memory?	❏	❏
Have you ever had a seizure?	❏	❏
Do you have frequent or severe headaches?	❏	❏
Have you ever had numbness or tingling in your arms, hands, legs, or feet?	❏	❏
Have you ever had a stinger, burner, or pinched nerve?	❏	❏
8. Have you ever become ill from exercising in the heat?	❏	❏
9. Do you cough, wheeze, or have trouble breathing during or after activity?	❏	❏
Do you have asthma?	❏	❏

	Yes	No
Do you have seasonal allergies that require medical treatment?	❏	❏
10. Do you use any special protective or corrective equipment or devices that aren't usually used for your sport or position (for example, knee brace, special neck roll, foot orthotics, retainer on your teeth, hearing aid)?	❏	❏
11. Have you had any problems with your eyes or vision?	❏	❏
Do you wear glasses, contacts, or protective eyewear?	❏	❏
12. Have you ever had a sprain, strain, or swelling after injury?	❏	❏
Have you broken or fractured any bones or dislocated any joints?	❏	❏
Have you had any other problems with pain or swelling in muscles, tendons, bones, or joints?	❏	❏

If yes, check appropriate box and explain below.

❏ Head   ❏ Elbow   ❏ Hip
❏ Neck   ❏ Forearm   ❏ Thigh
❏ Back   ❏ Wrist   ❏ Knee
❏ Chest   ❏ Hand   ❏ Shin/calf
❏ Shoulder   ❏ Finger   ❏ Ankle
❏ Upper arm   ❏ Foot

	Yes	No
13. Do you want to weigh more or less than you do now?	❏	❏
Do you lose weight regularly to meet weight requirements for your sport?	❏	❏
14. Do you feel stressed out?	❏	❏

15. Record the dates of your most recent immunizations (shots) for:
Tetanus: _____ Measles: _____
Hepatitis B: _____ Chickenpox: _____

FEMALES ONLY

16. When was your first menstrual period? _____
When was your most recent menstrual period? _____
How much time do you usually have from the start of one period to the start of another? _____
How many periods have you had in the last year? _____
What was the longest time between periods in the last year?

Explain "Yes" answers here: _____
_____
_____
_____
_____
_____
_____
_____

I hereby state that, to the best of my knowledge, my answers to the above questions are complete and correct.

Signature of Athlete: _____ Signature of parent/guardian: _____ Date: _____

© 1997 *American Academy of Family Physicians, American Academy of Pediatrics, American Medical Society for Sports Medicine, American Orthopaedic Society for Sports Medicine, and American Osteopathic Academy for Sports Medicine*

F I G U R E 14-1—*Continued*

Preparticipation physical evaluation. Reprinted from *Physician Sportsmed.*

Medical Conditions and Sports Participation

This table is designed to be understood by medical and nonmedical personnel. In the "Explanation" sections below, "needs evaluation" means that a physician with appropriate knowledge and experience should assess the safety of a given sport for an athlete with the listed medical condition. Unless otherwise noted, this is because of the variability of the severity of the disease or of the risk of injury among the specific sports, or both.

Condition	May participate
Atlantoaxial instability* (instability of the joint between cervical vertebrae 1 and 2)	Qualified Yes
Explanation: Athlete needs evaluation to assess risk of spinal cord injury during sports participation.	
Bleeding disorder*	Qualified Yes
Explanation: Athlete needs evaluation.	
Cardiovascular diseases	
Carditis (inflammation of the heart)	No
Explanation: Carditis may result in sudden death with exertion.	
Hypertension (high blood pressure)	Qualified Yes
Explanation: Those with significant essential (unexplained) hypertension should avoid weight and power lifting, body building, and strength training. Those with secondary hypertension (hypertension caused by a previously identified disease) or severe essential hypertension need evaluation.	
Congenital heart disease (structural heart defects present at birth)	Qualified Yes
Explanation: Those with mild forms may participate fully; those with moderate or severe forms, or who have undergone surgery, need evaluation.[†]	
Dysrhythmia (irregular heart rhythm)	Qualified Yes
Explanation: Athlete needs evaluation because some types require therapy or make certain sports dangerous, or both.	
Mitral valve prolapse (abnormal heart valve)	Qualified Yes
Explanation: Those with symptoms (chest pain, symptoms of possible dysrhythmia) or evidence of mitral regurgitation (leaking) on physical examination need evaluation. All others may participate fully.	
Heart murmur	Qualified Yes
Explanation: If the murmur is innocent (does not indicate heart disease), full participation is permitted. Otherwise, the athlete needs evaluation (see "Congenital heart disease" and "Mitral valve prolapse" above).	
Cerebral palsy*	Qualified Yes
Explanation: Athlete needs evaluation.	
Diabetes mellitus*‡	Yes
Explanation: All sports can be played with proper attention to diet, hydration, and insulin therapy. Particular attention is needed for activities that last 30 minutes or more.	
Diarrhea[§]	Qualified No
Explanation: Unless disease is mild, no participation is permitted because diarrhea may increase the risk of dehydration and heat illness. See "Fever" below.	
Eating disorders	
Anorexia nervosa, Bulimia nervosa	Qualified Yes
Explanation: These patients need both medical and psychiatric assessment before participation.	
Eyes	
Functionally one-eyed athlete, loss of an eye, detached retina, previous eye surgery or serious eye injury	Qualified Yes
Explanation: A functionally one-eyed athlete has a best-corrected visual acuity of <20/40 in the worse eye. These athletes would suffer significant disability if the better eye were seriously injured, as would those with loss of an eye. Some athletes who have previously undergone eye surgery or had a serious eye injury may have an increased risk of injury because of weakened eye tissue. Availability of eye guards approved by the American Society for Testing Materials (ASTM) and other protective equipment may allow participation in most sports, but this must be judged on an individual basis.	
Fever[§]	No
Explanation: Fever can increase cardiopulmonary effort, reduce maximum exercise capacity, make heat illness more likely, and increase orthostatic hypotension during exercise. Fever may rarely accompany myocarditis or other infections that make exercise dangerous.	
Heat illness, history of	Qualified Yes
Explanation: Because of the increased likelihood of recurrence, the athlete needs individual assessment to determine the presence of predisposing conditions and to arrange a prevention strategy.	
HIV infection[§]	Yes
Explanation: Because of the apparent minimal risk to others, all sports may be played that the state of health allows. In all athletes, skin lesions should be properly covered, and athletic personnel should use universal precautions when handling blood or body fluids with visible blood.	
Kidney: absence of one	Qualified Yes
Explanation: Athlete needs individual assessment for contact/collision and limited contact sports.	

FIGURE 14-2

Medical conditions and sports participation. Reprinted from *Physician Sportsmed.*

Medical Conditions and Sports Participation—*Continued*

Condition	May participate
Liver, enlarged Explanation: If the liver is acutely enlarged, participation should be avoided because of risk of rupture. If the liver is chronically enlarged, individual assessment is needed before contact/collision or limited contact sports are played.	Qualified Yes
Malignancy* Explanation: Athlete needs individual assessment.	Qualified Yes
Musculoskeletal disorders Explanation: Athlete needs individual assessment.	Qualified Yes
Neurologic	
History of serious head or spine trauma, severe or repeated concussions, or craniotomy Explanation: Athlete needs individual assessment for contact/collision or limited contact sports, and also for noncontact sports if there are deficits in judgment or cognition. Recent research supports a conservative approach to management of concussion.	Qualified Yes
Convulsive disorder, well controlled Explanation: Risk of convulsion during participation is minimal.	Yes
Convulsive disorder, poorly controlled Explanation: Athlete needs individual assessment for contact/collision or limited contact sports. Avoid the following noncontact sports: archery, riflery, swimming, weight or power lifting, strength training, or sports involving heights. In these sports, occurrence of a convulsion may be a risk to self or others.	Qualified Yes
Obesity Explanation: Because of the risk of heat illness, obese persons need careful acclimatization and hydration.	Qualified Yes
Organ transplant recipient* Explanation: Athlete needs individual assessment.	Qualified Yes
Ovary: absence of one Explanation: Risk of severe injury to the remaining ovary is minimal.	Yes
Respiratory	
Pulmonary compromise including cystic fibrosis* Explanation: Athlete needs individual assessment, but generally all sports may be played if oxygenation remains satisfactory during a graded exercise test. Patients with cystic fibrosis need acclimatization and good hydration to reduce the risk of heat illness.	Qualified Yes
Asthma Explanation: With proper medication and education, only athletes with the most severe asthma will have to modify their participation.	Yes
Acute upper respiratory infection Explanation: Upper respiratory obstruction may affect pulmonary function. Athlete needs individual assessment for all but mild disease. See "Fever" above.	Qualified Yes
Sickle cell disease Explanation: Athlete needs individual assessment. In general, if status of the illness permits all but high exertion, contact/collision sports may be played. Overheating, dehydration, and chilling must be avoided.	Qualified Yes
Sickle cell trait Explanation: It is unlikely that individuals with sickle cell trait (AS) have an increased risk of sudden death or other medical problems during athletic participation except under the most extreme conditions of heat, humidity, and possibly increased altitude. These individuals, like all athletes, should be carefully conditioned, acclimatized, and hydrated to reduce any possible risk.	Yes
Skin: boils, herpes simplex, impetigo, scabies, molluscum contagiosum Explanation: While the patient is contagious, participation in gymnastics with mats, martial arts, wrestling, or other contact/collision or limited contact sports is not allowed. Herpes simplex virus probably is not transmitted via mats.	Qualified Yes
Spleen, enlarged Explanation: Patients with acutely enlarged spleens should avoid all sports because of risk of rupture. Those with chronically enlarged spleens need individual assessment before playing contact/collision or limited contact sports.	Qualified Yes
Testicle: absent or undescended Explanation: Certain sports may require a protective cup.	Yes

*Not discussed in text of the monograph.

†Mild, moderate, and severe congenital heart disease are defined in 26th Bethesda Conference: Recommendations for determining eligibility for competition in athletes with cardiovascular abnormalities. January 6–7, 1994. *Med Sci Sports*. 1994;Exerc 26 (10 suppl):S246–253.

‡Well controlled

§AAP recommendation as indicated; see text for qualifications by other commentators.

Reprinted with permission from American Academy of Family Physicians, American Academy of Pediatrics (AAP) American Medical Society for Sports Medicine, American Orthopaedic Society for Sports Medicine, American Osteopathic Academy of Sports Medicine: Preparticipation Physical Evaluation, 2nd ed (monograph). Physician and Sportsmedicine, 1997, and American Academy of Pediatrics Committee on Sports Medicine and Fitness: Medical conditions affecting sports participation. *Pediatrics*. 1994;94:757–760.

FIGURE 14-2—*Continued*

Medical conditions and sports participation. Reprinted from *Physician Sportsmed.*

- Any organ enlargement (liver, spleen, or kidney) in an athlete will disqualify that person from sports until the underlying cause is determined.

- A diagnosis that is increasing is exercise-induced bronchospasm. Up to 20% of Olympic athletes report some level of exercise-induced bronchospasm. In some sports, this is less an issue than in others. It is important to recognize and treat this common problem.

- A hernia does not disqualify an athlete from participation but does require communication with the athlete and family.

- Loss of a paired organ was an immediate disqualification in the past. However, when tested in the courts, the decision has always sided with the athlete. To be proactive in such cases, the physician, school, and school district should draft a document informing all parties about the risks and consequences. All parties must sign the document to show that full disclosure has been made.

- It is very common to find evidence of past musculoskeletal injuries. All coaches and school health care professionals need to be aware of past injuries. It is important to ensure that the prior injury has been completely rehabilitated, because an incompletely healed injury puts the athlete at a high risk for further injury to that site or another site.

- Other less common problems may need further exploration either by clinical tests or counsel with the athlete and parents. These could include bloodborne pathogens, amenorrhea, eating disorders, recent acute illnesses, and history of heat illness.

After the examination, it is not advisable to offer assurances or guarantees regarding participation. Shaffer[7] suggests that the best response is that a review of the medical history and physical examination does not show any conditions that would make sports participation inadvisable.

Another issue is the managed care of high school athletes and some college athletes. The examining physician has no clinical obligations regarding follow-up of a condition found during the evaluation, other than informing the athlete and parents or guardians and recommending follow-up with the primary care physician if needed.

Unfortunately, many people view the preparticipation evaluation as a hassle and an inconvenience. The hours of preparation, number of volunteers to help, necessity of standing in line and arranging transportation to the session, examination of dozens (or hundreds) of athletes, and numerous reports and details all contribute to this opinion. However, this assessment screens for conditions that increase the risk of morbidity and mortality due to athletic participation and thus has an important purpose in the realm of sports medicine.

REFERENCES

1. Lombardo J. Sports medicine: a team effort. *Physician Sportsmed.* 1985;13:72–81.

2. Henderson JM. The team physician. In: *Principles and Practice of Primary Care Sports Medicine.* Philadelphia, Pa: Lippincott, Williams & Wilkins; 2001:Ch 18.

3. American Heart Association. Cardiovascular preparticipation screening of competitive athletes. *Circulation.* 1996;94:850–856.

4. American Heart Association. Cardiovascular preparticipation screening of competitive athletes: addendum. *Circulation.* 1998;97:2294.

5. American Academy of Pediatrics Committee on Sports Medicine and Fitness. Medical conditions affecting sports participation. *Pediatrics.* 1994;94:757–760.

6. American College of Sports Medicine. American College of Cardiologists, 26th Bethesda Conference: recommendations for determining eligibility for competition in athletes with cardiovascular abnormalities. *Med Sci Sports Exerc.* 1994;26:S223–S283.

7. Shaffer T. So you've been asked to be a team physician? *Physician Sportsmed.* 1976;4:53–67.

RESOURCES

American Academy of Family Physicians, American Academy of Pediatrics, American Medical Society for Sports Medicine, American Orthopaedic Society for Sports Medicine, and American Osteopathic Academy of Sports Medicine. Pre-participation physical evaluation. 2nd ed. *Physician Sportsmed.* 1997.

American Academy of Neurology. Practice parameter: the management of concussion in sports (summary statement). *Neurology.* 1997;48:581–585.

Bailes J. Management of athletic injuries of the cervical spine and spinal cord. *Neurosurgery.* 1991;29:491–497.

Cantu R, Bailes J, Wilberger J. Guidelines for return to contact of collision sports after a cervical spine injury. *Clin Sports Med.* 1998;17:138–146.

Garrett WE, Kirkendall DT, Squire DL, eds. *Principles and Practice of Primary Care Sports Medicine.* Philadelphia, Pa: Lippincott, Williams & Wilkins; 2001.

Grafe MW, Pal RG, Foster TE. The preparticipation sports examination for high school and college athletes. *Clin Sports Med.* 1997;16:569–589.

Knochel J. Heat stroke and related heat disorders. *Dis Monthly.* 1989;35:301–317.

Matheson G. *Sports Medicine Manual.* Calgary. International Olympic Committee; 1990.

McCrory P. Were you knocked out? A team physician's approach to initial concussion management. *Med Sci Sports Exerc.* 1997;29:S207–S212.

Mellion M. *Office Sports Medicine.* 2nd ed. Philadelphia, Pa: Hanley and Belfus; 1996.

Safran M, McKeag D, van Camp D, eds. *Manual of Sports Medicine.* Philadelphia, Pa: Lippincott-Raven; 1998.

chapter 15

Steroids and Other Ergogenic Aids

Robert J. Dimeff, MD, and Rick Kring, MS

INTRODUCTION

For more than 3000 years, athletes have used numerous agents and techniques to improve performance. Most of these agents have had little or no ergogenic (tendency to increase work output) effect. Many have been associated with serious short-term and long-term adverse effects. To understand why an elite athlete or a nonathlete would subject his or her body to the potential ill effects of these agents is important to the treatment and prevention of abuse of these drugs.

Numerous factors influence athletic performance. Cardiovascular fitness, muscular flexibility, and strength are key to success in sports. Systematic exercise training over a prolonged period is the most effective method for improving physical performance. Skills such as balance, muscle memory, reaction time, and eye-hand coordination are other important components in determining performance. Many aspects of skill are inherited; however, they can be influenced by training. General nutrition for training and competition, baseline psychologic makeup, and acute psychologic changes also highly affect performance. The ability of an athlete to mentally prepare for competition is often the difference between athletic success and failure. Proper rest allows the body time to recover from the stresses of training and competition, allows the athlete to be more alert and attentive, and improves reaction time. Genetic differences in size, strength, quickness, balance, coordination, muscle composition, and metabolic efficiency all play roles in athletic performance. Until recently, these differences were completely out of the athlete's control; however, with advances in recombinant DNA technology and genetic engineering, individual genetic limitations may be exceeded.

Performance-enhancing agents and techniques are other factors that play a role in athletic performance. These ergogenic aids include any physical, mechanical, nutritional, psychological, or pharmaceutical substance or treatment that either directly improves physiological variables associated with exercise performance or removes subjective restraints that may limit physiological capacity. These aids allow individuals to perform more work than they would otherwise be capable of performing. Most ergogenic aids do not result in substantial improvement in work output. At high levels of performance, however, large increases in training effort are required to prompt small improvement in performance. Therefore, a small increase in work output can make a large difference in results.[1]

Athletes use ergogenic agents in their desire to achieve the fame and fortune that accompany athletic success. Viewed in the context of a training program, ergogenic aids may simply be considered another part of the training regimen. In addition to athletes, a growing number of nonathletes are beginning to use ergogenic aids for cosmetic purposes. These individuals tend to be adolescent and young adult men, often of low self-esteem and poor self-confidence, who are taking drugs to develop larger muscles, appear leaner, and look more attractive to members of the opposite sex.[2]

Although many agents may affect performance by more than 1 mechanism, it is helpful to classify ergogenic aids according to their major effect:

1. Provide supplementary source of fuel.
2. Increase metabolism and/or transport of fuel to increase the available energy.
3. Remove waste products that may contribute to fatigue.
4. Increase the quality and efficiency of the work output.
5. Improve the efficiency of the nervous system input into the physiological systems.

In general, the type of sport determines the type of ergogenic aid an athlete uses. Sports that require substantial aerobic endurance, such as long-distance cycling, swimming, and running, lead to the use of agents that improve aerobic fitness. Sports that require strength and power, such as football, weightlifting, and sprinting, lead to the use of agents that improve muscular power.

More than $100 million a year are spent illegally on the black market in the United States on ergogenic aids. Up to $20 billion per year are spent in the United States on legal over-the-counter nutritional supplements. Of this sum, it is estimated that up to $800 million is spent on supplements claiming to improve athletic performance.[3] These agents are often sold by nutrition centers and mail order catalogs. Anabolic steroids are schedule III drugs, which carry large penalties for illegal distribution; this has led to a substantial increase in black market price. Ergogenic agents are described in Table 15-1.[4-58]

RECOGNITION OF ABUSE

The medical history is perhaps the most important factor in the identification of the person using performance-enhancing agents. Unfortunately, most athletes and potential users of ergogenic aids are young and healthy, rarely seek medical care, and thus are not usually detected by medical personnel. The best opportunity for discussion of this topic is at the time of the preseason and postseason physical examination. If the physical examination is performed in an open, group setting, little opportunity exists for confidential discussion. Having a separate private station will give the athlete the opportunity to discuss not only the use of ergogenic substances but also other pertinent health issues, such as drug and alcohol abuse, sexually transmitted disease, and human immunodeficiency virus (HIV).

The interview should begin with general questions regarding the athlete's overall health status, general nutrition, desire to gain or lose weight, and strength and conditioning programs. Specific questions can then be asked as guided by the patients' responses. A review of pertinent adverse effects may assist in identifying an athlete who denies but is suspected of ergogenic use.[7] Athletes who may be penalized for using performance-enhancing agents and techniques are less likely to admit abuse unless they are experiencing adverse effects. If the patient admits to using ergogenic techniques, obtain a thorough history, including names of agents, dates of use, frequency and volume of use, and potential side effects.[7]

The physical examination can be helpful in identifying the user of ergogenic aids. Users of anabolic-androgenic steroids (AAS) may have a sudden and dramatic increase in size, weight, and strength. Other findings on physical examination may include hypertension, tachycardia, cardiac hypertrophy, tender or nontender hepatomegaly, gynecomastia, testicular atrophy, alopecia, acne, and needle marks. Physical findings in the female user may also include vocal cord hypertrophy with deepening of the voice, alopecia, clitoromegaly, and breast tissue atrophy. Use of anti-estrogens have few obvious physical findings.[7]

Physical findings in users of human chorionic gonadotropin may include hypertension, water retention, gynecomastia, and needle marks. Decreased body fat and increased lean body mass and strength may be observed in users of growth hormone (GH). Acromegalic features and other physical findings are rare.

Athletes using erythropoietin, darbepoetin, and blood doping will have few physical findings. Indications of blood donation or transfusion such as hematoma, phlebitis, and puncture wounds in the antecubital fossa may be the only physical finding. After blood donation, aerobic performance may decline secondary to the phlebotomy-induced anemia, which may be noted by a coach or other person close to the training athlete.

Athletes using stimulants such as amphetamine, caffeine, ephedrine, and pseudoephedrine may be found to have tachycardia, hypertension, palpitations, anxiety, agitation, tremulousness, anorexia, and weight loss. Creatine users will often have large weight gain, with gradual weight loss over the course of 8 to 12 weeks after cessation of the supplement. Users of amino acid and protein supplements, glutamine, ribose, bicarbonate, and phosphate will have no obvious physical findings. Diuretic users may be found to have orthostatic hypotension and other findings consistent with dehydration.

Athletes using alcohol solely as an ergogenic aid will have few, if any, physical findings. Mood disturbance, sedation, and impairment of psychomotor skills may be present with acute alcohol use. Use of β-blockers by athletes may be manifest by hypotension, bradycardia, and bronchospasm. Long-term side effects of β-blockers are rarely seen in the athlete, as these medications are used only during the actual time of competition.

Routine laboratory investigations may uncover abnormalities suggestive of abuse of 1 or more of these techniques. Other testing may be required to fully evaluate the athlete. When ergogenic use is suspected, a variety of tests may be helpful.[7,26] The use of AAS may cause elevation of alanine aminotransferase (ALT), aspartate aminotransferase (AST), alkaline phosphatase, lactate dehydrogenase, and bilirubin levels. Follicle-stimulating hormone, luteinizing hormone, and natural testosterone will decrease. If a testosterone preparation is being used however, the testosterone level will increase significantly. Hypertriglyceridemia and hypercholesterolemia, with an increase in low-density lipoprotein cholesterol (LDL-C) and a decrease in high-density lipoprotein cholesterol (HDL-C), will be present. A sperm count may be necessary to evaluate testicular function. Chest roentgenogram, electrocardiogram, and echocardiogram may reveal nonspecific signs of left ventricular hypertrophy.

Blood doping, erythropoietin, and darbepoetin use will result in an increase in hemoglobin and hematocrit concentrations if the athlete is tested within 2 to 3 months of using these techniques. Creatine use may cause a temporary

TABLE 15-1

Ergogenic Agents

Agent	Mechanisms of Action	Benefits	Adverse Effects
Anabolic-androgenic steroids (AAS)[4-14]	Testosterone analogues, indirect or indirect stimulation of protein synthesis, anticatabolic effect	Increased lean body (muscle) mass, strength, aerobic capacity, and aggressive behavior	*General:* Liver enzyme elevation, cholestatic jaundice, peliosis hepatis and hepatic tumors (oral agents), fluid retention, hypertension, increased LDL-C, decreased HDL-C, concentric myocardial hypertrophy, acute myocardial infarctions, stroke, atrial fibrillation, and arterial thrombosis. *Males:* Reversible azoospermia and testicular atrophy, gynecomastia, acne, glucose intolerance, altered libido, priapism, alopecia, and scrotal pain *Females:* Vocal cord hypertrophy, male-pattern baldness, hirsutism, clitoromegaly, breast tissue atrophy, menstrual abnormalities, altered libido, acne, glucose intolerance, anxiety, panic disorder, psychosis, depression, mania, addiction, headaches, dizziness, nausea, anorexia, increased appetite, euphoria, muscle spasms, rash, dysuria, insomnia, transmission of infectious diseases (eg, hepatitis B and C, HIV) *Youth:* Possible premature closure of growth plates
Prohormones: dehydroepiandrosterone (DHEA; 3B-hydroxy-5-androstene-17-one); androstenedione (andros-4-ene-3,17-dione); 5-androstenediol (androst-5-ene-3B,17B-diol); 4-androstenediol (androst-4-ene-3B,17B-diol); 19-nor-4-androstenediol; androst-1-ene (17-hydroxyandrost-1-ene-3-one)[13-17]	Weak anabolic, androgenic, and estrogenic activity; convert to or elevate testosterone and estrogen levels; nor- prohormones metabolize into nortestosterone (nandrolone) rather than testosterone; androst-1—acts directly on androgen receptor and is not a precursor or form of testosterone	Similar to testosterone but to a lesser degree	Similar to testosterone but to a lesser degree

Continued

Ergogenic Agents—*Continued*

Agent	Mechanisms of Action	Benefits	Adverse Effects
Antiestrogens and aromatase inhibitor: clomiphene, aminoglutethimide, tamoxifen, testolactone, anastrozole[5,14,18-21]	Antiestrogens bind to estrogen receptors, thereby preventing estrogen transcription; aromatase inhibitors decrease estrogen production by blocking formation of aromatase enzyme	Used by AAS users to decrease estrogen levels, increase testosterone levels, and prevent gynecomastia and prostatic hypertrophy	Dizziness, insomnia, depression, headache, blurred vision, visual complaints, flu syndrome, nausea, vomiting, diarrhea, vasodilation, hypertension, peripheral edema, dyspnea, cough, pelvic pain, chest pain, bone pain, and rash
Human chorionic gonadotropin[5,10,14,22]	Structural resemblance to luteinizing hormone; stimulates testosterone production by Leydig cells of testes	Increase serum testosterone levels; used in conjunction with AAS to prevent or reverse testicular atrophy; used on withdrawal from an AAS cycle to "naturally" stimulate endogenous testosterone production	Due to increased testosterone level: water retention, hypertension, change in mood and libido, headaches, gynecomastia, and morning sickness
Growth hormone: somatropin, somatrem[5,10,14,23-25]	Increased intracellular transportation of amino acids and production of messenger RNA; stimulates lipolysis, increases sensitivity of fat to catecholamines, and inhibits glucose uptake and utilization by muscle cells; enhanced collagen synthesis	Increased protein synthesis and fat metabolism; preservation of muscle glycogen stores; decreased body fat; enhanced healing of musculoskeletal injuries; increased axial growth (if epiphyseal growth plates are open)	Probably minimal; theoretically gigantism and acromegaly; somatrem may cause antibody production because of extra amino acid
Stimulants: amphetamine, ephedra, ephedrine, phenylephrine, pseudoephedrine, β-agonists (eg, albuterol, isoetharine, terbutaline, metaproterenol, and clenbuterol), and caffeine[5,14,25-28]	Displace catecholamine into synaptic cleft; direct catecholamine agonist; inhibit catecholamine reuptake at synaptic cleft; inhibit degradation of catecholamine by monoamine oxidase	Improved speed, power, endurance, concentration, and fine motor coordination; elevated alertness and mood; improved self-confidence; decreased body weight and fat by appetite suppression, increased lipolysis, decreased glycogenolysis, and increased metabolic rate; increased bronchodilation; masked, delayed, or altered perception of fatigue	Headache, anxiety, nervousness, agitation, anorexia, gastrointestinal distress, insomnia, delirium, paranoia, hallucinations, hypertension, tachycardia, palpitations, cardiac arrhythmia, cerebrovascular accident, seizure, myocardial infarction

TABLE 15-1

Ergogenic Agents—*Continued*

Agent	Mechanisms of Action	Benefits	Adverse Effects
Blood doping and erythropoietin and darbepoetin[5,10,14,26,29-35]	Transfusion of donated packed red blood cells 1 to 7 days before competition; erythropoietin and darbepoetin directly stimulate erythrocyte-forming units in bone marrow to increase erythrocyte production, hemoglobin content, and release from marrow; also stimulate megakaryocyte production	Improved aerobic performance by: increased oxygen-carrying capacity of the blood, arterial-venous oxygen difference, and maximum oxygen consumption (VO2max); increased buffering capacity for metabolic wastes; decreased cardiac workload for a given aerobic performance, which also allows for a larger component of cardiac output to be diverted to skin for heat dissipation	Blood doping itself carries all potential complications of transfusion, including venous thrombosis, phlebitis, sepsis, transfusion reaction, delayed red blood cell destruction, and disease transmission, such as HIV and hepatitis B; blood doping, erythropoietin, and darbepoetin abuse may lead to hyperviscosity syndrome (headache, dizziness, vertigo, tinnitus, visual changes, angina, intermittent claudication, peripheral artery thrombosis, cerebrovascular accident, myocardial infarction, cardiac arrhythmia, and sudden death)
Protein and amino acid supplements[13,36-39]	Precursors for protein and muscle synthesis, including hemoglobin, myoglobin, metabolic enzymes and hormones, and antibodies; converted into glucose and tricarboxylic acid cycle precursors; oxidized to provide energy	Strength athletes require up to 2.2 g/kg/d, and aerobic athletes require up to 1.5 g/kg/g of protein; precursors for muscle hypertrophy associated with strength training; precursors for gluconeogenesis and tricarboxylic acid cycle intermediates during aerobic amino acids (leucine, isoleucine, and valine) are oxidized during aerobic exercise; some amino acids may increase growth hormone (GH) levels but without beneficial effects observed with actual GH administration; vegetarians may benefit from supplementation with lysine and methionine	Minimal; dehydration, gout, hypocalcemia from urinary calcium losses and renal and hepatic damage from excessive nitrogen load; excessive dietary protein may result in carbohydrate deficiency
β-hydroxy-β- methylbuterate[40,41]	Anticatabolic; prevents muscle breakdown from strength training	Possible increase in lean body mass and strength in young, previously untrained individuals beginning a strength-training program	Few; appears safe
Glutamine[38,42,43]	Most abundant amino acid in the body; substrate for nucleotide synthesis; accelerate muscle glycogen formation after intense exercise; regulate protein synthesis; enhancing immunity	Boosts immunity; may increase protein synthesis and/or decrease protein catabolism	Up to 20 g appears safe

TABLE 15-1

Ergogenic Agents—*Continued*

Agent	Mechanisms of Action	Benefits	Adverse Effects
Creatine monohydrate[44-47]	Increases muscle phosphocreatine concentration to improve adenosine triphosphate (ATP) resynthesis during and after anaerobic activities; may stimulate myofibrillar protein synthesis by enhancing uptake of amino acids into muscle	Increases muscle mass, maximal strength, and power during high-intensity, repetitive exercise	Appears safe; water retention and gastrointestinal disturbance most common; no scientific evidence to support anecdotal reports of cramping, muscle strains, hypertension, dehydration, or changes in renal function; avoid if there is preexisting renal dysfunction or if athlete is taking nephrotoxic agents to decrease kidney workload
Ribose[48,49]	Increases rate of adenine nucleotide restoration by preventing loss of or increasing synthesis; precursor of glucose, proteins, and nucleic acids; converted to pyruvate	May improve exercise tolerance in those with cardiac ischemia and those who are active in intense anaerobic exercise several times per week	Minimal complications with up to 60 g/d; diarrhea and decreased blood glucose levels
Sodium bicarbonate[50,51]	Proton sink, allowing for more rapid removal of lactic acid produced during exercise	May delay or prevent acidosis-induced muscle fatigue; decreases lactic acid levels, improves glycogenolysis and performance time in high-intensity, short-duration (40–90 s) exercise	Gastrointestinal gas, eructation, flatulence, and diarrhea; chronic bicarbonate use may result in electrolyte disturbances
Phosphate[10,52-54]	Increased concentration of 2, 3-diphosphoglycerate (2, 3-DPG) in erythrocytes to increase oxygen delivery at tissue level; increases phosphate-dependent glycolysis; proton sink; creatine phosphate and ATP precursor	Possible increase in aerobic performance; increased learning efficiency at altitude	Abdominal pain, nausea, vomiting, and diarrhea; chronic phosphate supplementation may result in hyperphosphatemia, causing osteomalacia and bone and joint pain
Diuretics[5,10,14,55]	Increase fluid loss	Rapid weight loss to get into a specific weight class; improve body image; reduce urine concentration of banned drugs	Dehydration and electrolyte abnormalities

increase in serum creatinine levels due to increased muscle content of creatine and laboratory misidentification of creatine as creatinine. This will usually reverse within 2 to 3 months. Bicarbonate use may cause metabolic alkalosis and hyperkalemia. Phosphate loading may lead to hyperphosphatemia and hypocalcemia. The use of diuretics may cause hypokalemia, hypercholesterolemia, hyper-

triglyceridemia, and hyperuricemia. Use of alcohol as an ergogenic aid may result in an increase in ALT, AST, and gamma glutamyltransferase (GGT). The use of human chorionic gonadotropin, GH, stimulants, amino acids and protein supplements, glutamine, ribose, narcotics, and β-blockers as ergogenic aids will result in no major abnormalities in laboratory values.

TABLE 15-1

Ergogenic Agents—*Continued*

Alcohol[10,55-58]	Central nervous system depressant; anxiolytic and antitremor effect in low doses	Anxiolytic and antitremor effect is ergogenic in sports such as archery and riflery, for which a steady hand is required for optimum performance	Acute use impairs accuracy, balance, steadiness, reaction time, complex and fine motor coordination, visual tracking, judgment, and information processing; decreases aerobic capacity with no change in muscle strength or endurance; may impair athletic performance the day after use
β-blockers[5,10,14,55]	Inhibit adrenergic stimulation	Anxiolysis, bradycardia, and antitremor effects may be ergogenic in sports requiring steadiness, such as archery, riflery, and golf	Decrease aerobic and anaerobic endurance and power, bronchospasm, hypotension, bradycardia, atrioventricular block, sleep disturbance, sexual dysfunction, and hypoglycemia

TREATMENT

Once an athlete is found to be using an ergogenic aid, treatment should be initiated. It is important to treat any severe side effects and to be prepared for the development of withdrawal effects. After cessation of use of AAS and, to a lesser extent, human chorionic gonadotropin, creatine, and GH, the athlete must realize that a substantial amount of body size and strength will be lost. In the case of AAS, major depression may be associated with withdrawal and will need to be addressed and treated. Fluoxetine hydrochloride (Prozac) has been successful in treating major depression associated with AAS withdrawal.[59] Treatment of athletes using blood doping, erythropoietin, or darbepoetin, which can cause hyperviscosity syndrome, may require phlebotomy, strict avoidance of dehydration, and close monitoring of the hematocrit concentration. Potassium replacement may be necessary to treat hypokalemia associated with diuretic use. Bradycardia and cardiac dysrhythmia associated with β-blocker use may require cardiac monitoring and treatment. The use and withdrawal of most other ergogenic aids generally require no other specific evaluation or treatment.

PREVENTION

Many of the prevention programs for ergogenic agents are modeled after programs designed to prevent abuse of drugs and alcohol. Success of such programs depends on involvement of the athlete, coaching staff, sports medicine personnel, physical therapists, athletic trainers, teachers, and parents. Role models, teaching, and policies all affect likelihood of use of these substances.

A proactive education program geared toward the athlete and persons having influence on the athlete is a deterrent to the use of ergogenic aids. Currently, at the college level, 76% of division I, 50% of division II, and 41% of division III schools have formal educational programs regarding use of ergogenic techniques.[26] Optimally such programs start at the elementary school level and continue through the high school, college, and professional ranks. These programs should present accurate information to the individual regarding potential risks and benefits associated with the use of these techniques. All groups should be educated to recognize the signs and symptoms of abuse in order to help identify the potential abuser. Particularly important is that all understand the healthy, legal, and ethical means for improving athletic performance.

Nutrition

Proper nutrition and hydration is essential during all phases of athletic performance. By educating athletes and those associated with them about proper nutrition, the use of ergogenic aids may be prevented. The main dietary goal is to supply adequate nutrition to optimize training. The metabolism of carbohydrates and fats during exercise provides most of the energy required for exercise. Fatigue is associated with a depletion of either glycogen or fat. Dietary intake should be equivalent in total calories (energy) and percentage of fat and carbohydrate that are utilized during the exercise activity. If glycogen and fat stores are depleted, protein resynthesis is also inhibited, leading to a loss of muscle mass and impaired performance.[60] Numerous studies have shown that a high-carbohydrate diet increases muscle glycogen stores and improves endurance performance.[37] Athletes should consume 5 to 10 g/kg/d of carbohydrate. Good sources of carbohydrates include breads, cereals, pastas, grain products, fruits and vegetables, and dairy products. Protein and amino acids provide only 5% to 10% of the energy during prolonged exercise.[37] The current US Recommended Daily Allowances (RDA) for protein is 0.8 g/kg/d. Athletes involved in prolonged endurance events require up to 1.5 g/kg/d of protein, whereas those involved in heavy-resistance weightlifting may require up to 2.2 g/kg/d of protein. Most athletes eating a normal Western diet consume up to 1.5 g/kg/d, and thus some athletes may need additional dietary protein.

Fat is an important energy source for the athlete involved in prolonged low-intensity exercise.[37,60] With moderate or heavy-intensity exercise of short duration, carbohydrate from muscle and liver glycogen is the main energy source. As the intensity of exercise decreases and the duration increases, a greater percentage of energy is derived from fat. With improved endurance training, general cellular and physiological adaptations result in improved fat use.[37] Recent studies have demonstrated improved performance in endurance runners consuming a high-fat diet: increased exercise time to exhaustion, deceased blood lactate accumulation, and improved aerobic activity performed at intensities at or below 80% of maximum oxygen consumption (VO2max).[60-63] Endurance runners consuming diets with up to 40% fat have improved lipid profiles compared with those consuming diets with 16% fat. The high-fat diet maintained favorable risk factors for coronary heart disease, whereas the 16% fat diet lowered apolipoprotein A-I and HDL-C levels and raised total cholesterol-to-HDL-C ratios. The high dietary fat intake did not change weight; body fat; heart rate; blood pressure; or triglycerides, total cholesterol, or LDL C levels. Increased fat intake has been shown to have no adverse effects on level of plasma interleukin 2 (IL-2), proinflammatory cytokines, cortisol, interferon gamma, and lipid peroxide.[63] In conclusion, athletes involved in regular endurance running may benefit from increased dietary fat intake of up to 40%.

Water is the most critical nutrient for an athlete during training and competition. Sweat losses, which are affected by overall conditioning and acclimatization, can range from 1.5 to 3 L/h. Because thirst is an inadequate indicator of fluid losses, it is important that oral hydration be maintained during training.[37] During exercise, 4 to 8 oz of cool water should be consumed every 15 to 20 minutes; 5% to 8% carbohydrate liquids may also be used. Carbohydrate liquids, in addition to providing hydration, will help preserve muscle glycogen stores and are most beneficial when the duration of exercise is more than 60 to 90 minutes.[37]

Pre-event nutrition

The goals of the pre-event meal are to ensure adequate carbohydrates, prevent dehydration, avoid gastrointestinal tract (GI) irritation, and provide a relatively empty stomach while avoiding hunger pangs. The meal should be pleasant and satisfying, of minimal bulk and low salt, provide adequate fluid of at least 16 oz, be composed of foods the athlete is accustomed to eating, and be consumed 2 to 5 hours before competition. If the athlete cannot consume a solid meal, a liquid carbohydrate meal may be consumed up to 60 minutes before the event. Carbohydrate feedings are generally to be avoided 15 to 60 minutes before exercise, as this may cause an increase in serum insulin level leading to hypoglycemia.[37] This hypoglycemia may decrease performance during high-intensity exercise, but appears to have little deleterious effect on performance during moderate-intensity exercise. Carbohydrate ingested immediately before a high-intensity exercise may improve performance due to an increase in carbohydrate bioavailability.

Carbohydrate loading is a dietary technique that may improve performance in endurance events, such as cross-country skiing, distance cycling, running, and swimming. This technique should be used only in well-trained athletes. Endurance may be improved in exercise that lasts more than 90 minutes by allowing muscle to store 2 to 3 times more glycogen than normal. The classic carbohydrate loading regimen[64] developed in the 1960s involves 3 days of intense exercise on an extremely low-carbohydrate (<10%) diet to deplete muscle glycogen stores. Days 4 to 6 are spent resting and consuming a high-carbohydrate (>80%) diet. The competition is then held on day 7 with consumption of a normal high-carbohydrate precompetition meal. This technique will increase muscle glycogen stores up to 3 times baseline; however, it is very strenuous and may lead to injury, fatigue, and irritability. The modified carbohydrate regimen[37] involves a moderate-carbohydrate (50%) diet on days 1 to 3, and a high-carbohydrate (>80%) diet on days 4 to 6 with a high-carbohydrate, precompetition meal. In association with this diet, exercise is tapered on days 1 through 5, with rest on day 6. The modified technique results in an increase in muscle glycogen stores similar to the classic regimen but appears to be safer and less strenuous.

Event nutrition

During sporting events that last less than 1 hour, water alone may be used. To prevent dehydration, the athlete should consume 4 to 8 oz of cool water every 15 to 20 minutes. Increased volumes are required in hot, humid weather, especially in the unacclimatized, less-trained athlete. Carbohydrate should be consumed during competition of greater than 60 minutes' duration. The carbohydrate will help maintain blood glucose and liver glycogen levels and spare muscle glycogen stores. The most effective carbohydrate supplements during exercise are the 5% to 8% carbohydrate solutions.[37] The glucose supplements are thought to be superior to fructose solutions, as the latter may cause a delay in gastric emptying, leading to GI distress. The minimal amount of carbohydrate needed for effectiveness is 22 g/h. Some experts recommend up to 250 g/h.[37] Solid carbohydrate sources are also beneficial but do not provide the necessary liquid to prevent dehydration. Compared with solids, liquid supplements provide both fluid and carbohydrate and have faster gastric emptying.

Severe hyponatremia has been reported in individuals consuming large volumes of water during endurance activities lasting more than 4 hours. Serum sodium levels below 120 mg/dL have been recorded, which potentially may lead to fatal cerebral edema. Hyponatremia has been reported in slow marathoners, ultramarathoners, triathletes, tennis players, football players in 2-a-day practices, and desert hikers who usually consume only water and actually maintain or gain weight during their activity.[65]

Postevent nutrition

After exercise, there occurs decreased muscle glycogen stores, increased proteolysis, negative muscle protein balance, and usually decreased weight due to dehydration.[66] As a result of these conditions the athlete may experience prolonged muscular soreness as well as decreased performance, muscle mass, and metabolic rate. An increase in proteolysis and a decrease in protein synthesis will occur for up to 24 hours. If training does not occur again within that time, protein synthesis can take place at a greater

rate than proteolysis. This may become a limitation in the competitive athlete who tends to overtrain or train too frequently.

The goals of postevent nutrition are to replace fluid losses and replenish glycogen stores.[37] The volume of fluid loss during competition can be calculated from the difference between pre-event and postevent weights. Close monitoring of weight, especially early in the sport season, should be practiced to minimize dehydration and fluid imbalance. For every 1 lb of weight lost, 16 oz of fluid should be consumed.

Three key factors need to be addressed to improve the rate of glycogen repletion. First, the rate of glycogen synthesis is highest immediately after exercise.[37,67] Second, adequate dietary carbohydrate availability is necessary to convert to muscle glycogen and to decrease proteolysis. Third, the athlete needs to establish a high insulin level to stimulate glycogen storage. At rest, insulin is anabolic in nature. After exercise, high insulin levels decrease proteolysis by more than 30%. Consumption of a combination carbohydrate and protein drink after exercise has been shown to increase insulin levels to a greater extent than equal numbers of calories of carbohydrates alone.[37,39,68] If the beverage is consumed immediately after training, glycogen synthesis will be up to 300% greater than if taken 2 hours after training. Thus, to maximize glycogen repletion, the athlete should consume protein and carbohydrate drink immediately after the workout. A beverage is consumed rather than whole food due to the rate of absorption and tolerance after exertion.[68] The optimal source of carbohydrate is glucose or a glucose polymer such as maltodextrin, and the optimal source of protein appears to be the rapidly absorbed whey hydrolysate. The postworkout beverage will provide fuel for recovery, increase insulin concentrations (allowing uptake of glucose, amino acids, and creatine into the muscles), improve glycogen repletion, stimulate protein synthesis, and provide a positive protein status. Approximately 75 g of carbohydrate and 25 g of protein should be consumed within the first hour after exercise and every 2 to 4 hours thereafter.

Equipment and Training

Good coaching will affect athletic performance. A good coach knows all facets of athletic participation, including use of sport-specific skills and proper technique; adequate adjustment of training programs; repetition in practice; appropriate rest and rehabilitation from training, competition, and injury; and mental preparation for the sport. A coach who is well versed in these techniques can give this knowledge to athletes to allow them to compete at peak form. Proper equipment is essential for use in practice and competition. The athlete, coaches, and trainers need to ensure that all equipment is in proper working condition and of high quality. Irregularities in the playing surface may lead to injury and should therefore be promptly repaired. Those involved in athletics need to be aware of the risk factors associated with practice and competition on improper surfaces and appropriately alter schedules. By maintaining high-quality athletic equipment and practice standards, an athlete will be better able to achieve excellence without the use of ergogenic aids.

Strength and Conditioning

As an adjunct to proper training, overall fitness is essential to maximize success in sports. There are 2 basic aspects of fitness: (1) anaerobic or muscle strengthening and (2) aerobic or cardiovascular conditioning. Depending on the sport involved, the amount of training in either of these areas may be altered. A well-trained strength and conditioning coach can help the athlete improve performance without the use of ergogenic substances. The goal of aerobic training is to provide sufficient cardiovascular overload to cause cardiac changes that improve efficiency. The goal of muscular conditioning is to provide sufficient resistance to overload muscles, allowing them to achieve their maximum tension-developing or force output capacity through the entire range of motion.

Psychological Techniques

Instruction on the psychologic aspect of training and competition can be extremely helpful in prevention of use of ergogenic aides.[69] Sports psychologists can make a tremendous difference in athletic performance. Optimum athletic performance requires optimum mental stimulation. If the level of stress is too low, performance declines; and if the level of stress is too great, anxiety develops, which interferes with performance. The level of stimulation required for optimum performance varies from athlete to athlete and from competition to competition within the same individual. This fluctuation may be altered with mental training. The ability to "psyche up" can be learned and will improve athletic performance in situations where stimulation is low. A variety of feedback techniques have been developed, which may work to relax the athlete in situations where the stimulation is too great. Techniques, such as biofeedback, rehearsal, imagery, and self-talk, may help the athlete in establishing the mental toughness required to succeed at a high level. With experience and proper psychologic instruction, the mental health of the athlete is stabilized, athletic performance is improved, and use of ergogenic aids is deterred.

Drug Testing

Drug testing is an important aspect of preventing use of ergogenic aids but is controversial, with strong proponents both for and against it. Before drug testing is instituted, rules should be established to govern how the results are to be used, and prevention and treatment programs established to avoid inconsistencies in the treatment of any given athlete. The concern about randomization of testing, whom to test, when to test, and just cause need to be addressed. Many ergogenic drugs and techniques cannot be detected through testing at this time, and newer drugs and techniques are constantly being developed.

Urine drug testing by mass spectrophotometry and gas chromatography with and without derivatization is the most commonly used method. The specimen is usually split into 2 samples so that if there is an appeal on the basis of laboratory error, the second specimen can then be tested to confirm the results. Although urine drug testing for AAS and metabolite abuse using mass spectrophotometry and gas chromatography is accurate, new steroids are being developed for which patterns are not known. For athletes using over-the-counter supplements, the purity of these compounds is unregulated by the US Food and Drug Administration, and thus possible contamination and inadvertent positive testing may occur.[70] Due to its distinct gas chromatography appearance, darbepoetin was easily identified on urine drug testing and resulted in numerous disqualifications at the 2002 Salt Lake City Winter Olympics Games.[26] Urine electropherography can also be used to detect exogenous erythropoietin abuse.[26] Monitoring for a decrease in the hemoglobin and hematocrit concentrations with serial blood work, detection of an elevated hematocrit concentration, or an abnormal result of mass spectrophotometry and gas chromatography urinalysis may be used to detect illicit methods of increasing hematocrit concentration.[26]

Abuse of GH may be detected by immunoassays, which can distinguish pituitary-derived GH from recombinant GH.[71] This requires a blood sample and can detect exogenous GH use within 24 hours of administration, making it valuable for out-of-competition testing. Measurement of increased levels of GH-sensitive substances, which are not affected by stress levels, may be used to detect illicit GH use up to 2 weeks after administration.[24] Increased GH levels with normal insulin-like growth factor (IGF) levels have been reported in Olympic medalists under stress, which normalized when competition stress was removed.[72] Additionally, measurement of urinary IGF-1 and IGF binding protein 2 and 3 levels may be used as a marker for GH abuse.[73] Hair analysis has been used to determine illicit used of AAS and stimulants and appears to correlate well with urine testing.[74]

National Collegiate Athletic Association (NCAA) policy requires testing for ergogenic aids at all championship events, but only division I and II football and division I track and field athletes are subject to year-round drug testing. Among colleges, 75% of division I and 43% of division II schools, but only 8% of division III schools, have drug testing programs. This discrepancy in drug testing is evident, as the use of illicit ergogenic aids is higher at the division III level than at the division I and II levels.[26]

The NCAA Ergogenic Program is described in Table 15-2.

Penalties

Although random drug testing is important in the prevention of the use of ergogenic aids, penalties contribute to effectiveness. The penalties should be unbiased, consistent, and harsh. The use of some of these agents carry major legal ramifications. If the penalty is minimal, the effectiveness of prevention of the use of ergogenic aids through education and drug testing will also be minimal.

NCAA penalties may include record stripping and temporary or lifetime ban from sports participation placing athletic careers in jeopardy. These types of penalties underscore the need for prevention.

TABLE 15-2

National Collegiate Athletic Association (NCAA) Ergogenic Program*

Banned agents
1. Anabolic-androgenic steroids
2. Blood doping
3. Diuretics
4. Urine manipulation agents
5. β-blockers when used in riflery competition
6. Peptide hormones and analogues, including human chorionic gonadotropin, corticotropin, human GH, erythropoietin, and releasing factors
7. Stimulants, including cocaine, amphetamine, amphetamine-like drugs, sympathomimetics, and β$_2$ agonists except for inhaled β-agonists—all inhaled β-agonists are permitted
8. Caffeine intake in which maximum urine concentration exceeds 15 µg/mL
9. Alcohol in riflery competition
10. Street drugs, including heroin, marijuana, and tetrahydrocannabinol (THC)
11. Cough and cold decongestants except for over-the-counter sympathomimetic agents, which are permitted
12. Intravenous administration of injestable anesthetics
13. Cocaine
Note: Topical anesthetics and local and intra-articular injections of injestable anesthetics not containing vasoconstrictor drugs are permitted.

Athletes tested
1. All NCAA athletes are subject to drug testing before, during, and after NCAA championship competitions as well as year-round and on-campus short-notice testing.
2. Method for selecting championships, institutions, and athletes to be tested is recommended by NCAA Competition Safeguards Committee and approved by Executive Committee.
3. Selection basis may include playing time, position, and financial aid status or may be entirely random.
4. First-, second-, and third-place finishers and other chance-selected athletes from the remaining field may be selected for drug testing.
5. During off-season, division I-A and I-AA football and division I men's and women's track and field athletes are subject to testing for anabolic-androgenic steroids and masking agents. All other athletes may be tested at NCAA championships and bowl events, possibly for the entire list of banned substances.
6. Individual schools may perform their own drug testing.

Penalties
1. First violation: Athlete is ineligible for all regular and postseason competitions for a minimum of 1 calendar year after positive test result; athlete must retest negative and have eligibility restored by NCAA Eligibility Committee.
2. Second violation (except for use of street drugs only): more severe penalty, including lifetime ban.
3. Second violation street drugs only: 1-year suspension; lifetime expulsion does not apply.

*From NCAA *Drug Education Handbook.*

REFERENCES

1. Coyle EF. Ergogenic aids. *Clin Sports Med.* 1984;3:7313–7342.

2. Buckley WE, Yesalis CE III, Friedl KE, Anderson WA, Streit AL, Wright JE. Estimated prevalence of anabolic steroid use among male high school seniors. *JAMA* 1988;260:3441–3445.

3. Green GA, Catlin DH, Starcevic B. Analysis of over the counter dietary supplements. *Clin J Sports Med.* 2001;11:254–259.

4. Bergink EW, Geelen JA, Turpijn EW. Metabolism and receptor binding of nandrolone and testosterone under in vitro and in vivo conditions. *Acta Endocrinol Suppl (Copenh).* 1985;271:31–37.

5. Hardman JG, Limbird LE, Gilman AG, eds. *Goodman and Gilman's The Pharmacological Basis of Therapeutics.* 10th ed. New York, NY: McGraw-Hill; 2001.

6. Haupt HA, Rovere GD. Anabolic steroids: a review of the literature. *Am J Sports Med.* 1984;12:469–484.

7. Johnson MD. Anabolic steroid use in adolescent athletes. *Pediatr Clin North Am.* 1990;37:1111–1123.

8. Matsumoto AM. Effects of chronic testosterone administration in normal men: safey and efficacy of high dose testosterone and parallel dose-dependent suppression of leuteinizing hormone, follicle-stimulating hormone, and sperm production. *J Clin Endocrinol Metab.* 1990;70:282–287.

9. Giorgi A, Weatherby RP, Murphy PW. Muscular strength, body composition and health responses to the use of testosterone enanthate: a double blind study. *J Sci Med Sport.* 1999;2:341–355.

10. Humes HD, Dupont HL, eds. *Kelley's Textbook of Internal Medicine.* 4th ed. Philadelphia, Pa: Lippincott Williams & Wilkins; 2000.

11. Bhasin S, Storer TW, Berman N. Testosterone replacement increases fat free mass and muscle size in hypogonadal men. *J Clin Endocrinol Metab.* 1997;82:407–413.

12. Vermeulen A, Goemaere S, Kaufman JM. Testosterone, body composition and aging. *J Endocrinol Invest.* 1999;22S:110–116.

13. Pipe A, Ayotte C. Nutritional supplements and doping. *Clin J Sports Med.* 2002;12:245–250.

14. *Physicians' Desk Reference.* 57th ed. Montvale, NJ: Medical Economics Co; 2003.

15. Morales AJ, Nolan JJ, Nelson JC, Yen Ss. Effects of replacement dose of dehydroepiandrosterone in men and women of advancing age. *J Clin Endocrinol Metab.* 1994;78:1360–1367.

16. Sundaram K, Kumar N, Monder C, Bardin CW. Different patterns of metabolism determine the relative anabolic activity of 19-norandrogens. *J Steroid Biochem Molec Biol.* 1995;53(1–6):253–257.

17. Corrigan B. DHEA and sport. *Clin J Sports Med.* 2002;12:236–241.

18. Burge MR, Lanzi RA, Skarda ST, Easton RP. Idiopathic hypogonadotropic hypogonadism in a male runner is reversed by clomiphene citrate. *Fertile Steril.* 1997;67:783–785.

19. Dony JM, Smals AG, Rolland R, Fauser BC, Thomas CM. Effect of lower versus higher doses of tamoxifen on pituitary-gonadal function and sperm indices in oligozoospermic men. *Andrologia.* 1985;17:369–378.

20. Martikainen H, Ruokonen A, Ronnberg L, Vihko R. Short-term effects of testolactone on human testicular steroid production and on the response to human chorionic gonadotropin. *Fertil Steril.* 1985;43:793–798.

21. Miller WR. Aromatase inhibitors: Where are we now? *Br J Anaesth.* 1996;4:415–417.

22. Voy RO. IOC bans human chorionic gonadotropin. *Sportsmediscope.* 1988;7:11.

23. Dean H. Does exogenous growth hormone improve athletic performance? *Clin J Sports Med.* 2002;12:250–253.

24. Sonksen PH. Insulin, growth hormone and sport. *J Endocrinol.* 2001;170:13–25.

25. Berlin I, Warot D, Aymard G. Pharmacodynamics and pharmacokinetics of single nasal (5mg and 10mg) and oral (50mg) doses of ephedrine in healthy subjects. *Eur J Clin Pharmacol.* 2001;57:447–455.

26. Green GA. Annual update on supplements and ergogenic aids. Presented at American Medical Society for Sports Medicine 12th Annual Meeting, San Diego, Calif, April 6, 2003.

27. Bouchard R, Weber AR, Geiger JD. Informed decision-making on sympathomimetic use in sports and health. *Clin J Sports Med.* 2002;12:209–225.

28. McKenzie DC, Stewart AB, Fitch KD. The asthmatic athlete, inhaled beta agonists, and performance. *Clin J Sports Med.* 2002;12:225–229.

29. American College of Sports Medicine position stand: blood doping as an ergogenic aid. *Med Sci Sports Exerc.* 1987;19:540–543.

30. Erslev AJ. Erythropoietin. *N Engl J Med.* 1991;324:1339–1344.

31. Jones M, Pedoe DST. Blood doping: a literature review. *Br J Sports Med.* 1989;23:84–88.

32. Once-weekly erythropoeses-stimulating protein enters market. *Am J Health Syst Pharm.* 2001;58:2120–2121.

33. Egrie JC, Browne JK. Development and characterization of novel erythropoesis stimulating protein (NESP). *Nephrol Dial Transplant.* 2001;16 (Suppl 3):3–13.

34. Macdougall IC. An overview of the efficacy and safety of novel erythropoesis stimulating protein (NESP). *Nephrol Dial Transplant.* 2001;16:14–21.

35. Kazlauskas R, Howe C, Fitch KD. Strategies for rhEPO detection in sport. *Clin J Sports Med.* 2002;12:229–236.

36. Blomstrand E, Hassmen P, Ekblom B, Newsholme EA. Administration of branched-chain amino acid during sustained exercise: effects on performance and on plasma concentration of some amino acids. *Eur J Appl Physiol Occup Physiol.* 1991;63:83–88.

37. Dimeff RJ. Sports nutrition. In: Johnson RJ, Lombardo JA, eds. *Current Review of Sports Medicine.* Philadelphia, Pa: Current Medicine Inc; 1994:201–221.

38. Garlick P. Assessment of the safety of glutamine and other amino acids. *J Nutr.* 2001;131:2556S–2561S.

39. Rasmussen BB, Tipton KD, Miller SL, Wolf SE, Wolfe RR. An oral essential amino acid-carbohydrate supplement enhances muscle protein anabolism after resistance exercise. *J Appl Physiol.* 2000;88:386–392.

40. Gallagher PM, Carrithers JA, Godard MP, Schulze KE, Trappe SW. Beta-hydroxy-beta-methylbutyrate ingestion: I. Effects on strength and fat free mass. *Med Sci Sports Exerc.* 2000;32:2109–2115.

41. Gallagher PM, Carrithers JA, Godard MP, Schulze KE, Trappe SW. Beta-hydroxy-beta-methylbutyrate ingestion: II. Effects on hematology, hepatic and renal function. *Med Sci Sports Exerc.* 2000;32:2116–2119.

42. Walsh NP, Blannin AK, Robson PJ, Gleeson M. Glutamine, exercise and immune function: links and possible mechanisms. *Sports Med.* 1998;26:177–191.

43. Ziegler T, Szeszycki EE, Estivariz CF, Puckett AB, Leader LM. Glutamine: from basic science to clinical applications. *Nutrition.* 1996;12(Suppl 11–12):S68–S70.

44. Smith SA, Montain SJ, Matott RD, Zientara GD, Jolesz FA, Fielding RA. Creatine supplementation and age influence muscle metabolism during exercise. *J Appl Physiol.* 1998;85:1349–1356.

45. Juhn MS, Tarnopolsky M. Oral creatine supplementation and athletic performance: a critical review. *Clin J Sports Med.* 1998;8:286–297.

46. Juhn MS, Tarnopolsky M. Potential side effects of oral creatine supplementation: a critical review. *Clin J Sports Med.* 1998;8:298–304.

47. Volek JS, Kraemer WJ, Bush JA, et al. Creatine supplementation enhances muscular performance during high-intensity resistance exercise. *J Am Diet Assoc.* 1997;97:765–770.

48. Lee H, Graeff R, Walseth T. Cyclic ADP-ribose and its metabolic enzymes. *Biochemie.* 1995;77:245–255.

49. Sahlin K, Broberg S. Adenine nucleotide depletion in human muscle during exercise: causality and significance of AMP deamination. *Int J Sports Med.* 1990;11:S62–S67.

50. McNaughton L, Thompson D. Acute versus chronic sodium bicarbonate ingestion and anaerobic work and power output. *J Sports Med Phys Fitness.* 2001;41:456–465.

51. Hollidge-Horvat MG, Parolin ML, Wong D, Jones NL, Heigenhauser GJ. Effect of induced metabolic alkalosis on human skeletal muscle metabolism during exercise. *Am J Physiol Endocrinol Metab.* 2000;278:E316–E329.

52. Cade R, Conte M, Zauner C. Effects of phosphate loading on 2, 3-diphosphoglycerate and maximal oxygen uptake. *Med Sci Sports Exerc.* 1984;16:263–268.

53. Kreider RB, Miller GW, Williams MH, Somina CT, Nasser TA. Effects of phosphate loading on oxygen uptake, ventilatory anaerobic threshold, and run performance. *Med Sci Sports Exerc.* 1990;22:250–256.

54. Goss F, Robertson R, Riechman S. Effect of potassium phosphate supplementation on perceptual and physiological responses to maximal graded exercise. *Int J Sport Nutr Exerc Metab.* 2001;11:53–62.

55. Wadler GI, Hainline B. *Drugs and the Athlete.* Philadelphia, Pa: FA Davis Co Publishers; 1989.

56. Bond V. Effects of small and moderate doses of alcohol on submaximal cardio-respiratory functions, perceived exertion and endurance performance in abstainers and moderate drinkers. *J Sports Med.* 1983;23:221–228.

57. Koller WC, Biary N. Effect of alcohol on tremors: comparison with propranolol. *Neurology.* 1984;34:221–222.

58. McNaughton L, Preece D. Alcohol and its effect on sprint and middle distance running. *Br J Sports Med.* 1982; 14:481–482.

59. Malone DA, Dimeff RJ. The use of fluoxetine in depression associated with anabolic steroid withdrawal: a case series. *J Clin Psychiatry.* 1992;53:130–132.

60. Pendergast DR, Horvath PJ, Leddy JJ, Venkatraman JT. The role of dietary fat on performance, metabolism, and health. *Am J Sports Med.* 1996;24:S53–S58.

61. Horvath PJ, Eagen CK, Fisher NM, Leddy JJ, Pendergast DR. The effects of varying dietary fat on performance and metabolism in trained male and female runners. *J Am Coll Nutr.* 2000;19:52–60.

62. Horvath PJ, Eagen CK, Ryer-Calvin SB, Pendergast DR. The effects of varying dietary fat on the nutrient intake in male and female runners. *J Am Coll Nutr.* 2000;19:42–51.

63. Venkatraman JT, Feng X, Pendergast DR. Effects of dietary fat and endurance exercise on plasma cortisol, prostaglandin E2, interferon-gamma and lipid peroxide in runners. *J Am Coll Nutr.* 2001;20:529–536.

64. Bergstrom J, Hermansen L, Holtman E, Saltin B. Diet, muscle glycogen and physical performance. *Acta Physiol Scand.* 1967;7:140–150.

65. Noakes T. Hyponatremia in distance runners: fluid and sodium balance during exercise. *Curr Sports Med Rep.* 2002;1:197–208.

66. MacDougall JD, Gibala MJ, Tarnopolsky MA, MacDonald JR, Interisano SA, Yarasheski KE. The time for elevated muscle protein synthesis following heavy resistance exercise. *Can J Appl Physiol.* 1995;20:480–486.

67. Roy BD, Tarnopolsky MA, MacDougall JD, Fowles J, Yarasheski KE. Effect of glucose supplement timing on protein metabolism after resistance training. *J Appl Physiol.* 1997;82:1882–1888.

68. van Loon L, Saris WH, Kruij Shoop M, Wagenmakers AJ. Maximizing postexercise muscle glycogen synthesis: carbohydrate supplementation and the application of amino acid or protein hydrolysate mixtures. *Am J Clin Nutr.* 2000;72:106–111.

69. Lynch GP. Athletic injuries in the practicing sports psychologist: practical guidelines for assisting athletes. *Sports Psychol.* 1988;2:161–167.

70. Catlin DH, Leder BZ, Ahrens B, et al. Trace contamination of over-the-counter androstenedione and positive urine test results for a nandrolone metabolite. *JAMA.* 2000;284:2618–2621.

71. Bidlingmaier M, Wu Z, Strasburger CJ. Test method: GH. *Best Pract Res Clin Endocrinol Metab.* 2000;14:99–109.

72. Armanini D, Faggian D, Scaroni C, Plebani M. Growth hormone and insulin-like growth factor I in a Sydney Olympic gold medallist. *Br J Sports Med.* 2002;36:148–149.

73. Kicman AT, Miell JD, Teale JD, et al. Serum IGF-I and IGF binding proteins 2 and 3 as potential markers of doping with human GH. *Clin Endocrinol.* 1997;47:43–50.

74. Dumestre-Toulet V, Cirimele V, Ludes B, Gromb S, Kintz D. Hair analysis of seven bodybuilders for anabolic steroids, ephedrine, and clenbuterol. *J Forensic Sci.* 2002;47:211–214.

RESOURCES

Drugs

Bahrke M, Yesalis C, ed. *Performance Enhancing Substances in Sport and Exercise.* Champaign, Ill: Human Kinetics Books; 2002.

Fuentes RJ, Rosenberg JM, Davis A, eds. *Athletic Drug Reference'96.* Durham NC: Clean Data Inc; 1996.

Duchaine D. *The Underground Steroid Handbook.* Venice, Calif: HLR Technical Books; 1988.

Duchaine D. *The Underground Steroid Handbook II.* Venice, Calif: HLR Technical Books; 1989.

World Anabolic Review 1996: Anabolic Steroid Handbook. Houston, Tex: MB Muscle Books; 1995.

Williams MH. *The Ergogenic Edge: Pushing the Limits of Sports Performance.* Champaign, Ill: Human Kinetics Books; 1998.

Yesalis CE, ed. *Anabolic Steroids in Sport and Exercise. 2nd ed.* Champaign, Ill: Human Kinetics Books; 2002.

Drug Testing Information

National Collegiate Athletic Association (NCAA) Drug Education Program, 6201 College Blvd, Overland Park, KS 66211-2422.
    Web site: www.ncaa.org.

US Olympic Committee (USOC) Drug Education Program, 1750 E Boulder St, Colorado Springs, CO 80909.
    Web site: www.olympic-usa.org.

Performance Improvement

Clark N. *Nancy Clark's Sports Nutrition Guidebook.* 2nd ed. Champaign, Ill: Human Kinetics Books; 1997.

Fleck SJ, Kraemer WJ. *Designing Resistance Training Programs.* 3rd ed. Champaign, Ill: Human Kinetics Books; 2003.

PART 4

Nutrition, Supplements, and Complementary and Alternative Medicine

chapter 16

Nutrition Screening and Assessment

Marie-Andree Roy, MSc, and Gordon L. Jensen, MD, PhD

INTRODUCTION

The prevalence of undernutrition among hospitalized patients has been documented and reported for more than 25 years.[1,2] It is well known that undernourished patients are at high risk of developing complications during their medical treatment.[3] Undernutrition has been associated with poor wound healing, compromised immune status, impairment of organ functions, and increased mortality.[4,5] In addition, increased use of health care resources is associated with undernutrition among older persons.[6]

Despite these observations, undernutrition still occurs in about one third of hospitalized or institutionalized adult patients.[7-9] The poor recognition and treatment of undernutrition in hospitalized patients has been linked to a lack of physician awareness.[10] A simple education program for practitioners can improve nutrition knowledge and result in better identification and appropriate intervention for undernourished patients.[10]

It is therefore essential that practitioners increase their awareness and recognition of undernutrition to provide optimal patient care. In the primary care setting, practical and reliable methods are required for nutrition screening and assessment. This chapter will describe general indicators of undernutrition syndromes and highlight practical nutrition assessment techniques suitable for routine clinical practice.

UNDERSTANDING UNDERNUTRITION SYNDROME

As new indicators of poor nutritional status have been identified, the definition of undernutrition has been refined. The differential diagnosis of undernutrition is complex and requires further classification and evaluation to determine underlying causes. There is no established gold standard to identify which individuals are undernourished or at risk of undernutrition. Classification of patients can be facilitated using these simple indicators of undernutrition:

- Weight loss and underweight status are the best validated indicators of undernutrition.
- Morphometric measures (measures of body size and composition) are helpful.
- Poor dietary intake, as revealed by diet records, patient recall, or food frequencies, can be useful.
- Laboratory indicators (albumin, prealbumin) of inflammatory response and possible undernutrition must be interpreted with caution.

Undernutrition can be categorized into 5 syndromes: wasting, sarcopenia, cachexia, protein-energy undernutrition (PEU), and failure to thrive.[11] To select helpful interventions and management, it is necessary to recognize the appropriate undernutrition syndrome. However, there may be overlap among undernutrition syndromes, and a given underlying condition may result in more than one type of syndrome. It is therefore important to recognize key characteristics for each syndrome.

Wasting

Poor dietary intake or assimilation with resulting loss of body cell mass is the common feature of wasting conditions.[12] In pure wasting (clinical marasmus) there are no manifestations of acute-phase metabolic response or underlying inflammatory condition. Resting energy expenditure is reduced, and visceral proteins are preserved. Increased extracellular fluid is therefore not observed.

Sarcopenia

The loss of muscle mass that occurs with aging is called sarcopenia.[12-14] Reduced physical activity and loss of strength are 2 common features that have been associated with sarcopenia. Whether this condition is an inevitable part of aging or a consequence of a sedentary lifestyle and/or poor nutritional status remains unclear. Since the relationship between undernutrition and sarcopenia is unknown, patients with this syndrome may or may not benefit from nutrition intervention. Experimental approaches that have resulted in increased skeletal muscle mass include administration of trophic factors, such as growth hormone and testosterone,[15,16] and resistance strength training.[17]

Cachexia

Cachexia develops when there is an underlying inflammatory process, injury, or condition. It is characterized by increased cytokine production that favors a catabolic state.[14] Resting energy expenditure is elevated, amino acids are exported from muscle to liver, gluconeogenesis is increased, and there is increased production of acute-phase proteins with a concomitant decline in the synthesis of proteins such as albumin.[18] Increased extracellular fluid will often result in edema, such that there may not be a decline in body weight despite erosion of body cell mass.

Protein-Energy Undernutrition

Protein-energy undernutrition is characterized by both clinical signs (physical signs such as weight loss, low body mass index, or BMI) and biochemical signs (low levels of albumin or other proteins) of insufficient energy and protein intake.[1,19] Many patients with inflammatory diseases will also have compromised dietary intakes. These patients represent a subtle overlap of wasting and cachexia syndromes. Note that, in routine clinical practice, many patients with only reduced albumin or prealbumin levels are often designated as having PEU, despite having only manifestations of an inflammatory response.

Failure to Thrive

Originally, failure to thrive was used to describe infants who did not achieve milestones in height, weight, or behavior. This term has since been extended to describe older persons who lose weight, exhibit decline in physical and/or cognitive functions, and demonstrate signs of hopelessness and helplessness.[20] The National Institute on Aging has described failure to thrive as "a syndrome of weight loss, decreased appetite and poor nutrition, and inactivity, often accompanied by dehydration, depressive symptoms, impaired immune function, and low cholesterol."[21] Failure to thrive does not readily encompass a single identifiable clinical syndrome, so some have proposed to abandon this term in favor of a group of potentially more treatable conditions: impaired physical functioning, undernutrition, depression, and cognitive impairment.[22]

NUTRITION ASSESSMENT

Nutrition assessment aims to evaluate the nutritional status of patients and to detect any suspected undernutrition syndromes. Because there is no single clinical or laboratory indicator of comprehensive nutritional status, it is necessary to gather information from many different sources, including historical, physical, anthropometric, dietary intake, and biochemical (laboratory) data.

Historical Data

Important historical elements that should be explored are listed in Table 16-1.

Weight history

One of the most important historical elements in determining the type of undernutrition syndrome is prior weight loss (including attempts at weight reduction). Clinical significance varies according to the amount of weight lost and the duration of the weight loss. A weight loss greater than 10% of body weight can affect clinical outcome.

TABLE 16-1

History and Physical Examination Elements for Undernutrition Syndromes*

History
Body weight
Medical and surgical conditions; chronic disease
Constitutional signs and symptoms
Eating difficulties and gastrointestinal complaints
Eating disorders
Medication use
Dietary practices and use of supplements
Influences on nutritional status
Physical examination
Body mass index (BMI)
Weight loss
Weakness or loss of strength
Peripheral edema
Hair examination
Skin examination
Eye examination
Perioral examination
Extremity examination
Mental status and nervous system examination
Functional assessment

*Further details on these elements can be found in Jensen GL.[26]

Medical-surgical history

Many chronic diseases and medical or surgical interventions are known to have an impact on nutritional status. In some instances, the treatment of these diseases may lead to dietary restrictions or limitations that compromise nutritional status.[23] Some disorders may precipitate undernutrition because they create the inability to ingest or absorb nutrients. In others, the burden of the disorder may lead to increased energy requirements. Undernutrition may, in turn, affect the course and treatment of specific acute and chronic diseases.[24]

Medication history

It is important to take a careful medication history. Many drugs can compromise nutritional status by interfering with food intake or with the absorption, metabolism, and excretion of nutrients.[25] Food and nutrients may also interact with drugs by altering their absorption, metabolism, and excretion.[26] Practitioners should be familiar with the potential nutrient interactions of drugs they commonly use to treat their patients. Table 16-2 describes some common drug-nutrient interactions. Many other interactions have been and are still being identified.

Dietary practice history

Dietary habits and food choices are determined by a variety of environmental, cultural, economic, and interpersonal and intrapersonal factors. Some of them are known to adversely affect food intake or assimilation, thus compromising nutritional status. It is therefore essential to obtain a thorough history of dietary practices when completing a nutrition assessment.

TABLE 16-2

Common Drug-Nutrient Interactions*

Drug	Nutrient Lost
Aluminum (magnesium hydroxide antacids)	Phosphate
Cholestyramine (bile resin)	Fat-soluble vitamins, folate
Omeprazole (acid-pump inhibitor)	Vitamin B_{12}
Methotrexate (chemotherapy agent, folate antagonist)	Folate
Isoniazid (antituberculotic, B_6 antagonist)	Pyridoxine
Coumadin	Vitamin K
Lasix (diuretic)	Calcium, potassium, magnesium, zinc

*Adapted with permission from Jensen GL.[26]

Physical Examination

Undernutrition can affect many organs and tissues resulting in physical signs. Key physical findings are weight loss (loss of body cell mass) and the presence of peripheral edema (hypoalbuminemia).[11] Parts of the body where cell replacement occurs at a high rate (eg, hair, skin, mouth, tongue) are most likely to show signs of undernutrition and should be closely examined. Important physical examination elements for undernutrition syndrome appear in Table 16-1. All the potential physical findings and deficiencies associated with these findings are beyond the scope of this chapter and are reviewed elsewhere.[26]

Anthropometric Data

Anthropometrics are simple and inexpensive physical measurements that provide an indirect assessment of body size and composition. When using anthropometry, the investigator compares measurements with standards (for the same sex and age) and/or with previous measurements taken on the same individual. Variations in the amount and proportion of measurements can be used in the detection of undernutrition and obesity. The most common anthropometric measurements include height, weight, skin folds, and circumferences.

Height

Height measurements are useful in the determination and interpretation of other anthropometric measurements and indexes. For individuals who are able to stand unassisted, height should be measured in an upright position using a wall-mounted stadiometer. For adults who are bedridden or wheelchair bound, height can be estimated by doubling the arm span measurement (from the patient's sternal notch to the end of the longest finger). Stature in the elderly can be estimated using knee height (measured with a caliper device).[27]

Men: Stature (cm) = $[2.02 \times$ Knee Height (cm)$] - (0.04 \times$ Age$) + 64.19$

Women: Stature (cm) = $[1.83 \times$ Knee Height (cm)$] - (0.24 \times$ Age$) + 84.88$

Weight

Actual weight and weight changes may be the most important elements in nutrition assessment. Actual body weight relative to height is often compared with ideal reference tables such as the Metropolitan Height and Weight Tables.[28] These tables suffer from limitations that include subjective interpretation of frame size and inadequate reference data for many population groups.

Body mass index, defined as weight in kilograms divided by height in meters squared, is a practical measure of body size and an indirect measure of body fatness. Unlike most other anthropometric measurements, BMI does not require the use of a reference table. The National Institutes of Health in 1998 released new guidelines for body size classification,[29] which are:

- BMI less than 18.5 is classified as underweight, at risk of undernutrition
- BMI 18.6 to 24.9: normal weight
- BMI 25 to 29.9: overweight
- BMI 30 or greater: obese

Skin folds and circumferences

Anthropometric measurements such as skin folds and circumferences have limited practical application in patient care settings because highly trained personnel are required to achieve acceptable reliability. The practitioner who wants to use them can find a detailed description of procedures in the National Health and Nutrition Examination Survey (NHANES) III Anthropometric Procedures video.[30]

Other body composition assessment tools

A variety of other high-technology body composition assessment tools are available, but they have mostly been used in research settings and are impractical for routine clinical use. These include water displacement, bioelectrical impedance analysis, dual-energy X-ray absorptiometry, computed tomography (CT), magnetic resonance imaging (MRI), total body counting of the naturally occurring potassium isotope, and air plethysmography. Table 16-3 lists these other tools.

Dietary Data

Dietary assessment can be used to detect inadequate or imbalanced food or nutrient intakes, which can lead to nutrient deficiencies. Dietary intakes alone do not provide adequate information on the nutritional status of individuals. They should be interpreted carefully and in combination with other indicators of nutritional status.

There are a number of approaches to estimating energy and nutrient intakes of individuals. These can be separated into 2 categories: prospective and retrospective methods. Each method can further be classified according to the degree of quantitative detail that is provided. Dietary intake instruments from both categories are subject to random (eg, mistake in estimation of portion size, poor recollection of past diet) and systematic (eg, misreporting of true intake, intraindividual and interindividual variability of true intake) errors.

To minimize random measurement errors, dietary assessment requires a highly trained investigator who follows a standardized data collection protocol. To increase

TABLE 16-3

Body Composition, Laboratory Studies, and Other Studies for Nutritional Syndromes*

Body composition studies
  Anthropometrics
  Bioelectrical impedance
  Water displacement
  Whole-body counting and isotope dilution techniques
  Air plethysmography
  Dual-energy X-ray absorptiometry (DXA)
  Computed tomography (CT) or magnetic resonance
    imaging (MRI)
Laboratory and other studies
  Albumin
  Prealbumin
  Transferrin
  Retinol-binding protein
  C-reactive protein
  Cholesterol
  β-carotene
  Cytokines
  Electrolytes, serum urea nitrogen, and creatinine
  Complete blood cell count with differential
  Total lymphocyte count
  Helper-suppressor T-cell ratio
  Nitrogen balance
  Urine 3-methylhistidine
  Creatinine height index (CHI)
  Prothrombin time/international normalized ratio (INR)
  Specific nutrients
  Skin testing-recall antigens
  Electrocardiogram
  Videofluoroscopy
  Endoscopic and X-ray studies of gastrointestinal tract
  Fat absorption
  Schilling test
  Indirect calorimetry

*Further details on these tests can be found in Jensen GL.[26]

the precision of the assessment—to decrease the effect of intraindividual variability in true dietary intake—repeated measures are often necessary (depending on the methods selected). The number of days of data collection required varies with the nutrient of interest.[31] Recent studies using the doubly labeled water method, a valid indicator of habitual energy intake, have shown that both prospective and retrospective methods tend to underestimate true energy intakes.[32]

The choice of dietary assessment method depends on the skills of the assessor, the feasibility in the context of

T A B L E   16-4

Dietary Assessment Methods*

Method	Classification	Procedure	Limitations of Method
Food record or diary	Prospective, quantitative	All food and beverages consumed are recorded.	Requires numerate and literate subjects; eating patterns may be modified; compliance decreases with longer time frames; underreporting common
24-hour recall	Retrospective, quantitative	All foods and beverages consumed in previous 24 h are reported to interviewer.	Requires trained interviewer; relies on memory; single recall unlikely to represent usual intake; underreporting common
Food Frequency Questionnaire (FFQ)	Retrospective, qualitative or quantitative	Subject self-reports (or reports to an interviewer) frequency of consumption from a list of food items.	Can be expensive; broad time frame, usually averaged over months; least accurate

*Adapted from Gibson RD. *Principles of Nutritional Assessment*. New York, NY: Oxford University Press; 1990.

clinical assessment, and the characteristics of the subject (eg, age, education). Table 16-4 describes some of the most popular dietary assessment methods.

Once the dietary data have been collected, the investigator typically enters all foods, beverages, and supplements into nutrient calculation software for analysis of the diet's nutritional value. Most nutrient calculation software compares values with standards such as the Recommended Dietary Allowances (RDA), which ease the investigator's task. A number of software programs are available, such as the Minnesota Nutrition Data System (NDS, Nutrition Coordination Center, University of Minnesota, Minneapolis, Minn), Nutritionist IV (First Databank, San Bruno, Calif), and ESHA Food Processor (ESHA, ESHA Research, Salem, Ore). Most of these tools use an underlying food and nutrient database that contains values derived from the US Department of Agriculture (USDA) National Nutrient Database and food manufacturers. The choice of software package depends on the accuracy of the underlying database, ease of use, available features, and cost.[33]

In the past, poor nutritional intake was defined as an average intake of energy and/or nutrients below a threshold level of the RDA (usually 66% or 75% of the RDA).[34] However, this is not an appropriate use of the RDA, and these numbers should now be interpreted with caution.[35] Comparison of dietary intakes to the RDA gives only an estimate of the risk of development of nutrient deficiencies, which increases with the duration of the low intake. A single measure indicating a nutrient intake under the recommended level does not mean that nutrition needs are not met for a specific patient.

The RDA have been updated and incorporated in a new set of reference values called the Dietary Reference Intakes (DRI), which have been designed to replace the former RDA.[35,36] The DRIs also include Adequate Intake (AI), Tolerable Upper Intake Level (UL), and Estimated Average Requirement (EAR). Adequate Intakes (AI) are used as the goal for individual intake when there is no associated RDA value for a specific nutrient.

The management of dietary data is time consuming and difficult to achieve in most clinical settings. For a routine dietary assessment, the 24-hour recall may be the easiest and most practical instrument to use. It provides an overview of the patient's dietary intakes and can guide further evaluation. However, it cannot be used to estimate usual intakes of individuals, since a single recall is likely to omit food consumed infrequently. For a more comprehensive dietary assessment, referral to a registered dietitian would be recommended.

Laboratory Data

Laboratory studies can be useful in the determination of a patient's nutritional status. Since many factors can affect laboratory results, it is often not possible to diagnose an undernutrition syndrome on the basis of a single test. Laboratories should therefore be used with other assessment data, such as clinical history and physical examination, to help confirm the diagnosis of an undernutrition syndrome.

Measures of changes in visceral protein status, such as serum albumin or prealbumin, should be obtained to evaluate any patient with a suspected undernutrition syndrome. Hypoalbuminemia has been commonly considered a sign of undernutrition. However, it should be interpreted with caution since it has been shown to lack specificity and sensitivity as an indicator of nutritional status.[37-39] Low albumin level is often associated with underlying injuries, disease, or inflammatory conditions. Prealbumin may better reflect short-term changes in protein status than albumin.[40] It otherwise suffers from the same limitations as albumin as an indicator of nutritional status, since it may also be confounded by response to injury, disease, or inflammation. Patients with low visceral protein levels may or may not be undernourished. Additional evidence suggesting loss of body cell mass or compromised dietary intake is required in supporting an undernutrition diagnosis. Table 16-3 lists a variety of laboratory and other tests used to evaluate nutritional disorders.

MULTI-ITEM NUTRITION SCREENING AND ASSESSMENT TOOLS

Nutrition screening is useful for detecting patients who are at risk of undernutrition, therefore promoting appropriate diagnosis and intervention. It can initially be undertaken to identify individuals who would require additional nutrition assessment.

Young and middle-aged adults typically do not require frequent nutrition screening unless disease or eating disorders are present. Older patients, particularly those who are homebound, frail, sick, or hospitalized, should be screened annually, since the prevalence of undernutrition is higher in this population.

The lack of any single screening measure that is a valid indicator of comprehensive nutritional status has precipi-tated the development of multi-item screening and assessment tools (Table 16-5). Some tools combine under-nutrition risk factors and/or clinical observations, for example, the Mini-Nutritional Assessment (MNA) and Subjective Global Assessment (SGA). These tools require the calculation of a total score, which classifies individuals into nutritional risk categories. Other screening and assessment tools incorporate clinical assessment data, such as anthropometrics, laboratories, and diagnoses, into predictive equations that determine the risk of adverse outcomes for an individual. Such tools include the Hospital Prognostic Index (HPI) and Prognostic Nutritional Index (PNI).

Patients in acute or long-term care settings have been studied extensively to identify indicators and predictors of nutritional status, whereas those in community settings have been subject to less investigation. It is unknown whether many of these tools have appropriate specificity and sensitivity to identify undernourished persons. It is also unclear whether subjects identified as high-risk are amenable to interventions that result in favorable outcomes.[41,42]

The SGA initially was developed for administration to hospitalized patients.[43] It combines scored parameters of medical history and physical examination. It divides

TABLE 16-5

Common Nutrition Screening and Assessment Tools and Properties*

Name of Tool	Purpose	Administration Method
Ambulatory Patients		
Mini-Nutritional Assessment Short-Form (MNA-SF)	Assess nutritional status	Trained clinician
Mini-Nutritional Assessment (MNA)	Assess nutritional status	Trained clinician
Nutrition Screening Initiative (NSI) Checklist	Encourage those at risk to seek help	Self-administered
Nutrition Screening Initiative—Level I Screen	Assess for further evaluation and intervention	Trained clinician
Nutrition Screening Initiative—Level II Screen	Collect diagnostic information for evaluation and intervention	Self-administered; trained clinician
Hospitalized Patients		
Subjective Global Assessment (SGA)	Assess nutritional status	Trained clinician
Nutrition Risk Index (NRI)	Predict operative complications	Predictive equation using laboratories and anthropometrics
Hospital Prognostic Index (HPI)	Predict sepsis and mortality	Predictive equation using laboratory and clinical data
Prognostic Nutritional Index (PNI)	Predict operative complications	Predictive equation using laboratory and clinical data
Prognostic Inflammatory and Nutritional Index (PINI)	Predict mortality and risk of complications	Predictive equation using laboratory data

*Adapted from Reuben DB, Greendale GA, Harrison GG.[55]

patients into 3 classes: class A indicating well nourished; class B, moderately (or suspected of being) malnourished; and class C, severely malnourished. It has shown good interrater reliability and is a useful predictor of postoperative complications.[3] It requires trained practitioners to administer it and provides a validated measure of nutritional risk.[3,43]

The MNA is a clinical tool designed to assess the nutritional status of older persons.[44-46] The MNA must be administered by a trained professional and consists of 18 items, including anthropometric, clinical, and dietary data. The first 6 items (also called MNA Short-Form) are used as a screening tool to identify possible malnourished patients.[47] A score of 11 or lower on the MNA Short-Form is a prompt to continue the assessment in order to confirm the diagnosis and plan further interventions. The MNA classifies older persons into 3 levels of nutritional status on a scale ranging from 0 to 30. A score of 24 or more indicates satisfactory nutritional status, a score of 17 to 23.5 indicates risk of undernutrition, and a score below 17 suggests PEU.

Extensive cross-validation studies have been completed on the MNA. Scores were significantly correlated with dietary intake and anthropometric and biological nutritional parameters.[48] It has also shown acceptable reliability, as indicated by its internal consistency and test-retest reproducibility.[49] Although the MNA is probably the most studied tool, its utility has been questioned.[50]

The Nutrition Screening Initiative (NSI) has developed 3 interdisciplinary nutrition risk-screening/assessment tools to aid in evaluation of the nutritional status of older persons.[51,52] The DETERMINE checklist was created to raise public awareness regarding nutritional concerns of older persons.[51,53] This self-report questionnaire is composed of 10 items and is intended to help identify potential nutritional risk factors. It is not intended to provide diagnostic assessment. The NSI Level I screen is a comprehensive tool intended for use by health care professionals and incorporates measures of height and weight as well as weight change, dietary habits, functional status, and living environment.[51] The NSI Level II screen encompasses all of the items from Level I but has additional laboratory and anthropometric measures as well as provision for more in-depth examination of depression and mental status as indicated.[51] The Level II screen requires more highly trained medical and nutrition professionals for administration and is suggested for use in the diagnosis of undernutrition. Testing of the DETERMINE checklist has suggested limited utility in identification of undernourished persons or those with compromised intake.[41,50,53,54] Selected items from the Level II screen have been associated with increased risk of functional limitation, use of health care resources, and hospital admissions.[6]

The NSI nutrition screening tools have been widely disseminated and are currently being used in capacities that far exceed those for which they were originally intended. More extensive testing is needed to clarify their valid clinical applications.[5,6,42,55]

SUMMARY

An understanding of clinical nutrition is crucial to the principles of preventive medicine and sound patient care. This chapter has introduced the undernutrition syndromes and highlighted some practical approaches to screening and assessment. The use of key historical elements and a systems approach to the physical examination are promoted. The lack of any single clinical or laboratory measure that provides a comprehensive assessment of nutritional status means that it is necessary to gather information from a variety of sources, including historical, physical examination, anthropometric, dietary intake, and biochemical means.

REFERENCES

1. Bistrian BR, Blackburn GL, Hallowell E, Heddle R. Protein status of general surgical patients. *JAMA.* 1974;230:858–860.

2. Bistrian BR, Blackburn GL, Sherman M, Scrimshaw NS. Therapeutic index of nutritional depletion in hospitalized patients. *Surg Gynecol Obstet.* 1975;141:512–516.

3. Detsky AS, Smalley PS, Chang J. Is this patient malnourished? *JAMA.* 1994;271:54–58.

4. Keys A, Brozel J, Henschel A, Mickelsen O, Taylor HL. *The Biology of Human Starvation.* Vols 1 and 2. Minneapolis, Minn: University of Minnesota Press; 1950.

5. Klein S, Kinney J, Jeejeebhoy K, et al. Nutrition support in clinical practice: review of published data and recommendations for future research directions. *JPEN.* 1997;21:133–156.

6. Jensen GL, Friedmann JM, Coleman CD, Smiciklas-Wright H. Screening for hospitalization and nutritional risks among community-dwelling older persons. *Am J Clin Nutr.* 2001;74:201–205.

7. Mowe M, Bohmer T. The prevalence of undiagnosed protein-calorie undernutrition in a population of hospitalized elderly patients. *J Am Geriatr Soc.* 1991;39:1089–1092.

8. Constans T, Bacq Y, Brechot JF, Guilmot JL, Choutet P, Lamisse F. Protein-energy malnutrition in elderly medical patients. *J Am Geriatr Soc.* 1992;40:263–268.

9. Burns JT, Jensen GL. Malnutrition among geriatric patients admitted to medical and surgical services in a tertiary care hospital: frequency, recognition, and associated disposition and reimbursement outcomes. *Nutrition.* 1995;11(suppl 2):245–249.

10. Roubenoff R, Roubenoff RA, Preto J, Balke CW. Malnutrition among hospitalized patients: a problem of physician awareness. *Arch Intern Med.* 1987;147:1462–1465.

11. Roubenoff R, Heymsfield SB, Kehayias JJ, Cannon JG, Rosenberg IH. Standardization of nomenclature of body composition in weight loss. *Am J Clin Nutr.* 1997;66:192–196.

12. Roubenoff R. The pathophysiology of wasting in the elderly. *J Nutr.* 1999;129(suppl 1S):256S–259S.

13. Rosenberg IH. Sarcopenia: origins and clinical relevance. *J Nutr.* 1997;127(suppl 5):990S–991S.

14. Roubenoff R. Inflammatory and hormonal mediators of cachexia. *J Nutr.* 1997;127(suppl 5):1014S–1016S.

15. Papadakis MA, Grady D, Black D, et al. Growth hormone replacement in healthy older men improves body composition but not functional ability. *Ann Intern Med.* 1996;124:708–716.

16. Snyder PJ, Peachey H, Hannoush P, et al. Effect of testosterone treatment on body composition and muscle strength in men over 65 years of age. *J Clin Endocrinol Metab.* 1999;84:2647–2653.

17. Evans WJ, Cyr-Campbell D. Nutrition, exercise, and healthy aging. *J Am Diet Assoc.* 1997;97:632–638.

18. Kushner I. Regulation of the acute phase response by cytokines. *Perspect Biol Med.* 1993;36:611–622.

19. Abbasi AA, Rudman D. Observations on the prevalence of protein-calorie undernutrition in VA nursing homes. *J Am Geriatr Soc.* 1993;41:117–121.

20. Braun JV, Wykle MH, Cowling WR III. Failure to thrive in older persons: a concept derived. *Gerontologist.* 1988;28:809–812.

21. Lonergan ET. *Extending life, enhancing life: a national research agenda on aging.* Washington DC: National Academy Press; 1991.

22. Sarkisian CA, Lachs MS. 'Failure to thrive' in older adults. *Ann Intern Med.* 1996;124:1072–1078.

23. Reuben DB, Moore AA, Damesyn M, Keeler E, Harrison GG, Greendale GA. Correlates of hypoalbuminemia in community-dwelling older persons. *Am J Clin Nutr.* 1997;66:38–45.

24. Riquelme R, Torres A, El-Ebiary M, et al. Community-acquired pneumonia in the elderly: a multivariate analysis of risk and prognostic factors. *Am J Respir Crit Care Med.* 1996;154:1450–1455.

25. Roe DA. *Geriatric Nutrition.* 3rd ed. Englewood Cliffs, NJ: Prenctice-Hall International Inc; 1992.

26. Jensen GL. Physician's Information and Education Resource. Philadelphia, Pa: American College of Physicians-American Society of Internal Medicine, Available at: www.pier.acponline.org/index.html. Accessed September 24, 2003.

27. Chumlea WC, Roche AF, Steinbaugh ML. Estimating stature from knee height for persons 60 to 90 years of age. *J Am Geriatr Soc.* 1985;33:116–120.

28. Society of Actuaries and Association of Life Insurance Medical Directors. *1979 Build Study.* Chicago, Ill: Metropolitan Life Insurance Company; 1980.

29. *Clinical Guidelines on the Identification, Evaluation, and Treatment of Overweight and Obesity in Adults.* Bethesda, Md: National Institutes of Health; 1998.

30. US Department of Health and Human Services, National Health and Nutrition Examination Survey. *NHANES III Anthropometric Procedures* [videotape]. Government Printing Office; 1988.

31. Nelson M, Black AE, Morris JA, Cole TJ. Between- and within-subject variation in nutrient intake from infancy to old age: estimating the number of days required to rank dietary intakes with desired precision. *Am J Clin Nutr.* 1989;50:155–167.

32. Trabulsi J, Schoeller DA. Evaluation of dietary assessment instruments against doubly labeled water, a biomarker of habitual energy intake. *Am J Physiol Endocrinol Metab.* 2001;281:E891–E899.

33. McCullough ML, Karanja NM, Lin PH, et al. Comparison of 4 nutrient databases with chemical composition data from the Dietary Approaches to Stop Hypertension trial. *J Am Diet Assoc.* 1999;99(suppl 8):S45–S53.

34. Institute of Medicine. *How Should the Recommended Dietary Allowances be Revised?* Washington, DC: National Academy Press; 1994.

35. Institute of Medicine. *Dietary Reference Intakes for Calcium, Phosphorus, Magnesium, Vitamin D, and Fluoride.* Washington, DC: National Academy Press; 1997.

36. Institute of Medicine. *Dietary Reference Intakes for Thiamin, Riboflavin, Niacin, Vitamin B6, Folate, Vitamin B12, Pantothenic acid, Biotin, and Choline.* Washington, DC: National Academy Press; 1998.

37. Doweiko JP, Nompleggi DJ. The role of albumin in human physiology and pathophysiology: III. Albumin and disease states. *JPEN.* 1991;15:476–483.

38. Rall C, Roubenoff R, Harris T. Albumin as a marker of nutritional and health status. In: Rosenberg IH, ed. *Nutritional Assessment of Elderly Populations: Measure and Function.* New York, NY: Raven Press; 1991.

39. Rothschild MA, Oratz M, Schreiber SS. Serum albumin. *Hepatology.* 1988;8:385–401.

40. Ingenbleek Y, Young V. Transthyretin (prealbumin) in health and disease: nutritional implications. *Annu Rev Nutr.* 1994;14:495–533.

41. Sahyoun NR, Jacques PF, Dallal GE, Russell RM. Nutrition Screening Initiative Checklist may be a better awareness/educational tool than a screening one. *J Am Diet Assoc.* 1997;97:760–764.

42. Rush D. Nutrition screening in old people: its place in a coherent practice of preventive health care. *Annu Rev Nutr.* 1997;17:101–125.

43. Detsky AS, McLaughlin JR, Baker JP, et al. What is subjective global assessment of nutritional status? *JPEN.* 1987;11:8–13.

44. Guigoz Y, Vellas B, Garry PJ. Assessing the nutritional status of the elderly: the Mini Nutritional Assessment as part of the geriatric evaluation. *Nutr Rev.* 1996;54:S59–S65.

45. Vellas B, Guigoz Y, Garry PJ, et al. The Mini Nutritional Assessment (MNA) and its use in grading the nutritional state of elderly patients. *Nutrition.* 1999;15:116–122.

46. MNA Mini-Nutritional Assessment [Nestle Nutrition Web site]. Available at: www.mna-elderly.com. Accessed February 28, 2003.

47. Rubenstein LZ, Harker JO, Salva A, Guigoz Y, Vellas B. Screening for undernutrition in geriatric practice: developing the short-form mini-nutritional assessment (MNA-SF). *J Gerontol A Biol Sci Med Sci.* 2001;56:M366–372.

48. Vellas B, Guigoz Y, Baumgartner M, et al. Relationships between nutritional markers and the mini-nutritional assessment in 155 older persons. *J Am Geriatr Soc.* 2000;48:1300–1309.

49. Bleda MJ, Bolibar I, Pares R, Salva A. Reliability of the mini nutritional assessment (MNA) in institutionalized elderly people. *J Nutr Health Aging.* 2002;6:134–137.

50. de Groot LC, Beck AM, Schroll M, van Staveren WA. Evaluating the DETERMINE Your Nutritional Health Checklist and the Mini Nutritional Assessment as tools to identify nutritional problems in elderly Europeans. *Eur J Clin Nutr.* 1998;52:877–883.

51. Nutrition Screening Initiative. *Nutrition interventions manual for professionals caring for older Americans.* Washington, DC; 1992.

52. American Academy of Family Physicians. Nutrition Screening Initiative. Available at: www.aafp.org/nsi. Accessed February 28, 2003.

53. Posner BM, Jette AM, Smith KW, Miller DR. Nutrition and health risks in the elderly: the nutrition screening initiative. *Am J Public Health.* 1993;83:972–978.

54. Boult C, Krinke UB, Urdangarin CF, Skarin V. The validity of nutritional status as a marker for future disability and depressive symptoms among high-risk older adults. *J Am Geriatr Soc.* 1999;47:995–999.

55. Reuben DB, Greendale GA, Harrison GG. Nutrition screening in older persons. *J Am Geriatr Soc.* 1995;43:415–425.

RESOURCES

American Academy of Physicians
Nutrition Screening Initiative
Web site: www.aafp.org/nsi

American Board of Nutrition
Web site: www.uab.edu/nusc/abn.htm

American College of Nutrition
Web site: www.am-coll-nutr.org

American Dietetic Association
Web site: www.eatright.org

American Society for Clinical Nutrition
Web site: www.faseb.org/ascn

American Society for Parenteral and Enteral Nutrition
Web site: www.clinnutr.org

Institute of Medicine, Food and Nutrition Board
Web site: www.nap.edu

Nestle Nutrition
Mini Nutritional Assessment
Web site: www.mna-elderly.com

chapter 17

Nutrition and Chronic Disease

Donald D. Hensrud, MD, MPH

For the two out of three adult Americans who do not smoke and do not drink excessively, one personal choice seems to influence long-term health prospects more than any other—what we eat.*

INTRODUCTION

As reviewed by the first US surgeon general's 1988 report on nutrition, and emphasized by continued research since publication of that report, nutrition can have a powerful impact on maintaining health and preventing disease. Nutritional factors are associated with 5 of the top 10 leading causes of death in the United States, and in 1990 it was estimated that more than 300,000 deaths per year were due to suboptimal diet and activity habits.[1]

This chapter will outline the relationships between nutrition and chronic diseases. Dietary factors that are important in the prevention of specific diseases will be discussed. The information in this chapter will be summarized by describing dietary patterns that are associated with an overall low risk of chronic disease. Dietary supplements will be primarily covered in Chapter 21, and the effects on disease risk of physical activity and obesity will be included in Chapters 13 and 18, respectively.

HYPERLIPIDEMIA AND CORONARY HEART DISEASE

Hypercholesterolemia is one of the major risk factors for coronary heart disease (CHD). Diet influences serum lipids and, in addition, there are dietary factors that influence CHD risk independent of serum lipids.

Dating back to experiments by Keys and Hegsted in the 1950s and 1960s, respectively, it has been known that saturated fat has the predominant dietary effect on raising serum total and low-density lipoprotein cholesterol (LDL-C). Individual saturated fatty acids vary in their propensity to raise LDL-C. The long-chain stearic acid (found in chocolate) has the least effect, and the shorter chain myristic acid (found in dairy products) has the greatest effect at usual levels of consumption. Dietary cholesterol also raises serum cholesterol, but to a lesser degree than does saturated fat. However, the effect of dietary saturated fat on increasing LDL-C is augmented in the presence of dietary cholesterol.

Most foods that have relatively large amounts of saturated fat also contain cholesterol. These include meat; full-fat dairy products, such as cheese, butter, and ice cream; and other foods derived from animal sources. Shrimp and lobster contain cholesterol, but very little saturated fat. Therefore, they do not raise serum cholesterol as much as would be expected. Tropical oils, including coconut and palm kernel oil, are derived from plants and, therefore, do not contain cholesterol. However, they contain relatively large amounts of saturated fat, which increases serum cholesterol. Tropical oils are added to processed foods not for health reasons, but because they increase shelf life and are solid at room temperature while melting at body temperature, which gives a good "mouth feel."

Trans–fatty acids, such as margarine and vegetable shortening, are vegetable oils that have been partially hydrogenated. This changes polyunsaturated fat, which is liquid at room temperature, to more closely resemble saturated fat, which is solid at room temperature. *Trans–fatty* acids also are found in low levels in meat and dairy products. *Trans fats* raise serum cholesterol, but not quite to the same degree as do saturated fats. They have additional disadvantages of lowering high-density lipoprotein cholesterol (HDL-C) and raising lipoprotein (a) cholesterol. In view of the increased recognition of these negative effects, food labels will be required to list the amount of *trans–fatty* acids in foods by 2006.

Polyunsaturated and monounsaturated fats lower serum cholesterol when substituted for dietary saturated fat. Monounsaturated fat has an additional advantage in being more resistant to oxidation. Potential disadvantages of polyunsaturated fat include susceptibility to oxidation, concerns about promotion of tumor growth, and increased thrombogenicity secondary to an increased ratio of omega-6 to omega-3 fatty acids. Most vegetable oils contain predominantly polyunsaturated fat. Olive oil, canola oil, nuts, and avocados are the major sources of monounsaturated fat.

Omega-3 fatty acids lower serum triglycerides in large doses, have a mild effect on lowering blood pressure, reduce the propensity for blood to clot, and affect immune function. Moreover, they appear to lower the risk of sudden cardiac death by decreasing the propensity to life-threatening cardiac arrhythmias. This has been observed in epidemiologic studies with as few as 2 servings per week of fish. Besides fish, flaxseed, walnuts, and canola and soybean oils are plant sources of omega-3 fatty acids, including α-linolenic acid. Supplementation with 1 g/d of omega-3 fatty acids containing almost 300 mg of eicosapentaenoic acid and 600 mg of docosahexaenoic acid was shown to decrease the risk of sudden death and overall mortality in a randomized trial among subjects who had recently suffered a myocardial infarction.[2] For these reasons, the American Heart Association has stated that patients with CHD, in conjunction with their physician, could consider supplementation with omega-3 fatty acids.[3]

Soluble fiber from oats, beans, or psyllium has lowered serum cholesterol 2% to 9% in subjects following a fat-modified diet.[4] The effect of soluble fiber on serum cholesterol diminishes as the saturated fat content of the diet decreases.

Garlic requires ingestion of relatively large amounts to have a very modest, if any, effect on lowering serum cholesterol. Garlic supplements may not work because the active ingredient, allicin, is not stable and is difficult to standardize. Soy products will lower serum cholesterol when substituted for meat, and soy protein has an independent cholesterol-lowering effect, possibly from phytoestrogens.[5] Nuts have been associated with a reduced risk of CHD in a number of studies. This may be because of their relatively high content of monounsaturated fat as well as α-linolenic acid in walnuts.

Elevated levels of blood homocysteine are associated with an increased risk of CHD, peripheral arterial disease, and deep venous thrombosis. Folic acid and, to a lesser extent, vitamins B_6 and B_{12} can lower homocysteine levels. The above relationships may help, in part, to explain the inverse association between vegetable and fruit intake and CHD.

Moderate consumption of alcohol has been associated with a reduced risk of CHD in many studies. Alcohol enhances fibrinolytic activity, decreases platelet aggregation, and increases HDL-C. However, this needs to be balanced in individual patients with the effects of increasing blood pressure and triglycerides. Moreover, excess alcohol consumption contributes to more than 100,000 deaths per year in the United States in addition to the social problems it incurs. Thus, for people who do not consume alcohol, it is not recommended that they start. For people who do drink, moderate consumption of up to 1 alcoholic drink per day for women and 2 drinks per day for men may reduce the risk of CHD. Although much media attention has been given to the specific benefits of red wine, most data suggest that it is primarily alcohol per se that is responsible for most of the benefits and that the type of alcohol (wine, beer, or spirits) is less important. In addition, people who consume wine have been shown to have healthier lifestyle habits.

Stanols and sterols are the plant equivalent of mammalian cholesterol. Plant stanols and sterols inhibit the absorption of dietary cholesterol by up to 10% to 15%, and this effect is additive to 3-hydroxy-3-methylglutaryl coenzyme A (HMG-CoA) reductase inhibitors (statins).[6] Currently, 2 forms of margarine are available on the market, and it is likely that more foods containing stanols and sterols will be available in the near future.

The third report of the National Cholesterol Education Program outlined the Therapeutic Lifestyle Change (TLC) diet, designed to treat hyperlipidemia and decrease the risk of CHD (Table 17-1).[7]

Epidemiologic evidence dating to the Seven Countries Study has suggested that there are 2 candidate diets for the optimum prevention of CHD: the traditional Asian diet and the Mediterranean diet. Both diets are high in plant products and low in animal products. Whereas both diets are low in saturated fat, the Asian diet is low in total fat, while the Mediterranean diet has a relatively high fat content. However, the major dietary fat in the Mediterranean diet is monounsaturated fat from olive oil.

The Lifestyle Heart Trial was a randomized, prospective study comparing a 10% fat vegetarian diet, exercise, and stress management with a control group receiving usual care.[8,9] Subjects following the vegetarian diet experienced slight regression of CHD, as demonstrated angiographically, at 1 year and 5 years. Subjects in the control group experienced progression of greater than

T ABLE 17-1

Therapeutic Lifestyle Change (TLC) Diet

Dietary Intake	Recommended Allowance
Total fat	25%–35%
Saturated fat	<7%
Monounsaturated fat	Up to 20%
Polyunsaturated fat	Up to 10%
Cholesterol	<200 mg/d
Fiber	20–30 g/d
Protein	Approximately 15%
Total calories	As needed to maintain desired weight

10% diameter stenosis of coronary arteries after 5 years and suffered more coronary events. These results were observed despite no use of lipid-lowering medications in the experimental group, whereas many subjects in the control group were placed on a regimen of these medications. Although it is not clear exactly which component of the program was primarily responsible, a low-fat, plant-based diet, along the lines of a traditional Asian diet, contributed to the improved outcome.

The Lyon Diet Heart Trial randomized subjects who had experienced a myocardial infarction to a Mediterranean diet or a usual-care control group.[10,11] The Mediterranean diet consisted of slightly more vegetables, fruits, legumes, fish, and bread. Less meat was consumed, and canola oil margarine was used in place of butter. At 2 years and again at 4 years of follow-up, subjects following the Mediterranean diet experienced lower cardiovascular and overall mortality, independent of traditional risk factors. Once again, it was not possible to determine what part of the diet was responsible for the benefit, although statistically the omega-3 fat content of the canola oil margarine was singled out. It is likely that the collective effect of the entire diet provided the benefit.

HYPERTENSION

Updated national guidelines now classify normal blood pressure as less than 120/80 mm Hg. Blood pressures of 120 to 139 mm Hg systolic and 80 to 89 mm Hg diastolic are now classified as prehypertension.[12] A more aggressive approach to blood pressure control will be necessary with this new classification, which makes preventive efforts increasingly important. There are 5 lifestyle measures that will lower blood pressure and presumably help prevent the development of hypertension.

In people who are overweight, weight loss is the most effective strategy for lowering blood pressure. Decreased consumption of alcohol may also have a substantial blood pressure–lowering effect in people who consume large amounts. Regular exercise has a modest effect on lowering blood pressure. People vary in their sensitivity to the effect of salt on their blood pressure, but this cannot be determined prospectively. Therefore, from both a preventive and therapeutic perspective, salt restriction should be recommended, although benefits may vary. Taste preferences for salt, similar to other foods, can change over time. As the salt content of the diet is reduced, people become more sensitive to the taste and therefore require less.

In 2 large randomized trials, the Dietary Approach to Stop Hypertension (DASH) diet was shown to lower blood pressure in people with hypertension and in people with blood pressure in the normal range.[13,14] This dietary approach consists of 8 to 10 servings of vegetables and fruits daily, a modest decrease in meat consumption, and substitution of low-fat for high-fat dairy products. In the first trial, subjects with hypertension experienced a mean decrease in blood pressure of 11.4/5.5 mm Hg compared with a control diet similar to a typical American diet. The second study showed that salt restriction had a small but significant additive effect on blood pressure when instituted in addition to the DASH diet. Because the DASH diet was effective in lowering blood pressure in those with prehypertension and in both blacks and whites, it appears to be an effective preventive strategy.

Dietary intake of calcium, magnesium, and potassium from food is associated with a modest decrease in blood pressure. However, data are not strong enough to recommend supplementation with these minerals. Instead, people should try to obtain these nutrients through diet, and the DASH diet contains generous amounts of each. Intermittent use of caffeine will temporarily raise blood pressure. Tolerance develops with daily use, so there is little effect from regular use of caffeine.

The data on nutrition and stroke are generally consistent with the data on hypertension. Dietary intake of vegetables, fruits, fish, and folate have been inversely related to the incidence of stroke. Light to moderate alcohol consumption may provide slight protection against ischemic stroke, the major type of stroke, and increases the risk of hemorrhagic stroke consistent with alcohol's blood-thinning effect. Heavy consumption increases the risk of all types of stroke.

DIABETES

The main risk factors for developing type 2 diabetes are a genetic predisposition, increased body weight, and a sedentary lifestyle. At least 80% of type 2 diabetics are overweight or obese. The risk of diabetes is further increased with upper body (abdominal) distribution of body fat.

Usually in the setting of a genetic predisposition, increased body weight leads to insulin resistance, which eventually manifests itself as impaired fasting plasma glucose (6.1 to 6.9 mmol/L [110 to 125 mg/dL]) and finally diabetes (fasting plasma glucose ≥7.0 mmol/L [126 mg/dL]). Physical activity improves insulin resistance and can delay or prevent the onset of diabetes. To a lesser extent, a diet high in fiber and low in glycemic index can also delay the onset of diabetes. Other aspects of diet composition (eg, low fat/high carbohydrate, high fat/low carbohydrate), independent of total calories, have little impact on the development of diabetes.

Thus, for primary prevention of diabetes, maintaining a normal body weight (BMI <25 kg/m^2) along with regular physical activity and dietary intake of fiber-containing foods is the optimum strategy to prevent type 2 diabetes mellitus. Total caloric intake is the most important dietary feature affecting body weight. However, because people with diabetes are at high risk of cardiovascular disease, it is prudent to also follow the previously described dietary recommendations for the prevention of hyperlipidemia and hypertension.

CANCER

Cancer is a multistage process involving activation of a precarcinogen to a carcinogen that can then initiate a cancer. Promotion of the clone of tumor cells will eventually result in a clinically significant cancer. Nutritional factors can interact in any of the steps of carcinogenesis to either increase or decrease risk. Nutritional factors that influence the development of cancer may differ from the factors that affect the progression of clinically established cancer.

Because of the complexities in studying diseases with such long preclinical and clinical stages, evidence from randomized trials on the association between cancer and nutritional factors is not common. Despite this, the consistency of evidence from epidemiologic, basic science, and animal studies reveals clues to the etiology of many cancers. For example, migration studies have demonstrated that when Japanese persons migrate to the United States, the risk of stomach cancer decreases and colon cancer increases to the rates of their adopted country within 1 to 2 generations. This is strong evidence of an environmental influence, which is likely diet. It has been estimated that about one third of all cancer mortality is related to diet.

Cancer is not one disease but many different diseases with the common feature of uncontrolled cell growth. Obesity is one of the few factors that appears to increase the risk of most cancers.[15] Vegetables and fruits, while being heterogeneous in their nutritional composition, provide protection against many cancers.[16] Each cancer has its own specific nutritional correlates, which will be discussed below.

Alcohol increases the risk of oral cancer, and the effect is synergistic with tobacco. Fruits and, to a less extent, vegetables may decrease the risk of oral cancer. Alcohol and smoking are also strong risk factors for esophageal cancer. Hot liquids such as tea and coffee may also increase risk.

Gastroesophageal reflux, which is more common in obesity, predisposes to Barrett esophagus and increases the risk of adenocarcinoma of the distal esophagus. Fruits and vegetables also decrease the risk of esophageal cancer. Salt and salted foods, including smoked or pickled food, increase the risk of gastric cancer, which may help explain the increased incidence in Japan. Alcohol may also increase risk. Fruit and vegetable consumption are protective against gastric cancer. Green tea, in particular, may be effective in gastric cancer prevention. Vitamin C and carotenoids are specific nutrients that may decrease risk, although the strength of the associations, as with many nutrients, has been less than whole foods.

Because of intercorrelations, it is difficult to determine the independent effect of saturated fat, red meat, and excessive total calorie intake on colorectal cancer, and all 3 factors may increase risk. Obesity increases risk, and physical activity decreases risk of colorectal cancer, consistent with their effect on energy balance. Alcohol increases the risk of colorectal cancer, possibly by affecting folate status. Folic acid decreases the risk of colorectal cancer, and attenuates the risk between alcohol and colorectal cancer. In the past, it was commonly believed that fiber was protective against colorectal cancer. In a closer examination of the data, however, the independent effect of fiber in protecting against colon cancer is not entirely clear, although fiber-containing foods appear to be protective. It may be that fiber is a marker for other protective substances in foods, such as folate, that provide benefit. Among the types of foods that contain fiber, vegetable consumption appears to show the most protection, followed by fruits and then grains.

Smoking is responsible for the vast majority of lung cancers. After controlling for smoking, vegetable and fruit intake appears to decrease risk. There have been 2 large randomized, controlled trials that observed an increased risk of lung cancer and overall mortality from beta carotene supplementation.[17,18] The exact reason for this has not been determined but could be due to the interference with absorption of other carotenoids or beta carotene acting as a pro-oxidant in high-oxygen environments. Regardless of the mechanism, this illustrates that individual micronutrients can have vastly different effects than the foods that contain them.

Alcohol appears to modestly increase the risk of breast cancer, which begins to increase with small amounts of consumption—just a few drinks per week. In contrast to common belief, dietary fat has little effect on the development of breast cancer. Vegetables and fruits provide only mild protection. Obesity increases risk, especially upper body fat distribution. Physical activity has a mild protective effect.

Red meat and dairy products along with their content of saturated fat have been associated with prostate cancer. Interestingly, calcium, primarily from dairy products, has been linked to aggressive forms of prostate cancer in some studies, possibly by lowering vitamin D levels. Vegetables, specifically legumes and lycopene-rich tomatoes, have been associated with reduced risk.

It is clear from the above that vegetables and fruits have protective effects on many cancers. Multiple agents operating through different mechanisms may be collectively responsible for these benefits. In addition to essential vitamins and minerals, there are many phytochemicals in vegetables and fruits, including flavonoids, indoles, isothiocyanates, lignans, terpenes, and others. While it is important to identify and understand the specific agents and their effects, it is not necessary for preventive intervention, that is, eating a variety and increased amounts of vegetables and fruits can be beneficial whether the individual nutrients and mechanisms are known or not.

Positive energy balance, obesity, alcohol, and components of animal products such as saturated fat and protein increase the risk of many cancers. Physical activity decreases the risk of some cancers and helps manage weight.

OSTEOPOROSIS

Osteoporosis is more common in women than men, although the incidence among men has risen in recent years, being present in more than one fourth of men aged 75. This increased incidence may be because men are living longer, and awareness and detection have improved. Risk factors for osteoporosis include low levels of physical activity, a slight body habitus, smoking, genetic influences, and hormonal factors such as premature menopause.

Nutritional factors that influence osteoporosis can be described based on their effect on calcium balance, bone density, or fracture risk. Calcium intake is well known to influence bone metabolism. An increased intake of calcium with adequate vitamin D will increase bone density up to a theoretic threshold. The intake of most people is below recommended levels of 1000 to 1500 mg/d during adult life. Adequate intakes of calcium and vitamin D early in life are important to help develop a high peak bone mass. In addition, calcium and vitamin D requirements are increased in the elderly.

It is not well recognized that calcium loss may have a greater impact on calcium balance than calcium intake. Animal protein, due to increased acid load, and salt promote increased calcium loss in the urine. Caffeine intake inhibits the absorption of calcium and has been associated with hip fracture. An adequate dietary intake of calcium can negate the effect of caffeine. Increased vitamin A intake has been linked to decreased bone density and increased risk of hip fracture. Excessive alcohol consumption also increases the risk of osteoporosis. Magnesium and phosphorus have relatively minor roles on bone density. Current nutrition recommendations appropriately focus on calcium and vitamin D intake, which is suboptimal for much of the population. However, it should be recognized that other nutritional factors, particularly protein and sodium, may also have a large influence on bone density and risk of osteoporosis.

EYE DISEASE

The risk of macular degeneration may be decreased by dietary intake of the carotenoids lutein and zeaxanthin and possibly other antioxidants. Lutein and zeaxanthin are found in corn; zucchini; egg yolks; and green, leafy vegetables. It has been suggested that the risk of developing cataracts is also related to these nutrients, but the evidence is not strong.

SUMMARY

In determining the relationship between nutrition and disease prevention, a reductionist approach has often been used, examining associations with individual micronutrients. In many cases, this has proved fruitful, such as the causal association between folate deficiency and neural tube defects. With most diseases, however, the association between specific nutrients is less strong than the effect of whole foods and dietary patterns. For example, a diet rich in vegetables and fruits has consistently been associated with a low risk for developing various diseases. This benefit is probably the composite effect of not only vitamins and minerals but also the literally hundreds of known phytochemicals as well as many undiscovered ones. The specific concentrations and combinations of these nutrients present in food may be part of this benefit.

The evidence discussed earlier for individual conditions describe disease-specific relationships. However, consistent features are apparent that can be translated into an overall pattern of eating associated with a low risk of chronic disease. As already mentioned, one of the most consistent lines of evidence involves eating a plant-based diet. For different reasons, almost all of the conditions discussed above are inversely related to consumption of a diet that is high in vegetables, fruits, whole-grain carbohydrates, and legumes. In addition, a diet high in animal products and saturated fat is directly associated with many of the above conditions. From a practical standpoint, these 2 changes often occur simultaneously; as the dietary intake of plant products increases, the intake of animal products usually decreases. Objectively, there is little health benefit and established risk to including meat, particularly red meat, in the diet; taste preference is the primary reason. In one study of 42,000 women, those in the quartile most closely following a diet with these features (vegetables, fruits, whole grains, low-fat dairy, and lean meat) experienced a 31% decrease in overall mortality.[19]

Other foods that are associated with decreased risk of disease are those high in monounsaturated fat, including olive oil, canola oil, and nuts; fish and other sources of omega-3 fats, such as canola oil, soybean oil, and walnuts; soy products; and tea. Moderate consumption of alcohol is beneficial primarily for heart disease and decreases overall mortality. However, alcohol use also increases blood pressure; triglyceride levels; and the risk of some cancers, accidents, homicide, and suicide. Dairy products, if consumed, should be reduced in fat and, although they may be beneficial because of their calcium content, they do not have health benefits on other diseases as great as commonly perceived by the general population. The intake of refined and processed foods, including those containing simple sugars, salt, refined flour, tropical oils, and *trans*–fatty acids, should be minimized as much as possible.

If one tries to define an optimum diet for prevention of chronic disease from among existing diets in the world, 2 candidate diets would be the traditional Asian diet and the Mediterranean diet, which were discussed earlier in relation to CHD. Common features of these diets are that they are predominantly composed of plant foods, with animal foods used as condiments. They also include many of the other beneficial foods mentioned earlier, such as soy products and tea in the Asian diet and fish in both diets. The main difference is that the Asian diet is a low-fat diet and the Mediterranean diet is a high-fat diet with most of the fat composed of olive oil, a monounsaturated fat. Neither one is clearly superior, which allows people increased flexibility and choice. Although there is not one Mediterranean diet and each of the diets among the countries bordering the Mediterranean have their own unique features, they share common elements, which also gives people flexibility and choice.

Using the aforementioned evidence, with the best examples of foods from societies around the world, it is possible to consume a diet based on individual taste preferences that is enjoyable and practical, and has the greatest likelihood of reducing the risk of chronic disease.

REFERENCES

1. McGinnis JM, Foege WH. Actual causes of death in the United States. *JAMA.* 1993;270:2207–2212.

2. Dietary supplementation with n-3 polyunsaturated fatty acids and vitamin E after myocardial infarction: results of the GISSI-Prevenzione trial. *Lancet.* 1999;354:447–455.

3. Kris-Etherton PM, Harris WS, Appel LJ, for Nutrition Committee, American Heart Association. Omega-3 fatty acids and cardiovascular disease: new recommendations from the American Heart Association. *Arterioscler Thromb Vasc Biol.* 2003;23:151–152.

4. Van Horn L. Fiber, lipids, and coronary heart disease: a statement for healthcare professionals from the Nutrition Committee, American Heart Association. *Circulation.* 1997;95:2701–2704.

5. Anderson JW, Johnstone BM, Cook-Newell ME. Meta-analysis of the effects of soy protein intake on serum lipids. *N Engl J Med.* 1995;333:276–282.

6. Nguyen T. The cholesterol-lowering effect of plant stanol esters. *J Nutr.* 1999;129:2109–2112.

7. Expert Panel on Detection, Evaluation, and Treatment of High Blood Cholesterol in Adults. Executive summary of the third report of the National Cholesterol Education Program (NCEP) Expert Panel on Detection, Evaluation, and Treatment of High Blood Cholesterol in Adults (Adult Treatment Panel III). *JAMA.* 2001;285:2486–2497.

8. Ornish D, Brown SE, Scherwitz LW, et al. Can lifestyle changes reverse coronary artery disease? The Lifestyle Heart Trial. *Lancet.* 1990;336:129–133.

9. Ornish D, Scherwitz LW, Billings JH, et al. Intensive lifestyle changes for reversal of coronary heart disease. *JAMA.* 1998;280:2001–2007 [published correction appears in *JAMA.* 1999;281:1380].

10. de Lorgeril M, Renaud S, Mamelle N, et al. Mediterranean alpha-linolenic acid-rich diet in secondary prevention of coronary heart disease. *Lancet.* 1994;343:1454–1459.

11. de Lorgeril M, Salen P, Martin JL, et al. Mediterranean diet, traditional risk factors, and the rate of cardiovascular complications after myocardial infarction. *Circulation.* 1999;99:779–785.

12. Chobanian AV, Bakris GL, Black HR, et al. The seventh report of the Joint National Committee on Prevention, Detection, Evaluation, and Treatment of High Blood Pressure. *JAMA.* 2003;289:2560–2572.

13. Appel LJ, Moore TJ, Obarzanek E, et al. A clinical trial of the effects of dietary patterns on blood pressure. *N Engl J Med.* 1997;336:1117–1124.

14. Sacks FM, Svetkey LP, Vollmer WM, et al. Effects on blood pressure of reduced dietary sodium and the Dietary Approaches to Stop Hypertension (DASH) diet. *N Engl J Med.* 2001;344:3–10.

15. Calle EE, Rodriguez C, Walker-Thurmond K, Thun MJ. Overweight, obesity, and mortality from cancer in a prospectively studied cohort of U.S. adults. *N Engl J Med.* 2003;348:1625–1638.

16. Byers T, Nestle M, McTiernan A, et al, for American Cancer Society 2001 Nutrition and Physical Activity Guidelines Advisory Committee. American Cancer Society guidelines on nutrition and physical activity for cancer prevention: reducing the risk of cancer with healthy food choices and physical activity. *CA Cancer J Clin.* 2002;52:92–119.

17. Alpha-Tocopherol, Beta Carotene Cancer Prevention Study Group. The effect of vitamin E and beta carotene on the incidence of lung cancer and other cancers in male smokers. *N Engl J Med.* 1994;330:1029–1035.

18. Omenn GS, Goodman GE, Thornquist MD, et al. Effects of a combination of beta carotene and vitamin A on lung cancer and cardiovascular disease. *N Engl J Med.* 1996;334:1150–1155.

19. Kant AK, Schatzkin A, Graubard BI, Schairer C. A prospective study of diet quality and mortality in women. *JAMA.* 2000;283:2109–2115.

chapter 18

Obesity

Donald D. Hensrud, MD, MPH

INTRODUCTION

Obesity has emerged as a major public health problem. The prevalence of obesity is increasing in almost all parts of the world[1] and in the United States has increased by more than one third over the past few decades. Obesity is much more than a cosmetic problem, as the associated health complications also are increasing. Obesity is responsible for greater health care costs than either smoking or problem drinking, according to some estimates.[2]

The results of treatment of obesity have generally been disappointing; almost all weight is regained within 5 years regardless of method, except bariatric surgery.[3] Therefore, strategies targeting the prevention of weight gain will be even more important in the future. The interface of obesity and prevention occurs at multiple levels. In primary prevention, clinicians try to prevent weight gain throughout life so obesity does not develop. In secondary prevention, there are screenings for overweight and obesity in clinical practice and appropriate interventions to promote weight loss and prevent the complications of established obesity. In tertiary prevention, health care providers seek to prevent patients' weight regain after successful weight loss.

EPIDEMIOLOGY AND HEALTH RISKS

In 1999 to 2000, nearly 64.5% of the US population was overweight and 30.5% was obese based on data from the National Health and Nutrition Examination Survey.[4] This survey, which measures height and weight among a random sample of Americans, has documented a progressive increase in body mass index (BMI) since the early 1970s. The Behavioral Risk Factor Surveillance Survey also has reported a progressive increase in obesity prevalence, but with lower point prevalence estimates, probably due to the nature of this survey, which is by self-report.[5] Class 3 obesity (BMI $\geq$40 kg/m^2) almost tripled in prevalence in just 10 years, from 0.8% in 1990 to 2.2% in 2000.[6] The prevalence of obesity has been steadily increasing among both sexes and all age and ethnic groups. Of particular concern is the rise of obesity among children and adolescents, which increased by twofold to threefold in the 2 decades before 2000.[7]

As overweight and obesity increase, a corresponding increase in associated adverse health conditions can be expected after a short lag time. Health complications of obesity include the following:

- Glucose intolerance and type 2 diabetes mellitus
- Hypertension
- Dyslipidemia (hypertriglyceridemia, low high-density lipoprotein cholesterol [HDL-C])
- Coronary heart disease
- Congestive heart failure
- Most cancers
- Osteoarthritis
- Respiratory problems (obstructive sleep apnea, restrictive lung disease, obesity-hypoventilation syndrome)
- Hepatobiliary problems (cholelithiasis, hepatosteatosis, and nonalcoholic hepatosteatitis)
- Menstrual irregularities
- Psychological distress and disorders
- Increased overall mortality

The prevalence of diabetes mellitus increased from 4.9% in 1990 to 7.9% in 2000.[5] The health consequences of obesity are not limited to adults. Type 2 diabetes mellitus, previously considered an adult disease, is now increasingly being diagnosed in adolescents. An estimated 300,000 people die each year due to obesity.[8]

The direct health care costs related to obesity have been estimated to be more than $50 billion[9] and may be as high as $90 billion.[10] Because of the high and increasing prevalence, health risks of developing associated comorbidities, health care costs, poor treatment results to date, and few current promising efforts in prevention, obesity may be the most important public health problem in the United States today.

CLASSIFICATION

Obesity is an excess of body fat resulting in adverse health effects. Direct and accurate measurement of body fat is impractical in clinical practice, so BMI is currently the standard for classifying obesity. Body mass index is defined as: Weight (kg)/Height^2 (m). In clinical practice, BMI can be obtained from a chart, calculated by an electronic medical record, or determined by the formula: 703 × Weight (lb)/Height^2 (in). Compared with standard weight-height tables of ideal body weights, BMI correlates better with percent body fat and health outcomes. However, similar to ideal body weight, BMI is a surrogate measure of body fat and does not take into consideration body composition. Someone with a high BMI and low percent body fat, such as a bodybuilder, may be classified as obese by BMI yet have relatively low health risks. For most of the population, BMI is a useful clinical parameter, as it correlates well with health outcomes, including overall mortality.

Overweight is defined as a BMI of 25 kg/m^2 or higher, and obesity is defined as a BMI equal to or greater than 30 kg/m^2 (Table 18-1).[11] The health risks of obesity also are influenced by distribution of body fat. Greater abdominal fat, as estimated clinically by the waist circumference, further increases the health risks associated with elevated weight independent of BMI. Use of the waist-to-hip ratio has given way to the waist measurement after it was demonstrated that the waist measurement alone correlates as well with adverse health conditions. A high waist measurement, indicative of abdominal fat distribution, is defined as a waist circumference greater than 88 cm (35 in) in women and more than 102 cm (40 in) in men. Actually, the relationship between increasing abdominal fat and health risks is probably continuous, but these values have been identified to aid in clinical classification.

Increased upper body or abdominal fat is associated with the metabolic syndrome (also known as syndrome X or insulin resistance syndrome). The main features of this syndrome are the constellation of abdominal fat distribution, glucose intolerance or diabetes, hypertension, dyslipidemia (high triglycerides and low HDL-C levels), and an increased risk of coronary heart disease. The association of abdominal fat distribution with these health risks appears to be due to increased visceral and subcutaneous abdominal fat leading to excess release of free fatty acids and insulin resistance.[12]

In summary, the health risks associated with obesity and, therefore, the importance of sustained weight loss increases with increasing BMI and waist circumference and is greatest in those with established comorbidities. Weight gain is often insidious; on average people gain just a few pounds per year throughout adult life. Yet, it is cumulative. For this reason, primary prevention is critically important. In addition, although the treatment of obesity and its comorbidities is challenging, secondary and tertiary preventive efforts through lifestyle changes in diet and exercise are even more vital.

ETIOLOGY AND RISK FACTORS

The development of overweight and obesity is extremely complex and involves genetic, physiological, nutritional, psychological, and environmental factors. Ultimately, however, it is the imbalance of energy intake being greater than energy expenditure that contributes to weight gain. The relatively rapid increase in obesity prevalence in recent years suggests environmental factors are predominantly responsible, or at least environmental changes on top of a permissive genetic background.

Nutritional factors related to obesity are relative to total energy expenditure. For example, even if a diet is high in fat and total calories (energy), a large amount of exercise such as performed by some athletes may prevent the development of obesity. Unfortunately, in developed

TABLE 18-1

Classification of Overweight and Obesity

Classification	BMI (kg/m^2)*	Obesity Class	Disease Risk	
			Low Waist Circumference	High Waist Circumference+
Underweight	<18.5		—	—
Normal	18.5–24.9		—	—
Overweight	25.0–29.9		Increased	High
Obesity	30.0–34.9	1	High	Very high
	35.0–39.9	2	Very high	Very high
Extreme obesity	≥40.0	3	Extremely high	Extremely high

*Body mass index (BMI) can be calculated as: Weight (kg)/Height^2 (m), or Weight (lb) × 703/Height^2 (in). Tables of weight, height, and BMI are also widely available.

+High waist circumference is defined as >102 cm (40 in) in men and >88 cm (35 in) in women.

societies, in contrast to developing countries, there are many technological advances that have resulted in decreasing total energy expenditure (eg, well-developed transportation systems, computers, remote controls, and other "step-saving" devices). Some have estimated that the predominant factor related to the increase of obesity in the United States in recent years is a decline of overall physical activity, distinct from exercise per se.[13] Other studies have suggested that physical activity is probably the most important factor in the primary prevention of weight gain and also preventing weight regain after weight loss.[14]

In examining the intake side of the energy balance equation, total calories consumed are clearly the most important factor. In general, people are poor judges of total calories in their diet. Studies in which normal-weight subjects have tried to accurately record dietary calories without trying to lose weight have shown people underes-

timate energy intake by approximately 20% on average, with studies reporting a wide range of estimates.[15] Obese subjects may underestimate energy intake to a greater degree, by up to 47% in one study of subjects refractory to weight loss.[16] This is probably not a conscious or intentional act. It may relate to the discrepancy between the appearance of the amount of food consumed and the caloric content (energy density of food), which will be discussed later. In addition, high-energy-dense foods are widely available for most of the population through the large number of restaurants, new processed food products, and efficient food transportation systems currently available.

Other factors may predispose to increased weight in an individual (Table 18-2). Two common beliefs among patients are that a low metabolic rate or underactive thyroid gland is largely responsible for weight gain. Less than 2% of all obesity is due to a metabolic, endocrine,

TABLE 18-2

Predisposing Factors to Obesity

Factor	Comment
Decreased physical activity	
Activities throughout the day	Major contributor to increasing obesity in United States
Exercise	Strongest effect is in preventing weight gain and weight regain after weight loss
Increased energy intake	
Various factors	Increased portion size; high-energy-dense foods, including fat, sugar, and processed foods; decreased intake of vegetables and fruits
Alcohol	Increases abdominal weight gain
Smoking cessation	Mean increase of 2.7–4.5 kg (6–10 lb)
Medications	
Corticosteroids	
Tricyclic and other antidepressants	
Pregnancy	Mean increase of 1.8–2.7 kg (4–6 lb) after each pregnancy
Endocrine/metabolic	Cause in <1%–2% of all obesity cases
Hypothyroidism	Weight gain usually only in long-standing hypothyroidism
Cushing syndrome	Characteristic fat deposition
Genetic conditions	Very rare
Prader-Willi syndrome	
Laurence-Moon-Biedl syndrome	
Other medical conditions	
Depression	
Physical limitations that limit activity	
"Yo-yo" dieting—gaining and losing weight multiple times	Does not result in sustained depression of metabolic rate and increased risk of weight gain despite popular belief

Reprinted with permission from *Conn's Current Therapy 2002*.[3]

or pure genetic abnormality. The major determinant of resting metabolic rate is lean body mass. With increasing total body weight, the absolute amount of lean body mass increases, as well as fat. Approximately 25% to 35% of excess weight is lean body mass. Therefore, obese persons have an increased resting metabolic rate relative to lean persons.

PRIMARY PREVENTION OF OBESITY

The lack of complete understanding regarding the etiology of obesity makes preventive efforts more difficult. Because the prevalence of obesity is increasing in all age, sex, and geographic groups, the factors causing this increase must be highly prevalent. Predisposing factors must ultimately operate on an individual level, and individuals should adopt behaviors conducive to a healthy body weight. However, the environment also will need to be changed, in part through public health efforts, to have a major impact in decreasing body weight on a population-wide basis. For example, community development should include ample opportunities for physical activity, such as walking and biking paths, neighborhoods that encourage local travel, buildings with stairs more conveniently located than elevators, physical activity in schools, and other initiatives. Nutrition interventions could include subsidizing low-energy-dense vegetables and fruits by the government and private sources. Development of palatable, low-energy-dense food products by the food industry may help. Economic incentives eventually may need to be employed, as the cost of obesity continues to increase.

Clinical practice often leaves little time for counseling patients, including on healthy weight. Less than 50% of physicians counsel obese patients on weight loss, and few physicians counsel on weight maintenance. However, because weight gain is so common and insidious, it is important to briefly give people advice on weight management, similar to other health promotion messages. For the general population, this could consist of reinforcement of current strategies that are helping to maintain weight, including prudent dietary habits and especially regular physical activity. In addition, most people can improve in these areas. Progressive advice can be provided as outlined in the following sections. It should be emphasized that these changes are consistent with other recommendations to reduce the risk of many different chronic diseases, including hyperlipidemia, hypertension, diabetes mellitus, cancer, and overall quality of life. Proactively addressing the predisposing factors in Table 18-2 may help prevent weight gain (eg, starting a regular physical activity program and considering bupropion treatment when quitting smoking).

NUTRITION AND PREVENTION AND TREATMENT OF OBESITY

Decreasing Caloric Intake

There are many different methods to decrease total intake of calories. Counting calories is the most obvious. For weight loss, a goal of 1200 to 1600 kcal/d is a general target. As mentioned previously, people tend to underestimate the number of calories they consume, so actual caloric intake is often greater than the goal. Counting fat grams is another method. Decreasing fat intake may help reduce overall caloric intake if baseline fat intake is high but will not work if nonfat calories are increased from such things as simple sugars. For example, low-fat yogurt with added sugar may contain a similar amount of calories as whole-milk yogurt. This may be one reason why low-fat diets have not been as successful as people had hoped. Limiting the consumption of specific high-calorie foods, the portion size, or the number of servings from food groups are other methods of decreasing total caloric intake and can be effective in individual patients. Whatever the method, a key point is that dietary changes should be approached as a sustained lifestyle change, as opposed to "going on a diet."

Energy Density

Energy density is the number of calories in a given amount—volume or weight—of food. Foods high in energy density have a relatively large number of calories in a small amount. These include not only high-fat foods but also high-sugar-containing and highly refined products. Using this concept, butter, meat, sugar cereals, soda, white bread, pretzels, and crackers are all high in energy density.

Foods that are low in energy density have a relatively small amount of calories in a large volume. In addition to small amounts of fat and simple carbohydrate, the major factor that lowers energy density is water. Fiber and air, which also contribute weight or volume, but not calories, to food have lesser effects on lowering energy density. Fruits and, in particular, vegetables are low-energy-dense foods. If individuals consume a diet high in low-energy-dense foods, they can achieve satiety by the bulk and volume of these foods, yet at a lower overall energy intake, thus promoting weight loss. For example, 1⅓ sticks of butter have the same number of calories as 10 to 11 heads of lettuce or 35 cups of green beans.

Energy density is the principle behind the Mayo Healthy Weight Pyramid (Fig 18-1).[17] Vegetables and fruits are at the bottom of the pyramid, and unlimited amounts of fresh or frozen forms of each are recommended. In each of the other food groups, a specific number of servings is recommended and healthy choices are emphasized. For example, in the carbohydrate category, whole grains are emphasized; in the protein and dairy category, fish, beans, and low-fat dairy products are encouraged; and in the fat category, monounsaturated fats are recommended. Daily physical activity, from lifestyle activities throughout the day as well as planned exercise, is an important component for weight management and health and is placed at the center of the pyramid. For weight loss, servings from each food group are recommended consistent with an initial caloric goal of 1200 kcal/d for women and 1400 kcal/d for men. For weight maintenance and prevention of weight gain, the principles of the Mayo Healthy Weight Pyramid also apply, with a greater number of servings from each group.

Meal Replacements

Meal replacements are categorized as a food for special use. They are designed to replace 1 or more meals, are nutritionally complete, and contain 200 to 400 calories. An increasing number of studies are showing they are safe and can be more effective than traditional calorie-restricted diets to promote weight loss.[18] Additional advantages include convenience and cost. Meal replacements should be considered for patients who are interested in this approach.

Very-Low-Calorie Diets

Very-low-calorie diets (VLCDs) contain 400 to 800 kcal/d and usually consist of a liquid high-protein drink. Initial

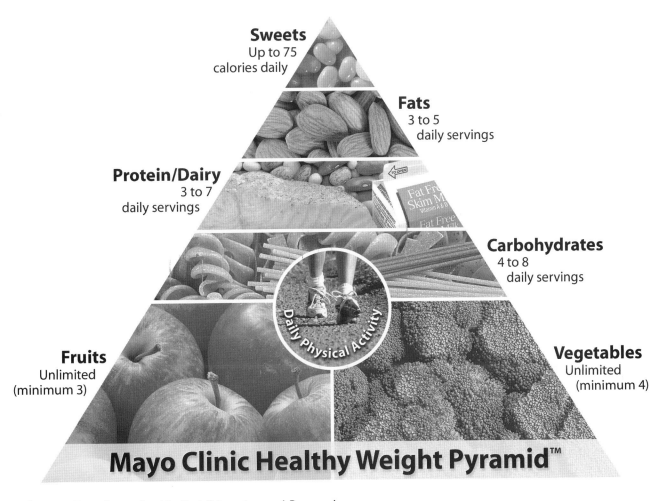

© Mayo Foundation for Medical Education and Research.

F I G U R E   18-1

weight loss is greater with VLCDs compared with less restrictive diets. However, the major challenge for the patient is making the transition back to real food. Weight regain often occurs at this transition time, particularly if patients revert to previous dietary habits. Long-term results are no better with VLCDs than with more conservative approaches.[19]

Popular Diets

A multitude of books on the market outline various diets and dietary programs. Some programs recommend consumption of only certain foods (eg, grapefruit diet). Other programs restrict the timing or combinations of foods consumed (eg, not eating fruit after lunch or not combining protein with carbohydrate). Whatever the type of program, if weight loss is to occur, energy intake must be reduced relative to energy expenditure.

A common current theme of popular diets is to limit total carbohydrate. The proposed theory behind this is that carbohydrate is broken down into glucose, which stimulates insulin production. Insulin is anabolic in that it prevents lipolysis and promotes glucose uptake into cells. Therefore, with a reduced carbohydrate intake, blood insulin concentrations will decrease and people will lose weight. Currently, few data support this theory or that low-carbohydrate diets are any more effective in long-term weight management than other approaches.[20]

Weight loss on a low-carbohydrate diet is probably due to 3 effects. First, initial weight loss is water loss, because stored glycogen is broken down. Second, a very-low-carbohydrate diet can produce ketosis, which is anorexigenic. Third and most important, by a reduction in carbohydrates, which should comprise 50% to 65% of total calories, a decrease in total energy intake occurs.[21]

If people are able to lose weight on a low-carbohydrate diet, it may be temporary if they do not continue following the diet. When they liberalize their diet to include more carbohydrate, weight gain often recurs, aided in part by restoration of glycogen stores. A real concern with many low-carbohydrate diets that is particularly relevant to prevention is that they are, by necessity, high in fat, which is often saturated fat. If people are able to continue consuming a low-carbohydrate, high-fat diet, there is no evidence it is safe long-term. The high intake of saturated fat (along with lack of consumption of beneficial foods such as many vegetables, fruits, and whole grains) raises concerns about increasing the risk of some chronic diseases.

PHYSICAL ACTIVITY AND PREVENTION AND TREATMENT OF OBESITY

Increased energy expenditure is the other half of the energy balance equation that affects body weight. Total physical activity consists of exercise and activities performed throughout the day. Exercise is the most efficient way to increase energy expenditure but requires planning, time, and in some cases equipment. Daily activities can be modified throughout the day to promote increased energy expenditure. Examples include:

- Walk to talk to an office colleague instead of using e-mail.
- Deliver things in person.
- Walk while talking on the cell phone.
- Take the stairs instead of the elevator.
- Park farther away from a destination.
- Find an excuse to walk somewhere.
- Walk during breaks or during lunch hour.
- Make a conscious effort to not use a television remote control.
- Don't ask children to do tasks rather than doing them oneself.
- Take a walk in the airport (not on the moving walkway!).
- Choose outdoor activities in the summertime.

Both exercise and modification of daily activities should be employed to maximize energy expenditure. Eventually people should try to reach the goal of at least 30 minutes of moderately vigorous physical activity most days of the week, either through exercise or activities throughout the day. Even a brief counseling message by a health care provider can lead to increased physical activity among patients. Health care providers should tailor recommendations to the individual based on his or her readiness to change, physical limitations, goals, schedule, and resources.

For people who are sedentary, recommendations for exercise should include choosing an enjoyable activity, making it a regular priority, and striving for consistency over time. Patients should start slowly and then gradually increase the frequency, duration, and intensity over time, probably in that order. Lack of time often is given as a reason for not exercising. However, the long-term health consequences of being sedentary are so severe that virtually everyone should examine his or her priorities and incorporate moderately vigorous physical activity into even the busiest schedule.

The health effects of physical activity and fitness independent of body weight should be emphasized to patients whether they are of normal weight or overweight. Adopting a physically active lifestyle will decrease the risk of developing or improve the treatment of many of the same conditions that are predisposed to by obesity, including hypertension, diabetes mellitus, and cardiovascular disease. There is evidence that obese people who are fit are at lower risk of dying than are thin people who are not fit.[22] Similar to healthy dietary habits, this underscores the fact that even if people are not able to reach their goal weight, their health will improve by adopting a regular habit of physical activity.

BEHAVIORAL MODIFICATION

An important aspect of the prevention and treatment of obesity is sustained lifestyle changes. Too many people approach weight management as "going on a diet," which has connotations of being restrictive, negative, and temporary. In addition, many people undertake an exercise program too vigorously. After enduring this for a time, people eventually revert to previous diet and activity habits with resultant weight regain. A common belief is if people can lose weight, they will be able to make the necessary adjustments to keep the weight off. However, this strategy has not been found to be effective.[23] In contrast to the common negative outlook on losing weight, if people are prepared to approach it with a positive attitude of making healthy, sustainable lifestyle changes, they may be more likely to succeed. Behavioral changes in lifestyle can be addressed through a formal behavioral modification program or individually.

Some features of behavioral modification techniques that can be used clinically are described in this section.

Assessment

Initial evaluation should involve measuring height, weight, and BMI, and assessing waist measurement by either gross inspection or measurement. For patients with a normal BMI and waist measurement, the clinician should provide advice regarding primary prevention through healthy diet and physical activity habits. For patients with an elevated BMI and/or waist measurement, health conditions related to excess weight should be noted.

If a patient has elevated BMI and waist measurements and obesity-related complications are present, a recommendation of specific weight loss strategies is fruitless if the patient is not interested. One method of assessing a patient's readiness to change is the Transtheoretical Model of Behavior Change, or stages of change. The stages in this model are precontemplation, contemplation, preparation, action, and maintenance. The importance of assessment using this tool is that the intervention strategy can be tailored to the patient's particular stage. If patients are in the precontemplation stage and are not interested in weight loss, brief written information can be provided, whereas if the patient is in the action stage, a plan of action and appropriate resources can be used. Further information regarding this model can be found in Chapter 6.

For patients ready to pursue weight loss, further information should be collected that can help formulate an appropriate plan. This can be collected in a focused interview or via a written questionnaire, which can save time. Information that should be collected includes the following:

- Weight history (minimum, maximum, and changes over time)
- Previous weight loss attempts and results
- Current and past exercise and activity habits
- Current and past dietary habits
- Triggers to eating
- Factors affecting weight (eg, sedentary job, physical limitations, medications)
- Medications and dietary supplements
- History of eating disorder
- Binging, purging, and use of laxatives or diuretics
- Family history of obesity
- Patient's understanding of reasons for increased weight
- Patient's initial goals
- Patient's expectations

Goal Setting

Goal setting gives patients something for which to strive. Goals should be specific, measurable, and achievable. In addition, goals should be process-oriented and not outcome-oriented. For example, many people have as their goal a specific amount of weight loss, but no goals on how to achieve that weight loss. Often, when people do not achieve a weight loss goal, they become frustrated and abandon further efforts. Examples of specific initial process goals are eating 1 more serving of vegetables each day or walking 15 minutes 3 days each week.

Self-monitoring

Self-monitoring techniques include diet records, an activity log, or a pedometer. Through self-monitoring techniques, patients can track their progress toward their goals and become more aware of current habits in the areas of physical activity and diet. Studies have demonstrated that people who keep diet and activity records are more successful at weight management.

Problem-solving Techniques

Problems should be expected during weight loss efforts. Many people experience certain triggers to eating, such as watching television, stress, or eating late at night. By using problem-solving techniques, patients can deal with problems much more effectively. First, the specific behavioral trigger, problem, or issue is written down. Then the barriers to changing that behavior are identified. Next, the benefits to changing the behavior are listed. Finally, potential solutions to the problem are outlined with specific goals for implementing the solution.

Cognitive Restructuring (Setting Appropriate Expectations)

Most people who attempt weight loss have unrealistic expectations. In one study in which 60 women lost an average of 18.45 kg (41 lb) over 6 months on a VLCD, only 7% reached a weight with which they were happy.[24] A realistic initial expectation is 5% to 10% loss of initial body weight. However, the primary goal of any weight loss program should be to improve health. If patients are making healthy changes in diet and physical activity habits but not losing weight, this is still successful and ideally should be appreciated by the patient as such.

Obesity can be psychologically distressing for many people. Poor body self-image, low self-esteem, frustration, social isolation, and depression are serious consequences. Bias and discrimination, including among physicians, are widespread toward obese individuals. Physicians and other health care personnel who deal with obesity should use appropriate sensitivity and empathy. In addition, the office environment should be set up to help obese subjects feel comfortable, such as location of the scale in a discreet place, appropriate furniture, and weight-sensitive reading and patient education materials.

PHARMACOTHERAPY FOR OBESITY

Currently there is no drug approved for prevention of weight gain. Metformin was studied in 3200 obese subjects (mean BMI, 34 kg/m^2) with glucose intolerance.[25] The primary outcome was the prevention of diabetes. After almost 3 years, subjects treated with metformin lost 2.1 kg and experienced a 31% reduction in the incidence of diabetes. However, in that same trial, lifestyle changes in diet and exercise were associated with a weight loss of 5.8 kg and a 58% lower incidence of diabetes. Lifestyle efforts remain the cornerstone for prevention of weight gain.

For secondary prevention (treatment of established obesity to promote weight loss and prevent the complications associated with increased weight), 3 medications are most commonly used. Indications for sibutramine and orlistat are a BMI greater than 30, or a BMI over 27 if complications from obesity are present. Phentermine was approved for short-term use 30 years ago, and there are little long-term data on efficacy or safety. Pharmacotherapy should always be used in conjunction with lifestyle changes in diet and physical activity.

The length of time that medications should be used to treat obesity is not entirely clear. Short-term studies have shown that when medications are stopped, weight regain occurs. Most experts feel that treatment should be continued indefinitely unless major changes in lifestyle will make weight maintenance likely. Long-term treatment of obesity with pharmacotherapy is consistent with treatment of other chronic conditions such as hypertension and hyperlipidemia.

Sibutramine

Sibutramine inhibits the reuptake of norepinephrine and serotonin, resulting in increased satiety. It is important to note that sibutramine does not primarily affect appetite. Only 7% of patients taking sibutramine experience anorexia. Patients should understand that it is important to be aware of satiety sensations when eating and to stop eating when they feel satisfied.

Patients should have reasonable expectations concerning the results of pharmacotherapy for weight loss. Overall, the mean amount of weight loss due to sibutramine is 3 to 5 kg more than placebo in studies with treatment greater than 6 months.[26] Although this weight loss may seem modest, it is independent of weight loss secondary to changes in diet and physical activity. Moreover, weight loss of 5% to 10% of initial body weight will improve many of the comorbidities associated with obesity, such as diabetes and hypertension.[11]

The most common side effects from sibutramine are usually mild and include headache, dry mouth, constipation, and insomnia, all of which occur in 6% to 13% more people than with placebo. The most important side effect of sibutramine is elevated blood pressure. Although the mean increase in blood pressure is only about 2 mm Hg systolic and diastolic, 10% of people experience an increase in diastolic blood pressure of 10 mm Hg greater than placebo. Blood pressure should be monitored closely in patients receiving sibutramine. The usual starting dosage of sibutramine is 10 mg daily. If people experience side effects, the dose can be decreased to 5 mg, and if adequate weight loss is not achieved, the dose can be increased to 15 mg.

Orlistat

Orlistat is an inhibitor of lipase and blocks the absorption of about one third of dietary fat that is absorbed. Treatment results in controlled studies longer than 6 months show a weight loss of 3 to 4 kg above placebo. Orlistat is not absorbed, so there are no systemic side effects. Gastrointestinal side effects, which occur in up to 20% of people, include oily stools and spotting, flatus, and fecal urgency. However, in about 50% of people who experience side effects, they last for less than a week, and in the second year of treatment side effects are no greater than with placebo. The dosage of orlistat is 120 mg 3 times daily with meals that contain fat. It is recommended that patients take a multivitamin daily at a time different from the orlistat.

Orlistat may be a reasonable choice for someone who is a candidate for pharmacotherapy but has hypertension that is difficult to control, whereas sibutramine may be an appropriate choice for someone with gastrointestinal problems or conditions, such as irritable bowel syndrome, that may be exacerbated by orlistat.

Dietary Supplements

Dietary supplements to promote weight loss are a billion-dollar industry. Because of the difficulty in achieving weight loss, promises of effortless weight loss, and ease of obtaining these products, they offer an attractive option for people trying to manage their weight. Unfortunately, very few data exist that any dietary supplements lead to large amounts of sustained weight loss. In addition, there are safety issues with some ingredients, particularly ephedra, which has now been taken off the market.[27] For these reasons, there is little rationale for people to use dietary supplements to promote weight loss.

TERTIARY PREVENTION OF WEIGHT REGAIN

Clues to the successful long-term treatment of obesity can be inferred from people who have lost weight and maintained that weight loss. The National Weight Control Registry is composed of people who have lost at least 13.5 kg (30 lb) and kept it off for at least 1 year. The mean amount of weight loss among subjects in this registry is 30 kg (66 lb), and they have kept it off an average of 5 years. When asked what was responsible for their beneficial results, 75% of subjects noted a triggering event that motivated them, more than 90% exercised regularly, and over 90% made some type of dietary change.[28] The type of dietary change varied; many limited the intake of certain foods, some limited portion size, and some counted calories. Subjects exercised, on average, 1 hour each day, with walking being the main form of exercise for more than 75% of subjects. Just as physical activity is one of the strongest factors in the primary prevention of weight gain, it is also one of the most important factors in weight loss maintenance. The strategies these subjects employed involved sustained lifestyle changes in the basic areas of nutrition and physical activity as opposed to a quick-fix diet or unrealistically stringent program.

Another study evaluated people who were successful in maintaining weight after weight loss ("maintainers") and compared them with people who regained the weight they lost. Maintainers were more likely to exercise regularly, use problem-solving techniques, have adequate social support, and make sustained dietary changes as opposed to eating diet foods.[29] Eating breakfast regularly and using self-monitoring techniques also have been associated with improved weight maintenance.

CRITERIA FOR SUCCESS

The obvious goal for prevention and treatment of obesity is to achieve a normal BMI. However, this can be difficult for many people to attain once overweight and obesity have developed. There are many other important measures of success in treatment of obesity, including the following[3]:

- Improved health habits
- Weight loss
- Long-term weight maintenance
- Prevention of weight gain
- Improvement in comorbidities of obesity
- Inches/centimeters lost
- Changes in body composition
- Quality of life (feeling better, improved ability to carry out activities of daily living)

Perhaps the most important of these is improved health. Adopting beneficial lifestyle habits in diet and physical activity will improve health independent of weight. Among patients who are overweight, this is important to counteract the major health risks associated with obesity. Among persons of normal weight, beneficial lifestyle habits in diet and activity will help prevent obesity and its associated health risks along with maintaining a good quality of life.

REFERENCES

1. World Health Organization. *Obesity: Preventing and Managing the Global Epidemic*. Geneva, Switzerland: World Health Organization; 2000.

2. Sturm R. The effects of obesity, smoking, and drinking on medical problems and costs. *Health Affairs*. 2002; 212:45–53.

3. Hensrud DD. Obesity. In: Rakel RE, Bope ET, eds. *Conn's Current Therapy 2002*. Philadelphia, Pa: WB Saunders Co; 2002:577–585.

4. Flegal KM, Carroll MD, Ogden CL, Johnson CL. Prevalence and trends in obesity among US adults, 1999–2000. *JAMA*. 2002;288:1723–1727.

5. Mokdad AH, Ford ES, Bowman BA, et al. Prevalence of obesity, diabetes, and obesity-related health risk factors, 2001. *JAMA*. 2003;289:76–79.

6. Freedman DS, Khan LK, Serdula MK, Galuska DA, Dietz WH. Trends and correlates of class 3 obesity in the United States from 1990 through 2000. *JAMA*. 2002;288:1758–1761.

7. Ogden CL, Flegal KM, Carroll MD, Johnson CL. Prevalence and trends in overweight among US children and adolescents, 1999–2000. *JAMA*. 2002;288:1728–1732.

8. Allison DB, Fontaine KR, Manson JE, Stevens J, VanItallie TB. Annual deaths attributable to obesity in the United States. *JAMA*. 1999;282:1530–1538.

9. Wolf AM, Colditz GA. Current estimates of the economic cost of obesity in the United States. *Obes Res*. 1998;6:173–175.

10. Finkelstein EA, Fiebelkorn IC, Wang G. National medical spending attributable to overweight and obesity: how much, and who's paying? *Health Affairs*. Available at: www.healthaffairs.org/WebExclusives/Finkelstein_Web_Excl_051403.htm. Accessed May 16, 2003.

11. *The Practical Guide to the Identification, Evaluation, and Treatment of Overweight and Obesity in Adults (NIH)*. Bethesda, Md: National Heart, Lung, and Blood Institute; 2000. NIH publication 00–4084.

12. Sheehan MT, Jensen MD. Metabolic complications of obesity: pathophysiologic considerations. *Med Clin North Am*. 2000;84:363–385.

13. Weinsier RL, Hunter GR, Heini AF, Goran MI, Sell SM. The etiology of obesity: relative contribution of metabolic factors, diet, and physical activity. *Am J Med*. 1998;105:145–150.

14. Leermakers EA, Dunn AL, Blair SN. Exercise management of obesity. *Med Clin North Am*. 2000;84:419–440.

15. Trabulsi J, Schoeller DA. Evaluation of dietary assessment instruments against doubly labeled water, a biomarker of habitual energy intake. *Am J Physiol Endocrinol Metab*. 2001;281:E891–E899.

16. Lichtman SW, Pisarska K, Berman ER, et al. Discrepancy between self-reported and actual caloric intake and exercise in obese subjects. *N Engl J Med*. 1992;327:1893–1898.

17. Hensrud DD, ed. *Mayo Clinic on Healthy Weight*. Rochester, Minn: Mayo Clinic; 2000.

18. Heymsfield SB, van Mierlo CAJ, van der Knaap HCM, Heo M, Frier HI. Weight management using a meal replacement strategy: meta and pooling analysis from six studies. *Int J Obes Metab Disord*. 2003;27:537–549.

19. Wadden TA, Foster GD, Letizia KA. One-year behavioral treatment of obesity: comparison of moderate and severe caloric restriction and the effects of weight maintenance therapy. *J Consult Clin Psychol*. 1994;62:165–171.

20. Foster GD, Wyatt HR, Hill JO, et al. A randomized trial of a low-carbohydrate diet for obesity. *N Engl J Med*. 2003;348:2082–2090.

21. Bravata DM, Sanders L, Huang J, et al. Efficacy and safety of low-carbohydrate diets: a systematic review. *JAMA*. 2003;289:1837–1850.

22. Lee CD, Blair SN, Jackson AS. Cardiorespiratory fitness, body composition, and all-cause and cardiovascular disease mortality in men. *Am J Clin Nutr*. 1999;69:373–380.

23. Hensrud DD, Weinsier RL, Darnell BE, Hunter GR. A prospective study of weight maintenance in obese subjects reduced to normal body weight without weight-loss training. *Am J Clin Nutr*. 1994;60:688–694.

24. Foster GD, Wadden TA, Vogt RA, Brewer G. What is a reasonable weight loss? Patients' expectations and evaluations of obesity treatment outcomes. *J Consult Clin Psychol*. 1997;65:79–85.

25. Knowler WC, Barrett-Connor E, Fowler SE, et al. Reduction in the incidence of type 2 diabetes with lifestyle intervention or metformin. *N Engl J Med*. 2002; 346:393–403.

26. Hensrud DD. Pharmacotherapy for obesity. *Med Clin North Am*. 2000;84:463–476.

27. Shekelle PG, Hardy ML, Morton SC, et al. Efficacy and safety of ephedra and ephedrine for weight loss and athletic performance: a meta-analysis. *JAMA*. 2003;289:1537–1545.

28. Klem ML, Wing RR, McGuire MT, et al. A descriptive study of individuals successful at long-term maintenance of substantial weight loss. *Am J Clin Nutr*. 1997;66:239–246.

29. Kayman S, Bruvold W, Stern JS. Maintenance and relapse after weight loss in women: behavioral aspects. *Am J Clin Nutr*. 1990;52:800–807.

RESOURCES

Brownell KD. *The LEARN Program for Weight Control 2000*. Dallas, Tex: American Health Publishing Co; 2000.

Hensrud DD, ed. *Mayo Clinic on Healthy Weight*. Rochester, Minn: Mayo Clinic; 2000.

Kushner R. *Roadmaps for Clinical Practice: Case Studies in Disease Prevention and Health Promotion—Assessment and Management of Adult Obesity: A Primer for Physicians*. Chicago, Ill: American Medical Association; 2003.

The Practical Guide to the Identification, Evaluation, and Treatment of Overweight and Obesity in Adults. Bethesda, Md: National Heart, Lung, and Blood Institute; 2000. NIH publication 00–4084.

chapter 19

Using Dietary Guidelines in Clinical Practice

Tim Byers, MD, MPH, and Amy Bode, MD, MSPH

INTRODUCTION

No shortage of guidelines intended to shape clinical practice exists. Clinical guidelines have proliferated in recent years to the point where it is increasingly difficult even to be aware of all the guidelines, let alone use them effectively to guide a practice. Nearly all aspects of clinical practice, from disease treatment to health promotion, have been reviewed by expert groups, with resulting advice in the form of a guideline that specifies both what to do and how to do it. Many different nutrition guidelines have been developed for general health promotion and for risk reduction of specific diseases.[1-4] Nutrition guidelines typically have been developed and targeted for the general public. However, these guidelines also affect medical practice when it comes to discussions about choices of food and physical activity in the setting of clinical disease management and prevention.

The scientific evidence that links nutrition to the causes of chronic diseases such as coronary artery disease, cancer, and diabetes is reviewed in Chapter 17. Even though these relationships are not yet completely understood, it is clear that there are many modifiable relationships between chronic diseases and factors such as body weight, physical activity, and diet. In this chapter, we will review the most important US consensus guidelines on nutrition, weight control, and physical activity. There are also important international dietary guidelines,[5,6] which in most instances generally agree with US guidelines.[1-4] Federal objectives have been set to define targets for clinical nutrition counseling. We will comment on the process of guideline development and how patients regard guidelines, and will offer some practical tips on how dietary guidelines can be incorporated into a busy clinical practice.

GUIDELINE DEVELOPMENT

Nutrition guidelines often are developed by governmental, professional, or private voluntary agencies. Guidelines for the provision of specific clinical services, such as those developed and promoted by the US Preventive Services Task Force,[7] are typically "evidence-based," meaning they have been developed by a specific formula in which the scientific evidence is summarized by *a priori* defined criteria. Those criteria tend to weigh the evidence from randomized, controlled trials quite heavily. In contrast, nutrition guidelines tend to be developed in a less quantitative way, usually emerging from an expert panel using a consensus development process.[1-6]

The use of an expert consensus approach to development of dietary guidelines is necessary because of the complexity of nutrition science. The evidence relating nutritional factors to health and disease comes from a wide range of types of studies. The clearest evidence of the approximate magnitude of nutritional effects on risk of chronic disease comes from the simplest of epidemiologic observations, such as international ecological studies and studies of the changing patterns of disease among migrants. Such observations are far from certain, however, in their conclusions of causation. Randomized, controlled trials are commonly regarded as a much more definitive design to support causal inference. However, randomized, controlled trials cannot easily test whole food or whole diet interventions; they usually study only individuals at high risk of disease over short periods of time, and they often examine only intermediate markers of disease risk. Trials, therefore, answer only narrow questions about the risk of chronic diseases; they usually cannot directly prove causation for the patterns of long-term diet, physical activity, or body weight that have been shown by observational studies to be strongly associated with risk of heart disease, cancer, and diabetes.[8]

SUMMARY OF MAJOR DIETARY GUIDELINES

Obesity

Guidelines for body weight have been consistent across various expert groups since 1998.[9] Overweight is defined as a body mass index (BMI; weight in kilograms divided by height in meters squared) between 25 and 29, and obesity as a BMI of 30 or greater. Both overweight and obesity are epidemic in the United States.[10] Concomitant with this epidemic of obesity has been an epidemic in diabetes mellitus.[11] Although trends in heart disease and cancer have been favorable in the past 1 to 2 decades, it is clear that more improvements would have been observed if we had not experienced the obesity epidemic.

Weight control has been extensively studied and written about, seemingly in every newsstand magazine. The simple conclusion of 3 decades of weight control research is that many different types of diets can be used to lose weight as long as energy intake is below output. All weight loss programs share 2 common features: short-term weight loss is assured as long as caloric (energy) intake is reduced, and long-term weight loss is virtually impossible without sustained physical activity.[9] Guidelines for an individual patient are less successful when they are tied to BMI goals, and more successful when they emphasize reachable goals. The objective is to embark on a program of sustained changes in nutrition and physical activity resulting in long-term weight control and improved health.

Physical Activity

The key guidelines for physical activity are summarized in Table 19-1. The US Department of Agriculture (USDA) and the American Cancer Society (ACS) recommend 30 to 45 minutes per day of moderate exercise for adults and 60 minutes per day for children. Only in the past decade have experts fully appreciated the importance of physical inactivity as a major risk factor for heart disease, diabetes, and several cancers.[12] Before the 1996 US surgeon general's report on physical activity and health, guidelines for physical activity were confusing and contradictory. Even today, however, there is not a complete consensus on the amount of activity needed to reduce the risk of specific diseases.

Regular physical activity is an essential element in lifetime weight control. Therefore, inasmuch as excess body weight increases the risk of heart disease, diabetes, and several cancers, physical inactivity is also a contributing

TABLE 19-1

Major US Advisory Group Recommendations on Daily Physical Activity and Nutrition

Class of Recommendation	US Dietary Guidelines[1]	American Heart Association[2]	American Cancer Society[3]	American Diabetes Association[4]
Physical activity (min/d)				
Children	60	NR*	60	NR
Adults	30	30–60	45	Increase
Selected nutrients (% of calories)				
Total fats	<30	<30	<30	NR
Polyunsaturated fats	NR	Replace saturates with polyunsaturates and monosaturates	NR	NR
Monounsaturated fats	NR			
Saturated fats	<10		Reduce	<7
Cholesterol (mg)	<300	<300	NR	<300
Carbohydrates	55–60	NR	NR	NR
Protein	10–15	15	NR	60–70**
Fiber (g/d)	25–30	Increase	Increase	15–20
Selected foods				
Breads/cereals (servings per day)	6–11	6+	Use whole grains	NR
Vegetables (servings per day)	3–5	3–5	3–5	3–5
Fruits (servings per day)	2–4	2–4	2–4	NR
Red meat (oz/d)	5–7	<5	Reduce	NR
Alcohol (drinks per day)	1–2	1–2	1–2	1–2

*NR = No recommendation.

**Combines calories from carbohydrates and monounsaturated fats.

cause. In the past decade, it has become more apparent that in addition to the role physical activity plays in preventing obesity, it also has effects on health independent of body weight. At every level of body weight, including obesity, physical activity is protective against heart disease. Colorectal cancers, postmenopausal breast cancer, and endometrial cancer are related to obesity and also, independent of obesity, to physical activity.[13] The dose-response effects of the frequency, intensity, and duration of physical activity are not completely described for all diseases, but it appears that the most important behavior is to move from the sedentary category, in which there is little or no physical activity, to at least moderate levels of activity, such as walking. For heart disease, there is an additional benefit from increasing activity to progressively higher levels of aerobic fitness. However, for cancer, diabetes, and heart disease, the greatest benefits of increasing physical activity are gained in the first steps. Substantial risk reduction accompanies even moderate levels of activity.[12,13]

Dietary Fats

The recommendations for dietary fats and other macronutrients are summarized in Table 19-1. For the past 15 years, the message about dietary fat in the United States has been dominated by the "total fat" dictum—to keep total fat intake under 30% of calories. This recommendation continues to be espoused by the USDA,[1] the American Heart Association (AHA),[2] and the ACS.[3] Emerging evidence in the past decade has caused many to question this message, however. The best current evidence points more to the types of fat in the diet as being important to health, and less to total fat intake.

For the prevention of heart disease, reduced consumption of saturated fats from animal foods is clearly more important than is reduction of total fats in the diet. Transfats, which are created in the processing of vegetable oils, behave much like saturated fats in increasing low-density lipoprotein cholesterol (LDL-C) levels. Conversely, monounsaturated fats and omega-3 fatty acids are neutral or have beneficial effects on the risk of heart disease.

The effects of total fats and/or specific types of fats on cancer risk are less clear than for heart disease. This may be because the relationships truly differ, or because for cancer there is not a validated intermediate marker of risk analogous to serum cholesterol. Most of the interest in the relationship of dietary fats with cancer risk has focused on breast, colorectal, and prostate cancers. The evidence that total fat intake is a cause of breast cancer is quite weak, whereas evidence is stronger for colon and prostate cancer.[3,5] It may well be true for cancer, as for heart disease, that types of fats (eg, saturated fats in particular) are more important than total dietary fat in enhancing risk. A good practical guideline for advising patients on fats in the diet is to use the AHA guidance to moderate fat intake, but to be particularly attentive to limiting intakes of saturated fats and trans-fats.[2]

Fruits and Vegetables

The recommendations for fruit and vegetable intake and other selected foods and their associated micronutrients are summarized in Table 19-1. The US Dietary Guidelines, as well as guidelines from the AHA, ACS, and the American Diabetes Association all recommend 5 to 9 servings of fruits and vegetables per day. Observational studies have shown that diets high in fruits and vegetables are associated with lower risk of heart disease and cancer.[1-4] Our understanding of the relationships between fruit and vegetable intake and cancer risk has not fundamentally changed over the past 20 years, although our understanding of the importance of fruits and vegetables for prevention of heart disease is more recent.[6] Nutritional effects on heart disease were assumed for many years to be affected only by lipids. In the past decade, however, the relationship between heart disease and other factors in the diet, such as fruit and vegetable intake, fiber, and the glycemic index of foods, has come to light.[2] The reasons for lower heart disease risk with more frequent consumption of fruits and vegetables is not yet known but may relate to specific vitamins (eg, folate effects on homocysteine levels) or to the joint effects of several phytochemical compounds in plants. The simple message of eating at least 5 servings of fruits and vegetables each day has been a sustaining message over the past decade.

Alcohol

The USDA, AHA, ACS, and the American Diabetes Association all recommend limiting alcohol intake to 1 drink per day for a woman and 2 drinks per day for a man. One alcoholic drink is equal to 140 g (5 oz) of red or white wine, 336 g (12 oz) of beer, or 42 g (1.5 oz) of distilled spirits. Consumption of 1 to 2 drinks of alcohol per day is sufficient to reduce the risk of heart disease. Although alcohol can increase cancer risk, there is little reason to believe that the low levels of intake sufficient to reduce heart disease risk will affect the risk of alcohol-induced cancers of the head and neck or liver cancer. Increased risk of breast cancer has been shown to occur at doses as low as 1 to 2 drinks per day, however.[3] Because alcohol offers both benefit and harm, guidelines for alcohol intake apart from the message of moderation have not been clear.[2,3] If alcohol is consumed, people should be encouraged to limit consumption to no more than 1 to 2 drinks per day, and for those who have previously had problems controlling their intake of alcohol, or for women at high risk of breast cancer in middle adult years, total abstinence may be the best choice.

Dietary Supplements

Dietary supplements include nutrients, vitamins, and minerals, as well as a wide variety of other compounds, including phytochemicals, hormones, and herbs. As a rule, dietary supplements should never replace whole foods. Nutritionists often express a concern that some people will choose to take multivitamins in preference to healthy foods, but there is little evidence that this trade-off frequently happens. In fact, users of vitamin supplement tend to have a healthier diet than do those who do not take supplements. There is little evidence that anyone eating a healthful diet can benefit from a multivitamin supplement, but some individual experts have recently recommended multivitamin supplements with folate for the general US population,[14] even though expert groups have not.[1-4]

Observational studies generally reveal weaker relationships between chronic diseases and measures of nutrients taken as supplements than they do for measures of nutrients derived from eating fruits and vegetables. Physicians should therefore be sure to educate patients that the benefits of fruits and vegetables in the diet are not reproduced by vitamin pills. Because high-dose nutrients can have adverse effects, physicians should also inform patients that if they choose to take multivitamins, it is best to choose moderate doses at the level of the Recommended Dietary Allowances.

The idea that a nutritional supplement is "natural" and therefore can be only beneficial, even in high doses, is incorrect. The experience of beta carotene's harm in large trials should be a sober reminder of our incomplete understanding of the potential for harm in high-dose nutritional supplements.[15] Vitamin E in large doses may be another example of a high-dose supplement that does more harm than good.[16] Although folic acid supplements have been recommended by some, it is important to remember that if folate deficiency does increase risk of heart disease and/or some cancers, this may be of only historical interest because the United States has been fortifying all grain products with folic acid since 1997. Selenium supplements are also commonly used because of the surprise findings of a randomized, controlled trial for skin cancer prevention, in which selenium was shown to be associated with reduced risk of lung, colorectal, and prostate cancers.[17] Whether these were chance findings or indications of a strong beneficial effect of selenium supplementation is now being assessed in new trials designed specifically for these end points.

DIETARY GUIDELINES FROM THE PATIENT'S PERSPECTIVE

Patients come to a medical encounter with information and advice on nutrition more from the media than from guideline statements. The public is increasingly confused and skeptical about nutrition information because of the seemingly ever-changing advice from experts in the media. Surprising findings about single foods or single nutrients make good headlines but add to the public's confusion. The USDA Food Guide Pyramid has been a constant image in the past decade, but despite the remarkable consistency in the observations that weight control and physical activity reduce risk of heart disease, diabetes, and many cancers, and that fruit and vegetable intake lowers risk of these same diseases, the media has tended to emphasize only the more startling, ironic, or food-specific findings. Add the public's confusion to the difficulty that patients have making lifestyle changes, and the problem becomes more challenging.

PRACTICAL ADVICE ON USE OF DIETARY GUIDELINES IN CLINICAL PRACTICE

Perhaps the most important and clinically useful fact about nutrition guidelines is that the nutritional factors that increase risk of heart disease, many cancers, and diabetes are extremely similar.[18] By controlling body weight, being physically active, limiting intake of saturated fats, and eating ample amounts of fruits and vegetables, people can simultaneously reduce the risk of many different chronic diseases. Physicians have not only the responsibility but also many opportunities to assist their patients in reducing their nutritional risk of chronic diseases. One of the Healthy People 2010 goals is to increase to 75% the inclusion of counseling on diet and nutrition in physician visits with patients who have cardiovascular disease, diabetes, or hyperlipidemia.[19] Here are 4 tips for the busy physician to incorporate nutritional messages into a busy practice:

1. Be brief.
2. Emphasize immediate benefits.
3. Become comfortable with uncertainty.
4. Use the office environment for nutrition education.

Be Brief

Since office visits are typically short, there is not time for long dietary assessments in clinical practice. To avoid long nutritional discussions many physicians simply ignore the topic of nutrition in talking with patients. It is important to realize, however, that patients come to the clinic having already seen, read, and discussed many messages about the very same nutrition topics the physician would address, including weight control, physical activity, saturated fats, and fruits and vegetables. The best role for the physician, even in a brief clinical encounter, is to validate the importance of key messages. This can be done in several time-efficient ways.

Opening conversation with an inquiry in common language about what the patient ate for breakfast or lunch is a good way to indicate your interest in nutrition. A discussion about nutrition and physical activity can also be integrated into the physical examination. The time when someone asks about breast or prostate cancer prevention is an opportune time to not only speak about the prevention of those diseases but also to point out the similarity in nutritional factors for cancers and heart disease. Women are very aware of the impact of breast cancer and men of prostate cancer, so both are often motivated to prevent these cancers via nutrition. However, patients do not always understand that heart disease is several times more common as a cause of death in both men and women than are either prostate or breast cancers. The 2 most important modifiable nutritional factors for breast cancer prevention (weight control and physical activity) are also major nutritional factors for heart disease prevention in women, and the most modifiable nutritional factor for prostate cancer (saturated fat intake) also influences heart disease risk in men.

Emphasize Immediate Benefits

Living to age 90 years instead of age 88 is not a strong motivator for most people in the middle of their lives. The advertising world knows that what sells is what people want now. Often lost in our zeal to prevent chronic diseases is the fact that there are many benefits to good nutrition that are much more immediate than are future reductions in morbidity and extensions of longevity. The increased energy, better sleep, and improved mood that come from regular physical activity, and the weight management and improved bowel function that come from eating healthy are more than just side effects of positive nutritional behaviors. These are immediate benefits that should be emphasized as motivators for behavior change.

Become Comfortable With Uncertainty

The public is increasingly confused and skeptical about nutrition information, in large part because of conflicting news stories about diet and health in the media, in which changing science tends to be overstated, and financial interests to sell particular foods, supplements, or diet books tend to emphasize the unusual. When there is scientific uncertainty, the right choice for one person might be the wrong choice for another. The physician's role in times of scientific uncertainty (as, for example, is currently the state for most nutritional supplements) is to both support the reasoned choices of patients and help patients include other proven factors in their behavioral plan. It is important to be clear in recommendations and to use simple written materials as backup. In many offices, the doctor can also rely on the skills of a registered dietitian, nurse, or medical assistant to strengthen and deepen advice to the patient, particularly when the patient would like specific counsel, such as menu planning or guidance on types of exercise.

Use the Office Environment for Nutrition Education

Advertisers know that attitudes and opinions are based on impressions. The office environment offers an excellent opportunity to provide positive impressions to patients about the links between food choices, weight control, physical activity, and health. In the year 2000, 72% of US adults reported going to an office or clinic sometime over the previous year.[20] The physician can be aided in addressing behavioral risk factors by manual or computerized support systems in the office. A brief medical office-based intervention using a touchscreen computer-assisted assessment of dietary self-management produced improvements in several measures of dietary behavior.[21] Systematic reminders, whether electronic or not, can prompt physicians to perform diet and exercise counseling.[22-24]

Making brochures available in waiting areas and posters in examination rooms is useful for prompting interest by patients in discussing nutrition issues. Even more effective, however, is beautiful artwork or photography depicting physically active people and healthy foods. Artwork and signage prompting patients to discuss nutrition with their providers can be an easy way to increase attention to these issues in the medical encounter.

SUMMARY

Clearly, the commonality in nutritional factors for the most common of the chronic diseases suggests that nutrition advice to patients need not be disease-specific. Obesity increases heart disease risk via its effects on blood pressure, lipids, and other ways. Physical activity reduces heart disease risk via its effects on obesity and by other mechanisms. Fatty acids that raise LDL-C, including saturated fats and trans-fats, increase heart disease risk, and fruits and vegetables and alcohol reduce heart disease risk. Because it is more common than other causes of death, heart disease prevention should be the principal clinical focus of nutritional prevention of chronic diseases. Fortunately, the nutritional factors for heart disease are virtually identical to those for cancers and diabetes, as are the nutrition guidelines. Emphasizing the 3-for-the-price-of-1 nature of the choices in foods and physical activity can be a powerful message in the clinical setting.

REFERENCES

1. US Department of Agriculture and US Department of Health and Human Services (2000). *Dietary Guidelines for Americans.* 5th ed. Washington, DC: US Government Printing Office; 2000. Home and Garden Bulletin No. 232.

2. Krauss RM, Eckel RH, Howard B, et al. American Heart Association scientific statement: American Heart Association Dietary Guidelines, Revision 2000: a statement for health care professionals from the Nutritional Committee of the American Heart Association. *Circulation.* 2000;102:2284–2299. .

3. Byers T, Nestle M, McTiernan A, et al. American Cancer Society Guidelines on nutrition and physical activity for cancer prevention: reducing risk of cancer with healthy food choices and physical activity. *CA Cancer J Clin.* 2002;52:92–119.

4. Franz MJ, Bantle JP, Beebe CA, et al. Evidence-based nutrition principles and recommendations for treatment and prevention of diabetes and related complications. *Diabetes Care.* 2002;25:148–198.

5. World Cancer Research Fund. *Food, Nutrition, and the Prevention of Cancer: A Global Perspective.* Washington, DC: American Institute for Cancer Research; 1997.

6. World Health Organization. *Diet, Nutrition, and the Prevention of Chronic Disease.* Geneva, Switzerland: World Health Organization; March 2003.

7. US Preventive Services Task Force. *Guide to Clinical Preventive Services.* 2nd ed. Baltimore, Md: Williams & Wilkins; 1996.

8. Byers T. What can randomized controlled trials tell us about nutrition and cancer prevention? *CA Cancer J Clin.* 1999;49:353–361.

9. National Institutes of Health, National Heart, Lung, and Blood Institute. Clinical guidelines on the identification, evaluation, and treatment of overweight and obesity in adults—the evidence report. *Obes Res.* 1998;6(suppl 2):51S.

10. Mokdad A, Serdula M, Dietz W, et al. The spread of the obesity epidemic in the United States, 1991–1998. *JAMA.* 1999;282:1519–1522.

11. Mokdad A, Ford E, Bowman B, et al. Diabetes trends in the US: 1990–1998. *Diabetes Care.* 2000;23:1278–1283.

12. *Physical Activity and Health: A Report of the Surgeon General.* Atlanta, Ga: US Department of Health and Human Services, Centers for Disease Control, National Center for Chronic Disease Prevention and Health Promotion; 1996.

13. International Agency for Cancer Research. *Weight Control and Physical Activity.* Lyon, France: IARC Press; 2002. IARC Handbook of Cancer Prevention No. 6.

14. Willett W. Goals for nutrition for the year 2000. *CA Cancer J Clin.* 1999;49:331–352.

15. Albanes D. Beta-carotene and lung cancer: a case study. *Am J Clin Nutr.* 1999;69:1345s–1350s.

16. Heart Outcomes Prevention Evaluation Study Investigators. Vitamin E supplementation and cardiovascular events in high-risk patients. *N Engl J Med.* 2000;342:154–160.

17. Clark LC, Combs GF Jr, Turnbull BW, et al. Effects of selenium supplementation for cancer prevention in patients with carcinoma of the skin: a randomized controlled trial. *JAMA.* 1996;276:1957–1963.

18. Deckelbaum et al. Summary of a scientific conference on preventive nutrition: pediatrics to geriatrics. *Circ.* 1999;100:450–456.

19. US Department of Health and Human Services and Office of Disease Prevention and Health Promotion. *Healthy People 2010: Understanding and Improving Health and Objectives for Improving Health.* Washington, DC: US Department of Health and Human Services; 2000.

20. Agency for Healthcare Research and Quality. *Evidence Report on the Efficacy of Interventions to Modify Dietary Behavior Related to Cancer Risk: Final Evidence Report.* Rockville, Md: Agency for Healthcare Research and Quality; 2001.

21. Glasgow RE, Toobart DJ, Hampson SE. Effects of a brief office-based intervention to facilitate diabetes dietary self-management. *Diabetes Care.* 1996;19:835–842.

22. Ockene IS, Hebert JR, Ockene JK, et al. Effect of training and a structured office practice on physician-delivered nutrition counseling: the Worcester-Area Trial for Counseling in Hyperlipidemia (WATCH). *Am J Prev Med.* 1996;12:252–258.

23. McPhee SJ, Bird JA, Fordham D, et al. Promoting cancer prevention activities by primary care physicians: results of a randomized, controlled trial. *JAMA.* 1991;266:538–544.

24. Ornstein SM, Garr DR, Jenkins RG, et al. Implementation and evaluation of a computer-based preventive services system. *Fam Med* 1995;27:260–266.

Vitamins and Minerals

Mandy C. Leonard, PharmD, BCPS

INTRODUCTION

Nutrients are entities that the body utilizes for growth, maintenance, and repair of tissues. Vitamins and select minerals are classified as nutrients. Vitamins are organic, non-energy-producing nutrients and are necessary for biochemical processes in the body. Since vitamins are not routinely manufactured endogenously or produced in sufficient amounts, they must be obtained from exogenous sources.

Vitamins are classified into 2 categories: fat-soluble (A, D, E, and K) and water-soluble (B complex and C). Fat-soluble vitamins are stored in the tissues in large amounts, whereas water-soluble vitamins must be consumed consistently to maintain adequate saturation of tissues as they are stored in the tissues only to a limited extent. Minerals are inorganic, non-energy-producing substances that are essential for enzymatic activities and specific hormonal regulation. Minerals are also classified into 2 categories: major and trace.

In medicine today, vitamin and mineral supplementation are mainly used therapeutically for treatment of deficiencies or for prevention of diseases or conditions associated with insufficient vitamin and mineral intake. Nutritional deficiencies in the United States are uncommon compared with other countries. When nutritional deficiencies occur in the United States, they are most likely due to (1) inadequate dietary intake (eg, food fads, eating disorders, and alcoholics), (2) increased metabolic requirements (eg, pregnancy and lactation), (3) poor absorption (eg, gastrointestinal disease, prolonged diarrhea, and cystic fibrosis), and/or (4) treatment with select medications (eg, broad-spectrum antibiotics, interactions, and parenteral nutrition).

In 2001, vitamins and minerals accounted for greater than $7.5 billion in annual sales in the United States.[1] Fifty percent of the US population are estimated to take a vitamin, mineral, or dietary supplement daily.[1] Data suggest that vitamins and minerals taken as dietary supplements may not be as beneficial as vitamins and minerals obtained from foods. Vitamins and minerals are not substitutes for food. Most people who consume vitamin and mineral supplements do not require additional supplementation beyond an adequate diet. Select patient populations (eg, elderly, nursing home patients, smokers, and teenagers) may not consume a balanced diet with an appropriate content of vitamins and minerals, and therefore supplementation may be appropriate.

DIETARY REFERENCE INTAKES[2,3]

Dietary reference intakes (DRI) have replaced the recommended dietary allowances (RDA) as the daily nutrient reference values from the Food and Nutrition Board of the Institute of Medicine, National Academy of Sciences. Dietary reference intakes describe categories of reference values that are quantitative approximations of nutrient intakes used for planning and evaluating diets for healthy individuals. The DRI include 4 reference categories: (1) Estimated Average Requirement (EAR), (2) RDA, (3) Adequate Intake (AI), and (4) Tolerable Upper Intake Level (UL).

Estimated Average Requirement

The EAR is defined as the intake value estimated to meet the requirement defined by a specific indicator of adequacy in 50% of an age- and sex-specific group. The EAR consists of levels to prevent deficiencies as well as levels linked to disease reduction. The EARs are used as the foundation for establishing RDA such that, if it is determined that an EAR cannot be established, an RDA is not provided.

Recommended Dietary Allowances

The RDA is defined as the intake value sufficient to meet the nutrient requirements of nearly all healthy individuals of an age-specific and sex-specific group. Unlike the multiple uses of RDA in the past, according to the new DRI structure, RDA are used only as a goal for individuals. The RDA are the recommended levels of essential nutrients required by healthy individuals to reach sufficient nutritional status.

Adequate Intake

The AI is defined as approximations of the mean nutrient intake that appears to sustain a nutritional state in a defined population. Adequate Intakes are used when data are lacking to calculate an EAR and, in turn, an RDA.

Tolerable Upper Intake Level

The UL is defined as the maximum level of daily nutrient intake that is not likely to pose risks of adverse effects to most individuals in a group. Additionally, the UL pertains to long-term daily use. Because of the increased interest in food fads and dietary supplements, ULs are helpful from a safety perspective. Importantly, if a UL is not established for a nutrient, this does not mean that there are no risks or adverse effects of high intake.

FOOD AND DIETARY SUPPLEMENT LABELING

The US Food and Drug Administration (FDA) does not use DRI values on food and dietary supplement labeling. The FDA uses percentage of daily values (%DV), which is based on DRI values, for nutrients in food and dietary supplements. The label should state "Nutrition Facts" or "Supplement Facts" and include serving size, servings per container, and, when established, the %DV, which may be rounded to the next whole number.[4] Vitamins are usually dosed at 50% to 150% of DRI values.[5]

LAWS AND REGULATIONS[6]

Vitamins and minerals are considered dietary supplements by the Dietary Supplement Health and Education Act (DSHEA) of 1994. The DSHEA defines dietary supplements as *vitamins*, *minerals*, herbs, botanicals, or amino acids used to supplement the diet to increase total dietary intake. The FDA is prohibited from regulating dietary ingredients in dietary supplements as food additives. Since October 1994, the FDA and Congress have officially not considered dietary supplements as drugs. The DSHEA allowed dietary supplements to be marketed in the United States without having to pass the stringent requirements imposed by the FDA for new drugs. However, some vitamins and minerals have prescription drug or nonprescription drug status (ie, manufacturers submitted data to the FDA for therapeutic claims as well as safety data).

VITAMINS

Fat-Soluble Vitamins

Vitamin A[7,8]

The vitamin A family consists of different forms of the vitamin known as retinoids (retinol or preformed vitamin A, retinal, and retinoic acid), carotenoids (lycopene and lutein), and provitamin A carotenoids (α-, β-, and γ-carotene). Geometric isomers (*cis-trans* configurations) exist for the various forms, and there are also other "generation" retinoids that have been synthesized from retinoic analogs. In the majority of tissues, all-*trans*-retinoic acid (tretinoin) is the active form of vitamin A. Furthermore, β-carotene is a precursor of retinol, and all *trans*-β-carotene is the most biologically active. For example, other provitamin A carotenoids such as α-carotene and β-cryptoxanthin are only 50% as potent as β-carotene.

Oral vitamin A requires fat to be absorbed, is readily absorbed from the gastrointestinal tract, and is stored predominantly in the liver (90%) and in other areas, including the retina.[3,7,9] In addition, retinol is better absorbed than most carotenoids. Absorbed beta carotene is mainly converted to retinoids by specific enzymes and pathways in the gut and, in general, is a relatively slow process. When released from the liver, retinol is bound to a specific carrier protein called retinol-binding protein (RBP) and to a second hepatic protein known as transthyretin, which is then transported to a target cell and released for activity.[10] Plasma concentrations of retinol can be maintained for months from liver stores; therefore, plasma concentrations are not an accurate measurement of a patient's vitamin A status. Low blood concentrations, on the other hand, imply depleted liver stores.[10,11]

Vitamin A is required for reproduction, cell division and differentiation, bone growth, immune function, gene expression, vision, and the integrity of mucosal and epithelial surfaces.[3,5,7-16] The different forms of vitamin A are responsible for different pharmacologic functions. Vitamin A is used to prevent and treat symptoms of vitamin A deficiency.[3,5,7-17] Vitamin A deficiency is uncommon, and most often due to malnutrition or chronic diseases that interfere with fat absorption. Vegetarians may be at increased risk of vitamin A deficiency since only animal-derived products contain preformed vitamin A. The symptoms of vitamin A deficiency include visual disturbances, respiratory infections, dryness and keratinization of the skin, genitourinary disturbances, and faulty bone formation.

The potential anticarcinogenic effects of vitamin A are not yet clear. There appears to be an inverse relationship of vitamin A intake and cancer morbidity and mortality.[7,11] Green and yellow vegetables, which are sources of vitamin A and beta carotene, can potentially decrease risk of lung cancer,[18] whereas other studies have demonstrated beta carotene and vitamin A supplements to not be protective against lung cancer. Patients taking beta carotene were found to have higher morbidity and mortality.[19,20]

When vitamin A intake is within recommended ranges, adverse reactions are rare.[3,5,7,9,11] However, vitamin A toxicity or hypervitaminosis A can occur when excessive amounts of the vitamin are consumed in the diet or in the form of supplementation. The toxicity occurs because the RBP capacity is exceeded and unbound retinol enters the circulation. The unbound retinol is then transported nonspecifically to cells and exerts a membranolytic action. A retinol plasma concentration greater than 100 µg/dL is usually diagnostic for hypervitaminosis A.

The signs and symptoms associated with acute toxicity are nausea, vomiting, headache, blurred vision, and lack of muscle coordination.[3,5,7,11] With long-term large doses of vitamin A, early symptoms of overdose may include fatigue, irritability, psychiatric changes mimicking severe depression, anorexia, nausea and vomiting, hepatic abnormalities, and reduced bone mineral density (including an increased risk of hip fracture). Symptoms may begin to occur with daily intakes of 50,000 IU in adults and 20,000 IU in children.[11] The UL for adults is based on the occurrence of hepatic abnormalities, specifically abnormal hepatic pathology[7] (Table 20-1). Most of the symptoms resolve within 1 week of withdrawal of the retinoid; however, skin changes can persist, and bone malformations may be permanent.

In general, beta carotene is relatively safe, with minimal side effects. However, when ingested in high doses for several weeks, beta carotene has been associated with the coloring of adipose tissue. This causes the skin, especially the palms of the hands or soles of the feet, to appear yellow and is known as carotenosis or carotenodermia, which is harmless and reversible when the use of beta carotene is discontinued.

Vitamin A should be used with caution during pregnancy since certain doses of retinol (eg, >10,000 IU/d) have been associated with fetal malformations.[7,9,14] Isotretinoin (Accutane), a vitamin A analog used for severe acne, is a known teratogen. Female patients of childbearing age who are receiving isotretinoin should therefore use an effective method of birth control and undergo a pregnancy test before initiation of therapy and periodically thereafter.

Cholestyramine (Questran), colestipol (Colestid), orlistat (Xenical), neomycin (oral), and mineral oil can decrease the absorption of vitamin A.[3,5,9,12] Either administration of a water-miscible formulation of vitamin A or separation of the doses by 2 hours can avert some of these drug interactions. Vitamin A stores in the body can be depleted by excessive alcohol consumption.[9] Vitamin E works as an antioxidant and may enhance the body's utilization of vitamin A.[3,7] Additionally, vitamin A may interfere with the effectiveness of chemotherapy, and large amounts of vitamin A may increase the hypoprothrombinemic effects of warfarin (Coumadin).[3,9]

Based on the Institute of Medicine's Food and Nutrition Board 2001 report, vitamin A activity is based on retinol activity equivalents (RAEs) where 1 RAE equals 1 µg of all-*trans*-retinol, 2 µg of supplemental all-*trans*-β-carotene, 12 µg of dietary all-*trans*-β-carotene, and 24 µg of other provitamin A carotenoids. The RAEs have replaced the previous term of *retinol equivalents* (REs).[3,5,7] The RDAs of vitamin A are listed as RAEs to encompass the different activities of retinol and provitamin A carotenoids.[7] The RDA for vitamin A for men and women is 900 µg/d (3000 IU) and 700 µg/d (2330 IU), respectively.[7] Most adults obtain adequate amounts of vitamin A from the diet, and supplementation with vitamin A products should be used only to treat vitamin A deficiency or for other reasonable preventive measures.[3,9,11] The median vitamin A content in the *diet* is 744 to 811 µg/d for men and 530 to 716 µg/d for women.[7] Additionally, the median intake from vitamin A *supplements* was approximately 1400 µg/d RAE for men and women. Dietary sources of vitamin A include whole eggs, whole milk, liver, fresh-water fish, grains, oils, green and yellow vegetables, carrots, and fruits.[7] Dietary sources of beta carotene include palm oil and yellow, orange, and green leafy vegetables. When needed, vitamin A is usually administered via the oral route as capsules, tablets, or solution containing 10,000 to 50,000 U.[3,12,21,22] If absorption is a problem, vitamin A may be administered in a water-miscible oral preparation or as an intramuscular injection. Vitamin A is also available in numerous combination products, including multivitamin supplements.

Vitamin D

Vitamin D is synthesized in the skin and is, therefore, truly not a nutrient.[23-25] The vitamin D family consists of calciferol, ergocalciferol (vitamin D_2), and cholecalciferol (vitamin D_3).[3,23-26] Cholecalciferol is the naturally occurring form of vitamin D, but ergocalciferol is also biologically active. Cholecalciferol and ergocalciferol can be obtained from the diet in animal- and plant-based foods; they are absorbed in the small intestines,[3,23-26] stored in the liver, and excreted in the bile. Ultraviolet (UV) rays trigger the synthesis of vitamin D in the skin. More specifically, cholecalciferol is formed from 7-dehydrocholesterol (provitamin D_3) in the skin after exposure to UV light. Vitamin D is stored in fat during periods of minimal sun exposure. In the liver, cholecalciferol is hydroxylated to calcifediol (25-hydroxyvitamin D_3 or 25-hydroxycholecalciferol) and then, in the kidneys, calcifediol is hydroxylated to calcitriol

TABLE 20-1
Dietary Reference Intakes for Fat-Soluble Vitamins*

Life Stage Group	Vitamin A,† µg/d		Vitamin D,‡ µg/d		Vitamin E,§ mg/d		Vitamin K, µg/d	
	RDA	UL	AI	UL	RDA	UL	AI	UL
Males								
9–13 y	**600**	1700	5	50	**11**	600	60	ND
14–18 y	**900**	2800	5	50	**15**	800	75	ND
19–30 y	**900**	3000	5	50	**15**	1000	120	ND
31–50 y	**900**	3000	5	50	**15**	1000	120	ND
51–70 y	**900**	3000	10	50	**15**	1000	120	ND
>70 y	**900**	3000	15	50	**15**	1000	120	ND
Females								
9–13 y	**600**	1700	5	50	**11**	600	60	ND
14–18 y	**700**	2800	5	50	**15**	800	75	ND
19–30 y	**700**	3000	5	50	**15**	1000	90	ND
31–50 y	**700**	3000	5	50	**15**	1000	90	ND
51–70 y	**700**	3000	10	50	**15**	1000	90	ND
>70 y	**700**	3000	15	50	**15**	1000	90	ND
Pregnancy								
≤18 y	**750**	2800	5	50	**15**	800	75	ND
19–30 y	**770**	3000	5	50	**15**	1000	90	ND
31–50 y	**770**	3000	5	50	**15**	1000	90	ND
Lactation								
≤18 y	**1200**	2800	5	50	**19**	800	75	ND
19–30 y	**1300**	3000	5	50	**19**	1000	90	ND
31–50 y	**1300**	3000	5	50	**19**	1000	90	ND

*RDA indicates Recommended Dietary Allowances in bold type; UL, Tolerable Upper Intake Level; AI, Adequate Intake; and ND, not determinable. Adapted from Institute of Medicine, Food and Nutrition Board.[7,23,32]

†Given as retinol activity equivalents (RAEs).

‡In the absence of adequate sunlight.

§Given as α-tocopherol.

(1,25-hydroxyvitamin D$_3$ or 1,25-dihydroxycholecalciferol), which is the active form of vitamin D. Because vitamin D requires hydroxylation by both the liver and kidneys, depending on hepatic or renal disease, different forms of vitamin D may need to be administered to patients.

Vitamin D is needed for calcium and phosphorus homeostasis.[3,5,9,23,26,27] Vitamin D in conjunction with the parathyroid hormone (PTH) and calcitonin maintain a constant extracellular calcium concentration to prevent hypocalcemia and hypercalcemia. Vitamin D increases calcium and phosphate absorption from the small intestine, mobilizes calcium from the bone, allows normal bone mineralization, and increases renal tubular reabsorption of calcium.[28] If calcium and phosphate homeostasis is not maintained, demineralization of the bone may occur. When serum calcium levels decrease, PTH levels increase, potentially leading to secondary hyperparathyroidism.

Vitamin D deficiency can be caused by inadequate dietary intake of calcium, limited exposure to sunlight, decreased capacity of the skin to synthesize vitamin D, and renal or liver disease.[3,5,9,23-26] Vitamin D deficiency leads to rickets (inadequate bone mineralization) in children and to osteomalacia (defect in bone mineralization) in adults. A deficiency in vitamin D can also cause osteoporosis, hearing loss, and tooth decay.

The adverse effects of hypervitaminosis D are predominantly due to hypercalcemia.[3,5,9,23-26,29] Vitamin D synthesized from UV rays in the skin is self-regulated. Prolonged exposure of the skin to sunlight does not produce an excess of vitamin D.[30] Excessive doses of supplemental vitamin D can, however, lead to disturbances in body calcium homeostasis. The initial signs of hypercalcemia include weakness, fatigue, gastrointestinal disturbances, irritability, and muscle or bone pain. Consequences that develop later include impaired renal function; decreased libido; and metastatic calcification in the kidneys, blood vessels, heart, and lungs.[3,15,23] The UL for vitamin D is based on risk of hypercalcemia[23] (see Table 20-1).

Cholestyramine, colestipol, orlistat, and mineral oil can decrease the absorption of vitamin D.[3,5,9,12] Separation of doses by 2 hours may avert some of these drug interactions. Carbamazepine (Tegretol), phenytoin (Dilantin), and phenobarbital (Luminal) induce hepatic isoenzymes and may reduce plasma concentrations of select vitamin D analogs; therefore, it has been suggested to administer 400 to 800 IU of vitamin D in these patients.[3,5,9,12,23] Patients receiving long-term or high-dose corticosteroids may require supplemental calcium as well as vitamin D.[9,23]

Based on the Institute of Medicine's Food and Nutrition Board 1997 report, 1 IU of vitamin D equals the biologic activity of 25 mg of cholecalciferol, and 1 µg of vitamin D is equal to 40 IU.[23] Due to the inconsistency in quantifying the amount of vitamin D required to maintain sufficient calcium concentrations and good bone health, as well as the wide variety of factors that affect exposure to sunlight, AIs rather than EARs or RDA are used for vitamin D. The AI of vitamin D for adults depends on age (see Table 20-1). An accurate estimate of vitamin D intake from the diet is difficult because of the high variability in vitamin D content of fortified foods. However, a median vitamin D intake from the *diet* in young women is 114 IU/d and in older women is 90 IU/d.[23] Vitamin D intake from *supplements* was similar for men, women, and children (median intake, 400 IU/d). Factors that suggest need for supplemental vitamin D include age greater than 50 years, limited exposure to sunlight, and fat malabsorption.[5,23,24] The majority of vitamin D intake is from fortified milk (400 IU/qt) and fortified breakfast cereal. However, other good sources of vitamin D are fish liver oils, liver, and eggs.[23]

Vitamin E
The vitamin E family consists of tocopherols (α, β, γ, and δ) and tocotrienols (α, β, γ, and δ).[3,5,9,11,12,31,32] Naturally occurring vitamin E is RRR-α-tocopherol (formerly D-α-tocopherol) and synthetic vitamin E is all-*rac*-α-tocopherol (formerly DL-α-tocopherol). Each form of vitamin E has its own biological activity, with all-*rac*-α-tocopherol having approximately 50% of the relative activity of RRR-α-tocopherol.

Vitamin E is absorbed (20% to 60%) in the gastrointestinal tract, distributed to the circulation by the lymphatic system, and stored in the liver.[3,9,11,31-33] Vitamin E forms are not interconvertible in humans. RRR-α-tocopherol is better absorbed than all-*rac*-α-tocopherol and is the only form of vitamin E maintained in the plasma. The normal range for plasma tocopherols is 6 to 14 µg/mL, but levels may not correlate with total body stores of vitamin E. Levels below 5 µg/mL are indicative of deficiency.[3,11,32] Vitamin E deficiency is not common but can occur in patients with fat absorption disorders.[3,5,9,11,12,31-34] The primary symptom of vitamin E deficiency is peripheral neuropathy. Other symptoms include dry skin and hair, poor wound healing, bruising, anemia, ataxia, muscle weakness, and reproduction failure.

Vitamin E has many important functions in the body but primarily functions as an antioxidant.[3,5,9,11,12,31-34] Vitamin E maintains integrity of the cell membrane by preventing oxidation of polyunsaturated fatty acids. As an antioxidant, vitamin E may prevent (1) select cancers; (2) cardiovascular disease; (3) development of advanced age-related macular degeneration and visual acuity loss; (4) muscle injury; and (5) further decline in Alzheimer disease.[3,5,9,11,12,31-35] The data regarding the use of vitamin E for the above indications remain unclear. For example, observational studies demonstrate that patients who consume select doses of vitamin E have a lower incidence of heart disease and have lower mortality from heart disease. However, prospective, randomized clinical trials have not confirmed these observations.[36-39] Four large, double-blind, randomized intervention trials of vitamin E for the prevention of myocardial infarction produced mixed results. Even though doses of vitamin E varied in the 4 trials, current data appears insufficient to recommend use of vitamin E supplements for prevention of heart disease.[32]

Vitamin E is relatively nontoxic.[3,11,31,32] Symptoms that may be experienced by patients taking excessive doses are headache, gastrointestinal disturbances, diplopia, and muscle weakness. The UL for vitamin E is based on the incidence of hemorrhagic effects[32] (see Table 20-1). Cholestyramine, colestipol, orlistat, and mineral oil can decrease the absorption of vitamin E.[3,5,9,12] Either administration of a water-miscible formulation of vitamin E or separation of the doses by 2 hours can avert some drug interactions. Low levels of selenium may contribute to vitamin E depletion. Higher doses of vitamin E ($\geq$400 U/d) can cause an increase in clotting time; therefore, caution should be used in patients receiving anticoagulants or before surgical procedures.[3,5,9,12,32] Vitamin E antioxidant properties may reduce the effectiveness of chemotherapy.[9]

The EARs and RDA for vitamin E are based on α-tocopherol from food, fortified food, and multivitamins.[32] Only α-tocopherol is considered for DRI values, because other tocopherols and tocotrienols are not well absorbed in the gastrointestinal tract and converted to α-tocopherol in the body. The RDA for vitamin E is 15 mg/d (22 IU) for adults[32] (see Table 20-1). Since most nutrition labels do not differentiate between the different forms of vitamin E, vitamin E activity is often expressed as RRR-α-tocopherol equivalents (α-TEs). One α-TE equals 1 mg of RRR-α-tocopherol (all-*rac*-α-tocopherol 0.74, β-tocopherol 0.5, γ-tocopherol 0.1, α-tocotrienol 0.3). One USP unit of vitamin E equals 670 µg of the RRR-α-tocopherol and 450 µg of all-rac-α-tocopherol.[32] The median vitamin E intake from *food and supplements* is 9 mg/d of α-TEs.[32] Vitamin E is found in nuts, soy beans, green leafy vegetables, wheat germ oil, whole wheat, and whole grain cereals.[32] Current diets appear to provide adequate amounts of vitamin E to avoid deficiency and related symptoms.[3,9,11] However, people with malabsorption may need vitamin E supplementation. The dose of vitamin E depends on the condition being prevented or treated, but usually adult doses range from 200 to 800 U daily. Vitamin E is typically administered via tablets and capsules containing 100 to 1000 U.[3,12,21,22] The water-miscible solution is 50 U/mL. Vitamin E is also contained in multivitamin preparations.

Vitamin K

Vitamin K and related compounds are known as quinones or naphthoquinone derivatives.[3,7,9,11,40] Examples of quinones are: phylloquinone (K_1; phytonadione), menaquinone (K_2), menadione (K_3), menadiol acetate (K_4; menadiol sodium diphosphate), and 4-amino-2-methyl-1-napthol (K_5). Phylloquinone is the most potent form of vitamin K. Menaquinone is produced by intestinal flora, whereas menadione and menadiol acetate are synthetic.

As with the other fat-soluble vitamins, vitamin K requires fat to be absorbed properly.[3,7,9,11,40,41] Vitamin K is fairly well absorbed from the small intestines, is stored in the liver, and is then distributed to a variety of tissues. Compared with other fat-soluble vitamins, vitamin K is stored in minute amounts. The normal plasma range for vitamin K is 80 to 120 µg/mL.[7]

Vitamin K has 2 main essential functions in the body[3,7,9,11,12,40-43]: (1) as a coenzyme for the synthesis and activation of certain clotting factors and (2) for the creation of other proteins in the plasma, kidney, and bone (eg, osteocalcin and matrix G_{la} protein). Vitamin K deficiency most often occurs from inadequate nutrition, malabsorption syndromes, extended parenteral nutrition, or destruction of intestinal flora.[3,7,9,11,12,40-43] Factors contributing to vitamin K deficiency are prolonged hospitalization, chronic liver disease, renal insufficiency, drugs that destroy intestinal flora, and drugs that interfere with vitamin K activity. A deficiency of vitamin K or abnormalities in the hepatic synthesis of clotting proteins result in hypoprothrombinemia and a prolonged prothrombin time (PT).[3,7,9,11,40] Therefore, the diagnostic test for vitamin K deficiency is the PT.

Vitamin K is relatively nontoxic.[7,11] Since there have been no reports of adverse effects from the consumption of high amounts of vitamin K, there is no UL established (see Table 20-1). However, adverse reactions have occurred when administered intravenously. Bile acid sequestrants, mineral oil, and orlistat can interfere with the absorption of vitamin K.[3,5,9,12] These medications and the administration of oral vitamin K should be separated by at least 2 hours. Vitamin K antagonizes the effects of warfarin; therefore, patients receiving warfarin should be consistent in their dietary intake and supplementation of vitamin K or when using any medication that interferes with vitamin K.[43] When select antibiotics are taken, vitamin K-producing intestinal microflora are destroyed.

The AI of vitamin K is 120 µg/d for men and 90 µg/d for women[7] (see Table 20-1). It is estimated that the median *dietary and supplemental* intake of vitamin K in the United States for men and women is 93 to 119 µg/d and 82 to 90 µg/d, respectively.[7] Sources of vitamin K include green leafy vegetables, plant oils and margarine, dairy products, and liver.[7] The dose of vitamin K depends on patient-specific factors as well as the severity of the deficiency.

Water-Soluble Vitamins

Thiamin (vitamin B₁)

Thiamin's main functions include energy metabolism and nerve conduction, as well as normal aerobic metabolism.[3,5,44-47] Thiamin combines with adenosine triphosphate (ATP) and the enzyme thiamin diphosphokinase to form TPP. The active form of thiamin, TPP serves as a coenzyme in carbohydrate metabolism. Thiamin is well absorbed from the gastrointestinal tract, is carried by portal blood to the liver, and is minimally bound to plasma proteins.[3,5,44-47] Orally, thiamin is used for the treatment and prophylaxis of thiamin deficiency syndromes, including beriberi, peripheral neuritis associated with pellagra, and neuritis of pregnancy.[9,45] Thiamin can be used via injection when the oral route is not feasible.

Thiamin deficiency, or beriberi, may be due to numerous factors, including the following: (1) inadequate intake, (2) decreased absorption, (3) defective transport, (4) impaired biosynthesis of TPP, (5) increased requirement, and (6) enhanced loss of thiamin.[12,44,46] Patients vulnerable to this deficiency include those with chronic alcoholism and adults with a high carbohydrate intake mainly from unenriched white rice (eg, Asian countries). Deficiency occurs in alcoholics because alcohol impairs thiamin absorption and storage, and alcoholics may already have a nutritionally poor diet. Other patients vulnerable to thiamin deficiency include patients receiving long-term dialysis, patients receiving parenteral nutrition, and patients with hypermetabolic states. Thiamin deficiency can cause cardiac failure, muscle weakness, peripheral and central neuropathy, and gastrointestinal malfunction.[44-46] Furthermore, notable laboratory findings include increased pyruvate and lactate.

Beriberi is divided into 2 categories: infantile and adult. Infantile beriberi, although rare in developed countries, usually affects infants between the ages of 2 and 3 months and is divided into 3 categories: cardiac beriberi, aphonic beriberi, and pseudomeningitic beriberi. Adult beriberi can affect both children and adults, and is also divided into 3 categories: dry beriberi, wet beriberi, and Wernicke-Korsakoff syndrome. Dry beriberi is characterized by peripheral neuropathy of the distal segments of limbs and results in muscle tenderness. Wet beriberi consists of peripheral neuropathy but is also characterized by edema, tachycardia, cardiomegaly, congestive heart failure, and abnormal electrocardiograms. Wernicke-Korsakoff syndrome, with symptoms ranging from ophthalmoplegia, nystagmus, and ataxia to severely impaired memory, cognitive function, and coma, is most often seen in alcoholic persons but can also be associated with long-term dialysis and parenteral glucose administration.

Orally, thiamin may cause dermatitis and other hypersensitivity reactions, whereas intravenous preparations may cause tingling, pruritus, nausea, and hypotension.[44] There is no evidence of thiamin toxicity by oral administration (Table 20-2). Large intravenous doses (>400 mg) may cause nausea, lethargy, anorexia, and mild ataxia. Thiamin requirements are variable and depend on select influences such as levels of strenuous activity, pregnancy, lactation, febrile conditions, hyperthyroidism, and those experiencing adolescent growth.[44-46] The DRI values for thiamin are based on the age and sex of the individual (see Table 20-2). A healthy diet should be ensured before adding oral supplementation to a patient's daily regimen. Dietary sources of thiamin include enriched and fortified cereal grains, brewer's yeast, organ meats, lean cuts of pork, legumes, and seeds and nuts.[44] Thiamin is available over-the-counter orally as a tablet (50, 100, and 250 mg) and by prescription as an injection (100 and 200 mg/mL).[3,12,21,22] Thiamin is found also in combination multivitamin products.

Riboflavin (vitamin B₂)

Riboflavin is converted to the coenzyme, riboflavin 5-phosphate (flavin mononucleotide [FMN]), which is then converted to another coenzyme, flavin adenine dinucleotide (FAD).[3] Both FMN and FAD are the active forms of riboflavin and bind to flavoprotein enzymes, which catalyze oxidation-reduction reactions in cells.[12,48] Riboflavin facilitates metabolism, plays a critical role in energy production, and is necessary for growth and reproduction.[12,45] Riboflavin is readily absorbed in the upper gastrointestinal tract.[3,44,45,49] The extent of riboflavin absorption is increased when the nutrient is administered with food and is decreased in patients with hepatitis, cirrhosis, or biliary obstruction. Although FAD and FMN are distributed into body tissues, concentrations are low and little is stored, thereby creating the need for daily intake.

Most individuals receive adequate riboflavin from dietary sources, but riboflavin deficiency may occur in alcoholic or elderly persons, infants, patients receiving probenecid, and individuals with nutritionally deficient diets. Riboflavin deficiencies primarily affect the skin, eyes, and mucous membranes of the gastrointestinal tract. Some symptoms of riboflavin deficiency include sore throat; angular stomatitis; glossitis; cheilosis; seborrheic dermatitis of the face; red, tearing, and itchy eyes; anemia; and neuropathy.[3,12,44,45,49] Riboflavin has also been used in the treatment of microcytic anemia and management of acne, migraine headaches, and muscle cramps.

Oral contraceptives increase the need for riboflavin, whereas tricyclic antidepressants inhibit the absorption of riboflavin.[12,48,49] Probenecid inhibits gastrointestinal absorption and renal tubular secretion of riboflavin. Select antibiotics can destroy normal gastrointestinal flora, which decreases the production of riboflavin.

TABLE 20-2

Dietary Reference Intakes for Water-Soluble Vitamins*

Life Stage Group	Thiamin, mg/d		Riboflavin, mg/d		Niacin,† mg/d		Pantothenic Acid, mg/d		Pyridoxine, mg/d	
	RDA	UL	RDA	UL	RDA	UL	AI	UL	RDA	UL
Males										
9–13 y	0.9	ND	0.9	ND	12	20	4	ND	1.0	60
14–18 y	1.2	ND	1.3	ND	16	30	5	ND	1.3	80
19–30 y	1.2	ND	1.3	ND	16	35	5	ND	1.3	100
31–50 y	1.2	ND	1.3	ND	16	35	5	ND	1.3	100
51–70 y	1.2	ND	1.3	ND	16	35	5	ND	1.7	100
>70 y	1.2	ND	1.3	ND	16	35	5	ND	1.7	100
Females										
9–13 y	0.9	ND	0.9	ND	12	20	4	ND	1.0	60
14–18 y	1.0	ND	1.0	ND	14	30	5	ND	1.2	80
19–30 y	1.1	ND	1.1	ND	14	35	5	ND	1.3	100
31–50 y	1.1	ND	1.1	ND	14	35	5	ND	1.3	100
51–70 y	1.1	ND	1.1	ND	14	35	5	ND	1.5	100
>70 y	1.1	ND	1.1	ND	14	35	5	ND	1.5	100
Pregnancy										
≤18 y	1.4	ND	1.4	ND	18	30	6	ND	1.9	80
19–30 y	1.4	ND	1.4	ND	18	35	6	ND	1.9	100
31–50 y	1.4	ND	1.4	ND	18	35	6	ND	1.9	100
Lactation										
≤18 y	1.4	ND	1.6	ND	17	30	7	ND	2.0	80
19–30 y	1.4	ND	1.6	ND	17	35	7	ND	2.0	100
31–50 y	1.4	ND	1.6	ND	17	35	7	ND	2.0	100

Continued

T A B L E 20-2

Dietary Reference Intakes for Water-Soluble Vitamins*—*Concluded*

Life Stage Group	Folate,‡ µg/d		Cyanocobalamin, µg/d		Biotin, µg/d		Vitamin C, µg/d	
	RDA	UL	RDA	UL	AI	UL	RDA	UL
Males								
9–13 y	300	600	1.8	ND	20	ND	45	1200
14–18 y	400	800	2.4	ND	25	ND	75	1800
19–30 y	400	1000	2.4	ND	30	ND	90	2000
31–50 y	400	1000	2.4	ND	30	ND	90	2000
51–70 y	400	1000	2.4	ND	30	ND	90	2000
>70 y	400	1000	2.4	ND	30	ND	90	2000
Females								
9–13 y	300	600	1.8	ND	20	ND	45	1200
14–18 y	400	800	2.4	ND	25	ND	65	1800
19–30 y	400	1000	2.4	ND	30	ND	75	2000
31–50 y	400	1000	2.4	ND	30	ND	75	2000
51–70 y	400	1000	2.4	ND	30	ND	75	2000
>70 y	400	1000	2.4	ND	30	ND	75	2000
Pregnancy								
≤18 y	600	800	2.6	ND	30	ND	80	1800
19–30 y	600	1000	2.6	ND	30	ND	85	2000
31–50 y	600	1000	2.6	ND	30	ND	85	2000
Lactation								
≤18 y	500	800	2.8	ND	35	ND	115	1800
19–30 y	500	1000	2.8	ND	35	ND	120	2000
31–50 y	500	1000	2.8	ND	35	ND	120	2000

*RDA indicates Recommended Dietary Allowances; UL, Tolerable Upper Intake Level; AI, Adequate Intake; and ND, not determinable. Adapted from Institute of Medicine, Food and Nutrition Board.[32,44]

†Given as niacin equivalents (NEs).

‡Given as dietary folate equivalents (DFEs).

The DRI values for riboflavin vary based on individual's age and sex[44] (see Table 20-2). Riboflavin can be found in milk, eggs, cheese, organ meats, green leafy vegetables, and whole grain and enriched cereals and breads.[45] Riboflavin is available over-the-counter as 50- and 100-mg tablets[3,12,21,22] and is present in multivitamin preparations.

Niacin (vitamin B₃)

The family of vitamin B_3 includes niacin (nicotinic acid or pyridine-3-carboxylic acid) and niacinamide (nicotinamide). Additionally, the amino acid, tryptophan, is converted to niacin in the body. This conversion depends on patient-specific factors and can vary greatly. Niacin, niacinamide, and tryptophan are precursors of the coenzymes nicotinamide adenine dinucleotide (NAD) and nicotinamide adenine dinucleotide phosphate (NADP), which act as hydrogen carrier molecules. [15,44,45,50,51]

Niacin and niacinamide are well absorbed from the gastrointestinal tract and are distributed into the tissues of the body.[3,9,44,45,50] They are hepatically metabolized to metabolites (eg, nicotinuric acid, *N*-methylnicotinamide, and *N*-methylniacinamide) and are excreted in the urine. A deficiency of niacin can be detected by measuring niacin metabolites in the urine. Even though niacin and niacinamide are related and identical in their role as vitamins, they are handled differently by cells and produce different pharmacologic responses. For example, niacin affects lipids, but niacinamide does not.

Niacin is required for lipid metabolism, tissue respiration, and glycogenolysis.[3,5,9,44,45] Niacin causes peripheral prostaglandin-mediated vasodilation and an increase in histamine-mediated gastric motility. It affects the fibrinolytic system, glucose tolerance, synthesis of very-low-density lipoprotein cholesterol (VLDL-C) and low-density lipoprotein cholesterol (LDL-C) in the liver, and lipolysis in adipose tissue.

Niacin deficiency or pellagra may be seen in alcoholic individuals and in patients with conditions that disrupt tryptophan pathways.[3,5,9,44,45,50] Pellagra causes redness and swelling of the tongue, mental symptoms, cutaneous infections, gastrointestinal disturbances, and dermal lesions. The polyneuritis and cheilosis of pellagra are associated with thiamin and riboflavin deficiency, and these nutrients should be supplemented accordingly.

Niacin is used alone or in combination with other medications for the management of primary hypercholesterolemia, mixed dyslipidemia, and hypertriglyceridemia.[3,9,44,45,50] At adequate doses, niacin lowers LDL-C and triglycerides and increases high-density lipoprotein cholesterol (HDL-C). Niacinamide appears to have no beneficial effect on lipids.

Niacin, given in small doses, is rarely toxic.[3,9,44,45,50] The UL for niacin is based on the flushing effect of niacin[44] (see Table 20-2), which is due to vasodilation of cutaneous blood vessels in the face, neck, and chest.

Vasodilation can occur within 20 to 60 minutes of administration depending on the formulation (ie, immediate-release compared with extended-release). Premedication with aspirin may alleviate the flushing. Other side effects of niacin are burning sensation, vomiting, dizziness, headache, hyperglycemia, and hypotension. Niacin can increase uric acid levels and exacerbate gout. Abnormal results of liver function tests may occur with high-dose and long-term niacin therapy. Niacin therapy should be discontinued if liver function transaminase levels exceed 3 times the upper limit of normal. Severe hepatotoxicity, hepatitis, and the need for liver transplant have been reported. Niacin is contraindicated in patients with hepatic disease, active peptic ulcer disease, or severe hypotension. A new preparation of sustained-release niacin (Niaspan) has been developed and appears to be associated with less hepatotoxicity than other formulations of modified-release niacin.

Cholestyramine and colestipol can decrease the absorption of niacin.[9] Niacin may cause insulin resistance, and doses of hypoglycemic medications may need to be adjusted or the niacin avoided in diabetic patients.[3,9,45] Long-term therapy with isoniazid may interfere with the conversion of dietary tryptophan to niacin, resulting in the need for niacin supplementation.[3] The combination therapy of niacin and a 3-hydroxy-3-methylglutaryl coenzyme A (HMG-CoA) reductase inhibitor may increase the risk of myopathy.[9] Transdermal nicotine patches may increase likelihood of flushing and headache in patients taking niacin. Niacin may enhance the hypotensive effect of ganglionic-blocking drugs.

Because tryptophan is converted to niacin and contributes to niacin intake, DRIs are in niacin equivalents (NE).[3,44] One NE is equal to 1 mg of niacin, which is equal to 60 mg of tryptophan. The RDA for niacin is based on the urinary excretion of niacin metabolites. The RDA for men and women is 16 mg NEs/d and 14 mg NEs/d, respectively[44] (see Table 20-2). Niacin and nicotinamide are administered orally.[3,9] As a dietary supplement, niacin, 10 to 20 mg daily, is used. For prevention and treatment of pellagra, the adult dosage of niacin is 300 to 500 mg/d. For hyperlipidemia, various doses and forms of niacin have been used. Niacin therapy is usually initiated at 125 mg twice daily and slowly titrated to 1.5 to 3 g/d. There are 2 forms of niacin: crystalline (regular- or immediate-release) and modified (sustained-, extended-, or time-release). Immediate-release formulations are available in 50 to 500 mg, and sustained-release niacin (Niaspan) is available in 500-, 750-, and 1000-mg tablets.[3,12,21,22] Niacinamide is available as 100-, 250-, and 500-mg tablets. Dietary sources of niacin include meats (especially red meat), beans, and fortified foods, whereas milk and eggs contain tryptophan.[44,50] Niacin is frequently used with other B vitamins in vitamin B complex formulations.[3,12,21,22]

Pantothenic acid (vitamin B₅)

Pantothenic acid is present in all cells and is a precursor of CoA.[3,12,22] Coenzyme A is a cofactor in enzyme-catalyzed reactions involved in acetylcholine synthesis, such as the metabolism of fats, carbohydrates, and proteins.[52,53] Pantothenic acid is used for the rare occurrence of vitamin B₅ deficiency.[9,22,45] It usually is added to B complex vitamin products since patients at risk of vitamin B₅ deficiency are most likely at risk of other nutrient deficiencies. Dexpanthenol (Panthoderm) is also available as a topical formulation and can be used for relief of pruritus and mild eczema.[21] There are no known adverse reactions to pantothenic acid in normal doses.[9,12,44] In large doses (10 to 20 g/d), diarrhea may occur. Symptoms of deficiency include somnolence, fatigue, headache, tingling of the hands and feet ("burning feet" syndrome), muscle weakness of the legs, and increased susceptibility to infections.[3,9,44] Blood levels less than 100 µg/dL are indicative of pantothenic acid deficiency.

For adults, the AI for pantothenic acid is 5 mg/d[13,44,45] (see Table 20-2). Topical dexpanthenol can be used once or twice daily. Pantothenic acid is widespread in many foods and is most abundant in eggs, liver, fish, poultry, whole grain breads and cereals, and legumes.[12] Pantothenic acid is available as an oral formulation (calcium pantothenate) and can be found over-the-counter in 100-, 218-, and 545-mg strengths.[3,12,21,22] Dexpanthenol is also available as an over-the-counter topical cream (2% Panthoderm).

Pyridoxine (vitamin B₆)

Vitamin B₆ is made up of a group of biologically related compounds, the pyridines:[14,15,44,45,54,55] pyridoxine, pyridoxal, and pyridoxamine. These compounds usually are referred to as a single entity: pyridoxine. Pyridoxal phosphate (PLP) and pyridoxamine phosphate (PMP) are the active coenzyme forms of pyridoxine. Pyridoxal phosphate is multifaceted and acts as a coenzyme in numerous functions, including the metabolism of protein, carbohydrates, and fat. Pyridoxine is involved in the conversion of tryptophan to niacin or serotonin and may also modify the actions of steroid hormones. Other functions of pyridoxine include gluconeogenesis, erythrocyte metabolism and function, and immune function.

Although pyridoxine deficiency is rare, patients with other vitamin B deficiencies are presumed to also lack pyridoxine.[14,15,45,54] Pyridoxine deficiency may also occur in alcoholism, malabsorption, and drug interactions. Signs and symptoms of deficiency include seborrheic dermatosis, glossitis, cheilosis, irritability, depression, confusion, and peripheral neuropathy. Pyridoxine is used as prophylaxis in patients receiving isoniazid to prevent the development of peripheral neuritis and also to manage symptoms associated with isoniazid overdose. Drug-induced deficiencies have been noted with other vitamin B₆ antagonists, such as hydralazine, penicillamine, and

cycloserine. Therefore, when these drugs are used for an extended period, pyridoxine should be taken in combination. Although there are no supporting clinical trials, pyridoxine supplementation has been reported to be beneficial in alleviating premenstrual syndrome (PMS) symptoms.[9,14]

In high doses, pyridoxine may be toxic and has a UL of 100 mg/d in adults[12,14,44,55] (see Table 20-2). Symptoms of pyridoxine toxicity include tingling sensation of the hands and feet, decreased coordination, and stumbling gait.

The RDA for pyridoxine is 1 to 1.7 mg/d in males and 1 to 1.5 mg/d for females[44] (see Table 20-2). The best sources of pyridoxine include brewer's yeast, wheat germ, liver, peanuts, legumes, potatoes, and bananas.[44] Supplemental doses of pyridoxine are available over-the-counter as tablets (25-, 50-, 100-, 250-, 500-mg and 20-mg enteric coated tablets) and by prescription as an injectable (100 mg/mL).[3,12,21,22]

Folate (vitamin B₉)

Folate, also known as folic acid and pteroylglutamic acid, is necessary for the production and maintenance of new cells, especially during times of rapid cell division (eg, pregnancy).[12,14,56-58] It is required in the synthesis of DNA, RNA, and normal red blood cells. In the body, folic acid is converted to the active form, tetrahydrofolic acid, of which niacin and vitamin C are necessary components. Dietary sources of folate are polyglutamates, which must be converted to the monoglutamate form for absorption. Dietary folate is readily absorbed through the proximal part of the small intestine and stored in the liver. The primary circulating form, N-5-methyltetrahydrofolate, is extensively bound to plasma proteins, with any excess being eliminated by the kidneys. Supplements generally provide more absorbable folic acid than what is found in food. Greater than 2% of folic acid is degraded daily; therefore, a continuous supply is required. If this supply is not achieved, deficiency leading to anemia may occur within 6 months.

Folic acid is used for the prevention and treatment of folic acid deficiency as well as in the treatment of megaloblastic anemia and the prevention of neural tube defects.[5,14,15,44,56] Initial signs of deficiency include diarrhea, loss of appetite, weight loss, weakness, glossitis, headache, heart palpitations, and irritability. Adults with advanced folate deficiency often acquire anemia, while infants and children can experience slow growth rates. Folic acid deficiency is most often due to inadequate intake or absorption, and to increased requirement and excretion. Deficiency causes decreased serum folate levels, decreased erythrocyte folate concentrations, increased homocysteine levels, and megaloblastic changes in the bone marrow ultimately leading to megaloblastic anemia. The onset of anemia is gradual and may not be evident until anemia is moderate or severe.

More recently, folic acid has been used to decrease homocysteine levels, for the purpose of possibly reducing risk of coronary artery disease.[5,44,59-63] Studies have shown moderate hyperhomocysteinemia may be an independent risk factor for coronary, cerebral, and peripheral atherosclerotic disease.

Pregnancy, a time of increased metabolic rate and cell turnover, often requires an increase in folic acid intake, especially during the third trimester, to prevent birth defects.[5,14,64] A deficiency occurs in up to one third of all pregnancies worldwide, and 4% of pregnancies in the United States have a folate deficiency. Folate deficiency increases eightfold with multiple gestations, teenage pregnancies, and closely spaced pregnancies.

Caution should be used when giving folic acid to patients with undiagnosed anemia since folic acid can mask the diagnosis of pernicious anemia (vitamin B_{12} deficiency).[5,15,44,62] If folic acid is given without concurrent administration of vitamin B_{12} to a patient with pernicious anemia, the hematologic aspect of anemia will improve, but the folic acid will not be able to prevent the progression of neurologic damage.

There have been documented drug interactions with folic acid; however, short-course therapy with the causative agent does not appear to require folic acid supplementation, whereas long-term or high doses generally may require supplementation.[3,5,14,58] Oral contraceptives, sulfasalazine (Azulfidine), trimethoprim (Proloprim), and methotrexate can all interact with folic acid. There are 2 ways phenytoin and folic acid can interact. First, phenytoin may inhibit folic acid absorption, leading to megaloblastic anemia. Second, folic acid may increase phenytoin metabolism, resulting in decreased phenytoin serum concentrations. Additionally, folinic acid (Leucovorin) is a reduced form of folic acid that bypasses the antifolate activity of methotrexate and is usually administered to "rescue" the antifolate effects of methotrexate.

Folic acid is nontoxic, even at large doses, due to its water solubility and rapid excretion; however, a UL has been established at 1000 µg/d for most patients.[3,5,12,44] The RDA of folic acid for adults is 400 µg with adjustments required for pregnant and lactating women (see Table 20-2). The fortification of cereal grains became mandatory in the United States as of January 1, 1998.[44,65] The highest amount of folate can be found in organ meats, green vegetables, eggs, and some fresh fruits.[44] Folic acid can be found over-the-counter as 0.4- and 0.8-mg tablets.[3,12,21,22] In addition, folic acid is also available by prescription as 1-mg tablets and as a 5-mg/mL injection. Folic acid is found in numerous multivitamin and prenatal vitamin products.

Cyanocobalamin (vitamin B₁₂)

Vitamin B_{12} occurs in many forms and is categorized as a cobalamin.[5,12,14,44,45,66,67] Cyanocobalamin is used in vitamin B_{12} preparations since it remains active upon storage. Cyanocobalamin is active in all cells; is essential for normal blood formation and neurologic function; and is involved in fat, protein, and carbohydrate metabolism as well as in the synthesis of DNA.

Cyanocobalamin is consumed and released from food; bound to gastric intrinsic factor; and carried to the ileum, where it interacts with a receptor on the mucosal cell surface to cause absorption leading to transport into the circulation. Adequate intrinsic factor, bile, and sodium bicarbonate are all required for transport. Cyanocobalamin deficiency is rarely due to a deficient diet but more often due to a defect in the absorption process. The liver stores approximately 50% of cyanocobalamin after absorption, and the remainder is dispersed to other tissues. Any excess cyanocobalamin is excreted in the urine.

Vitamin B_{12} is used for prevention and treatment of deficiency.[5,12,44,45,66] Patients with cyanocobalamin deficiency initially present with anemia (pernicious anemia) or neurologic changes. Symptoms include fatigue, loss of appetite, peripheral neuropathy, poor blood clotting, and easy bruising. Cyanocobalamin deficiency may occur in malabsorption, in decreased secretion of intrinsic factor, after gastric bypass, or with a vegan diet. In healthy individuals, cyanocobalamin stores are maintained, and deficiency can take up to 3 years to manifest.

In initial stages of pernicious anemia, therapy focuses on correcting the deficiency and reversing the sequelae.[58] Pernicious anemia is caused by a cobalamin malabsorption; therefore, subcutaneous or intramuscular vitamin B_{12} supplementation is administered. Subcutaneous supplementation is also used in gastric bypass patients. Since up to 80% of the vitamin is excreted in the urine, initial doses should be large, ranging from 100 to 1000 µg. Doses can then be tapered to maintenance of dosing once monthly for life. There are limited adverse drug reactions and drug interactions with cyanocobalamin.

The RDA of cyanocobalamin for men and women is 2.4 µg/d, with adjustments due to growth, pregnancy, and lactation[12,44] (see Table 20-2). Organ meats, liver, eggs, milk, chicken, cheese, and fortified cereals are sources.[44] Cyanocobalamin is not available in fruits, vegetables, or grains. The oral form of cyanocobalamin is available over-the-counter as tablets (100-, 500-, 1000-, and 5000-µg) and lozenges (100-, 250-, and 500-µg).[3,12,21,22] Parenteral formulations of cyanocobalamin are available by prescription (100- and 1000-µg/mL) and should be administered intramuscularly or by deep subcutaneous injection. An intranasal gel (Nascobal) is available by prescription and provides 500 µg/0.1 mL.

Biotin

Biotin is an essential vitamin and must be obtained from exogenous sources. Biotin is an essential cofactor of 4 carboxylases, each with a critical role in the metabolism of fats and carbohydrates.[44,45,68,69] Two biotin enzymes, pyruvate carboxylase and acetyl CoA carboxylase, are essential for gluconeogenesis, while the other 2 biotin enzymes, propionyl-CoA carboxylase and 3-methyl-crotonyl CoA carboxylase, are required for propionate metabolism and the catabolism of branched chain amino acids. When ingested, biotin is quickly absorbed from the gastrointestinal tract and eliminated in the urine.

Biotin is specifically used for prevention and treatment of biotin deficiency.[12,45,68,69] Symptoms of deficiency include hair loss, exfoliative dermatitis, anorexia, nausea, numbness of the extremities, and muscle pain. Biotin deficiency is rare, since the nutrient is readily available in the diet as well as synthesized by intestinal bacteria. Select diabetic persons may have an abnormality of pyruvate carboxylase, and individuals consuming numerous raw eggs are at risk of biotin deficiency. Avidin, a component of raw egg whites, may prevent biotin absorption. Biotin deficiency may contribute to seborrheic dermatitis and brittle nails. Biotin has been used to promote healthy hair and fingernails. Even with long-term, high-dose therapy, biotin toxicity has not been reported.[12,45]

The AI for biotin in adults is 30 µg/d[44] (see Table 20-2). Biotin is readily available in most foods, including organ meats, egg yolk, fish, nuts, bananas, grapefruit, and strawberries.[12,44,45] Biotin is available over-the-counter, alone and in combination, as well as by prescription.[3,21,22]

Vitamin C

Vitamin C is a water-soluble vitamin and refers to both ascorbic acid and its oxidized form, dehydroascorbic acid (DHAA).[3,9,32,45,70,71] Ascorbic acid is the functional and most abundant form of the vitamin in the body. Ascorbic acid is readily absorbed after oral administration; however, the absorption is saturable and dose-dependent. When doses exceed 1000 mg, absorption is decreased by approximately 50%. Ascorbic acid is widely distributed in body tissues, minimally protein bound, metabolized to inactive metabolites, and excreted in the urine. When the body is saturated with ascorbic acid, it is excreted unchanged in the urine. A urine excretion test may be used to determine vitamin C deficiency. Vitamin C, an antioxidant, provides reducing equivalents for biochemical oxidation-reduction reactions and is a cofactor for reactions requiring reduced iron or copper metalloenzyme.[3,15,32,70] Vitamin C is needed for collagen synthesis and maintains the integrity of connective tissue, osteoid tissue, and dentin. Vitamin C is also an electron donor of at least 8 human enzymes.

Vitamin C is used in the prevention and treatment of vitamin C deficiency.[3,9,32,45,70,71] If vitamin C deficiency is not treated, scurvy may result. Symptoms of scurvy include myalgia, weakness, irritability, anemia, hemorrhage, hyperkeratotic follicles (corkscrew hairs), gingivitis, and loosening of teeth. Vitamin C deficiency is primarily due to an improper diet. Deficiencies may also occur in individuals with gastrointestinal diseases, acute and chronic inflammatory diseases, or patients undergoing surgery. Additionally, patients who are pregnant or lactating, have diarrhea, or experience cold or heat stressors may require increased supplementation. Prolonged use of high-dose vitamin C may increase the metabolism of the vitamin, causing deficiency when the intake is reduced to normal. Large doses during pregnancy may result in scurvy in neonates.

Vitamin C has been used for several clinical reasons:[3,9,32] as an antioxidant in combination with beta carotene, vitamin E, and zinc in high-risk patients to prevent progression of age-related macular degeneration; to decrease risk of developing select cancers; and for prevention and treatment of the common cold. Some data support the use of high doses for decreasing common cold symptoms by 1 to 1.5 days; however, these high doses may also cause adverse effects. Clear evidence to support use of vitamin C in these clinical situations remains controversial.

In general, vitamin C is nontoxic.[3,5,9,32,45,70] The reason for the relatively low toxicity is saturation of absorption and renal excretion of the unchanged vitamin. The most common adverse effect when vitamin C is taken in large quantities or megadoses is gastrointestinal disturbances such as nausea, diarrhea, and abdominal cramps. These effects occur because intestinal absorption of vitamin C is saturable and the unabsorbed vitamin C has osmotic effects. Since oxalic acid is a metabolite of ascorbic acid catabolism, hyperoxaluria and kidney stones may also occur, especially in patients with preexisting renal disease. Hemolysis has also been reported in patients with glucose-6-phosphate-deficiency taking high-dose vitamin C supplementation. The UL for vitamin C for adults is 2000 mg/d[32] (see Table 20-2).

The concurrent use of vitamin C and cholestyramine should be separated, since both ascorbic acid absorption and bile acid-binding capacity may be affected.[5] In addition, salicylates inhibit the uptake of ascorbic acid by leukocytes and platelets; however, data are lacking to support that this leads to vitamin C deficiency.[3] Large amounts of vitamin C may reduce the anticoagulant action of warfarin.[5,9] The concomitant use of vitamin C and iron, particularly ferric iron, increases the amount of iron absorbed from the gastrointestinal tract.[3,5,9] The potential acidification of the urine by ascorbic acid may affect the urine excretion of other medications.[5,15] Individuals who smoke tobacco require more vitamin C (100 to 125 mg/d) than nonsmokers due to increased turnover of the vitamin and increase in oxidative stress.[3,5,32,70] Nonsmokers exposed to secondhand smoke may require additional vitamin C, although no specific value has been recommended.

Vitamin C doses greater than or equal to 250 mg/d have been associated with false-negative results for detecting stool occult blood.[5,9] The RDA for vitamin C for men and women is 90 mg/d and 75 mg/d, respectively[32] (see Table 20-2). Dietary sources of vitamin C include citrus fruits, tomatoes, cauliflower, broccoli, spinach, and potatoes.[32] For therapy, dietary deficiencies should be corrected and then, if needed, supplemental vitamin C administered.[3,9,15,45] The dose of vitamin C depends on the condition being prevented or treated. For treatment of scurvy, 100 to 250 mg of vitamin C is administered orally or parenterally once to twice daily, which usually restores functions of vitamin C in a few days and reverses the signs and symptoms in 1 to 2 weeks. Ascorbic acid is usually administered orally; however, parenteral solutions may be administered in conditions that impair adequate absorption from the gastrointestinal tract. Vitamin C is commercially available in tablet (immediate- and extended-release), capsule (immediate- and extended-release), lozenge, solution, and prescription injection (500 mg/mL).[3,12,21,22] Vitamin C is contained in most multivitamin preparations.

MINERALS

Minerals are inorganic, non–energy-producing substances and are essential for enzymatic activities and specific hormonal regulation. Minerals are a component of a variety of organic and inorganic compounds in the body. In addition, the concentration of each mineral is dependent on specific body tissues. A balanced diet is needed to obtain minerals and to maintain a proper mineral balance. Minerals have been associated with adverse reactions and toxicity as well as interactions, specifically nutrient-nutrient interactions.

Minerals are classified into 2 categories: major (required by the body in larger amounts) and trace (required by the body in minute amounts). Examples of major minerals are phosphorus, the second most plentiful mineral in the body; calcium; and magnesium. Trace minerals include iodine and iron. Tables 20-3 and 20-4 provide information pertaining to minerals.[3,7,13-15,23,32,72]

SUMMARY

In humans, nutrients such as vitamins and minerals are required for biochemical and enzymatic activities, as well as specific hormonal regulation. Humans do not have the ability to produce or do not produce sufficient quantities of these nutrients, and therefore, they must be obtained exogenously via the diet or supplementation. They are best obtained through a balanced diet. Furthermore, the majority of people consuming supplemental vitamins and minerals generally acquire adequate quantities from a proper diet. However, due to a poor diet, food fads, pregnancy and lactation, select disease states, or concurrent drug therapy, vitamin and/or mineral supplementation may be needed to prevent or treat deficiencies. Similar to prescription drugs, vitamins and minerals have the potential for adverse reactions and interactions. Health care professionals need to be knowledgeable about DRIs for these nutrients, including the ULs. In addition, patients need to be educated to read all labels carefully prior to administration. The total daily intake of vitamins and minerals from all supplements should be determined. Finally, this chapter was a brief overview of vitamins and minerals, therefore, the reader is directed to the Institute of Medicine, Food and Nurition Board, DRI Reports for an in-depth review of these nutrients.

TABLE 20-3

Major Minerals[3,13-15,24,73,74]

Mineral	Function	Deficiency State	Sources	Life Stage Group	RDA/AI	UL	Special Considerations	Toxicity
Calcium, mg/d	Important for normal cardiac function, muscle and nerve function, blood coagulation, and maintenance of teeth and bones	Arm and leg muscle spasms (eg, tetany), heart palpitations, softening of bones, brittle bones, rickets, poor growth, osteoporosis, tooth decay, and depression	Milk and milk products, yogurt, cheese, oysters, salmon, collard greens, spinach, ice cream, cottage cheese, kale, broccoli, and oranges	Males and females: 9–18 y 19–50 y >50 y Pregnancy and lactation: ≤18 y 19–50 y	(AI) 1300 1000 1200 1300 1000	2500 2500 2500 2500 2500	Exercise-induced or anorexia nervosa–induced amenorrheic women have reduced net absorption of calcium.	Mineral imbalances, gastrointestinal atony, renal failure, kidney stones, and psychosis
Magnesium, mg/d	Required for many enzymatic processes, muscle and nerve function, and maintenance of teeth and bones	Heart failure and other cardiac disorders, hypertension, hypokalemia, nervousness, kidney damage and stones, irritability, and muscle spasms	Brown rice, nuts, green leafy vegetables, grains, seeds, wheat germ, beans, whole grains, peas, bananas, oranges, and strawberries	Males: 9–13 y 14–18 y 19–30 y >30 y Females: 9–13 y 14–18 y 19–30 y >30 y Pregnancy: ≤18 y 19–30 y 31–50 y Lactation: ≤18 y 19–30 y 31–50 y	(RDA) 240 410 400 420 240 360 310 320 400 350 360 360 310 320	350 350 350 350 350 350 350 350 350 350 350 350 350 350	None	Osmotic diarrhea, cardiac disturbances, hypotension, and respiratory failure
Phosphorus, mg/d	Key component of DNA, RNA, acid-base balance, energy production, and maintenance of teeth and bones	Bone fractures, irritability, weakness, blood cell disorders, gastrointestinal tract disorders, and renal dysfunction	Protein-rich foods such as meats, fish, and dairy products; legumes, nuts, and cereals	Males and females: 9–18 y 19–70 y >70 y Pregnancy: ≤18 y 19–30 y 31–50 y Lactation: ≤18 y 19–30 y 31–50 y	(RDA) 1250 700 700 1250 700 700 1250 700 700	4000 4000 3000 3500 3500 3500 4000 4000 4000	None	Rare, except in renal failure Inhibits calcium absorption

*RDA indicates Recommended Dietary Allowances; AI, Adequate Intake; and UL, Tolerable Upper Intake Level.

TABLE 20-4
Trace Minerals*

Mineral	Function	Deficiency State	Sources	Life Stage	RDA/AI	UL	Special Considerations	Toxicity
Chromium, µg/d	Participates in glucose metabolism by enhancing effects of insulin	Glucose intolerance and peripheral neuropathy	Brewer's yeast, liver, whole grain cereals, beer, poultry, and spices	Males: 9–13 y	(AI) 25	ND	None	Nausea and vomiting, ulcers, convulsions, kidney and liver damage, and coma
				14–50 y	35	ND		
				>50 y	30	ND		
				Females: 9–13 y	21	ND		
				14–18 y	24	ND		
				19–50 y	25	ND		
				>50 y	20	ND		
				Pregnancy: ≤18 y	29	ND		
				19–50 y	30	ND		
				Lactation: ≤18 y	44	ND		
				19–50 y	45	ND		
Copper, µg/d	Critical component of numerous essential enzymes, bone formation, and hematopoiesis	Anemia; leukopenia; skeletal defects; Menkes syndrome, an inherited copper deficiency that occurs in male infants (1 in 50,000 live births)	Organ meats, oysters, whole grains, nuts, shellfish, and dark-green leafy vegetables	Males and females: 9–13 y	(RDA) 700	5000	Zinc inhibits absorption of copper. Molybdenum increases copper urinary excretion, which can lead to deficiency.	Nausea, vomiting, and diarrhea. Quantities in grams may result in copper-induced hemolytic anemia and anuria (Wilson disease).
				14–18 y	890	8000		
				>18 y	900	10,000		
				Pregnancy: ≤18 y	1000	8000		
				19–50 y	1000	10,000		
				Lactation: ≤18 y	1300	8000		
				19–50 y	1300	10,000		
Fluoride, mg/d	Inhibits initiation and progression of dental caries and stimulates new bone formation	Predisposition to dental caries and osteoporosis, although some authorities do not consider fluoride an essential mineral because a deficiency state, reversed by the mineral alone, has not been induced	Grains, vegetables, seafood, seaweed, cheese, tea, coffee, and fluoridated water	Males: 9–13 y	(AI) 2	10	None	Fluorosis, mottling, pitting of permanent teeth, skeletal changes (eg, exostosis of spine)
				14–18 y	3	10		
				>18 y	4	10		
				Females: 9–13 y	2	10		
				>13 y	3	10		
				Pregnancy and lactation: ≤18 y	3	10		
				19–50 y	3	10		

Continued

T A B L E 20-4
Trace Minerals*—*Continued*

Mineral	Function	Deficiency State	Sources	Life Stage	RDA/AI	UL	Special Considerations	Toxicity
Iodine, µg/d	Provides substrate for synthesis of thyroid hormones, thyroxine, and triiodothyronine, which are crucial for normal growth and development	*Moderate deficiency:* Colloid goiter (although most of these cases remain euthyroid) *Severe deficiency:* Endemic myxedema among adults and endemic cretinism among infants	Seafood, iodized salt, eggs, dairy products, and drinking water	Males and Females: 9–13 y 14–18 y >18 y Pregnancy: ≤18 y 19–50 y Lactation: ≤18 y 19–50 y	(RDA) 120 150 150 220 220 290 290	600 900 1100 900 1100 900 1100	ULs may not apply to individuals with autoimmune thyroid disease, previous deficiency, or nodular goiter due to increased sensitivity for adverse effects of excess iodine.	Brassy taste, increased salivation, gastric irritation, and acneiform skin lesions
Iron, mg/d	Essential constituent of blood (hemoglobin) and muscle (myoglobin) and important for transport of oxygen	Iron deficiency anemia with pallor of skin and tissue, weakness, fatigue, shortness of breath, heart palpitations, deformed nails, and headaches	Meat, fish, beans, spinach, molasses, kelp, brewer's yeast, broccoli, and seeds	Males: 9–13 y 14–18 y >18 y Females: 9–13 y 14–18 y 19–50 y >50 y Pregnancy: ≤18 y 19–50 y Lactation: ≤18 y 19–50 y	(RDA) 8 11 8 8 15 18 8 27 27 10 9	40 45 45 40 45 45 45 45 45 45 45	Vitamin C enhances iron absorption. Vegetarians should supplement or eat foods high in vitamin C due to a twofold greater iron requirement.	Vomiting, diarrhea, headache, and damage to the intestine Hemochromatosis is a potentially fatal but treatable hereditary disorder.

Continued

T A B L E 20-4
Trace Minerals*—Continued

Mineral	Function	Deficiency State	Sources	Life Stage	RDA/AI	UL	Special Considerations	Toxicity
Manganese, mg/d	Necessary for enzymatic processes, muscle and nerve function, and synthesis of cholesterol and fatty acids in the liver	Manganese deficiency has not been documented in the clinical literature. One case reported transient dermatitis, hypocholesterolemia, and increased alkaline phosphatase levels.	Seeds, unrefined grains, tea, beans, legumes, and other vegetables	Males: 9–13 y 14–18 y >18 y Females: 9–13 y 14–18 y >18 y Pregnancy: ≤18 y 19–50 y Lactation: ≤18 y 19–50 y	(AI) 1.9 2.2 2.3 1.6 1.6 1.8 2.0 2.0 2.6 2.6	 6 9 11 6 9 11 9 11 9 11	Individuals with hepatic disease may be at increased risk of adverse effects from excess manganese intake.	Rarely, neurologic symptoms resembling Parkinson or Wilson disease
Molybdenum, µg/d	Enzyme component for specific oxidases and xanthine dehydrogenase	Rarely, tachycardia, headache, nausea, vomiting, disorientation, and coma (sulfite intoxication syndrome)	Milk, beans, peas, cereals, and bread	Males and females: 9–13 y 14–18 y >18 y Pregnancy and lactation: ≤18 y 19–50 y	(RDA) 34 43 45 50 50	 1100 1700 2000 1700 2000	Copper-deficient individuals could be at increased risk of molybdenum toxicity.	Goutlike syndrome (increased levels of uric acid and xanthine oxidase)
Selenium, µg/d	Antioxidant that regulates thyroid hormones and reduction and oxidation of molecules (eg, vitamin C)	Rarely, muscle weakness, muscle pain and tenderness, and cardiomyopathy of Keshan disease	Seafood and organ meats	Males and females: 9–13 y >13 y Pregnancy: ≤18 y 19–50 y Lactation: ≤18 y 19–50 y	(RDA) 40 55 60 60 70 70	 280 400 400 400 400 400	Selenium is toxic and supplementation is usually not needed.	Dermatitis, alopecia, diseased nails, dental defects, depression, and peripheral neuropathy

Continued

T A B L E 20-4

Trace Minerals*—Concluded

Mineral	Function	Deficiency State	Sources	Life Stage	RDA/AI	UL	Special Considerations	Toxicity
Zinc, mg/d	Involved in wound healing, normal skin hydration, taste and smell, regulation of gene expression and growth; also serves as cofactor in >70 different enzymes	Anorexia, apathy, depression, growth retardation, dysosmia, delayed sexual maturation, hypogonadism and hypospermia, alopecia, immune disorders, dermatitis, anemia, night blindness, hypogeusia, and impaired wound healing	Meat, liver, eggs, seeds, whole grains, peanuts, cheese, and other plant sources	Males: 9–13 y 14–18 y >18 y Females: 9–13 y 14–18 y >18 y Pregnancy: ≤18 y 19–50 y Lactation: ≤18 y 19–50 y	(RDA) 8 11 11 8 9 8 12 11 13 12	 23 34 40 23 34 40 34 40 34 40	Vegetarians should supplement or eat foods high in zinc due to twofold greater requirement.	Lowered copper retention, nausea, vomiting, tachycardia, hypotension, and headaches

*RDA indicates Recommended Dietary Allowances; AI, Adequate Intake; UL, Tolerable Upper Intake Level; ND, not determinable; and NA, not applicable.

Adapted from references 3, 7, 13–15, 32, and 72.

REFERENCES

1. Chavis LM. Pharmacy-based consulting in dietary supplements. *J Am Pharm Assoc.* 2001;41:181–191.

2. Yates AA, Schlicker SA, Suitor CW. Dietary reference intakes: the new basis for recommendations for calcium and related nutrients, B vitamins, and choline. *J Am Diet Assoc.* 1998:98;699–706.

3. McEvoy GK, Miller JL, Snow EK, Welsh OH, eds. *American Hospital Formulary Service Drug Information Book.* Bethesda, Md: American Society of Health-System Pharmacists; 2002.

4. Commission on Dietary Supplement Labels. *Report of the Commission on Dietary Supplement Labels.* Washington, DC: US Government Printing Office; November 1997.

5. Huckleberry Y, Rollins CJ. Prevention of nutritional deficiencies. In: Berardi RR, DeSimon EM, Newton GD, Oszko MA, Popovich NG, Rollins CJ, eds. *Handbook of Nonprescription Drugs: An Interactive Approach to Self-Care.* 13th ed. Washington, DC: American Pharmaceutical Association; 2002:451–492.

6. Parisian S. Center for food safety and applied nutrition (CFSAN) 51–112. In: *FDA: Inside and Out.* Front Royal, Va: Fast Horse Press; 2001:chap 3.

7. Institute of Medicine, Food and Nutrition Board. *Dietary Reference Intakes: Vitamin A, Vitamin K, Arsenic, Boron, Chromium, Copper, Iodine, Iron, Manganese, Molybdenum, Nickel, Silicon, Vanadium, and Zinc.* Washington, DC: National Academy Press; 2001.

8. Ross AC. Vitamin A and retinoids. In: Shils ME, Olson JA, Shike M, Ross AC, eds. *Modern Nutrition in Health and Disease.* 9th ed. Baltimore, Md: Williams & Wilkins; 1999:305–328.

9. Jellin JM, Gregory P, Batz F, Hitchens K, eds. *Pharmacist's Letter/Prescriber's Letter: Natural Medicines Comprehensive Database.* 3rd ed. Stockton, Calif: Therapeutic Research Faculty; 2000.

10. Sitren HS. Vitamin A. In: Baumgartner TG, ed. *Clinical Guide to Parenteral Micronutrition.* 3rd ed. Deerfield, Ill: Fugisawa USA Inc; 1997:403–426.

11. Marcus R, Coulston AM. Fat-soluble vitamins: vitamins A, K, and E. In: Hardman JG, Limbird LE, eds. *Goodman & Gilman's: The Pharmacological Basis of Therapeutics.* 10th ed. New York, NY: McGraw-Hill; 2001:1753–1762.

12. Pelton R, La Valle JB, Hawkins EB, Krinsky DL, eds. *Drug-Induced Nutrient Depletion Handbook.* 2nd ed. Hudson, Ohio: Lexi-Comp Inc; 2001.

13. Chessman KH, Teasley-Strausburg KM. Assessment of nutrition status and nutrition requirements. In: DiPiro JT, Talbert RL, Yee GC, Matzke GR, Wells BG, Posey LM, eds. *Pharmacotherapy: A Pathophysiologic Approach.* New York, NY: McGraw-Hill; 2002.

14. McCarter DN, Holbrook J. Vitamins and minerals. In: Herfindal ET, Gourley JR, eds. *Textbook of Therapeutics: Drug and Disease Management.* 7th ed. Baltimore, Md: Lippincott Williams & Wilkins; 2000.

15. Beers MH, Berkow R, eds. *The Merck Manual of Diagnosis and Therapy.* 17th ed. Whitehouse Station, NJ: Merck Research Laboratories; 1999.

16. Bates CJ. Vitamin A. *Lancet.* 1995;345:31–35.

17. De Pee S, West CE. Dietary carotenoids and their role in combating vitamin A deficiency: a review of the literature. *Eur J Clin Nutr.* 1996;50(suppl 3):S38–S53.

18. Koo LC. Diet and lung cancer 20+ years later: more questions than answers? *Int J Cancer.* 1997;suppl 10:22–29.

19. Albanes D, Heinoinen OP, Taylor PR, et al. Alpha-tocopherol and beta-carotene supplement and lung cancer incidence in the Alpha-Tocopherol, Beta-Carotene Cancer Prevention Study: effects of base-line characteristics and study compliance. *J Natl Cancer Inst.* 1996;88:1560–1570.

20. Redlich CA, Blaner WS, Van Bennekum AM, et al. Effect of supplementation with beta-carotene and vitamin A on lung nutrient levels. *Cancer Epidemiol Biomarkers Prev.* 1998;7:211–214.

21. *2002 Drug Topics RedBook.* Montvale, NJ: Thomson Medical Economics; 2002.

22. *MICROMEDEX Healthcare Series.* 115th ed. Greenwood Village, Colo: MICROMEDEX; 2002.

23. Institute of Medicine, Food and Nutrition Board. *Dietary Reference Intakes: Calcium, Phosphorus, Magnesium, Vitamin D, and Fluoride.* Washington, DC: National Academy Press; 1997.

24. Holick MF. Vitamin D. In: Shils ME, Olson JA, Shike M, Ross AC, eds. *Modern Nutrition in Health and Disease.* 9th ed. Baltimore, Md: Williams & Wilkins, 1999:329–346.

25. Sitren HS. Vitamin D. In: Baumgartner TG, ed. *Clinical Guide to Parenteral Micronutrition.* 3rd ed. Deerfield, Ill: Fugisawa USA Inc; 1997:427–444.

26. Marcus R. Agents affecting calcification and bone turnover: calcium, phosphate, parathyroid hormone, vitamin D, calcitonin, and other compounds. In: Hardman JG, Limbird LE, eds. *Goodman & Gilman's: The Pharmacological Basis of Therapeutics.* 10th ed. New York, NY: McGraw-Hill; 2001:1715–1752.

27. DeLuca HF, Zierold C. Mechanisms and functions of vitamin D. *Nutr Rev.* 1998;56:S4–S10.

28. Malluche HH, Mawad H, Koszewski NJ. Update on vitamin D and its newer analogues: actions and rational for treatment on chronic renal failure. *Kidney Int.* 2002;62:367–374.

29. Fraser DR. Vitamin D. *Lancet.* 1995;345:104–107.

30. Veith R. Vitamin D supplementation, 25-hydroxyvitamin D concentrations and safety. *J Am Clin Nutr.* 1999;69:842–856.

31. Traber MG. Vitamin E. In: Shils ME, Olson JA, Shike M, Ross AC, eds. *Modern Nutrition in Health and Disease.* 9th ed. Baltimore, Md: Williams & Wilkins; 1999:347–362.

32. Institute of Medicine, Food and Nutrition Board. *Dietary Reference Intake: Vitamin C, Vitamin E, Selenium, and Carotenoids.* Washington, DC: National Academy Press; 2000.

33. Sitren HS. Vitamin E. In: Baumgartner TG, ed. *Clinical Guide to Parenteral Micronutrition.* 3rd ed. Deerfield, Ill: Fugisawa USA Inc; 1997:445–464.

34. Meydani M. Vitamin E. *Lancet.* 1995;345:170–175.

35. Stampfer MJ, Hennekens CH, Manson JE, Colditz GA, Rosner B, Willett WC. Vitamin E consumption and the risk of coronary disease in women. *N Engl J Med.* 1993;328:1444–1449.

36. ATBC (Alpha-Tocopherol, Beta Carotene) Cancer Prevention Study Group. The effect of vitamin E and beta carotene on the incidence of lung cancer and other cancers in male smokers. *N Engl J Med.* 1994;330:1029–1035.

37. Stephens NG, Parsons A, Schofield PM, Kelly F, Cheeseman K, Mitchinson MJ. Randomised controlled trial of vitamin E in patients with coronary disease: Cambridge Heart Antioxidant Study (CHAOS). *Lancet.* 1996;347:781–786.

38. GISSI-Prevenzione Investigators. Dietary supplementation with n3 polyunsaturated fatty acids and vitamin E after myocardial infarction: results of the GISSI-Prevenzione Trial. *Lancet.* 1999;354:447–455.

39. The Heart Outcomes Prevention Study Investigators. Vitamin E supplementation and cardiovascular events in high-risk patients. *N Engl J Med.* 2000;342:154–160.

40. Olson RE. Vitamin K. In: Shils ME, Olson JA, Shike M, Ross AC, eds. *Modern Nutrition in Health and Disease.* 9th ed. Baltimore, Md: Williams & Wilkins; 1999:363–380.

41. Sitren HS. Vitamin K. In: Baumgartner TG, ed. *Clinical Guide to Parenteral Micronutrition.* 3rd ed. Deerfield, Ill: Fugisawa USA Inc; 1997:465–482.

42. Shearer MJ. Vitamin K. *Lancet.* 1995;345:229–234.

43. Ansell J, Hirsh J, Dalen J, et al. Managing oral anticoagulant therapy. *Chest.* 2001;119(suppl 1):22S–38S.

44. Institute of Medicine, Food and Nutrition Board. *Dietary Reference Intakes for Thiamin, Riboflavin, Niacin, Vitamin B6, Folate, Vitamin B12, Pantothenic acid, Biotin, and Choline.* Washington, DC: National Academy Press; 1998.

45. Marcus R, Coulston AM. Water-soluble vitamins: the vitamin B complex and ascorbic acid. In: Hardman JG, Limbird LE, eds. *Goodman & Gilman's: The Pharmacological Basis of Therapeutics.* 10th ed. New York, NY: McGraw-Hill; 2001:1753–1762.

46. Tanphaichtir V. Thiamin. In: Shils ME, Olson JA, Shike M, Ross AC, eds. *Modern Nutrition in Health and Disease.* 9th ed. Baltimore, Md: Williams & Wilkins; 1999:381–390.

47. Sitren HS, Bailey LB, Cerda JJ. Thiamin (vitamin B_1). In: Baumgartner TG, ed. *Clinical Guide to Parenteral Micronutrition.* 3rd ed. Deerfield, Ill: Fugisawa USA Inc; 1997:483–498.

48. Sitren HS, Bailey LB, Cerda JJ. Riboflavin (vitamin B_2). In: Baumgartner TG, ed. *Clinical Guide to Parenteral Micronutrition.* 3rd ed. Deerfield, Ill: Fugisawa USA Inc; 1997:499–514.

49. McCormick DB. Riboflavin. In: Shils ME, Olson JA, Shike M, Ross AC, eds. *Modern Nutrition in Health and Disease.* 9th ed. Baltimore, Md: Williams & Wilkins; 1999:391–400.

50. Cevantes-Laurean D, McElvaney NG, Moss J. Niacin. In: Shils ME, Olson JA, Shike M, Ross AC, eds. *Modern Nutrition in Health and Disease.* 9th ed. Baltimore, Md: Williams & Wilkins; 1999:401–412.

51. Bailey LB, Sitren HS, Cerda JJ. Niacin (vitamin B_3). In: Baumgartner TG, ed. *Clinical Guide to Parenteral Micronutrition.* 3rd ed. Deerfield, Ill: Fugisawa USA Inc; 1997:515–530.

52. Plesofsky-Vig N. Pantothenic acid. In: Shils ME, Olson JA, Shike M, Ross AC, eds. *Modern Nutrition in Health and Disease.* 9th ed. Baltimore, Md: Williams & Wilkins; 1999:423–432.

53. Bailey LB, Sitren HS, Cerda JJ. Pantothenic acid (vitamin B_5). In: Baumgartner TG, ed. *Clinical Guide to Parenteral Micronutrition.* 3rd ed. Deerfield, Ill: Fugisawa USA Inc; 1997:549–562.

54. Leklem JE. Vitamin B_6. In: Shils ME, Olson JA, Shike M, Ross AC, eds. *Modern Nutrition in Health and Disease.* 9th ed. Baltimore, Md: Williams & Wilkins; 1999:413–422.

55. Bailey LB, Caudill MA. Pyridoxine (vitamin B_6). In: Baumgartner TG, ed. *Clinical Guide to Parenteral Micronutrition.* 3rd ed. Deerfield, Ill: Fugisawa USA Inc; 1997:563–578.

56. Herbert V. Folic acid. In: Shils ME, Olson JA, Shike M, Ross AC, eds. *Modern Nutrition in Health and Disease.* 9th ed. Baltimore, Md: Williams & Wilkins; 1999:433–446.

57. Bailey LB, Caudill MA. Folic acid. In: Baumgartner TG, ed. *Clinical Guide to Parenteral Micronutrition.* 3rd ed. Deerfield, Ill: Fugisawa USA Inc; 1997:611–628.

58. Sacher RA. Pernicious anemia and other megaloblastic anemias. In: Rakel RE, Bope ET, eds. *2002 Conn's Current Therapy.* Philadelphia, Pa: WB Saunders Co; 2002:366–369.

59. Boushey CJ, Beresford SA, Omenn GS, Motulsky AG. A quantitative assessment of plasma homocysteine as a risk factor for vascular disease: probable benefits of increasing folic acid intakes. *JAMA.* 1995;274:1049–1057.

60. Morrison HI, Schaubel D, Desmeules M, Wigle DT. Serum folate and risk of fatal coronary heart disease. *JAMA.* 1996;274:1893–1896.

61. Rimm EB, Willett WC, Hu FB, et al. Folate and vitamin B_6 from diet and supplements in relation to risk of coronary heart disease among women. *JAMA.* 1998;279:359–364.

62. Eikelboom JW, Lonn E, Genest J, Hankey G, Yusuf S. Homocyst(e)ine and cardiovascular disease: a critical review of the epidemiologic evidence. *Ann Intern Med.* 1999;131:363–375.

63. Hung J, Beilby JP, Knuiman MW, Divitini M. Folate and vitamin B-12 and risk of fatal cardiovascular disease: cohort study from Busselton, Western Australia. *BMJ.* 2003;326:131.

64. Antony AC. Megaloblastic anemias. In: Hoffman R, Benz EJ, Shattil SJ, Furie B, Cohen HJ, Silberstein LE, McGlave P, eds. *Hematology: Basic Principles and Practice.* 3rd ed. New York, NY: Churchill Livingstone Inc; 2000:446–485.

65. Quinlivan EP, Gregory JF. Effect of food fortification on folic acid intake in the United States [comment]. *Am J Clin Nutr.* 2003;77:221–225.

66. Weir DG, Scott JM. Vitamin B_{12} 'Cobalamin.' In: Shils ME, Olson JA, Shike M, Ross AC, eds. *Modern Nutrition in Health and Disease.* 9th ed. Baltimore, Md: Williams & Wilkins; 1999:447–458.

67. Bailey LB, Caudill MA. Cyanocobalamin (vitamin B_{12}). In: Baumgartner TG, ed. *Clinical Guide to Parenteral Micronutrition.* 3rd ed. Deerfield, Ill: Fugisawa USA Inc; 1997:579–596.

68. Mock DM. Biotin. In: Shils ME, Olson JA, Shike M, Ross AC, eds. *Modern Nutrition in Health and Disease.* 9th ed. Baltimore, Md: Williams & Wilkins; 1999:459–466.

69. Bailey LB, Caudill MA. Biotin. In: Baumgartner TG, ed. *Clinical Guide to Parenteral Micronutrition.* 3rd ed. Deerfield, Ill: Fugisawa USA Inc; 1997:597–610.

70. Jacob RA. Vitamin C. In: Shils ME, Olson JA, Shike M, Ross AC, eds. *Modern Nutrition in Health and Disease.* 9th ed. Baltimore, Md: Williams & Wilkins; 1999:367–384.

71. Bailey LB, Sitren HS, Cerda JJ. Ascorbic acid (vitamin C). In: Baumgartner TG, ed. *Clinical Guide to Parenteral Micronutrition.* 3rd ed. Deerfield, Ill: Fugisawa USA Inc; 1997:531–548.

72. Cada DJ, Covington TR, Generali JA, Hussar DA, Lasagna L, Selevan JR, eds. *Drug Facts and Comparisons.* St Louis, Mo: Facts and Comparisons; 2003.

chapter 21

Herbs and Other Dietary Supplements

Mandy C. Leonard, PharmD, BCPS

INTRODUCTION

In 1990, 1 of every 3 people in the United States used at least one form of alternative medicine, including dietary supplements.[1] The percentage of the US population consuming dietary supplements rose from 4.9% in 1990 to 17.6% in 1997.[2] Still, no formal process is in place to monitor or determine the exact use of dietary supplements in the United States.[3] A survey noted that less than 40% of alternative therapies used were disclosed by patients to their physicians.[2] Other studies note this same trend in managed care populations and in diverse ethnic backgrounds.[4,5] Dietary supplements are used by patients to treat not only self-limiting conditions but also serious conditions and diseases. Therefore, health care professionals need to know which dietary supplements are potentially beneficial and safe as well as which are ineffective and harmful for patients to use.

DEFINITIONS

Conventional medicine is defined as "medicine practiced by holders of MD or DO degrees and by their allied health professionals," such as physical therapists, psychologists, pharmacists, and registered nurses.[6] *Complementary and alternative medicine* (CAM), as defined by the National Center for Complementary and Alternative Medicine (NCCAM), is a "group of diverse medical and health care systems, practices, and products that are not presently considered to be part of conventional medicine."[6] More specifically, complementary medicine is used together with conventional medicine. An example of a complementary therapy noted by NCCAM is aromatherapy to help lessen a patient's discomfort after surgery. Different from complementary medicine, *alternative medicine* is used in place of conventional medicine. An example of an alternative therapy noted by NCCAM is using a special diet to treat cancer instead of undergoing surgery, radiation, or chemotherapy that has been recommended by a conventional doctor. Another defini-

tion for alternative medicine is "interventions neither taught widely in medical schools nor generally available in US hospitals."[1]

Dietary supplements are defined in the Dietary Supplement Health and Education Act of 1994 and are summarized in Table 21-1.[7] Herbal medicines are considered to be dietary supplements.

Homeopathy is defined as a healing system based on the use of minute doses of specially prepared natural substances for pharmacologic effects.[8,9] Homeopathy differs from herbal medicine,[8,9] although both practices incorporate plants and botanicals as therapy. Whereas herbal medicine uses active constituents derived from natural substances for the desired pharmacologic properties, homeopathy uses only minute doses. Homeopathy is claimed to be effective for treatment of symptomatic ailments, including allergies, colds, arthritis, headaches, insomnia, and menopause. A homeopathic substance is chosen to elicit symptoms similar to those the patient is suffering. An example is the use of *Allium cepa* (an onion

TABLE 21-1

Definition of Dietary Supplements From DSHEA*

Product (other than tobacco) intended to supplement the diet that bears or contains 1 or more of the following dietary ingredients: vitamin, mineral, amino acid, *herb,* or *other botanical*

Dietary substance for use to supplement the diet by increasing the total dietary intake

or

Concentrate, metabolite, constituent, extract, or combination of any ingredient described above

and

Intended for ingestion as a capsule, powder ..., and not represented as a conventional food or as a sole item of a meal or the diet

*Data from Parisian S.[7]

compound) to treat the watery eyes associated with seasonal allergic rhinitis.[10]

REASONS FOR USE

Dietary supplements, including herbs, are used for many reasons. First, many people may be disappointed by results of conventional medicine. An example is some women choosing herbal supplements, such as black cohosh (*Cimicifuga racemosa*), *dong quai* (*Angelica sinensis*), evening primrose oil (EPO, *Oenothera* species), and phytoestrogens, to manage postmenopausal symptoms because of side effects of hormone replacement therapy.[11,12] Also, alternative medication philosophies and practices have existed for centuries, with documented indications and reported cures.[9,13] Some people question the safety or fear the long-term effects of conventional medications. Patients are exposed continually to reports of adverse reactions and interactions with prescription medications. Herbs and other natural medicines are often used in place of established standards of care or pharmacotherapy because of the perceived benign safety profile.[14] Many diseases lack effective treatments and cures. Alternative medications may be used in these diseases in combination with conventional therapy or as the last line of therapy. Many people believe that herbal and other alternative medicines are safer than conventional medicines because they are derived from nature.[15] People relate the word *nature* with being innocent and wholesome, not artificial or synthetic.[16] People may perceive medicine derived from herbs as "person-friendly."[16] Some persons use alternative medicines because of peer influences and a desire to have autonomy. Family and friends are often the reason why people try alternative medicine.[17] Finally, persons may be influenced by false or unsupported claims from the herbal industry. Statements often are made by herbal and alternative medicine manufacturers without evidence-based medicine to support the efficacy and safety of products.

LAWS AND REGULATIONS

The Food, Drug, and Cosmetic Act of 1906 prohibited all adulterated (ie, errors with manufacturing and compounding) and misbranded (eg, false claims or labeling) drugs.[7] At that time, drugs did not have to be proved safe or effective to be marketed and sold in the United States. The Federal Food, Drug, and Cosmetic Act of 1938 stated that all drugs must be proved safe.[7] The impetus for this act was more than 100 deaths associated with elixir-of-sulfanilamide, which contained an unsafe additive similar to automobile antifreeze.[13] At that time, herbal supplements were considered foods and were therefore not permitted to make any direct or indirect therapeutic claims. In 1958, the Delaney Amendment permitted the

US Food and Drug Administration (FDA) to regulate food additives.[7,9] Four years later, the Kefauver-Harris Amendment declared that all drugs marketed in the United States after 1962 must be proved both safe and effective.[7,9] The Rogers-Proxmire Amendment, passed in 1976, defined the scope of foods to include vitamins, minerals, or other ingredients for use by humans to supplement the diet or increase total dietary intake.[7,9] Herbal supplements were deemed to be *other ingredients*, which therefore gave the FDA some regulative authority over them. Over the next 15 years, the herbal industry and the FDA went to court many times. The FDA argued that certain herbs were contaminated and unsafe. The herbal industry argued that the FDA abused its regulatory authority. In 1994, herbal medicines became specifically exempt from FDA regulations.

For more than 20 years, the FDA had regulated dietary supplements as foods. However, in 1994, the Dietary Supplement Health and Education Act (DSHEA) was passed. This act defined dietary supplements as vitamins, minerals, herbs, botanicals, or amino acids used to supplement the diet to increase total dietary intake.[7,18] The FDA is prohibited from regulating dietary ingredients in dietary supplements as food additives. In other words, dietary supplements became no longer subject to premarket safety evaluations. Since October 1994, the FDA and the US Congress have officially not considered dietary supplements as drugs. The DSHEA allowed herbal supplements to be marketed in the United States without having to pass the stringent requirements imposed by the FDA for new molecular entities (drugs).[7,14]

The burden of proof that a dietary supplement is adulterated or unsafe, however, is the responsibility of the FDA. For example, in May 2000, the FDA imposed an import alert for plants of the family Aristolochiaceae because of concerns about potential adulteration as well as the potential for nephrotoxicity and carcinogenicity.[19] Two reports had occurred in the United States of serious kidney disease associated with products containing aristolochic acid, but many more reported cases had taken place in Europe.[20,21] After further investigation, these cases were found to be caused by *Aristolochia fangchi* inadvertently being substituted for *Stephania tetrandra* and *Magnolia officinalis* in Chinese herb products used for weight loss.[21] Another example took place in 2000 when the FDA warned consumers that despite previous recalls of products marketed as dietary supplements that contained tiratricol, a potent thyroid hormone that may cause serious events, including myocardial infarctions and strokes, the products were still reaching the public.[22] Similarly, in March 2002, the FDA issued a consumer and health care provider advisory on the use of kava (*Piper methysticum*) after reports that 11 patients who had consumed products containing kava contracted liver failure and had undergone liver transplantation. Canada and some European countries removed kava from the market.[23]

The DSHEA permits "third-party" literature about a product or substance with specific guidelines. First, the literature cannot promote one manufacturer. Second, the literature must present a balanced view of the available, scientific data such that the information is truthful and not misleading. Third, the literature must appear physically separate from the product with no appended materials, such as stickers. Dietary supplements are permitted to have statements or claims regarding the ability of the product to alter structure and function, but not to have statements or claims regarding managing diseases. Any product that makes a disease claim is considered by the FDA to be a drug. For example, a package of St John's wort (*Hypericum perforatum*) can state that it enhances mood but cannot state that St John's wort treats depression. Similarly, a saw palmetto product can state that saw palmetto maintains a healthy prostate but cannot claim the product treats benign prostatic hyperplasia (BPH). Additionally, all dietary supplements must have the following warning about the structure and function claim: "This statement has not been evaluated by the Food and Drug Administration. This product is not intended to diagnosis, treat, cure, or prevent any disease." The definition of disease was changed or clarified in 2000.[24,25] The current definition of *disease* is "damage to an organ, part, structure, or system of the body such that it does not function properly (eg, cardiovascular disease), or a state of health leading to such (eg, hypertension);" except that diseases resulting from essential nutrient deficiencies (eg, scurvy, pellagra) are not included in this definition.[26] If an herbal supplement is being used for a disease, the manufacturer and the packaging are *not* permitted to make therapeutic or disease claims. Examples of diseases that are not permitted under DSEHA are Alzheimer's disease and other senile dementia; arteriosclerotic diseases in coronary, cerebral, or peripheral blood vessels; and osteoporosis. Examples of disease claims that are not permitted are "prevents irregular heartbeat" and "maintains healthy lungs in smokers." Additionally, disease claims cannot be made in the name of the product (eg, "Hepatacure," "Carpaltum," or "Circu-Care") or in the use of pictures or symbols (eg, heart symbol or electrocardiogram tracings).[24,26]

Conditions associated with natural states are not considered diseases. A condition is considered to be an impaired function of an organ or system due to particular normal physiologic process, such as common or minor symptoms of life stages. If an herbal supplement is being used for a condition, the manufacturer is permitted to make therapeutic or disease claims. However, if the product claims that it "has an effect on an *abnormal* condition associated with a natural state or process, or if the abnormal condition is uncommon or can cause significant or permanent harm," the statement would be considered an implied disease claim. Examples of allowed conditions and statements for which structure and function claims can be made under DSHEA are absentmindedness and mild memory problems associated with aging; premenstrual syndrome (PMS) and normal healthy attitude during PMS; support for menopausal women (hot flashes); and appetite suppressant and weight loss if not linked to obesity.[26]

The DSHEA established the Office of Dietary Supplements (ODS) of the National Institutes of Health (NIH).[7] The ODS received funding to collect, compile, conduct, and coordinate scientific research on dietary supplements.

STANDARDIZATION

The FDA does not regulate the manufacturing process of dietary supplements. Unlike for prescription drugs, product quality standards such as Good Manufacturing Practices do not exist for dietary supplements. This lack of standardization has resulted in many problems.[14,27] Good Manufacturing Practices require products such as drugs and foods to meet specific quality standards, to be manufactured and compounded appropriately, and to be labeled accurately as to correct ingredients and doses. The names and chemical components of supplements differ from product to product, thereby making identification of ingredients difficult. Recent regulations state that all ingredients and quantities must be listed as well as the source (eg, leaves, stem, root, or flower). However, the responsibility lies with the manufacturer to ensure that the ingredients on the label are consistent and accurate with what it is manufacturing.

Recently, chromatographic analytical methods for some herbal supplements (eg, echinacea root, garlic, ginger root, and ginkgo leaf extract) have been reviewed and published in the *American Herbal Pharmacopeia*, by the Institute for Nutraceutical Advancement (INA), and in the *United States Pharmacopeia* (*USP*).[28] However, it is important to keep in mind that the active constituents of many herbs are not known. For example, many manufacturers standardize St John's wort according to the hypericin content, but hypericin is only one of the proposed active ingredients of St John's wort.[14] Standardization is also difficult because many constituents may be working additively or synergistically to produce the effects,[29] and one dietary supplement product proved to be safe and effective may not be compared with another similar herbal product on the market. Furthermore, the concentration and quality of the herbal ingredients can be affected by environmental conditions, such as temperature, rainfall, altitude, and soil. Additionally, dietary supplements derived from plants may contain a wide range of US-banned pesticides or microorganisms.[27,30,31] Finally, standardization is difficult because dietary supplements may not contain any active ingredients, and some dietary supplements contain contaminants.[13,27,30,32-39]

Due to the lack of product and quality assurance standards for dietary supplements, as well as reports of inactive ingredients or contaminants, 3 organizations offer third-party fee-for-service certification for dietary supplements (Table 21-2).[40-43] One of the organizations, ConsumerLab.com, has tested hundreds of popular supplements and found that as many as 25% do not pass the evaluations.[44] For example, most vitamin B products tested well, whereas ginseng products tested poorly. With lack of federal mandates, these certification programs most likely will be important only to dietary supplement manufacturers who consider certification as a helpful marketing tool. Another drawback is that patients may not understand the meaning of certification seals (ie, the dietary supplements with seals are guaranteed only for quality and not for safety and efficacy).

SAFETY

Much of the safety of herbal products is unknown. Reports of adverse reactions and interactions for dietary supplements, including herbal medicines, are scarce. The information needed to determine the occurrence and actual risk of adverse reactions and interactions is not frequently available or is difficult to evaluate because the contents of natural medicines are not standardized.[17,45,46] Other factors that complicate the assessment of adverse reactions and interactions with natural products are as follows: (1) failure of patients to tell health care providers of concomitant use of natural products, (2) incomplete or inaccurate product information, (3) multiple ingredients, (4) product adulteration, and (5) product misidentifica-

tion. Additionally, few clinical data in the medical and scientific literature document and describe the occurrence of adverse reactions and interactions.[47]

Adverse Reactions

All medicinal agents, including prescription and dietary supplements, have the potential to cause unexpected or unwanted effects and toxicity. Age, sex, race, and concurrent disease state can influence the risk of experiencing an adverse reaction. Recognition of an adverse reaction associated with an herbal medicine may be challenging because patients do not always disclose the use of herbs, and health care providers may not routinely screen for adverse reactions caused by herbs or other dietary supplements. In a recent study involving 11 poison control centers in the United States, one third of all adverse events associated with dietary supplements were linked to harmful outcomes such as seizures, coma, myocardial infarctions, arrhythmias, coagulation disorders, hepatic disease, anaphylaxis, and death.[17] Ginkgo (*Ginkgo biloba*) has been reported to cause spontaneous bleeding in the anterior chamber of the eye, bilateral subdural hematoma, and subarachnoid hemorrhage.[48-50] St John's wort has been documented to cause photosensitivity and hypomania.[11,51] *Ma huang* (ephedra or ephedrine alkaloid), known to be a powerful central nervous system stimulant, has been associated with serious adverse events such as seizures, strokes, myocardial infarctions, and death. *Ma huang* and products containing *ma huang* are considered by many to be unsafe. Additionally, the FDA has proposed limits on the use of ephedrine-containing products

TABLE 21-2

Dietary Supplement Product Certification/Seals*

Certifying Organization	Web Site	Evaluation Process	Criteria Evaluated
United States Pharmacopeia (USP)	www.usp.dsvp.org	USP Verified Dietary Supplement evaluation done at manufacturer's request for a fee	Purity (free of contaminants), document review (accurate labeling), standards (*USP*s Good Manufacturing Practices)
ConsumerLab.com	www.consumerlab.com	Randomly selects products or done at manufacturer's request for a fee	Purity (free of contaminants), therapeutic dose of active ingredient (as defined by ConsumerLab)
NSF International	www.nsf.org	Done at manufacturer's request for a fee	Purity (free of contaminants), document review (accurate labeling), standards (NSF's Good Manufacturing Practices)

*Data from *Washington Post*,[40,41] Traynor K,[42] and Palacioz K.[43]

as a maximum of 8 mg per dose and 24 mg/d for no longer than 1 week. Patients with cardiovascular disorders, thyroid disease, or diabetes should avoid the use of *ma huang*.[47] Because of lack of data and the potential severity of possible adverse reactions, most herbal medicines should be avoided during pregnancy and lactation, in children, and in persons with serious medical conditions.[11-13]

Manufacturers of dietary supplements are not required to maintain or track adverse reactions associated with their products (reporting is voluntary). In 1998, the American Association of Poison Control Centers received approximately 7000 reports of adverse reactions associated with dietary supplements.[14] Adverse reactions associated with dietary supplements can be reported to the FDA using the same vehicle as prescription drugs (the FDA's MedWatch Program) or the Special Nutritionals Adverse Event Monitoring System (SN/AEMS). Unlike the MedWatch database, the SN/AEMS database can be viewed and searched online to locate reported adverse reactions. In contrast to the reports in the MedWatch database, the reports in the SN/AEMS are not validated and verified for quality such as incomplete or missing information. The FDA estimates that less than 1% of serious adverse events associated with dietary supplements are reported to that agency.[52] Therefore, the FDA Center for Food Safety and Applied Nutrition is in the process of developing a new procedure for monitoring and assessing adverse drug reactions associated with dietary supplements.[53] The center's Adverse Event Reporting System is expected to be completely functional by mid-2003.

Drug-Dietary Supplement or Drug-Herb Interactions

Dietary supplements have been documented to interact with prescription and nonprescription drugs. Additionally, dietary supplements can interact with other dietary supplements. Most of the reported drug interactions with dietary supplements or herbs are anecdotal or single case reports, and they frequently lack relevant information to determine a causal relationship.[46,54-56] Just as drug-drug interactions can be caused by pharmacokinetic or pharmacodynamic processes, interactions between drugs and herbs also can be caused by both mechanisms. An example of a pharmacokinetic drug-herb interaction is St John's wort causing decreased cyclosporine levels by inducing the cytochrome P-450 3A4 isoenzyme or modulating P-glycoprotein.[11,12] There are reports of transplant recipients whose concomitant use of St John's wort was associated with subtherapeutic levels of cyclosporine.[57] Another example, although technically not a dietary supplement, is grapefruit juice inhibiting the cytochrome P-450 3A4 isoenzyme and decreasing the metabolism of certain 3-hydroxy-3-methylglutaryl coenzyme A (HMG CoA) reductase inhibitors (specifically, atorvastatin calcium

[Lipitor], fluvastatin sodium [Lescol], and simvastatin [Zocor]), thereby placing the patient at an increased risk of toxicity related to these drugs.[58,59] Because predicting which patients are at greatest risk of this interaction due to multiple factors (eg, genetic polymorphisms of the cytochrome enzymes and different concentration and/or components of grapefruit juice) is difficult, patients should minimize use of grapefruit juice while receiving specific HMG CoA reductase inhibitors.[58,59]

An example of a pharmacodynamic drug-herb interaction is ginkgo increasing the risk of bleeding in a patient receiving warfarin therapy. Ginkgo has been documented to inhibit platelet activating factor.[60] Conversely, patients taking *Oriental* ginseng (*Panax ginseng*) and warfarin concomitantly can experience a decreased international normalized ratio (INR).[61] Another herb documented to decrease INR in patients concurrently receiving warfarin treatment is green tea (*Camellia sinensis*). Dried green tea leaves contain a substantial amount of vitamin K, and, therefore, consuming large amounts may antagonize the effects of warfarin.[62]

Many of the proposed drug-herb interactions as well as those reported in the literature are between herbs and blood modifiers or other cardiovascular agents. Table 21-3 summarizes documented and potential interactions between herbs and blood modifiers,[11-13,27,63-67] and Table 21-4 lists documented and potential interactions between herbs and cardiovascular medications.[11-13,27,63-67] Persons receiving these medications and considering concomitant use of supplements or herbal products will find review of these tables and information helpful. Similarly, use of select natural medicines should be discontinued before surgery because of potential additive effects, such as increased risk of bleeding or sedation or interactions with anesthetic agents (Table 21-5).[68] Finally, certain supplements, such as echinacea (*Echinacea* species), have immune-modulating properties,[11-13,63-65] and therefore these natural products should be avoided in patients receiving immunosuppressants, such as cyclosporine, and in those with diseases involving the immune system, such as cancer, multiple sclerosis, and autoimmune disorders. Other supplements with immune-modulating properties include:

- Alfalfa
- Asian (*Panax*) ginseng
- Astragalus
- Cat's claw
- Coenzyme Q$_{10}$
- Dehydroepiandrosterone (DHEA)
- Garlic
- Goldenseal
- Grape seed extract
- Melatonin
- Siberian ginseng

TABLE 21-3

Select Interactions Between Dietary Supplements and Blood Modifiers*

Medication	Dietary Supplement (Reason for Interaction)
Anticoagulants/ Antiplatelets	Acerola (reduces anticoagulant activity)
	Agrimony (vitamin K constituents)
	American ginseng, Siberian ginseng (reduces platelet aggregation)
	Arnica (coumarin constituents)
	Bilberry (antiaggregation effect on platelets)
	Bogbean (hemolytic activity)
	Boldo (coumarin constituents)
	Capsicum (increases fibrinolytic activity)
	Cayenne (reduces platelet aggregation and increases fibrinolytic activity)
	Celery (coumarin constituent)
	Chlorella (vitamin K constituents)
	Dong quai (coumarin constituents)
	English chamomile (coumarin constituents)
	European mistletoe (agglutinating activity)
	Fenugreek (coumarin constituents)
	Feverfew (reduces platelet aggregation and increases fibrinolytic activity)
	Fish oils (decreases platelet adhesiveness)
	γ-Linolenic acid (contained in borage seed oil)
	Garlic (inhibits platelet aggregation and increases fibrinolytic properties)
	Ginger (inhibits platelet aggregation)
	Ginkgo leaf extract (inhibits platelet activating factor)
	Goldenseal (possesses coagulant activity)
	Horse chestnut seed (coumarin constituents)
	Panax ginseng (inhibits platelet aggregation)
	Passionflower (coumarin constituents)
	Plantain (vitamin K constituents)
	Red clover (coumarin constituents)
	Stinging nettle (vitamin K constituents)
	Sweet clover (contains dicoumarol)
	Vitamins C and E (inhibits platelet aggregation and adhesiveness)
	Vitamin K (antagonism)
	Willow bark (salicylate constituent)
Heparin	Goldenseal (possesses coagulant activity)
Warfarin (Coumadin)	Acerola (reduces anticoagulant activity)
	Angelica (inhibits platelet aggregation)
	Anise (coumarin constituents)
	Chlorella (vitamin K constituents)
	Coenzyme Q$_{10}$ (vitamin K constituents)
	Devil's claw (inhibits platelet aggregation)
	Dong quai (contains coumarin derivatives)
	Fenugreek (coumarin constituents)
	Feverfew (reduces platelet aggregation and increases fibrinolytic activity)
	Garlic (inhibits platelet aggregation and increases fibrinolytic properties)
	Ginger (inhibits platelet aggregation)
	Ginkgo leaf extract (inhibits platelet activating factor)
	Panax ginseng (diminished platelet adhesiveness)
	Papain (increases international normalized ratio)
	St John's wort (induces cytochrome P-450 2C9)
	Vitamins C, E, and K

*Data from references 11–13, 27, and 63–67.

T A B L E 21-4

Select Interactions between Dietary Supplements and Cardiovascular Agents*

Medication	Dietary Supplement (Reason for Interaction)
Antiarrhythmics	Aloe latex (possible loss of intestinal potassium leading to decrease in serum potassium)
Antihypertensives	Devil's claw (additive effects)
	European mistletoe (additive effects)
	Fish oils (additive effects)
	Ginger (additive or decreased effects)
	Goldenseal (decreased effects)
	Hawthorn (additive effects)
	Licorice (decreased effects)
	Stinging nettle (interferes with effects)
	Yohimbe (interferes with effects)
Calcium channel blockers	*Dong quai* (synergistic effects)
	Ginger (increases calcium uptake by heart muscle)
	Grapefruit juice (additive effects)
	St John's wort (interferes with metabolism)
Carvedilol (Coreg)	Grapefruit juice (increases bioavailability)
Coronary vasodilators	Hawthorn (additive effects)
Digoxin (Lanoxin)	Aloe (possible loss of intestinal potassium leading to decrease in serum potassium)
	Digitalis (additive effects)
	Ephedra (dysrhythmias)
	Hawthorn (increases cardiac toxicity)
	Licorice (loss of serum potassium)
	Pectin (affects absorption)
	Psyllium (decreases absorption)
	Siberian ginseng (increases digoxin levels)
	St John's wort (decreases effects)
HMG CoA reductase inhibitors (atorvastatin, fluvastatin, simvastatin)	Grapefruit juice (inhibits gut cytochrome P-450 3A4)
Potassium-depleting diuretics	Licorice (additive effects)
Thiazide diuretics	Ginkgo leaf extract (decreases effects)

*Data from references 11–13, 27, and 63–67. HMG CoA indicates 3-hydroxy-3-methylglutaryl coenzyme A.

EFFICACY

Most data about efficacy of natural products is historical and anecdotal and not rooted in evidence-based medicine.[11-13,27,63-65] Although some methodologically sound clinical trials evaluating dietary supplements have been described in the literature, a number of trials contain flaws and deficiencies.[14,27] Many trials have had a small sample size and are not powered sufficiently to detect a difference between treatment groups. Other trials were not conducted for a sufficient time for the disease state being treated or for the active ingredients to produce an effect (eg, glucosamine and chondroitin may take as long as 4 to 6 weeks to have an effect in osteoarthritis).[69] The natural product used in a clinical trial may not completely be identified or standardized. Problems may be present with

TABLE 21-5

Dietary Supplements to Discontinue Use Before Surgery*

Dietary Supplement	No. of Days Before Surgery to Discontinue Use	Reason
Echinacea	No data	Potential for immunosuppression
Ephedra (*ma huang*)	1	Potential for cardiac adverse effect
Garlic	7	Increased risk of bleeding
Ginkgo	3	Increased risk of bleeding
Ginseng	7	Increased risk of bleeding; potential for hypoglycemia
Kava	2	Potential for increased sedation
St John's wort	5	Potential for numerous drug-herb interactions
Valerian	No data	Potential for increased sedation

*Data from Ang-Lee et al.[68]

the placebo that is used (ie, some herbs have a distinct smell or taste). Natural products often are compared only with placebo and not with drugs that are considered part of the standard of care. The outcomes reported in trials for alternative medicines have less rigorous or defined end points than those investigated, reported, and expected for drugs (eg, garlic trials report the effects on the lipid profile but not the effects on morbidity and mortality).

SELECTED HERBS

In 2001, ginkgo, echinacea, and garlic were the top-selling herbs in the mainstream market in the United States.[70] The top 3 selling herbs in 1999 were ginkgo, St John's wort, and ginseng.[71]

Ginkgo[11–13,63–67]

Ginkgo is used in a wide variety of conditions and diseases, such as memory impairment, dementia, and mood changes. The major classes of active ingredients are the ginkgolides and bilobalides (also known as terpenes) and the flavonoids. Even though the chemical components of the ginkgo have distinctive intrinsic pharmacologic properties, they may work synergistically to produce more potent pharmacologic effects. Ginkgo is reported to possess antioxidant and neuroprotective properties. Ginkgo is possibly effective when used in persons with Alzheimer's vascular or mixed dementia. Studies report that ginkgo can stabilize or improve several measures of cognitive function and social functioning. Outcome studies have not yet verified ginkgo's effect on disease progression, and it has not been directly compared with conventional treatment of dementia. German practitioners consider ginkgo to be the treatment of choice for dementia and for age-related memory dysfunction.

Common adverse effects associated with ginkgo are hypersensitivity reactions, gastrointestinal disturbances, and bleeding. Additionally, seizures have been reported in children. Ginkgo exhibits the potential for enhanced effect on platelet-activating factor when taken concurrently with antiplatelet or anticoagulant medication. Use of ginkgo should be discontinued at least 36 hours before elective surgery.

The recommended dosage for dementia is 120 to 240 mg administered orally in 2 or 3 divided doses. Most clinical trials have used a standardized ginkgo biloba leaf extract. A ginkgo product that contains at least 24% flavone glycosides and 6% terpenes generally is recommended.

Echinacea[11–13,29,63–65,67]

Persons most often use Echinacea in an attempt to prevent and treat upper respiratory tract infections. The applicable parts of the plant (*Echinacea angustifolia, Echinacea pallida,* and *Echinacea purpurea*) for therapeutic use are roots and above ground parts. Echinacea is thought to possess antiviral activity and stimulatory effects on the immune system. Echinacea may be effective for decreasing the symptoms associated with the common cold and flu. Published results of clinical trials indicate a reduction in the duration and severity of symptoms when echinacea therapy is initiated at the onset of symptoms and continued for 7 to 10 days. Conversely, use of echinacea for the prevention of the common cold and flu appears ineffective. Various echinacea products and formulations were used in the clinical trials.

Common adverse effects associated with echinacea include gastrointestinal disturbances, fever, unpleasant taste, and dizziness. Additionally, allergic reactions including anaphylaxis, urticaria, and angioedema have occurred in patients taking echinacea. Patients at higher risk of these allergic reactions may be individuals allergic to ragweed, daisies, and marigolds, as well as patients with atopy. Echinacea may interfere with immunosuppression pharmacotherapy such as cyclosporine; may exacerbate some conditions, such as multiple sclerosis; or may interfere with certain immune disorders, such as human immunodeficiency virus (HIV) infection. Echinacea should be taken for no longer than 8 consecutive weeks due to potential effects on the immune system. Use of echinacea should be discontinued before elective surgery.

The recommended dose of echinacea depends on the formulation. Adulteration and standardization is a common problem with many commercially available echinacea products.

Garlic[11-13,63-66]

Garlic (*Allium sativum*) is used in a wide variety of conditions and diseases, such as hypercholesterolemia, hypertension, and diabetes. The principle active ingredient in garlic is allicin, a sulfur-containing compound that gives garlic its characteristic odor. Allicin is enzymatically formed from alliin. The alliin content of natural garlic varies approximately by 10-fold; therefore, the quantity of allicin released is influenced by specific manufacturing processes. The exact mechanism for garlic's lipid-lowering effect is not known; however, some theories state that garlic affects cholesterol absorption, synthesis, and metabolism. There are conflicting data from trials regarding the use of garlic for the management of patients with hypercholesterolemia. A few well-designed clinical trials have demonstrated garlic having no beneficial effect on the lipid profile. However, most data show that garlic modestly improves total cholesterol, low-density lipoprotein cholesterol (LDL-C), and triglyceride levels. When used for 4 to 25 weeks, garlic lowers total cholesterol levels by 4% to 12%. Garlic has been shown also to lower blood pressure by 2% to 7% after 4 weeks of therapy.

Common adverse effects associated with garlic include gastrointestinal disturbance, garlic odor, sweating, lightheadedness, and allergic reactions. Potential for increased risk of bleeding exists when garlic is taken concurrently with warfarin, and for enhanced antiplatelet effect when taken concurrently with antiplatelet agents. Due to possible increased risk of bleeding, garlic should be discontinued 1 to 2 weeks before elective surgery. Garlic also increases risk of hypoglycemia when taken concurrently with hypoglycemic agents.

The recommended dosage of garlic for the management of hypercholesterolemia is 600 to 900 mg orally per day, usually divided and administered 3 times a day. A garlic product that releases at least 0.6% allicin generally is recommended. Some odorless products appear to be ineffective (because they lack active ingredient).

Asian or Oriental Ginseng[11-13,63-65,67]

There are numerous types of ginseng. The 3 most common types are Asian or Oriental ginseng (*Panax ginseng*), Siberian ginseng (*Eleutherococcus senticosus*), and American ginseng (*Panax quinquefolius*). Each type of ginseng has a unique and distinct mechanism of action, efficacy and safety profile, and recommended dose. *Panax ginseng* is used mainly to combat stress, enhance immune function, improve concentration and memory, and increase physical and athletic endurance. The active ingredients are thought to be the ginsenosides Rg1 and Rb1. These ginsenosides have opposing pharmacologic activity. Ginsenoside Rg1 possesses central nervous system–stimulating properties and increases blood pressure, whereas ginsenoside Rb1 possesses central nervous system–suppressing properties and lowers blood pressure. *Panax ginseng* also can affect the immune system, by stimulating activity of natural killer cells. *Panax ginseng* is possibly effective in improving memory, although the data are conflicting. It may be more effective, however, in enhancing memory when used in combination with ginkgo leaf extract. Additionally, *Panax ginseng* is possibly effective for enhancing athletic performance in healthy individuals.

Common adverse effects associated with the use of *Panax ginseng* are insomnia, mastalgia, palpitations, hypertension, hypotension, hypoglycemia, edema, headache, and decreased appetite. Skin reactions may occur with high doses and prolonged use. A "ginseng abuse syndrome" has been reported after both short- and long-term use of *Panax ginseng* and is manifested by hypertension, nervousness, insomnia, estrogenic effects, skin eruptions, edema, and diarrhea. Use of *Panax ginseng* with antiplatelet or anticoagulant drugs should proceed with caution because of an increased risk of bleeding. Of interest is a case report of *Panax ginseng* causing a diminished response to warfarin. Patients undergoing elective surgery should discontinue Asian ginseng 7 days preoperatively to avoid an increased risk of bleeding. *Panax ginseng* may lower blood glucose levels and, therefore, should be used with caution in diabetic patients. It also may alter immune function and should be avoided in patients who are receiving immunosuppressive therapy or who have autoimmune disorders.

The dose of *Panax ginseng* varies based on the condition being prevented or treated. It usually is taken as the root powder, as a tea (ginseng tea bags have approximately 1500 mg of ginseng root), or as capsules (root extract).

Soy/Phytoestrogens[11-13,63-65,72]

Soy is used in women to manage menopausal symptoms and prevent osteoporosis and cardiovascular disease after menopause. Soybeans and soy food have the highest amount of isoflavones. In the intestines, isoflavones release phytoestrogens (genistein, daidzein, and glycitein), which are structurally related to estradiol and work like a selective estrogen receptor modulator (SERM). In premenopausal women with normal estrogen levels, phytoestrogens are thought to possess antiestrogenic properties, whereas in postmenopausal women with low estrogen levels, phytoestrogens appear to possess weak estrogenic properties. Phytoestrogens are thought to have select therapeutic effects and decreased adverse effects due to a stronger affinity for the estrogen β-receptor (heart, vasculature, bone, and bladder) than the estrogen α-receptor (breast and uterus). Phytoestrogens may be effective in lowering cholesterol by decreasing total cholesterol, LDL-C, and triglyceride levels. They also may help prevent osteoporosis (with varying results in bone mineral density scores) and reduce hot flashes in postmenopausal women.

The most common adverse effects associated with soy use are gastrointestinal disturbances, such as nausea, bloating, and constipation, and allergic reactions, such as skin rash and itching. In asthmatics, inhaled soy dust and soy hull aeroallergen may trigger asthma symptoms. Because data are unreliable about the effects of soy in patients with breast cancer, a history of breast cancer, or a family history of breast cancer, pharmacotherapy with soy should be avoided or used with caution in these individuals.

The amount of soy that needs to be ingested each day varies depending on the disease or condition being prevented or treated. A typical daily dosage of soy to lower cholesterol is 20 to 50 g. For preventing osteoporosis, a daily intake of 40 g is needed, and for reducing the number and severity of hot flashes, a daily intake of 20 to 60 g is needed. The typical Western diet contains a small amount of phytoestrogens compared with Asian diets. Adult soy products containing at least 6.25 g of soy protein per serving are permitted by the FDA to be labeled for cholesterol reduction when used with a diet low in saturated fat and cholesterol.

Saw Palmetto[11–13,63–65,67,73–75]

Saw palmetto extract (*Serenoa repens*) is used in men to treat the symptoms of BPH. The applicable part of the plant is the ripe fruit, and saw palmetto extract is a mixture of fatty acids, long-chain alcohols, and plant sterols. Saw palmetto is thought to block conversion of testosterone to dihydrotestosterone; however, the exact mechanism of action of saw palmetto in suppressing symptoms of BPH is poorly understood. Saw palmetto improves BPH symptom scores and measurements of urine flow but has not been shown to affect the size of the prostate or prostate specific antigen (PSA) levels.

Common adverse effects associated with saw palmetto are headache and gastrointestinal disturbances. Combination products containing saw palmetto have been associated with a variety of adverse effects, including

cholestatic hepatitis and decreased ejaculatory volume. Saw palmetto may interfere with hormonal and contraceptive pharmacotherapy, and it should be avoided during pregnancy due to its antiandrogen and antiestrogenic activity.

The recommended dosage of saw palmetto is 160 mg twice a day or [320 mg once a day administered orally if a lipophilic extract.] Saw palmetto brewed teas or other hydrophilic preparations may not contain an adequate amount of active components.

St John's Wort[11–13,63–65,67,76,77]

People use St John's wort (*Hypericum perforatum*) for a number of reasons, but primarily because of depression and anxiety. Even though the chemical components of St John's wort have unique pharmacologic properties, they may work additively to produce the pharmacologic effects. The 2 major active components of St John's wort are hypericin, which in vitro inhibits catechol *O*-methyltransferase and monoamine oxidase, and hyperforin, which inhibits the reuptake of serotonin, γ-aminobutyric acid (GABA), and L-glutamate. Data have suggested that St John's wort is superior to placebo, possibly as effective as low-dose tricyclic antidepressants (TCAs), and possibly as effective as selective serotonin reuptake inhibitors (SSRIs) for the treatment of mild to moderate depression. However, problems have been noted in published trials to date, including: (1) too short a treatment duration, (2) inadequate doses of comparative medications, (3) nonuniform selection of the study populations, and (4) variability of the products available on the market, which confound comparisons and extrapolations to the clinical setting.

Common adverse reactions associated with the use of St John's wort are insomnia, restlessness, irritability, gastrointestinal upset, dizziness, vivid dreams, paresthesias, photosensitivity or phototoxicity, hypomania, and mania. To avoid resultant insomnia, St John's wort usually is taken in the morning. St John's wort is an inducer of the cytochrome P-450 3A4 isoenzyme and may therefore decrease levels and/or effectiveness of a variety of medications. Concurrent use of St John's wort with medications that increase serotonin levels should be avoided to prevent serotonergic side effects and the development of serotonin syndrome. Examples of medications that increase serotonin levels include sumatriptan (Imitrex) and other 5-hydroxytryptamine$_1$ agonists, sertraline (Zoloft) and other SSRIs, tramadol (Ultram), and nefazodone (Serzone). Patients receiving quinolones, sulfonamides, and tetracyclines should avoid the use of St John's wort because of the increased risk of photosensitivity reactions. Patients scheduled for elective surgery should discontinue St John's wort 5 days preoperatively to decrease the potential for drug interactions.

In most trials evaluating the use of St John's wort for the treatment of mild to moderate depression, a dosage of 300 mg administered orally 3 times a day of a standardized extract containing 0.3% hypericin or 5% hyperforin was used.

Valerian[11-13,63-65,78]

Valerian (*Valeriana officinalis*) is mainly used by patients who have insomnia or anxiety. The pharmacologic properties of valerian are due to multiple constituents possessing hypnotic and spasmolytic properties. Valerian (400 to 900 mg) usually is taken approximately 2 hours before bedtime to treat insomnia. Studies evaluating valerian for use in sleep disorders have shown improvement in subjective parameters, such as sleep latency, quality of sleep, and global functioning. Valerian may be as effective as low-dose benzodiazepines but may not relieve insomnia as quickly.

Common adverse reactions of valerian are headache, nausea, nervousness, vivid dreams, and palpitations. Hepatotoxicity has been noted with long-term use, and therefore chronic use is not recommended. Many valerian extract products have a high alcohol content. Patients taking valerian should use caution when driving or operating machinery. Patients concurrently taking valerian and ingesting other sedating medications, alcohol, and dietary supplements should use caution owing to enhanced therapeutic and adverse effects. Valerian should be discontinued before elective surgery because of the potential for additive sedation.

Black Cohosh[11-13,63-65]

Black cohosh (*Cimicifuga racemosa*) is primarily used in women to manage menopausal symptoms, premenstrual syndrome (PMS), and dysmenorrhea. Select constituents of black cohosh have been shown to bind to estrogen receptors and decrease the secretion of luteinizing hormone in women.

Common adverse effects associated with the use of black cohosh are gastrointestinal disturbances, headache, and weight gain. Black cohosh should be avoided in pregnancy due to reports of miscarriages. Because of possible estrogenic properties, black cohosh should be avoided in estrogen receptor–positive breast cancer, uterine cancer, and thromboembolic disorders.

For menopausal symptoms, a typical dosage of black cohosh used in the clinical studies was 40 to 80 mg administered orally twice a day. Black cohosh should not be confused with blue cohosh, which is toxic.

Kava[11-13,63-65,67,79-82]

Kava (*Piper methysticum*) is taken in a variety of conditions, including anxiety, stress, and sleep disorders. The active ingredients in kava are kavalactones, also known as kavapyrones. Kava possesses anxiolytic, sedative, anesthetic, and analgesic properties, but the exact mechanism of action for these effects is unknown. Kava may be effective for the short-term treatment of anxiety, as it demonstrates comparable efficacy to that of low-dose benzodiazepines.

Common adverse effects associated with the use of kava include gastrointestinal disturbances, headache, dizziness, rash, and enlarged pupils. Hepatotoxicity has been reported. Kava should not be used in conjunction with alcohol, nor used for longer than 4 weeks. The long-term use of high-dose kava can result in a pellagra-like syndrome known as kava dermopathy and consisting of dry, flaky skin; reddened eyes; and discoloration of the skin and nails. The sedative properties of kava warrant caution in patients receiving related medications or when driving or operating heavy machinery. Similarly, kava should be discontinued at least 24 hours before elective surgery to avoid the risk of additive sedative effects.

The dosage of kava usually taken for anxiety is 100 mg administered orally 3 times a day.

Milk Thistle[11-13,63-65]

Milk thistle (*Silybum marianum*) is taken to relieve gastrointestinal complaints, protect the liver, and help with liver disease and damage. The active ingredient of milk thistle, silymarin, is derived from an extract of the fruit and the seed. Silymarin is composed of 4 flavolignans: silibinin (silybin), isosilybinin, silichristin, and silidianin. This extract appears to have antioxidant and hepatoprotective properties. Silymarin may prevent liver damage from chemicals, drugs, and mushroom toxins. Milk thistle may have beneficial effects, such as improved hepatic transaminase levels and the time to reach normal levels in liver disease caused by alcoholism, as well as improved liver function tests, hastened recovery, and decreased length of hospital stay in patients with liver disease caused by either acute or chronic hepatitis.

Common adverse effects associated with milk thistle include a laxative effect and allergic reactions, especially in patients with allergies to ragweed, marigolds, and daisies. Milk thistle appears to have no known drug interactions.

Most studies of milk thistle have used a product containing a standardized silymarin extract (70%) at a daily dosage of 200 to 400 mg (calculated as silibinin content). For treatment of mushroom poisoning, an intravenous milk thistle (silibinin) product has been used successfully but is unavailable in the United States.

Evening Primrose Oil[11-13,63-65]

Evening primrose oil (*oenothera* species) is used in premenstrual syndrome, mastalgia, menopausal symptoms, and rheumatoid arthritis, as well as a number of other conditions. Evening primrose oil (EPO) is obtained from plant seeds and contains 2% to 16% γ-linolenic acid, 65% to 80% linoleic acid, and vitamin E. γ-Linolenic acid is a precursor to select prostaglandins (PGE_1 and PGE_2) and is the constituent most likely responsible for the anti-inflammatory effects of EPO. Evening primrose oil has demonstrated efficacy in the management of mastalgia and rheumatoid arthritis.

Common adverse effects from the use of EPO include nausea, soft stools, and headache. Evening primrose oil should be avoided in pregnancy due to the potential for related complications. Schizophrenic patients receiving phenothiazine medications should avoid or use EPO with caution due to the risk of lowering seizure threshold. Due to its γ-linolenic acid component, EPO has an increased risk of bleeding in patients receiving concomitant antiplatelet and anticoagulant medications.

The recommended doses of EPO depend on the condition being treated. Dosages of EPO used for management of mastalgia have ranged from 3 to 4 g/d, and for PMS range from 2 to 4 g/d.

Grape Seed[11,12,63–65]

Grape seed (*Vitis vinifera*) extract is taken for the management of venous insufficiency, varicose veins, peripheral vascular disease, and wound healing. It also is a dietary source of supplemental essential fatty acids and tocopherol (vitamin E). The pharmacologic properties of grape seed are likely due to oligomeric proanthocyanidins or procyanidins that possess antioxidant and antilipoperoxidant activity. Grape seed oil is high in essential fatty acids and tocopherol. Adverse reactions or drug interactions with grape seed extract have not been demonstrated.

The usual daily dosage for grape seed extract ranges from 75 to 300 mg administered orally.

Bilberry[11–13,63–65]

Bilberry (*Vaccinium myrtillus*) is taken in a wide variety of conditions, such as gastrointestinal disturbances, visual disturbances, cardiovascular disorders, diabetes, and arthritis. Differences exist between the active constituents and pharmacologic properties of bilberry fruit and bilberry leaf extract. The bilberry fruit and the bilberry leaf extract are usually taken in the form of a tea. The fruit of bilberry contain tannins, anthocyanosides, and flavonoids. Data suggest that bilberry fruit can be used for acute diarrhea and for improving visual acuity, specifically night vision and night contrast sensitivity. The leaves of bilberry contain tannins, polyphenols, flavonoids, and chromium. Some data suggest that bilberry leaf extract lowers blood glucose levels and may lower triglyceride levels. Patients taking hypoglycemic medications and

bilberry leaf extract concurrently should therefore be monitored closely for hypoglycemia.

Common adverse effects from the use of bilberry fruit and leaf extract appear minimal, although reports in animals of anemia, jaundice, and even death resulting from chronic intoxication suggest avoidance of long-term use. Bilberry may affect platelet function and should be used with caution in patients receiving antiplatelet or anticoagulant medications.

Yohimbe[11–13,63–65]

Yohimbe (*Pausinystalia yohimbe*) has been used in sexual dysfunction, cardiovascular disorders, and diabetes. The active ingredient in yohimbe is obtained from the bark and is called yohimbine. Yohimbine is an α_2-adrenergic receptor blocker, and possesses the ability to block monoamine oxidase (MAO), calcium channels, and peripheral serotonin receptors. Clinical trials have shown mixed results for the efficacy of yohimbine in the treatment of male sexual dysfunction. Yohimbe has not been compared directly with other available prescription agents for erectile dysfunction.

Common adverse effects associated with yohimbe use are hypertension, tachycardia, gastrointestinal disturbances, and symptoms of central nervous system stimulation. Yohimbe should be avoided in patients with cardiovascular disease, diabetes, depression, BPH, and kidney and liver disease. It also is contraindicated in patients receiving other α_2-adrenergic blocking medications. Yohimbe may cause additive effects and an increase in side effects in patients receiving MAO inhibitors. Finally, this supplement should be avoided in patients receiving sympathomimetic drugs because of the potential for hypertensive crisis.

The FDA does not consider yohimbine effective or safe for nonprescription use in the United States. Yohimbine is available as a prescription drug in the United States as a 5.4-mg tablet.

Coenzyme Q$_{10}$[11,13,63–65,83–86]

Coenzyme Q_{10}, formerly called ubiquinone, is taken in a number of diseases and conditions, including congestive heart failure (CHF), mitochondrial cytopathies, angina, hypertension, immune deficiency, and chronic fatigue. Coenzyme Q_{10} is a cofactor for a variety of metabolic pathways, such as the production of adenosine triphosphate (ATP). Its popularity as a dietary supplement stems from its role in the production of ATP as well as its properties as a membrane stabilizer and an antioxidant. The proposed mechanism of action for the use of coenzyme Q_{10} in CHF is replacement of coenzyme Q_{10}, which is thought to be deficient in CHF. The effectiveness of coenzyme Q_{10} in CHF has not been demonstrated to be attributable to an improved ejection fraction or exercise tolerance. Coenzyme Q_{10} is possibly effective for improving angina symptoms, improving immune function, lowering blood pressure and blood glucose, and slowing the functional decline in Parkinson's disease.

Common adverse effects that have been associated with the use of coenzyme Q_{10} are gastrointestinal disturbances, decreased blood pressure, and, in high doses, elevated serum aminotransferase levels. Select oral hypoglycemic agents and select HMG CoA reductase inhibitors may reduce serum coenzyme Q_{10} levels. Oral hypoglycemics inhibit enzymes that produce coenzyme Q_{10}, and HMG CoA reductase inhibitors block the synthesis of mevalonic acid, which is a precursor to not only cholesterol but also coenzyme Q_{10}. Coenzyme Q_{10} may decrease the effectiveness of warfarin because of structural similarity of coenzyme Q_{10} to vitamin K.

Dietary sources of coenzyme Q_{10} are oily fish, organ meats, and whole grains. As a dietary supplement, the recommended dosages of coenzyme Q_{10} vary from 50 to 100 mg daily in divided doses.

Melatonin[11-13,63-65,87,88]

Melatonin (*N*-acetyl-5-methoxytryptamine) has been taken most often for management of sleep disturbances and jet lag. It also has been used in Alzheimer's disease, management of benzodiazepine withdrawal in the elderly, and as an adjunctive therapy during chemotherapy and radiation therapy. Melatonin is a substance manufactured endogenously in the pineal gland. The secretion of melatonin depends on environmental light and darkness. Light suppresses melatonin secretion, and darkness induces melatonin secretion. Melatonin levels are low during the day and increase at night around 9 to 10 PM, peaking between 2 and 4 AM. The level of melatonin in the body is thought to decrease with increasing age. Melatonin affects the circadian rhythm, sleep patterns, and endocrine secretions. Melatonin may be effective in decreasing symptoms associated with jet lag, especially for travelers flying across 5 or more time zones; for managing sleep disorders associated with circadian rhythm (eg, blind entrainment); and for treating insomnia in elderly patients. The drug may possibly be effective as adjuvant therapy for cancer and for benzodiazepine withdrawal in the elderly. Melatonin has not been found effective for improving sleep in workers who rotate shifts or who work exclusively at night.

Common adverse effects associated with melatonin include headache, dizziness, gastrointestinal disturbances, daytime fatigue, drowsiness, and reduced alertness. Drowsiness may be experienced 30 minutes after melatonin administration and may persist for 60 minutes or more. Consequently, persons should be advised not to drive a vehicle for 4 to 5 hours after taking melatonin. Melatonin has been reported to induce dysphoria in patients with depression. Women trying to conceive should avoid the use of high-dose melatonin due to pos-

sible contraceptive effects. The effects of long-term administration of exogenous melatonin on the endogenous production of melatonin by the pineal gland are not known. Melatonin is hepatically metabolized primarily and should therefore be used with caution or avoided in patients with liver impairment. The concurrent use of melatonin with fluvoxamine maleate (Luvox) significantly increases melatonin concentrations. Melatonin in conjunction with medications or dietary supplements that have sedative properties may produce additive therapeutic and adverse effects. Melatonin may alter immune function and, therefore, should be avoided in patients receiving immunosuppressive therapy or in patients with autoimmune disorders.

The usual dosage of melatonin for sleep disturbance is 0.3 to 5 mg administered orally 30 to 60 minutes before bedtime. The usual dosage of melatonin for jet lag is 5 mg administered orally at bedtime for 1 week beginning 3 days before the flight.

Flaxseed[11-13,63-65,89,90]

People use flaxseed (*Linum usitatissimum*) for constipation, to manage hypercholesterolemia, and to relieve gastrointestinal disturbances. Flaxseed oil also is taken for arthritis symptoms and weight loss, and as a dietary supplement of α-linolenic acid. Flax contains fiber, α-linolenic acid (a polyunsaturated fatty acid and precursor to omega-3 fatty acid), and lignans. A study of the ingestion of flaxseed-containing muffins demonstrated a 4.6% decrease in total cholesterol levels and a 7.6% decrease in LDL-C levels but no effect on high-density lipoprotein cholesterol (HDL-C) levels. Flaxseed is possibly effective as a bulk-forming laxative due to its soluble fiber content. The fiber in flaxseed also may be responsible for its potential to lower blood glucose levels.

In patients with inadequate fluid intake, intestinal blockage may occur with the use of flaxseed. Anaphylactic episodes resulting from flaxseed hypersensitivity have been reported. The administration of flaxseed and other oral medications should be separated by at least 2 hours, because the fiber component of flaxseed can impair the absorption. Whether flaxseed oil affects platelet aggregation is unclear; therefore, patients should be monitored when taking flaxseed and receiving antiplatelet or anticoagulant medications.

For patients taking flaxseed for the purpose of preventing disease, flaxseed meal (3 to 6 tablespoons per day) can be incorporated into a low-saturated-fat, high-fiber diet, or flaxseed oil (1 to 2 tablespoons) may be substituted for other vegetable oils.

Fish Oils (Omega-3 Fatty Acids)[11,12]

Fish oils have been used in the management of hypertension, hyperlipidemia, hypertriglyceridemia, coronary heart disease, and rheumatoid arthritis. Fish oils contain long-chain, omega-3 fatty acids, which compete with arachidonic acid in the cyclooxygenase and lipoxygenase pathways. Fish oils affect very low-density lipoproteins and have been found to reduce triglyceride levels by as much as 20% to 50%. Additionally, fish oils decrease cholesterol absorption and synthesis and may increase HDL-C levels. Fish oils also may be effective in reducing mortality after myocardial infarction, lowering systolic and diastolic blood pressure, preventing cyclosporine-induced hypertension and nephrotoxicity, and relieving morning arthritic symptoms.

Common side effects of fish oils are belching, halitosis, heartburn, nausea, and soft stools. The long-term use of fish oils may result in vitamin E deficiency because of resultant reduced absorption or increased utilization by tissues of vitamin E. Many fish oil products also have a high content of vitamins A and D. Fish oils should be used with caution in persons receiving anticoagulant or antiplatelet medications, patients receiving antihypertensive medications or prone to hypotension, and aspirin-sensitive patients, as fish oils can decrease pulmonary function.

Dosing of fish oil is usually 1 to 2 g/d for management of hypertriglyceridemia and 4 g/d for hypertension. Fish oils are obtained from a number of marine species, such as mackerel, herring, tuna, salmon, cod liver, and halibut. In healthy individuals, fish oils are best obtained by consuming these types of fish 2 or more times per week. Commercially available fish oil products vary in terms of the amounts of specific omega-3 fatty acids.

Glucosamine Sulfate[11–13,63–65,69,91,92]

Glucosamine sulfate (2-amino-2-deoxyglucose sulfate) is used for management of osteoarthritis. Glucosamine is needed for the synthesis of glycoproteins, glycolipids, and glycosaminoglycans, which are constituents in cartilage, synovial fluid, and other body parts. Glucosamine can influence production of chondrocytes in cartilage and synoviocytes in synovial tissue. Glucosamine is the building block for cartilage glycosaminoglycans. Glucosamine has been found to be superior to placebo and as effective as nonsteroidal anti-inflammatory drugs (NSAIDs) for the treatment of osteoarthritis, although a longer time is needed for glucosamine to produce beneficial effects.

Side effects associated with glucosamine include gastrointestinal disturbances, drowsiness, headache, and hyperglycemia. Effects from long-term exposure (>3 years) are not known. Diabetic patients taking glucosamine should monitor themselves for hyperglycemia. Importantly, glucosamine sulfate differs from glucosamine hydrochloride, with the sulfate and hydrochloride forms providing 47.8% and 81.3% of active glucosamine, respectively. The sulfate form has been used in most clinical trials, and whether the sulfate form is required to

produce beneficial effects is unclear. Glucosamine and chondroitin often are combined in supplements; however, no data support this combination being superior to either individual component.

The recommended dosage of glucosamine sulfate for osteoarthritis is 500 mg administered orally 3 times a day.

Chondroitin (Chondroitin 4- and 6-sulfate)[11–13,63–65,69,91,93]

Chondroitin sulfate is used for management of osteoarthritis. Chondroitin sulfate is a glycosaminoglycan reported to block enzymes that break down cartilage and stimulate the formation of new cartilage. Chondroitin is obtained from shark and bovine cartilage or is manufactured synthetically. Chondroitin has been found to be superior to placebo and likely to be effective in reducing symptoms of osteoarthritis as an adjunct to analgesics and NSAIDs. The addition of chondroitin to analgesics and NSAIDs may allow a dose reduction for those agents. Data are mixed regarding the use of chondroitin alone vs NSAIDs for reducing the symptoms of osteoarthritis. A longer time (up to 3 months) is needed for chondroitin to produce beneficial effects.

Adverse effects associated with the use of chondroitin are gastrointestinal disturbances, edema, and euphoria, and little data are known about effects of long-term use. Patients receiving antiplatelet and anticoagulant medications in conjunction with chondroitin should be monitored routinely.

The recommended dosage of chondroitin for osteoarthritis is 200 to 400 mg administered orally 2 or 3 times a day, or 1200 mg administered orally once a day.

S-adenosyl-L-methionine (SAMe)[11–13,63–65,94,95]

S-adenosyl-L-methionine (SAMe) is used for the treatment of depression, osteoarthritis, liver disorders, migraines, fibromyalgia, and sleep modulation. This naturally occurring molecule is produced by a reaction between methionine and ATP. It acts as a substrate for many biological reactions, such as transmethylation, transsulfuration, and polyamine synthesis. The commercial product is produced by yeast cell cultures. For the treatment of depression, SAMe has been found to be superior to placebo and possibly as effective as TCAs. Also, SAMe has demonstrated superior efficacy to placebo and similar efficacy to NSAIDs for decreasing the symptoms associated with osteoarthritis. A longer time is needed for SAMe to produce beneficial effects than with NSAIDs. Some information suggests SAMe may help to restore hepatic function in conditions such as intrahepatic cholestasis and cirrhosis.

Side effects associated with the use of SAMe are generally gastrointestinal. It has been suggested that SAMe exacerbates hyperhomocystinemia and increases a patient's risk of thrombosis, but further study is needed to determine any relationship. When SAMe is used with antidepressants, the risk of additive serotonergic effects and serotonergic-like effects may be increased. In patients with bipolar disorder, SAMe should be avoided, to prevent precipitating manic episodes.

The recommended dosage for the treatment of depression is 400 mg orally 3 to 4 times per day. For osteoarthritis, the recommended dosage is 200 mg 2 to 3 times a day, and for liver disease it is 1200 to 1600 mg/d in divided doses.

Caffeine[11,64–65,96–103]

Caffeine is used as a stimulant and diuretic, and as an analgesic for headaches. Caffeine is a methylxanthine entity and is structurally related to theophylline. Caffeine stimulates the central nervous system, cardiovascular system, and skeletal musculature. Caffeine is likely to be effective for enhancing mental alertness as well as for treatment of headaches in conjunction with analgesics. Caffeine and caffeine-containing herbs are contained in many dietary supplements used for weight loss. Table 21-6 outlines the caffeine content of select beverages, foods, nonprescription and prescription drugs, and dietary supplements.

Caffeine doses in excess of 250 mg/d have been associated with side effects such as heart palpitations and sleep disturbances. Additionally, caffeine use has been associated with nervousness, restlessness, headache, nausea, vomiting, tremor, hypertension, and diuresis. Caffeine withdrawal symptoms, particularly headaches, are common in persons abruptly stopping intake after long-term use.

DIETARY SUPPLEMENT REFERENCES

There is a wealth of information available on dietary supplements. The question is: How much of the information is reliable and comes from reputable sources or references?[14,104] Health care professionals need to know reputable resources for alternative and herbal medicine and be able to direct patients to appropriate, reliable sources of information written in lay language (Table 21-7).

A variety of textbooks and tertiary databases are available on alternative medicines. Reliable tertiary references for data on natural products should be referenced. Examples of reliable and reputable general references are *Natural Medicine's Comprehensive Database* and *The Review of Natural Products*. Other sources are select secondary references that index citations and articles pertaining to natural products and alternative medicine. The National Library of Medicine's MEDLINE database does not routinely index citations and articles pertaining to herbal medicine. Therefore, a clinician may conclude that no data are available when a MEDLINE search on an herbal product gives no results. Examples of databases that should be used to enhance a MEDLINE search are:

1. EMBASE: 9 million records dating from 1974 from more than 4000 international journals, with citations and abstracts for CAM not contained in MEDLINE
2. International Pharmaceutical Abstracts (IPA): more than 400,000 records from over 750 international journals, with citations and abstracts from articles not found in any other database
3. Iowa Drug Information Service (IDIS): records from more than 200 journals, with index records to articles about drugs and drug therapy in humans

A medical library can be helpful for accessing these secondary references. Many medicine, pharmacy, and nursing journals publish original research and review articles on dietary supplements and alternative medicine. Additionally, both peer-reviewed and non–peer-reviewed journals specifically dedicated to natural products, such as *Alternative Medicine Review, European Journal of Herbal Medicine, Complementary Therapies in Medicine,* and *HerbalGram,* are available.

Patients can obtain information regarding dietary supplements from many sources, including the Internet, magazines, and health food stores. Most information on the Internet appears to be anecdotal stories from individuals or unsubstantiated claims and materials from dietary supplement manufacturers. A study recently noted that comments to patients from health food store employees regarding the use of St John's wort for depression were potentially detrimental to their health.[105] The clinician can greatly help patients by directing them to more reliable information sources.

TABLE 21-6

Caffeine Content of Select Beverages, Foods, Drugs, and Dietary Supplements*

Beverage or Food	Caffeine, mg	Medications	Caffeine, mg
Coffee (5 oz)		Over-the-counter	
Decaffeinated, instant	1–5	Anacin	32
Decaffeinated, brewed	2–5	Anacin Maximum Strength	32
Instant	30–120	Goodie's Extra Strength	32.5
Brewed, percolator	40–170	Vanquish	33
Espresso (1.5-2 oz)	50–100	BC Powder Original Formula	33.3
Brewed, automatic drip	60–180	BC Powder Arthritis Strength	38
		Midol Maximum Strength	
		Menstrual	60
Tea (5 oz)		Excedrin Aspirin Free	65
Brewed, US brands	20–90	Excedrin Migraine	65
Instant	25–50	Excedrin Extra Strength	65
Brewed, imported brands	25–110	NoDoz, Vivarin	200
Iced (12 oz)	67–76		
		Prescription	
Soft drinks and other beverages (12 oz)		Cafcit (caffeine citrate)	20 mg/mL
7Up	0	Norgesic	30
Sunkist Orange	0	Darvon Compound 65	32.4
Ginger ale	0	Fiorinal	40
Root beer (most brands)	0	Fiorinal with codeine	40
Snapple Tea (8 oz)	5–21	Fioricet with codeine	40
Elements by Snapple (8 oz)	32	Fioricet, Esgic	40
Diet Pepsi	36	Esgic Plus	40
Pepsi Cola	38.4	Butalbital Compound	40
Dr. Pepper and			
Sugar-free Dr. Pepper	39.6	Norgesic Forte	60
Coca-Cola/Diet Coke	45.6	Cafergot, Ergaf, Wigraine,	
		Cafatine tablets and	
		suppositories	100
Mountain Dew	54	Caffeine and sodium benzoate	121–125
Jolt (12 oz)	72		
Red Bull (12 oz)	115	Dietary supplements	
		Green tea (1 cup)	8–80
Chocolate		Black tea	10–110
Milk chocolate (1 oz)	1–15	Oolong tea	12–55
Chocolate milk (8 oz)	2–7	Guarana (1–2 capsules or tablets)	200–1000
Cocoa beverage (5 oz)	2–20	Guarana (1 cup of tea)	50
Chocolate ice cream (2/3 c)	4.5	Mate	Variable
Dark chocolate, semisweet (1 oz)	5–35	Cola nut	Variable
Chocolate pudding, instant (1/2 c)	5.5		
Chocolate cake (1/16 of 9-in cake)	13.8		
Baker's chocolate (1 oz)	26		

*Data from references 11, 64, 65, and 96–103.

TABLE 21-7

Alternative Medicine References*

Name	Web Site	Comments
Natural Medicine Comprehensive Database	www.naturaldatabase.com	From the *Pharmacists' Letter* Both print and Web-based version available Information on >250 herbs (names, uses, efficacy, safety, mechanism of action, adverse effects, interactions, doses) Web-based version contains patient education leaflets on herbs Referenced
The Review of Natural Products	www.drugfacts.com	From *Facts and Comparisons* Both print and CD-ROM available Information on >300 herbs (names, history, chemistry, pharmacology, interactions, toxicology) Referenced
The Professional's Handbook of Complementary and Alternative Medicine		Print version Information on >300 herbs (names, source, chemical components, uses, mechanism of action, adverse reactions, interactions, contraindications, dosage, and administration) Patient-friendly version available Referenced (select)
National Center for Complementary and Alternative Medicine (NCCAM)	www.nccam.nih.gov	Exploring CAM practices in the context of rigorous science Training CAM researchers Disseminating information to public and health care professionals Health information, research, training, clinical trials
International Bibliographic Information on Dietary Supplements (IBIDS) Database	www.ods.od.nih.gov	From ODS at NIH Published, international literature on vitamins, minerals, and botanicals >676,000 scientific abstract citations 3 databases available: (1) full IBIDS, (2) peer-reviewed citations only, and (3) IBIDS for consumers
Computer Access to Research on Dietary Supplements (CARDS) Database	www.ods.od.nih.gov	From ODS at NIH Federally funded research projects on dietary supplements
HerbMed	www.herbmed.org	From the Alternative Medicine Foundation Inc Abstracts from National Library of Medicine's PubMed Information on >120 herbs (efficacy, warnings, preparations, mixtures, mechanism of action)
The Herbs Index	www.mywebmd.com	Monographs written in lay language Not referenced or lacks citations
The Natural Pharmacist	www.tnp.com	From Prima Communications Inc Information on >100 herbs (uses, efficacy, dose, adverse effects, interactions)
American Botanical Council	www.herbalgram.org	Education and research organization dedicated to disseminating scientific-based information promoting the safe and effective use of medicinal plants and phytomedicines Publishes the quarterly journal *Herbalgram* Produces *HerbClip,* which provides critical reviews of articles covering research, regulation, marketing, and responsible use of medicinal plants

*CAM indicates complementary and alternative medicine; ODS, Office of Dietary Supplements; and NIH, National Institutes of Health.

REFERENCES

1. Eisenberg DM, Kessler RC, Foster C. Unconventional medicine in the United States: prevalence, costs and patterns of use. *N Engl J Med.* 1993;328:246–252.

2. Eisenberg DM, Davis RB, Ettner SL, et al. Trends in alternative medicine use in the United States, 1990–1997. *JAMA.* 1998;280:1569–1575.

3. Chavez ML. With resurgence in use of herbal remedies, unanswered questions take on greater urgency [editorial]. *J Am Pharm Assoc.* 2000;40:349–351.

4. Bennett J, Brown CM. Use of herbal remedies by patients in a health maintenance organization. *J Am Pharm Assoc.* 2000;40:353–358.

5. Dole EJ, Rhyne RL, Zeilmann CA, Skipper BJ, McCabe ML, Dog TL. The influence of ethnicity on use of herbal remedies in elderly Hispanics and non-Hispanic whites. *J Am Pharm Assoc.* 2000;40:359–365.

6. National Center for Complementary and Alternative Medicine. What is complementary and alternative medicine (CAM)? Available at: www.nccam.nih.gov/health/whatiscam/#d6. Accessed April 2, 2003.

7. Parisian S. Center for Food Safety and Applied Nutrition (CFSAN). In: *FDA: Inside and Out.* Front Royal, Va: Fast Horse Press; 2001:51–112.

8. Tyler VE. Herbal medicine is not homeopathy. *J Am Pharm Assoc.* 1996;NS36:37.

9. Miller LG, Murray WJ, eds. *Herbal Medicinals: A Clinician's Guide.* Binghamton, NY: Pharmaceutical Products Press; 1998.

10. Bormeth A. Assisting the patient who uses homeopathic medicines. *US Pharmacist.* April 2002:32–34.

11. Jellin JM, Gregory P, Batz F, Hitchens K, eds. *Pharmacist's Letter/Prescriber's Letter Natural Medicines Comprehensive Database.* 3rd ed. Stockton, Calif: Therapeutic Research Faculty; 2000.

12. DerMarderosian A, Beutler JA, eds. *The Review of Natural Products.* St Louis, Mo: Facts and Comparisons; 2003.

13. Fetrow CW, Avila JR, eds. *Professional's Handbook of Complementary & Alternative Medicines.* 2nd ed. Springhouse, Pa: Springhouse Corporation; 2001.

14. Miller LG, Hume A, Harris IM, et al. White paper on herbal products. *Pharmacotherapy.* 2000;20:877–891.

15. Landis NT. Consumers want details about prescription drugs; many use 'alternative' medicines. *Am J Health Syst Pharm.* 1999;56:307.

16. Kaptchuk TJ, Eisenberg DM. The persuasive appeal of alternative medicine. *Ann Intern Med.* 1998;129:1061–1065.

17. Palmer ME, Haller C, McKinney PE, et al. Adverse events associated with dietary supplements: an observational study. *Lancet.* 2003;361:101–106.

18. Blumenthal M, ed. *The Complete German Commission E Monographs: Therapeutic Guide to Herbal Medicines.* Boston, Mass: American Botanical Society; 1998.

19. Robin K. New FDA advisory and AHPA trade recommendation on aristolochia. *HerbalGram.* 2001;52:56.

20. US Food and Drug Administration. FDA warns consumers to discontinue use of botanical products that contain aristolochic acid [consumer advisory]. April 11, 2001. Available at: www.cfsan.fda.gov/%7Edms/addsbot.html. Accessed April 2, 2003.

21. Nortier JL, Martinez MM, Schmeiser HH, et al. Urothelial carcinoma associated with the use of a Chinese herb (*Aristolochia fangchi*). *N Engl J Med.* 2000;342;1686–1692.

22. US Food and Drug Administration. FDA warns against consuming dietary supplements containing tiratricol [FDA Talk Paper]. November 21, 2000. Available at: www.cfsan.fda.gov/~lrd/tptriac.html. Accessed April 2, 2003.

23. Hepatic toxicity possibly associated with kava-containing products—United States. Germany, and Switzerland, 1999–2002. *MMWR Morb Mortal Wkly Rep.* 2002;51:1065–1067.

24. US Food and Drug Administration. Regulations on statements made for dietary supplements concerning the effect of the product on the structure or function of the body [Docket No. 98N-0044]. 65 *Federal Register* 1000-150 (2000) (codified at 21 CFR Pt 101-93).

25. US Food and Drug Administration. Regulations in statements made for dietary supplements concerning the effect of the product on the structure or function of the body [Docket No. 98N-0044]. 63 *Federal Register* 23623–23632 (1998).

26. Israelsen LD, Blumenthal M. FDA issues final rules for structure/function claims for dietary supplements under DSHEA. *HerbalGram.* 2000;48:32–38.

27. De Smet P. Herbal remedies. *N Engl J Med.* 2002;347:2046–2056.

28. McGriffin M. Issues of quality: analyzing herbal materials and the current methods of validation. *HerbalGram.* 2001;53:44–49.

29. Grant KL. Patient education and herbal dietary supplements. *Am J Health Syst Pharm.* 2000;57:1997–2003.

30. Problems with dietary supplements. *Med Lett.* 2002;44:84–86.

31. Boullata JI, Nace AM. Safety issues with herbal medicine. *Pharmacotherapy.* 2000;20:257–269.

32. Hasagawa GR. Uncertain quality of dietary supplements: history repeated. *Am J Health Syst Pharm.* 2000;57:951.

33. Gurley BJ, Gardner SF, Hubbard MA. Content versus label claims in ephedra-containing dietary supplements. *Am J Health Syst Pharm.* 2000;57:963–969.

34. Cui J, Garle M. Eneroth P, Bjorkem I. What do commercial ginseng preparations contain [letter]? *Lancet.* 1994;344:134.

35. Hahm H, Kujawa J, Augsburger L. Comparison of melatonin products against *USP*'s nutritional supplements standards and other criteria. *J Am Pharm Assoc.* 1999;39:27–31.

36. US Food and Drug Administration. Herbsland company recalls Ancom anti-hypertensive compound tablets [press release]. January 17, 2003. Available at: www.fda.gov/oc/po/firmrecalls/herbsland01_03.html. Accessed April 2, 2003.

37. US Food and Drug Administration. Natural Organics, Inc., cooperates on the recall of digestive aid dietary supplements because of supplements possible *Salmonella* contaminated raw material supplied by American Laboratories, Inc. Available at: www.fda.gov/oc/po/firmrecalls/natorg5-01.html.

38. Slifman NR, Obermeyer WR, Aloi BK, et al. Contamination of botanical dietary supplements by digitalis lanata. *N Engl J Med.* 1998;339:806–811.

39. Blumental M. Industry alert: plantain adulterated with digitalis. *HerbalGram.* 1997;40:28–29.

40. Seals of approval: what do they mean? *Washington Post.* November 16, 2002. Available at: www.washingtonpost.com/wp-dyn/articles/A64961-2002Nov16.html.

41. Packer-Tursman J. Certified, to a point: seals will gauge supplements' purity, not safety, efficacy. *Washington Post.* November 19, 2002. Available at: www.washingtonpost.com/wp-srv/health/daily/graphics/supplements_111902.html.

42. Traynor K. Dietary supplement bottles may bear new certification mark. Available at: www.ashp.org/news/ShowArticle.cfm?id=3213.

43. Palacioz K. Dietary supplements' seals of approval. *Pharmacists Lett Prescribers Lett.* 2003;19:190112.

44. Cooperman T, Obermeyer W. Do all supplements contain what their labels say they contain? *US Pharmacist.* October 2002:68–74.

45. Vaes LPJ, Chyka PA. Interactions of warfarin with garlic, ginger, ginkgo, or ginseng: nature of the evidence. *Ann Pharmacother.* 2000;34:1478–1482.

46. Tatro DS. Drug interactions with herbal products. *Review of Natural Products* [newsletter]. July 1999.

47. Klepser TB, Klepser ME. Unsafe and potentially safe herbal therapies. *Am J Health Syst Pharm.* 1999;56:125–138.

48. Rosenblatt M, Mindel J. Spontaneous hyphema associated with ingestion of Ginkgo biloba extract [letter]. *N Engl J Med.* 1997;336:1108.

49. Rowin J, Lewis JL. Spontaneous bilateral subdural hematoma associated with chronic Ginkgo biloba ingestion. *Neurology.* 1996;46:1775–1776.

50. Vale S. Subarachnoid haemorrhage associated with Ginkgo biloba [letter]. *Lancet.* 1998;352:36.

51. Schneck C. St. John's wort and hypomania. *J Clin Psychiatry.* 1998;59:689.

52. Walker AM. The relation between voluntary notification and material risk in dietary supplement safety. Food and Drug Administration Docket 00N-1200, 2000. Available at: www.fda.gov/ohrms/dockets/00n1200.

53. Levy S. FDA to launch ADR reporting system for dietary supplements. *Drug Top.* September 16, 2002:20.

54. Blumenthal M. Interactions between herbs and conventional drugs: introductory considerations. *HerbalGram.* 2000;49:52–63.

55. Fugh-Berman A. Herb-drug interactions. *Lancet.* 2000;355:134–138.

56. Scott GN, Elmer GW. Update on natural products-drug interactions. *Am J Health Syst Pharm.* 2002;59:339–347.

57. Ruchitzka F, Meier PJ, Turina M, Luscher TF, Noll G. Acute heart transplant rejection due to Saint John's wort. *Lancet.* 2000;355:548–549.

58. Kane GC, Lipsky JJ. Drug-grapefruit interactions. *Mayo Clin Proc.* 2000;75:933–942.

59. Lilja JJ, Kivisto KT, Neuvonen PJ. Grapefruit juice increases serum concentrations of atorvastatin and has no effect on pravastatin. *Clin Pharmcol Ther.* 1999;66:118–127.

60. Matthews MK Jr. Association of *Ginkgo biloba* with intracerebral hemorrhage [letter]. *Neurology.* 1998;50:1933–1934.

61. Janetzky K, Morreale AP. Probable interaction between warfarin and ginseng. *Am J Health Syst Pharm.* 1997;54:692–693.

62. Taylor JR, Wilt VM. Probable antagonism of warfarin by green tea. *Ann Pharmacother.* 1999;33:426–428.

63. *Physicians' Desk Reference for Herbal Medicines.* 2nd ed. Montvale, NJ: Medical Economics Co; 2000.

64. Robbers JE, Tyler VE. *Tyler's Herbs of Choice.* 2nd ed. Binghamton, NY: Hawthorn Herbal Press; 1999.

65. Tyler VE, ed. *The Honest Herbal: A Sensible Guide to the Use of Herbs and Related Remedies.* 4th ed. Binghamton, NY: Hawthorn Herbal Press; 1999.

66. Heck AM, DeWitt BA, Lukes AL. Potential interactions between alternative therapies and warfarin. *Am J Health Syst Pharm.* 2000;57:1221–1230.

67. Ernst E. The risk-benefit profile of commonly used herbal therapies: ginkgo, St. John's wort, ginseng, echinacea, saw palmetto, and kava. *Ann Intern Med.* 2002;136:42–53.

68. Ang-Lee MK, Moss J, Yuan C. Herbal medicines and perioperative care. *JAMA.* 2001;286:208–216.

69. Chavez ML. Glucosamine sulfate and chondroitin sulfates. *Hosp Pharm.* 1997;32:1275–1285.

70. Blumenthal M. Herb sales down in mainstream market, up in natural food stores. *HerbalGram.* 2002;55:60.

71. Blumenthal M. Herb sales down 3% in mass market retail stores; sales in natural food stores still growing, but at a lower rate. *HerbalGram.* 2000;49:68.

72. Umland EM. Cauffueld JS, Kirk JK, Thomason TE. Phytoestrogens as therapeutic alternatives to traditional hormone replacement therapy in postmenopausal women. *Pharmacotherapy.* 2000;20:981–990.

73. McQueen CE, Shields KM. Alternative therapies for benign prostatic hyperplasia. *Alternative Med Alert.* 2001;1:25–32.

74. Barrette EP. Saw palmetto for benign prostatic hyperplasia: an update. *Alternative Med Alert.* 2002;5:96–99.

75. Chavez ML, Chavez PI. Saw palmetto. *Hosp Pharm.* 1998;33:1335–1361.

76. Barrette EP. St. John's wort for depression. *Alternative Med Alert.* 2000;3:97–101.

77. Burstein AH. St. John's wort and drug interactions. *Pharmacist's Dietary Supplement Alert.* 2000;1:28–30.

78. Marcolina ST. Valerian root for insomnia. *Alternative Med Alert.* 2002;5:77–80.

79. Pepping J. Kava: *Piper methysticum. Am J Health Syst Pharm.* 1999;56:957–960.

80. Ring M, Alschuler M. Kava: curing or causing anxiety. *Alternative Med Alert.* 2002;5:89–93.

81. Blumenthal M. Kava safety questioned due to case reports of liver toxicity. *HerbalGram.* 2002;55:26–32.

82. Hepatitis associated with kava ingestion. *Alternative Med Alert.* 2001;4:60.

83. Greenberg S, Frishman WH. Co-enzyme Q_{10}: a new drug for cardiovascular disease. *J Clin Pharmacol.* 1990;30:596–608.

84. Fuke C, Krikorian SA, Couris RR. Coenzyme Q10: a review of essential functions and clinical trials. *US Pharmacist.* 2000:28–41.

85. Khatta M, Alexander B, Krichten CM, Fisher ML, Fruenberger R, Robinson SW. The effect of coenzyme Q_{10} in patients with congestive heart failure. *Ann Intern Med.* 2000;132:636–640.

86. L-carnitine and coenzyme Q_{10}. *Alternative Med Alert.* 2001;4:S1–S2.

87. Herxheimer A, Petrie KJ. Melatonin for the prevention and treatment of jet lag. *Cochrane Database Syst Rev.* 2002;2:CD001520.

88. Burstein A. Melatonin for shift work insomnia. *Pharmacist's Dietary Supplement Alert.* 2000;1:33–36.

89. Szapary PO, Bloedon LT. Flaxseed and flaxseed oil in the management of hypercholesterolemia (part I). *Alternative Med Alert.* 2001;4:140–143.

90. Szapary PO, Bloedon LT. Flaxseed and flaxseed oil for cardiovascular disease: beyond lowering cholesterol (part II). *Alternative Med Alert.* 2002;5:25–29.

91. Hulisz DT. Safety and efficacy of glucosamine and chondroitin in osteoarthritis. *US Pharmacist.* 2001:40–52.

92. Kolasinski SL. Glucosamine for the treatment of osteoarthritis. *Alternative Med Alert.* 2001;4:73–77.

93. Klepser T, Nisly N. Chondroitin for the treatment of osteoarthritis pain. *Alternative Med Alert.* 2000;3:85–89.

94. Fetrow CW. S-adenosyl-L-methionine (SAMe) and depression. *Pharmacist's Dietary Supplement Alert.* 2000;1:1–4.

95. Fetrow CW, Avila JR. Efficacy of the dietary supplement S-adenosyl-L-methionine. *Ann Pharmacother.* 2001;35:1414–1425.

96. Cada DJ, Covington TR, Generali JA, et al, eds. *Drug Facts and Comparisons.* St Louis, MO: Facts and Comparisons; 2003.

97. Crismon ML, Canales PL. Drowsiness. In: Berardi RR, DeSimone EM, Newton GD, et al, eds. *Handbook of Nonprescription Drugs: An Interactive Approach to Self-care.* 13th ed. Washington, DC: American Pharmaceutical Association; 2002:986–992.

98. Caffeine content in some foods and beverages. Available at: www.softcom.net/users/westa/caffcont.htm.

99. Center for Science in the Public Interest. Caffeine content of foods and drugs. Available at: www.cspinet.org/new/cafchart.htm. Accessed April 2, 2003.

100. Caffeine content of beverages, foods, and drugs. Available at: www.holymtn.com/tea/caffeine_content.htm Accessed April 2, 2003.

101. How much caffeine? Available at: www.myhealth2000.com/tools2/caffeine/table.lasso.

102. What are the ingredients of Red Bull® energy drink? Available at: www.redbull.com/product/ingredients/ingredients01.html.

103. Guarana. Available at: www.gnc.com/health_notes/herb/guarana.htm.

104. Walker JB. Evaluation of the ability of seven herbal resources to answer questions about herbal products asked in drug information centers. *Pharmacotherapy.* 2002;22:1611–1615.

105. Glisson JK, Rogers HE, Abourashad EA, Ogletree R, Hufford CD, Khan I. Clinic at health food store? Employee recommendations and product analysis. *Pharmacotherapy.* 2003;23:64–72.

chapter 22

Complementary and Alternative Medicine

Brent A. Bauer, MD, and Milt Hammerly, DMD

INTRODUCTION

A great deal has been written about the topic of complementary and alternative medicine (CAM) since Dr David Eisenberg's oft-quoted initial study[1] in 1993 suggested that 30% of the US population was using some form of CAM. A subsequent survey in 1997 showed that, by then, 40% of the US population was using CAM and that use and expenditures had increased by 25% and 45%, respectively.[2]

Subsequently, there have been numerous studies,[3-5] both in general populations across the United States as well as within specific disease populations, suggesting usage rates between 20% and 80%. The wide variety of results obtained reflects the major difficulty in identifying a single definition of what constitutes a CAM therapy.

Eisenberg's initial definition identified CAM primarily by what it is not (ie, CAM was defined as those modalities or therapies not widely taught in medical schools, not widely available in hospitals, and not covered by insurance reimbursement). However, in the decade since that original publication, much has changed. In fact, at least two thirds of US medical schools now have some form of CAM education incorporated into their curriculum.[6] Many hospitals have actually opened and incorporated CAM centers as a means of trying to increase patient satisfaction and capture market share. In addition, the insurance industry has steadily been providing greater coverage for a wider range of CAM modalities.

Thus, Eisenberg's definition of CAM no longer holds. Some authors have made a distinction between complementary practices and alternative practices. Complementary practices are those that are used in conjunction with conventional medicine while alternative therapies are used in place of conventional therapy. However, most CAM users do not forgo conventional treatment, but simply incorporate CAM modalities in addition. Therefore, this distinction may not be clinically useful.

Another problem with trying to define this realm is that the field is not static. Some modalities may start out on the "alternative" end of the spectrum and gradually move into complementary or even mainstream usage. For example, this appears to be the case with acupuncture, which now has a growing body of evidence of efficacy in pain management, decrease in postoperative nausea, and other areas.[7] What is CAM today may not be CAM tomorrow.

In the end, all descriptions, definitions, and attempts at bracketing this intriguing realm have their pluses and minuses. The more detail one tries to incorporate into the definition, the more one finds CAM therapies that resist such categorization. At this time, simplicity may be most beneficial, and a definition offered by Steven Strauss, MD, director of the National Center for Complementary and Alternative Medicine (NCCAM), may be best. He states, "CAM is defined as health care practices that are not an integral part of conventional medicine."[8] This has the advantages of being comprehensive and nonjudgmental.

Although exact definitions may be problematic, the definition provided by Strauss allows one to identify most of the commonly used modalities and therapies that the average physician would recognize as CAM. The NCCAM has divided the realm of CAM into 5 broad domains. These include alternative medical systems, mind-body interventions, biologically based therapies, manipulative and body-based methods, and energy therapies (Table 22-1).[9]

PREVENTIVE MEDICINE IMPLICATIONS

Regardless of the definition used, it is clear that a large proportion, if not a majority, of American citizens currently are using or at least are interested in using CAM. This means that every physician will encounter patients in his or her practice who are consuming products or trying therapies that may have either beneficial or harmful effects. This also means that there is a potential chance of interactions with medications or therapies prescribed in the conventional setting. The effects of CAM may range from the relatively innocuous (eg, aromatherapy to help relieve stress) to the potentially toxic (eg, comfrey tea for

TABLE 22-1

Major Domains of CAM*

Major CAM Domains	Common Examples
Alternative medical systems	*Ayurveda,* traditional Chinese medicine, acupuncture, homeopathy, naturopathy
Mind-body interventions	Meditation, spiritual healing, art or music therapy
Biologically based therapies	Dietary supplements, including herbs and high-dose vitamins
Manipulative and body-based therapies	Chiropractic, massage
Energy therapies	*Qi gong,* therapeutic touch, magnetic therapy

*Adapted from National Center for Complementary and Alternative Medicine Web site. Available at: http://altmed.od.nih.gov. Accessed April 4, 2003. CAM indicates complementary and alternative medicine.

chronic stomach problems) to the potentially confounding (eg, the interaction of St John's wort with numerous pharmaceutical agents). For these reasons, every physician, regardless of practice, will need to become familiar with at least a rudimentary understanding of the CAM practices most commonly used in the United States. Physicians interested in a preventive approach to health should pay particular attention to their patients' use of these various products and/or therapies, as the preventive setting may lend itself to an open discussion and education between patient and physician.

Unfortunately, much of the realm of CAM does not lend itself easily to the traditional Western concept of research. For example, the use of randomized, placebo-controlled, double-blind trials as the gold standard immediately runs into difficulties when applied to the discipline of acupuncture. In traditional Chinese medicine, acupuncture is applied only after a practitioner has had a chance to examine the patient, paying particular attention to pulse diagnosis, tongue diagnosis, and other key aspects of the medical history and physical examination findings. Individual acupuncture points (based on that person's unique constellation of findings) would then be employed. It is quite possible for several different patients with the same Western diagnosis to receive different acupuncture points for treatment. Such individualized treatment complicates a traditional research protocol where standardization and reproducibility are considered paramount.

The advent of the National Institutes of Health NCCAM has led to numerous studies being funded over the past 10 years, which are now reaching the quality and stature of traditional scientific research. This growing body of knowledge is finally allowing some statements to be made about the pros and cons of various modalities. The rigorous investigation of CAM, although still in its relative infancy, should bring increasing clarity and direction to physicians and patients in the years to come.

To facilitate the patient-physician dialogue, several of the most commonly encountered CAM therapies are discussed in the following sections. A brief history of the modality or medical system is included along with some basic theoretical background information. This is followed by a listing of conditions that the therapy is commonly used to treat. Finally, the evidence behind these modalities is included where available.

ACUPUNCTURE

Background

Acupuncture has been part of traditional Chinese medicine for at least 2500 years. It involves the insertion of thin, sterile, steel needles superficially into specific locations (acupuncture points) on the body. Once inserted, needles may be manipulated manually or with electrical current. Some practitioners also warm the skin over acupuncture points using smoldering herbs, a practice known as moxibustion. Needles are left in place for a varying amount of time but usually somewhere between 20 and 30 minutes.

Theory/Mechanism of Action

Acupuncture theory holds that there are channels of energy (meridians) that flow throughout the body. This energy (*Qi,* pronounced "chee") needs to flow freely throughout the body to maintain health. The concept of balance and its importance in maintaining health is exemplified by the ideals of *yin and yang,* often symbolized by the familiar circular symbol. Practitioners of traditional Chinese medicine use a variety of techniques (eg, pulse diagnosis, tongue diagnosis) to identify patterns of imbalance of the *Qi.* Acupuncture needles are then inserted at well-defined key points to free the flow of *Qi.*

Commonly Used to Treat

In the United States, acupuncture has been growing in popularity since the mid-1980s. Although initially primarily used to treat pain, more recent experience suggests that patients are seeking acupuncture for an expanding cadre of symptoms and illnesses.

Evidence

The NIH conducted a consensus conference in 1997 to evaluate efficacy of acupuncture based on existing studies. The panel acknowledged the difficulties in conducting acupuncture research but noted "promising results have emerged, for example, showing efficacy of acupuncture in adult postoperative and chemotherapy nausea and vomiting and in postoperative dental pain. There are other situations, such as addiction, stroke rehabilitation, headache, menstrual cramps, tennis elbow, fibromyalgia, myofascial pain, osteoarthritis, low back pain, carpal tunnel syndrome, and asthma, in which acupuncture may be useful as an adjunct treatment or an acceptable alternative or may be included in a comprehensive management program."[7]

Recent studies (subsequent to the NIH Consensus Conference) have found mixed results. One of these found a modest benefit of acupuncture for osteoarthritis of the knee.[10] However, a Cochrane Review found no evidence of benefit for a number of signs and symptoms in patients with rheumatoid arthritis who were treated with acupuncture.[11] It is intriguing that there is a growing body of neuroimaging work that seems to lend credence to the connection between certain acupuncture points and corresponding brain cortices.[12,13]

Preventive Practice Applications

When practiced by licensed and competent practitioners, acupuncture is relatively safe. Minor adverse events have been reported (eg, bent or broken needles, bleeding). More serious events are extremely rare (eg, pneumothorax, infection). The use of disposable needles has largely eliminated the potential for hepatitis transmission. Drowsiness is a common side effect of acupuncture treatments for some patients and, therefore, patients should be cautioned about driving immediately after such a treatment. Drowsiness may be most noticeable after the first experience with such treatment.

Although there may be a limited role for acupuncture as a primary preventive tool based on existing data, patients who adhere to a traditional Chinese medicine philosophy may use it to help maintain "balance" in their bodies. It is important to counsel patients who are considering acupuncture therapy to find licensed and reputable practitioners. They should be instructed to make sure that sterile, disposable needles are used. The patient should be encouraged to set realistic treatment goals and to assess the efficacy of the treatment periodically. If no benefit is noted after 3 or 4 weeks, alternative interventions should be considered.

CHIROPRACTIC

Background

Chiropractic medicine has been defined as "a major school of Western medicine that focuses on the spine as integrally involved in maintaining health, providing primacy to the nervous system as the primary coordinator for function, and thus, health, in the body." Maintenance of optimal neurophysiological balance in the body is accomplished by correcting structural or biomechanical abnormalities or disk relationships through chiropractic adjustment.[14] Chiropractics was founded in the late 19th century by Daniel David Palmer, a self-educated healer who developed the theory that spinal dysfunction was the basis of all disease.

Theory/Mechanism of Action

Chiropractic theory is largely based on the premise that the relationship between the structural integrity of the spinal column and function in the human body is a significant determinant of health. Misalignments (or subluxations) within the spine can affect the function of nerves, which in turn can cause disorders in the organs served by that nerve. The basic chiropractic techniques involve manual maneuvers that typically apply thrust to the spine.

Commonly Used To Treat

Chiropractics is frequently used to treat musculoskeletal disease and symptoms such as low back pain, head and neck pain, whiplash injuries, or muscular headaches. Chiropractic treatment is also applied variably by different practitioners to various illnesses ranging from asthma to infantile colic.

Evidence

Studies of chiropractics to date have shown mixed results. One study reported the results of spinal manipulation therapy for a group of patients with low back pain.[15] No significant improvement in measured outcomes was noted. However, this study has been criticized by chiropractic practitioners because of methodologic issues. Of note, the treated group did require less physical therapy and significantly fewer medications. Another study found benefit in range of motion in gait in patients with Parkinson's disease who received manipulative treatment.[16]

Preventive Practice Applications

There is limited evidence at this time to suggest a preventive role for chiropractic treatment in regard to health maintenance or promotion. Physicians practicing clinical prevention should be aware that their patients may be interested in or already using this popular treatment. Risks are limited, but patients should be cautioned to avoid aggressive manipulation of the cervical spine. Rare incidents of dissection of the vertebral arteries have occurred.[17] Patients seeking care from a chiropractor should search for licensed individuals with good reputations. The patient should be encouraged to set reasonable expectations for the therapy and clear end points to help assess whether the therapy has been effective.

MASSAGE THERAPY

Background

Massage is defined as the "systematic manual or mechanical manipulations of the soft tissues of the body by such movements as rubbing, kneading, pressing, rolling, slapping, and tapping for therapeutic purposes such as promoting circulation of the blood and lymph, relaxation of muscles, relief of pain, restoration of metabolic balance, and other benefits both physical and mental."[18] Massage therapy has been a component of many cultural systems, with initial references dated to Chinese texts from 3000 BC. There are numerous types of massage, including Swedish massage, sports massage, shiatsu, reflexology, trigger point therapy, myofascial release, and Rolfing. Each type varies primarily by the degree of pressure applied or the body region focus.

Theory/Mechanism of Action

There are multiple theories and postulated mechanisms regarding the effect of massage on the body. One such proposed mechanism for pain relief associated with massage is the gate control theory. At the most basic level, the mechanics of massage may aid in enhancing venous blood return and may, therefore, have some effect on reduction of edema. It also has been postulated that the stretch of tissues that occurs during massage could lead to activation of receptors in the skin and subcutaneous tissues with secondary physiological effects. The psychological effects of massage are complex but generally result in relaxation.[19]

Commonly Used to Treat

Many patients seek massage therapy for the simple benefit of feeling good. Others use massage to treat anxiety and stress, aches and pains, fibromyalgia, lymphedema, low back pain, and insomnia. There is also a growing recognition of the utility of massage therapy in hospital practices, where it is used for both patients and their caregivers.[20]

Evidence

Massage therapy has been shown to be effective for decreasing stress and anxiety.[21-23] There is also suggested benefit of massage in patients with fibromyalgia.[24] A systematic review by Ernst suggested efficacy for low back pain.[25]

Preventive Practice Applications

Physicians practicing preventive medicine will encounter patients who are using massage therapy as part of their overall health and well-being management strategy.

The potential benefits of stress reduction and/or anxiety reduction can have a positive impact on overall health. Application of massage therapy to specific conditions (eg, insomnia, low back pain) may also be a useful adjunct in caring for patients.

To help guide patients to qualified massage therapists, consider directing them to the American Massage Therapy Association (AMTA) web site (www.amta massage.org/home.htm). The AMTA notes that there are now 23 states and the District of Columbia that have licensure regulation for massage therapy.[26] The association suggests that patients seek therapists who have graduated from an accredited massage therapy school (with 500 hours minimum suggested). The National Certification for Therapeutic Massage and Body Work examination is an additional credential that is available.

Massage therapy is a relatively safe intervention when practiced by competent and trained individuals. Some care should be taken with particularly aggressive forms of massage therapy when osteoporosis or severe arthritis is present. Some patients report mild muscle soreness or aches following massage, more commonly with the more aggressive forms of massage.

MEDITATION

Background

Meditation is defined as "to train, calm, or empty the mind, often by achieving an altered state, as by focusing on a single object."[27] It also has been described as self-regulation of attention. Meditation is a mind-body medicine modality that has been a component of many major religions and has been practiced for centuries. Analogous to the situation with massage therapy, there are numerous types of meditation, including transcendental, mindfulness, prayerful, and focused meditation.

Theory/Mechanism of Action

The field of mind-body medicine and meditation, in particular, received a great deal of interest in the 1970s as a result of Herbert Benson's work on the physiological responses to meditation. This ultimately led to the concept of the "relaxation response."[28] Benson's original work showed that individuals who performed 20 minutes of deep relaxation twice a day showed a 50% decrease in catecholamine production over a 24-hour period.

Commonly Used to Treat

Patients use meditation to reduce stress and anxiety associated with daily life. Specific applications include migraine headaches, irritable bowel syndrome, and chronic pain.

Evidence

A study of 2000 people who practiced transcendental meditation found that, over 5 years, their health care utilization dropped significantly.[29] A Canadian study looked at the effects of a meditation program on mood and symptoms of stress in individuals receiving outpatient cancer treatment.[30] The patients who practiced meditation experienced less mood disturbance and fewer symptoms of stress. The authors concluded that this program was effective in decreasing mood disturbance and stress symptoms for up to 6 months in both male and female patients with a wide variety of cancer diagnoses, stages of illness, and educational background, and with disparate ages.[30] A meta-analysis of the current literature on relaxation training in patients with cancer also showed significant positive effects for treatment-related symptoms (nausea, pain, blood pressure, and pulse rate). Relaxation training also had a significant effect on depression, anxiety, and hostility. The authors stated according to these results, relaxation training should be implemented into routine clinical use for patients with cancer receiving "acute" medical treatment.[31]

Preventive Practice Applications

Meditation is an increasingly popular CAM modality that patients can incorporate into their health promotion activities. Some use it routinely as a means to decrease stress, focus attention, and promote general well-being. Others use it to seek relief from physical or psychological symptoms. In either case, there is mounting evidence to suggest that meditation can play a helpful role. Fortunately, meditation is relatively easy to learn and practice, and the risks are negligible.

SUMMARY

There are literally thousands of other CAM modalities, with new ones seeming to appear as fast as new Web sites can be created to expound their virtues. The brief discussions here on a few of the more common ones will, we hope, promote further interest in learning more about other modalities as patients inquire about them. Since the realm of CAM is vast, the questions complex, and the research exploding, it is challenging to find reliable information to use in counseling patients. The Resources section at the end of the chapter lists some of the most useful and reliable Web sites. These are recommended because of their adherence to an evidence-based approach, up-to-date information, and reliability. All of the Web sites listed in the Resources section may be accessed without cost and can be an excellent set of resources for the clinician who needs real-time information to help counsel a patient. One proprietary site that deserves mention is Natural Standard (www.naturalstandard.com). Although this site requires a modest yearly fee, it provides a regularly updated and growing compendium of monographs regarding many CAM therapies. Evidence is ranked as to the level of support that exists for the efficacy of a therapy. Information is displayed in an easy-to-navigate fashion.

These are just some of the ever-increasing plethora of Internet resources related to CAM. Quantity, of course, does not necessarily correlate with quality, and there are a distressing number of sites that appear authoritative but are little more than advertising fronts. By developing familiarity with a few of the more reliable ones, a clinician should be able to rapidly find reliable information. This, in turn, should allow increased opportunity for patients to learn about CAM therapies they are considering. By providing evidence-based information and by addressing CAM questions openly and honestly, physicians and other caregivers can help patients make informed decisions. Because CAM has potential risks and benefits, it will require a commitment from patients and physicians working together to ensure that the best choices are ultimately made.

REFERENCES

1. Eisenberg DM, Kessler RC, Foster C, Norlock FE, Calkins DR, Delbanco TL. Unconventional medicine in the United States: prevalence, costs, and patterns of use. *N Engl J Med.* 1993;328:246–252.

2. Eisenberg DM, Davis RB, Ettner SL, et al. Trends in alternative medicine use in the United States, 1990–1997: results of a follow-up survey. *JAMA.* 1998;280:1569–1573.

3. Palinkas LA, Kabongo ML. The use of complementary and alternative medicine by primary care patients: a SURF*NET study. *J Family Pract.* 2000;49:1121–1130.

4. Rao JK, Mihaliak K, Kroenke K, Bradley J, Tierney WM, Weinberger M. Use of complementary therapies for arthritis among patients of rheumatologists. *Ann Intern Med.* 1999;131:409–416.

5. Richardson MA, Sanders T, Palmer JL, Greisinger A, Singletary SE. Complementary/alternative medicine use in a comprehensive cancer center and the implications for oncology. *J Clin Oncol.* 2000;18:2505–2514.

6. Wetzel MS, Eisenberg DM, Kaptchuk TJ. Courses involving complementary and alternative medicine at US medical schools. *JAMA.* 1998;280:784–787.

7. *Acupuncture.* Vol 15. NIH Consensus Statement. Bethesda, Md: National Institutes of Health (NIH); 1997:1–34.

8. Strans SE. Complementary and alternative medicine: challenges and opportunities for American medicine. *Academic Medicine.* 2000;75(6):572–573.

9. What is complementary and alternative medicine (CAM)? [National Center for Complementary and Alternative Medicine Web site]. Available at: http://altmed.od.nih.gov/health/whatiscam. Accessed April 4, 2003.

10. Singh BB, Berman BM, Hadhazy V, et al. Clinical decisions in the use of acupuncture as an adjunctive therapy for osteoarthritis of the knee. *Alternative Ther Health Med.* 2001;7:58–65.

11. Casimiro L, Brosseau L, Milne S, Robinson V, Wells G, Tugwell P. Acupuncture and electroacupuncture for the treatment of RA. *Cochrane Database Syst Rev.* 2002;(3):CD003–788.

12. Wu MT, Sheen JM, Chuang KH, et al. Neuronal specificity of acupuncture response: a fMRI study with electroacupuncture. *Neuroimage.* 2002;16:1028–1037.

13. Cho ZH, Chung SC, Jones JP, et al. New findings of the correlation between acupoints and corresponding brain cortices using functional MRI. *Proc Natl Acad Sci USA.* 1998;95:2670–2673.

14. Jonas WB, Levin JS, eds. *Essentials of Complementary and Alternative Medicine.* Philadelphia, Pa: Lippincott, Williams & Wilkins; 1999.

15. Andersson GB, Lucente T, Davis AM, Kappler RE, Lipton JA, Leurgans S. A comparison of osteopathic spinal manipulation with standard care for patients with low back pain. *N Engl J Med.* 1999;341:1426–1431.

16. Wells MR, Giantinoto S, D'Agate D, et al. Standard osteopathic manipulative treatment acutely improves gait performance in patients with Parkinson's disease. *J Am Osteopath Assoc.* 1999;99:92–98.

17. Assendelft WJ, Bouter LM, Knipschild PG. Complications of spinal manipulation: a comprehensive review of the literature. *J Family Pract.* 1996;42:475–480.

18. Beck M. *Milady's Therapy and Practice of Therapeutic Massage.* Albany, NY: Milady's Publishing Co; 1994.

19. American College of Physicians Physicians' Information and Education Resource. Massage Therapy. www.pier.acponline.org/physicians/alternative/camdi433.html. Accessed September 26, 2003.

20. Rexilius SJ, Mundt C, Erickson MM, Agrawal S. Therapeutic effects of massage therapy and handling touch on caregivers of patients undergoing autologous hematopoietic stem cell transplant. *Oncology Nurs Forum.* 2002;29:E35–E44.

21. Ferrell-Tory AT, Glick OJ. The use of therapeutic massage as a nursing intervention to modify anxiety and the perception of cancer pain. *Cancer Nurs.* 1993;16:93–101.

22. Cady SH, Jones GE. Massage therapy as a work place intervention for reduction of stress. *Percept Mot Skills.* 1997;84:157–158.

23. McDonald G. Massage as a respite intervention for primary care givers. *Am J Hosp Palliative Care.* 1998;15:43–47.

24. Brattberg G. Connective tissue massage in the treatment of fibromyalgia. *Eur J Pain.* 1999;3:235–244.

25. Ernst E. Massage therapy for low back pain: a systemic review. *J Pain Symptom Manage.* 1999;17:65–69.

26. American Massage Therapy Association Web site. Available at: www.amtamassage.org/becometherapist/starting.htm. Accessed April 14, 2003.

27. *The American Heritage Dictionary of the English Language.* 4th ed. Boston, Mass: Houghton Mifflin & Co; 2000.

28. Benson H, Beary J, Carol M. The relaxation response. *Psychiatry.* 1974;37:37–46.

29. Orme-Johnson DW. Medical care utilization and the Transcendental Meditation programme. *Psychosomatic Med.* 1987;49:493–507.

30. Carlson LE, Ursuliak Z, Goodey E, Angen M, Speca M. The effects of a mindfulness meditation-based stress reduction program on mood and symptoms of stress in cancer outpatients: 6-month follow-up. *Supportive Care Cancer.* 2001;9:112–123.

31. Luebbert K, Dahme B, Hasenbring M. The effectiveness of relaxation training in reducing treatment-related symptoms and improving emotional adjustment in acute non-surgical cancer treatment: a meta-analytical review. *Psycho-oncol.* 2001;10:490–502.

RESOURCES

American Cancer Society. Making treatment decisions: Complementary and alternative therapies.
  Web site: www.cancer.org/docroot/ETO/ETO_5.asp?sitearea=ETO. (An excellent source of information, especially relating to cancer.)

Complementary/Integrative Medicine Education Resources, University of Texas M. D. Anderson Cancer Center.
  Web site: www.mdanderson.org/departments/cimer. (Focused on CAM and its applications to cancer but also has information that can be helpful to individuals without cancer.)

National Cancer Institute, Office of Cancer Complementary & Alternative Medicine.
  Web site: www3.cancer.gov/occam. (Contains much background information regarding CAM treatments for cancer.)

National Center for Biotechnology Information, National Library of Medicine Pub Med.
  Web site: www.ncbi.nlm.nih.gov/entrez/query.fcgi?db=PubMed&orig_db=PubMed&cmd_current=Limits&pmfilter_Subsets=Complementary+Medicine. (This search engine limits results within PubMed to articles in the CAM field.)

National Center for Complementary and Alternative Medicine.
  Web site: http://nccam.nih.gov. (There is a great deal of general information on CAM, along with links to additional sources of information. It is a helpful place to start for the novice in CAM who wishes to understand the field in more detail.)

PART 5

Personal Safety and Prevention in Age-Related Groups

chapter 23

Safety in the Home and Automobile

Barbara J. Messinger-Rapport, MD, PhD, and Patrick T. Baker, MSHS, OTR/L, CDRS

INTRODUCTION

Although we tend to associate the gains in health and longevity attained during the 20th century to the great technological developments, such as vaccines, surgical antiseptics, and antibiotics, it is important to acknowledge the contribution of relatively low-technology interventions within the home to the tremendous gains in individual health during the previous century. Pressure to transform personal hygiene practices and improve individual cleanliness began in the late 1800s and blossomed during the 20th century. Health officials targeted poor sanitation, crowding, and inadequate ventilation in private residences to reduce both infectious disease and fire hazards. Cities instituted "water works" to pipe filtered water directly into the home. The US Food and Drug Administration began to regulate the use of insecticides and fungicides on cotton and vegetable fields so that clothing and foods would be safer. Home products also had to be designed to meet certain safety standards. For instance, sleepwear was regulated in the latter half of the century to reduce the morbidity and mortality of home fires. The results of improvements in home and food safety and personal hygiene during the past century were improved child health and a two-thirds decrease in the number of accidental deaths at home in all age groups.

Nonetheless, safety issues in and around the home continue to contribute to morbidity and mortality. Most poisonings occur in the home, and 62% are unintentional. Accidents are the leading cause of death in children and adults under 45 years old, and most accidents in children under the age of 5 years occur in the home.[1]

Additionally, the automobile, which evolved during the 20th century as the primary means of transportation for most adults, is associated with a large number of fatalities. The youngest and oldest drivers are at the highest risk of fatal injury. Motor vehicle accidents (MVAs) account for most accidental deaths from age 5 years until approximately age 75, when fall-related deaths become the leading cause of accidental death.[2]

Thus, the need for preventive measures in and around the home is still important in the 21st century. Physicians play a vital role in recommending preventive health measures to their patients, particularly by identifying persons at high risk of home-related and vehicular injuries and by providing appropriate counseling and referral.

INDOOR HOME ENVIRONMENT

Infection Control

Features of substandard housing contribute to the spread of infectious disease, particularly through crowding. In some cases, infectious disease is spread by lack of safe drinking water, absence of hot water for washing, ineffective waste disposal, pests (insects and rodents), and inadequate food storage. Adults and children living in temporary housing or shelters are particularly susceptible to infectious complications of substandard housing. These complications include transmission of an assortment of respiratory tract and gastrointestinal infections. Long-term-care facilities provide a milieu for transmitted respiratory tract and gastrointestinal infections as well. Transplant recipients and other immunocompromised patients are at risk from aspergillosis in the home or in institutions, or from direct contact with hay, barns, compost, and decaying vegetable matter. Although there is not an issue in general for immunocompetent hosts *Stachybotrys atra,* a mold found in damp ceilings and basements, it has been associated with acute episodes of pulmonary hemorrhage in infants and children, although the strength of this association is disputed.

Improved industrial refrigeration techniques and the ability to transport large quantities of produce to distant locations have resulted in the availability of food products in the home from across the United States and from all over the world. Newly recognized foodborne pathogens have emerged from the globalization of the food supply. For instance, individuals may acquire brucellosis by eating unpasteurized cheese, which they did not need to travel to the Mediterranean to buy; they may have brought it home from a buffet in a specialty restaurant or from a local supermarket. In 1998, a multistate outbreak of shigellosis was traced to imported parsley. During 1997 and 1998 in the United States, outbreaks of cyclosporiasis were associated with mesclun (mixed types of lettuce), basil or basil-containing products, and Guatemalan raspberries.[3] The most common foodborne infectious agent may be the calicivirus (a Norwalk-like virus). *Escherichia coli* 0157:H57 gained notoriety in 1993, when it resulted in 501 cases of illness due to consumption of contaminated ground beef. This bacterial strain, now well known, recurs periodically across the United States. It typically is associated with consumption of a variety of contaminated foods and also was implicated in an outbreak in children after a trip to a petting farm. More information on specific foodborne pathogens and outbreaks can be found on the Web site of the US Centers for Disease Control and Prevention (CDC) at www.cdc.gov.

Other important foodborne pathogens that can cause illness in the home include *Listeria* and *Salmonella*. Listeria can be found in soft cheese, unpasteurized dairy products, and meats such as hot dogs, turkey franks, and deli meats, even when properly refrigerated. Leftover cooked food such as hot dogs should be reheated to steaming hot before consumption, particularly by immunocompromised or pregnant persons. *Salmonella* often is found in eggs and poultry and requires food handling precautions. All knives, cutting boards, bowls, and hands should be washed in hot soapy water before preparation of the next food course. Immunocompromised persons should avoid soft-boiled or runny eggs and should confine themselves to well-cooked egg products. Recipes (generally found now only in older cookbooks) calling for raw eggs, such as Caesar salad, homemade mayonnaise, or tapioca, should be avoided.

Scombroid poisoning and ciguatera are the 2 most common foodborne illnesses in the United States associated with seafood. Scombroid poisoning is a toxin-associated illness that occurs after consuming dark-meat fish, such as tuna, mackerel, skipjack, and bonito, but not uncommonly after other types of fish (bluefish, mahimahi, marlin, salmon, and trout), and is due to bacterial overgrowth with *Vibrio, Proteus, Klebsiella, Clostridium, E coli, Salmonella,* and *Shigella.* The contamination usually occurs during inadequate refrigeration at sea, often off the coast of Central America, and is not necessarily the fault of the vendor or consumer. These bacteria decarboxylate histidine, which is naturally present in the muscle of dark-meat fish, and produce high levels of histamine and other toxins. Symptoms occur within 1 hour of ingestion of the contaminated food. Poisoning may be mistaken for an allergic reaction. Patients receiving isoniazid may be more vulnerable to scombroid poisoning. Ciguatera is caused by several distinct neurotoxins occurring in a variety of tropical fishes, such as barracuda, moray eel,

amberjack, and certain types of grouper, mackerel, parrot fish, and red snapper. Large, predatory fish concentrate the toxin in their organs and flesh, and thus are considered most risky to human health. Fish containing ciguatera toxin do not taste, smell, or appear unusual. Cooking, marinating, freezing, or stewing of the fish does not destroy the toxins. Prevention is by avoiding consumption of high-risk fish. Additional infectious illnesses are associated with ingestion of seafood, particularly if raw or undercooked. These illnesses include hepatitis A, anisakiasis (roundworm), and *Vibrio* species, usually *parahaemolyticus.* Immunocompromised individuals, particularly those with liver disease, are susceptible to *Vibrio vulnificus.* Further information on control of foodborne and other infectious diseases can be found in the *Control of Communicable Diseases Manual.*[4]

Household pets can carry and transmit a variety of illnesses. The young, old, and immunosuppressed are the most susceptible to infection. Transmission of infection can occur in the home, on petting farms, and even during contact with pets during pet therapy in hospitals and nursing homes. Although immunocompromised patients are not necessarily advised to give away their dogs and cats, they are advised to take precautions. Only a person who is not immunocompromised should empty the kitty litter (because of the risk of toxoplasmosis) or clean the fish tank (which may contain *Mycobacterium marinum*). Immunocompromised patients should not own any reptiles, including iguanas, turtles, and lizards, because of the risk of *Salmonella* infection. If contact is made with reptiles at home or at a petting zoo, hands should be washed immediately after contact; children too small to wash their hands properly should have their hands washed for them. Toxocariasis (visceral larva migrans) is not acquired by petting dogs (or less likely cats), but instead by ingesting soil contaminated by the infected animal feces. Children who ingest soil, or any persons who eat unwashed raw vegetables may acquire this illness. Table 23-1 lists these and other pathogens and diseases associated with common animals.

Chronic Disease

Epidemiologic studies have linked substandard housing to an increased risk of chronic illness, particularly pulmonary disease. Damp, cold, and moldy housing is associated with asthma and other chronic respiratory symptoms, even after accounting for income, social class, smoking, crowding, and unemployment.[5] Water intrusion, overcrowding, and inadequate ventilation all increase interior moisture; this, in turn, nurtures mites, roaches, respiratory viruses, and molds, contributing to further respiratory illness.

Exposure to toxic substances in the home may cause chronic illness. Secondhand inhalation of tobacco increases the risk of asthma complications and develop-

TABLE 23-1

Diseases Associated With Household Animals

Pathogen/Disease	Birds, Fowl	Reptile*	Cats Dogs
Viral			
Newcastle disease	Yes	No	No
Rabies	No	No	Yes
Bacterial			
Capnocytophaga canimorsus†	No	No	Yes
Cat scratch	No	No	Yes
Pasteurellosis	Yes	No	Yes
Psittacosis	Yes	No	No
Q fever	No	No	Yes
Salmonellosis	Yes	Yes	No
Fungal			
Cryptococcosis	Yes	No	No
Dermatophytosis	No	No	Yes
Parasitic			
Toxocariasis	No	No	Yes
Toxoplasmosis	No	No	Yes

*Turtles, iguanas, and lizards.

†Formerly DF-2, cause of fulminant postsplenectomy sepsis resulting from dog bite or scratch.

ment of lung cancer. Moderately elevated levels of carbon monoxide from poorly functioning heating systems cause headache; higher levels result in acute intoxication. Lead exposure from ingestion of leaded paints or of water through leaded conduits causes neurodevelopmental abnormalities in children and may be associated with hypertension as well as central nervous, hematologic, and renal system diseases in adults. Although most elevated blood lead levels (BLLs) in adults are acquired in the workplace, exposure in the home can occur during renovation of old homes or from hobbies such as working with stained glass or refinishing furniture. Asbestos from deteriorating insulation can cause chronic lung disease, mesothelioma, and lung cancer. Residential exposure to radon within structural defects in basements can contribute to lung cancer.

Older adults are particularly susceptible to effects of both heat and cold. Cold weather is associated with an increased incidence of fatal and nonfatal coronary events, particularly with known cardiovascular disease.[6] Extreme heat is a risk for elderly individuals, young children, and persons with mental illness and chronic diseases. In the past 20 years, more people in this country died of extreme heat than from hurricanes, lightning, tornadoes, floods, and earthquakes combined. Even young and healthy individuals can succumb to heat if they participate in strenuous physical activities during hot weather.

Air-conditioning is the number one protective factor against heat-related illness and death. If a home is not air-conditioned, people can reduce their risk of heat-related illness by spending time in public facilities that are air-conditioned. Physicians should have a lower threshold for suspecting dehydration and other heat-related illness in their older patients in the appropriate setting. Assistance for low-income households with their heating or cooling needs may be available through federal block grants in their community, such as the Low-Income Home Energy Assistance Program (LIHEAP) administered by the Department of Health and Human Services.

Fires, Burns, and Electrical Injuries

Each year, fire and burn injuries are responsible for a high degree of morbidity. Death rates due to fire are highest in older adults and in very young children. Although mortality from fires and burns is low overall, it is the third leading cause of injury-related death in children aged 1 through 9 years. Reduction in fire-related deaths involves addressing both the causes of fire and the prevention of injury from fire. Cigarettes are a major cause of residential fires and are the leading cause of death resulting from residential fires. A common scenario is the delayed ignition of a sofa, chair, or mattress by a lit cigarette, dropped by a smoker whose cognition is impaired by alcohol or medication. Although "fire-safe" cigarettes have been technically feasible for more than 10 years, they have not been marketed.[7] Flammable holiday decorations or garments (eg, Christmas tree, homemade Halloween costumes) are other potential sources of home fires.

Cooking equipment (eg, ranges, toaster ovens, deep-oil fryers, hot plates, and pressure cookers) is the leading cause of home fires reported to US fire departments. The most common cause of such fires is unattended cooking, that is, food and utensils forgotten on the stove. Older adults who are cognitively impaired are at high risk of these incidents.

Asphyxiation from smoke inhalation is the cause of 75% of deaths due to residential fires. Half of residential fires and 60% of fire deaths occur in homes without a working smoke detector. Standard alarm-type smoke detectors have been shown to greatly reduce the risk of death due to residential fires. There are also special smoke-detector devices with a flashing strobe light or vibrator for the deaf. Although legislation requires working smoke detectors in all existing homes, such laws are not readily enforceable. Community programs to distribute smoke detectors to high-risk homes may decrease mortality and injury from residential fires. Sprinkler systems have been proposed for new homes, but few jurisdictions require them at present. The CDC recommends that every home have a multipurpose fire extinguisher and that each household member practice an escape route in case of a fire.

Although house fires account for almost all unintentional fire- and burn-related deaths in children, most hospital admissions for heat-related injury in children involve scald burns. Recommendations by physicians and community health programs to lower the temperature of water heaters to 48.9°C (120°F) are successful in inducing homeowners to lower their water-heater settings. Water heaters usually leave the factory set at 60°C to 65.6°C (140°F to 150°F). The lower temperature increases the time before a full-thickness burn forms from 2 seconds at 65.6°C (150°F) to 30 seconds at 54.5°C (130°F) and 10 minutes at 48.9°C (120°F). Scald burns in the home, particularly of children, can be nearly eliminated by maintaining the water heater at a maximum of 51.7°C (125°F).

Electrical injuries inside the North American home tend to be low-voltage (110 V), alternating current (AC) exposure. Typical scenarios of such injuries include a homeowner manipulating electrical wires, or a child handling, biting, or sucking on an electrical cord. Injuries may include damage to the central nervous system, cardiac arrhythmias including cardiac arrest, fractures of long bones or vertebrae (occurring from intense muscle contraction or secondary blunt trauma, such as a fall from a ladder), and cutaneous injuries. Internal organs are not generally damaged by electrical current but can be affected by secondary blunt trauma. Acute renal failure may follow rhabdomyolysis or hypovolemia in severe cases.

Firearms in the Home

Death rates for gun-related injuries rise during childhood and peak in young adulthood. Homicide is the leading cause of death in African Americans aged 15 to 34 years, with 85% to 90% of these deaths from firearm use. Firearm-related death is the second leading cause of death in African American children aged 10 to 14 years. Death rates from firearm use decline in all ethnic groups in middle age but rise after age 65 years, reflecting a rise in the suicide rate in older white men.[8] Firearms account for 60% of all suicides and about 72% of homicides. Members of households with a new gun purchase are at about twice the risk of suicide or homicide compared with households without a gun purchase matched for age, sex, and neighborhood. The risk is highest during the first year but persists at least 5 years.[9] There is also more attention being drawn to guns in households of adults with dementia. In one study of 106 consecutive patients referred to a memory clinic, 60% of households had firearms.[10] Of those households with firearms, 45% of guns were kept loaded, 17% were unloaded, and the status of the remaining 38% was unknown.[10]

Handguns account for the majority of deaths and injuries due to firearms in the United States. Depending on the region of the country and the survey technique, between 15% and 30% of all homes contain at least one handgun. Most homicides occur on impulse during interpersonal conflict. The American Academy of Pediatrics (AAP) recommends that physicians educate families with young children and adolescents about the risk of having guns, although the effectiveness of this approach is unknown. The academy's position is that the most reliable and effective measure to prevent firearm-related injuries in children and adolescents is the absence of guns from the children's home and community.[11] There are also many safety devices available in the consumer market, which vary in terms of their ease of operation, cost, and the type of injuries they may prevent. These include loaded-chamber indicators, manual thumb safeties, grip safeties, magazine disconnectors, drop safeties, built-in locks, trigger locks, lockboxes, and personalized handguns. The AAP encourages legislation requiring trigger locks, lockboxes, and other safe storage of guns until guns are removed from the environment of children. Further study is needed to evaluate the effectiveness of these and other safety interventions in reducing firearm injuries and deaths.

Special Concerns for Children in the Home

Childhood respiratory conditions are a major cause of morbidity. Between 500 and 2500 excess hospitalizations per 100,000 young children as a result of respiratory infections can be directly attributed to parental smoking.[12] Reduction in parental smoking would benefit both the parents and the children in the home. Asthma is a common respiratory condition of childhood and is felt to be associated with damp homes (with its concomitant burden of house dust mites). Data are not as clear on whether a decrease in house mites reduces asthma, possibly because improving ventilation and decreasing dampness in homes is expensive and difficult. The Childhood Asthma Prevention Study (CAPS) trial may shed light on this issue after it is completed.[13] Interestingly, children living on farms may have a lower prevalence of atopy and asthma than other children, although it is not clear whether the protective mechanism is associated with farm animals or other related exposures.[14]

Most adults with lead poisoning acquire it through their occupation, but most children with elevated BLLs are exposed to lead at home. Although the prevalence of elevated BLLs (level ≥10 µg/dL) dropped from 77.8% to 4.4% in the past 3 decades, prevalence varies across the country and even within states. In Ohio, for example, the proportion of children with elevated BLLs ranges from 1.3% to 27.3% depending on the county.[15] In 1998, the CDC and the AAP endorsed universal screening in areas where 27% of the housing was built before 1950 and in populations in which the proportion of 1- and 2-year-old children with elevated BLLs is at least 12%. At-risk children are typically poor, non-Hispanic black, urban children living in older homes.[16] Sources of lead include lead pipes, peeling lead paint, surrounding soil from past exposure to industrial toxins and lead-based gasoline, and most recently certain candies and alternative remedies. Hispanic children given greta (lead oxide) for intestinal illness or azarcon (lead tetroxide) for infant colic have been found to have elevated lead levels. Ghasard, a brown powder used as a tonic, and paylooah, a Southeast Asian yellowish-red powder or paste used for fever, also contain quantities of lead. Some imported candies such as tamarind, a fruit or tree pulp from the tropics and Mexico, may contain toxic levels of lead; lead is also found in certain imported candy wrappers.[17]

Drug ingestion is the most common form of poisoning in children. Legislation requiring child-resistant containers for medications and other hazardous substances introduced in 1970 in the United States and in 1976 in Britain resulted in reduced mortality and morbidity associated with poisoning in children in both countries. On the other hand, warning labels have been singularly ineffective in reducing the incidence of poisoning. Many pediatricians recommend that syrup of ipecac and activated charcoal be kept in any home with preschool children, to be used when a child ingests a hazardous substance and after consultation with a poison control center.

Poisoning or toxic reaction to household plants is another safety concern, although few domestic plants are highly toxic. Plant exposures are the fourth most common cause of poisoning, and 86% involve children. The 5 most common plant exposures leading to poisoning are listed in Table 23-2.[18] Two other plants not on that list deserve mention, however. Phorandendron (mistletoe) placed in the home during the holiday season has little white berries with numerous toxins, including cardiac glycosides and sympathomimetics. Ingestion may produce severe gastroenteritis and cardiovascular collapse. *Datura stramonium* (jimsonweed) has been used as a hallucinogenic agent by teenagers and young adults. Additionally, toxic plant resin (such as poison ivy and poison oak) can be carried inside on dog and cat fur and transmitted to susceptible persons, causing allergic contact dermatitis. Toxic outside plants such as rhododendron and wisteria are less of a target to exploring children but can still be problematic.

Special Concerns for Older Adults in the Home

Elderly adults living at home with functional impairments from chronic disease including arthritis, osteoporosis, stroke, and cognitive impairments are at risk of functional decline and substantial morbidity. Home adaptation (Table 23-3) may help elderly adults age in place with a longer and higher quality of life. Adaptive equipment can be ordered from a variety of elder care catalogs, or purchased at pharmacies, medical supply companies, or even department stores. Few

T A B L E   23-2

Common Plant Exposures Leading to Poisoning*

Name	Common Name	Exposure	Symptoms
Philodendron	Philodendron	Ingestion of leaves or berries	Most ingestion is asymptomatic. Some persons have minor burning in mouth and throat. Rarely, laryngeal edema with airway compromise, or esophageal erosions occur.
Dieffenbachia	Dumbcane	Ingestion of leaves or stems; contact with sap	Most ingestion is asymptomatic. Some have minor burning in mouth and throat; some have nausea, vomiting, and diarrhea. Symptoms can last for days. Rarely, mouth and tongue swell. Contact with sap may cause dermatitis.
Euphorbia pulcherrima	Poinsettia	Touching or ingesting sap	Rarely toxic. Occasionally the person may have skin blistering, or nausea, vomiting, diarrhea, and abdominal pain.
Capsicum annum	Christmas pepper	Contact with the fruit or seeds	Irritant to skin and mucous membranes. Abdominal pain and cramping may occur from ingestion.
Ilex	Holly	Ingestion of berries	Nausea, vomiting, diarrhea, and abdominal pain. Ingestion of 20–30 berries can be fatal in a small child.

*From *Vet Hum Toxicol.* 1996;38:289–298.[18]

T ABLE 23-3

Adaptation of the Home for Elderly or Severely Impaired

Area/Activity	Problem	Cause	Intervention
Bathroom	Narrow doorway Transfer to tub or toilet Falls	Limited mobility (arthritis in low back, hips, and knees; wheelchair-bound)	Remove door (use curtain) Raised toilet seat, side bars, grab bars, tub bench, transfer bench Rubber mat, handheld shower nozzle
	Hot-water burns	Increased susceptibility	Lower water temperature to 50°C (120°F) or less
	Poor dental hygiene	Poor dexterity, diminished saliva, caries	See dentist routinely for prophylaxis and extraction Mouth rinses without alcohol Sugar-free candy as needed
Bedroom	Dressing	Poor dexterity	Assistive devices: dressing stick, sock aid, button/zipper aid, long shoehorn
	Falls from bed	Problems with mobility, balance	Move bed against wall, lower height of bed to reduce injury from falls; transfer handle at edge of bed Light switch by bed
	Tripping against furniture	Visual impairment	Nightlight; remove or tack down sliding rugs; furniture should be without sharp corners
	Emergency calls	Cannot reach phone	Lifeline personal help button, cordless phone
Kitchen	Fire and/or burn injury	Inattentiveness to stove	Disable stove (family should contact utility company), substitute microwave
	Falls	Balance problems	Nonskid wax Never stand on a chair
	Access	Arthritis in neck and shoulders	Adjust height of counters, cupboards, drawers Foot lever for fridge
	Managing utensils	Stroke, arthritis	Adaptive cutlery, plate guard, scoop dish
	Dysphagia	Stroke	Dysphagia cup; supplements such as Thick-it
	Identification of utensils	Vision (presbyopia, cataracts, macular degeneration)	Adequate lighting, utensils with brightly colored handles, reduce glare
Living room	Access to chairs	Problems with mobility, balance (hips, back, knees)	Elevate seats, seat lift chair
	Falls	Problems with mobility, balance, visual impairment	Relocate furniture, eliminate sharp corners and unnecessary cords, remove or tack down sliding rugs Remove raised doorway thresholds
Telephone	Access	Limited mobility	Cordless phone, answering machine
	Hearing ring	Presbycusis	Speaker phone, headset
	Dialing numbers	Arthritic hands	Preset numbers, large buttons, voice-activated dialing
Steps	Mobility	Arthritis or stroke affecting back, hips, and knees	Stair glide, lift, ramp Keep second walker or wheelchair at top or bottom of stairs Bedside commode
	Falls	Balance problems (neuromuscular diseases, arthritis)	Handrails at least one side; nail down or remove loose rugs
	Vision	Low vision	Adequate lighting; mark edge of steps with bright-colored tape for contrast; use low-shine linoleum
Homemaking	Laundry: location and access	Limited mobility (lower extremity)	Move machines to main floor; carry laundry in bag on stairs; use cart, use laundry service
	Mail access	Poor dexterity and mobility	Move mail basket to door; adaptive box
	Housekeeping	Arthritis and poor endurance	No-bend dustpan, lightweight all-surface sweeper; commercial housekeeping
	Thermostat	Poor vision and dexterity	Large-print numbers, remote controlled thermostat

Continued

TABLE 23-3

Adaptation of the Home for Elderly or Severely Impaired—*Concluded*

Area/Activity	Problem	Cause	Intervention
Safety	Managing door locks	Poor dexterity in hands	Hook/chain, remote-controlled, lever and crank handles
	Hearing fire alarms	Presbycusis	Blinking lights, vibrating surfaces
	Dark hallways	Low vision	Nightlights, install additional lighting
	Fire	Limited mobility (lower extremity)	Kitchen safety Assess safety of portable heater in winter Multipurpose fire extinguisher Practice escape route
	Emergency (any type)	Limited mobility or dexterity	Activate emergency system (knowledge of 911); place phones in each room; use cell phone; rent Lifeline service
Leisure	Hearing TV, radio	Presbycusis	Amplifier; closed captioning; hearing aids
	Changing channels	Arthritis/poor manual dexterity	Simple remote control with large buttons, voice-activated remote
	Reading	Poor dexterity	Book holder
		Vision problems (presbyopia, low vision, glare sensitivity)	Magnifying glass, large-print books, appropriate light source, "talking" books or newspaper
	Computer	Poor manual dexterity, glare sensitivity	Adaptive keyboard with larger keys, glare protection
	Outdoor activity	Skin and eye sensitivity	Sunglasses, hat with large brim, sun block Skin moisturizer without alcohol or water
	Travel (local or remote)	Medical condition	Medical bracelet or necklace; list of medications, allergies, and medical problems

studies have evaluated the effect of interventions such as home adaptation on preventing functional decline in frail, elderly persons. One recent study demonstrated that a "prehabilitation" program targeting mobility, balance, and home environmental hazards could slow the decline in physically frail elderly individuals.[19] Those who were rated as severely disabled or cognitively impaired (score below 24/30 on Folstein Mini-Mental State Examination, or MMSE) benefited less than those who were rated as moderately disabled. In individuals qualifying for home health care after an acute illness, targeting physical function and psychosocial needs in a multi-modal restorative home care program resulted in improved functioning.[20]

More than 60% of persons who die of injuries sustained in falls are older than 65 years old. Falls are the leading cause of accidental death in adults 75 years and over.[2] Hazards in the home are an important risk factor for falls and fall-related injuries, as are a history of prior falls, cognitive impairment, chronic illness, balance and gait impairment, low body mass index, female sex, general physical frailty, and certain medications such as diuretics and psychotropics.[21-23] Prevention of falls in older adults has been most successful with the use of multimodal pro-

grams. In one study, a combined intervention of a home health care nurse, physical therapist, medication adjustment, exercise program, and behavioral modification decreased the risk of falling by 31%.[24]

Reducing the risk of injury from falls is another approach. Osteoporosis prevention and management in at-risk individuals is important. Another approach to the prevention of fracture, particularly hip fracture, is the use of protective hip pads, which was shown to reduce the risk of fracture (but not falls) among nursing home residents by at least 60%.[25]

Drug safety is a special concern of older adults. Drugs with antihistaminic, anticholinergic, antimuscarinic, or any sedative effects can cause confusion in older adults. Consideration should be given to prescribing medications with minimal toxic effects when taken in higher doses than prescribed. This approach may limit accidental overdose because of low vision, confusion about instructions, or cognitive impairment resulting in accidental ingestion. Although only 5% of suicides involve overdoses of antidepressants, appropriate consideration should be taken regarding prescription of large quantities of antidepressant medications to depressed older adults, given the high rate of suicide in older adults, particularly white men.[8]

TABLE 23-4

Diseases Associated With Outdoors*—*Continued*

Disease/Agent	Reservoir	Locations	Particular Susceptibility	Symptoms
Giardia lamblia	Contaminated water or food; peak prevalence in the spring	Backcountry; day care (fecal incontinence)	HIV	Diarrhea, weight loss May be asymptomatic, self-limited, or chronic
Cryptosporidium	Contaminated water (drinking or swimming)	Backcountry; dairy farms; day care (fecal incontinence)	HIV without ART	Watery diarrhea, headache, fever
Cyclospora cayetanensis	Contaminated food and water	Sporadic cases, associated with imported foodstuff, eg, Guatemalan raspberries	HIV	Diarrhea, fatigue
Sporotrichosis schenckii	Thorny plants, hay, decaying wood, sphagnum moss	Landscapes, Christmas tree farms, rose gardens	Alcoholism, diabetes, chronic emphysema, HIV	Cutaneous lesions, regional lymphadenopathy Pulmonary infection mimics TB
Strongyloidiasis	Soil or material contaminated with feces; direct skin penetration	Appalachia; southeast United States	Immunocompromised, especially steroid-dependent COPD or asthma	Eosinophilia; skin inflammation; larva currens, GI symptoms, cough
Lyme (*Borrelia burgdorferi*)	Gut of infected deer tick *Ixodes pacificus*	90% cases in 9 states (Mass, Conn, RI, NJ, NY, Pa, Minn, Wis, Md)		Fever, rash early; carditis and neurologic deficits late
Rocky Mountain spotted fever (*Rickettsia rickettsii*)	Dog tick (eastern and south central states) or wood tick (western mountain states)	Spring, early summer		Rash, fever, fatigue, myalgias, focal neurologic deficits
Hantavirus	Rodents (mainly by inhaled rodent excreta)	Mainly Calif, Wash, Tex, NM		Hemorrhagic cardiopulmonary syndrome; epidemic hemorrhagic fever
West Nile virus	Bird-mosquito-bird cycle	Northeastern US since 1999; Aug and Sept	Elderly persons more susceptible to neurologic complications	Myalgias, mild febrile illness; encephalitis; meningoencephalitis
Rabies	Bats, raccoons, skunks, coyotes; unvaccinated dogs, cats, ferrets		HIV-positive individuals have suboptimal response to vaccination	Invariably fatal unless postexposure prophylaxis given
Pfiesteria piscicida	Estuaries, East Coast fish	Swimming; eating local fish	Fishers; laboratory workers	CNS, cutaneous toxicity
Bites	Scorpion	Southern US and Calif		Neurotoxin
	Spider	Black widow: firewood, outhouses Brown spider: inside homes in Midwest, south central US Funnel-web: basements		Local, systemic, or allergic reactions. Black widow: latrodectism; brown recluse: viscerocutaneous loxoscelism

T A B L E 23-4
Diseases Associated With Outdoors*—*Concluded*

Disease/Agent	Reservoir	Locations	Particular Susceptibility	Symptoms
Bites *(concluded)*	Snake	Usually *Viperidae* (rattlesnakes in Southwest), occasionally coral snakes (eastern US)		Neurotoxin
"Killer bee" Africanized honey bee		Texas since 1990	Increased risk of anaphylaxis in persons with atopy, particularly young men	Massive stings, seldom death Local and toxic systemic reactions

*HIV indicates human immunodeficiency virus; ART, antiretroviral therapy; COPD, chronic obstructive pulmonary disease; TB, tuberculosis; GI, gastrointestinal; CNS, central nervous system; and US, United States.

OUTDOOR ENVIRONMENT

Exposure to infectious and toxic agents outside the home depends on the activity and the geography. As with exposures to infectious agents in food, travel is not a prerequisite to acquiring unusual infections. A list of both unusual infections that can be acquired outside the home are listed in Table 23-4. A variety of less common diseases, such as insectborne encephalitides other than West Nile, tickborne illness such as babesiosis, tularemia, Colorado tick fever, and borreliosis, or foci of plague in the Southwest in rodents or prairie dogs are not included but can be found in references such as the *Control of Communicable Diseases Manual.*[4]

Nonoccupational pesticide exposure may cause illness in vulnerable populations (children, women of reproductive age), but the extent is not well defined. The CDC's National Center for Environmental Health (NCEH) monitors confined animal feeding operations (CAFOs), particularly off-farm transport of waste-associated nutrients, trace elements, heavy metals, antibiotics, microbes, and antimicrobial-resistance genes. It also conducts follow-up studies of surface water contamination proximal to CAFOs. Other activities of the NCEH include studying a possible association between lupus and environmental contaminants in Arizona, and the relationship between air quality and pediatric asthma.[26]

Pedestrians

In the year 2000, approximately 4600 pedestrians died of traffic-related injuries, and another 180,000 were injured.[8] Fatal injuries occur disproportionately among pedestrians who are young, elderly, or intoxicated. Children are at greatest risk, particularly those who live on streets with high traffic volumes and density, few pedestrian-control devices, few alternatives to the street for play, and a high density of curbside parking. Ethnic differences also exist. African American pedestrians have a fatality rate twice as high as the national average. Alaskan natives and American Indians have fatality rates nearly 3 times as high. Although there has been a 40% reduction in pedestrian fatality over the past 20 years,[8] the reduction is probably not due to preventive efforts. The reduction is largely due to the decrease in outdoor activity over the past 2 to 3 decades. Children who do walk and play outside benefit from environmental modifications: diversion of high-volume traffic from residential areas, lower speed limits, and narrower streets. Counseling regarding road crossing and playing behavior may decrease the rate of accidents as well.[27]

Elderly pedestrians are at increased risk of injuries compared to their younger adult counterparts. Their elevated risk results from visual and auditory impairments; cognitive impairments, particularly regarding the ability to process simultaneous input; and musculoskeletal, cardiac, and neurologic conditions that interfere with walking. Certain aspects of the traffic environment may increase the risk in elderly adults. These include the allowance of a right turn at a red light, which allows cars to turn while pedestrians may be crossing, and walk signals that do not anticipate the reduced speed of an older walker. There is no evidence that programs directed toward either drivers or elderly pedestrians have any long-term benefit in reducing the number of pedestrian injuries among older adults. However, elderly pedestrians may benefit from the same "traffic-calming" programs that help decrease child pedestrian injury and death.

Cycling

Over the past 2 to 3 decades, participation in cycling has declined, as has participation by children in other outdoor activities. In the year 2000, there were approximately 740 deaths due to cycling accidents, and about 660,000 cycling-related injuries treated in emergency departments. Children 5 to 15 years old have the highest injury rates. Alcohol is involved in perhaps up to 50% of all bicycle-related injuries and deaths.[8]

Decreasing death and injury from cycling may require multiple approaches. Helmets decrease the risk of head and brain injuries by 60% to 90%, according to numerous studies. Despite these statistics, fewer than 20% of children and adults use helmets all or most of the time. If universally worn by children, helmets would prevent 135 to 155 deaths, 39,000 to 45,000 head injuries, and 18,000 and 55,000 injuries of the scalp and face, respectively, each year.[28] Other approaches to risk reduction, such as separate lanes for bicycles, are appealing but have not thus far been shown to decrease the risk of injury. Traffic-calming interventions, to decrease pedestrian injury and fatality, would concomitantly improve safety for cyclists.

Motorcycles

Motorcycle fatalities have decreased over the past 2 decades, but remain a major problem. In 2000 there were 2700 motorcyclist fatalities and 197,000 nonfatal injuries, with the highest fatality rates among 20- to 40-year-old black men.[8] The US age-adjusted fatality rates declined by 56% from 1981 to 1998, but among African Americans fatality declined by only 32%. Most serious or fatal injuries involve the head. Other injury sites common in motorcyclists include the neck and lower extremities.

Helmet use is strongly associated with a decreased probability and severity of injury in a motorcycle accident.[29] Alcohol and illicit drugs appear to be associated with motorcycle accidents, particularly in motorcyclists not wearing a helmet. Drug and alcohol counseling and efforts at reducing use of these substances may indirectly decrease motorcycle crash and injury rates.

Boating

Both the US Coast Guard and the National Transportation Safety Board recommend that boaters wear personal flotation devices (life vests). However, very few adults—approximately 14%—who participate in recreational boating actually wear these vests. Among drowning victims, about 85% were not wearing life vests, and an estimated 85% of those persons might have survived had they worn the vests. Recent alcohol use also is associated with 25% to 50% of persons who drown.[30] Therefore, counseling boaters about avoidance of alcohol consumption and the benefits of life vests is encouraged. Although

it seems reasonable to believe that the ability to swim may provide protection from drowning, the size of the benefit is unknown. Exposure to aquatic environments, risk-taking behavior, and alcohol use appear to be the strongest predictors of risk of drowning.[31]

Special Concerns of Children Outside the Home

Each year in the United States, emergency departments treat more than 200,000 children aged 14 and younger for playground-related injuries. Although 75% of nonfatal injuries related to playground equipment occur on public playgrounds, 70% of deaths from playground-related injuries occur on home playgrounds. The 2 most frequent causes of death in these cases are strangulation and falls.[32]

Drowning is second only to MVAs as the leading cause of injury-related death for children.[26] Access to unsupervised or inadequately supervised swimming pools is associated with drownings in older children. Half of drownings in young children occur at the child's own home. For infants, the bathtub is a common site for drowning. Alcohol is a major contributing factor in up to 50% of drownings among adolescent boys.[33]

Lightning

Lightning injuries affect 800 to 1000 persons each year, with 75 to 150 deaths per year.[34] Although lightning strikes always are generated by and connected to a thundercloud, lightning can strike up to 10 miles away from the edge of a thunderstorm. Farmers used to be the ones most often struck by lightning, but recreation-related lightning injuries are now more frequent. Also, while most lightning injuries occur outside, injury can occur within the home, for instance, while using the telephone or working on plumbing. In these situations, the effect of energy from ground current transmitted into the structure along wires or pipes finds a person a better conduit to ground. Preventive counseling by physicians can include advice to seek shelter in a substantial building or a completely enclosed metal vehicle during an electrical storm, and to avoid being the highest object, close to a high object, or connected to one during a storm. Outdoor or at-risk activity should not be resumed until 30 minutes after the last flash of lightning or sound of thunder.[35]

Natural Disasters

The greatest natural disaster in US history occurred on September 8, 1900, when a hurricane struck Galveston, Tex, killing more than 6000 people. Fortunately, hurricane forecasting, emergency response plans, evacuation procedures, and training of public health workers improved during the 20th century. In 1992, although Hurricane

Andrew caused an estimated $20 billion in property damage in Florida and Louisiana, the human toll was 41. The loss of human life from natural disasters such as floods, tornadoes, hurricanes, forest fires, and earthquakes has been greatly reduced. On a national level, the CDC's Division of Emergency and Environmental Health Services (EEHS) provides national leadership for coordinating, delivering, and evaluating emergency and environmental health services. Emergencies include natural disasters as well as civil strife, famine, and acts of terrorism. The EEHS established and maintains the National Pharmaceutical Stockpile Program, designed to ensure the rapid deployment of lifesaving pharmaceuticals in the event of terrorist attacks. Adequate preparation is key to reducing morbidity and mortality from natural disasters.

Physicians should know the emergency procedures established in their communities and remind homeowners to prepare a personal family action plan. Typical recommendations include keeping emergency supplies on hand, such as extra food, water, and battery-operated radios and flashlights. Persons should be encouraged to heed evacuation orders and follow the suggested routes. The health department of each state provides a health response network for assistance during natural and manmade disasters. Links are available from the CDC Web site to each state health department and include documents to download and 24-hour emergency phone numbers. They are useful for physicians and for all concerned individuals.

After a natural disaster, individuals should return to their homes only when public announcements indicate the area is considered safe. Downed power lines should be reported to the utility company. Typical hazards include structural damage, live electrical wires, gas leaks, and contaminated water and food supplies. The weeks after a natural disaster are usually physically and emotionally draining. Stress management techniques are helpful, including reminders to patients to rest. While some sleeplessness, anxiety, anger, hyperactivity, mild depression, or lethargy is normal, extreme or prolonged symptoms may need to be treated or referred appropriately.

AUTOMOBILE SAFETY

Despite the proliferation of motor vehicles and the increase in number of miles traveled during the past century, motor vehicle safety has improved. The annual death rate has declined from 18 per 100 million vehicle miles traveled (VMT) in 1925 to 1.7 per 100 million VMT—a 90% decrease.[36] Systematic motor vehicle safety efforts during the past 40 years have had a major impact in motor vehicle safety improvement. Safety features implemented in vehicles over the years include headrests, energy-absorbing steering wheels, shatter-resistant windshields, and safety belts. Environmental changes include better delineation of curves, use of breakaway sign and utility poles, improved illumination, addition of barriers

separating oncoming traffic lanes, and guardrails. Front air bags and, in some vehicles, side air bags have been implemented to supplement seat belts. Legislative issues involving vehicle inspections, driver licensing and testing, and driving while intoxicated (DWI) have made the roads safer as well. Changes in health education that may contribute to reduced morbidity and mortality after a motor vehicle crash include development and dissemination of Advanced Trauma Life Support (ATLS).

However, MVAs are still the leading cause of death due to injury in children and in young and middle-aged adults. Motor vehicle crashes are also the third leading cause of years of potential life lost before age 65 years, behind cancer and heart disease. In 2000, there were 43,354 motor vehicle fatalities, and 3.36 million persons injured in MVAs.[8] There are some regional and vehicular factors, with higher motor vehicle death rates in the Southeast and in scattered western states. The highest rates of vehicular fatalities are in the youngest and oldest drivers, their passengers, and in all who drive under the influence of alcohol (DWI) or as a passenger of a car driven by someone under the influence.

Medical Conditions

Medical conditions may compromise driving ability and/or increase the fatality rate in adults of all ages. Many chronic medical conditions and visual problems can alter driving ability, as can medications and surgical procedures. Selected medical and surgical conditions that may affect driving are listed in Table 23-5.

Alcohol Use

Approximately 40% of motor vehicle fatalities are associated with the use of alcohol.[37] Intoxicated drivers have an increased risk of injury because their driving skills are impaired, they are less likely to use seat belts, and are more likely to speed than are nonintoxicated drivers. The risk of a fatal or nonfatal injury from a motor vehicle crash increases with the severity of the alcohol-related problem.

There has been a multidisciplinary effort over the years to reduce alcohol-related injuries. Interventions include increased penalties for DWI, changes in attitudes of law enforcement personnel and the courts, and changes in the attitudes of the public due to grassroots efforts such as Mothers Against Drunk Driving. In 2000, a national conference developed a set of best practices of emergency care for the alcohol-impaired patient.[38] This conference identified paramedics, nurses, and physicians as critical links to optimal care for the patient who was DWI. Goals for emergency physicians involved screening for use of alcohol, providing brief intervention for patients who screen positive for alcohol, being aware of state laws and need to report alcohol use problems in accordance with these laws,

TABLE 23-5

Selected Common Conditions or Illnesses That Affect Driving*

Condition	Specific Problem	Limitation to Driving
Vision	Acuity	Varies between states, usually 20/40 or 20/50. Assessment by DRS if best-corrected VA <20/70. More than half the states permit bioptic lenses mounted on glasses; safety has not been established.
	Cataracts	No restriction if standards for VA and field of vision are met
	Monocular vision	Should not drive for 3 mo after loss of binocular vision. May then drive if remaining eye has adequate VA and mirrors are placed on both sides of vehicle.
	Poor night vision	Physician can recommend that patient not drive at night or in low-light conditions (eg, storms)
	Postsurgical	Usually 4 wk after any surgery that affects vision
	Hemianopia or quadrantanopia	Requires on-road assessment performed by DRS; may require rehabilitation and vehicular adaptation
Hearing	Deafness	May require additional external mirror. In general, no restriction.
Cardiac	Rhythm disorder (ventricular tachycardia, ventricular fibrillation, or nonsustained ventricular tachycardia)	Symptom-free for 3–6 mo depending on condition and intervention
	Pacemaker placement	1 wk if ECG shows normal sensing and capture and patient no longer experiences presyncope or syncope
Central nervous system disease	Stroke with sensory, motor, visual, or cognitive impairment	Requires on-road assessment performed by DRS; may require rehabilitation and vehicular adaptation. Stroke patients with aphasia but demonstrated safe driving ability may require exemption from written examination.
	Transient ischemic attack	No driving until medical assessment and appropriate treatment
	Seizure disorder	Depends on state laws. In general, no driving until seizure-free for 3 mo. Shorter period with physician approval, longer period with unfavorable modifiers (alcohol and/or drug abuse, structural brain lesion, noncorrectable metabolic condition).
	Narcolepsy	Driving cessation upon diagnosis. Resumption after effective treatment. Consider objective scoring tool such as Epworth Sleepiness Scale.
Musculoskeletal	Cervical spine limitations	May require special wide-angle mirrors and training in use
	Thoracic spine limitations	May require special wide-angle mirror, raised seat, and seat-belt adaptation, plus training in use
	Loss of extremity	Cannot use artificial limbs on foot pedals (no sensory feedback). Patient may require specialized hand controls in place of pedals, plus training in use.

*DRS indicates driver rehabilitation specialist; VA, visual acuity; and ECG, electrocardiogram. From Wang C, Kosinski C, Schwartzberg J, Shanklin A. *The Physician's Guide to Assessing and Counseling Older Drivers.* Washington, DC: National Highway Traffic Safety Administration; 2003. Available at: www.ama-assn.org/go/olderdrivers.

advocating for appropriate public policy, and working to improve care of patients with alcohol use problems.[38]

In 2001, the CDC released a systematic review of blood alcohol concentrations (BAC) and motor vehicle injury, and strongly recommended lowering the BAC laws from 0.1% to 0.08%. States were expected to comply by October 2003 or risk losing federal highway construction funds.[39] Brief screening for and counseling of high-risk drinkers by physicians or nurse practitioners have been

shown to be effective in reducing alcohol intake.[40] Patients who are found to be alcohol dependent and driving or have an alcohol-related injury should be referred for counseling and alcohol-dependency treatment.

Efforts to reduce alcohol-related auto injuries have had some success. The number of alcohol-related deaths decreased by one third to about 17,500 over the past 20 years. However, decreasing alcohol-associated injury and death remains an ongoing challenge. Despite the multiple interventions, the number of deaths has only stabilized or even increased lately in some states.

Young Drivers and Passengers

Among the resident population, the 2 age groups of highest risk to traffic safety are the 15- to 24-year-olds and individuals over 70 years of age. The 15- to 24-year-olds are estimated to make up about 14% of the population, but account for about 24% of traffic fatalities.

The primary safety issues related to drivers between the ages of 15 and 24 years are inexperience, immaturity, and risk taking. Accidents in younger drivers are associated with alcohol and high speeds. The risk of accidents in newly graduated drivers transporting persons under the age of 20 years is particularly high.[41] The restriction of new drivers from transporting young passengers would reduce fatalities in this age group by 7% to 42%.[42]

Effective methods to restrain dangerous, impulsive, and/or risky behaviors have traditionally concentrated on law enforcement, license restriction or denial, or other aversive controls. The effectiveness of these approaches is limited by the resources that communities can devote to them. The National Highway and Traffic Safety Association has a variety of research initiatives and programmatic activities directed at younger drivers. Physicians can contribute by counseling young drivers regarding alcohol use, seat belts, minimizing distraction in the vehicle such as multiple passengers, and observation of posted speed limits. Physicians also can counsel adults to place their children younger than 12 years in the back seat with proper restraints.

Minority subgroups appear to have increased morbidity and mortality from auto accidents. A study examining motor vehicle fatality rates found that, although black and Hispanic male teenagers travel fewer vehicle miles than their white counterparts, they are nearly twice as likely to die in a motor vehicle crash. Per vehicle mile, black children aged 5 through 12 years face a risk of dying in a motor vehicle crash that is almost 3 times as great as white children.[43] In 2001, some 771,000 African Americans were treated for motor vehicle injuries, at a rate of 20 per 1000 persons compared with 7 per 1000 persons for whites.[8] Reasons for this difference are unclear but may reflect differences in restraint use (safety belts and position of infant seats), vehicle condition, road surface, alcohol use, and vehicular speed.

Older Drivers and Passengers

The US Census Bureau reported an increase in population by about 17.7% overall during the years from 1981 to 1998. During that time, the older segment of the population grew almost twice as fast as the general population. The 12.7% of the US population over the age of 65 years accounts for approximately 11% of motor vehicle injuries and 19% of all motor vehicle deaths. Although the crash involvement of older drivers is low compared with other age groups, the fatality rate increases sharply with age in older subgroups, whether the analysis is per driver or per mile driven (Figs 23-1 to 23-3).

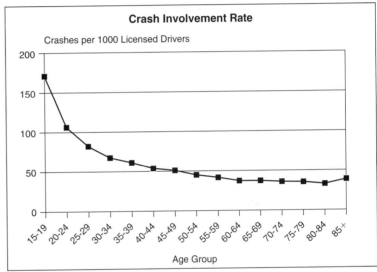

FIGURE 23-1

Older adults have a low crash involvement rate. Age is in years.

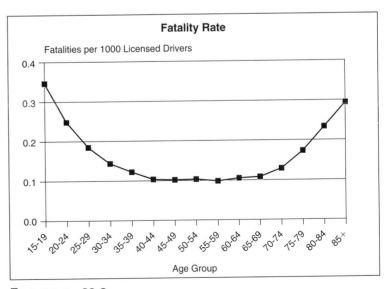

FIGURE 23-2

Fatality rate is high in oldest and youngest drivers.

Accidents in older drivers are, in contrast with younger adults, generally associated with low speeds and the absence of alcohol. Accidents involving older adults are more likely to involve multiple vehicles, occur at an intersection, during the day, and close to home.[44] However, it is important to remember that although the prevalence of driving difficulties increases with age, "at-risk" and "older" are not synonymous. Visual, cognitive, and physical problems can occur at any age and complicate the driving task. Similarly, old age alone does not equal poor driving. The increased fatality of crashes in older adults compared with younger adults is attributed to their frailty, decreased bone density, increased potential for multiorgan failure and sepsis resulting from a trauma, and the increased morbidity and mortality of a head injury in an older person compared with a young or middle-aged adult. Trauma research shows that older adults are 5 to 6 times more likely to die of a comparable injury than are younger adults with the same degree of injury.[45]

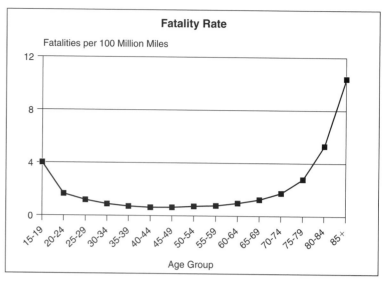

FIGURE 23-3

Fatality rate per mile driven is highest in oldest drivers. From National Highway Traffic Safety Administration. *Older Road User Research Plan.* Washington, DC: National Highway Traffic Safety Administration. Available at: www.nhtsa.dot.gov/PEOPLE/injury/olddrive/pub/Chapter1.html. Accessed January 25, 2003.

Effect of aging on driving ability

Age-related social, biological, and medical changes that occur with aging may influence driving patterns, skills, and ultimately safety. Driving is an important instrumental activity of daily living (ADL) in the United States because of the lack of alternative transportation as well as the symbolic nature of driving as a display of independence, financial means, and personality. As the number of older individuals increases, so does the number of older drivers. Currently, fewer older women drive than do older men. Some women permitted their skills to lapse or relinquished their license over the years; many never learned to drive at all. However, the proportion of women who drive is increasing, and as the current baby boomers age, all older men and women are expected to be licensed. Much of the research on aging and driving has focused on sensory and motor changes, including vision, hearing, mobility, and reaction time.

Approximately 90% of the information required for driving is acquired visually. Changes in visual function with age include decreased static and dynamic visual acuity, decreased temporal fields, decreased resistance to glare, and reduced vision in low luminescence. Dynamic visual acuity (the ability to discriminate an object when there is relative movement between the object and observer) and lateral-motion detection decline earlier and more rapidly than static vision Most studies have failed to show a consistent relationship between vision and recorded crashes, however. It is possible that many of the studies did not take into account the complexity of visual functioning and relied on only one particular test of vision. Static vision alone, for instance, is used in most states' visual assessment for license renewal but is not a particularly good predictor of crashes.

Hearing impairments begin around age 40 years and increase sharply after age 60. Although one would assume that hearing loss would decrease perception of traffic patterns and driving risks, research outcomes are again mixed regarding the association between impaired hearing and injury. Individuals with hearing loss tend to compensate for their disability with increased visual attentiveness, which may lower their driving risk to baseline. Trunk and neck mobility, range of motion of extremities, and strength all decline with age, and reaction time and motor response times increase with age. It is controversial whether proprioception declines with age. Although there are age-related decrements in the sensory, central processing, and motor components of reaction time, these changes do not appear to greatly affect driving risk in otherwise healthy older drivers.

Central processing skills, which decline with age, include performance on divided attention tasks and the ability to focus selectively and to switch attention. More recent research, however, has focused on higher levels of functioning, such as perception rather than sensory processing, and attention rather than reaction times or motor speed. The useful field of view, for instance, measures the area in the visual field over which information can be acquired during a brief glance and thus incorporates both sensory input and perception. This test has been found in one study to be the strongest predictor of vehicle crashes rather than direct measurements of ocular health or visual functioning.

Evidence suggests that the skills putatively relevant to safe driving do deteriorate with age. However, the physiological changes that occur with age are both complex and variable across time and among individuals. A deficit in one area may be compensated for by increased skill in another area. Older drivers can thus maintain their skill and safety by both conscious and subconscious adaptation.

Adaptive strategies

Older drivers tend to reduce their exposure by driving less and by avoiding driving in situations that are generally believed to be more difficult (eg, rain, night, heavy traffic, rush hour). Adults with visual or cognitive impairments are particularly noted to self-regulate.[46] Other adaptations are social in nature. Older couples sometimes direct and assist each other in driving. The passenger, often the wife, may often navigate, read signs, assist in hazard detection, and remind the driver of tasks. It has never been proved, however, that this "pilot-navigator" adaptation decreases the risk associated with a driver who has decreased cognitive ability.

Medical illness and older adults

Medically compromised drivers make up a substantial subset of drivers who crash, especially when the crash involves an older driver. Identifying those older adults whose abilities have been compromised to an unsafe level, rather than targeting the entire older population, is both appropriate and more likely to be effective. Chronic medical illness is more commonly seen in older adults (see Table 23-5).

A potentially high-risk group of older drivers are those with a dementing illness. Alzheimer's disease, the most common form of dementia, has a prevalence of 3% in adults aged 65 to 74 years and increases to 47% by age 85.[47] Earliest cognitive symptoms include difficulties in recent memory, word finding, naming, orientation, and concentration. Over time, information processing becomes slow, and there are attentional deficits, disturbances in executive function, impairments in language, perception, and praxis. Both social and occupational functioning are involved. Although driving risk may be minimal very early in the disease, driving ability declines over time in all persons with Alzheimer's disease. Many patients will, however, continue to drive too long after the onset of their illness.

Although it is generally well accepted that demented patients who drive, as a group, pose substantial safety problems, clear guidelines for identification and evaluation of the at-risk drivers within this group are lacking.

The diagnosis itself, or the score on the Folstein MMSE, are not adequate predictors and should not prejudice the licensing bureau against the nearly one third of drivers with a dementing illness who are competent to drive in the early stages of their illness.

Assessing and counseling the impaired older driver

An older person who is suspected of having difficulty driving needs a thorough but targeted history and examination. History should include changes in habits or personality, chronic medical conditions and medication use, alcohol use, prior history of accidents and/or DWI, and functional limitations in any ADL or instrumental ADL. Physical examination should include vision, hearing, range of motion and strength, neurological integrity, cognition, and pain. Adjunct studies may include a metabolic workup for dementia and targeted imaging studies.

A formal driving evaluation program run by a certified occupational therapist can measure the effect of specific cognitive or physical deficits on driving. Medicare does reimburse for this type of program under specific diagnoses and with a prescription. Recommendations of the occupational therapist may include resumption of driving with no restrictions, having the vehicle fitted with adaptive equipment, a rehabilitation program, or refraining from driving. Each physician should also know the laws of his or her state. For example, during the last decade, California has included Alzheimer's disease under the "lapse of consciousness" heading, requiring a report of the diagnosis to the Bureau of Motor Vehicles in that state.

It is difficult to counsel a patient regarding driving behavior. Persons who relinquish driving privileges suffer a sense of loss. Driving cessation threatens self-esteem and personal dignity. It also implies social disability and dependency. If one spouse must stop driving and the other spouse never learned to drive or no longer drives, the mobility of the family unit may be threatened. Preventive counseling for a couple might include suggesting that they share the driving to maintain their skill level.

The resources at the end of the chapter contain Web sites with information useful in assessing and counseling older drivers.

SUMMARY

The challenges of home and auto safety in the 21st century are many but perhaps can be condensed for physician purposes to the following:

1. The need to maintain safety while teaching independence to children (poisoning, fires and burns, drowning, car accidents).

2. The need for ongoing counseling of young adults regarding risky behavior (eg, high speeds) and alcohol intake plus encouragement of use of appropriate protective items (life vest, helmets, safety belts, etc) to reduce accidents while cycling, walking, swimming, boating, and driving. Counseling may need to be adapted to the ethnic and cultural setting (ie, African American, Alaskan native, American Indian, and Hispanic groups with higher injury rates than the national average). Counseling directed toward injury reduction should also include queries regarding access to weapons.

3. Support of traffic-calming programs to reduce road speed, divert high-volume traffic from residential areas, and have narrower streets to reduce injury in pedestrians and cyclists, both children and adults.

4. The imperative to maintain the quality of life in the growing population of older adults while preserving mobility and independence in the home and community.

The role of the health care provider regarding these challenges is to identify and selectively target those who are at risk within their patient population. Brief focused counseling may be effective for some. For others, appropriate referral to medical specialists or to community resources for services is critical.

Acknowledgments: Stephen P. Hayden, MD, Robin K. Avery, MD, and Mary E. Hujer, MSN, RN, provided assistance.

REFERENCES

1. Murphy S. *Deaths: Final Data for 1998. National Vital Statistics Reports.* Hyattsville, Md: National Center for Health Statistics; 2000. Available at: www.cdc.gov/nchs/products/pubs/pubd/nvsr/48/48-19.htm. Accessed March 14, 2003.

2. Hoyert D, Arias E, Smith B, Murphy S, Kochanek K. *Deaths: Final Data for 1999. National Vital Statistics Reports.* Hyattsville, Md: National Center for Health Statistics; 2001:1–116.

3. Centers for Disease Control and Prevention. Achievements in public health, 1900–1999: safer and healthier foods. *MMWR Morbid Mortal Wkly Rep.* 1999;48:905–913.

4. American Public Health Association. *Control of Communicable Diseases Manual.* 17th ed. Washington, DC: American Public Health Association; 2000.

5. Peat JK, Dickerson J, Li J. Effects of damp and mold in the home on respiratory health: a review of the literature. *Allergy.* 1998;53:120–128.

6. Danet S, Richard F, Montaye M, et al. Unhealthy effects of atmospheric temperature and pressure on the occurrence of myocardial infarction and coronary deaths: a 10-year survey: the Lille-World Health Organization MONICA project (Monitoring trends and determinants in cardiovascular disease). *Circulation.* 1999;100:E1–7.

7. Barillo D, Brigham P, Kayden D, Heck R, McManus A. The fire-safe cigarette: a burn prevention tool. *J Burn Care Rehabil.* 2000;21:162–164.

8. Centers for Disease Control. *Web-based Injury Statistics Query and Reporting System.* Atlanta, Ga: Office of Statistics and Programming, National Center for Injury Prevention and Control; 2003.

9. Cummings P, Koepsell TD, Grossman D, Savarino J, Thompson RS. The association between the purchase of a handgun and homicide or suicide. *Am J Public Health.* 1997;87:974–978.

10. Spangenberg KB, Wagner MT, Hendrix S, Bachman DL. Firearm presence in households of patients with Alzheimer's disease and related dementias. *J Am Geriatr Soc.* 1999;47:1183–1186.

11. American Academy of Pediatrics. Firearm-related injuries affecting the pediatric population. *Pediatrics.* 2000;105:888–895.

12. Peat JK, Keena V, Harakeh Z, Marks G. Parental smoking and respiratory tract infections in children. *Paediatr Respir Rev.* 2001;2:207–213.

13. Mihrshahi S, Peat JK, Webb K, et al. The Childhood Asthma Prevention Study (CAPS): design and research protocol of a randomized trial for the primary prevention of asthma. *Controlled Clin Trials.* 2001;22:333–354.

14. Downs SH, Marks GB, Mitakakis TZ, Leuppi JD, Car NG, Peat JK. Having lived on a farm and protection against allergic diseases in Australia. *Clin Exp Allergy.* 2001;31:570–575.

15. Centers for Disease Control and Prevention. Blood lead levels in young children—United States and selected states, 1996–1999. *MMWR Morbid Mortal Wkly Rep.* 2000;49:1133–1137.

16. Centers for Disease Control and Prevention. Update: Blood lead levels—United States, 1991-1994. *MMWR Morbid Mortal Wkly Rep.* 1997;46:141–146.

17. Centers for Disease Control and Prevention. Childhood lead poisoning associated with tamarind candy and folk remedies—California, 1999-2000. *MMWR Morbid Mortal Wkly Rep.* 2002;51:684–686.

18. Krenzelok E, Jacobsen T, Aronis J. Plant exposures: a state profile of the most common species. *Vet Hum Toxicol.* 1996;38:289–298.

19. Gill T, Baker D, Gottschalk M, Peduzzi P, Allore H, Byers A. A program to prevent functional decline in physically frail, elderly persons who live at home. *N Engl J Med.* 2002;347:1068–1074.

20. Tinetti ME, Baker D, Gallo WT, Nanda A, Charpentier P, O'Leary J. Evaluation of restorative care vs usual care for older adults receiving an acute episode of home care. *JAMA.* 2002;287:2098–2105.

21. Tinetti M, Doucette J, Claus E, Marottoli RA. Risk factors for serious injury during falls by older persons in the community. *J Am Geriatr Soc.* 1995;43:1214–1221.

22. Tinetti ME, Doucette J, Claus E. The contribution of predisposing and situational risk factors to serious fall injuries. *J Am Geriatr Soc.* 1995;43:1214–1221.

23. Ensrud KE, Blackwell M, Mangione C, et al. Central nervous system-active medications and risk for falls in older women [comment]. *J Am Geriatric Soc.* 2002;50:1629–1637.

24. Tinetti M, Baker D, Garrett P, Gottschalk M, Koch M, Horwitz R. Yale FICSIT: risk factor abatement strategy for fall prevention. *J Am Geriatr Soc.* 1993;41:315–320.

25. Kannus P, Parkkari J, Niemi S, et al. Prevention of hip fracture in elderly people with use of a hip protector. *N Engl J Med.* 2000;343:1506–1513.

26. National Center for Environmental Health. *Fact Book 2000.* Atlanta, Ga: Centers for Disease Control and Prevention; 2000.

27. Cross D, Stevenson M, Hall M, et al. Child pedestrian injury prevention project: student results. *Prev Med.* 2000;30:179–187.

28. Centers for Disease Control and Prevention. *Bicycle Helmet Usage and Head Injury Prevention. Revised Final FY 1999 Performance Plan and FY 2000 Performance Plan 2000; Section X: Injury Prevention and Control.* Atlanta, Ga: Centers for Disease Control and Prevention; 2001. Available at: www.cdc.gov/od/perfplan/2000x.htm.

29. Rowland J, Rivara F, Salzberg P, Soderberg R, Maier R, Koepsell T. Motorcycle helmet use and injury outcome and hospitalization costs from crashes in Washington State. *Am J Public Health.* 1996;86:41–45.

30. Howland J, Hingson R. Alcohol as a risk factor for drownings: a review of the literature (1950-1985). *Accident Analysis Prev.* 1988;20:19–25.

31. Howland J, Hingson R, Mangione TW, Bell N, Bak S. Why are most drowning victims men? Sex differences in aquatic skills and behaviors. *Am J Public Health.* 1996;86:93–96.

32. Tinsworth D, McDonald J. *Special Study: Injuries and Deaths Associated with Children's Playground Equipment.* Washington, DC: US Consumer Product Safety Commission; 2001.

33. Alcohol use and aquatic activities—United States, 1991. *MMWR Morbid Mortal Wkly Rep.* 1993;42:675, 681–683.

34. Cooper MA. Emergent care of lightning and electrical injuries. *Semin Neurol.* 1995;15:268–278.

35. Cooper MA, Holle R, Lopez R. Recommendations for lightning safety. *Acad Emerg Med.* 2002;9:172–174.

36. Centers for Disease Control and Prevention. Motor-vehicle safety: a 20th century public health achievement. *MMWR Morbid Mortal Wkly Rep.* 1999;48:369–374.

37. Centers for Disease Control and Prevention. Notice to readers: alcohol involvement in fatal motor-vehicle crashes—United States, 1999–2000. *MMWR Morbid Mortal Wkly Rep.* 2001;50:1064–1065.

38. National Highway Traffic Safety Administration. *Developing Best Practices of Emergency Care for the Alcohol Impaired Patient: Recommendations from the National Conference.* Washington, DC: US Department of Transportation; 2001. Publication DOT HS 809 281. Available at: www.nhtsa.dot.gov/people/ injury/alcohol/EmergCare. Accessed January 7, 2002.

39. Centers for Disease Control and Prevention. Motor-vehicle occupant injury: strategies for increasing use of child safety seats, increasing use of safety belts, and reducing alcohol-impaired driving. *MMWR Morbid Mortal Wkly Rep.* 2001;50(RR07):1–13.

40. Ockene JK, Adams A, Hurley TG, Wheeler EV, Hebert JR. Brief physician- and nurse practitioner-delivered counseling for high-risk drinkers: does it work? *Arch Intern Med.* 1999;159:2198–2205.

41. Chen LH, Baker SP, Braver ER, Li G. Carrying passengers as a risk factor for crashes fatal to 16- and 17-year-old drivers [comment]. *JAMA.* 2000;283:1578–1582.

42. Chen LH, Braver ER, Baker SP, Li G. Potential benefits of restrictions on the transport of teenage passengers by 16- and 17-year-old drivers. *Injury Preven.* 2001;7:129–134.

43. Baker SP, Braver ER, Chen LH, Pantula JF, Massie D. Motor vehicle occupant deaths among Hispanic and black children and teenagers. *Arch Pediatr Adolesc Med.* 1998;152:1209–1212.

44. Centers for Disease Control and Prevention. *Older Adult Drivers.* Atlanta, Ga: National Center for Injury Prevention and Control; 2002.

45. Mandavia D, Newton K. Geriatric trauma. *Emerg Med Clin North Am.* 1998;16:257–274.

46. Ball K, Owsley C, Stalvey B, Roenker DL, Sloane ME, Graves M. Driving avoidance and functional impairment in older drivers. *Accident Analysis Prev.* 1998;30:313–322.

47. Evans D, Funkenstein H, Albert M, et al. Prevalence of Alzheimer's disease in a community population of older persons: higher than previously reported. *JAMA.* 1989;262:2551–2556.

RESOURCES

The following Web sites provide useful information about older drivers.

Alzheimer's Association, "Driving" (signs of unsafe driving and tips for caregivers on how to prevent persons with Alzheimer's disease from driving).
www.alz.org/FamCare/DaytoDay/Driving.htm

American Academy for Ophthalmology, policy statement: vision requirements for driving.
www.aao.org/aao/member/policy/driving.cfm.

American Automobile Association. (useful information for elderly drivers).
www.seniordrivers.org/home/toppage.cfm.

American Medical Association, *The Physician's Guide to Assessing and Counseling Older Drivers.*
www.ama-assn.org/go/olderdrivers.

Association for Driver Rehabilitation Specialists. (fact sheets for patients with functional limitations of different types).
www.aded.net.

Insurance Institute for Highway Safety. (information on crashes and fatalities; licensure renewal procedures for each state).
www.hwysafety.org.

National Highway and Traffic Safety Association. (tracks crashes and fatalities; issues reports on older driver problems).
www.nhtsa.dot.gov.

National Motorist Association, position statement on elderly drivers.
www.motorists.org/issues/elderly/elderly.html.

Compilation of transportation sites and sources.
www.umtri.umich.edu/tdc/trans.html.

chapter 24

Travel: Risks and Prevention

Abinash Virk, MD, DTMH

INTRODUCTION

In recent decades, international air travel increased by an average of 3% per year, reaching a peak of nearly 699 million international tourist arrivals in 2000. Although most people travel to Europe, many travel from the industrialized world to the developing world each year. Since the terrorist attacks of September 11, 2001, in the United States, international travel has decreased by 0.6%. The decrease has been primarily to the Americas, followed by South Asia and the Middle East.[1] The top 3 tourist destinations in the world are France, Spain, and the United States. Of countries that carry a higher risk of travel-related illnesses, China, Mexico, the Russian Federation, and Greece are the most popular. Although countries in Southeast Asia, South Asia, and Africa have fewer total numbers of travelers, most countries in these regions pose a higher infectious and noninfectious disease risk.

During 2001, approximately 30 million persons traveled from the United States to international locations. Of these, 80% traveled for leisure or to visit friends or relatives and just over 30% traveled for business or a convention.[2] There was a 6% decrease in international travel from the United States in 2002. Nearly 4 million US residents traveled to Mexico and the same number to the Caribbean and Canada. More than 3.5 million US residents traveled to Asia and 1.5 million each to South America and Central America. Close to 200,000 persons traveled to Africa from the United States in 2002. Therefore, approximately 6 to 8 million persons travel annually from the United States to areas where the risk of infectious or other diseases is high.

This chapter outlines risks and preventive strategies for problems encountered during international travel. Infectious and noninfectious conditions, including insectborne or foodborne infections, vaccine-preventable diseases, and other travel-related diseases such as deep vein thrombosis (DVT), will be covered.

TRAVEL-RELATED RISKS AND ASSESSMENT

Travel risks include both infectious and noninfectious conditions. Between 20% and 70% of travelers to developing countries report some illness associated with their travel.[3,4] Traveler's diarrhea (TD) and upper respiratory tract infections are the most common infectious diseases acquired during travel.[5,6] More lethal diseases such as malaria, typhoid, and yellow fever occasionally occur and are mostly due to lack of appropriate preventive measures before travel. Infectious diseases account for less than 1% of all deaths while traveling. Although, clearly, the risks of acquiring infectious diseases or other conditions are higher for those traveling from developed countries to developing countries, persons traveling from developing countries are also at risk of conditions such as DVT during travel.

Travel-related risks vary with host factors, destination factors, type and purpose of travel, and accommodations and budget during travel. Host factors such as age, medical illnesses, and behavioral factors should be considered in assessing a traveler's risk. For instance, the incidence of TD is highest among children less than 2 years and the 20- to 29-year age group.[7] Similarly, dehydration resulting from TD is much more likely among the very young or the elderly. Underlying chronic medical illnesses have an impact on events while traveling. Accidents, including motor vehicle accidents, plane crashes, homicides, and drowning, are the most common preventable cause of death, responsible for 25% of deaths overseas.[8,9] The risk of injuries while overseas is higher in all age groups and is highest among persons aged 35 to 44 years. Mexico and the Americas account for most of the reported injuries among American travelers.

Many overseas deaths (50% to 60%), however, are from natural causes, with cardiovascular events being the most common.[8,9] Hence, evaluation of a preexisting disease can decrease potential problems (morbidity or

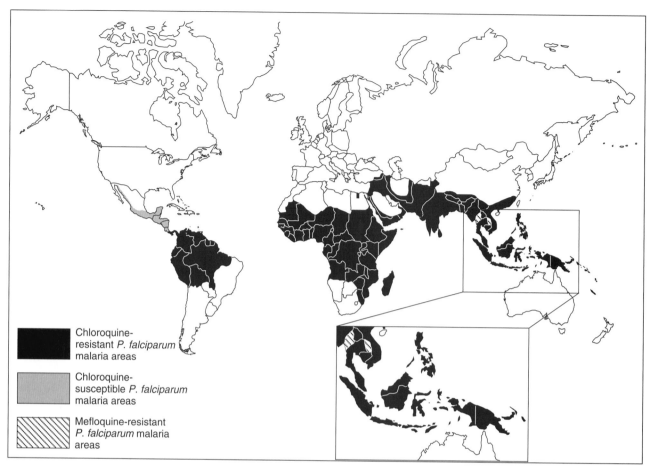

FIGURE 24-1

Travel destinations for US residents. Black areas indicate chloroquine-resistant malaria areas; light gray, chloroquine-susceptible malaria areas; and stipple-effect, mefloquine-resistant areas. Data adapted from International Trade Administration, Office of Travel and Tourism Industries, US Department of Commerce.[2]

mortality) while traveling. Preexisting diseases that are important to identify and address include asthma; diabetes; immunocompromised states such as human immunodeficiency virus (HIV) infection, acquired immunodeficiency syndrome (AIDS), or organ transplantation; predisposition to DVT; blood dyscrasias; and asplenia. In addition, some underlying medical conditions can place a person at higher risk of side effects from vaccines or medications being administered for prevention. A particular vaccine may be contraindicated in some medical conditions leading to an inability to protect the traveler. Administering the vaccine may cause vaccine strain disease, such as yellow fever virus vaccination in an immunocompromised host.

A traveler's behavior plays a critical role in disease acquisition. Poor insight into behaviors such as food habits, extensive outdoor exposure, or sexual exposure pose an increased risk from these modes of transmission of diseases. Counseling before travel about these and other routes of transmission may help decrease the risk.

The risk of a particular disease may vary among or within countries. For example, the risk of malaria is higher in some malaria-endemic countries as opposed to others.[10] Ethnicity factors should also be considered for assessment and prevention of disease risk. In addition, the risk of disease acquisition is also cumulative over time, as seen with malaria, typhoid, hepatitis, and diarrhea.[5]

The type and purpose of travel affect disease acquisition. The primary purposes of international travel are leisure (62%), business (18%), health care delivery, missionary work, and to visit friends or relatives. Business travel usually poses less risk than travel such as backpacking in rural locations. However, the risk will vary with activities undertaken; a businessman who regularly jogs during his frequent trips to South Asia may be at similar risk of a dog bite as the backpacker. Business travelers suffer different travel-related problems such as stress from frequent and long travel, separation from family and home environment, frequent time changes, and having to conduct business in a foreign country.[11,12] In addition, business travelers or other frequent travelers are at a higher risk of developing low back pain or other musculoskeletal complaints from sitting in airplanes or from carrying luggage.[12] Health care workers going for health care delivery in developing countries are subjected to occupational hazards such as needlesticks (hepatitis, HIV), tuberculosis exposure, or other disease exposure. People who visit friends or relatives comprise a completely different risk group; these are often immigrants returning to home countries. Most immigrants lack an understanding regarding their risk of diseases such as malaria or typhoid and are at increased risk of acquiring these diseases.[10,13] They tend to live with local families, eat less carefully, and not take precautions against preventable diseases.

A pretravel preventive approach must include a detailed medical history, including the factors discussed above. Based on the information obtained, individualized preventive strategies (vaccination, medications, and advice) for a safe trip can be made. Pretravel assessment and advice should be completed 6 to 12 weeks before travel and preferably 6 months before expatriation for longer than 4 weeks. Although not ideal, short-term travelers can still benefit from vaccination or medications (eg, hepatitis A vaccine or γ-globulin for hepatitis A protection) even if departure is within 24 hours.

TRAVEL-RELATED INFECTIOUS DISEASES AND THEIR PREVENTION

Insectborne Diseases

Malaria

Approximately 3% of travelers report fever, with malaria being the most common cause. Approximately 125 million persons travel annually into areas with malaria risk. Regions of risk include Africa, the Indian subcontinent, Southeast Asia, Central and South America, Hispaniola (Haiti and the Dominican Republic), the Middle East, and Oceania (Fig 24-1).[14] The estimated incidence of malaria in West Africa is 24 cases per 1000 travelers per month of stay compared with 0.1 case per 1000 travelers per month in Central America.[15] Annually, 10,000 to 30,000 cases of malaria are estimated to occur among travelers returning to developed countries from risk areas. Despite underreporting, an increase in imported malaria has been observed over the last decade.[16] In the United States, about 1500 malaria cases are reported annually. Of these, 40% to 60% are caused by *Plasmodium falciparum* and most are acquired in Africa.[15] It is important to note that half of the imported malaria occurs among visitors of friends or relatives. *P falciparum* malaria-related mortality among nonimmune travelers from developed countries varies from 0.6% to 3.8%.[17] Key factors in malaria-related mortality are severity of disease, extremes

in age, inappropriate chemoprophylaxis for the region visited, noncompliance with prophylaxis, delay in seeking medical care after onset of symptoms, delay in diagnosis, misdiagnosis, or inappropriate therapy.[18,19]

Risks of malaria acquisition are travel to rural areas, adventure tourism, prolonged travel (expatriates), no or inappropriate chemoprophylaxis, and noncompliance with prophylaxis or mosquito bite prevention. Visitors of friends or relatives often do not seek pretravel advice because of lack of understanding of individual risk.[20] Very young children, elderly persons, and pregnant women are at risk of severe malaria. Elderly individuals with malaria have a cerebral complication rate and case fatality rate 3 and 6 times greater, respectively, than do younger persons. Antimalarial chemoprophylaxis is significantly associated with a lower case fatality rate and frequency of cerebral complications.[21] Pregnant women in whom malaria develops carry a risk of spontaneous abortion, stillbirth, and low birth weight, with an associated risk of maternal or neonatal death. Pregnant women should be advised to postpone travel to malaria-risk areas. The risk of malaria decreases with increasing altitudes; it is rarely seen above 2000 m.

Prevention of malaria. Preventive measures are best addressed by the physician reviewing the following factors before travel:

- Assess the risk of infection and obtain details of the individual's activities and itinerary.
- Provide education and advice on methods of preventing mosquito bites (discussed at the end of this section).
- Identify the most suitable chemoprophylactic therapy.
- Make sure the patient is aware of malaria symptoms and the need to seek medical help in case of fever during travel or after return home.

Malaria chemoprophylaxis. The specific antimalarial drug used for chemoprophylaxis depends on the risk of acquiring malaria, drug resistance pattern in the area of travel, medical contraindications, cost of the drug, and availability of medical care while overseas. See Tables 24-1 and 24-2.

Chloroquine-susceptible malaria. Areas with chloroquine-susceptible malaria include Mexico, Central America, Haiti, the Dominican Republic, and certain parts of China and the Philippines. A regimen of chloroquine is started a week before entering the malaria-endemic area, taken weekly while there, and continued for 4 weeks after leaving the area. Chloroquine is efficacious and safe, can be used in pregnancy, and has few major side effects. Gastrointestinal adverse effects are the most common and usually tolerable. Taking the medication with food can help

TABLE 24-1

Antimalarial Chemoprophylaxis Based on Patterns of Malaria Drug Resistance

Chloroquine-susceptible Malaria	Chloroquine-resistant		Chloroquine- and Mefloquine- resistant	Doxycycline-resistant
	P vivax	**P falciparum**		
First-line Preventive Medications in These Zones				
Chloroquine	Mefloquine		Doxycycline	Atovaquone plus proguanil (Malarone)
Alternatives for Prevention				
Atovaquone plus proguanil (Malarone) or doxycycline	Malarone, doxycycline, or chloroquine plus proguanil		Malarone or chloroquine plus proguanil	None

TABLE 24-2

Antimalarial Dosing, Efficacy, and Contraindications

Antimalarial Drug	Formulation	Efficacy, %	Dosing Schedule	Safety	Use During Pregnancy	Side Effects	Contra-indications
Mefloquine	Tablets	90–100	1 tablet every week: 1–3 wk before travel, weekly during travel, and 4 wk after return	Yes	Yes but caution during first trimester (no safety data)	Neuro-psychiatric side effects, cardiac arrhythmias	Depression, psychiatric diagnosis, seizures, cardiac arrhythmias, hypersensitivity reaction
Chloroquine	Tablets and suspension	For use in chloroquine-sensitive areas only	1 tablet every week: 1 wk before, weekly, and 4 wk after return reaction	Yes	Yes	Nausea, dyspepsia, tinnitus, retinopathy	Retinopathy, hypersensitivity
Doxycycline	Tablets	77–99	1 tablet daily with food starting 2 d before travel, daily, and 4 wk after return	Yes	No	Gastro-intestinal (GI) side effects, esophageal reaction, ulcers, yeast vaginitis, phototoxicity	Not for children <8 y of age, previous hypersensitivity
Atovaquone plus proguanil (Malarone)	Tablets	99	1 tablet daily with food starting 2 d before travel, daily, and 7 d after return	Yes	No	GI side effects, occasional rash	Previous hypersensitivity reaction to either atovaquone or proguanil

tolerance. The drug can exacerbate psoriasis and, therefore, should be used with caution in persons with psoriasis. Hydroxychloroquine (Plaquenil) is prescribed at a dose of 400 mg (310-mg base) once weekly on the same day.

Chloroquine-resistant malaria.   Chloroquine-resistant malaria refers primarily to *P falciparum* malaria and is

prevalent in Africa, South Asia, South America, and the Middle East. *Plasmodium vivax* resistance to chloroquine has been reported from West Papua (formerly Irian Jaya) in Indonesia. Mefloquine, doxycycline, atovaquone and proguanil hydrochloride (Malarone), or chloroguanide, or, rarely, the combination of chloroquine and proguanil are medications used for prophylaxis of chloroquine-resistant malaria. The decision regarding which of these to use depends on duration of travel, contraindications, patient's affordability, and adverse effects. Mefloquine is effective (>95% protection) and has been used for a long time. Because of its long half-life (13 to 30 days), it has a convenient weekly dosing similar to chloroquine, making it easier for longer-duration travel. It is approximately $10 per tablet in the United States and is cost-effective for persons planning trips longer than 6 weeks compared with a daily tablet of Malarone, which costs approximately $5 per tablet. Approximately 20% to 40% of persons taking mefloquine report mild side effects of nausea, strange dreams, insomnia, mood changes, transient dizziness, and headaches. However, neuropsychiatric side effects such as acute anxiety, depression, hallucinations, paranoia, restlessness, or confusion can occur in 1 in 10,000 to 13,000 persons taking the prophylactic dose.[15,17] Less commonly mefloquine can cause paresthesias, postmalarial neurologic syndrome, and seizures. These side effects are more likely in females and may not be correlated with blood levels.[22] Mefloquine should be avoided in persons relying on fine motor skills, such as airline pilots, machine operators, and drivers. Because of the potential of confusion with mefloquine, it is best avoided in situations in which development of confusion may place the traveler in severe harm, such as scuba divers or those at risk of altitude sickness. Recently, there have been reports of traveler fatalities caused by cardiac arrhythmias resulting from use of halofantrine for treatment of malaria while simultaneously receiving mefloquine chemoprophylaxis. Travelers with cardiac abnormalities or those receiving mefloquine for malaria prophylaxis should be warned against the use of halofantrine while overseas.[23]

Alternatives for mefloquine are Malarone and doxycycline. Malarone is safe, and studies have shown minimal severe side effects during treatment or prophylaxis.[24,25] Malarone is an equally efficacious antimalarial prophylactic drug to mefloquine in nonimmune travelers.[25,26] It is best used for short stays, for patients with contraindications to mefloquine and/or doxycycline, and as standby therapy for malaria in persons receiving other chemoprophylactic regimens. Standby therapy involves taking an additional drug along for the treatment of proven or highly suspected acute malaria while overseas despite receiving prophylaxis with another agent. Having standby medications is best suited for expatriates in countries with poor availability of malaria therapy and who have a clear understanding of when and how to use them.

Doxycycline is another alternative for chloroquine-resistant malaria chemoprophylaxis and is equally efficacious (90% to 95%) and inexpensive (approximately $0.15 per tablet).[21,27] Doxycycline is an alternative for persons with mefloquine contraindications and those who cannot afford Malarone. Doxycycline is available worldwide, unlike Malarone. It may offer limited protection against TD; however, increased antimicrobial resistance

limits that advantage.[28] Cautions include gastrointestinal side effects, such as esophageal irritation or ulcers because of the tablet's low pH; phototoxicity; and the possibility of *Candida* (yeast) vaginitis in women. These adverse effects can be lessened by taking the drug with food and water, use of sunscreen, and avoiding use in women who are prone to vaginitis or, alternatively, providing them with self-treatment education and medications for yeast vaginitis.

Of the drugs available for prophylaxis for chloroquine-resistant malaria, only mefloquine can be potentially used in pregnancy. However, stillbirths (0.8%) and spontaneous abortions have been associated with mefloquine use during the first 4 months of pregnancy.[29]

Chloroquine and mefloquine-resistant malaria.
Currently known areas of both chloroquine and mefloquine *P falciparum* malaria resistance are along the Thai-Cambodia and Thai-Myanmar border areas. Chloroquine and mefloquine-resistant *P vivax* malaria has been reported from Myanmar and Papua New Guinea. For these locations, prophylactic options include Malarone and doxycycline. Protective efficacy of Malarone against *P vivax* is approximately 84%.[30]

To prevent the morbidity and mortality of imported cases of acute malaria, all travelers should be advised of common symptoms of malaria. Any fever during *and within a few weeks after* travel to a malaria-endemic area should prompt appropriate investigation irrespective of complete compliance with prophylaxis. Travelers who acquire malaria abroad often present with nonspecific symptoms such as fever, chills, headache, myalgia, and abdominal symptoms. Patients should be advised to inform the examining physician of their travel history. Rapid assessment and diagnoses is essential to lower morbidity and mortality rates.[31]

Dengue fever
Dengue, a flavivirus, is the most common mosquitoborne disease in the world. Dengue fever is characterized by sudden onset of fever, headaches, joint pain, muscle pain, nausea, vomiting, and rash. There are 4 different serotypes of the virus. Acquiring dengue fever does not confer immunity against the other 3 serotypes. A prior dengue infection places a person at risk of dengue hemorrhagic syndrome or dengue shock syndrome during a subsequent dengue reinfection. Dengue seropositivity rates among travelers returning from dengue-prevalent areas with or without symptoms range from 4.3% to 19%.[32] The highest risk area for travelers is Southeast Asia or Western Indonesia.[33] The risk of acquisition increases with duration of stay (expatriates). Patient education on methods of personal protective measures is very important. Currently, there is no vaccine; however, some are being studied.

Other insectborne diseases

Although vaccines and chemoprophylactic drugs are available against some diseases, travelers should be advised about other diseases due to insect bites as well as prevention techniques appropriate for the risk in their area of travel. Japanese encephalitis and yellow fever are mosquitoborne and are discussed under the section dealing with vaccine-preventable illnesses. *Rickettsia africae*, a tickborne disease common in Africa, causes a febrile illness with a bite site eschar. Other insect-transmitted diseases such as *Bartonella* infection, Lyme disease, or tickborne encephalitis need personal protective measures.

Personal protective measures are as follows:

- Avoid being outdoors during the peak periods of insect activity (dawn, dusk, and early evening).
- Prompt removal of attached ticks can prevent infection.
- Long-sleeved shirts and long pants (tucked into the socks) are advised.
- Mosquito nets should be used in the bedroom. Most of these can be purchased from hardware, camping, sporting goods, or military surplus stores. Mosquito bed nets can be pretreated with permethrin to provide additional protection. This is advisable for expatriates, backpackers, or those camping in high-risk areas.
- Use insect repellents as directed.

Application of insect repellents

Mosquitoes preferentially bite adults, males, larger bodies, and younger persons. Mosquitoes bite during both daytime (*Aedes* spp) and nighttime (*Anopheline* spp). Repellents that contain deet (N,N-diethyl-methyl-toluamide or N,N-diethyl-3-methylbenzamide) have been well studied and are more effective than non–deet-containing products.[34,35] They are effective against mosquitoes, ticks, chiggers, and fleas. Typically, insect repellents with deet concentrations of 20% to 30% are adequate for both adults and children. These provide protection for up to 5 hours, whereas products with lower concentrations such as 10% or less protect for 1 to 2 hours. No additional protection is gained with concentrations beyond 50%. Duration of protection varies with ambient temperature, amount of perspiration, water exposure, abrasive removal, and other factors.[36] Deet-containing repellents have been in use since the 1940s. Overall, deet is an extremely safe product.[37] Cases of encephalopathy were reported with use in children less than 8 years of age, but this was not substantiated in a study that reviewed 9086 cases of deet exposure. Rash and eye irritation can occur. Animal studies do not demonstrate teratogenicity or oncogenicity.[34] Deet-containing products were found to be safe in pregnant women, without adverse effects on the fetus.[38]

Plant-derived insect repellents such as citronella or soy-derived products provide repellency for less than 45 minutes. Permethrin, an insecticide, can be sprayed or impregnated into clothing, shoes, bed nets, and camping gear. When properly done and combined with a deet-containing repellent on the skin, this is very effective in preventing insect bites.[34,39]

General principles of use of deet-containing insect repellents include the following:

- Apply on exposed skin and on clothing. Avoid use on plastic items, such as a wristwatch band.
- Apply sunscreen first on the skin, followed by a repellent with deet. (Insect repellents may decrease the sun protection factor (SPF) by 33%. Therefore, a higher-SPF sunscreen should be applied next over a deet-containing product.)
- Product directions regarding the use of deet products should be followed carefully:
- Avoid application on or near the eyes or mouth.
- Avoid applying to children's hands to prevent contact with their eyes or mouth.
- Wash off the repellent as soon as it is not needed.

Foodborne and Waterborne Diseases (Non-vaccine-preventable Diseases)

Travelers' diarrhea

Traveler's diarrhea is the most common health problem experienced by travelers to developing countries. Between 20% and 70% of travelers to developing countries experience diarrhea resulting in an astonishing 7 million cases annually.[40] Traveler's diarrhea is defined by the passage of 3 or more unformed stools over 24 hours with or without nausea or vomiting.[40] The mean duration of incapacitation is 17 to 21 hours, although TD may last up to 7 days.[41] Prior short-term travel to high-risk areas does not result in immunity against TD. Continued exposure to enteropathogens in developing countries may be necessary for any immunity to develop.[42]

Causative agents differ among countries, with bacterial pathogens being the most common cause worldwide. Enterotoxigenic *E coli* is the most common organism worldwide and usually causes a mild, self-limiting disease.[43,44] Other bacteria causing TD include *Campylobacter, Shigella, Salmonella*, and *Aeromonas* organisms. *Campylobacter* is particularly common in Thailand, in winter, and has a high rate of fluoroquinolone resistance. In approximately 40% of cases, no pathogen is identified, but the disease may still respond to empiric antimicrobial therapy, suggesting a bacterial cause.[45] Some TD is viral, such as rotavirus or Norwalk. Amebiasis and giardiasis are more common with prolonged stays in developing countries, rural travel, or hiking.

Pretravel advice regarding TD for travelers going to developing countries includes preventive education on safety of food and water, advising self-management of TD while overseas, and primary prophylaxis in a select group of patients. Vaccines currently have a limited role in TD prevention.

Risk factors for TD include drinking iced beverages or water from an unknown source, eating precut fruit or ice cream, eating at small restaurants, or eating with a local family.[46,47] The cool, moist quality of salads, lasagna, quiches, cheese (indigenous cheeses, especially soft cheeses, may not be pasteurized), and mayonnaise provide an ideal environment for growth of microorganisms and should be avoided. Dry foods (breads) and hot, processed, and cooked foods are considered safer. Boiled water, hot drinks made with boiled water, and canned and bottled carbonated drinks are considered safe to drink. Swimming pools may not be properly chlorinated. Fresh or salt water may be contaminated by animal waste, sewers, or rivers that join them, so drinking water from these sources is not advised. Other sources of water (tap, wells) are considered contaminated in developing countries.[48,49]

Host factors influence the likelihood of TD. The highest incidence of TD is observed in children and young adults, and is less common in the elderly. Achlorhydria, congenital or iatrogenic, is a risk factor for enteric infections. Immunocompromised travelers or those with inflammatory bowel disease (Crohn disease or ulcerative colitis) are at higher risk of acquiring TD, experience worse symptoms from TD, and are more likely to develop a complication of TD. Primary prophylaxis of TD with either a quinolone (ciprofloxacin 500 mg/d) or bismuth subsalicylate is best restricted to immunocompromised hosts (transplant recipients, persons with advanced AIDS), patients with inflammatory bowel disease, or those on a critical trip who cannot afford to be disabled for a day. Ciprofloxacin offers approximately 90% protection against TD compared with 65% protection with bismuth subsalicylate.[42] Primary prophylaxis with ciprofloxacin is more appropriate for severely immunocompromised hosts, whereas bismuth subsalicylate is better for those at average risk.

Empiric self-treatment of TD during travel. Although meticulous attention to food sources may decrease the risk of TD, many travelers find it hard to follow food and water precautions. Therefore, education regarding self-treatment of TD is important. In mild cases, water, juice, and other liquids can accomplish fluid replacement. For severe TD, oral rehydration therapy may be required. Antibiotics for treatment of TD decrease the duration and severity of diarrhea.[40] An increase in antimicrobial resistance limits the usefulness of trimethoprim-sulfamethoxazole and doxycycline. Fluoroquinolones (ciprofloxacin, norfloxacin, levofloxacin, ofloxacin)

are the most studied and recommended self-treatment drugs for TD.[50] They are active against most common TD pathogens except *Campylobacter,* which has increasing quinolone resistance worldwide. A 3-day course is equally as effective as a 5-day course for TD when promptly started for moderate or severe diarrhea.[51] A single dose of a quinolone (ciprofloxacin, 750 mg, or levofloxacin, 500 mg) is effective for mild diarrhea.[52] Antibiotics are more effective when used in conjunction with loperamide hydrochloride.[52,53] Antimotility agents such as loperamide or atropine and diphenoxylate hydrochloride are safe in mild to moderate TD and reduce stool frequency and duration of illness. Their use alone in mild diarrhea may be adequate. Antimotility drugs should be avoided with acute, bloody, or severe diarrhea and in children less than 12 years of age because of the risk of ileus or toxic megacolon. Bismuth subsalicylate exerts its antidiarrheal effects via both antimicrobial and antisecretory properties. It is not as efficacious as antibiotics but may be helpful in mild diarrhea. An effective alternative to quinolones is azithromycin (500 mg orally once a day for 3 days, or 1000 mg as a single dose). It is equally active against TD pathogens as is ciprofloxacin and more active against *Campylobacter.*[54] Azithromycin offers an advantage over quinolones for children and pregnant women.

Vaccine-Preventable Diseases

A wide range of vaccines is available in preventing travel-related diseases. Factors to consider in vaccine recommendations are:

- Travel destination—some vaccine-preventable diseases are more prevalent in some geographic areas than others.

- Disease acquisition risk—prior immunity to a disease, immune status (compromised or not), planned activities, and duration of potential exposure.

- Host factors—individual risk from the vaccine itself (immune status, prior immunity, or pregnancy) and affordability.

Immunizations for international travel can be classified as routine immunizations, required immunizations, and recommended travel vaccines. See Tables 24-3 through 24-5. General information regarding routine vaccinations is covered in Chapter 50.

Routine vaccinations for travelers

Influenza. Influenza is nonseasonal in the tropics and occurs during the winter in the Northern and Southern Hemisphere. The influenza vaccine should be recommended to all travelers aged 50 years and older, particularly those with chronic cardiopulmonary diseases,

TABLE 24-3

Routine Adult Vaccinations That May Need Updating Before International Travel

Vaccine	Ideal and Minimum Time Needed to Complete Vaccination Before Travel	Indications	Healthy Adults		Risk Groups	
			18–65 y	>65 y	Pregnant Women	Immuno-compromised Persons*
Tetanus-diphtheria	Ideal: none for routine booster; 3 mo if primary series is needed	All travelers should be up-to-date in case of accidental injury	Vaccinate if <10 y since booster; primary series if not done previously	Vaccinate if >10 y since booster; primary series if not done previously	Vaccinate if >10 y since booster, preferably after first trimester	Vaccinate if >10 y since booster
Measles, mumps, and rubella (MMR)	Ideal: none for routine second-dose measles Minimum: at least 4 weeks before departure if first dose ever	All nonimmune travelers to endemic areas	Vaccinate if patient is not immune or has not completed 2 doses of MMR for persons born after 1957	Vaccinate if patient is not immune or has not completed 2 doses of MMR for persons born after 1957	Contraindicated	Contraindicated
Pneumococcal	Ideal: no time limitation Minimum: at least 2–4 wk for immunity to develop	Prolonged travel to countries with high pneumococcal resistance†	Vaccination not required	Vaccinate	Vaccinate if indicated	Vaccinate
Influenza	Minimum: at least 2 wk before exposure	During winter in Northern and Southern hemispheres, and year-round in tropics	Vaccination optional	Vaccinate	Vaccinate after first trimester	Vaccinate
Varicella	Minimum: at least 4–8 wk before travel if possible	If no evidence of varicella immunity and plan to have close contact with local populations	Vaccinate if nonimmune by medical history and serologic findings	Vaccinate if nonimmune by medical history and serologic findings	Contraindicated	Contraindicated

*Immunocompromised persons include those receiving high-dose steroids (20 mg/d for >3 weeks), chemotherapy, on immunosuppressive regimens for transplantation or other diseases, congenital or acquired immunodeficiency states, including HIV or AIDS.

†Chronic diseases such as chronic obstructive lung disease, chronic heart or renal failure, chronic liver disease (cirrhosis), diabetes mellitus, and asplenia.

chronic renal disease, and diabetes. Younger travelers going to developing countries may benefit as well. The influenza vaccine should be advised before all ship cruises because of the association of influenza with cruises. For those allergic to eggs and unable to take the influenza vaccine, a prescription of amantadine hydrochloride, rimantadine hydrochloride, or oseltamivir could be considered for prophylaxis should an outbreak occur on the cruise ship.

Measles, mumps, and rubella.   Measles, mumps, and rubella (MMR) are common in developing countries where MMR may not be part of routine childhood immunizations. Travelers to developing countries should have immunity against these diseases.

Pneumococcal.   The pneumococcal vaccination should be considered for all healthy adults older than 65 years and to those of any age with chronic cardiopulmonary diseases, chronic liver or renal disease, asplenia, or diabetes. This is particularly important for those traveling for prolonged periods to countries with high penicillin resistance among the pneumococci, such as South Korea; Japan; China, including Hong Kong and Taiwan; Vietnam; Spain; and South Africa.[55]

Tetanus and diphtheria. Tetanus and diphtheria are prevalent in most developing countries, and outbreaks have been reported in Eastern Europe, the former Soviet Union, England, the Netherlands, and the United States. If indicated, a tetanus-diphtheria booster should be completed before all travel to prevent the need of a booster or tetanus immunoglobulin in case of an injury overseas. If the traveler was never previously vaccinated, the primary series should be completed before travel. The vaccine is safe but may give rise to local pain and swelling at the injection site.

Varicella vaccine. Primary varicella (chickenpox) is a disease not only of children but also of adults in developing countries. It is important to verify immunity by a definite history of disease or by serologic findings in patients with unclear medical histories.

Recommended travel vaccines

Cholera. Cholera is endemic in the Indian subcontinent, Southeast Asia, the Middle East, North and East Africa, and Latin America. The risk to average travelers is extremely low. Persons working in refugee camps with an active cholera epidemic, military personnel, missionaries, or health care workers going to an endemic area are at greater risk and may warrant vaccination. The older cholera vaccine is not available in the United States. Efficacy of the newer cholera vaccines ranges between 60% and 100%; however, these are also currently unavailable in the United States.

Hepatitis A. Hepatitis A is endemic everywhere except North America, Western Europe, Great Britain, Scandinavia, Japan, Australia, and New Zealand. Anyone traveling to parts of the world other than these areas is advised to receive the hepatitis A vaccine. The available hepatitis A vaccines are highly immunogenic and are safe in both adults and children. The immune response to the hepatitis A vaccine is primarily humoral, similar to that induced by natural infection. By 4 weeks after vaccination, protective antibodies develop in 94% to 100% of immunocompetent adults and in 97% to 100% of immunocompetent persons aged 2 to 18 years.[56,57] With 2 doses, immunity can be expected to last between 15 and 20 years.[58] Ideally, patients should be vaccinated at least 4 weeks before departure, but even immediately before leaving is helpful.

Hepatitis B. Countries in South America, Africa, Asia, and the South Pacific have a high prevalence of hepatitis B. A large numbers of travelers are at potential risk of acquiring hepatitis B while traveling. The risk increases with injuries, sexual exposure, or dental or medical emergencies requiring hospital care overseas. In one study, approximately 45% of travelers required dental or medical care that placed them at increased risk. The vaccine is extremely safe and effective and is recommended for persons traveling for short or long trips. The risk is much lower for short-term travel but can be high if high-risk activities are planned. All long-term (>4 weeks) travelers, health care workers, missionaries, executives taking multiple international trips to developing countries, and visitors of friends or relatives should be vaccinated.

Japanese B encephalitis. Japanese B encephalitis is a mosquito-transmitted viral encephalitis endemic in Asia (Southern China, Korea, Japan, the Indian subcontinent, and Southeast Asia). The disease is more prevalent in the rural areas where both the pig reservoir and the mosquito vector are present. There are seasonal variations in some countries, whereas it occurs year round in others. The vaccine is efficacious, providing 80% to 90% protection. It is recommended for anyone staying in an endemic area for longer than 4 weeks or for those planning a shorter trip entirely in the rural areas during the transmission season. It is a 3-dose vaccine schedule requiring 14 days minimum to complete, but after the last dose an additional 7 to 10 days of having ready access to medical care is advised before travel because of the possibility of a delayed allergic reaction. The risk of an allergic reaction increases in persons with a history of urticaria, asthma, allergic rhinitis, or multiple allergies. The risk of a hypersensitivity reaction is estimated to be 0.8 and 6.3 per 100,000 doses.[59] Side effects of the vaccine include malaise, fever, headache, myalgia, and swelling at the injection site. Personal protective measures against mosquitoes should be emphasized, particularly for short-term travelers who may not be at high enough risk to warrant the vaccine.

Poliovirus. Polio is endemic in some countries in Asia and Africa. It has reached near eradication in many previously endemic regions of the world. As of 2003, only 7 countries are considered endemic: India, Pakistan, Nigeria, Egypt, Afghanistan, Niger, and Somalia. Boosting prior immunity with the inactivated poliovirus vaccine is important before travel to an endemic area. The primary series should be completed for patients who have not had it. The oral vaccine is associated rarely with paralytic poliomyelitis and, therefore, is not used anymore in the United States.

Rabies. Rabies is endemic in the Indian subcontinent, China, Southeast Asia, the Philippines, parts of Indonesia, Latin America, Africa, and the former Soviet Union. Preexposure rabies vaccination is advised for persons planning to expatriate to endemic countries; those going for longer than 4 to 8 weeks, especially if primarily rural

TABLE 24-4

Recommended Travel Immunizations

Vaccine	Ideal and Minimum Time Needed to Complete Vaccination Before Travel	Indications	Healthy Adults	Risk Groups	
				Pregnant Women	Immuno-compromised Persons*
Hepatitis A	Ideal: 4 wk for short-term travel; 6 mo for expatriation. Minimum: day before departure	Nonimmune persons traveling to areas endemic for hepatitis A (Asia, Africa, Central and South America, Caribbean, East Europe, Russian Federation and the Independent States); check serologic findings before vaccination in immigrants returning to home country	Vaccinate	Vaccinate if risk exceeds any risk from vaccine; category C	Vaccinate; if no seroconversion occurs after 4 wk in immuno-compromised people, consider hepatitis A immunoglobulin before departure
Combined hepatitis A and hepatitis B (*Twinrix*)	Ideal: 6 mo Minimum: 21 d before departure with a booster in 12 mo	Those meeting both hepatitis A and hepatitis B vaccine indications	Vaccinate	Vaccinate if risk exceeds any risk from vaccine; category C	Vaccinate but check hepatitis A serologic findings before departure
Hepatitis B	Ideal: 6 mo Minimum: complete 3 doses in 3 mo (0, 1, 2 mo) or 21 d (0, 7, 21 d) with a booster in 12 mo	Travelers who anticipate high-risk activities, people planning to travel for >4 wk, business personnel with multiple international trips annually	Vaccinate	Vaccinate	Vaccinate
Typhoid	Ideal: 4 wk Minimum: 2 wk for protection	Travel to developing countries in Asia, Africa, and Latin America, especially if longer than 2–3 wk or 1-wk travel to high-risk areas (eg, Indian subcontinent)	Vaccinate	Oral live vaccine is contraindicated; injectable vaccine is relatively contraindicated Vaccinate if risk of disease is higher than vaccine risk	Oral live vaccine is contraindicated; injectable vaccine may be used but may have lower efficacy
Rabies	Ideal: 6 weeks for full immunity Minimum: 21 d when 3 doses are accelerated	Long-term travelers to areas where rabies is a threat (see text), or short-term travelers who are likely to have animal contact in enzootic areas	Vaccinate	Vaccinate only if risk is considered high	Vaccinate
Japanese encephalitis	Ideal: 2 mo. Minimum for 3 doses: 24 d	Travel to endemic areas for >4 wk, especially to rural areas	Vaccinate	Contraindicated	Vaccinate, but efficacy may be low
Tickborne virus (not available in United States)		Expatriates to endemic areas (eg, Eastern European countries, Independent States of Russia)	Vaccinate	Contraindicated	Vaccinate

Continued

T A B L E 24-4

Recommended Travel Immunizations—*Concluded*

Vaccine	Ideal and Minimum Time Needed to Complete Vaccination Before Travel	Indications	Healthy Adults	Risk Groups	
				Pregnant Women	Immuno-compromised Persons*
Poliovirus	No specific time limit before travel if previously vaccinated; 3–12 mo if no previous primary series was given	Travelers to endemic areas—African and Asian countries only Due to near-worldwide eradication, recommendations are likely to change with continued eradication	Booster with inactivated poliovirus vaccine if primary series was completed >10 y ago Give primary series if primary series was not completed	Live oral vaccine contraindicated, but injectable poliovirus vaccine advised if risk is high	Live oral vaccine contraindicated, but injectable poliovirus vaccine advised
Cholera (currently unavailable in United States)	4 wk	Health care delivery, missionary, or military workers in endemic and epidemic areas	Vaccinate for high-risk exposure as indicated	Contraindicated	Contraindicated

*Immunocompromised persons include those receiving high-dose steroids (20 mg/d for >3 weeks), chemotherapy, or immunosuppressive regimens due to transplantation or other diseases, or persons with congenital or acquired immunodeficiency states, including HIV or AIDS.

travel is anticipated; those planning to work with animals; spelunkers; or persons who travel to these areas many times a year and run outdoors. It is a very safe and effective 3-dose vaccine. Preexposure vaccination reduces the postexposure rabies doses, if needed, to 2 (day of bite and 3 days later) and precludes the need for rabies immunoglobulin. Protective immunity can be expected to last for 3 to 5 years. A contraindication is hypersensitivity to a previous dose. Side effects include urticaria, pruritus, and malaise.

Tickborne encephalitis. Tickborne encephalitis is a tick-transmitted virus that is endemic in Austria, the Czech Republic, Slovakia, Germany, Hungary, Poland, Switzerland, the former Soviet Union, and the northern part of the former Yugoslavia and other forested areas in Europe. The vaccine is not available in the United States. Persons planning to stay long term in these countries who expect extensive exposure in wooded areas may need to consider the vaccine and receive it in the destination country.

Typhoid. Foodborne transmission of *Salmonella typhi* is not uncommon in some countries in South America, Western Africa, and the Indian subcontinent, which has the highest risk.[60] In the United States, 2 vaccines are used: a live, attenuated, oral vaccine and an inactivated, injectable

one. The oral vaccine is extremely safe and only rarely may cause mild gastric upset. Its efficacy is approximately 70% to 96% and it lasts for approximately 5 years. Because it is a live, attenuated, bacterial vaccine, it is contraindicated in immunocompromised persons and pregnant women. The efficacy of the injectable vaccine is approximately 60% to 72%, and it lasts for 2 years. It has minimal side effects compared with the previously available killed, whole-cell, heat-inactivated, phenol-preserved, injectable vaccine.

Required travel vaccines

The term *required* implies that entry to a certain country requires proof of vaccination. This is mandated and monitored by the World Health Organization (WHO). It is imposed to prevent the spread of a particular disease beyond its current endemicity into another country. It is also for the protection of the individual traveling into the endemic area.

Yellow fever. The *Aedes* spp mosquito transmits yellow fever, which is prevalent in parts of tropical Africa and South America. Yellow fever is an acute viral hemorrhagic disease and can be prevented by avoiding mosquito bites and by vaccination before travel to endemic areas. The vaccine is highly immunogenic and confers more

TABLE 24-5

Required Travel Immunizations

Vaccine	Ideal and Minimum Time Needed to Complete Vaccination Before Travel	Indications	Healthy Adults		Risk Groups	
			18–65 y	>65 y	Pregnant Women	Immuno-compromised Persons*
Yellow fever	Ideal: 4 wk Minimum: 10 d	Countries where yellow fever is endemic (equatorial Africa and South America) and there is a yellow fever vaccine requirement for entry	Vaccinate	Vaccinate There is a potential risk of vaccine strain-related yellow fever in elderly persons, especially those >70 y	Contraindicated Should be used only if travel to endemic areas is unavoidable and risk of infection is high	Contraindicated Can vaccinate HIV-positive patients if travel is unavoidable and immune status is preserved (CD4 T cells >200/mm^3)
Meningococcal (Quadrivalent: A, C, Y, and W135)	Ideal: 4 wk for immunity to develop	Travelers to Hajj/Umra and "meningitis belt"† during dry season from December to June; students living in dormitories in United States and other countries	Vaccinate	Vaccinate	Vaccinate if risk of infection is high	Vaccinate, but immune response may be low

*Immunocompromised persons include those receiving high-dose steroids (20 mg/d for >3 weeks), chemotherapy, or immunosuppressive regimens due to transplantation or other diseases, or those with congenital or acquired immunodeficiency states, including HIV or AIDS.

†"Meningitis belt" of Africa consists of the following countries: Burkina Faso, Cameroon, Central African Republic, Chad, Côte D'Ivoire, Djibouti, Ethiopia, Gambia, Ghana, Guinea, Guinea Bissau, Mali, Niger, Nigeria, Senegal, Sudan, Somalia, and Togo.

than 94% protection against the disease. It is a live, viral vaccine that can be received only from WHO-approved yellow fever vaccination centers. It is contraindicated in persons with impaired immune function (eg, HIV or AIDS, pregnancy, or congenital or [acquired immuno-compromise]). The vaccine must be received no less than 10 days before the planned date of entry and is valid for 10 years. Vaccine administration is documented and stamped on the appropriate page of the *International Certificate of Vaccination*.

Meningococcal.   Epidemics of *Neisseria meningitidis* occur during the winter dry season in the "meningitis belt" of Africa. Meningococcal vaccination is required for entry into some of the countries in this belt. Epidemics of meningitis have also occurred annually during travel to the hajj pilgrimage in Saudi Arabia. Meningococcal

vaccination may be required to obtain a visa and entry into Saudi Arabia. Although meningococcal vaccination is not required by WHO, students traveling for study abroad may be required to have the vaccine to meet school entry requirements.

Travel-related Sexually Transmitted Diseases

International spread of sexually transmitted diseases (STDs) is well documented in the medical literature. The incidence of travel-related STD is estimated to be approximately 5%, but this varies with STD prevalence at destination and the number of exposures. Anywhere from 5% to 60% of travelers engage in casual sex while abroad, and less than half use condoms.[61] This estimate may be even higher among long-term travelers. Risk factors for casual sex during travel include male sex, single status, age less than 20 years, traveling without a partner, recent history of multiple sexual partners, and history of recent illicit drugs or alcohol abuse. Gonorrhea and chlamydia are the most common STDs seen. Others include HIV, trichomoniasis, herpes simplex, hepatitis B and C, and human papillomavirus. Travelers should be counseled about safe-sex practices, such as to carry condoms with them from their home country, since availability or reliability of condoms (for both males and females) in developing countries might be limited, and to avoid alcohol or drug abuse. They also should be advised of the risks and symptoms of STD. Currently, hepatitis B is the only preventable STD with effective vaccination.

Conditions With Special Needs for Travel

Diabetes mellitus

Metabolic dysregulation is a clinically significant problem for diabetic patients, especially those receiving insulin who are traveling across multiple time zones. Diabetic patients carry an increased risk of acquiring travel-related illnesses, diabetic complications, and complications related to glycemic control. Pretravel health assessment is essential and general pretravel advice should be stressed. In addition, foot care and glycemic control, particularly the prevention of hypoglycemia, should be advised. Avoidance of hypoglycemia should be the goal during transit, and allowance of somewhat higher blood glucose levels can be acceptable until arrival at the destination. Diabetic individuals should monitor blood glucose levels more frequently while traveling. Patients receiving oral hypoglycemic agents or once-daily insulin therapy should maintain the prescribed interval between doses. Those receiving sliding-scale insulin should adjust insulin needs according to blood glucose levels. For those receiving 12-hour insulin therapy, a detailed discussion of time zones with planning of all doses and glucose monitoring should be undertaken. For long flights, it is advisable to keep the dose time on the departure location time until arrival at the destination. Diabetic patients should carry with them their medications, snacks, capillary glucose monitor, test strips, and a letter with their medical diagnosis wherever they go. They should also wear an emergency medical bracelet. A hot climate, increased physical activity, or changes in diet increase the likelihood of development of hypoglycemia. Therefore, monitoring closely for signs of hypoglycemia and keeping a snack close by are advised.[62]

Human immunodeficiency virus

Travel for immunologically intact HIV-positive patients (CD4+ T cells >200 cells/mm^3) is not any riskier than for non–HIV-infected persons. However, the risk of acquiring infections and the severity, frequency, and difficulty in management of infections increases with declining immune status (CD4+ T-cell count).[63] If the CD4+ T-cell count is below 200 cells/mm^3, the risk of infections, lack of adequate immune response to protective vaccines, and risk of disease from live virus vaccines should affect the decision to travel.[64] Irrespective of travel, the HIV-positive patient should be immunized against hepatitis A, hepatitis B, influenza, and pneumococcal disease. Depending on the destination, additional vaccines such as Japanese encephalitis or rabies may be required. Live, viral vaccines (yellow fever, MMR, oral poliovirus, and varicella) are contraindicated. However, in some situations where the patient's CD4 count is high (>200 cells/mm^3), the risk of natural disease is high, and travel is unavoidable, yellow fever vaccine may be considered. Travelers with HIV infection should take with them enough antiretroviral medications, as they may not be readily available worldwide. They should also be advised to be more meticulous about what they consume, as they are more likely to acquire food-borne and waterborne diseases. Although travel-related risks exist, studies show low levels of prophylactic measures undertaken by HIV-positive patients, underscoring the need to review future travel plans with such patients.[65]

Pregnancy

In general, healthy pregnant women carrying a single fetus can travel. The safest travel time is during the second trimester and probably until the 36th week.[66] Most airlines restrict travel for pregnant women after the 36th week of pregnancy, and some international carriers may restrict travel after the 35th week of gestation. Flying is restricted beyond 32 weeks for complicated pregnancies.[67] Women with a high-risk pregnancy (those with medical comorbidities or obstetric risk factors such as multiparity or preeclampsia) should avoid travel if possible. Women with sickle-cell disease or severe anemia should avoid air travel. Vaccinations for the pregnant traveler are based on the risk-benefit assessment of a travel-related illness and the vaccine itself. Live, viral vaccines are contraindicated in pregnancy. Both the mother and fetus are at increased risk of malaria morbidity and mortality. In addition, there are limited options for antimalarial prophylaxis available for pregnant women. Therefore, pregnant women are advised against travel to malaria-endemic countries. Pregnant women are also at an increased risk of TD because of lowered gastric acidity. Fluoroquinolones are contraindicated in pregnancy. Other risks to pregnant women include early labor (if >25 weeks gestation) and DVT. Pretravel advice should focus on identifying and counseling key risk factors in the pregnant traveler. Pregnant women should carry their medical history and blood group information when they travel.

Other Travel-related Risks and Advice

Deep vein thrombosis

There is a small association of DVT with long flights, and this association is much higher in persons with risk factors for DVT. In one study, 25% of patients with DVT had undertaken a journey of more than 4 hours' duration in the 4 weeks before presentation.[68] Deep vein thrombosis is more likely to occur in individuals over 40 years of age, with additional risk factors such as previous DVT, malignant or chronic diseases, hormone therapy, recent lower limb injury, recent surgery, having a femoral catheter, prothrombotic predisposition, pregnancy, and obesity. It is estimated that in approximately 10% of long-haul airline travelers DVT develops in the calf, although not all affected persons have symptoms.[69] Regular leg exercises and short walks along the aisles are recommended on long flights. Excess alcohol should be avoided, as it can lead to dehydration. Because DVT involves venous stasis, aspirin plays a minimal role in prevention. For those with risk factors, below-knee compression stockings with 20-mm Hg pressure should be advised. Therapy with low-molecular-weight heparin may be needed for high-risk patients such as those with previous DVT.[70,71]

Travel insurance

All travelers should be advised on travel insurance, including air evacuation insurance. Medicare and most insurance policies may not provide coverage for health services received outside the United States. Travel medical insurance is particularly important for persons with underlying medical conditions, prolonged travel, and high-risk travel (backpacking, hiking, rural travel).

SUMMARY

International travel is important for leisure, business, and learning. It has some attendant risks to the traveler that can easily be identified and minimized using an individualized approach. Detailed knowledge of the traveler's medical history and itinerary will likely provide the best guide for preventive advice against the infectious and noninfectious hazards of international travel.

REFERENCES

1. Tourism Highlights 2002. World Tourism Organization. Available at: www.world-tourism.org. market_research/facts&figures/latest_data/Mje.%20Highlights%202002%20INGLES.pdf. Accessed March, 28, 2003.

2. International Trade Administration, Office of Travel and Tourism Industries, US Dept of Commerce. 2001 Profile of U.S. Resident Travelers Visiting Overseas Destinations. Available at: www.tinet.ita.doc.gov. Accessed April 11, 2003.

3. Ryan ET, Kain KC. Health advice and immunizations for travelers. *N Engl J Med.* 2000;342:1716–1725.

4. Kemmerer TP, Cetron M, Harpar L, Kozarsky PE. Health problems of corporate travelers: risk factors and management. *J Travel Med.* 1998;5:184–187.

5. Hill DR. Health problems in a large cohort of Americans traveling to developing countries. *J Travel Med.* 2000;7:259–266.

6. Leder K, Sundararajan V, Weld L, et al. Respiratory tract infections in travelers: a review of the GeoSentinel surveillance network. *Clin Infect Dis.* 2003;36:399–406.

7. Pitzinger B, Steffen R, Tschopp A. Incidence and clinical features of traveler's diarrhea in infants and children. *Pediatr Infect Dis J.* 1991;10:719–723.

8. Hargarten SW, Baker TD, Guptill K. Overseas fatalities of United States citizen travelers: an analysis of deaths related to international travel. *Ann Emerg Med.* 1991;20:622–626.

9. MacPherson D, Guérillot F, Streiner DL, Ahmed K, Gushulak BD, Pardy G. Death and dying abroad: the Canadian experience. *J Travel Med.* 2000;7:227–234.

10. Phillips-Howard PA, Radalowicz A, Mitchell J, Bradley DJ. Risk of malaria in British residents returning from malarious areas. *BMJ.* 1990;300:499–503.

11. Striker J, Luippold RS, Nagy L, Liese B, Bigelow C, Mundt KA. Risk factors for psychological stress among international business travelers. *Occup Environ Med.* 1999;56:245–252.

12. Liese B, Mundt KA, Dell LD, Nagy L, Demure B. Medical insurance claims associated with international business travel. *Occup Environ Med.* 1997;54:499–503.

13. Schlagenhauf P, Steffen R, Loutan L. Migrants as a major risk group for imported malaria in European countries. *J Travel Med.* 2003;10:106.

14. World Health Organization. World malaria situation in 1994. *Wkly Epidemiol Rec.* 1997;72:269–276.

15. Steffen R, Fuchs E, Schildknecht J, et al. Mefloquine compared with other malaria chemoprophylactic regimens in tourists visiting east Africa. *Lancet.* 1993;341:1299–1303.

16. Bradley D. Prophylaxis against malaria for travellers from the United Kingdom: Malaria Reference Laboratory and the Ross Institute. *BMJ.* 1993;306:1247–1252.

17. Kain KC, Keystone JS. Malaria in travelers: epidemiology, disease, and prevention. *Infect Dis Clin North Am.* 1998;12:267–284.

18. Kain KC, MacPherson DW, Kelton T, Keystone JS, Mendelson J, MacLean JD. Malaria deaths in visitors to Canada and in Canadian travellers: a case series. *CMAJ.* 2001;164:654–659.

19. Kain KC, Harrington MA, Tennyson S, Keystone JS. Imported malaria: prospective analysis of problems in diagnosis and management. *Clin Infect Dis.* 1998;27:142–149.

20. dos Santos CC, Anvar A, Keystone JS, Kain KC. Survey of use of malaria prevention measures by Canadians visiting India. *CMAJ.* 1999;160:195–200.

21. Schwartz E, Potasman I, Rotenberg M, Almog S, Sadetzki S. Serious adverse events of mefloquine in relation to blood level and gender. *Am J Trop Med Hyg.* 2001;65:189–192.

22. Andersen SL, Oloo AJ, Gordon DM, et al. Successful double-blinded, randomized, placebo-controlled field trial of azithromycin and doxycycline as prophylaxis for malaria in western Kenya. *Clin Infect Dis.* 1998;26:146–150.

23. Sudden death in a traveler following halofantrine administration: Togo, 2000. *MMWR Morb Mortal Wkly Rep.* 2001;50:169–170, 179.

24. van Riemsdijk MM, Sturkenboom MC, Ditters JM, Ligthelm RJ, Overbosch D, Stricker BH. Atovaquone plus chloroguanide versus mefloquine for malaria prophylaxis: a focus on neuropsychiatric adverse events. *Clin Pharmacol Ther.* 2002;72:294–301.

25. Overbosch D, Schilthuis H, Bienzle U, et al. Atovaquone-proguanil versus mefloquine for malaria prophylaxis in nonimmune travelers: results from a randomized, double-blind study. *Clin Infect Dis.* 2001;33:1015–1021.

26. Shanks GD, Gordon DM, Klotz FW, et al. Efficacy and safety of atovaquone/proguanil as suppressive prophylaxis for *Plasmodium falciparum* malaria. *Clin Infect Dis.* 1998;27:494–499.

27. Ohrt C, Richie TL, Widjaja H, et al. Mefloquine compared with doxycycline for the prophylaxis of malaria in Indonesian soldiers: a randomized, double-blind, placebo-controlled trial. *Ann Intern Med.* 1997;126:963–972.

28. Arthur JD, Echeverria P, Shanks GD, Karwacki J, Bodhidatta L, Brown JE. A comparative study of gastrointestinal infections in United States soldiers receiving doxycycline or mefloquine for malaria prophylaxis. *Am J Trop Med Hyg.* 1990;43:608–613.

29. Nosten F, Vincenti M, Simpson J, et al. The effects of mefloquine treatment in pregnancy. *Clin Infect Dis.* 1999;28:808–815.

30. Kain KC, Shanks GD, Keystone JS. Malaria chemo-prophylaxis in the age of drug resistance: I. Currently recommended drug regimens. *Clin Infect Dis.* 2001;33:226–234.

31. Casalino E, Le Bras J, Chaussin F, Fichelle A, Bouvet E. Predictive factors of malaria in travelers to areas where malaria is endemic. *Arch Intern Med.* 2002;162:1625–1630.

32. Jelinek T. Dengue fever in international travelers. *Clin Infect Dis.* 2000;31:144–147.

33. Jelinek T, Muhlberger N, Harms G, et al. Epidemiology and clinical features of imported dengue fever in Europe: sentinel surveillance data from TropNetEurop. *Clin Infect Dis.* 2002;35:1047–1052.

34. Fradin MS. Mosquitoes and mosquito repellents: a clinician's guide. *Ann Intern Med.* 1998;128:931–940.

35. Fradin MS, Day JF. Comparative efficacy of insect repellents against mosquito bites. *N Engl J Med.* 2002;347:13–18.

36. Centers for Disease Control and Prevention (CDC). *Health Information for International Travel, 2001–2002.* Atlanta, Ga: CDC; 2002.

37. Osimitz TG, Grothaus RH. The present safety assessment of deet. *J Am Mosq Control Assoc.* 1995;11:274–278.

38. McGready R, Hamilton KA, Simpson JA, et al. Safety of the insect repellent N,N-diethyl-M-toluamide (DEET) in pregnancy. *Am J Trop Med Hyg.* 2001;65:285–289.

39. Young GD, Evans S. Safety and efficacy of DEET and permethrin in the prevention of arthropod attack. *Mil Med.* 1998;163:324–330.

40. Lima AA. Tropical diarrhoea: new developments in traveller's diarrhoea. *Curr Opin Infect Dis.* 2001;14:547–552.

41. Steffen R, Collard F, Tornieporth N, et al. Epidemiology, etiology, and impact of traveler's diarrhea in Jamaica. *JAMA.* 1999;281:811–817.

42. Ericsson CD. Travelers' diarrhea: epidemiology, prevention, and self-treatment. *Infect Dis Clin North Am.* 1998;12:285–303.

43. Jiang ZD, Lowe B, Verenkar MP, et al. Prevalence of enteric pathogens among international travelers with diarrhea acquired in Kenya (Mombasa), India (Goa), or Jamaica (Montego Bay). *J Infect Dis.* 2002;185:497–502.

44. Adachi JA, Jiang ZD, Mathewson JJ, et al. Enteroaggregative *Escherichia coli* as a major etiologic agent in traveler's diarrhea in 3 regions of the world. *Clin Infect Dis.* 2001;32:1706–1709.

45. Ansdell VE, Ericsson CD. Prevention and empiric treatment of traveler's diarrhea. *Med Clin North Am.* 1999;83:945–973.

46. Herwaldt BL, de Arroyave KR, Roberts JM, Juranek DD. A multiyear prospective study of the risk factors for and incidence of diarrheal illness in a cohort of Peace Corps volunteers in Guatemala. *Ann Intern Med.* 2000;132:982–988.

47. Daniels NA, Neimann J, Karpati A, et al. Traveler's diarrhea at sea: three outbreaks of waterborne enterotoxigenic *Escherichia coli* on cruise ships. *J Infect Dis.* 2000;181:1491–1495.

48. Kelly P, Baboo KS, Ndubani P, et al. Cryptosporidiosis in adults in Lusaka, Zambia, and its relationship to oocyst contamination of drinking water. *J Infect Dis.* 1997;176:1120–1123.

49. Beller M, Ellis A, Lee SH, et al. Outbreak of viral gastroenteritis due to a contaminated well: international consequences. *JAMA*. 1997;278:563–568.

50. Ericsson CD, Johnson PC, Dupont HL, Morgan DR, Bitsura JA, de la Cabada FJ. Ciprofloxacin or trimethoprimsulfamethoxazole as initial therapy for travelers' diarrhea: a placebo-controlled, randomized trial. *Ann Intern Med*. 1987;106:216–220.

51. DuPont HL, Ericsson CD, Mathewson JJ, DuPont MW. Five versus three days of ofloxacin therapy for traveler's diarrhea: a placebo-controlled study. *Antimicrobial Agents Chemother*. 1992;36:87–91.

52. Ericsson CD, DuPont HL, Mathewson JJ, West MS, Johnson PC, Bitsura JA. Treatment of traveler's diarrhea with sulfamethoxazole and trimethoprim and loperamide. *JAMA*. 1990;263:257–261.

53. Adachi JA, Ostrosky-Zeichner L, DuPont HL, Ericsson CD. Empirical antimicrobial therapy for traveler's diarrhea. *Clin Infect Dis*. 2000;31:1079–1083.

54. Khan WA, Seas C, Dhar U, Salam MA, Bennish ML. Treatment of shigellosis: V. Comparison of azithromycin and ciprofloxacin: a double-blind, randomized, controlled trial. *Ann Intern Med*. 1997;126:697–703.

55. Song JH, Lee NY, Ichiyama S, et al. Spread of drug-resistant *Streptococcus pneumoniae* in Asian countries: Asian Network for Surveillance of Resistant Pathogens (ANSORP) Study. *Clin Infect Dis*. 1999;28:1206–1211.

56. Van Damme P, Thoelen S, Cramm M, De Groote K, Safary A, Meheus A. Inactivated hepatitis A vaccine: reactogenicity, immunogenicity, and long-term antibody persistence. *J Med Virol*. 1994;44:446–451.

57. Prevention of hepatitis A through active or passive immunization: recommendations of the Advisory Committee on Immunization Practices (ACIP). *MMWR Morb Mortal Wkly Rep Recomm Rep*. 1999;48(RR-12):1–37.

58. Maiwald H, Jilg W, Bock HL, Loscher T, Sonnenburg F. Long-term persistence of anti-HAV antibodies following active immunization with hepatitis A vaccine. *Vaccine*. 997;15:346–348.

59. Takahashi H, Pool V, Tsai TF, Chen RT. Adverse events after Japanese encephalitis vaccination: review of post-marketing surveillance data from Japan and the United States: the VAERS Working Group. *Vaccine*. 2000;18:2963–2969.

60. Mermin JH, Townes JM, Gerber M, Dolan N, Mintz ED, Tauxe RV. Typhoid fever in the United States, 1985–1994: changing risks of international travel and increasing antimicrobial resistance. *Arch Intern Med*. 1998;158:633–638.

61. Matteelli A, Carosi G. Sexually transmitted diseases in travelers. *Clin Infect Dis*. 2001;32:1063–1067.

62. Gill GV, Redmond S. Insulin treatment, time-zones and air travel: a survey of current advice from British diabetic clinics. *Diabet Med*. 1993;10:764–767.

63. Wilson ME, von Reyn CF, Fineberg HV. Infections in HIV-infected travelers: risks and prevention. *Ann Intern Med*. 1991;114:582–592.

64. Castelli F, Patroni A. The human immunodeficiency virus-infected traveler. *Clin Infect Dis*. 2000;31:1403–1408.

65. Orlando G, Galimberti L, Visona R, et al. Effect of international travel on HIV-positive patients' health. Paper presented at 8th Conference of International Society of Travel Medicine; 2003; New York, NY.

66. Samuel BU, Barry M. The pregnant traveler. *Infect Dis Clin North Am*. 1998;12:325–354.

67. World Health Organization. Travellers with special needs. Available at: www.who.int/ith/chapter02_03.html. Accessed June 20, 2003.

68. Ferrari E, Chevallier T, Chapelier A, Baudouy M. Travel as a risk factor for venous thromboembolic disease: a case-control study. *Chest*. 1999;115:440–444.

69. Scurr JH, Machin SJ, Bailey-King S, Mackie IJ, McDonald S, Smith PD. Frequency and prevention of symptomless deep-vein thrombosis in long-haul flights: a randomised trial. *Lancet*. 2001;357:1485–1489.

70. Geroulakos G. The risk of venous thromboembolism from air travel. *BMJ*. 2001;322:188.

71. Giangrande PLF. Thrombosis and air travel. *J Travel Med*. 2001;7:149–155.

chapter 25

The Adolescent

Ellen S. Rome, MD, MPH

INTRODUCTION

Adolescence encompasses the period of rapid physical and psychological growth and development that differentiates the child from the adult. Years spanned usually range from 12 through 21 years of age, However, the hormonal changes of puberty can start as young as 8 years old, and the "adolescent mindset" may last well into the fourth decade of life or longer! Theories of adolescence have evolved over time, moving away from the view of the teen years as a time of "storm and stress," with raging hormones and uncontrolled behaviors.[1,2] More recent theories have seen "normal" adolescence as far less tempestuous, with the typical teen negotiating this transitional time with relatively little major disruption or sustained high-risk behavior, building his or her own identity, maintaining relationships with parents and family, and developing new relationships and skill sets.[3,4] Using this perspective, problem behaviors should be seen as a red flag that a teen needs more help or interventions. Moreover, successful interventions with this group are likely to have important payoffs later in productivity in the community, prevention of health problems, and reduced cost to society.[3,5]

The tasks of adolescence can be seen in terms of early adolescence from ages 11 to 14 years, (2) middle adolescence from 15 to 17 years, and (3) late adolescence from 18 to 21 years (Table 25-1). In early adolescence, the defining question for emotional and physical well-being is, Am I normal? In the early teens, the adolescent may feel like a character in *Alice in Wonderland,* wondering if body parts are too big or too small, and how he or she measures up to peers.

By middle adolescence, the question changes to, Am I liked? Here, the adolescent shifts from a focus on family to increased importance of peers, with inordinate amounts of time and energy put into appearance by both boys and girls. The clothing and cosmetics industries certainly have taken advantage of this phenomenon, targeting teens as primary consumers.

By late adolescence, peers become less important than the one-on-one relationship with a significant other, with the question shifting from, Am I liked? to Am I loved? If an adolescent is challenged with a pregnancy, depression, school failure, or especially substance abuse, the normal tasks of adolescence may come to a halt, with the teen getting stuck at whatever developmental stage he or she was in at the time of the stress. For instance, the substance-abusing teen may not develop the ability to think abstractly and instead is able only to think of the here and now. The pregnant and parenting teen may not be able to achieve emotional and financial separation from her family, whom she now needs to help with the myriad aspects of care for her own child. These tasks may be completed later. The parenting teen may become the head of her own household in her 20s, or the drug-addicted teen may recover (usually with some sort of intervention) and move on to a productive adulthood.

THE ADOLESCENT INTERVIEW

An agenda of preventive health should be advanced well before adolescence. Health maintenance visits from birth onward should help educate parents and families on issues of safety, appropriate diet and exercise, role modeling healthy relationships, cigarettes, alcohol, and substance abuse. As the child reaches adolescence, the clinician should carve out time with the adolescent alone to address issues that the teen may find difficult to discuss with a parent in the room.

How one establishes confidentiality can be critical. In the worst-case scenario, the parent may feel left out of the equation and bar access to the child. In the best-case scenario, both the adolescent and the parent feel empowered to make healthy choices, with the clinician as a bridge of communication when needed or appropriate. Adolescents will share personal health information best when confidentiality *plus* the limits of confidentiality are clearly delineated.[6] There is no single right way to establish confidentiality, and it may take practice to establish

T A B L E 25-1

Tasks of Adolescence

Task	Early (11–14 y)	Middle (15–17 y)	Late (18–22 y)
Body image	Adjusting to pubertal changes	"Trying out" different images	Integration of a satisfying body image
Central question	Am I normal?	Am I liked?	Am I loved?
Independence	Emotional break from parents; prefers friends to family; needs privacy and approval	Ambivalence about separation; peak of parental conflict	Integration of independence
Sexual drives	Sexual curiosity	Social experimentation	Beginning of intimacy
Relationships	Unisex peer group; crushes on adults	Begins heterosexual peer group; multiple adult role models	Intimate relationship more important than peers
Career plans	Vague and unrealistic; economically dependent	Moving from vague to specific; economically dependent to independent	Specific, tangible; economically independent
Conceptualization	Concrete thoughts; monosyllabic answers	Self-centered; experimentation	Abstract thought (not achieved by all); future oriented
Value system	Testing of the parents' moral system	Moral development begins	Incorporation of own values and beliefs

T A B L E 25-2

HEADS Examination (Obtaining a Psychosocial History)

Home: How is home? Who lives at home? What happens when there is an argument at home?

Education: What grade are you in? How are your grades this year? How were your grades last year?

Activities: What do you like to do for fun? What do you do for exercise? Do you do any after-school activities? Are you in a gang? Do you carry a weapon/gun? Are there guns in your home?

Drugs/depression: Do your friends smoke? Do you smoke? How long does a pack last you? For how long have you smoked? Do your friends drink alcohol? Do you drink alcohol? How much? How often? Have you ever gotten sick? Blacked out? Passed out? Do your friends use drugs? Have you ever used drugs? Which ones? How often? Have you ever been depressed? Ever to the point of wanting to hurt yourself? Have you tried? Have you ever wished you were dead? Have you ever thought, I'm going to kill myself? If so, have you had a plan? What was it?

Sex: Have you ever had sex? With how many partners? What did you use for protection? If condoms, did you use them sometimes, all the time, or none of the time? What was your second method of contraception? Have you or a partner had any STDs? Any pregnancies? (Or have you gotten anyone pregnant?) Have you ever had to swap sex for food, clothing, drugs, or shelter? Sexually, has anyone ever done anything to you that made you uncomfortable? Are you attracted to guys, girls, or both?

confidentiality artfully. A clinician might say, " I would like to take some time alone with your parents if they have any worries or concerns that they wish to discuss with me alone. Then I will take some time alone with you, to give you time to address any worries or health concerns that you may have. Anything I talk about with your parents privately will be kept confidential, meaning I will not share with you their private concerns; in the same way, anything we talk about without a parent will be kept confidential. However, if you tell me something life-threatening or dangerous, I will have to tell you that we need to talk to your parents about this." When possible, the clinician should try to talk to the parent (or parents) first before taking time alone with the adolescent; thus, the teen sees that the parent's private

concerns are kept confidential. If the teen is interviewed before the parent, the adolescent may feel that you are then reporting the conversation to the parent. Such subtleties build trust with patient and parents while continuing to reinforce healthy messages.

Once confidentiality has been established, the clinician can obtain a psychosocial history by asking the HEADS questions (Table 25-2).[7] These questions should not be asked with the parent present and then repeated without the parent in the room, as it implies that it is okay not to tell the whole truth with a parent in the room, but that "another truth" exists outside of the parents' hearing. These questions can be asked while performing the physical examination, before the examination, or after. Timing of questions can be clinically useful. If you ask a young teen if he smokes while listening to his lungs, he may think that you will know just by doing your examination, prompting him to answer truthfully!

Patients in early and middle adolescence are more likely to talk about their own risk behaviors if they have already admitted to having friends who engage in risk behaviors. Accordingly, ask about friends' use of cigarettes, drugs, or other risk behaviors before asking the adolescent about whether they have engaged in the risk behavior. If an adolescent girl tells you that all of her friends smoke but that she has not tried cigarettes, you can informally build skills using role-play, by asking her what she tells friends when they are smoking and want her to smoke, too. If she cannot think of an appropriate response, you can provide her with several responses, such as "No thanks, I like my lungs the way they are" or "I choose not to smoke." If a teenage girl's sibling has become a teen parent, she is at greater risk of having her own baby in her teens.[8] If the teenager has not yet initiated sexual activity, the provider should ask what the teen's views on sex are. How old does he think he should be before starting? Which methods of contraception would she plan to use to keep herself safe? If she replies, "condoms," the provider can then ask about what second method she wishes to use to avoid pregnancy, stating that with condoms alone, pregnancies still occur, and that to stay pregnancy free, she will need to use 2 methods of protection all the time. When the clinician asks about home, if an adolescent states that he lives with mom, the clinician should ask how often he sees dad, and is that enough? After the provider asks what happens when there is an argument in the home, if an adolescent says that it is fine except when dad drinks, the provider should follow up with, "What happens when dad drinks?" If a teenager reports that grades this year are worse than last year, the provider should ask the teen why he or she thinks that change has happened. School failure can be a red flag for depression, a learning disability or attention deficit disorder that had not been detected previously, trouble at home, a drug habit, or other psychosocial problems.

Continuity of care helps build trust with both patient and parents. Trust, in turn, helps to reinforce healthy messages, to empower teens to be their own best health care consumer and advocate for health, to build skills, and to enhance motivation to change when problem behavior already exists. Barriers to care include not feeling comfortable in a setting, lack of knowledge of available services, cost, lack of transportation, and perceived lack of confidentiality.

MORTALITY IN ADOLESCENTS

Understanding adolescent development is essential to preventive medicine, as the adolescent's main risks of morbidity and mortality are behaviorally related. The leading causes of mortality among inner-city African American males are motor vehicle accidents, followed by homicide and suicide; for white teenaged males and Caucasian and minority females, the leading causes of death are motor vehicle accidents, suicide, and homicide.

Motor Vehicle Accidents

Two of 5 deaths among adolescents in the United States are caused by motor vehicle accidents.[9] In 2001, more than 30% of teens who died in motor vehicle accidents had ridden with a driver who had been drinking alcohol.[10] Per miles driven, teens 16 to 19 years of age are 4 times more likely than older drivers to crash.[11] Unsupervised teenaged drivers carrying teen passengers have a higher crash risk, with that risk increasing with the number of teen passengers.[12] Adolescent male drivers represent the highest risk group.[13]

Developmental factors put teens most at risk; the adolescent sense of invulnerability may lead teens to underestimate the dangers of hazardous situations. Moreover, they have less experience coping with such situations once in them.[14] Adolescents are also more likely to run red lights, speed, and make illegal turns. They are more likely to ride with an intoxicated driver and to drive after using alcohol and drugs.[14]

One effective means of decreasing motor vehicle fatalities has been the use of mandatory seat belt laws. Adolescents remain the group least likely to wear seat belts.[10,15] After consuming alcohol, they are even less likely to wear seat belts.[16] Since most of those deaths occur later at night, clinicians should consider counseling parents about these risks and suggesting the idea of a "car curfew," a time at which the car needs to be back home. Repeated emphasis of the "don't drink and drive" message from parents, school, community, physicians, and the media may lower the risks.

Violence

Violence is a major cause of morbidity and mortality in the adolescent age group. In 2001, nearly 17.5% of students carried a weapon in the month before being surveyed, and 5.7% had carried a gun in that past month.[10] In the 12 months before the survey, 4% of students had been treated by a doctor or nurse for injuries sustained in a physical fight, and 6.6% had missed school at least one day in the prior month because of feeling unsafe at school or in transit between home and school.[10] In 2001, more than 10% of female students and approximately 5% of male students reported having been forced to have sexual intercourse, and 9.5% of students had been hit, slapped, or physically hurt on purpose by their boyfriend or girlfriend that year.[10]

Children and adolescents who witness violence or are victims themselves show increased risk of academic underachievement, depression, and post-traumatic stress disorder.[17] According to social learning theory, learning emerges through repeated observations of others' behavior; youth learn about violence through what they experience and what they see around them. Vulnerability to these social influences depends on the individual's personality, attitudes, knowledge, and beliefs. Risk factors for perpetuating violence include exposure to violence in the home, even if it occurred when the teen was a young child.

Another risk factor occurs when parents rely on corporal punishment for discipline; parents who teach that might is right should not be surprised when their now physically grown adolescent strikes back or strikes his or her own child. The American Academy of Pediatrics (AAP), in response to studies noting the link between corporal punishment and subsequent violence as adults, published a position statement encouraging pediatricians to counsel parents about alternatives to corporal punishment from childhood onward.[18,19]

A third risk factor for adolescent violence is exposure to violence through television, with young children particularly vulnerable. Violent mainstream productions have been shown to produce measurable short-term effects on adolescents.[17]

Anticipatory guidance about violence prevention should have its groundwork laid in childhood. From preschool onward, bullying should not be tolerated in the school or in the community. Since the fatal shootings at Columbine High School in Littleton, Colo, many schools have adopted a zero tolerance toward expressed intent to hurt or kill. If a student's words, "I'm going to kill you," are brought to the attention of a school administrator or teacher, responses can range from suspension to having the police come and take the adolescent to the station for a formal investigation of intent and educational intervention. The United States has the highest homicide rate of any developed country and the easiest access to guns, thereby lending support to a zero tolerance policy. However, teens most at risk of violence are often those not attending school, and poverty and low socioeconomic status are associated with the highest rates of violent death.[17]

Other parental interventions can include removing handguns from the house, limiting TV viewing time from infancy onward, and role modeling alternatives to violence. Clinicians can ask adolescents during an office visit if they carry any kind of weapon, helping the teens understand that they are more likely to be injured just by carrying the weapon. Adolescents who arm themselves as self-protection may place themselves in more risky situations because of an illusion of safety combined with the their own personal illusion of invincibility.[17,20]

Concrete skills building can be useful in preventing the cycle of violence, especially during early and middle adolescence. To ascertain risk, the provider can use the FISTS mnemonic (Table 25-3), then follow up with questions such as, "What else might you have said in that situation to avoid the fight?" If the adolescent cannot think of alternatives, the clinician can offer other strategies, such as "In similar situations, it might be useful to try looking the other person in the eye and say, 'This isn't worth fighting about.' or 'I don't want to fight you.' What else could you say if someone was trying to pick a fight with you?" In this way, the clinician gives the teen a chance to practice these skills out loud, with repetition working toward mastery.

Table 25-4 outlines strategies for teaching teenagers warning signs of a potentially violent partner. Antiviolence curricula in schools can teach conflict resolution, anger management, and prevention of dating violence, with most programs building skills through role-plays and active learning. Peer mediation programs also have been successful in some school systems.

Depression and Suicide

If substance abuse, school truancy, driving under the influence of alcohol, and violent behavior to others are

---

TABLE 25-3

FISTS Mnemonic: Screening Tool for Risk of Violence-Related Injury*

Fighting: How many fights have you been in over the past year? When was your last fight? If a recent fight has occurred, how did it start? Who else was there? Why did you choose to fight at that time? What could you do differently?

Injuries: Have you ever been hurt in a fight? Have you ever injured anyone else in a fight?

Sex: Has your partner ever hit you? Have you ever hit or hurt your partner? Have you ever been forced to have sex against your will? Do you think that couples can stay in love when one partner makes the other one feel afraid?

Threats: Have you ever been threatened by someone who carried a weapon? What happened? Has anything changed since then to make you feel safer? What are ways you can help yourself feel safer?

Self-defense: Have you ever carried a weapon as self-defense? What do you do when someone tries to pick a fight with you?

*Adapted from Alpert E, Sege R, Bradshaw Y, for the Association of American Medical Colleges. Interpersonal violence and the education of physicians. *Acad Med.* 1997;72(suppl):S41–S50.

seen as *acting-out behaviors*, then issues of mental health, including eating disorders, cutting oneself, depression, and suicide, can be considered *acting in*, or *quietly disturbed behaviors*.[21] In 2001, more than 28% of students felt so sad or hopeless almost daily for at least 2 weeks in a row that they had stopped doing their usual activities; 19% of students had seriously considered attempting suicide, and 8.8% of American youth admitted to having attempted suicide in the year before being surveyed.[10] Estimates show that 1 in 10 teens contemplate suicide annually, about 0.5 million annually in the United States alone.[22] Girls tend to attempt suicide more often than boys, but boys choose more violent methods, thus making their suicide completion rate higher. As US surgeon general, David Satcher announced in 2001 a national campaign to prevent suicide, urging that suicide risk screening become part of every primary care practice.

Depressed children and adolescents are more likely to present with somatic complaints—headaches, abdominal pain, malaise, and fatigue (often with frequent school absenteeism)—than with a more direct complaint of depression. Signs for depression in this age group (Table 25-5) are nonspecific markers of a teen in distress and may point the clinician to ask more focused questions about depression.

SEXUALITY, SEXUALLY TRANSMITTED DISEASES, AND PREGNANCY

Of the 15 million new cases of sexually transmitted disease (STD) occurring in the United States each year, adolescents account for one fourth, and two thirds occur in the age group 25 years or younger.[23] Responsible sexual behavior among adolescents is one of the 10 leading health indicators of the national health objectives for 2010. In 2001, just over 45.5% of high school students had ever had sexual intercourse, with 42.1% of sexually active students reporting not using a condom at last sexual intercourse.[10] Over the decade 1991 to 2001, fewer high school students reported having sex, and adolescent rates of gonorrhea, teen pregnancy, and birth rates have similarly declined.[24-26] These positive trends in health outcomes are most likely the result of the combined efforts of parents and families, schools, health care providers, religious organizations, media, and government agencies. One factor that may account for the declining teen pregnancy rates is that fewer teens are having sex at all. In addition, adolescents who do engage in intercourse have a declining pregnancy rate, most likely because of better contraceptive use and possibly less frequent sexual activity.

Birth rates among teenagers have also steadily decreased between the years 1991 and 2001. Greater declines were seen for 15- to 17-year-old teens than for teens aged 18 to 19 years. The largest decline occurred in black teens aged 15 to 17 years. In 1997 among adolescents, more than 55% of pregnancies ended in live birth, 29% in induced abortions, and 15% in fetal loss.[27] Four of 5 teen births are first births.[28]

Factors that predict the increased likelihood of early sexual activity include being African American, being male, living in a low-income family, and living with unsupportive parents who do not supervise the child or

TABLE 25-4

Teaching Teens: Warning Signs of Potentially Violent Partner*

Wants to get serious quickly
Will not take "no" for an answer
Is possessive or jealous; wants to know where the partner is at all times
Wants to choose the partner's friends and activities
Blames the victim: "You make me so mad!"
Apologizes for outbursts and promises never to do it again
May participate in other risky behaviors: drinking, drugs, cigarettes, gangs, or guns

*Adapted from *Adolesc Health Update.* 1999;12:1–8.[17]

TABLE 25-5

Red Flags for Depression in the Adolescent

Recurrent somatic complaints
Headaches
Abdominal pain
Nausea/vomiting
Fatigue/malaise
Chest pain
School failure or declining grades
Anhedonia (loss of pleasure in situations and events)
A dysfunctional family
Divorce or separation of parents
Disordered eating
Loss of friends; social isolation
Insomnia or hypersomnolence
Prior suicide attempt or attempts
Substance/alcohol use (may be self-medication)
Prior traumatic experience (global or personal)
Abuse (physical, emotional, sexual)
Loss of concentration
Low self-esteem
Decreased attention to personal hygiene
Bouts of crying or irritability

TABLE 25-6

Characteristics of Effective Sex and HIV Education Programs*

1. Focus on reducing 1 or more sexual behaviors that lead to unintended pregnancy, HIV, or other STDs.
2. Are grounded in theory that has been demonstrated to influence other health-related behaviors and identify specific important sexual antecedents to be targeted.
3. Deliver and consistently reinforce a clear message on abstinence and using condoms and other forms of contraception if sexually active (abstinence *plus* contraceptive counseling).
4. Provide basic, accurate information about the risks of adolescent sexual activity and about ways to avoid intercourse or use methods of protection against pregnancy and STDs.
5. Include activities that address societal pressures that influence sexual behavior.
6. Provide examples and build skills in communication, negotiation, and refusal.
7. Actively engage participants and use teaching methods that personalize the information.
8. Incorporate behavioral goals, teaching methods, and materials that are appropriate for the age, sexual experience, and culture of the student.
9. Last a sufficient time (eg, more than a few hours).
10. Select teachers or peer leaders who believe in the program and the message and then provide these teachers or leaders with adequate training.

*HIV indicates human immunodeficiency virus; STD, sexually transmitted disease. Adapted from Kirby D.[33]

adolescent's activities.[3,29] Other factors include low expectations for school achievement, lack of engagement in school activities, less religiosity, having an external locus of control rather than an internal one, use of drugs and alcohol, and being easily influenced by peers in similar situations.[3,30,31] From the Add Health survey data, these demographic factors play only a minor role in explaining teenage sexual activity, with tremendous variance between individual racial, ethnic, and income groups.[32]

Because healthy sexuality, including intercourse, is an expected part of adulthood, the approach to sexual risk behaviors differs from addressing substance abuse or smoking, where the goal is never to start or to quit if started. Accordingly, even a delay in initiation of sexual activity is considered a valid and worthwhile goal. In 15- to 17-year-olds, for instance, virginity pledges delayed sexual intercourse by an average of 18 months.[32] These findings, however, did not generalize to all groups, ages, and ethnic groups. Pledges worked best when not all adolescents in the school endorsed the behavior; a virginity pledge gave participants a shared group identity that set them apart from their peers.[32] Such pledges carry some risk, in that teens who break their pledge are one third less likely than non-pledgers to use contraceptives once they become sexually active.[32] To prevent such outcomes, current theory proposes that contraceptive counseling should accompany education on virginity pledges, even when it might appear at first glance that the teens will not need such counseling.

Other factors that delay initiation of sexual activity include connectedness to parents, peer relationships, and culture. When teens live with both parents, they are less likely to engage in sex, more likely to use contraception when they have sex, and less likely to become pregnant or cause a pregnancy.[33] When a teen's peers obtain poor grades, feel disconnected from school, and participate in other risky behaviors, the teen is more likely to engage in sexual activity or other risk behaviors. Culture also affects adolescent sexuality. For example, Hispanic families may be more accepting of early childbearing than are non-Hispanic, white families.[33]

To encourage the development of sexual health in adolescent patients, clinicians can provide education on abstinence as a healthy choice combined with contraceptive counseling for those patients who choose to engage in sex. Other topics for education include negotiation of "no" or sexual limit setting, prevention of STDs including human immunodeficiency virus (HIV), and pregnancy prevention. Components of effective sex and HIV education programs can be found in Table 25-6. If a provider feels ill-equipped to discuss contraceptive options, referral sources can be used. Not asking the questions, thereby avoiding the discussion, is a major error to avoid in promotion of sexual health. Communication between families and children or adolescents builds decision-making skills in the adolescent. Parents, however, may feel unsure of themselves in initiating or continuing conversations on sexuality, abstinence, or contraceptive counseling. When parents explicitly state their values and express their goals for their children and adolescents, the adolescents are less likely to engage in the behavior than when the value is merely implied and not spoken aloud. Single parents should also be counseled to keep their own dating practices separate from their children's lives.

TOBACCO, ALCOHOL, AND SUBSTANCE ABUSE

Use of cigarettes, alcohol, and drugs typically begins in adolescence and can have a long-term impact on the physical and mental health of past and present users.

A longitudinal evaluation begun in 1975 at the University of Michigan, called Monitoring the Future, annually surveys American adolescents, college students, and young adults and documents trends in use of illicit and licit drugs.[34] Since 1991, the survey has included a nationally representative sample of 8th and 10th graders as well as 12th graders. Estimates in 2001 show that more than one half of American youth tried an illicit drug by the time they finished high school, more than one third had tried inhalants by 8th grade, and 3 of 10 students had used an illicit drug other than marijuana by the end of 12th grade. Nearly two thirds of US teenagers have tried cigarettes by 12th grade, and 30% of 12th graders are current smokers. By eighth grade, nearly 4 of 10 students have tried cigarettes, and 1 in 8 has become a current smoker.

Use of smokeless tobacco also declined considerably in the last few years[10,34] but cigars have become more popular, with 15.2% of students in the Youth Risk Behavior Survey noting cigar use in the month before the survey.[10] The purchase of cigarettes continues to be easy; more than two thirds of students who purchased or attempted to buy cigarettes in a store or gas station during the 30 days before the survey had not been asked to show proof of age.[10]

Four of 5 students have consumed more than a few sips of alcohol by the end of high school, with 51% having done so by eighth grade. Nearly two thirds of 12th graders and almost one fourth of 8th graders in 2001 report having been drunk at least once. According to the Youth Risk Behavior Survey, 78.2% of students had drunk at least one alcoholic beverage in their lifetime, and 29.9% had consumed at least 5 alcoholic drinks on at least one occasion in the month before the survey.[10]

Marijuana use peaked in 1979 at 51% of 12th graders, reached as low as 22% in 1992, and approximates 39% in 12th graders in 2001. Marijuana remains a highly accessible drug, with little perceived risk and falling rates of personal disapproval of use among 10th and 12th graders.[34]

In 2001, the primary drug showing an increase in use was Ecstasy (methylenedioxymethamphetamine, or MDMA), which had been rising sharply since 1998.[34] Also known as "E," "X," "the love drug," and other names, Ecstasy is a stimulant drug that became popular in the late 1990s at "raves," or all-night parties often featuring loud, technopop music. In 2001, 5% of 8th graders, 8% of 10th graders, and 12% of 12th graders had already tried Ecstasy, and since 1998 Ecstasy use has doubled among American adolescents.[34] Other drugs noted to be on the rise are anabolic steroids.[34] Steroids are particularly prevalent among youth in the Southeast, and steroid users also are likely to experiment with marijuana and alcohol.

Some drugs are less commonly used. Heroin use has decreased among 10th and 12th graders; after showing a sharp rise in the late 1990s, heroin use without a needle (snorting or smoking) became popular.[34] Use of this drug by 8th graders had started to taper in 2000, with the 10th and 12th graders' rates first declining in 2001. Virtually all decreases in use reflected decreased use of heroin without needles. The perceived risk of heroin use remains high. Another drug showing declined use in 2001 was lysergic acid diethylamide (LSD), although perceived risk of this drug has not increased.[34] Use of inhalants (solvents and aerosols such as glue and nail polish remover) peaks in younger adolescents and tends to decline as they get older. In 2001, 14.7% of students had sniffed glue, breathed the contents of aerosol spray cans, or inhaled paints or sprays to get high during their lifetime.[10] Use of cocaine powder decreased significantly among 10th graders in 2001, with both crack and powdered cocaine use modestly trending downward.[34] In the Youth Risk Behavior Survey, 9.4% of students reported ever using any form of cocaine.[10] Methamphetamines had been used at least once by 9.8% of students, and heroin in any form had been used by 3.1% of students.[10]

In screening for alcohol and drug abuse problems, the clinician will find the CRAFFT questions for adolescents helpful (Table 25-7). By counseling parents, clinicians can be instrumental in helping to identify a problem and in getting the adolescent to recognize and deal with the problem in a useful way. Parents may ask when to perform a drug test. In general, a confidential history will elicit most necessary information. If the adolescent states that he or she is using marijuana or other drugs, the drug test is not necessary and may actually be counterproductive if the test is negative but the history confirms use. If the adolescent denies use and the parent insists on a drug test, the adolescent must still consent to being tested. Clear-cut indications to perform a drug test include the comatose adolescent or teen with clearly altered mental state in the emergency room or office setting, and when ordered by a court or a school as part of a contract.

OBESITY

Obesity has its antecedents in childhood, with patterns of eating learned from parents first, then from families, peers, and society. Treatment of obesity is one of the most difficult challenges that a patient, family, and clinician can face. Prevention of obesity is highly dependent on family dynamics, role modeling of proper eating habits at home and elsewhere, biological factors, and availability of appropriate food choices. The term *obesity* usually has negative connotations for the patient and family; discussions can be framed in terms of overweight for height, to help teenagers feel empowered to make changes without feeling further stigmatized. Obesity is defined as body weight for height at greater than 120% of normal for age and sex, or approximately at or above the 95th percentile on body mass index (weight in kilograms divided by height in meters squared).[35]

In 2001, although 10.5% of students were overweight (14.2% of boys, 6.9% of girls), 29.2% of students thought

T A B L E 25-7

CRAFFT Questions*

Have you ever ridden in a **C**ar driven by someone (including yourself) who was high or had been using drugs or alcohol?

Do you ever use alcohol or drugs to **R**elax, feel better about yourself, or fit in?

Do you ever drink alcohol or use drugs **A**lone?

Do you ever **F**orget things you did while using alcohol or drugs?

Do your **F**amily or friends ever tell you that you should cut down on your drinking or drug use?

Have you ever gotten in **T**rouble from drinking or using drugs?

*Adapted from Knight JR, Schner LA, Bravende TD, et at. A new brief screen for adolescent substance abuse. *Arch Pediatr Adolesc Med.* 1999; 153:591–596.

they were overweight (34.9% of girls, 23.3% of boys), with no differences across racial and ethnic lines. Almost 50% of students had been trying to lose weight in the 30 days before being surveyed (62.3% of girls, 28.8% of boys). Less than 25% of students had eaten at least 5 servings of fruits and vegetables daily, and only 16.4% of students drank at least 3 glasses of milk per day.[10] Weight control strategies used in the 30 days before the survey included exercising (68.4% of girls, 51% of boys); restricting food, eating food with fewer calories, or eating low-fat food (58.6% of girls, 28.2% of boys); fasting for at least 24 hours (19.1% of girls, 7.6% of boys); diet pills, powders, or liquids without a doctor's advice (12.6% of girls, 5.5% of boys); and vomiting or use of laxatives (7.8% of girls, 2.9% of boys).

In the office setting, adolescents should be asked about eating habits and exercise. If disordered eating (overeating and undereating) is noted, appropriate interventions and follow-up should occur. The clinician must be careful not to create (or at least aid and abet) an eating disorder through negative or punitive uses of words, especially with younger children. The focus should be on strategies to increase physical activity, healthy eating, weight control behaviors, sources of social support, and issues of weight-related stigmatization or self-esteem. Adequate calcium intake also should be discussed. Discussion on how to make healthy choices at school lunch, in fast-food restaurants, and when fending for oneself at home can be useful. Teens also can be educated on simple rules, such as no food in front of the television or computer, as they are more likely to eat more than they planned. Emotional eating—eating when bored, angry, or in another emotional state—can be addressed, with the teen encouraged to

recognize patterns and try an alternate behavior (draw a picture, write in a journal, call a friend, or do 5 sit-ups) instead of heading to the refrigerator. Encouraging families to eat healthy meals together more consistently through the week may also help.

PREVENTIVE SERVICES

The concept of prevention of disease and psychosocial risk in adolescent health care led to the development of several guidelines in the 1990s. The Guidelines for Adolescent Preventive Services (GAPS) were developed by the American Medical Association's Division of Adolescent Health.[36] Bright Futures Guidelines for Health Supervision of Infants, Children, and Adolescents was sponsored by the Maternal and Child Health Bureau of the Health Resources and Services Administration and the Medicaid Bureau of the Health Care Financing Administration.[37] The AAP's Recommendations for Pediatric Preventive Health Care[38,39] are similar to those found in Bright Futures. The development process for each of these guidelines started with a literature review, followed by a cost-benefit analysis and ultimately a consensus opinion of a panel of experts in the field.[40] The guidelines outline the aspects of the medical history and physical examination, appropriate laboratory evaluations for the different age groups, and health guidance or advice on healthy lifestyles and developmental issues relevant to the different aged youth.

In Bright Futures and the AAP guidelines, early history and physical examinations are recommended for youth aged 11 to 21 years.[37,38] In contrast, GAPS recommends an annual visit with a history obtained to screen for the major developmental changes that take place during adolescence, but with an actual physical examination recommended only once each in early, middle, and late adolescence.[36] This latter recommendation of infrequent physical examinations has led to much controversy among pediatricians and other clinicians, and some insurance companies have refused to cover the annual visit based on the GAPS requirement for only 3 physical examinations.[41-43] Furthermore, clinicians feared that parents would not bring their adolescents for yearly visits given that GAPS mandated a physical only 3 times in adolescence, missing the point that most medical dangers of adolescence stem from behavioral choices rather than the onset of disease.

The GAPS algorithm consists of:

Gathering information

Assessing further the level of risk

Problem identification (eg, determining whether the adolescent sees the behavior as a problem and to what extent that person is willing to change)

Solutions, including self-efficacy and solving barriers

The annual visit is geared to addressing biomedical and psychosocial aspects of health, with preventive services designed to be age and developmentally appropriate. According to GAPS, physicians should establish office policies regarding confidential care for adolescents and how parents are to be involved in that care. Annual health guidance is designed to help adolescents better understand their own physical, psychosocial, and psychosexual development; become actively involved in their own health care; prevent injuries; achieve healthy eating and exercise habits; and avoid or cease cigarette, drug, and alcohol use (including anabolic steroids). Health guidance also is intended to screen adolescents for risky behaviors, STDs, depression and suicidal thoughts or intent, history of abuse, and learning or school problems. Tuberculosis screening is recommended for all adolescents who were exposed to active tuberculosis. These include adolescents who have run away or lived on the streets, incarcerated youth, those living in an area with a high prevalence of the disease, or individuals working in health care settings. Annual blood pressure screening is recommended, along with Papanicolaou tests for girls older than 18 years and for all sexually active girls.

Bright Futures emphasizes asking questions differently for the early, middle, and late stages of adolescence.[37,40] In contrast to GAPS, Bright Futures and the AAP guidelines specifically outline aspects of the physical examination that need to be evaluated.

INFLUENCE OF MEDIA

The media represents a pervasive influence on today's youth. The average child learns to work a mouse or remote control earlier than how to tie a shoe. Between ages 2 and 18 years, American youth watch or listen to a daily average of 6½ hours of media, ranging from television to video games, movies, radio, computer, and the Internet.[44,45] By age 18 years, the average American adolescent will have viewed 200,000 acts of violence on television alone, or 10,000 acts of violence per year, and heard 14,000 sexual references on television per year, with only 170 of these dealing with birth control, self-control, or abstinence.[44,46] Over 4 decades, research (longitudinal studies, cross-sectional analyses, laboratory experiments, meta-analyses, and government reports) has found a direct causative link between media violence and real-life violence.[44,46-48] The media can be seen as a "superpeer," making behaviors seem normative. Music videos and the Internet are also seen as being a part of the "superpeer" network. The clinician can exert a powerful influence by advising the adolescent and the parents to limit total media time to 1 or 2 hours per day as per the AAP's recommendations.[49] The clinician should further counsel parents to watch movies and television shows with their adolescents, and to place televisions and computers outside adolescents' rooms in public areas of the house, where they can monitor what their children are viewing.

ROLE OF THEORY: FRAMING INTERVENTIONS

According to social learning theory, learning emerges through repeated observations of others' behavior; youth learn about violence through what they experience and what they see around them. Vulnerability to these social influences depends on the individual's personality, attitudes, knowledge, and beliefs. Individuals with an internal locus of control, who believe that they can actively influence their environment, are less vulnerable than individuals with an external locus of control, who believe that "life happens to them." Applying social learning theory, aggressive video game characters can serve as models for aggressive behavior, with "winning" the game associated with more frequent violent behaviors.[50]

With respect to drug use, knowledge of perceived risks and benefits of each drug can be used to shape interventions. Because the adverse consequences of one drug may not generalize to a different drug, many young persons' beliefs and attitudes will be drug-specific.[51] "Generational forgetting," or the rediscovery of a drug without parents' or adults' knowledge of the adverse consequences, has resulted in the resurgence of some drugs that were popular in the 1960s.

Prochaska's[52] stages of change theory also can be used to shape interventions (Fig 25-1). This theory postulates that individuals move through a finite set of phases: from precontemplation, to contemplation, to action, and then maintenance. Relapse can occur anywhere along the path, setting the cycle in motion again. With respect to substance abuse, precontemplation might mean that the teenaged patient has not considered cessation of drug use. The first intervention, then, should be getting that patient

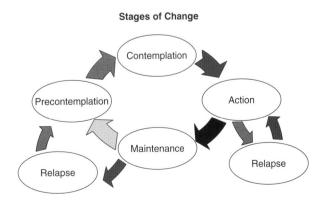

Stages of Change

FIGURE 25-1

Stages of change.

to think about quitting, or reach the contemplation phase. Once there, the clinician can work with the teen to make a concrete plan for quitting, complete with short-term and long-term rewards. Ideally, the quit date should be set fairly close to the visit, using school holidays or other markers of time in a teen's life. Close follow-up is essential, to ascertain whether action steps were taken, to reinforce positive changes, and to help prevent relapse.

Parents' perceptions of risk to themselves or to their children can have drastic effects on adolescent risk behaviors. "Do as I say, not as I do" tends not to work, because children live, or model, what they learn. Parents who drank alcohol or used drugs in high school or college may underestimate the risks, not realizing the higher potency of marijuana today compared with when they were young and experimenting. They also may be unaware of the addictive potential of marijuana and other drugs,[53] or of the polygenic nature of alcoholism and other drug addictions.[54]

SUMMARY

Clinicians need to take the time to ask developmentally appropriate questions, detect problems ideally before they occur, react to already existent problems, and ensure adequate follow-up. Knowledge of community resources plus barriers to care can be used to deliver timely care and ensure appropriate interventions. Helping adolescents develop the knowledge, skills, and motivation to make healthy choices is paramount. This places risk reduction into a lifelong perspective for both the adolescent and his or her family. Above all, assisting adolescents build self-esteem and an optimistic view of one's own future can help create a future generation of healthy adults.[55,56]

REFERENCES

1. Hall GS. *Adolescence: Its Psychology and Its Relations to Physiology, Anthropology, Sociology, Sex, Crime, Religion and Education.* New York, NY: D Appleton and Co; 1904.

2. Dryfoos J. *Adolescents at Risk.* New York, NY: Oxford University Press; 1990.

3. Burt MR. Reasons to invest in adolescents. *J Adolesc Health.* 2002;31:136–152.

4. Offer D. The mystery of adolescence. *Adolesc Psychol.* 1987;14:7–27.

5. Hamburg BA, Takanishi M. Preparing for life: The critical transition of adolescence. *Am Psychol.* 1989;44:825–827.

6. Ford CA, Millstein SG, Halpern-Felsher BL, Irwin CE. Influence of physician confidentiality assurances on adolescents' willingness to disclose information and seek future health care: a randomized controlled trial. *JAMA.* 1997;278:1029–1134.

7. Goldenring JM, Cohen E. Getting into adolescent heads. *Contempy Pediatr.* 1988; July:75–90.

8. East PL, Felice ME. Pregnancy risk among the younger sisters of pregnant and child-bearing adolescents. *J Dev Behav Pediatr.* 1992;13:128–136.

9. Insurance Institute for Highway Safety. Fatality facts: teenagers (as of November 2002). Available at: www.iihs.org/safety_facts/fatality_facts/teens.htm. Accessed March 29, 2003.

10. Grunbaum JA, Kann L, Kinchen SA, et al. Youth risk behavior surveillance—United States, 2001. *MMWR Surveill Summ.* 2002;51:1–62.

11. National Highway Traffic Safety Administration, US Dept of Transportation. Traffic safety facts 2000: speeding. Available at: www-nrd.nhtsa.dot.gov/pdf/nrd-30/NCSA/TSF2000/2000spdfacts.pdf. Accessed April 1, 2002.

12. Chen L, Baker SP, Braver ER, Li G. Carrying passengers as a risk factor for crashes fatal to 16- and 17-year old drivers. *JAMA.* 2000;283:1578–1582.

13. Centers for Disease Control and Prevention. Youth risk behavior surveillance—United States, 2001. *MMWR Surveill Summ.* 2002;51(SS-04):1–64.

14. Jonah BA, Dawson NE. Youth and risk: age differences in risky driving, risk perception, and risk utility. *Alcohol Drugs Driving.* 1987;3:13–29.

15. National Center for Injury Prevention and Control, Centers for Disease Control and Prevention. Web-based Injury Statistics Query and Reporting System (WISQARS) @online:. Available at: www.cdc.gov/ncipc/wisquars. Accessed Aug 27, 2002.

16. National Highway Traffic Safety Administration, US Dept of Transportation. Traffic safety facts 2000: young drivers. Available at: www-nrd.nhtsa.dot.gov/pdf/nrd-30/NCSA/TSF2000/2000ydrive.pdf. Accessed April 1, 2002.

17. Sege RD. Adolescent violence. *Adolesc Health Update.* 1999;12:1–8.

18. American Academy of Pediatrics, Committee on Psychosocial Aspects of Child and Family Health. Guidance for effective discipline. *Pediatrics.* 1998;101:723–728.

19. Strauss MA, Sugarman DB, Giles-Sims J. Spanking by parents and subsequent antisocial behavior of children. *Arch Pediatr Adolesc Med.* 1997;151:761–767.

20. Canada G. *Fist, Stick, Knife, Gun: A Personal History of Violence in America.* Boston, Mass: Beacon Press; 1995.

21. Resnick MD, Chambliss SA, Blum RW. Health and risk behaviors of urban adolescent males involved in pregnancy. *Fam Soc J Contem Hum Serv.* 1993;74:366–374.

22. Hagman J. Diagnosis and treatment of depression in adolescence. *Adolesc Health Update.* 2001;13:1–8.

23. Braverman PK. Sexually transmitted diseases. *Adolesc Health Update.* 2001;14:1–12.

24. Centers for Disease Control and Prevention (CDC). *Sexually Transmitted Disease Surveillance, 2000.* Atlanta, Ga: CDC; 2001.

25. Ventura SJ, Mosher WD, Curtin SA, Abma JC. Trends in pregnancy rates for the United States, 1976–97: an update. *Nat Vital Stat Rep.* 2001;49:1–12.

26. Martin JA, Park MM, Sutton PD. Births: preliminary data for 2001. *Nat Vital Stat Rep.* 2002;50:1–20.

27. MacDorman MF, Minino AM, Strobino DM, Guyer B. Annual summary of vital statistics—2001. *Pediatrics.* 2002;110:1037–1052.

28. National Center for Health Statistics. Teenage births in the United States: state trends, 1991–2000, an update. *Nat Vital Stat Rep.* 2002;50:1120.

29. Moore KA, Miller BC, Glei D, Morrison DR. *Adolescent Sex, Contraception, and Childbearing: A Review of Recent Research.* Washington, DC: Child Trends; 1995.

30. Jessor SL, Jessor R. Transition from virginity to nonvirginity among youth: a social-psychology study over time. *Dev Psychol.* 1975;11:473.

31. Brown RT. Adolescent sexuality at the dawn of the 21st century. In: *Adolescent Medicine: State of the Art Reviews.* Vol 11. Philadelphia, Pa: Hanley & Belfus Inc; 2000:19–34.

32. Dailard C. Recent findings from the 'Add Health' Survey: teens and sexual activity. *The Guttmacher Report on Public Policy.* August 2001;4(4):1–3.

33. Kirby D. *Emerging Answers: Research Findings on Programs to Reduce Teen Pregnancy.* Washington, DC: National Campaign to Prevent Teen Pregnancy; 2001:1–186.

34. Johnston LD, O'Malley PM, Bachman JG. *Monitoring the Future: National Results on Adolescent Drug Use. Overview of Key Findings, 2001.* Bethesda, Md: National Institute on Drug Abuse, US Dept of Health and Human Services; 2001:1–16.

35. Carnegie Council on Adolescent Development. *Turning Points: Preparing American Youth for the 21st Century.* Washington, DC: Carnegie Council on Adolescent Development; 1983.

36. Elster AB, Kuznets NJ. *Guidelines for Adolescent Preventive Services (GAPS): Recommendations and Rationale.* Baltimore, Md: Williams & Wilkins; 1992.

37. Green M, ed. *Bright Futures: Guidelines for Health Supervision of Infants, Children and Adolescents.* Arlington, Va: National Center for Education in Maternal and Child Health; 1994.

38. American Academy of Pediatrics, Committee on Practice and Ambulatory Medicine. Recommendations for pediatric preventive health care. *Pediatrics.* 1995;96:373–374.

39. American Academy of Pediatrics, Committee on Psychosocial Aspects of Child and Family Health. *Guidelines for Health Supervision III.* Elk Grove Village, Ill: American Academy of Pediatrics; 1997.

40. Fisher M. Adolescent health assessment and promotion in office and school settings. In: *Adolescent Medicine: State of the Art Reviews.* Vol 10. Philadelphia, Pa: Hanley & Belfus, Inc; 1999:71–86.

41. Joffe A. Filling in the gaps through research. *Arch Pediatr Adolesc Med.* 1997;151:121–122.

42. Knishkowy B, Palti H. GAPS (Guidelines for Adolescent Preventive Services): where are the gaps? *Arch Pediatr Adolesc Med.* 1997;151:123–128.

43. Copperman S. GAPS (AMA Guidelines for Adolescent Preventive Services). *Arch Pediatr Adolesc Med.* 1997;151:957–958.

44. American Academy of Pediatrics, Committee on Public Education. Media violence. *Pediatrics.* 2001;108:1222–1226.

45. Henry J Kaiser Family Foundation. *Kids and Media at the New Millennium: A Kaiser Family Foundation Report.* Menlo Park, Calif: Henry J Kaiser Family Foundation; 1999.

46. Strasburger VC, Donnerstein E. Children, adolescents, and the media in the 21st century. In: *Adolescent Medicine: State of the Art Reviews.* Vol 11. Philadelphia, Pa: Hanley and Belfus Inc; 2000;51–68.

47. Husemann LR. Television violence and aggressive behavior. In: Pearl D, Bouthilet L, Lazar J, eds. *Television and Behavior: Ten Years of Scientific Progress and Implications for the Eighties.* Vol 2. Rockville, Md: National Institute of Mental Health; 1982.

48. Strasburger VC, Donnerstein E. Children, adolescents, and the media: issues and solutions. *Pediatrics.* 1999;103:129–139.

49. American Academy of Pediatrics. *Media Matters: A National Media Education Campaign.* Elk Grove Village, Ill: American Academy of Pediatrics; 1997.

50. Bensley L, Van Eenwyk J. Video games and real-life aggression: review of the literature. *J Adolesc Health.* 2001;29:244–257.

51. Johnston LD, O'Malley PM, Bachman JG. *Monitoring the Future National Survey Results on Drug Use, 1975–2000: Secondary School Students.* Vol 1. Bethesda, Md: National Institute on Drug Abuse; 2001. NIH Publication No. 01–4924.

52. Prochaska JO, DiClemente CC. Transtheoretical therapy: toward a more integrative model of change. *Psychotherapy.* 1982;19:276–288.

53. Rodriguez de Fonseca F, Rocio M, Carrera A, et al. Activation of corticotropin-releasing factor in the limbic system during cannabinoid withdrawal. *Science.* 1997;276:2050–2052.

54. Comerci GD, Shwebel R. Substance abuse: an overview. In: *Adolescent Medicine: State of the Art Reviews.* Philadelphia, Pa: Hanley & Belfus, Inc; 2000:70–101.

55. Loewenson PR, Blum RW. The resilient adolescent: implications for the pediatrician. *Pediatr Ann.* 2001;30:76–80.

56. Resnick MD, Bearman PS, Blum RW, et al. Protecting adolescents from harm: findings from the National Longitudinal Study on Adolescent Health. *JAMA.* 1997;278:823–832.

RESOURCES

American Academy of Pediatrics, 141 Northwest Point Blvd, Elk Grove Village, IL 60007-1098; 847 434-4000.
Web site: www.aap.org.

North American Society for Pediatric and Adolescent Gynecology, 1015 Chestnut St, Suite 1225, Philadelphia, PA 19107-4302; 215 955-6331.
Web site: www.nspag.org.

Society for Adolescent Medicine, 1916 Copper Oaks Circle, Blue Springs, MO 64015; 816 224-8010.
Web site: www.adolescenthealth.org.

Substance Abuse and Mental Health Services Administration (SAMHSA), National Mental Health Information Center; 800 789-2647.
Web site: www.mentalhealth.org. (Fact sheets for children and teens in crisis.)

chapter 26

Aging and the Geriatric Patient

Carolyn Welty, MD, and Robert M. Palmer, MD

INTRODUCTION

Thirteen percent of the US population is 65 years or older and consumes 30% of the health care budget. By 2040, these percentages will increase to 22% and 50%, respectively.[1] The oldest old are the fastest growing portion of the population. Between 1990 and 2000, the number of persons 65 years and older increased by 12%, but a 23% increase occurred in those aged 75 to 84 years and a 38% increase in those aged 85 and older.[2]

The older population has the highest prevalence of chronic disease and physical disability. The 5 leading causes of death in adults older than 65 years are (1) heart disease, (2) malignant neoplasm (lung, colorectal, breast), (3) cerebrovascular disease, (4) chronic obstructive pulmonary disease, and (5) pneumonia and influenza.

A major purpose of preventive health care of older patients is to prevent premature death and disability by reducing risk factors and detecting treatable diseases. Doing so may compress morbidity such that the final decline to death is reduced into the last few years of life.[3] However, with advances in treatment of chronic diseases, a concern is that older persons will live longer but with a greater burden of disease and disability. Recent studies and trends dispute this concern. A study of college alumni demonstrated an 8-year delay in disability in those with lower health risk.[4] However, the gains are not uniform across demographic groups. Minorities and individuals with less education have higher mortality due to cardiovascular disease, diabetes, cancer, and lung disease, conditions that are also associated with major disability.[5] One goal of the national Healthy People 2010 initiative is to eliminate this discrepancy.[6]

Currently, 80% of those aged 65 years and older have at least one chronic disease, and two thirds of those over age 80 are living with a disability. However, older adults are becoming healthier, with a decline in prevalence of disability over the past 20 years.[7] Although the reasons for these improving trends are uncertain, improved detection and treatment of diseases is an important contributing factor. The process of identifying older patients who could benefit from multidimensional interventions is comprehensive geriatric assessment.

GERIATRIC ASSESSMENT

Comprehensive geriatric assessment involves the evaluation of the functional status and the physical, psychosocial, and environmental factors affecting the health of an older person. *Functional status* refers to the older person's ability to function in the physical, mental, and social activities of daily life. Many health problems in older adults are not known to the primary care provider, and as much as 50% of those may be treatable.[8] Clinicians face the difficult task of completing a comprehensive evaluation of a geriatric patient in a timely and efficient manner. Streamlined methods to screen older patients rely on validated and easily administered assessment tools to identify functional impairments or disabilities as well as common geriatric syndromes.[9-11] Table 26-1 summarizes screening tools to detect common geriatric syndromes. Adapted from a number of other sources,[9,10,12,13] these tools can be administered by a trained office assistant. More detailed evaluation is warranted when the screen suggests the presence of functional impairments that could lead to disability.

Support services in the community can act as an extended or virtual interdisciplinary team for the clinician. These include, among others, the Area Agency on Aging, Adult Protective Services, and the Alzheimer's Association (see Resources at the end of the chapter). Community-based services are funded by federal and state programs. Senior centers offer activities that include education, recreation, health, nutrition, information, and access. Many senior centers include activities such as arts, crafts, movies, music, and trips; others offer counseling, meals, transportation, employment placement, and health screenings.[14] Primary and secondary prevention are also components of geriatric assessment.[15-17] The US Preventive Services Task Force has made recommendations for preventive care for persons aged 65 years and older (Table 26-2).[18]

TABLE 26-1

Screening for Geriatric Syndromes*

Syndrome/Problem	Initial Screens (Use 1)	Follow-up Testing if Screening Result Is Abnormal
Hearing impairment	Whisper test[†] or audioscope	Audiogram
Visual impairment	Ask about ability to read newsprint *or* watch television *or* Ask patient to read newsprint *or* Use Snellen chart *or* Jaeger visual acuity card	Referral to ophthalmologist or optometrist
Dementia	Patient remembers 3 items after 1 min or clock drawing test[†]	MMSE; see Figure 26-1
Depression scale[†]	Does patient feel sad or blue?	GDS; see Table 26-3
Falls	Has patient fallen in the past year?	Document basic and instrumental ADL; see Table 26-5 for further evaluation
Mobility or gait disorders	Timed Get-up-and-go Test[†]	Evaluate fall risk and consider referral to physical therapy
Urinary incontinence	Has patient ever involuntarily lost urine and gotten wet?	See text for further evaluation
Failure to thrive or malnutrition	If weight of patient <45 kg (<100 lb), ask patient if he or she lost 10% of weight in past 6 mo without trying	Further evaluation
Polypharmacy	Ask patient to bring in all medications, including over-the-counter drugs, herbs, and vitamins	See Table 26-6
Lack of social support	Ask if patient has someone to help if he or she is sick or disabled	If yes, document. If no, investigate further.

*MMSE indicates Mini-Mental State Examination; GDS, Geriatric Depression Scale; and ADL, activities of daily living.
†Described in text.

DETAILED GERIATRIC SCREENING

Hearing Impairment

Hearing impairment is the fourth most prevalent disability in older adults. Studies show that 24% of persons aged 65 to 74 years, up to 40% of those older than 75 years, and 70% of nursing home residents have substantial hearing impairment.[19] Questionnaires and simple performance measures effectively screen for hearing loss or its effects in elderly patients. In the whisper test, the examiner stands 0.6 m (2 ft) behind the patient and whispers a short string of numbers (3 to 6) while the patient's ears are covered one at a time. A more sensitive tool is an audioscope, which can quantify the level of hearing loss. The Hearing Handicap Inventory for the Elderly—Screening Version, a questionnaire that asks about disability related to hearing problems,[20] is self-administered but is not validated in cognitively impaired patients.

Part of the hearing loss with age is due to a defect in central auditory processing that is not corrected by simple amplification and that requires more rehabilitation. The longer this defect is established, the harder the adjustment to hearing aids for the older adult. Even when hearing loss is detected, the older adult may be unlikely to use a hearing aid. Thus, it is important to screen patients early to prevent social and psychological impairment, and to improve likelihood of the patient's acceptance and compliance with a hearing aid.

Visual Impairment

Visual loss is a common problem, with estimates of 10% of people aged 55 to 84 years and 20% of persons aged 85 and older having severe visual impairment.[21] Diabetic retinopathy, glaucoma, and cataracts are 3 treatable and common causes of visual loss in the elderly population. A useful initial screen for visual impairment is to ask whether a person has difficulty viewing television or reading the newspaper. Screening for visual impairment is performed with the Snellen eye chart, which patients read from 20 ft away using corrective lenses if needed. Handheld cards such as the Rosenbaum Pocket Vision Screener are useful alternatives for testing near and distant vision. The card is held 14 in from the patient's eyes. Inability to read better than 20/50 with correction is clinically important and indicates the need for a more detailed evaluation or referral. A meta-analysis showed no benefit in community screening

T A B L E 26-2

Periodic Health Examination for Adults Aged 65 Years and Older*

Type of Intervention	Recommendation for Preventive Care
Screening	1. Height and weight measurement
	2. Measurement of blood pressure
	3. Fecal occult blood test and/or sigmoidoscopy
	4. Mammogram plus clinical breast examination (women <70 years of age)
	5. Papanicolaou test (women <70 years of age)
	6. Vision screening
	7. Assess for hearing impairment
	8. Assess for problem drinking
Counseling	
Substance use	1. Tobacco cessation
	2. Avoid alcohol and drug use while driving, swimming, boating, etc[†]
Diet and exercise	1. Limit fat and cholesterol intake; maintain energy balance; emphasize eating grains, fruits, and vegetables
	2. Adequate calcium intake
	3. Regular physical activity[†]
Injury prevention	1. Wear lap and shoulder seat belts
	2. Wear a bicycle, motorcycle, or all-terrain vehicle helmet[†]
	3. Fall prevention
	4. Smoke detector in home[†]
	5. Safe storage or removal of firearms from home[†]
	6. Hot water heater temperature less than 120°F to 130°F
	7. Cardiopulmonary resuscitation training for household members
Dental health	1. Regular visits to dental care provider[†]
	2. Floss and brush with fluoride toothpaste daily[†]
Sexual behavior	Prevention of sexually transmitted disease: avoid high-risk sexual behaviors[†]; use condoms[†]
Immunizations	1. Pneumococcal vaccine
	2. Influenza vaccine
	3. Tetanus-diphtheria boosters

*Adapted from US Preventive Services Task Force18 and National Library of Medicine. Available at: www.hstat.nlm.nih.gov/hq/ Hquest/db/local.gcps.cps/screen/Browse/s/38534/cmd/HF/action/GetText?IHR=TIII4. Accessed February 6, 2003.

[†]The value of clinician counseling in influencing this behavior is unproved.

of older adults for visual problems using questions about vision,[22] but the studies included in the analysis did not link screening to any physician evaluation or counseling.

Dementia

Cognitive dysfunction in old age may have numerous causes, but dementia is the most common cause seen in elderly patients in outpatient settings. The diagnosis of dementia requires documentation of a decline in cognition from an established baseline that includes memory impairment, substantial impairment in social or occupational functioning, and at least one of the following: language impairment, apraxia, visuospatial deficits, and decreased executive functioning; as well as significant impairment in social or occupational functioning. The prevalence of dementia is estimated to be as high as 6% to 10% at age 65 years,[23] and by age 85, largely due to Alzheimer's disease, 30% to 50%.[24] Despite the high prevalence of dementia and the associated social, psychological, and economic implications of what is termed a "silent" epidemic, routine screening of all older adults is not currently recommended. The US Preventive Services Task Force finds insufficient evidence to recommend for or against routine screening because of the poor predictive value of current screening and the risk of erroneously diagnosing an incurable disease. Detection through clinical screening is invaluable because cognitive impairment is common, complicates the medical care of an older patient, and often is associated with a treatable condition such as depression. The Public Health Service does recommend testing for dementia when a patient has been found to have a decline in function or a family concern has been expressed.

Although most causes of dementia are not curable, they are treatable when appropriately diagnosed. Adverse drug reactions, depression, thyroid disorders, vitamin B_{12} deficiency, calcium abnormalities, subdural hematoma, neurosyphilis, and even primary neoplasm all can present with symptoms of dementia, which can be improved by appropriate treatment. Even dementias that generally are considered to be incurable, such as Alzheimer's and vascular dementia, may be improved by treatment with cholinesterase inhibitors and treatment of vascular risk factors. Early detection of dementia also allows both the patient and the family to plan for the future while the patient is still capable of making decisions.

Mild cognitive impairment affects 5% to 40% of middle-aged and older adults. Mild cognitive impairment likely represents the earlier stages of a dementing illness. Older persons with mild cognitive impairment progress to dementia at a rate as high as 15% per year as compared with healthy controls, who progress at a rate of 1% to 2% per year.[25] Those with mild cognitive impairment have objective evidence of memory loss but are not disabled by their cognitive dysfunction, as are individuals with dementia. Currently, there is no specific treatment of mild cognitive impairment, and the natural history of this condition is poorly characterized. However, treatment of atherosclerosis risk factors, particularly hypertension, may play an important role in delaying progression to dementia. An Italian study showed that mild cognitive impairment without dementia was correlated with a history of stroke and heart failure.[26] Clinical trials of drug interventions in mild cognitive impairment are in progress.[27]

Detection of dementia can be accomplished through interviews with the patient or caregivers and supplemented by the use of simple screening tests. One test asks the person to remember 3 items and to recall them in 3 minutes. Older people without dementia can recall at least 2 of the items. In the clock drawing test, the person is asked to draw a clock with its 12 numbers and then to draw the hands to read a specific time (usually 11:10).[28] Although various scoring systems exist for this test,[29] a simple interpretation is to consider the test result negative (normal) if all numbers are arranged and hands placed appropriately, and abnormal (positive) if numbers and hands are not correct. An abnormal result suggests the need for further testing. The Mini-Mental State Examination (Fig 26-1) is the most common of the brief tests used to detect and quantify degree of cognitive impairment. With this test, a standard cutoff of 24 of 30 items is considered consistent with dementia. Cutoff points are higher for educated people and lower for uneducated or illiterate people. Following the diagnosis of dementia, appropriate evaluation and treatment are indicated.[24]

Depression

The prevalence of major depression in elderly people is 1% to 3% among community dwellers, 12% to 15% in patients at primary care clinics, 10% to 15% in hospitalized patients, and 12% to 16% in nursing home residents. However, the prevalence of depressive symptoms in these settings is much higher: 15%, 20%, 20% to 25%, and 30% to 40%, respectively.[30] Depression is common in patients with stroke, heart disease, and other chronic medical illnesses. Depression can be a primary diagnosis or secondary due to numerous causes. Alcohol abuse is often unrecognized in elderly persons and can be a contributory factor to depression, as can other geriatric syndromes, such as falls and weight loss. In 1997 the NIH Consensus Panel on Diagnosis and Treatment of Depression in Late Life recommends early recognition of depression. With appropriate diagnosis and treatment there can be improvement in quality of life, decrease in morbidity and mortality, better overall level of functioning, and independence.[31] The US Preventive Services Task Force 2002 update on depression agrees that there is sufficient evidence to recommend screening for depression in adults, in settings that assure appropriate diagnosis, treatment, and follow-up.[32] One group of older adults needing screening for depression are caregivers for a disabled spouse. Depression is prevalent in this group. A study has shown that older adults who report "caregiver strain" had a 63% higher mortality than did the noncaregiving controls.[33] A common screen for depression is the Geriatric Depression Scale (GDS), which was designed to be self-administered (Table 26-3). However, simply asking a person if he or she feels sad or depressed may be as predictive of depression as the GDS.[34] The GDS is not accurate for a person with dementia.

Functional Ability

Falls and gait disorders are related to functional ability. Decline in functional ability may be the first sign of serious underlying disease. Functional ability usually is divided into 2 categories: basic activities of daily living (ADL) and instrumental ADL (Table 26-4). Basic ADL include ability to bathe, dress, transfer from bed to chair, use the toilet, maintain continence, and eat without assistance. Instrumental ADL include tasks such as ability to independently take medications, perform household chores, shop, prepare meals, use the telephone, handle finances, and manage personal transportation needs. Validated and reliable questionnaires evaluate a person's ability to perform ADL and instrumental ADL.[35, 36] It is important to both detect and prevent functional disability. Once a person is disabled, recovery of independent ADL function is unlikely. The US Preventive Services Task Force recommends counseling patients on sustaining physical activity throughout life. In elderly individuals, exercise is important to maintain functional ability.

Maximum Score	Score	Item
		Orientation
5	( )	What is the (year) (season) (date) (day) (month)?
5	( )	Where are we: (state) (county) (town) (hospital) (floor)?
		Registration
3	( )	Name 3 objects: Take 1 second to say each. Then ask the patient to name all 3 after you have said them. Give 1 point for each correct answer. Repeat them until patient learns all 3 (for later testing).
		Attention and Calculation
5	( )	Subtract serial 7s. Give 1 point for each correct answer. Stop after 5 answers. Alternatively, ask patient to spell *world* backward.
		Recall
3	( )	Ask for the 3 objects mentioned above. Give 1 point for each correct answer.
		Language
9	( )	Point to a pencil and watch and ask for their names. (2 points)
		Repeat the following: no ifs, ands, or buts. (1 point)
		Follow a 3-stage command: Take a paper in your right hand, fold it in half, and put it on the floor. (3 points)
		Read and obey the following: Close your eyes. (1 point)
		Write a sentence. (1 point)
		Copy a simple design. (1 point)
30	___	Patients score

FIGURE 26-1

Mini-Mental State Examination. From Folstein MF, Folstein SF, McHugh PR. Mini-Mental State: a practical method for grading the cognitive state of patients for the clinician. *J Psychiatr Res.* 1975;12:189.

A prospective study demonstrated that individuals who maintained physical activity had less decline in mobility even in persons with chronic diseases.[37]

Falls

The incidence of falls in those 65 years of age and older is 30% to 35% per year. Older adults should be asked if they have fallen in the past year. Risk factors for falls include taking of certain drugs (eg, psychoactive); use of more than 4 prescription drugs; impaired cognition, strength, balance, or gait; use of an assistive device; arthritis; impaired ADL; depression; and increasing age, particularly over 80 years. Falling is most often caused by the accumulated effect of multiple predisposing and situational factors. Amelioration of these factors has been shown to reduce the occurrence of falling. Screening older patients for risks of recurrent falling is warranted given the combination of disease burden, available screening tools, and effective risk intervention therapies.

The examination of a person who has fallen or is at risk of falls includes the following[38,39]:

- Reevaluation of any acute or chronic medical condition
- Reevaluation of medications
- Examination of vision balance, and muscle strength in the lower extremities
- Evaluation of mental status
- Examination of peripheral nerve, extrapyramidal, and cerebellar function
- Assessment of the cardiovascular system, including a check for postural hypotension, defined as a decrease of 20 mm Hg or more in systolic blood pressure in 1 minute going from the supine to standing position
- Tests of gait and mobility

A study that targeted patients with at least one risk factor for falling and that provided a combination of medication adjustment, behavioral instructions, and an

TABLE 26-3

Geriatric Depression Scale (Short Form)*

Choose the best answer for how you felt over the past week.

1. Are you basically satisfied with your life?	YES / **NO**
2. Have you dropped many of your activities and interests?	**YES** / NO
3. Do you feel that your life is empty?	**YES** / NO
4. Do you often get bored?	**YES** / NO
5. Are you in good spirits most of the time?	YES / **NO**
6. Are you afraid that something bad is going to happen to you?	**YES** / NO
7. Do you feel happy most of the time?	YES / **NO**
8. Do you often feel helpless?	**YES** / NO
9. Do you prefer to stay at home, rather than going out and doing new things?	**YES** / NO
10. Do you feel you have more problems with memory than most?	**YES** / NO
11. Do you think it is wonderful to be alive now?	YES / **NO**
12. Do you feel pretty worthless the way you are now?	**YES** / NO
13. Do you feel full of energy?	YES / **NO**
14. Do you feel that your situation is hopeless?	**YES** / NO
15. Do you think that most people are better off than you are?	**YES** / NO

Count the number of answers in bold; score greater than 5 indicates probable depression.

*From Sheikh JI, Yesavage JA. Geriatric Depression Scale (GDS): recent evidence and development of a shorter version. *Clin Gerontol.* 1986;9:165.

TABLE 26-4

Activities of Daily Living (ADL)

Basic ADL	Instrumental ADL
Going to the toilet	Using telephone
Feeding	Traveling
Dressing	Shopping
Transferring, eg, from bed to chair	Preparing meals
Physical ambulation	Housework
Bathing	Taking medicine
Continence	Managing money

*Adapted from Katz S[35] and Lawton MP, Brody EM.[36]

exercise program, based on the patient's risk factors, reduced the incidence of falls by 30% in 1 year.[40] Table 26-5 summarizes assessment and management of older persons at risk of falls.

Mobility and Gait Disorders

Mobility and gait disorders are the most important factor in falls. Numerous tests of gait and mobility have been validated. In the Timed Get-up-and-go Test, the person is asked to rise from an armchair, walk 3 m, turn, walk back, and sit while being observed and timed. A cutoff of more than 14 seconds predicts those who are more likely to fall.[41] People who have difficulty with this maneuver can be further evaluated, and other risk factors for falls can be addressed. Referral to physical therapy to address mobility issues can be very useful.

Urinary Incontinence

Urinary incontinence is a widespread problem for older adults, affecting more than 13 million people in the United States. The prevalence of incontinence is estimated to be 15% to 35% in community-dwelling older adults, but 50% or higher in homebound elderly and nursing home residents. Incontinence is a major factor in long-term institutionalization. The social cost in terms of quality of life is substantial. The concern about accidents may limit activities outside the home, and embarrassment can cause the older person to avoid social interactions.

Incontinence is not a normal part of aging. Less than half of people who have urinary incontinence consult their health care provider. In many cases, urinary incontinence can be treated or at least improved. Thus, inquiring about incontinence is an important first step.[42] The initial evaluation of incontinence includes the history, outlining details about the pattern and frequency of incontinence, comorbid medical conditions, medications, and functional status. The physical examination should include pelvic, rectal, and focused neurologic assessments. Additional basic studies are urinalysis and determination of postvoid residual urine volume.[43]

Nutrition

A U-shaped relationship exists between weight and mortality, with higher mortality at both higher and lower ends of weight. Increased weight is associated with chronic diseases, including diabetes, cardiovascular disease, arthritis, gout, and gallbladder disease. However, in the

TABLE 26-5

Recommended Components of Clinical Assessment and Management for Older Persons Living in the Community and at Risk of Falling*

Assessment and Risk Factor	Management
Circumstances of previous falls[†]	Changes in environment and activity to reduce likelihood of recurrent falls

Medication use
    High-risk medications (eg, benzodiazepines, other sleeping medications, neuroleptics, antidepressants, anticonvulsants, or class IA antiarrhythmics) [†,‡,§]
    ≥4 medications[§]
	Review and reduction of medications

Vision[†]
    Acuity <20/60
    Decreased depth perception
    Decreased contrast sensitivity
    Cataracts
	Ample lighting without glare; avoidance of multifocal glasses while walking; referral to ophthalmologist

Postural blood pressure (after ≥5 min in a supine position, immediately after standing, and 1 min after standing), defined as ≥20 mm Hg drop in systolic pressure, with or without symptoms[§], either immediately or after 1 min of standing	Diagnosis and treatment of underlying cause, if possible; review and reduction of medications; modification of salt restriction; adequate hydration; compensatory strategies (eg, elevation of head of bed, rising slowly, or dorsiflexion exercises); pressure stockings; pharmacologic therapy if above strategies fail

Balance and gait[‡,§]
    Patient's report or observation of unsteadiness
    Impairment on brief assessment (e.g, the Get-up-and-go Test or performance-oriented assessment of mobility)
	Diagnosis and treatment of underlying cause, if possible; reduction of medications that impair balance; environmental interventions; referral to physical therapist for assistive devices and for gait and progressive balance training

Targeted neurologic examination
    Impaired proprioception[†]
    Impaired cognition[†]
    Decreased muscle strength[‡,§]
	Diagnosis and treatment of underlying cause, if possible; increase in proprioceptive input (with assistive device or appropriate footwear that encases the foot and has low heel and thin sole); reduction of medications that impede cognition; awareness on part of caregivers of cognitive deficits; reduction of environmental risk factors; referral to physical therapist for gait, balance, and strength training

Targeted musculoskeletal examination: examination of legs (joints and range of motion) and feet[†]	Diagnosis and treatment of underlying cause, if possible; referral to physical therapist for strength, range of motion, and gait and balance training and for assistive devices; use of appropriate footwear; referral to podiatrist

Targeted cardiovascular examination[‡]
    Syncope
    Arrhythmia (if there is known cardiac disease, an abnormal electrocardiogram, and syncope)
	Referral to cardiologist; carotid-sinus massage (in the case of syncope)

Home-hazard evaluation after hospital discharge[‡,§]	Removal of loose rugs and use of night-lights, nonslip bath mats, and stair rails; other interventions as necessary

*Adapted from Tinetti ME.[38]

[†]Recommendation of this assessment is based on observational data that the finding is associated with an increased risk of falling.

[‡]Recommendation of this assessment is based on 1 or more randomized controlled trials of a single intervention.

[§]Recommendation of this assessment is based on 1 or more randomized controlled trials of a multifactorial intervention strategy that included this component.

older adult, being overweight has less relationship to mortality than in middle age. Instead, weight loss is a major risk factor for mortality, stronger for unintentional weight loss, but also present for intentional weight loss.[44] The benefit of the energy reserve that the extra weight provides an older person in the event of illness may outweigh the risk of weight-related chronic diseases. Malnutrition is a major problem in the older adult, estimated to be up to 15% in outpatients and as high as 60% in hospitalized or chronically institutionalized elderly.[45] Weight loss and malnutrition are clearly related to increased morbidity and mortality. Weight loss may indicate underlying disease but also may relate to social, economic, and psychological factors. Contributing factors to malnutrition can include functional disability that limits access to stores, lack of funds for food, depression, loneliness, and isolation.

In addition to assessing the elderly patient for over-weight or underweight, the practitioner should look for common deficiencies. The National Health and Nutrition Survey III showed that the average intake of calcium in persons aged 70 years and older is approximately 700 mg/d,[46] substantially lower than the 1500 mg/d recom-mended for the older adult. Calcium supplements usually are required to achieve the appropriate intake. Vitamin D deficiency is found in 30% to 50% of homebound, nonin-stitutionalized elderly persons. Lack of sunlight, use of sunscreens, and decreased intake of vitamin D–fortified food, such as milk, contributes to this deficiency. Vitamin D receptors are found on muscle cells, and a few studies have suggested that vitamin D deficiency may contribute to risk of falls.[47] Vitamin B_{12} deficiency is one of the most common vitamin deficiencies, present in 5% to 15% of the elderly population.[48] In most cases, vitamin B_{12} deficiency is due not to pernicious anemia, but to poor absorption of protein-bound vitamin B_{12}. The serum vitamin B_{12} level may be in the low range of normal, but the diagnosis of vitamin B_{12} deficiency may be deter-mined by finding elevated levels of serum homocysteine and methylmalonic acid in the absence of renal impair-ment. Conversely, vitamin B_{12} levels can be low while serum homocysteine and methylmalonic acid levels are normal, indicating that the person does not have deficiency of vitamin B_{12} at the tissue level.

Adverse Drug Reactions and Polypharmacy

Adverse drug reactions (ADR) are common in the older adult. Studies of hospitalized older adult patients suggest a prevalence of ADR in 10% to 18% of hospitalized patients, whereas 3% to 10% of hospital admissions are related to adverse effects of drugs. Adverse drug reactions are 2 to 3 times more common in older adults. Whether adverse drug reactions are more common simply because of age or because of increased comorbid conditions and increased drug use is not clear. Older persons are taking, on average, 4.5 medicines per day. The estimated risk of an adverse drug reaction is 15% in persons taking 2 drugs per day, and as high as 50% to 60% in those taking 5 drugs daily.[49] The issue of polypharmacy is not simply the number of drugs prescribed but whether they are being prescribed appropriately for the older adult and in appro-priate dosages. Rates of inappropriate drug prescribing have ranged from 14% to 27% in the community and as high as 35% in hospitalized patients.[50]

Contributing to the problem of polypharmacy are issues of duplicate drug prescriptions and continuing drugs that are no longer needed.[50] Often the older adult is seeing more than one physician, with one doctor pre-scribing medications unbeknownst to the other provider. It is important to ask patients to bring in all their prescribed and over-the-counter medications as well as vitamin and herbal supplements. Table 26-6 describes steps the physi-cian can take to decrease risks of adverse drug reactions.

In addition to overprescribing, there is evidence of underprescribing of effective medications.[51] Older adults often do not receive medications that have been shown to be beneficial either as secondary or tertiary prevention of disease. These medications include β-blockers and cholesterol-lowering drugs for treatment of coronary artery disease (CAD), angiotensin-converting enzyme (ACE) inhibitors as therapy for congestive heart failure, antiplatelet drugs for stroke and CAD, and warfarin for atrial fibrillation. Antidepressants also are under-prescribed, particularly in the nursing home population. Thus, the physician must individualize each patient's prescriptions and weigh the competing risks of polypharmacy vs the benefits of specific drugs.

TABLE 26-6

Reducing Polypharmacy and Adverse Drug Reactions

1. Review all medications, including over-the-counter products and medications.
2. Where practical, use drugs that treat more than one condition.
3. Consider effects of comorbidity.
4. When initiating therapy with new medication, choose agents whose pharmacokinetic properties in elderly patients are known.
5. If patients require multiple medications, try to avoid drugs that are inhibitors or inducers of cytochrome P-450 hepatic metabolism and drugs that are highly bound to albumin.
6. When maintenance dose of medication is not established, "start low and go slow."
7. Use lower-than-usual maintenance doses of medications that are renally excreted.
8. Try to prescribe medications given once or twice daily.
9. Review all medications with patient and family, and provide written instructions.
10. Consider adverse drug effects when new or unexplained medical problems develop.

Social Support

Lack of social support can contribute to numerous problems of aging, including depression, weight loss and failure to thrive, and noncompliance with treatments. The socially isolated older adult has an increased risk of cognitive decline.[52] Lack of appropriate social support may contribute to self-neglect and the potential for financial or physical abuse. The older adult when in good health may be able to manage daily activities without assistance, but in the face of an intercurrent illness, a functional decline often occurs. Thus, it is important to ask whom the patient could turn to if unable to care for himself or herself. An essential component of caring for the older adult living with disability or chronic disease is knowing who are the person's caregivers and what are their resources. For many patients and caregivers, these resources are already marginal, and any stress to the support system can be important. Connecting the patient and the caregiver to community resources may avert a crisis in care. Patients and caregivers can obtain assistance from local social service agencies and information from the local Office on Aging or the Area Agency on Aging.

OTHER PREVENTIVE CARE ISSUES

End of Life

Many elderly people see death not as a failure of care, but rather a normal part of life. They do not fear dying as much as the pain, disability, and dependency that may occur at the end of life. The Study to Understand Prognoses and Preferences for Outcomes and Risks of Treatment (SUPPORT) showed that the dying process in the hospital is frequently painful and distressing.[53] Family members of dying patients often state that their loved one would have preferred comfort to prolongation of life. However, other patients wanted treatment even if it made them uncomfortable. Thus, knowing a person's values and beliefs long before the final illness is important.

The Patient Self-Determination Act mandates that persons be informed of their rights regarding medical treatment decisions in the event they become incapable of making decisions. Advance directives can take a variety of forms. Most states have statutes regarding durable power of attorney for health care. This document allows the individual to designate a person to make medical decisions in the event the person is not capable of making those decisions. Some states also have statutes regarding living wills. These documents allow a person to state that he or she does not want life-sustaining treatment in the event of terminal disease or permanent unconscious state. Each state has its own regulations regarding withholding or withdrawing care and may have special regulations regarding removal of feeding tubes. The Patient Self-Determination Act applies only to patients admitted to hospitals, home health agencies, and nursing homes. A study from SUPPORT suggested that having advance directives did not help end-of-life decision making, but one third of the families of patients who had advance directives found they did help.[54]

Optimally, advance directives are discussed before a person is hospitalized or placed in a nursing home. The primary care provider who has known the patient and the patient's medical problems is often the appropriate person to start the process. Deciding advance directives is a process and usually cannot be done in 1 visit. Encouraging patients to designate a durable power of attorney for health care is a good place to begin. This decision gives patients an opportunity to start a discussion with their families about end-of-life care. Advance directives should be reviewed periodically, or whenever a major change in the older person's health occurs, such as at the time of elective surgery or after recovery from an acute hospitalization.

Immunizations

Despite a 50% decrease in the age-adjusted death rate for pneumonia and influenza in the past 50 years, these conditions remain a leading cause of death and account for 3% of all deaths (as they did in 1950).[55] Immunization rates for these conditions have improved but still remain low.[56] Missed opportunities for pneumococcal vaccination occur during hospitalization or on admission to nursing homes. When pneumococcal vaccination status is unknown, the vaccine in most instances should still be given. The risk of repeated vaccinations is generally small, primarily being increased swelling at the injection site.

The US Preventive Services Task Force recommends diphtheria-tetanus (dT) vaccination, although the actual incidence of tetanus is small, and a diphtheria outbreak has not occurred in this country for years. However, the level of immunity for both these diseases is low in older adults. Another missed opportunity for immunization is when an older adult receives a tetanus shot after an injury, rather than a dT vaccination. However, a slightly increased risk of local reaction occurs with the dT vaccination compared with tetanus vaccination alone.

Screening for Cancer and Cardiovascular Risk Factors

Often preventive health care is not undertaken in older adults because of misconceptions by physicians and patients about life expectancy. Figure 26-2 shows the life expectancy of older men and women. At 75 years of age, the average American will have 10 more years of life. Given this fact, appropriate screening for cancer and reducing risk factors for cardiovascular disease can have a substantial impact on morbidity and mortality in many individuals.

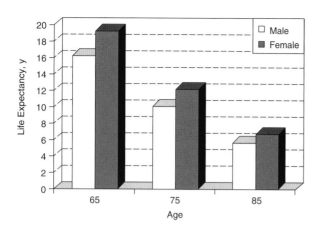

Life expectancy of elderly persons in the United States. Adapted from Arias E. United States life tables, 2000. *Natl Vital Stat Rep.* 2002;51:1–38.

The medical prognosis of persons over age 75 years varies. Furthermore, some older persons may be cognitively intact and others may have dementia. Thus, physicians must individualize preventive care to meet the needs and concerns of each patient and to take into account life expectancy, medical issues and condition, and mental status. Importantly, preventive screening and modification of risk factors should be considered in individuals likely to have 5 or more years of life.

The second leading cause of death in older adults, after cardiovascular disease, is cancer. In addition to knowing when and which elderly patients to screen for cancer, the clinician often must determine when it is appropriate to stop screening. Since cancer screening is targeted to detect cancer years in advance of clinical disease, limiting screening to those with at least a 5-year life expectancy appears prudent. For many individuals, this will occur at approximately age 85 years, but, in addition to age, comorbid conditions may lower life expectancy thereby suggest stopping screening at an earlier age. Discussion of and guidelines for screening of common cancers in older adults are addressed in the chapters devoted to each of these entities.

For women, the American Geriatrics Society recommends mammography screening as long as life expectancy is at least 4 years and the cervical Papanicolaou ("Pap") test every 1 to 3 years until age 70. After age 70, cervical Pap test screening can stop as long as the woman has had 2 negative Pap test results a year apart. However, screening should be continued for women who have continuing risk factors, although the American Geriatrics Society's consensus statement recognizes that high-risk subgroups of older adults are not well defined.[57]

Cardiovascular disease and stroke are among the most common causes of death in older adults. Treatment of hypertension decreases cardiovascular mortality, reduces risk of stroke, and may decrease risk of dementia. The benefits of treating isolated systolic hypertension in elderly patients are well established. Problems that arise with treatment of hypertension in elderly individuals are polypharmacy, adverse drug interactions, and postural hypotension with attendant risk of falls. Some concern exists that excessive lowering of diastolic blood pressure may negate the benefits of controlling systolic blood pressure.[58] Although the relative risk reduction of treatment of hypercholesterolemia in elderly adults is lower than that for younger adults, the absolute number of deaths attributed to elevated cholesterol level is higher because the prevalence of CAD increases with age. Treatment of elevated cholesterol levels in elderly patients with known heart disease is well established. Uncertainty remains whether patients over age 75 years without known CAD should have routine screening of serum lipid levels and treatment of elevated cholesterol levels for primary prevention.[59]

Fear of stroke with its resultant disability and loss of independence is a major concern for many older Americans. Screening for and treating hypertension, using aspirin in high-risk persons, and lowering cholesterol are all means of reducing the risk of stroke. Screening for carotid artery disease is more controversial. Enthusiasm for carotid endarterectomy in the United States is undergoing resurgence because of recent studies that have shown the benefit of surgical treatment of symptomatic carotid artery disease. Carotid endarterectomy also shows benefits in asymptomatic but high-risk patients. However, these studies were performed in highly selected patients, there was significant surgical mortality, and the studies were conducted before it became commonplace to give aggressive medical treatments for reduction of cardiovascular risk. One recommendation is to consider carotid endarterectomy for asymptomatic but severe carotid stenosis only if the institution's surgical mortality is less than 3% and the patient's life expectancy is at least 5 years.[60]

SUMMARY

Preventive health care in the older adult population is as important as in young or middle-aged adults. The high prevalence of diseases such as cancer and cardiovascular disease suggests that the clinician could greatly decrease a patient's morbidity and mortality through appropriate screening and intervention. For many older adults, the goals of prevention are early detection of functional decline and prevention of its progression, optimizing functional ability, and maintaining quality of life. Preventive practices are based on comorbid conditions, life expectancy, and a person's personal preferences and concerns.

REFERENCES

1. Rice DP, Feldman JJ. Living longer in the United States: demographic changes and health needs of the elderly. *Milbank Mem Fund Q.* 1983;61:362–396.

2. Hetzel L, Smith A. *The 65 Years and Over Population: 2000 Census 2000 Brief.* Washington, DC: US Census Bureau; 2001. Publication C2KBR/01–10.

3. Fries JF. Aging, natural death, and the compression of morbidity. *N Engl J Med.* 1980;303:130–135.

4. Fries J, Vita A, Terry R, et al. Aging, health risk, and cumulative disability. *N Engl J Med.* 1998;338:1035–1041.

5. Wong MD, Shapiro MF, Boscardin WJ, Ettner SL. Contribution of major diseases to disparities in mortality. *N Engl J Med.* 2002;347:1585–1592.

6. US Dept of Health and Human Services. *Healthy People 2010: Understanding and Improving Health.* 2nd ed. Washington, DC: Government Printing Office; November 2000.

7. Manton KG, Gu X. Changes in the prevalence of chronic disability in the United States black and nonblack population above age 65 from 1982 to 1999. *Proc Natl Acad Sci USA.* 2001;98:6354–6359.

8. Stults BM. Preventive health care for the elderly. *West J Med.* 1984;141:832–845.

9. Foley KT, Palmer RM. Evaluation of the frail elderly: tools for office practice. *Hosp Med.* 1996;32:21–29.

10. Lachs MS, Feinstein AR, Cooney LM Jr, et al. A simple procedure for general screening for functional disability in elderly patients. *Ann Intern Med.* 1990;112:699–706.

11. Moore AA, Siu AL. Screening for common problems in ambulatory elderly: clinical confirmation of a screening instrument. *Am J Med.* 1996;100:438–443.

12. Moore AA, Siu A, Partridge JM, Hays RD, Adams J. A randomized trial of office-based screening for common problems in older person. *Am J Med.* 1997;102:371–378.

13. Palmer RM. Geriatric assessment. *Med Clin North Am.* 1999;83:1503–1523.

14. Anetzberger GJ. Community resources to promote successful aging. *Clin Geriatr Med.* 2002;18:611–626.

15. Palmer RM, ed. Successful aging: preventive gerontology. *Clin Geriatr Med.* 2002;18(3).

16. Zylstra RG, Standridge JB, Frame PS. US Preventive Services Task Force: highlights of the 1996 report. *Am Fam Physician.* 2000;61:1089–1104.

17. Goldberg TH, Chavin SI. Preventive medicine and screening in older adults. *J Am Geriatr Soc.* 1997;45: 344–354.

18. US Preventive Services Task Force. *Guide to Clinical Preventive Services: Report of the U.S. Preventive Services Task Force.* 2nd ed. Baltimore, Md: Williams & Wilkins; 1996.

19. Jerger J, Chmiel R, Wilson N, Luchi R. Hearing impairment in older adults: new concepts. *J Am Geriatr Soc.* 1995;43:928–935.

20. Ventry I, Weinstein B. The hearing handicap inventory for the elderly: a new tool. *Ear Hear.* 1982;3:128–134.

21. Watson GR. Low vision in the geriatric population: rehabilitation and management. *J Am Geriatr Soc.* 2001;49:317–330.

22. Lee AG. Community screening for visual impairment in older people. *J Am Geriatr Soc.* 2001;49:673–675.

23. Kukull WA, Bowen JD. Dementia epidemiology. *Med Clin North Am.* 2002;86:573–590.

24. Morris JC. Clinical presentation and course of Alzheimer Disease. In: Terry RD, Katzman R, Bick KL, Sisodia SS, eds. *Alzheimer Disease.* 2nd ed. Philadelphia, Pa: Lippincott, Williams & Wilkins; 1999.

25. Petersen RC, Doody R, Kurz A, et al. Current concepts in mild cognitive impairment. *Arch Neurol.* 2001;58: 1985–1992.

26. Di Carlo A, Baldereschi M, Armaducci L, et al. Cognitive impairment without dementia in older people: prevalence, vascular risk factors, impact on disability: the Italian Longitudinal Study on Aging. *J Am Geriatr Soc.* 2000;48:775–782.

27. Sherwin BB. Mild cognitive impairment: potential pharmacological treatment options. *J Am Geriatr Soc.* 2000;48:431–441.

28. Shulman K, Shedletsky R, Silver I. The challenge of time: clock drawing and cognitive function in the elderly. *Int J Geriatr Psychiatry.* 1986;1:135–140.

29. Brodaty H, Moore CM. The Clock Drawing Test for dementia of the Alzheimer's type: a comparison of three scoring methods in a memory disorders clinic. *Int J Geriatr Psychiatry.* 1997;12:619–627.

30. Mulsant BH, Ganguli M. Epidemiology and diagnosis of depression in late life. *J Clin Psychiatry.* 1999;60(suppl 20):9–15.

31. Lebowitz BD, Pearson JL, Schneider LS, et al. Diagnosis and treatment of depression in late life: consensus statement update. *JAMA.* 1997;278:1186–1190.

32. US Preventive Services Task Force. Screening for depression: recommendations and rationale. *Ann Intern Med.* 2002;136:760–764.

33. Schulz R, Beach SR. Caregiving as a risk factor for mortality: the Caregiver Health Effects Study. *JAMA.* 1999;282:2215–2219.

34. Mahoney J, Drinka TJK, Abler R, et al. Screening for depression: single question versus GDS. *J Am Geriatr Soc.* 1994;42:1006–1008.

35. Katz S. Assessing self-maintenance: activities of daily living, mobility, and instrumental activities of daily living. *J Am Geriatr Soc.* 1983;31:721–727.

36. Lawton MP, Brody EM. Assessment of older people: self-maintaining and instrumental activities of daily living. *Gerontologist.* 1969;9:279–285.

37. Visser M, Pluijm SMF, Stel VS, Bosscher RJ, Deeg DJH. Physical activity as a determinant of change in mobility performance: the Longitudinal Aging Study Amsterdam. *J Am Geriatr Soc.* 2002;50:1774–1781.

38. Tinetti ME. Preventing falls in elderly person. *N Engl J Med.* 2003;348:42–49.

39. American Geriatrics Society, British Geriatrics Society, and American Academy of Orthopaedic Surgeons Panel on Falls Prevention. Guidelines for the prevention of falls in older persons. *J Am Geriatr Soc.* 2001;49:664–672.

40. Tinetti ME, Baker DI, McAvay G, et al. A multifactorial intervention to reduce the risk of falling among elderly people living in the community. *N Engl J Med.* 1994;331:821–827.

41. Podsiadlo D, Richardson S. The timed "Up and Go" test: a test of basic functional mobility for frail elderly persons. *J Am Geriatr Soc.* 1991;39:142–148.

42. Resnick NM. Initial evaluation of the incontinent patient. *J Am Geriatr Soc.* 1990;38:311–316.

43. Fantl JA, Newman DK, Colling J, et al. *Clinical Practice Guideline Update on Urinary Incontinence in Adults: Acute and Chronic Management.* 2nd ed: Agency for Health Care Policy and Research, Public Health Service, US Dept of Health and Human Services; 1996.

44. Wedick NM, Barrett-Connor E, Knoke JD, Wingard DL. The relationship between weight loss and all-cause mortality in older men and women with and without diabetes mellitus: the Rancho Bernardo Study. *J Am Geriatr Soc.* 2002;50:1810–1815.

45. Reuben DB, Greendale GA, Harrison GG. Nutrition screening in older persons. *J Am Geriatr Soc.* 1995;43:415–425.

46. National Center for Health Statistics. Dietary intake of macronutrients, micronutrients and other dietary constituents: United States, 1988–1994. *Vital Health Stat.* 2002;11:56.

47. Gloth FM, Tobin JD. Vitamin D deficiency in older people. *J Am Geriatr Soc.* 1995;43:822–828.

48. Stabler SP. Screening the older population for cobalamin (vitamin B12) deficiency. *J Am Geriatr Soc.* 1995;43:1290–1297.

49. Schwartz JB. Geriatric clinical pharmacology. In: Humes HD, ed. *Kelley's Textbook of Internal Medicine.* 4th ed. Philadelphia, Pa: Lippincott, Williams & Wilkins; 2000.

50. Hanlon JT, Schmader KE, Ruby CM, Weinberger M. Suboptimal prescribing in older inpatients and outpatients. *J Am Geriatr Soc.* 2001;49:200–209.

51. Rochon PA, Gurwitz JH. Prescribing for seniors: neither too much nor too little. *JAMA.* 1999;282:113–115.

52. Bassuk SS, Glass TA, Berkman LF. Social disengagement and incident cognitive decline in community-dwelling elderly persons. *Ann Intern Med.* 1999;131:165–173.

53. Lynn J, Teno J, Phillips RS, Wu AW, Desbiens N, Harrold J, for the SUPPORT investigators. Perceptions by family members of the dying experience of older and seriously ill patients: Study to Understand Prognoses and Preferences for Outcomes and Risks of Treatments. *Ann Intern Med.* 1997;126:97–106.

54. Teno J, Lynn J, Wenger N, et al, for the SUPPORT investigators. Advance directives for seriously ill hospitalized patients: effectiveness with the Patient Self-Determination Act and the SUPPORT intervention: Study to Understand Prognoses and Preferences for Outcomes and Risks of Treatment. *J Am Geriatr Soc.* 1997;45:500–507.

55. Collen MF. Vicissitudes of preventive medicine and a new challenge. *Methods Information Med.* 2002;41:224–229.

56. Pneumococcal and influenza vaccination levels among adults aged > or = 65 years: United States, 1993. *MMWR Morbid Mortal Wkly Rep.* 1996;45:853–859.

57. American Geriatric Society. Screening for cervical carcinoma in older women. *J Am Geriatr Soc.* 2001;49:655–657.

58. Smulyan H, Safar ME. The diastolic blood pressure in systolic hypertension. *Ann Intern Med.* 2000;132:233–237.

59. Messinger-Rapport B. Should hypercholesterolemia be treated in patients older than 65? *Cleveland Clin J Med.* 1999;66:393–394.

60. Brott T, Toole JF. Medical compared with surgical treatment of asymptomatic carotid artery stenosis. *Ann Intern Med.* 1995;123:720–722.

RESOURCES

For Health Care Professionals

Agency for Healthcare Research and Quality. Web site: www.ahrq.gov

American Geriatrics Society. Web site: www.americangeriatrics.org

National Institute on Aging. Web site: www.nia.nih.gov

For Patients and Families

National Family Caregivers Association. Web site: www.nfcacares.org.

National Institute of Aging, on-line directory. Web site: www.aoa.dhhs.gov.

National Safety Council. Web site: www.nsc.org.

Senior Scope. Web site: www.seniorscope.com.

Today's Caregiver magazine. Web site: www.caregiver911.com.

PART 6

Aspects of Prevention Unique to Gender

chapter 27

Unique Aspects of Mental Health in Women

Lilian Gonsalves, MD, and Gita P. Gidwani, MD

INTRODUCTION

Women's health has seen many changes during the century, particularly in the last 30 years, reflecting social, cultural, and economic transition in the lives of women. In the last 10 years, the field of women's health has been confronted by a host of new challenges and opportunities in the United States, such as a rapidly changing health care delivery system driven by cost containment and reduced public health expenditures. In the last half of the 20th century, there was a dramatic rise in the labor force participation of women in the United States. Women in the United States today spend, on average, more time in the workplace over their lifetime than they do parenting dependent children. In 1950, 30% of women age 16 years or older worked outside the home. In 1994, this figure rose to 59%. More women with children are employed outside the home. Less than 40% of women with children under age 6 years worked in the labor force in 1975 vs 65% in 1997.[1] Women today are increasingly confronted with having the dual roles of simultaneously caring for young children and elderly parents, as women are more likely than men to be caretakers of their aging parents. Along with later marriage and childbearing, there has been a rise in single-parent households, primarily due to rising divorce rates and an increase of childbearing outside of marriage.[2]

The role of women in society was changed by the women's movement of the 1960s. Women are now in positions of power in the media and government, throughout the workforce, and in the medical and legal professions. In fall 1990, Dr Bernadine Healy was appointed the first female director of the National Institutes of Health (NIH). During her tenure she established the Office of Women's Health and instituted a nationwide research effort called The Women's Health Initiative, a 15-year, $625 million NIH study, the largest clinical research study of women and their health ever undertaken in the United States or elsewhere.

Complicating the issue of women's health care is lack of or inadequate health insurance for many low-income women in the United States. Often, women hold part-time employment where health care insurance is not provided, or they are unable to work because of child care responsibilities. With inadequate health insurance coverage, low-income women are less likely to age in good health. Employment provides access to income, health care benefits, and social support, while also leading to expansion of opportunities for building knowledge, skills, self-esteem, and alternative sources of reward and satisfaction, thereby promoting health.[2]

An awareness by health care providers of mental health issues unique to women as well as the knowledge about symptoms, signs, setting, and underpinnings in which they occur can lead to early detection and prevention of more severe morbidity. Conditions that may affect women include stress (see Chapter 8), depression, mood disorders related to the menstrual cycle and childbirth, alcoholism, and violence.

WOMEN AND DEPRESSION

The treatment of depression in women is a substantial public health concern. Women constitute two thirds of patients suffering from common depressive disorders. Women's risk of depression exceeds that of men by 2:1.[3] The onset of depression in women peaks between the ages of 25 and 44 years, making women most at risk of depression during their childbearing years.

This difference may relate to female role socialization, producing maladaptive coping styles that increase the risk of depression. Social stressors, such as unequal household burdens, fragile or nonexistent support systems, and mixed messages of what a woman is "supposed to be," can all cause stress and strain. Social structures also have made women emotionally and economically dependent. Women have also been socialized to view their relationship with others as central to their lives. Contemporary women fulfill multiple social roles, and trying to balance these roles may result in emotional strain and burden, increasing the risk of depression. Seeking help, however, is not as threatening to the feminine image. Women do report depressive symptoms more readily and are more likely to seek help. For 5% to 10% of women, fluctuating levels of hormone related to the menstrual cycle (eg, the premenstruum, postpartum, and perimenopause) can trigger depression.

MOOD DISORDERS

Premenstrual Dysphoric Disorder

Although the name premenstrual dysphoric disorder (PMDD) is relatively new, the condition has been recognized since ancient times. Pliny the Elder, born in AD 23, wrote in his *Historia Naturalis* that: "On the approach of a woman in this state, milk will turn sour, seeds which are touched by her become sterile, grafts writhe away . . . her very look, even, will dim the brightness of mirrors, blunt the edge of steel, and take the polish from ivory." It was not until the 1930s that the syndrome was more officially recognized by Frank,[4] who coined the term *premenstrual tension syndrome*. Twenty years later, the simpler term, *premenstrual syndrome* (PMS) was commonly used. In the late 1970s and early 1980s, considerable concern was expressed about methodological issues, including unsophisticated methods of patient selection, open uncontrolled studies, and retrospective rating of symptoms. In 1987, criteria for late luteal phase dysphoric disorder (LLPDD) were proposed and published in the appendix of the *Diagnostic and Statistical Manual of Mental Disorders, Revised Third Edition* (*DSM-III-R*).[5] In the early 1990s the DMS-IV Work Group on LLPDD had a relatively large number of studies to review, leading to the work group recommending a change in name from LLPDD to premenstrual dysphoric disorder. In the late 1990s, based on a panel of experts, and the evidence, PMDD became a distinct clinical entity.

Common symptoms of PMDD include depressed mood, anxiety, affective lability, anger, irritability, decreased interest in usual activities, difficulty concentrating, decreased energy, appetite changes, hypersomnia, insomnia, a sense of being overwhelmed, and physical symptoms such as breast tenderness, bloating, and headache. Five or more of these symptoms must be present during the last week of the luteal phase; must remit for several days after the onset of menses; and must interfere with school work, social activities, or relationships to make a diagnosis of PMDD. The symptoms cannot be an exacerbation of another psychiatric disorder, such as major depression. The symptoms also must be confirmed by prospective daily ratings for a minimum of 2 consecutive symptomatic menstrual cycles (Table 27-1).

Using the above stringent criteria, PMDD affects 2.5% to 5% of women of reproductive age,[7] although approximately 75% of women have some symptoms of

TABLE 27-1

Summary of Premenstrual Dysphoric Disorder Criteria*

A. Symptoms must occur during the week before menses and remit a few days after onset of menses. Five of the following symptoms must be present and at least one must be (1), (2), (3), or (4).
  1. Depressed mood or dysphoria
  2. Anxiety or tension
  3. Affective lability
  4. Irritability
  5. Decreased interest in usual activities
  6. Concentration difficulties
  7. Marked lack of energy
  8. Marked change in appetite, overeating, or food cravings
  9. Hypersomnia or insomnia
  10. Feeling overwhelmed
  11. Other physical symptoms (ie, breast tenderness, bloating)
B. Symptoms must interfere with work, school, usual activities, or relationships
C. Symptoms must not merely be an exacerbation of another disorder
D. Criteria A, B, and C must be confirmed by prospective daily ratings for at least two consecutive symptomatic menstrual cycles

*Used with permission from the American Psychiatric Association.[6]

premenstrual dysphoria. Although the precise etiology of PMDD is unclear, evolving consensus suggests PMDD to be an abnormal response to normal ovarian function, rather than any hormonal imbalance.[8] Reproductive hormones often affect noradrenergic, serotonergic, and dopaminergic neuronal pathways, and the dysregulation of the serotonergic symptom appears to play a particularly substantial role in the pathophysiology of PMDD.

Clinical evaluation should include medical, gynecologic, and psychiatric history, with particular attention to mood changes during pregnancy and the postpartum period. The clinician should ask about substance use. It is often necessary to assess the spouse and family members to determine whether interpersonal and situational stressors play a role. The question, "What brings you to treatment now?" is important. Physical examination should include a pelvic examination, and laboratory studies should include thyroid function tests, a complete blood cell count, and testing of estrogen and progesterone levels. A patient record rating her symptoms for the next 2 or 3 menstrual cycles is helpful.

A stepwise approach to management of PMDD is outlined in Table 27-2.

For less severe forms of PMDD, it is beneficial to recognize and validate the patient's symptoms; educate the woman; and promote regular exercise and avoidance or

TABLE 27-2

Therapy for Premenstrual Dysphoric Disorder

First-step treatments
    Education and lifestyle modifications
        Diet modifications
        Exercise
    Somatic treatments
        Acetaminophen
        Diuretics
        Nonsteroidal anti-inflammatory drugs
Second-step treatments
    Hormonal therapies
        Oral contraceptives (mild symptoms)
        Gonadotropin-releasing hormone analogs or
        danazol (severe or refractory symptoms)
    Psychotropic drugs
        Selective serotonin reuptake inhibitors
        Anxiolytics
Third-step treatment
    Psychotherapy

minimization of caffeine, salt, and sugar. Symptoms of bloating can be treated with low doses of diuretics. Non-steroidal anti-inflammatory drugs are beneficial for headaches and breast tenderness. More than 30 studies describe the efficacy of selective serotonin reuptake inhibitors (SSRIs) for the treatment of premenstrual symptoms. Fluoxetine and sertraline are the only SSRI medications currently approved by the US Food and Drug Administration (FDA) for the treatment of PMDD.[9,10] Paroxetine and citalopram also are beneficial, as demonstrated by small studies.[11,12] Of the tricyclic agents, clomipramine has been shown to be effective in PMDD at low doses, such as 25 to 75 mg/d throughout the cycle.[13] Alprazolam and buspirone have shown to be effective in controlled trials.[14,15] The response to anxiolytics is less than with SSRIs. Selective serotonin reuptake inhibitors are the treatment of choice for prominent mood symptoms, tearfulness, anxiety, anger, and irritability. Intermittent luteal-phase dosing with fluoxetine or sertraline has been shown to be beneficial in women with PMDD.[16,17] Hormonal therapies, although appealing, have not proved to be effective, especially oral contraceptives and progesterone. Gonadotropin-releasing hormone (GnRH) agonists and danazol both have been used to eliminate the menstrual cycle and have led to significant reductions in PMDD symptoms.[18] These drugs should not be prescribed alone for longer than 6 months because of the risk of osteoporosis. Psychotherapy to work through issues of poor communication, anger and hostility, control, passivity, and marital strain is necessary to reduce

stress and premenstrual dysphoria, and to prevent a feeling of "my hormones take me over."

Postpartum Mood Disorders

The postpartum period carries a risk of new onset of psychiatric disorders or substantial worsening of pregravid mood and anxiety disorders. Postpartum mood disorders usually begin after delivery and can range in severity from rather mild subsyndromal episodes (eg, the blues) to unipolar and bipolar affective psychosis. To treat or not to treat is an important question for women in their childbearing years. Both alternatives can threaten the health and safety of the mother and offspring during pregnancy and the postpartum period, particularly if the woman wants to breast-feed. Although precise causes of postpartum mood disorders remain unknown, various studies have suggested that the abrupt change in estrogen and progesterone levels is responsible for central neurotransmitter dysregulation.

Maternity blues affect 50% to 80% of women in the first 3 postpartum weeks, but the condition often gets better without treatment. The mood disturbance is usually mild and transient, lasting from a few hours to a few days. Typical symptoms include low mood, crying, anxiety, insomnia, and irritability.

Some (10% to 15%) new mothers experience postpartum depression,[19] beginning approximately 3 to 4 weeks after delivery. Symptoms are more serious and persistent than the blues and are similar to major depression. They include depressed mood, loss of interest, changes in appetite and sleep, fatigue, guilt, difficulty concentrating, and suicidal ideation. Symptoms may be accompanied by prominent agitation, such as not wanting to be left alone with the baby, fear of harm coming to the baby, constantly checking the baby, and making phone calls to the pediatrician for reassurance.

Although postpartum psychosis is a rare condition, occurring in 1 to 2 of 2000 postpartum women, it is a severe illness with the propensity to escalate rapidly to suicide or infanticide. Symptoms usually begin within 3 to 5 days post partum and include agitation, confusion, bizarre behavior, paranoid delusions, and sleep disturbances.

Over the last decade, several studies have described either *new* onset of panic attacks, obsessive-compulsive symptoms, or worsening of preexisting symptoms during the puerperium. Patients with postpartum panic attacks or intrusive obsessive thoughts (frequently of harming an infant or of something bad happening to the baby) should be treated similarly to nonpuerperal patients who suffer from these disorders. It is an error to dismiss these symptoms of anxiety as normative.

Risk factors include a history of affective disorder before or during pregnancy, heightened sensitivity to shifts in hormonal milieu such as PMDD or sensitivity to oral contraceptives, family history of affective disorders, and history of postpartum thyroid dysfunction.[20] Ten percent of women with postpartum depression have no prior disorder. Twenty-five percent have a prior history of depression, and 50% have a prior history of postpartum depression. Psychosocial stressors include stressful life events, bereavement, prior pregnancy losses, unplanned pregnancy, primiparity, single-parent status, or poor spousal or social support.[21]

Diagnosis of Postpartum Depression

Negative cognitions, faulty interactions with the baby, or neurovegetative features, such as disturbances in sleep, appetite, and weight, in addition to worsening postpartum mood changes should alert the physician to the presence of an underlying disorder. The 6-week postpartum visit provides a good opportunity to screen for postpartum mood disorder.

A detailed medical and psychiatric history screening for prior mood or thought disorders is critical in diagnosing postpartum depression. Important to assess are previous pregnancies and outcomes, family history of psychiatric illnesses and stressful life events, and quality of the marital relationship. An anemia profile and thyroid function test are helpful to rule out organic causes of symptoms. The Edinburgh Postnatal Depression Scale is a self-report scale of 10 items helpful for screening and monitoring worsening of symptoms.[22]

Self-limiting subsyndromal blues generally respond to reassurance and rest. Mild to moderate cases of postpartum depression may resolve with reassurance, support, psychoeducation, and group or interpersonal psychotherapy. More severe cases respond to antidepressants.[23] All antidepressants cross the placental barrier and are excreted in breast milk. Hence, the decision to treat a depressed pregnant or breast-feeding woman is not risk free. The risk of fetal exposure to psychotropic medications must be weighed carefully against the potential adverse effects of untreated depression on both the mother and fetus.[24]

The infants of women who had received fluoxetine, citalopram, sertraline, paroxetine, or fluvox during pregnancy have been studied.[25-32] No study to date has revealed an increased risk of teratogenicity in the population exposed to SSRIs compared with individuals who have not had such exposure. More than 400 infants of women who were given tricyclic antidepressants during pregnancy have been evaluated without evidence for increased risk of congenital malformation.[25] Fluoxetine and sertraline are the preferred antidepressants for the depressed pregnant mother. The use of benzodiazepines is discouraged, especially in the first trimester, because of reported cases of cleft palate.[25] If an antipsychotic medication is needed, a high-potency antipsychotic, such as haloperidol, is recommended. The use of lithium in the first trimester as a mood stabilizer may be appropriate. The small absolute risk of cardiovascular malformations associated with lithium exposure during the first trimester is approximately 1 in 2000.[33]

Most case reports and series have reported no adverse effects in nursing infants whose mothers were receiving antidepressants, and the serum concentration of antidepressants and the metabolites were undetectable.[34-37] Although the total number of cases reported is small, concern for infant safety remains. Sertraline and paroxetine are the preferred antidepressants for breast-feeding mothers. Checking the infant blood level for antidepressants and their metabolites is also recommended.

Perimenopause and Mood Disorder

The World Health Organization defines perimenopause as the period (2 to 8 years) preceding menopause and the 1-year period after final menses. Perimenopause, also known as "menopausal transition," represents the passage from reproductive to nonreproductive life. Perimenopause usually begins in a woman's 40s, the mean age being 47 years. Many studies have shown that women going through menopause have no greater chance of facing a severe depression than they do at other times in their lives. However, evidence is growing that suggests that perimenopause may be a time of increased risk of depressive symptoms, both for women with a history of primary depression and for those without such a history.[38,39] The Massachusetts Women's Health Study, a 5-year prospective cohort, assessed 2565 subjects between the ages of 45 and 55 years, using semistructured interviews.[40] Information was gathered on sociodemographic status, social supports, lifestyle, physical health, health care utilization, menstrual status, and depressive symptoms. Results indicate that a long period of perimenopause correlated with increased physical symptoms and depression. Rates of depression decreased as women became postmenopausal.

Helene Deutsch[41] has described menopause as "the rose vanishes from the cheek" and "a woman's last traumatic experience as a sexual being." A perimenopausal woman may experience the stresses of midlife, including the empty nest syndrome, widowhood, divorce, illness, loss of youth, or death of parents. Women entering menopause are at risk of losing their role of childbearing and child rearing. Those women who are too engaged or overinvolved with their children may feel isolated and suffer depressive symptoms when their nest empties. Other women entering menopause describe a newfound freedom, increased energy level, and increased pleasure in sexual activities. For them, menopause marks entry into a new prime of life.

The evaluation of women in their perimenopausal years should include inquiries about changes in menstrual cycle, physical and mental health symptoms, and measurement of the thyroid-stimulating hormone level to rule out thyroid disease as a cause for symptoms. The timing of the depressive symptoms is critical in the perimenopause. Perimenopausal status may be confirmed by investigation of serum levels of follicle-stimulating hormone (FSH) and estradiol on day 2 or 3 of the cycle. Estrogen replacement therapy can improve subjective well-being and quality of life during the perimenopause. Alternative medications such as the serotonin reuptake inhibitors, vitamin E, soy products, and avoidance of caffeine and alcohol may prove beneficial.

WOMEN AND ALCOHOLISM

In 1993, the National Institute on Alcohol Abuse and Alcoholism (NIAAA) estimated that nearly 6 million American adult women met the diagnostic criteria for current alcohol abuse or alcohol dependence.[42] Kessler et al,[3] in the National Comorbidity Study, a population-based representative sample of individuals 15 to 54 years old in the United States, noted that substance abuse disorders were more prevalent in men than in women, with the ratio ranging from 2:1 to 3:1. Recent data, however, suggest that the gender gap between both adolescent girls and boys and older women and men may be narrowing in terms of substance abuse.[43]

Clear differences exist with respect to how women and men metabolize and use alcohol. The clinical presentation, course, and medical consequences are also different for women compared with men. Jones and Jones[44] were the first to report that even with single doses of alcohol under standard conditions, nonalcoholic women obtained a much higher blood alcohol level than did men. The differences related to the body water content, lower average body weight, lower concentration of gastric alcohol dehydrogenase, and hormonal fluctuations with the menstrual cycle. In recognition of these differences, the National Institute on Alcohol Abuse and Alcoholism has defined at-risk drinking for women as more than 7 drinks (either 12 ounces of beer, 5 ounces of wine, or 1.5 ounce of liquor) per week or 3 drinks per occasion, compared to 14 drinks per week or 4 drinks per occasion for men.[45] These facts may also explain why women, although they start drinking and begin their pattern for alcohol abuse at a later age than men do, present for alcohol treatment at approximately the same age as men. The rapid development for alcoholism or "telescoping" of the disease is an important consideration when treating women.[46]

Women with alcohol problems are more likely to see their primary care physicians with symptoms such as insomnia and anxiety, whereas men often enter alcohol treatment through drunk-driving rehabilitation and employee assistance programs. Women are better able to conceal their drinking, more often drink alone at home, are more likely to attribute their drinking to a traumatic event, and often view their drinking as self-medication. Childless, separated, or divorced women are more at risk than married women. Women who are not married but living with a partner are 50% more likely to drink heavily than are married women.[47] Divorced, widowed, unemployed women in their midlife, especially after their children leave, are at higher risk. There has been some speculation that women currently employed in historically male-dominated professions (eg, medicine, law, or business) are at increased risk of alcohol problems.

Psychiatric comorbidity is also an important consideration in women who drink excessively. There is a higher prevalence of affective disorders and eating disorders in women alcoholics.[48] Also, compared with alcoholic men, alcoholic women have death rates 50% to 100% higher and die more frequently of suicide, cirrhosis of the liver, alcohol-related accidents, and cardiac disease.

A special problem of concern to women is the fetal alcohol syndrome and fetal alcohol effects. Fetal alcohol syndrome occurs in 0.33 cases per 1000 live births.[49] Alcohol causes fetal damage by interfering with maternal nutrition and being directly toxic to fetal cellular growth and metabolism. The fetal alcohol syndrome is characterized by growth retardation, facial malformation, mental retardation, and neurobehavioral effects, such as poor coordination, irritability in infancy, and hyperactivity in childhood. Fetal alcohol syndrome costs nearly one third of $1 billion a year and is among the leading causes of mental retardation in the Western world. One drink daily appears to increase the risk of congenital malformations, especially in the first trimester. Six drinks of hard liquor per day during pregnancy poses a serious risk of fetal alcohol syndrome.

To diagnose alcoholism in women, physicians should have a high incidence of suspicion for depression and cross-addiction to sedative hypnotics, should routinely ask women about alcohol intake, and particularly should query pregnant women about alcohol use. The CAGE questionnaire[50] is a simple, accurate, fast, and nonjudgmental screening tool. CAGE is an acronym for the following 4 questions:

1. Have you tried to *C*ut down on your drinking?
2. Do you get *A*nnoyed when people criticize your drinking?
3. Do you feel *G*uilty about your drinking?
4. Do you ever need an *E*ye opener, that is, a drink in the morning on waking up?

Two or more affirmative answers identify 80% to 90% of those who have a drinking problem and require further evaluation.

WOMEN AND VIOLENCE

Violence against women is an important health issue and is growing at an alarming rate. In the United States, more than 700,000 women are sexually assaulted each year, or 1 woman every 45 seconds. Sixty-one percent of female rape victims are under 18 years of age. Most sexual assaults are committed by a friend, acquaintance, intimate partner, or family member. Each year, 2 to 4 million women are battered, 1500 are killed, and 1.8 million elderly women are mistreated. Twenty-two percent of women experience physical or sexual abuse before age 18, and 21% suffer such abuse during adulthood.[51] Alcoholism and drug abuse are much higher in women who have been victimized. Higher rates of depression and psychiatric disorders are commonly found in victims of interpersonal violence, and those who have a history of being sexually abused as children.

The mental health impact of violence is substantial in that once victimized, a woman can never again feel quite as invulnerable. Post-traumatic stress disorder may occur, in which symptoms include reexperiencing the trauma with flashbacks and disturbing dreams. Hypervigilance, insomnia, hopelessness, helplessness, self-defeating behaviors, and difficulty maintaining intimate relationships are core features of victimized adult women. Feelings of detachment, psychic numbing, and amnesia about the situation are examples of behaviors that help women avoid reexperiencing the trauma.

Battery is found in all walks of life; all socioeconomic levels; and all educational, racial, and age groups. An accurate history is best obtained when a woman is approached alone, in private, and in a supportive therapy climate. Questions should be asked directly about the details, duration, frequency, and severity of injury. If the woman is vague or evasive, the clinician should gently probe and use open-ended general questions, then move on to more specific terms. Abused women tend to be high users of emergency room services, where a high index of suspicion should be maintained for women exhibiting abrasions or contusions of the head, face, back, and arms. Vague somatic symptoms, headaches, pelvic pain, multiple miscarriages or abortions, use of minor tranquilizers or sleep medications, and alcohol abuse are other possible clues. Abused women are more likely to be beaten when pregnant.

PREVENTIVE STRATEGIES

Health builds or diminishes over decades of life. Prevention of the common women's issues and medical conditions, described in this chapter, needs to begin early and be continued with vigilance throughout the life span. Primary care physicians have numerous opportunities to build a physician-patient relationship with women based on trust, respect, and a willingness to listen, and to encourage the female patient to take an active role in health awareness, prevention, and healthy lifestyle. The health care professional, by inquiring about and discussing mental health and lifestyle, can often convince women to schedule regular times for themselves, share responsibilities, have good sleep hygiene, be involved in activities, exercise regularly, and follow an appropriate diet. Changes then may set a good example for their children, and health issues in their offspring can be addressed early, such as prevention of smoking.

Career frustrations through women's professional lives can cause severe and chronic symptoms. The "lexan* ceiling," rather than the glass ceiling, is a strong barrier, and men of good conscience can help take it down together with women.[52] In this way, women in midlife may be encouraged to take second chances to return to school, begin new careers, and start new endeavors.

Alcoholic women face many barriers to treatment, including fear of abandonment by her partner, fear of loss of children, financial dependency, lack of child care during treatment, and exclusion of pregnant women from treatment programs. Many alcohol programs are male oriented, in which women feel uncomfortable. Self-help groups, such as Alcoholics Anonymous and Women For Sobriety, are useful, as are female alcohol counselors who are recovered alcoholics. The physician also can direct female patients to treatment programs tailored to women's needs. All primary care physicians should carefully screen women with vague complaints of insomnia and anxiety, to prevent the underdiagnosis of alcohol disorders in women. Alcohol is the leading preventable cause of birth defects. Good prenatal care therefore emphasizes and promotes abstinence from alcohol during pregnancy.

Health care providers working with women victims of violence should be educated to take a careful history and be clear in their own beliefs that nothing justifies violent abuse. C. Everett Koop, former US surgeon general, said, "Battery is the single most significant cause of injury to women in this country. . . . [N]o woman is obliged to accept a beating and suffer because of it." Practitioners can be a productive resource to women, by being aware of and recommending available local legal services, shelters, welfare services, telephone hotlines, social service organizations, and community mental health centers. A helpful list of resources is listed at the end of this chapter.

Lastly, women should ask how we can build a better world for ourselves and our daughters. Our voices must be heard at the local, state, and federal levels through letters to congressmen and opinions expressed in local newspapers and the radio. Such endeavors will only ensure responsible health care for women and a fuller measure of life for all women in the 21st century.

---

*Lexan is a glass look-alike, stronger than steel and bulletproof.

REFERENCES

1. Killien MG. Women and employment: a decade review. *Ann Rev Nursing Res.* 2001;19:87–123.

2. Strobino DM, Grason H, Minkovitz C. Charting a course for the future of women's health in the United States: concepts, findings and recommendations. *Soc Sci Med.* 2002;54:839–848.

3. Kessler RC, McGonagle KA, Zhao S, et al. Lifetime and 12-month prevalence of *DSM-III-R* psychiatric disorders in the United States: results from the National Comorbidity Survey. *Arch Gen Psychiatry.* 1994;51:8–19.

4. Frank RT. The hormonal causes of premenstrual tension. *Arch Neurol Psychiatry.* 1931;26:1053.

5. American Psychiatric Association. *Diagnostic and Statistical Manual of Mental Disorders, Revised Third Edition.* Washington, DC: American Psychiatric Association; 1987.

6. American Psychiatric Association. *Diagnostic and Statistical Manual of Mental Disorders, Fourth Edition.* Washington, DC: American Psychiatric Association; 1994.

7. Reid PL. Premenstrual syndrome. *N Engl J Med.* 1991;324:1208–1210.

8. Schmidt PJ, Nieman LK, Danaceau MA, et al. Differential behavioral effects of gonadal steroids in women with and in those without premenstrual syndrome. *N Engl J Med.* 1998;338:209–216.

9. Steiner M, Steinberg S, Stewart D, et al, for Canadian Fluoxetine/Premenstrual Dysphoria Collaborative Study Group. Fluoxetine in the treatment of premenstrual dysphoria. *N Engl J Med.* 1995;332:1529–1534.

10. Yonkers KA, Halbreich U, Freeman E, et al, for Sertraline Premenstrual Dysphoric Collaborative Study Group. Symptomatic improvement of premenstrual dysphoric disorder with sertraline treatment: a randomized controlled trial. *JAMA.* 1997;278:983–988.

11. Yonkers KA, Gullion C, Williams A, Novak K, Rush AJ. Paroxetine as a treatment for premenstrual dysphoric disorder. *J Clin Psychopharmacol.* 1996;16:3–8.

12. Wikander I, Sundblad C, Andersch B, et al. Citalopram in premenstrual dysphoria: is intermittent treatment during luteal phases more effective than continuous medication throughout the menstrual cycle? *J Clin Psychopharm.* 1998;18:390–398.

13. Sundblad C, Modigh K, Andersch B, et al. Clomipramine effectively reduces premenstrual irritability and dysphoria: a placebo-controlled trial. *Acta Psychiatr Scand.* 1992;85:39–47.

14. Harrison WM, Endicott J, Nee J. Treatment of premenstrual dysphoria with alprazolam: a controlled study. *Arch Gen Psychiatry.* 1990;47:270–275.

15. Rickels K, Freeman E, Sondheimer S. Buspirone in treatment of premenstrual syndrome. *Lancet.* 1989;1:777.

16. Steiner M, Korzekwa M, Lamont J, Wilkins A. Intermittent fluoxetine dosing in the treatment of women with premenstrual dysphoria. *Psychopharmacol Bull.* 1997;33:771–774.

17. Halbreich U, Smoller J. Intermittent luteal-phase sertraline treatment of dysphoric premenstrual syndrome. *J Clin Psychiatry.* 1997;58:399–402.

18. Muse KN, Cetel NS, Futterman LA. The premenstrual syndrome: effects of medical ovariectomy. *N Engl J Med.* 1984;44:317–318.

19. O'Hara MW, Swain AM. Rates and risk of postpartum depression—a meta-analysis. *Int Rev Psychiatry.* 1996;8:37–54.

20. O'Hara MW. Social support, life events, and depression during pregnancy and the puerperium. *Arch Gen Psychiatry.* 1986;43:569–573.

21. O'Hara MW. *Postpartum Depression: Causes and Consequences.* New York, NY: Springer-Verlag; 1995:168–194.

22. Cox JL, Holden JM, Sagovsky R. Detection of postnatal depression: development of the 10-item Edinburgh Postnatal Depression Scale. *Br J Psychiatry.* 1987;150:782–786.

23. Stowe ZN, Casarella J, Landry J, et al. Sertraline in the treatment of women with postpartum major depression. *Depression.* 1995;3:49–55.

24. Wisner KL, Zarin DA, Holmboe ES, et al. Risk-benefit decision making for treatment of depression during pregnancy. *Am J Psychiatry.* 2000;157:1933–1940.

25. Altshuler LL, Cohen L, Szuba MP, Burt VK, Gitlin M, Mintz J. Pharmacologic management of psychiatric illness during pregnancy: dilemmas and guidelines. *Am J Psychiatry.* 1996;153:592–606.

26. McElhatton PR, Garbis HM, Elefant E, et al. The outcome of pregnancy in 689 women exposed to therapeutic doses of antidepressants: a collaborative study of the European Network of Teratology Information Services (ENTIS). *Reprod Toxicol.* 1996;10:285–294.

27. Chambers CD, Johnson KA, Dick LM, Felix RJ, Jones KL. Birth outcomes in pregnant women taking fluoxetine. *N Engl J Med.* 1996;335:1010–1015.

28. Loebstein R, Koren G. Pregnancy outcome and neurodevelopment of children exposed *in vitro* to psychoactive drugs: the Motherisk experience. *J Psychiatry Neurosci.* 1997;22:192–196.

29. Nulman I, Rovet J, Stewart DE, et al. Neurodevelopment of children exposed in utero to antidepressant drugs. *N Engl J Med.* 1997;336:258–262.

30. Goldstein DJ, Sundell KL, Corbin LA. Birth outcomes in pregnant women taking fluoxetine. *N Engl J Med.* 1997;336:872–873.

31. Kulin NA, Pastuszak A, Sage SR, et al. Pregnancy outcome following maternal use of the new selective serotonin reuptake inhibitors: a prospective controlled multicenter study. *JAMA.* 1998;279:609–610.

32. Ericson A, Kallen B, Wiholm B. Delivery outcome after the use of antidepressants in early pregnancy. *Eur J Clin Pharmacol.* 1999;55:503–508.

33. Cohen LS, Friedman JM, Jefferson JW, Johnson EM, Weiner ML. A reevaluation of risk of in utero exposure to lithium. *JAMA.* 1994;271:146–150.

34. Wisner KL, Perel JM, Findling RL. Antidepressant treatment during breast-feeding. *Am J Pschiatry.* 1996;153:1132–1137.

35. Stowe ZN, Owens MJ, Landry JC, et al. Sertraline and desmethylsertraline in human breast milk and nursing infants. *Am J Psychiatry.* 1997;154:1255–1260.

36. Stowe ZN, Cohen LS, Hostetter A, et al. Paroxetine in human breast milk and nursing infants. *Am J Psychiatry.* 2000;157:185–189.

37. Burt VK, Suri R, Altshuler L, Stowe Z, Hendrick VC, Muntean E. The use of psychotropic medications during breastfeeding. *Am J Psychiatry.* 2001;158:1001–1009.

38. Schmidt PJ, Roca CA, Bloch M, Rubinow DR. The perimenopause and affective disorders. *Semin Reprod Endocrinol.* 1997;15:91–100.

39. Burt VK, Altshuler LL, Rasgon N. Depressive symptoms in the perimenopause: prevalence, assessment, and guidelines for treatment. *Harv Rev Psychiatry.* 1998;6:121–132.

40. Avis NE, McKinlay SM. A longitudinal analysis of women's attitudes toward the menopause: results from the Massachusetts Women's Health Study. *Maturitas.* 1991;13:65–79.

41. Deutsch H. The menopause. *Int J Psychoanal.* 1984;65:55–62.

42. National Institute on Alcohol Abuse and Alcoholism. *Eighth Special Report to the U.S. Congress on Alcohol and Health.* Washington, DC: US Dept of Health and Human Services; 1993.

43. Substance Abuse and Mental Health Services Administration. *Household Survey on Drug Abuse: Population Estimates, 1996.* Washington, DC: Office of Applied Studies, US Substance Abuse and Mental Health Services Administration; 1997.

44. Jones BM, Jones MK. Women and alcohol: intoxication metabolism and the menstrual cycle. In: Greenblatt M, Schuckit MA, eds. *Alcoholism Problems in Women and Children.* New York, NY: Grune & Stratton; 1976.

45. National Institute on Alcohol Abuse and Alcoholism. *The Physician's Guide to Helping Patients With Alcohol Problems.* Washington, DC: US Government Printing Office; 1995.

46. Piazza NJ, Vrbka JL, Yeager RD. Telescoping of alcoholism in women alcoholics. *Int J Addict.* 1989;24:19–28.

47. Richman JA, Rospenda KM. Gender roles and alcohol abuse: costs of noncaring for future physicians. *J Nerv Ment Dis.* 1992;180:619–626.

48. Sinha R, O'Malley SS. Alcohol and eating disorders: implications for alcohol treatment and health services research. *Alcohol Clin Exp Res.* 2000;24:1312–1319.

49. Floyd RL, Davis MK, Martin ML, et al. Fetal alcohol syndrome: public health importance. *Child Health.* 2001;343–350.

50. Ewing JA. Detecting alcoholism: the CAGE questionnaire. *JAMA.* 1984;252:1905–1907.

51. Wyshak G. Violence, mental health, substance abuse—problems for women worldwide. *Health Care Women Int.* 2000;21:631–639.

52. Dickstein LJ. Primary prevention and practical techniques to encourage mental wellness. *Primary Care.* 2002;29:199–210.

RESOURCES

Depression and Mood Disorders

American College of Obstetricians and Gynecologists, 409 12th St SW, Washington DC 20024-2188; 800 673-8444.
Web site: www.acog.org. (For educational pamphlets on depression and other subjects related to women's health.)

Depression After Delivery Inc, 91 E Somerset St, Raritan, NJ 08869; 800 944-4773 (4PPD).
Web site: www.depressionafterdelivery.com.

Depression and Bipolar Support Alliance, 730 N Franklin St, Suite 501, Chicago, IL 60610-7224; 312 642-0049.
Web site: www.dbsalliance.org.

Healthy Mother, Healthy Babies Coalition, 121 N Washington, Suite 300, Alexandria, VA 22314; 703 836-6110.
Web site: www.hmhb.org.

National Alliance for the Mentally Ill, 2107 Wilson Blvd, Suite 300, Arlington, VA 22201; 703 524-7600.
Web site: www.nami.org.

National Foundation for Depressive Illness Inc, PO Box 2257, New York, NY 10611; 800 239-1265. Web site: www.depression.org.

Postpartum Support International (PSI); 805 967-7636.
Web site: www.postpartum.net.

Women's Health Information Line, 1289 Deming Way, Madison, WI 53717-1955; 800 222-4767. (For information on premenstrual syndrome and hormone replacement therapy.)

Alcoholism

National Clearinghouse for Alcohol and Drug Information, PO Box 2345, Rockville, MD 20852; 800 729-6686.

Web site: www.health.org.

National Council on Alcoholism and Drug Dependence Inc, 12 W 21st St, 8th Floor, New York, NY, 10010, 800 622-2255 (NCA-CALL).

Web site: www.ncadd.org. (Materials on alcoholism, fetal alcohol syndrome.)

National Institute on Drug Abuse; treatment referral hotline 800 662-4357.

Web site: www.nida.nih.gov. (For drug treatment facilities in local communities.)

Self-help groups: Alcoholics Anonymous (AA), Al-Anon, Adult Children of Alcoholics, Narcotics Anonymous, Women For Sobriety. (Listings of meetings can be obtained from headquarters offices, with telephone numbers listed in local directories. Also check the Internet for these organizations' Web sites.)

Violence

Childhelp USA, 15757 N 78th St, Scottsdale, AZ 85260. Child abuse hotline 800 422-4453.

Web site: www.childhelpusa.org.

Domestic Violence Center; 800 799-7233.

Legal Aid societies. Phone numbers are listed in local telephone directories.

National Organization for Women (NOW), 733 15th Street NW, Washington, DC 20005.

Web site: www.now.org.

Books

Altshuler LL, Cohen LS, Moline ML, Kahn DA, Carpenter D, Docherty JP. *The Expert Consensus Guideline Series: Treatment of Depression in Women 2001*. Postgraduate Medicine Special Report. New York, NY: McGraw-Hill; 2001.

Healy B. *A New Prescription for Women's Health: Getting the Best Medical Care in a Man's World*. New York, NY: Viking Penguin; 1995.

O'Hara MW. *Postpartum Depression: Cause and Consequences*. New York, NY: Springer-Verlag; 1995.

Sheehy G. *The Silent Passage: Menopause*. New York, NY: Pocket Books/Simon & Schuster; 1993.

chapter 28

Contraception and Prenatal Care

Shakuntala Kothari, MD, Pelin Batur, MD, and Julie Elder, DO

INTRODUCTION

This chapter is divided into two sections. The first section addresses contraception, and the second, prenatal care.

CONTRACEPTION

In the United States, approximately 35 million women currently use contraception, while 95% of all sexually active women have used contraception at some point during their lives.[1,2] Contraception offers both noncontraceptive health benefits and protection against unwanted pregnancies. Adverse side effects, inconvenience, and cost, however, cause many women to discontinue contraception. The improper use of contraception has led to an estimated 1 million unplanned pregnancies in the United States annually, with half of these unwanted pregnancies ending in abortion.[3] The introduction of newer contraceptive agents has provided more options for effective birth control. These newer agents tend to have fewer side effects, which may ultimately improve patient compliance and satisfaction.

Many effective contraceptive methods are available to women that provide both contraceptive and noncontraceptive benefits. The best contraceptive option for a woman is the method with which she feels the most comfortable and the one that best suits her lifestyle. Education about the various forms of contraception is essential. Contraceptive choices should be individualized, which, in turn, improves patient satisfaction and compliance and reduces the rate of unwanted pregnancies.

Oral Contraceptives

Types

For women, combined estrogen and progestin oral contraceptive pills (OCPs) are the second most popular contraceptive choice after sterilization.[4] Used for more than 40 years in the United States, OCPs contain both estrogen and progestin. They exert their contraceptive effect by suppressing gonadotropins, inhibiting ovulation, and thickening cervical mucus, thereby making sperm entry difficult. Despite the theoretical 0.1% failure rate, the true failure rate is actually 3% due to incorrect use.

The 2 estrogen compounds available in the United States are ethinyl estradiol (EE) and mestranol (Tables 28-1 to 28-3). Ethinyl estradiol is the most commonly used, while mestranol is a prodrug that is converted to EE by the liver. Mestranol products must contain at least 50 μg, since lower doses have diminished efficacy. Doses of EE have more variability, with current pills containing on average 30 to 35 μg. Pills containing less than 50 μg EE are referred to as low-dose, while newer products containing 20 to 25 μg are called ultra-low dose. This contrasts to the early OCP preparations, which contained up to 80 to 100 μg of EE. Ultra-low-dose pills are used for symptom control and contraception during the menopause transition, as well as for patients who do not tolerate higher doses due to side effects.

Progestins were created in the 1940s. Testosterone-derived progestins bind to the androgen receptor and have varying degrees of androgenic activity. Adverse metabolic effects of highly androgenic progestins (eg, levonorgestrel) include reduction in serum high-density lipoprotein cholesterol (HDL-C), increased low-density lipoprotein cholesterol (LDL-C), and glucose intolerance. More selective progestins, also called third-generation progestins (eg, norgestimate, desogestrel), were developed with structural changes to lower their androgen activity. The efficacy of OCPs containing these newer progestins is similar to that of the older formulations. Compared with levonorgestrel-containing pills, third-generation pills have less effect on carbohydrate and lipid metabolism and are more effective in reducing acne and hirsutism in hyperandrogenic women (Table 28-4). However, limited data are available comparing the third-generation progestins with other second-generation progestins such as norethindrone or ethynodiol diacetate. Compared with levonorgestrel, these other second-generation progestins are less androgenic.[5]

TABLE 28-1

Monophasic FDA-Approved Oral Contraceptive Regimens[*]

Dose and Brand	Manufacturer	Dose and Brand	Manufacturer
50 μg mestranol and 1.0 mg norethindrone		35 μg EE and 0.25 mg norgestimate	
Necon 1/50	Watson	Ortho-Cyclen	Ortho-McNeil
Nelova 1/50 M	Warner Chilcott	30 μg EE and 0.15 mg desogestrel	
Norinyl 1/50	Searle		
Ortho-Novum 1/50	Ortho-McNeil	Apri	Duramed
50 μg EE and 1.0 mg ethynodiol diacetate		Desogen	Organon
		Ortho-Cept	Ortho McNeil
Demulen 1/50	Searle	30 μg EE and 3.0 mg drospirenone	
Zovia 1/50	Watson		
50 μg EE and 0.5 mg norgestrel		Yasmin	Berlex
		30 μg EE and 0.15 mg levonorgestrel	
Ovral-28 (-28)	Wyeth-Ayerst		
Ogestrel	Watson	Levlen	Berlex
50 μg EE and 1.0 mg norethindrone		Levora	Watson
		Nordette	Wyeth-Ayerst
Ovcon 50	Bristol-Myers Squibb	30 μg EE and 1.5 mg norethindrone acetate	
35 μg EE and 1.0 mg ethynodiol diacetate		Loestrin 1.5/30	Parke-Davis
Demulen 1/35	Searle	30 μg EE and 0.3 mg norgestrel	
Zovia 1/35	Watson		
35 μg EE and 1.0 mg norethindrone		Lo/Ovral	Wyeth-Ayerst
		Low-Ogestrel	Watson
Necon 1/35	Watson	20 μg EE and 0.15 mg desogestrel (days 1–21)	
Nelova 1/35	Warner Chilcott		
Norinyl 1/35	Searle	Mircette	Organon
Nortrel 1/35	Barr	20 μg EE and 0.1 mg levonorgestrel	
Ortho-Novum 1/35	Ortho-McNeil		
35 μg EE and 0.5 mg norethindrone		Alesse	Wyeth-Ayerst
		Aviane	Duramed
Brevicon	Searle	Levlite	Berlex
Modicon	Ortho-McNeil	20 μg EE and 1.0 mg norethindrone acetate	
Necon 0.5/35	Watson		
Nelova 0.5/35	Warner Chilcott	Loestrin 21 1/20	Parke-Davis
Nortrel 0.5/35	Barr		
35 μg EE and 0.4 mg norethindrone			
Ovcon 35	Bristol-Myers Squibb		

[*]FDA indicates Food and Drug Administration; EE, ethinyl estradiol.

The use of third-generation OCPs has become a source of some controversy due to reports of increased risk of deep venous thrombosis compared with second-generation pills.[6] Given this concern, it appears reasonable to prescribe OCPs containing a less androgenic second-generation progestin, such as norethindrone, when starting a patient on a regimen of OCPs for the first time. Women using a third-generation progestin who are doing well and have no complications do not need to change preparations. Starting treatment with a third-generation progestin for a first-time OCP user is appropriately reserved for women with increased androgenic traits such as hirsutism or acne.

T A B L E 28-2

Biphasic and Triphasic Approved Oral Contraceptive Regimens

Biphasic

Brand	Manufacturer	Dosage*
Mircette	Organon	20 μg EE and 0.15 mg desogestrel days 1–21; 10 μg EE days 24–28
Necon 10/11	Watson	35 μg EE days 1–21; 0.5 mg norethindrone days 1–10 and 1.0 mg days 11–21
Ortho Novum 10/11	Ortho-McNeil	35 μg EE days 1–21; 0.5 mg norethindrone days 1–10 and 1.0 mg days 11–21

Triphasic

Brand	Manufacturer	Dosage*
Cyclessa	Organon	25 μg EE; 0.1 mg desogestrel days 1–7, 0.125 mg days 8–14, 0.150 mg days 15–21
Estrostep	Parke-Davis	20 μg EE and 1.0 mg norethindrone acetate days 1–5; 30 μg EE and 1.0 mg norethindrone acetate days 8–14; 35 μg EE and 1.0 mg norethindrone acetate days 13–21
Ortho Novum 7/7/7	Ortho-McNeil	35 μg EE; 0.5 mg norgestimate days 1–7, 0.75 mg days 8–14, 1.0 mg days 15–21
Ortho Tri-Cyclen	Ortho-McNeil	35 μg EE; 0.18 mg norgestimate days 1–7, 0.215 mg days 8–14, 0.25 mg days 15–21
Tri-Levlen	Berlex	30 μg 0.05 mg days 1–6, 40 μg 0.075 mg days 7–11, 0.125 mg days 12–21
Tri-Norinyl	Searle	35 μg EE; 0.5 mg norgestimate days 1–7, 1.0 mg days 8–16, 0.5 mg days 17–21
Triphasil	Wyeth-Ayerst	30 μg EE and 0.05 mg levonorgestrel days 1–6; 40 μg EE and 0.075 mg levonorgestrel days 7–11; 30 μg EE and 0.125 mg levonorgestrel days 12–21
Trivora	Watson	30 μg EE and 0.05 mg levonorgestrel days 1–6; 40 μg EE and 0.075 mg levonorgestrel days 7–11; 30 μg EE and 0.125 mg levonorgestrel days 12–21

*EE indicates ethinyl estradiol.

T A B L E 28-3

Progestin-Only Approved Oral Contraceptive Regimens

Brand	Manufacturer	Dose
Micronor	Ortho-McNeil	0.35 mg norethindrone
Nor-QD	Watson	0.35 mg norethindrone
Ovrette	Wyeth-Ayerst	0.075 mg norgestrel

T A B L E 28-4

Progestins for Oral Contraceptives by Type

Progestin	Type
First generation	No longer used
Second generation*	Norgestrel
	Ethynodiol diacetate
	Norethindrone
	Levonorgestrel
Third generation	Norgestimate
	Desogestrel
Spironolactone derivative	Drospirenone

*Second-generation progestins are thought to be more androgenic than are third-generation progestins.

Multiphasic OCP preparations were introduced in the late 1970s in an attempt to further lower total steroid dosage. No trial has found significant differences between triphasic, biphasic, and monophasic OCPs relative to bleeding pattern, symptoms, or efficacy.[7] Because most clinical studies have evaluated monophasic formulations, this is often the preferred regimen. The choice of progestin often plays a more important role in patient satisfaction than does the phasic formulation of the pill.

Progestin-only OCPs, also referred to as "the mini-pill," are available for those who cannot tolerate estrogen because of history of heart disease, thromboembolism, or other medical reasons. Unfortunately, these pills are associated with more breakthrough bleeding and lower contraceptive efficacy than are combination pills. In fact, a backup contraceptive method must be used for 2 days if a woman is more than 3 hours late taking a dose. A backup method is also recommended monthly at midcycle to improve efficacy. These pills are most often used in lactating women.

Medroxyprogesterone acetate (Depo-Provera) is an injectable progestin-only contraceptive. In contrast to the mini-pill, it is one of the most effective forms of contraception, with a theoretical and actual effectiveness of 99.7%. Intramuscular injections of 150 mg result in contraception for 3 months. Some women using progestin-only contraceptives may experience depression, weight gain, or acne. Therefore, women with a predisposition to these conditions may prefer another form of birth control. Progestin-only contraceptives have recently been linked to reversible decreases in bone density.[8,9] How these agents impact a woman's risk of osteoporosis is presently uncertain. For this reason, women using these forms of contraception should consume at least 1200 mg/d of calcium.

Drug interactions

Various drugs may influence the metabolism of OCPs. Contraceptive efficacy may be reduced when coadministered with antimicrobials (eg, penicillins, tetracyclines, griseofulvin, rifampin), anticonvulsants (eg, phenytoin, carbamazepine, felbamate, topiramate), anti-human immunodeficiency virus (HIV) protease inhibitors, and nonprescription and herbal products. The incidence of accidental pregnancy in women taking these medications with OCPs is unknown, but women using the lowest-dose preparations may be at higher risk. This is an important consideration, given the large number of ultra-low-dose regimens available on the market[10] (Tables 28-1 to 28-3).

Breakthrough bleeding also is possible with use of both OCPs and herbal products. For example, women taking OCPs and St John's wort (*Hypericum perforatum*) may experience bleeding irregularities 1 week after starting to take St John's wort, with regular cycles returning when the herbal treatment is stopped.[11]

Benefits

The safety profile of OCPs has been demonstrated in millions of women, with similar mortality rates noted between users and nonusers.[12,13] In fact, taking OCPs is considered safer than pregnancy. Most women are unaware of the noncontraceptive benefits of OCPs, including decreased risk of dysmenorrhea, anemia, acne, hirsutism, ectopic pregnancy, benign breast disease, endometrial cancer, pelvic inflammatory disease, and ovarian cysts.[14] Another benefit includes a 50% decrease in ovarian cancer risk, including those associated with mutations in the BRCA genes.[15,16] Similarly, studies have demonstrated an 18% to 40% reduction in colorectal cancer risk in OCP users.[17,18] Oral contraceptive pills provide a consistent dose of estrogen and, in turn, may lead to a higher peak bone mass and overall increase in bone density.[19] This benefit has been reported with ultra-low-dose formulations, although the positive effect increases with higher doses and longer duration of use. A 25%

reduction in hip fractures has been demonstrated.[20] Oral contraceptives containing third-generation progestins improve serum lipoprotein profiles by increasing HDL-C and decreasing LDL-C. However, whether these changes significantly affect the risk of cardiovascular disease is unclear.[21]

Risks

The benefits of OCP use must be considered in the setting of some potential risks. An increase in cardiovascular events associated with higher-dose OCPs prompted the development of low-dose OCPs. Studies of healthy, non-smoking women using OCPs with less than 50 μg/d of estrogen have found no increased risk of myocardial infarction (MI).[22] However, an increased risk of MI has been seen in cigarette-smoking OCP users over the age of 35 years.[23] Whether other cardiovascular risk factors, such as hypertension, dyslipidemia, diabetes, and/or obesity, increase MI risk in OCP users is unclear.

Studies consistently show a twofold to sixfold increased risk of venous thromboembolism (VTE) in OCP users,[24] although the baseline incidence of VTE in otherwise healthy women is low. Concerns are emerging about the third-generation progestins possibly further increasing this thromboembolism risk, compared with the second-generation progestins.[25,26] Risk factors for VTE include increasing age, obesity, family history, surgery, and factor V Leiden mutation. Patients with this mutation have a six-fold to sevenfold increased baseline VTE risk, which is amplified to 35-fold with OCP use. Women with a documented history of unexplained VTE and/or VTE associated with pregnancy should be advised to avoid OCPs.

Many women will have a mild increase in blood pressure with use of OCPs, although the blood pressure usually remains in the normal range. The risks of pregnancy in hypertensive women must be weighed against the risks of OCPs. Low-dose OCPs can be safely used in otherwise healthy women with well-controlled hypertension. Women older than 35 years with hypertension who smoke or have end-organ vascular disease should not use OCPs. Blood pressure should be closely monitored several months after starting OCPs and monitored yearly thereafter.

Studies evaluating the relationship of OCPs and stroke are difficult to interpret since they are small, do not differentiate between stroke types (thromboembolic vs hemorrhagic), and do not control for major risk factors. Most evidence suggests no increased risk of stroke with OCP use, except in women who are smokers.[27,28] Past studies using older, high-dose OCPs have shown an increased risk of stroke, whereas studies of low-dose OCPs have not demonstrated an increased risk.[29] The risk of stroke from OCP use in patients with migraine is not clear.

Evidence evaluating a link between breast cancer and hormone exposure has been inconsistent. A meta-analysis including 53,000 women with breast cancer and 100,000 controls found the relative risk of breast cancer diagnosis in current users of OCPs to be 1 in 24.[30] After discontinuation of OCPs, this risk decreased, and it returned to baseline after 10 years. Breast cancers occurring in women taking OCPs tended to be less advanced. On the other hand, a large case-control study found that among women aged 35 to 64 years, current or former OCP use was not associated with a significantly increased risk of breast cancer.[31] In women with a first-degree relative affected by breast cancer, high-dose OCPs may further increase risk, although the newer low-dose formulations have not been shown to have this same effect.[32] Women with a BRCA1 or BRCA2 mutation must weigh the concern over a possible increase in breast cancer risk with the potential reduced risk of ovarian cancer. These patients should consider discussing OCP safety with a geneticist or a women's health or medical breast specialist.

When OCPs are used for longer than 8 years, 30 to 125 additional cases of cervical cancer per 100,000 women may occur. However, OCP users may have more unprotected sexual encounters, leading to an increased exposure to the human papillomavirus, a known risk factor for cervical cancer. The possibility of a slight increased risk of cervical cancer associated with OCPs needs to be compared with the approximate 50% reduction in the risks of ovarian and endometrial cancer. One model estimated that of 100,000 women, 44 fewer reproductive cancers would occur among OCP users compared with nonusers.[33]

Intrauterine Devices

Intrauterine devices (IUDs) have been a popular form of birth control for centuries because they are safe, convenient, and highly effective. In the United States, only copper and hormone-releasing IUDs are approved for use. These include the copper T380A (Paragard), the levonorgestrel IUD (Mirena), and the progesterone T (Progestasert). The levonorgestrel IUD, followed closely by the T 380A, is the most effective form of reversible contraception available. The 7-year cumulative pregnancy rate with these 2 IUDs ranges from 1.1% to 1.6% (with the levonorgestrel being more effective).[34] This can be compared with a 10-year pregnancy rate after a tubal ligation of 1.9%, making these IUDs the most effective form of reversible contraception.[35] Intrauterine devices prevent fertilization by inhibiting conception and implantation, rather than acting as an abortifacient. At the site of the IUD, a sterile inflammatory reaction occurs, which is toxic to sperm and ova. The copper in the T 380A enhances the local inflammatory reaction in the endometrium. The progestin secreted by the progesterone T and levonorgestrel IUDs cause glandular atrophy of the endometrium as well as thickened cervical mucus.

Types

T 380A (copper) IUD.   The T 380A (Paragard) IUD is composed of a fine copper wire wound around a T-shaped polyethylene frame containing barium sulfate. With perfect use (in which the patient routinely checks the strings to ensure expulsion has not occurred), the likelihood of pregnancy in the first year is 0.6%, compared with 0.5% to 0.8% with typical use. This IUD is effective for 10 years. The main advantage of IUD contraception is seen in women who cannot use hormonal methods of contraception. The disadvantages of this IUD include heavy menses and dysmenorrhea, usually during the first year. Although the average monthly menstrual blood loss is increased by up to 55%, most women do not become anemic.[36]

Levonorgestrel IUD.   The levonorgestrel-releasing intrauterine system (Mirena) is composed of a T-shaped polyethylene frame containing 52 mg of levonorgestrel, releasing 15 μg daily. With perfect use, the probability of pregnancy in the first year is 0.1%, compared with 0.1% to 0.2% with typical use. This IUD is effective for up to 5 years. Its main advantage is a decrease in menstrual blood loss and dysmenorrhea by 40% to 50%, with a mean increase in hemoglobin of 1.2 g/dL within 5 years of use. In fact, amenorrhea is the most common reason for discontinuation. The levonorgestrel IUD can be a very effective treatment of menorrhagia and may potentially decrease the risk of pelvic inflammatory disease. It does cause elevated serum concentrations of progestin. Therefore, in progestin-sensitive patients (ie, those with depression, weight gain, and acne), side effects may occur.[37]

Progesterone T.   The Progestasert System is a T-shaped frame made of ethylene vinyl acetate copolymer with titanium dioxide, barium sulfate, and a silicone oil base. The stem contains 38 mg of progesterone, with 65 μg released daily, although there is no increase in serum progesterone. With perfect use, the probability of pregnancy in the first year is 1.51%, compared with 2.0% with typical use. This IUD is effective for 1 year only. The main advantages, similar to those of the levonorgestrel IUD, include a decrease in both menstrual blood loss and dysmenorrhea. The major disadvantage is the need for yearly replacement.

Inert IUDs.   These IUDs are composed of materials such as plastic and stainless steel. Although not approved for use in the United States, they are used throughout the world. These IUDs do not need to be replaced; however, they are less effective and many practitioners replace them with newer IUDs.

Contraindications

Intrauterine devices are contraindicated in women with any of the following:

1. Uterine anatomical abnormalities such as bicornuate uterus, cervical stenosis, or distorting leiomyomata. In these patients, insertion will be difficult and there is an increased risk of expulsion. Nondistorting leiomyomata are not a contraindication to IUD use.

2. Active, recent (within the last 3 months), or recurrent pelvic infections such as those associated with postpartum endometritis or sexually transmitted diseases (STDs). A remote history of pelvic inflammatory disease (PID) with subsequent pregnancy is not a contraindication to IUD placement, given that the patient is no longer at risk of STDs.

3. Pregnancy. Insertion of an IUD can lead to miscarriage and increases the risk of septic abortion.

4. Undiagnosed abnormal uterine bleeding. Irregular bleeding may be mistakenly attributed to the IUD after insertion.

5. Immunocompromised state. These women are at increased risk of PID. The IUD is not recommended for use in women at risk of HIV.

6. Wilson disease or copper allergy. Although no adverse event related to copper has been reported in these patients, hormone-releasing IUDs are preferred. The copper released daily by the T 380A is less than that consumed in an average daily diet.

Indications

Nulliparous women in monogamous relationships can safely use IUDs, although higher rates of expulsion may be seen than in multiparous women.[38] Controversy does exist over whether tubal infertility is associated with IUD use, especially with greater than 6 years of IUD use.[39] When contraceptive failure occurs with IUDs, approximately half will be ectopic. One study of the levonorgestrel IUD found an overall incidence of 1 ectopic pregnancy per 1000 users annually. This rate is not significantly different from the rate of ectopic pregnancies in sexually active women not using contraception.[40]

Public perception

Some patients appear fearful of IUDs due to earlier infectious complications with the Dalkon Shield IUD used in the 1970s. The braided, multifilament tail of this particular IUD allowed bacteria to ascend to the upper genital tract.[41] Other IUDs have not been associated with the same high rate of infectious complications.[42] The progesterone IUDs may decrease PID risk by altering cervical mucus. The T 380A does not provide protection against STDs, so there will be an increased risk of PID if a T380A user is exposed to STDs.

Barrier Methods

Physical and chemical barrier methods of contraception have been used for centuries. Barrier methods can be used in conjunction with other forms of contraception to prevent the passage of sperm and provide protection against STDs. Although efficacy depends on consistency and correctness of use, barrier methods are advantageous because they may be used intermittently and lack systemic side effects.[43]

Condoms

An Italian anatomist who depicted a linen sheath used to prevent the spread of syphilis first described the male condom in the 16th century.[44] The male condom has grown in popularity throughout the centuries and today is an important public health tool, especially in the prevention of HIV transmission. The male condom fits over the erect penis and serves as a barrier to sperm and infections. Latex provides better protection against STDs than "natural skin" condoms made from lamb's intestines. When used correctly, condoms can provide a 3% failure rate; however, the actual failure rate is closer to 14%.[45] The Food and Drug Administration (FDA) approved the female condom in 1993. This condom is a polyurethane sheath that has 2 flexible rings. One ring lies in the closed end of the sheath, allowing the condom to be inserted and be kept in place vaginally. The other ring is attached externally to the sheath and provides some protection to the perineum. A silicone-based nonspermicidal lubricant is on the inside of the condom. The efficacy of the female condom is similar to that of the male condom, although data are limited.[43]

Diaphragm

The diaphragm is a rubber cup that is inserted into the vagina to cover the cervix. The outer rim is thin and flexible and provides a spring coil that allows the diaphragm to stay in place in the upper vagina. Women must be fitted for a diaphragm based on the distance between the posterior vaginal fornix and the posterior aspect of the pubic symphysis arch. Most women use diaphragms that measure 65 to 80 mm. Diaphragms must be refitted annually, after a vaginal delivery, or after a large change in weight. Diaphragms are used with spermicidal jellies or creams to ensure the highest contraceptive efficacy. Insertion should occur no more than 6 hours before intercourse, and the diaphragm should be left in place for 6 to 24 hours afterward. After each use, the diaphragm should be washed with soap and water and allowed to air-dry.[43] The success rate for the diaphragm method of contraception depends on the fit and proper use. Pregnancy rates with the diaphragm vary from 1% to 28.9%.[46]

Cervical cap

The cervical cap is a fitted latex device that covers the cervix and stays in place by suction and anatomical placement. The cap can be left in place for up to 48 hours and does not require the use of spermicide. Spermicide is recommended, however, to improve efficacy rates, although additional amounts are not needed for repeated acts of intercourse.[43] Failure rates range from 6% to 20% and can vary depending on proper fit, correct placement, and dislodgment of the cap during intercourse.

Sponge

The sponge is dampened with water and fits against the cervix, releasing nonoxynol 9 during intercourse. The sponge is sold over the counter, does not require fitting, and provides 24 hours of protection, even during multiple acts of coitus. A large study of 1439 women found the failure rate to be as high as 17%.[47] Efficacy of the sponge method of contraception varies depending on user characteristics. The sponge has not been produced in the United States since 1995; however, it will likely be remarketed in the future.

Spermicides

Spermicides are chemical barrier agents that can be used alone or with other contraceptive methods. Nonoxynol 9 and octoxynol are the only FDA-approved spermicides, and most forms in the United States contain nonoxynol 9. Spermicides come in various forms, including gels, foams, creams, suppositories, and tablets and can be purchased without a prescription. Efficacy rates vary depending on the consistency and correctness of use. The Centers for Disease Control and Prevention (CDC) recently released a statement indicating that frequent use of nonoxynol 9 may lead to an increase in the transmission of HIV and should not be used for STD prevention. The CDC also does not recommend use of condoms lubricated with nonoxynol 9 because of higher cost, a shorter shelf life, and association with urinary tract infections in women.[48] In addition, some users of spermicides may develop allergic reactions or sensitivities to the ingredients.

Newer Contraceptive Agents

Yasmin is a monophasic, low-dose OCP that contains EE and drospirenone, a progestin analogue of spironolactone.[49] Drospirenone is the only progestin on the market

possessing both antimineralocorticoid and antiandrogenic properties. Yasmin's 99% efficacy is similar to that of most other OCPs.[50] Yasmin helps to improve acne, seborrhea, and hirsutism and provides good weight stability due to its antiandrogenic diuretic properties. As a result, it may benefit those with severe premenstrual symptoms such as bloating.[51,52] An 8-month study of women taking OCPs compared weight gain in women taking Yasmin vs EE and levonorgestrel (0.15 mg). Yasmin users lost an average of 0.8 kg, whereas women taking EE and levonorgestrel gained an average of 0.7 kg.[53] Each Yasmin pill contains 3 mg of drospirenone, the equivalent to 25 mg of spironolactone, a potassium-sparing diuretic. Therefore, the serum potassium level should be monitored during the first month of therapy. Yasmin should be used with caution in women taking medications that predispose to hyperkalemia, such as other potassium-sparing diuretics, angiotensin-converting enzyme (ACE) inhibitors, aldosterone antagonists, and nonsteroidal anti-inflammatory medications. Yasmin is contraindicated in women with renal, hepatic, or adrenal insufficiency.

Ortho Evra is the first FDA-approved transdermal contraceptive patch, which delivers 20 μg EE and 150 μg norelgestromin per 24 hours.[54] Norelgestromin is the metabolite of norgestimate, the same third-generation progestin found in Ortho-Cyclen and Ortho Tri-Cyclen. Three clinical trials of Ortho Evra have been conducted worldwide involving 4578 women. Compared with daily OCPs, Ortho Evra had similar contraceptive efficacy and menstrual cycle control, with the added benefit of improved compliance.[55] Ortho Evra users weighing more than 90 kg (198 lb) were noted to have more unintended pregnancies, suggesting that it may be less effective above this weight and therefore should be used with caution in these women. Breast tenderness, headache, skin irritation, and nausea, in decreasing order, were the most commonly reported side effects. Whether the risk of VTE differs with this contraceptive patch compared with OCPs is not known.

Ortho Evra should be started on the first day a woman begins her menstrual period or on the first day of withdrawal bleed in OCP users. A new patch is applied weekly, on the same day of the week, for 3 consecutive weeks. The fourth week is patch-free, and withdrawal bleeding is expected during this time. No more than a 1-week, hormone-free interval should occur between dosing cycles. The patch is applied to clean, dry skin of the buttocks, upper outer arm, lower part of the abdomen, or upper torso excluding the breasts. The patch should not be placed on skin that is red or irritated, or in an area rubbed by tight clothing. Oils, creams, or cosmetics near or around the patch should be avoided. The patient should be encouraged to enjoy her usual physical activities, including sauna, whirlpool, and swimming, without fear of the patch becoming loose or falling off. Experience with more than 70,000 Ortho Evra patches revealed that 4.7% of patches were replaced because they either fell off or were partly detached. If the patch detaches, a new one should be applied immediately. Supplemental adhesives or wraps should not be used. A patch that is loose or detached for less than 1 day should immediately be replaced with a new one. As long as it is replaced within 24 hours, no backup contraception is needed. If the patch is detached for more than 24 hours, or if the patient is unsure how long the patch has been detached, contraceptive efficacy cannot be guaranteed. The detached patch cycle should be discontinued, and a new patch cycle should be started immediately by applying a new patch. Ortho Evra comes in packs of 3 patches, and single replacement patches are available.

Lunelle is the first monthly, injectable combination hormone containing medroxyprogesterone acetate and estradiol cypionate. Medroxyprogesterone acetate (Depo-Provera), the other injectable birth control method, is a progestin-only formulation, given intramuscularly every 3 months. Efficacy rates of Depo-Provera and Lunelle are comparable. Lunelle is effective for contraception during the first cycle of use. The first injection is given within the first 5 days of menses, with subsequent injections given 28 to 30 days thereafter. If more than 33 days have passed since the last injection, pregnancy must be ruled out before another injection is given. Patients who are switching to Lunelle from OCPs should receive their first injection within 7 days of the last active pill.

Unexpected pregnancies in Lunelle users are uncommon and not shown to cause congenital malformations. Lunelle is comparable to Ortho-Novum 777 in efficacy, although Lunelle users are more likely to experience irregular bleeding at the end of the first year.[56] Weight gain of 1.8 kg (4 lb) during the first year and an additional 0.9 kg (2 lb) during the second year was the most common adverse event leading to discontinuation. Lunelle is comparable in cost to other OCPs; however, an office visit to administer the injection may increase its overall cost. Lunelle is an excellent option for women with issues of compliance. In October 2002, prefilled syringes of Lunelle were recalled due to concerns about subpotency. Lunelle packaged in standard vials was not affected by this recall and is still available for use.

NuvaRing is a contraceptive vaginal ring that releases 120 μg of etonogestrel and 15 μg of EE daily. The vaginal ring is colorless, odorless, 5.0 cm (2 in) in diameter, 4 mm in cross-sectional diameter, and easily inserted vaginally by most women. The ring is left in place for 3 weeks, with withdrawal bleed occurring during the fourth, ring-free week. NuvaRing will actually continue to inhibit ovulation for up to 5 weeks if a woman forgets to remove the ring after the third week of use. Although not recommended if a cystocele, rectocele, or uterine prolapse

is present, NuvaRing is an excellent, convenient choice for most women.[57]

A recent study compared cycle control and tolerability of NuvaRing to that of a standard OCP containing 30 μg of EE and 150 μg of levonorgestrel. Although both groups experienced withdrawal bleeding, NuvaRing users had less frequency of irregular bleeding and greater likelihood of normal intended bleeding patterns. Both groups had good tolerability, although NuvaRing users had a higher incidence of vaginal discomfort, vaginitis, and ring-related events.[58] NuvaRing has similar efficacy to OCPs; however, if the ring is left out of the vagina for more than 3 hours during the first 3 weeks of the cycle, efficacy cannot be guaranteed. To maintain the highest contraceptive efficacy, the user should rinse NuvaRing with warm water and reinsert it in the vagina within 3 hours.

Emergency Contraception

Postcoital or emergency contraception refers to the prevention of pregnancy within 72 hours after unprotected intercourse, including women who have had failure of another contraceptive method, such as a broken condom. Despite known efficacy and low potential for side effects, many patients are not prescribed emergency contraception due to lack of physician knowledge or comfort with its use. The most commonly prescribed regimens have included one of the following:

- EE, 2.5 mg, twice daily for 5 days
- EE, 100 μg, and levonorgestrel, 0.5 mg, repeated in 12 hours
- Levonorgestrel, 0.75 mg, repeated in 12 hours

More recently, the FDA approved specific emergency contraceptive kits. The Preven Kit contains a pregnancy test to exclude pregnancy before taking the hormones, which include 50 μg of EE and 0.25 mg of levonorgestrel. The patient takes 2 pills, and repeats this regimen in 2 hours. Plan B is a similar kit but contains progestin only, leading to less nausea and vomiting compared with regimens that also contain estrogen.[59] One tablet is taken, then repeated in 12 hours. Both regimens have similar efficacy in preventing pregnancy, generally reducing the number of pregnancies by 89%. Plan B taken in the first 24 hours can prevent 95% of expected pregnancies.

The antiprogestin mifepristone (RU-486), 600 mg in 1 dose, has higher efficacy than the above regimens, as well as a lower incidence of side effects.[60] However, the drug is not FDA approved for emergency contraceptive use in the United States, only for termination of early pregnancy. Although not commonly used in the clinical setting, a copper IUD placed within 120 hours of unprotected intercourse can also be used as emergency contraception.

PRENATAL CARE

Clinicians who provide health care to women of child-bearing years have the opportunity to positively affect pregnancy outcomes through prenatal care. To be truly "preventive," prenatal care should begin before pregnancy, as preconception care.[61] The goal of periconception care is to identify medical and social conditions that may put the mother or fetus at risk and to intervene before the critical period of organogenesis has occurred.[62] The components of preconception care include risk assessment, specific interventions, and patient education that promotes a healthy lifestyle.

Risk Assessment

The components of a periconceptional risk assessment should include history: medical/surgical, family, infection, obstetric/gynecologic, environmental, nutrition, and male partner's/paternal.[63] At the first prenatal visit, preconception laboratory evaluation screening should be performed for blood type/antibody, anemia, rubella, cervical dysplasia, syphilis, gonorrhea, chlamydia, asymptomatic bacteriuria, hepatitis B virus (HBV), and HIV.[64] If, at the first visit, the date of the last menstrual period is unknown or does not correlate with the uterine size, obstetrical ultrasonography should be used to establish the estimated date of confinement. Routine early ultrasound (in the first trimester) has been shown to reduce the rate of induction for post-term pregnancy, presumably because of better gestational age determination. Although this knowledge may decrease the cost of care associated with induction, fetal outcome has not been shown to improve.[65]

The purpose of the preconception evaluation is to detect conditions that merit management to optimize health outcomes of mother and fetus. Such conditions include rhesus isoimmunization and gestational diabetes. If anti-D is given at the appropriate time and at the appropriate dose, the risk of developing rhesus isoimmunization is decreased to 0.1%.[66] The nonsensitized RhD-negative women should receive anti-D immunoglobulin at approximately 28 weeks of gestation, and again within 72 hours after the delivery of an RhD-positive infant. She should also receive immunoglobulin after any pregnancy loss, as well as after any invasive procedure such as amniocentesis. Although the evidence is not strong, many providers also offer prophylaxis for a threatened miscarriage, second- or third-trimester bleeding, or abdominal trauma.[67]

Women with diabetes mellitus type 1 or 2 should try to achieve good glucose control before becoming pregnant. Sulfonylureas and other oral medications for diabetes are best avoided during pregnancy, so advanced planning for conception is important. Screening for gestational diabetes (GDM) should be offered to women between 24 and 28 weeks of gestation or earlier if the woman has particular risk factors such as previous gestational diabetes or fetal macrosomia. Blood glucose measurement is obtained 1 hour after a 50-g load of glucose. If this initial test is greater than 7.8 mmol/L (140 mg/dL), the woman is offered a 3-hour 100-g glucola challenge for confirmation. The test is considered positive if more than 1 of the serum levels is abnormal compared with standardized levels: fasting, 5.8 mmol/L (105 mg/dL); 1-hour, 10.5 mmol/L (190 mg/dL); 2-hour, 9.2 mmol/L (165 mg/dL); and 3-hour, 8.0 mmol/L (145 mg/dL).[68] In 50% of women whose test results are judged to be positive, overt diabetes will develop within 20 years.

Infections in Pregnancy

Estimates show that up to 50% of all pregnant women receive antibiotics at some point during the course of their pregnancy. These antibiotics are given for a variety of conditions. The most common bacterial infection encountered in pregnancy is urinary tract infection. Asymptomatic bacteriuria is a common occurrence in pregnancy and, because of the hormonal and structural changes that occur in the genital urinary tract as a result of pregnancy, predisposes the woman to the development of pyelonephritis. Screening for asymptomatic bacteriuria should be conducted at the first prenatal visit. When detected, asymptomatic bacteriuria should be treated and then followed up with repeated surveillance cultures of the urine as the pregnancy progresses.

Group B streptococci are a common cause of bacteriuria post partum. Infection with this organism is often secondary to colonization of the genital tract. Intrapartum antibiotic treatment of women colonized with group B streptococci reduces neonatal infection.[69] According to the American College of Obstetricians and Gynecologists (ACOG), screening for group B streptococcal colonization may be carried out by either the risk-based or the screening-based method. In the risk-based method, all women with risk factors are treated in labor with penicillin, without regard to a culture result. These include women in preterm labor, with an intrapartum temperature greater than 38°C, or prolonged rupture of membranes. In the screening-based method, all women at approximately 35 weeks receive a screening culture, and if it is positive for group B streptococci, the patients are treated in labor. Group B streptococcal bacteriuria during pregnancy should be treated at the time of diagnosis.[70] Penicillin G is the drug of choice for intrapartum prophylaxis. Intravenous clindamycin is used for women allergic to penicillin.[71]

Maternal infections with *Neisseria* gonorrhea can be transmitted to the infant in utero, during delivery, or post partum and may lead to conjunctivitis in the newborn. Transmission of syphilis from the mother to the fetus may similarly occur, leading to possible stillbirth or neonatal disease. Consequently, diagnosis of these infections should be considered in the prenatal period and managed appropriately.

Specific viral infections are of particular concern in the prenatal period due to their potential for leading to devastating health consequences for the fetus. Cytomegalovirus (CMV), rubella, varicella zoster, and herpes simplex are infections that have potential for placental transmission of disease and teratogenesis. Toxoplasmosis is another infection that may be transmitted transplacentally, leading to major health issues in the fetus, although this infection does not cause fetal malformation. Routine serologic screening for CMV and toxoplasmosis are not recommended by ACOG.[72] Women should be counseled, however, to prevent exposure to these conditions. To limit exposure to CMV, a woman should practice universal precautions with thorough hand washing when around young children and immunocompromised individuals. To avoid toxoplasmosis infection, women should avoid eating or preparing raw or uncooked meat, wear gloves when gardening, and avoid exposure to cat litter.[61] Treatment of herpes simplex infections in pregnant women is difficult because acyclovir cream and tablets are contraindicated in pregnancy, except in life-threatening situations. When active herpes simplex lesions are present at the time of delivery or rupture of membranes, cesarean delivery should be performed.[73,74] Routine cesarean deliveries are not indicated, however, for women with a history of prior genital herpes when active lesions are not present.

All women of childbearing age should be questioned about immunization and exposure history regarding rubella, varicella, and hepatitis B because of the potential impact of these infections on the health of the fetus. Congenital rubella syndrome occurs when a mother contracts rubella during the first trimester of pregnancy and transmits the infection to the fetus. The American Academy of Pediatrics Committee on Infectious Disease 2000 and the Advisory Committee on Immunization Practices recommend that all reproductive-aged women be assessed for rubella susceptibility during physical examinations, family planning visits, and STD screening. Women who have not received at least one dose of the vaccine or who are nonimmune by serologic testing should be given the measles-mumps-rubella (MMR) vaccine.[75,76] The rubella vaccine is contraindicated for pregnant women. Women should not attempt pregnancy for 3 months after rubella immunization.

Clinicians should also screen women for varicella before conception or simply immunize nonpregnant women who have no prior history of varicella infection.[77] Varicella infection in pregnancy can have serious consequences for the mother in the form of varicella pneumonia.[78] Neonatal varicella is associated with a high morbidity rate because of immaturity of the neonatal immune system and lack of maternal antibodies.[72] Women should be advised to avoid conception for at least 1 month after varicella vaccination.

People who acquire hepatitis B infection as infants or young children have a 25% risk of death due to HBV-related liver cancer or cirrhosis. Chronic HBV infection occurs in up to 90% of infants born to mothers who are hepatitis B e antigen positive.[79] All women of childbearing age should, therefore, be offered the hepatitis B vaccination series.

Most women who transmit HIV infection to their fetus are asymptomatic. Vertical transmission results in approximately a 30% chance of fetal infection from an untreated HIV-positive mother.[80] A regimen of zidovudine given antenatally and intrapartum to the mother and the newborn reduced the risk of transmission by approximately two thirds.[81] All sexually active women should be offered HIV testing.

Medications in Pregnancy

During the periconception evaluation, all medications the patient takes, including over-the-counter medications and herbal preparations, should be reviewed with her. The therapeutic regimen should be to avoid any potential teratogenic effects of medication. The FDA has outlined category ratings for drugs, which are based on the degree of available information regarding risk to the fetus and potential benefit to the mother. These ratings can be used to decide whether specific medications should be continued or stopped during pregnancy. Categories (A, B, C, D, and X) have been assigned and are explained as follows[82]:

Category A drugs are those for which controlled studies have shown no risk to the fetus in any trimester of pregnancy. Examples include potassium supplements, levothyroxine, multivitamins, and folic acid.

Category B encompasses drugs in which well-controlled human studies are not available but animal reproduction studies have been conducted and have not been found to demonstrate a fetal risk, or in which animal reproduction studies have shown an adverse effect that was not demonstrated in well-controlled studies in pregnant women. Examples of drugs in this category include meclizine, sucralfate, ranitidine, chlorpheniramine, clotrimazole, clindamycin, erythromycin, acetaminophen, many narcotic agents, some nonsteroidal anti-inflammatory agents, prednisone, and insulin.

Category C drugs are ones in which either studies in animals have revealed adverse effects on the fetus and there exist no controlled studies in women, or studies in both women and animals are not available. These drugs are used only if the potential benefit justifies the potential risk to the fetus. Examples include diphenhydramine, ketoconazole, isoniazid, acyclovir, vancomycin, codeine, albuterol, labetalol, atenolol, verapamil, digoxin, haloperidol, heparin, furosemide, omeprazole, theophylline, and zidovudine.

Category D drugs are those in which there is evidence of human risk, but the benefits from use in pregnant women may be acceptable if potential benefits outweigh potential risk. Examples include sulfonamides, tetracyclines, ACE inhibitors, phenytoin, amitriptyline, diazepam, lorazepam, lithium, and warfarin.

Category X drugs are those in which studies in animals or humans have demonstrated fetal abnormalities or there is evidence of fetal risk based on human or animal experience, or both. The risks of these drugs in pregnant women clearly outweigh any possible benefits and are therefore contraindicated in pregnancy. Examples include isotretinoin, thalidomide, lovastatin, coumarin derivatives, oral contraceptives, and the MMR vaccine.

Management of Chronic Medical Conditions in Pregnancy

Asthma

Asthma is one of the most common medical illnesses likely to occur in women of childbearing age. Approximately 1% of pregnancies are complicated by asthma.[83] One third of patients experience improvement of asthma during pregnancy, one third experience deterioration, and one third have no change in severity.[84] The risk of untreated and undertreated asthma in pregnancy is far greater than the risk of any of the medications used to treat asthma.[85] The therapy for an asthma exacerbation is very similar to the treatment in the nonpregnant individual. First-line agents are the β-adrenergic inhaled agonists as well as inhaled corticosteroids. Theophylline is a third-line agent, and its clearance decreases in the third trimester. During severe asthma attacks, endotracheal intubation is preferable to use of epinephrine, as epinephrine impairs placental blood flow. Terbutaline may be used as an alternative to epinephrine in such situations.[86]

Chronic hypertension

Women planning pregnancy who are receiving pharmacologic treatment of chronic hypertension should be treated with medications that may be used safely throughout gestation. Both ACE inhibitors and angiotensin II receptor antagonists should be discontinued. For patients who require drug therapy for moderate to severe hypertension, the drug of choice is methyldopa, for which maternal and fetal safety after the first trimester is well documented. Because of the physiologic nadir of blood pressure during the second trimester of pregnancy, medications can often be discontinued. Alternative agents for the treatment of

chronic hypertension in pregnant women include β-blockers and calcium channel blockers.[87]

Diabetes mellitus

Poor control of diabetes in early pregnancy is associated with pregnancy loss and major congenital malformations such as caudal regression syndrome and cardiac defects. Congenital anomalies due to maternal hyperglycemia are the leading cause of death in infants of diabetic mothers.[88] Optimal control of diabetes mellitus is essential during preconception and pregnancy. It is important to establish baseline renal function, rule out proliferative retinopathy, diagnose peripheral and autonomic neuropathies, and identify and treat hypertension.[89]

Oral hypoglycemic agents must be discontinued, as they cross the placenta and have no role in treatment of diabetes during pregnancy. Insulin should be used to maintain strict glycemic control along with diabetic nutritional education. In general, insulin dosage requirements are often less in the first trimester because of maternal loss of glucose to the developing fetus. In the second trimester, the "diabetogenic stress" of pregnancy begins and insulin requirements increase. Tight control with potential maternal hypoglycemia does not pose a risk to the fetus, as insulin does not cross the placenta. However, maternal hyperglycemia is to be avoided if possible because of resultant fetal insulin production and macrosomic complications.[90]

Thromboembolic disorders

Risk factors for antenatal deep vein thrombosis (DVT) include a prior history of DVT or pulmonary embolism, prolonged bed rest, obesity, and obstetrical complications including cesarean delivery, as well as inherited coagulation disorders.[91] Patients who have had recurrent thromboembolic events, recurrent pregnancy losses, or a family history of thromboembolic disease should be evaluated before pregnancy for hypercoagulable thrombophilias such as antithrombin III deficiency, protein C and S deficiencies, factor V Leiden mutation, and anticardiolipin antibody syndrome.[83]

The ACOG has published clinical management guidelines for prevention and management of VTE during pregnancy. Recommended prophylactic heparin regimens during pregnancy include both unfractionated and low-molecular-weight heparin.[92,93] Unlike heparin, warfarin freely crosses the placenta and is associated with warfarin embryopathy and should be avoided during pregnancy. Patients who are receiving warfarin therapy should be switched to a heparin regimen before conception or as soon as pregnancy is diagnosed.[94] Suspected DVT and/or pulmonary embolism in the pregnant patient needs to be vigorously evaluated, as the risk of maternal hypoxemia and potential death far outweighs the radiation exposure risk or medication treatment risk to the fetus.[95]

Seizure disorders

Seizure disorders are the most common serious neurologic complications of pregnancy. Preconception issues focus on the risk of medications used to treat seizure disorders and the effect of pregnancy on seizure control. The patient's history, diagnostic studies, and medication use should ideally be reviewed before pregnancy. Monotherapy is the goal when medication is necessary, as most of antiepileptic medications are classified as category D drugs. The decision to stop or change medications should be made in consultation with a neurologist, as approximately 40% of women with seizure disorders will have more frequent seizures during pregnancy.[83] Women with epilepsy are at increased risk of developmental and congenital abnormalities in their offspring. Women with seizure disorders should take adequate amounts of folic acid before conception to reduce the risks of specific drug-related neural tube disorders.[96]

Genetic Counseling and Risk Assessment

Patients with a specific indication for genetic testing such as maternal age greater than 35 years, family history of a genetic disease, or history of a previously affected pregnancy should be referred for genetic counseling. Once genetic risk has been assessed, couples may make informed decisions regarding reproduction and prenatal genetic evaluation through amniocentesis or chorionic villus sampling.[61] Amniocentesis is an established and safe procedure usually performed at approximately 16 weeks of gestation. The procedure is performed through ultrasound-guided, transabdominal insertion of a needle into the amniotic fluid. About 5% to 10% of total amniotic fluid volume can be safely removed, which approximately equals 1 mL of fluid for each week of gestation. Severe maternal injury resulting from amniocentesis is rare, and the estimated risk of spontaneous abortion due to amniocentesis at 15 weeks or later is 0.5% or less.[97,98]

Chorionic villus sampling is a technique for removing a small sample of placental tissue for performing chromosomal, metabolic, or DNA studies. The procedure is generally performed in the first trimester via transabdominal or transcervical ultrasound guidance. Although this procedure offers the advantage of first-trimester prenatal diagnosis, the procedure-related risk of pregnancy loss is 0.5% to 1.0% higher than that for amniocentesis.[97]

Women should be counseled regarding a screening test for neural tube defects known as the maternal serum α-fetoprotein assay. The test is performed between the 15th and 20th weeks of gestation. Abnormal results are further evaluated by ultrasonography and amniocentesis.[99]

Specific Aspects of Patient Education

An increased demand for iron exists for a pregnant woman because of maternal blood volume expansion, fetal iron needs, and blood loss during delivery.[1] However, iron supplementation has not been proved in controlled trials to improve either maternal or fetal clinical outcomes.[100]

Periconceptional supplementation with folic acid can reduce risk of neural tube defects by more than two thirds.[61,101] The US Preventive Services Task Force recommends folic acid supplementation of 0.4 to 0.8 mg/d beginning at least 1 month before conception and continuing through the first trimester. Women with a history of a prior pregnancy affected by a neural tube defect should take 4 mg/d.[61,64]

Maternal alcohol use is now the leading known cause of mental retardation. Fetal alcohol syndrome outranks both Down syndrome and spina bifida in prevalence. Children of mothers who drink alcohol during pregnancy are smaller in weight, height, head circumference, and palpebral fissure width.[62,102] Alcohol use should be discontinued completely during pregnancy.

Smoking should be discontinued during pregnancy. Guidelines from ACOG advocate use of the 5-step "Ask, Advise, Assess, Assist, Arrange" clinical practice guideline adapted from the US Public Health Service. Advice on the use of nicotine replacement in pregnancy is cautionary and should be used during pregnancy only if the benefits of smoking cessation outweigh the risk of nicotine replacement and potential concomitant smoking.[61,103]

Counseling pregnant women about passenger restraints has been shown to increase their use.[104] Use of seat belts should therefore be encouraged, and patients should be instructed on their proper placement.

Current medical evidence shows both mother and fetus benefit substantially when the mother maintains physical fitness during pregnancy. Women are advised to continue their prepregnancy activity level when they become pregnant.[93,105] Absolute contraindications to exercise during pregnancy include pregnancy-induced hypertension, premature rupture of membranes, preterm labor during the prior or current pregnancy, incompetent cervix or cerclage, persistent second-trimester or third-trimester bleeding, and intrauterine growth retardation.[83]

REFERENCES

1. Forrest JD, Singh S. The sexual and reproductive behavior of American women, 1982–1988. *Fam Plann Perspect.* 1990;22:206–214.

2. Forrest JD. Has she or hasn't she? U.S. women's experience with contraception. *Fam Plann Perspect.* 1987;19:133.

3. Rosenberg MJ, Waugh MS, Long S. Unintended pregnancies and use, misuse and discontinuation of oral contraceptives. *J Reprod Med.* 1995;40:355–360.

4. Piccinino LJ, Mosher WD. Trends in contraceptive use in the United States: 1982–1995. *Fam Plann Perspect.* 1998;30:4–10, 46.

5. Phillips A, Hahn DW, McGuire JL. Preclinical evaluation of norgestimate, a progestin with minimal androgenic activity. *Am J Obstet Gynecol.* 1992;167(pt 2):1191–1196.

6. Vandenbroucke JP, Rosendaal FR. End of the line for "third-generation-pill" controversy? *Lancet.* 1997;349:1113–1114.

7. Van Vliet HA, Grimes DA, Helmerhorst FM, Schulz KF. Biphasic versus monophasic oral contraceptives for contraception. *Cochrane Database Syst Rev.* 2003(2);CD003283.

8. Scholes D, Lacroix AZ, Ott SM, et al. Bone mineral density in women using depot medroxyprogesterone acetate for contraception. *Obstet Gynecol.* 1999;93:233–238.

9. Cromer BA, Blair JM, Mahan JD, et al. A prospective comparison of bone density in adolescent girls receiving depot medroxyprogesterone acetate (Depo-Provera), levonorgestrel (Norplant), or oral contraceptives. *J Pediatr.* 1996;129:671–676.

10. Dickinson BD, Altman RD, Nielsen NH, Sterling ML. Drug interactions between oral contraceptives and antibiotics. *Obstet Gynecol.* 2001;98(pt 1):853–860.

11. Yue QY, Bergquist C, Gerden B. Safety of St John's wort (*Hypericum perforatum*). *Lancet.* 2000;355:576–577.

12. Hatcher RA, Guillebaud MA. The pill: combined oral contraceptives. In: Hatcher RA, Trussell J, Stewart F, et al, eds. *Contraceptive Technology.* New York, NY: Ardent Media; 1998:405–466.

13. Beral V, Hermon C, Kay C, Hannaford P, Darby S, Reeves G. Mortality associated with oral contraceptive use: 25 year follow up of cohort of 46 000 women from Royal College of General Practitioners' oral contraception study. *Br Med J.* 1999;318:96–100.

14. Speroff L, Glass RH, Kase NG. Oral contraception. In: Mitchell C, ed. *Clinical Gynecologic Endocrinology and Infertility.* Baltimore, Md: Williams & Wilkins; 1999:867–945.

15. Narod SA, Risch H, Moslehi R, et al, for Hereditary Ovarian Cancer Clinical Study Group. Oral contraceptives and the risk of hereditary ovarian cancer. *N Engl J Med.* 1998;339:424–428.

16. Modan B, Hartge P, Hirsh-Yechezkel G, et al. Parity, oral contraceptives, and the risk of ovarian cancer among carriers and noncarriers of a BRCA1 or BRCA2 mutation. *N Engl J Med.* 2001;345:235–240.

17. Fernandez E, La Vecchia C, Balducci A, Chatenoud L, Franceschi S, Negri E. Oral contraceptives and colorectal cancer risk: a meta-analysis. *Br J Cancer.* 2001;84:722–727.

18. Franceschi S, La Vecchia C. Oral contraceptives and colorectal tumors: a review of epidemiologic studies. *Contraception.* 1998;58:335–343.

19. Pasco JA, Kotowicz MA, Henry MJ, Panahi S, Seeman E, Nicholson GC. Oral contraceptives and bone mineral density: a population based study. *Am J Obstet Gynecol.* 2001;184:249–250.

20. Michaelsson K, Baron JA, Farahmand BY, Persson I, Ljunghall S. Oral-contraceptive use and risk of hip fracture: a case-control study. *Lancet.* 1999;353:1481–1484.

21. Godsland IF, Crook D, Simpson R, et al. The effects of different formulations of oral contraceptive agents on lipid and carbohydrate metabolism. *N Engl J Med.* 1990;323:1375–1381.

22. Chasan-Taber L, Stampfer MJ. Epidemiology of oral contraceptives and cardiovascular disease. *Ann Intern Med.* 1998;128:467–477.

23. Rosenberg L, Palmer JR, Lesko SM, Shapiro S. Oral contraceptive use and the risk of myocardial infarction. *Am J Epidemiol.* 1990;131:1009–1016.

24. Cardiovascular disease and steroid hormone contraception: report of a scientific group. Geneva, Switzerland: World Health Organization; 1998. WHO Technical Report Series, No. 877. Available at: www.who.int/reproductive-health/hrp/progress/46/news46.pdf. Accessed January 27, 2003.

25. Spitzer WO, Lewis MA, Heinemann LA, Thorogood M, MacRae KD, for Transnational Research Group on Oral Contraceptives and the Health of Young Women. Third generation oral contraceptives and risk of venous thromboembolic disorders: an international case-control study. *Br Med J.* 1996;312:83–88.

26. Effect of different progestogens in low oestrogen oral contraceptives on venous thromboembolic disease: World Health Organization Collaborative Study of Cardiovascular Disease and Steroid Hormone Contraception. *Lancet.* 1995;346:1582–1588.

27. Vandenbroucke JP, Rosing J, Bloemenkamp KW, et al. Oral contraceptives and the risk of venous thrombosis. *N Engl J Med.* 2001;344:1527–1535.

28. Venous thromboembolic disease and combined oral contraceptives: results of international multicentre case-control study: World Health Organization Collaborative Study of Cardiovascular Disease and Steroid Hormone Contraception. *Lancet.* 1995;346:1575–1582.

29. The use of hormonal contraception in women with coexisting medical conditions: ACOG Practice Bulletin No. 18, July 2000. *Int J Gynaecol Obstet.* 2001;75:93–106.

30. Collaborative Group on Hormonal Factors in Breast Cancer. Breast cancer and hormonal contraceptives: collaborative reanalysis of individual data on 53 297 women with breast cancer and 100 239 women without breast cancer from 54 epidemiological studies. *Lancet.* 1996;347:1713–1727.

31. Marchbanks PA, McDonald JA, Wilson HG, et al. Oral contraceptives and the risk of breast cancer. *N Engl J Med.* 2002;346:2025–2032.

32. Grabrick DM, Hartmann LC, Cerhan JR, et al. Risk of breast cancer with oral contraceptive use in women with a family history of breast cancer. *JAMA.* 2000;284:1791–1798.

33. Coker AL, Harlap S, Fortney JA. Oral contraceptives and reproductive cancers: weighing the risks and benefits. *Fam Plann Perspect.* 1993;25:17–21, 36.

34. Sivin I, Schmidt F. Effectiveness of IUDs: a review. *Contraception.* 1987;36:55–84.

35. Sivin I, Stern J, for International Committee for Contraception Research (ICCR). Health during prolonged use of levonorgestrel 20 micrograms/d and the copper TCu 380Ag intrauterine contraceptive devices: a multicenter study. *Fertil Steril.* 1994;61:70–77.

36. Milsom I, Andersson K, Jonasson K, Lindstedt G, Rybo G. The influence of the Gyne-T 380S IUD on menstrual blood loss and iron status. *Contraception.* 1995;52:175–179.

37. Faundes A, Alvarez F, Diaz J. A Latin American experience with levonorgestrel IUD. *Ann Med.* 1993;25:149–153.

38. Duenas JL, Albert A, Carrasco F. Intrauterine contraception in nulligravid vs parous women. *Contraception.* 1996;53:23–24.

39. Doll H, Vessey M, Painter R. Return of fertility in nulliparous women after discontinuation of the intrauterine device: comparison with women discontinuing other methods of contraception. *Br J Obstet Gynaecol.* 2001;108:304–314.

40. Trussell J. Contraceptive efficacy. In: Hatcher RA, Trussell J, eds. *Contraceptive Technology.* 17th ed. New York, NY: Irvington Publishers; 1998.

41. Lee NC, Rubin GL, Ory HW, Burkman RT. Type of intrauterine device and the risk of pelvic inflammatory disease. *Obstet Gynecol.* 1983;62:1–6.

42. Toivonen J, Luukkainen T, Allonen H. Protective effect of intrauterine release of levonorgestrel on pelvic infection: three years' comparative experience of levonorgestrel- and copper-releasing intrauterine devices. *Obstet Gynecol.* 1991;77:261–264.

43. Gilliam M, Derman R. Barrier methods of contraception. *Clin Obstet Gynecol.* 2000;27:841–858.

44. Potts M, Diggory P. *Textbook of Contraceptive Practice.* 2nd ed. New York, NY: Cambridge University Press; 1984.

45. Cates W Jr, Stone KM. Family planning, sexually transmitted diseases and contraceptive choice: a literature update. Part I. *Fam Plann Perspect.* 1992;24:122–128.

46. Lane M, Arceo R, Sobrero AJ. Successful use of the diaphragm and jelly by a young population: report of a clinical study. *Fam Plann Perspect.* 1976;8:81–86.

47. Derman R. Cervical caps. In: Corson S, Derman R, Tyrer L, eds. *Fertility Control.* Boston, Mass: Little Brown & Co; 1985.

48. Centers for Disease Control and Prevention/Division of STD Prevention (DSTDP)/STD Treatment. Nonoxynol-9 spermicide contraception use—United States, 1999. *Morb Mortal Wkly Rep.* 2002;51:389–392.

49. Krattenmacher R. Drospirenone: pharmacology and pharmacokinetics of a unique progestogen. *Contraception.* 2000;62:29–38.

50. Yasmin—an oral contraceptive with a new progestin. *Med Lett Drugs Ther.* 2002;44:55–57.

51. Ludicke F, Johannisson E, Helmerhorst FM, Campana A, Foidart J, Heithecker R. Effect of a combined oral contraceptive containing 3 mg of drospirenone and 30 microg of ethinyl estradiol on the human endometrium. *Fertil Steril.* 2001;76:102–107.

52. Mansour D. Yasmin—a new oral contraceptive, a new progestogen: the reasons why. *Eur J Contracept Reprod Health Care.* 2000;5(suppl 3):9–16.

53. Oelkers W, Foidart JM, Dombrovicz N, Welter A, Heithecker R. Effects of a new oral contraceptive containing an antimineralocorticoid progestin, drospirenone, on the rennin-aldosterone system, body weight, blood pressure, glucose tolerance, and lipid metabolism. *J Clin Endocrinol Metab.* 1995;80:1816–1821.

54. Ortho Evra—a contraceptive patch. *Med Lett Drugs Ther.* 2002;44:8.

55. Audet MC, Moreau M, Koltun WD, et al. Evaluation of contraceptive efficacy and cycle control of a transdermal contraceptive patch vs an oral contraceptive: a randomized controlled trial. *JAMA.* 2001;285:2347–2354.

56. Kaunitz AM, Garceau RJ, Cromie MA, for Lunelle Study Group. Comparative safety, efficacy, and cycle control of Lunelle monthly contraceptive injection (medroxyprogesterone acetate and estradiol cypionate injectable suspension) and Ortho-Novum 7/7/7 oral contraceptive (norethindrone/ethinyl estradiol triphasic). *Contraception.* 1999;60:179–187.

57. Mulders TM, Dieben TO. Use of the novel combined contraceptive vaginal ring NuvaRing for ovulation inhibition. *Fertil Steril.* 2001;75:865–870.

58. Bjarnadoltir R, Tuppurainen M, Killick S. Comparison of cycle control with a combined contraceptive vaginal ring and oral levonorgestrel/ethinyl estradiol. *Am J Obstet Gynecol.* 2002;186:389–395.

59. Task Force on Postovulatory Methods of Fertility Regulation. Randomized controlled trial of levonorgestrel vs the Yuzpe regimen of combined oral contraceptives for emergency contraception. *Lancet.* 1998;352:428–433.

60. Webb AM, Russell J, Elstein M. Comparison of Yuzpe regimen, danazol, and mifepristone (RU486) in oral postcoital contraception. *BMJ.* 1992;305:927.

61. Barash JH, Weinstein LC. Preconception and prenatal care. *Primary Care.* 2002;29:519–542.

62. Morrison EH. Update in maternity care: periconception care. *Primary Care.* 2000;27:1–12.

63. Reynolds HD. Preconception care: an integral part of primary care for women. *J Nurse Midwifery.* 1998;43:445–458.

64. US Preventive Services Task Force. *Guide to Clinical Preventive Services.* 2nd ed. Baltimore, Md: Williams & Wilkins; 1996:112, 241, 270, 291, 315, 331, 355, 367, 430, 479.

65. Neilson JP. Ultrasound for fetal assessment in early pregnancy (Cochrane Review). *Cochrane Database Syst Rev.* 2000(2);CD000182.

66. Prevention of Rh D alloimmunization: ACOG Practice Bulletin No. 4, May 1999. In: *2001 Compendium of Selected Publications.* Washington, DC: American College of Obstetricians and Gynecologists; 2001:1048–1055.

67. Crowther CA, Keirse MJ. Anti-D administration in pregnancy for preventing rhesus alloimmunisation (Cochrane Review). *Cochrane Database Syst Rev.* 2001(2);CD000020.

68. National Diabetes Data Group. Classification and diagnosis of diabetes mellitus and other categories of glucose intolerance. *Diabetes.* 1979;28:1039–1057.

69. Smaill F. Intrapartum antibiotics for Group B streptococcal colonisation (Cochrane Review). *Cochrane Database Syst Rev.* 2000(2);CD000115.

70. Prevention of perinatal group B streptococcal disease: a public health perspective. *MMWR Morb Mortal Wkly Rep.* 1996;45(RR-7):1–24.

71. American Academy of Pediatrics Committee on Infectious Diseases, Committee on Fetus and Newborn. Revised guidelines for prevention of early onset Group B streptococcal (GBS) infection. *Pediatrics.* 1997;99:489–496.

72. Perinatal viral and parasitic infections: ACOG Practice Bulletin No. 20, September 2000. In: *2001 Compendium of Selected Publications.* Washington, DC: American College of Obstetricians and Gynecologists; 2001:1008–1010.

73. Landy HJ, Grossman JH. Herpes simplex virus. *Obstet Gynecol Clin North Am.* 1989;16:495–511.

74. Prober CG, Corey L, Brown ZE, et al. The management of pregnancies complicated by genital infections with herpes simplex virus. *Clin Infect Dis.* 1992;15:1031–1038.

75. Watson JC, Hadler SC, Dykewicz CA, et al. Measles, mumps, and rubella-vaccine use and strategies for elimination of measles, rubella and congenital rubella syndrome, and control of mumps: recommendations of the Advisory Committee on Immunization Practices (ACIP). *MMWR Morb Mortal Wkly Rep.* 1998;47:1–57.

76. Rubella. In: Pickering LK, ed. *2000 Red Book: Report of the Committee on Infectious Disease.* Elk Grove Village, Ill: American Academy of Pediatrics; 2000:498.

77. Prevention of varicella: update recommendations of the Advisory Committee on Immunization Practices (ACIP). *MMWR Morb Mortal Wkly Rep.* 1999;48:1–5.

78. Gibbs RS, Sweet RL. Maternal and fetal infectious disorders. In: Creasy RK, Resnik R, eds. *Maternal-Fetal Medicine.* Philadelphia, Pa: WB Saunders Co; 1999:680–682, 685.

79. Hepatitis B. In: Pickering LK, ed. *2000 Red Book: Report of the Committee on Infectious Disease.* Elk Grove Village, Ill: American Academy of Pediatrics; 2000:289.

80. Butler KM. Mother-to-infant transmission of human immunodeficiency virus infection. *AIDS Updates.* 1993;6:1–10.

81. Conner EM, Sperling RS, Gelber R, et al. Reduction of maternal-infant transmission of human immunodeficiency virus type 1 with zidovudine treatment. *N Engl J Med.* 1994;331:1173–1180.

82. Cefalo RC, Moos MK. *Preconceptional Health Promotion: A Practical Guide.* Rockville, Md: Aspen Publishers; 1988.

83. Leuzzi RA, Scoles KS. Preconception counseling for the primary care physician. *Med Clin North Am.* 1996;80:337–374.

84. Schatz M, Harden K, Forsythe A, et al. The course of asthma during pregnancy, postpartum, and with successive pregnancies: a prospective analysis. *J Allergy Clin Immunol.* 1988;81:509–517.

85. Barron W, Leff A. Asthma in pregnancy an editorial: *Am Rev Respir Dis.* 1993;147:510–511.

86. Dattel BJ, Gillogley KM. Respiratory complications. In: Niswander KR, Evans AT, eds. *Manual of Obstetrics.* 5th ed. Boston, Mass: Little, Brown & Co; 1996:83–89.

87. National High Blood Pressure Education Program Working Group report on high blood pressure in pregnancy. *Am J Obstet Gynecol.* 2000;183:S1–S22.

88. Cousins L. Congenital anomalies among infants of diabetic mothers. *Am J Obstet Gynecol.* 1983;147:333–338.

89. Leuzzi RA, Scoles KS. Preconception counseling for the primary care physician. *Med Clin North Am.* 1996;80:337–374.

90. Evans AT, deVeciana M, Benbarka MM. Endocrine disorders. In: Niswander KR, Evans AT, eds. *Manual of Obstetrics*. 5th ed. Boston, Mass: Little, Brown & Co; 1996:121–151.

91. Barbour LA, Pickard J. Controversies in thromboembolic disease during pregnancy: a critical review. *Obstet Gynecol*. 1995;86:621–633.

92. Frey KA. Preconception care by the nonobstetrical provider. *Mayo Clin Proc*. 2002;77:469–473.

93. American College of Obstetrics and Gynecology. Clinical management guidelines for obstetrician-gynecologists. *ACOG Pract Bull*. 2000;19:1–10.

94. Ginsberg JS, Hirsh J. Use of anticoagulants during pregnancy. *Chest*. 1989;95:S156–S160.

95. Ginsberg JS, Hirsh J, Rainbow AJ, Coates G. Risk to the fetus of radiologic procedures used in the diagnosis of maternal venous thromboembolic disease. *Thromb Haemost*. 1989;61:189–196.

96. Delgado-Escuetta A, Janz D. Consensus guidelines: Preconception counseling, management, and care of the pregnant woman with epilepsy. *Neurology*. 1992;42:149–160.

97. Antepartum care. In:. *Guidelines for Perinatal Care*. 4th ed. Elk Grove Village, Ill: American Academy of Pediatrics and American College of Obstetricians and Gynecologists; 1997:65–92.

98. American College of Obstetricians and Gynecologists (ACOG). *Antenatal Diagnosis of Genetic Disorders*. Washington, DC: ACOG; 1987. ACOG Technical Bulletin No. 108.

99. Reed BD, Ratcliffe S, Sayres W. Maternal serum alpha-fetoprotein screening. *J Fam Pract*. 1988;27:20, 22, 26.

100. Mahomed K. Iron and folate supplementation in pregnancy (Cochrane Review). *Cochrane Database Syst Rev*. 2000(2);CD001135.

101. Enkin M, Keirse M, Neilson J, et al. *Dietary Modification in Pregnancy: A Guide to Effective Care in Pregnancy and Childbirth*. New York, NY: Oxford University Press; 2000:38–46.

102. Day NL, Richardson GA, Geva D, et al. Alcohol, marijuana, and tobacco: effects of prenatal exposure on offspring growth and morphology at age six. *Alcohol Clin Exp Res*. 1994;18:786–794.

103. Lumley J, Oliver S, Waters E. Interventions for promoting smoking cessation during pregnancy (Cochrane Review). *Cochrane Database Syst Rev*. 2000(4);CD001055.

104. Pearlman MD, Phillips ME. Safety belt use during pregnancy. *Obstet Gynecol*. 1996;88:1026–1029.

105. Clapp JF III. Exercise during pregnancy: a clinical update. *Clin Sports Med*. 2000;19:273–286.

chapter 29

Preventing Low Bone Mass, Osteoporosis, and Fractures

Andrea L. Sikon, MD, and Holly L. Thacker, MD

INTRODUCTION

Osteoporosis is a systemic skeletal disease that is characterized by diminished bone strength (ie, loss of bone density, microarchitecture, and mineralization).[1] Forty percent to 60% of a person's bone mass is acquired during the adolescent years. Bone mineral density (BMD) peaks in the third decade of life and then begins to decline gradually. This age-related decline in BMD is accelerated in women by changes that accompany postmenopause. Secondary causes such as endocrine and genetic disorders as well as drugs also can lead to an excessive loss of BMD in both women and men.

Osteoporosis generally begins when osteoclastic bone resorption exceeds osteoblastic bone formation. This imbalance results in a loss of trabeculation. Bones then become thin and weak, progressively losing their ability to withstand the impact of normal activities of daily living and/or increasing the risk of fracture during falls. This excessive loss of BMD and altered quality of bone distinguishes normal age-related changes from the disease of osteoporosis.[2]

According to recent estimates from the National Osteoporosis Foundation (NOF), 44 million Americans have either osteoporosis or osteopenia, low bone mass that is not yet at a level considered to be osteoporosis.[3] The prevalence is expected to increase to 61 million by 2020.[4] Of the 10 million Americans estimated to have osteoporosis today, 2 million are men and 8 million are women.[3] An additional 34 million Americans are estimated to have osteopenia.[3]

Osteoporosis results in approximately 1.5 million low-trauma fractures each year.[3] The lifetime risk of symptomatic fracture of the spine, hip, or distal radius in people aged 50 and older is 6% to 40% for women and 3% to 13% for men depending on demographic variation.[4,5]

IMPLICATIONS, CONSEQUENCES, AND COSTS

Fractures are associated with major financial, physical, and psychosocial burdens for the affected individuals, their families, and society as a whole. Fractures cause pain and disfigurement, leading to disability with loss of independence. Almost one third of patients with osteoporosis require nursing home care in the year after hip fracture, during which their mortality rate alarmingly increases by 10% to 20%.[5] Men have a higher mortality rate than women do after a fracture. Of those men and women who survive, half will require a gait assistance device.[3]

Whereas women aged 50 to 70 years are more likely to experience wrist fractures, vertebral fractures increase during the sixth decade of life. Hip fractures increase during the end of the seventh decade and throughout the eighth decade. Pelvic and rib fractures can occur throughout postmenopause.[5] Vertebral compression fractures and the resulting kyphosis cause disfigurement that not only carries major psychosocial implications but also directly affects other parts of the body, such as the pulmonary and gastrointestinal systems.

Approximately $17 billion is spent each year to medically treat osteoporotic fractures.[3] That cost is likely to increase as the incidence of fractures due to osteoporosis rises with the age of the general population. Such estimates do not include the indirect costs, such as lost wages for the caregiver.[3,5]

CLASSIFICATION

Osteoporosis can be classified as primary or secondary. Primary osteoporosis can be further classified as type 1 or type 2. *Primary type 1 osteoporosis* is estrogen dependent and involves mainly trabecular (cancellous) bone loss.

Type 1 accounts for the accelerated bone loss that occurs during menopause, which occurs in at least 50% of menopausal women. The spine and calcaneus are composed mainly of trabecular bone. Although only approximately 20% of the total skeleton is made up of trabecular bone, the majority of catabolism and remodeling occurs in these sites.[6]

Primary type 2 osteoporosis, which is referred to as senile osteoporosis, involves cortical (compact) bone loss and affects both sexes. The distal radius is composed of mainly cortical bone, although the ratio can have considerable individual variation, as does the hip with its mixed composition of cortical and trabecular bone.[6]

Secondary osteoporosis results from other disorders or use of certain medications. The many causes, both disease and drug related, are outlined in Tables 29-1 and 29-2. Secondary causes of osteoporosis are most prevalent in men and premenopausal women. Although exact numbers and causes vary according to the specific population studied, greater than 50% of premenopausal women with osteoporosis can be found to have secondary causes, most commonly including hypoestrogenemia (associated with premenopausal amenorrhea), excess production of thyroid hormone, and use of steroids or anticonvulsant medications. Secondary causes can be found in 30% to 60% of men with osteoporosis and most commonly include hypogonadism, steroid use, and alcoholism.[5,7]

Anticonvulsant agents such as phenytoin (Dilantin), carbamazepine (Tegretol), and barbiturates can reduce the hydroxylation of vitamin D. Therefore, they can decrease levels of circulating active vitamin D, calcium absorption, and bone mass. Such drugs cause a form of osteomalacia and high-turnover osteoporosis, which is characterized by hypocalcemia, hypocalciuria, hypophosphatemia, reduced serum 25-hydroxyvitamin D, elevated serum parathyroid hormone (PTH), and alkaline phosphatase.[7]

Catabolic glucocorticoids inhibit gut absorption of calcium, increase calcium loss through the kidney, inhibit bone formation and repair, and increase bone catabolism. Glucocorticoids induce diffuse bone loss, with some predilection for trabecular bone over cortical bone. Although loss occurs most rapidly in the first 6 to

T A B L E   29-1

Secondary Causes of Osteoporosis*

Endocrine Disorders	Gastrointestinal Disease	Genetic Disorders	Marrow-Related Disorders	Organ and Tissue Transplantation	Miscellaneous Causes
Acromegaly	Alcohol-related diseases	Hypophosphatasia	Amyloidosis	Bone marrow	Ankylosing spondylitis
Adrenal atrophy in Addison's disease	Celiac disease	Osteogenesis imperfecta	Hemochromatosis	Heart	Chronic obstructive pulmonary disease
Cushing's syndrome	Chronic active hepatitis		Hemophilia	Kidney	
Eating disorders	Chronic cholestatic diseases		Leukemia	Liver	Congenital porphyria
Endometriosis	Gastrectomy		Lymphoma	Lung	Epidermolysis bullosa
Gonadal insufficiency (primary and secondary)	Inflammatory bowel disease		Mastocytosis		Hemophilia
Hyperpara thyroidism	Jejunoileal bypass		Multiple myeloma		Idiopathic hypercalciuria
Hyperprolactinemia	Malabsorption syndromes		Pernicious anemia		Idiopathic scoliosis
Hyperthyroidism	Pancreatic insufficiency		Sarcoidosis		Multiple sclerosis
Hypogonadism	Parenteral nutrition		Sickle cell anemia		Rheumatoid arthritis
Nutritional disorders	Primary biliary cirrhosis		Thalassemia		
Tumor secretion of parathyroid hormone-related peptide	Severe liver disease				
Type 1 diabetes mellitus					

*Reprinted with permission from Fitzpatrick LA.[7]

12 months of treatment, the risk of fracture increases with higher doses and prolonged duration of therapy. Reported minimum causative doses are variable, but doses as small as 2.5 mg/d of prednisone have been implicated in causing significant bone loss.[8] The American College of Rheumatology suggests that prophylactic therapy for osteoporosis be initiated for individuals receiving prednisone doses of 5 mg/d or higher for more than 3 months or lower doses for 6 months.[8] Overdoses of thyroid replacement hormone have also been linked with decreased bone mass, as has intrinsic hyperthyroidism.[4,5]

Calcium is absorbed throughout the intestine but mainly in the duodenum. Any disease process that interferes with this absorption process can lead to osteoporosis. Processes that can cause secondary hyperparathyroidism include disruption of vitamin D metabolism or absorption (eg, gluten enteropathy), kidney disorders, and liver disease and may contribute to diminished bone mass. Primary hyperparathyroidism is a fairly common disorder that occurs in 1 of every 500 to 1000 individuals.[9] This condition is usually asymptomatic and often discovered during a workup for incidentally noted elevated levels of serum calcium.

Despite major advances in the understanding of the pathogenesis of osteoporosis and new diagnostic tools and treatments, it is not possible to fully predict clinically who will develop this disease. Consequently, several risk indexes have been developed to help identify those who are at an increased risk of osteoporosis and thus guide screening. One recent study suggested that an effective method is the Osteoporosis Self-assessment Tool (OST) calculated from age and weight: 0.2 × (Weight in kilograms − Age in years). Although simple, the index performed equally to its more complex counterparts. A score of less than 2 predicted 90% of the cases of osteoporosis with an 88% sensitivity

T A B L E   29-2

Drugs Associated With Bone Loss*

Aluminum
Anticoagulants
Anticonvulsants
β-carotene
Cigarette smoking
Cytotoxic drugs
Excessive alcohol
Excessive vitamin A
Glucocorticoids and adrenocorticotropin
Gonadotropin-releasing hormone agonists
Heparin
Lithium
Tamoxifen (in the premenopausal patient)

*Reprinted with permission from Fitzpatrick LA. Secondary causes of osteoporosis. *Mayo Clin Proc.* 2002;77:453–468.[7]

(95% confidence interval) in predicting BMD in the femoral neck. This does not mean, however, that individuals with obvious risk factors such as a prior fracture or a family history of maternal hip fracture despite a high OST score should not have BMD testing, as these indexes are only predictive, not definitive.[10]

Although genetics plays an important role in determining peak bone mass, other risk factors to consider are inadequate daily intake of calcium and vitamin D, failure to maintain a normal body weight, lack of daily weight-bearing exercises, smoking, excessive alcohol intake, and inadequate concentrations of sex hormones.[4] Interestingly, several studies in adolescent populations have suggested that high consumption of soda pop is linked with bone fracture. This association has not been definitively established, nor is it well understood. One hypothesis suggests that the high phosphorus content in soda induces a secondary hyperparathyroidism or causes some other interference with calcium metabolism.[11]

Osteoporosis can affect individuals across ethnic origins and those in both sexes, although it occurs more frequently in women and affects the races variably. White females have the highest osteoporotic fracture risk. Asian women tend to have low levels of BMD, yet also a 40% to 50% lower risk of hip fracture than do white women.[12] A shorter hip axis may contribute to the lower hip fracture rate observed in people of Asian descent. Compared with white women, African American women have greater levels of BMD and one half the incidence of fractures. Although African-American women have lower fracture rates than women from other ethnic origins, their fracture rates have been shown to be much higher than previously expected. After menopause, the rate of bone loss and risk of fracture become less disparate with those of women from other ethnic origins. These findings support the practice of screening nonwhite women for this disease.[13]

Common risk factors for osteoporosis include the following:

- Family history of fracture or osteoporosis
- White or Asian ethnicity
- Weight less than 127 lb
- Surgical and/or premature menopause
- Long-term use of glucocorticoids and hormonal therapy that increases hypogonadal states
- Smoking
- Lack of physical activity
- Excess alcohol consumption
- Low intake of calcium and vitamin D

QUANTIFICATION OF BONE DENSITY

Bone loss is clinically silent until a manifestation of osteoporosis (eg, fracture) is experienced. Thus, the identification of risk factors and the measurement of bone density are currently the best available methods for determining a patient's probability of developing this condition.

Bone density is one of the strongest correlates to fracture outcome, although it is not the sole determinant, and accounts for approximately 70% of total bone strength.[5,14] Bone mineral density cannot be fully equated with bone strength, as it does not reflect the number of trabecular bridge links.[14] Other factors that confer an increased rate of fracture include risks of falling and trauma.

Different techniques exist to measure bone density. Dual-energy X-ray absorptiometry (DXA) is the current method of choice for quantifying BMD. Central DXA is the gold standard; however, other techniques also exist. Alternatives include quantitative CT and measuring bone density at a single peripheral site, such as with heel ultrasound or forearm and finger DXA. These peripheral-site alternatives to central DXA are appealing because of their lower cost and portability. Central DXA, however, remains the most extensively validated test for prediction of fracture outcomes and is the only method that can be used to monitor response to treatment.[8,15]

The site of measurement is important because peak BMD and rates of loss can vary among different skeletal sites in the same individual. Thus, the number of sites that are measured affects the likelihood of diagnosing osteoporosis. Early menopause accelerates bone loss in the lumbar spine, which is later followed by decreases in the hips. However, BMD tends to become more homogeneous with age, and thus the variability in measuring at different sites in older individuals becomes less disparate in predicting fracture risk.[16]

Dual-energy X-ray Absorptiometry

For central DXA testing, at least 2 sites of the central skeleton should be measured, including the lumbosacral spine and hip (femoral neck, trochanter, and total hip). The same machine should be used for all repeat testing for accurate comparisons, as results can vary among machines from different manufacturers. Osteophyte formation and scarring at sites of prior vertebral compression fractures can falsely elevate central spine density measurements. A newer DXA technology called lateral vertebral assessment (LVA) is now available for the quantitative assessment of vertebral fractures. This is particularly helpful in assessing patients who have lost 3.81 cm (1.5 in) or more from their historically captured maximum height. With high-resolution fan-beam technology, newer DXA bone density devices can be used to evaluate for the presence of vertebral fractures with an accuracy that approaches that of standard lateral plain films. Lateral vertebral assessment has the advantage over standard X-ray examination of exposing the patient to a much lower dose of radiation. It also has the convenience of being performed at the same time as DXA testing, thus eliminating the need for a referral for plain films.

Bone mineral density results are reported in T and Z scores. The T score is the difference in number of standard deviations (SDs) between an individual's BMD measurement and that of the mean value for young women at peak bone mass. The Z score is the difference in number of SDs between an individual's BMD measurement and an age-matched group. According to the World Health Organization (WHO), a T score of −1 to −2.4 SD is considered to qualify as a diagnosis of osteopenia, meaning reduced bone mass but not at a level determined to be osteoporosis. A T score of less than or equal to −2.5 SD qualifies as osteoporosis[5] (Table 29-3). The current values that are used to translate BMD measurements into T scores and their subsequent correlation in defining a diagnosis of osteopenia or osteoporosis are based on data from postmenopausal white women. This limits the applicability of these current definitions to nonfemale, nonwhite populations and is a much-needed focus for further research.

As previously mentioned, the assessment of osteoporosis needs to be guided by not only the BMD measurement but also by the overall risk assessment to maximize the ability to predict fracture risk. Only a few randomized controlled prospective studies have been performed to further define these issues. The National Osteoporosis Risk Assessment (NORA) Study is one such study, which presently has the largest longitudinal research database of osteoporosis risk factors in postmenopausal women and includes a much more diverse set of women than in other studies.[13] The expense associated with obtaining a central DXA scan limits its use as a screening tool in the general population. This has led to recent guidelines that better define who should be screened based on risk of osteoporosis.

Ultrasound of the Heel

Some prospective studies suggest that for hip fracture, quantitative ultrasound of the heel approaches the predictive ability of DXA-derived T scores. However, these studies included only women over age 65 years. The other peripheral measures—forearm and finger density as measured by DXA—do not have value for predicting hip fractures at this time. Other limitations of peripheral bone density testing include the following:

TABLE 29-3

World Health Organization Criteria for Diagnosis of Bone Status by Central DXA

Definition	T Score
Normal	>−1.0 SD
Osteopenia/low bone mass	−1.0 SD to −2.4 SD
Osteoporosis	≤−2.5 SD
Severe osteoporosis	≥−2.5 SD plus fracture

- Lack of precision with peripheral bone scanning is not useful in monitoring osteoporosis therapy.
- Lack of sensitivity by peripheral bone density scanners misses a considerable portion of patients with low BMD.
- The WHO bases its diagnostic criteria for osteoporosis on central measurements of bone density, not peripheral measurements.

The potential for substantial cost savings makes heel ultrasound an option to consider; however, patients with abnormal findings or normal peripheral results with major risk factors should still undergo central DXA.[16]

Quantitated Computed Tomography

Quantitated computed tomography (QCT) is the only current method that measures true volumetric BMD, in grams per cubic centimeter (as opposed to measuring apparent BMD in grams per square centimeter via DXA). Quantitated computed tomography is calculated by comparing the density of the studied area on the CT scan with the density of the standard. This option is not commonly used, however, because of higher expense compared with DXA, higher dose of radiation, and lower reproducibility.

Bone Turnover Tests

Tests of bone turnover markers in serum and urine are being researched for application in the clinical setting. Although they can reveal short-term changes in bone turnover, they have yet to be proved to predict bone mass or fracture risk. No one biochemical marker correlates well with the DXA scan.[5] However, in selected situations (eg, continuing glucocorticoid use or where markers are known to be elevated), serial markers can be followed to monitor the effect of antiresorptive medication to prevent or treat osteoporosis. Measurable biochemical changes can occur as early as 3 months after treatment with antiresorptive medication is initiated.

Guidelines for Screening

Osteoporosis screening is more important now than ever because new treatments are available to prevent and treat the disease. Bone densitometry using DXA of the lumbar spine and hip can be used to select patients for therapy. T scores calculated from DXA of the hip provide the best data for determining whether a patient is at high risk of a fracture.

The National Osteoporosis Foundation (NOF) and Medicare have issued recommendations on who should be screened with DXA based on a patient's age, the presence of risk factors, a prior history of fracture, and the presence of potential secondary causes. The NOF recommends BMD testing for all postmenopausal women under age 65

who have 1 or more additional risk factors for osteoporotic fracture besides menopause. All women aged 65 and older, regardless of ethnicity and risk factors, should be tested. Although an older woman with a fragility fracture may not need a DXA scan to justify pharmacologic therapy, DXA may be used to obtain a baseline T score with which to compare future results and judge efficacy of treatment. Criteria for routine screening with a BMD test include the following:

- All women regardless of ethnicity by age 65 years
- Men beginning around age 70 years (no definitive guidelines)
- Any person with previous fractures, a family history of osteoporosis, and/or other risk factors for fracture
- Any male or female with a disease or condition that is treated with an agent known to cause bone loss (eg, glucocorticoids and hormonal therapy that increases hypogonadal states)
- Any man or woman with an unexplained fracture

The US Preventive Services Task Force now recommends that all women aged 65 years and older and those aged 60 and older with risk factors be screened for osteoporosis by measuring BMD, which is consistent with recommendations issued in 1999 by the NOF.[17,18] Current data indicate that only approximately 12% of women 65 years and older have undergone BMD measurement.[4] For women aged 65 years and older, Medicare reimburses for densitometry at 24-month intervals. Bone mineral density may need to be monitored more frequently during glucocorticoid treatment (every 6 to 12 months). Many clinicians measure BMD every 24 months in persons with bone loss to monitor the effectiveness of antiresorptive medication.

PRIMARY PREVENTION

Modification of Risk Factors

The first step in the primary prevention of osteoporosis involves identifying high-risk patients and altering any modifiable risk factors, including nutrition and lifestyle habits. A primary focus on proper nutrition, physical activity, and calcium intake in childhood and adolescence is the foundation of osteoporosis and fracture prevention.[5] Not only can peak BMD be maximized during one's younger years, but good dietary and exercise habits will help maintain bone health throughout one's lifetime.

Nutrition

As a person ages, calcium absorption decreases and the rate of bone turnover increases. Men, premenopausal women, and postmenopausal women who are receiving hormone therapy (HT) should ingest 1000 to 1200 mg/d of calcium. Postmenopausal women who are not receiving HT should ingest 1500 mg/d of calcium. Patients should be educated to maximize their daily dietary intake of calcium, which they can accomplish by eating calcium-rich foods and taking a calcium supplement. Most women do not get sufficient calcium from their diets and thus do benefit from calcium supplements. Although there are many formulations of calcium available on the market, calcium citrate may be best suited for older women. Calcium citrate may be taken on a full or empty stomach, does not require gastric acid for absorption, and therefore can be absorbed in the presence of achlorhydria or a proton pump inhibitor. Calcium supplementation is contraindicated in persons with a history of hypercalcemia. Calcium is not contraindicated in those with a history of nephrolithiasis. Recent studies have supported that a low-calcium diet in such persons promotes a negative calcium skeletal balance.[19]

Supplemental vitamin D, 600 to 800 IU/d, is recommended for postmenopausal women, especially those with low levels of sun exposure. At least 400 to 600 IU/d of vitamin D is recommended for men. An adequate calcium and vitamin D intake has been proved to increase BMD and decrease fracture rates in postmenopausal women. In a trial of more than 3000 postmenopausal women (mean age, 84 years), 18 months' supplementation with calcium (1500 mg/d) and vitamin D (800 IU/d) was associated with a 44% reduction in the incidence of hip fracture.[20] Another study showed that 2 years of supplementation with vitamin D in the form of calcitriol (1,25-dihydroxy-cholecalciferol) increased BMD of the spine by approximately 2% in postmenopausal women.[21]

Lifestyle factors

Ingestion of more than 760 mg of caffeine a day (the equivalent of 4 or more cups of coffee) may decrease calcium absorption and increase calciuresis and the relative risk of hip fracture by 20% in older women.[22] Persons at risk of osteoporosis are generally advised to drink no more than 2 cups of caffeinated beverages per day. Excessive alcohol intake has been shown to decrease BMD in the radius and spine of older women.[23] Smoking also is associated with reduced bone mass, perhaps because nicotine alters hepatic metabolism of estrogen. Excessive consumption of alcohol and tobacco use decreases BMD; the avoidance of these lifestyle behaviors constitutes an important preventive measure. Alcohol intake should be limited to less than 56 g/d, and smoking should be eliminated.

Exercise is another key modifiable factor. The importance of gravitational force in stimulating the bone remodeling process—and thus its ability to maintain BMD—was perhaps most strikingly noted in studies of astronauts in space. Such studies showed that in astronauts significant hypercalciuria developed and BMD decreased despite daily strenuous activity.[24] Repeated studies have shown significant declines in BMD and

increased concentrations of urinary calcium, phosphorus, and serum calcium in healthy adults undergoing periods of bed rest. Regular weight-bearing exercise can help reverse these changes by stimulating bone remodeling and help maintain BMD.

Muscle strengthening not only stimulates the bone remodeling process but also helps minimize the risk of falls by increasing mobility and stability. In longitudinal studies, weight-bearing exercise such as walking and weight lifting with light weights (2.25 kg) improved bone mass in postmenopausal women.[25,26] The Nurses Health Study showed in part that postmenopausal women who engaged in more leisure-time activity such as walking and regular exercise had a significantly lower risk of hip fractures than those who did not.[27] Results from the prospective Study of Osteoporotic Fractures Research Group showed that postmenopausal women who stood for less than 4 hours each day increased their risk of hip fracture by 70%.[22] Daily walking has not only been associated with a decreased risk of hip fractures, but regular physical activity is also associated with numerous psychological benefits in adults of all ages.[27]

Women with osteoporosis who are at increased risk of falling should consider wearing hip protector pads. Recent data suggest that hip protector pads worn at the time of a fall significantly decrease the incidence of hip fractures.[28]

IDENTIFICATION OF SECONDARY CAUSES

Review of systems to guide the workup

The cost of a comprehensive exclusion of all possible secondary causes of osteoporosis is prohibitive as well as unnecessary. However, knowledge that the incidence of secondary causes is higher in men, perimenopausal women, and persons with Z scores more than 1.5 SD below the mean may prompt further investigations in these patients. A review that uncovers a history of anorexia, low calcium and vitamin D intake, use of steroids and anticonvulsant medications, low activity level, smoking status, excessive alcohol use, amenorrhea, and low estrogen in women or low testosterone in men also may help to direct evaluations. Studies evaluating the yield of specific laboratory screening to reveal secondary causes are limited, and results have been variable. One limitation is that many studies have been based on populations from subspecialty clinics and thus may reflect a probable higher prevalence of underlying causes by preselection. One study that assessed postmenopausal women in whom osteoporosis recently was diagnosed but who had no prior histories of a potentially causative illness found that up to one third had a secondary cause. A cost-effectiveness analysis in this study suggested that initial screening in postmenopausal women without other known risk factors for osteoporosis, consisting of serum calcium, serum PTH, 24-hour urinary calcium excretion, and thyrotropin measurements in those receiving thyroid replacement therapy, would yield a diagnostic rate of previously undiagnosed cases of 85%.[29] This workup, which should be tailored to a patient's needs, may also involve measuring phosphorus, alkaline phosphatase, and vitamin D levels, and, in men, testosterone. The Study of Osteoporotic Fractures was a large prospective evaluation of various risk factors for hip fracture in postmenopausal women. Participants who received thyroid hormone had a 60% increase in osteoporosis; however, correlation with respective thyroid function tests was not performed, and respective thyrotropin levels were therefore unknown.[22] Due to the high prevalence of hypothyroidism in postmenopausal women, care must be taken to avoid an overdose of thyroid replacement, which can significantly accelerate bone loss.[30]

PHARMACOLOGIC TREATMENT

There are many new pharmacologic treatments that can prevent or manage osteoporosis including estrogens, bisphosphonates, selective estrogen receptor modulators (SERMs), calcitonin-salmon, and exogenous PTH.

When to Initiate Pharmacologic Treatment for Prevention of Osteoporotic Fractures

The NOF recommends "initiating therapy to reduce fracture risk in women with BMD T-scores of less than −2 SD below the mean in the absence of risk factors and in women with T-scores less than −1.5 if other risk factors are present."[17,31] Currently no guidelines exist for determining if and when to offer pharmacologic therapy to those with low bone mass but with T scores less than −1 to −1.4, and therapy for total prevention in those at high risk of fracture but with normal BMD. Similarly, no direct head-to-head comparative trials are available to help direct which medical treatment to initiate.[32] Thus, risk profiling and individualization are key in selecting pharmacotherapy for persons with established osteoporosis or persons with low bone mass and increased risk of fracture.

Estrogen/hormonal therapy (HT)
The onset of menopause brings a period of accelerated bone loss. Hormonal therapy, initiated no later than 5 years after onset of menopause, can not only treat perimenopausal symptoms but also improve BMD. Estrogen inhibits cytokine-induced osteoclast activation, which decreases bone resorption.

Hormonal therapy with estrogen, initiated near the time of menopause, decreases the risk of osteoporotic

fractures by approximately 50%.[31] In osteoporotic women, HT can increase mean vertebral bone mass by more than 5% and reduce vertebral fracture rate by 50% to 80%, with a 25% decrease in nonvertebral fractures after 5 years of use.[17,31] The Women's Health Initiative (WHI), a recent prospective randomized controlled trial, showed a statistically significant decrease in the number of hip fractures after a 5-year follow-up among women receiving HT, an impressive result given that the women were not preselected as having osteoporosis.[26,33]

The dose of estrogen used to prevent osteoporosis in most clinical studies is 0.625 mg/d.[34,35] Conjugated estrogens (0.625 mg/d) with or without progesterone increased spine and hip BMD and decreased bone turnover markers in elderly postmenopausal women.[36] Similar results were found in a substudy from the Health, Osteoporosis, Progestin, and Estrogen (HOPE) Trial, a large, randomized, placebo-controlled trial with low-dose estrogen regimens of 0.3 mg/d or 0.45 mg/d. Both regimens prevented BMD loss in the spine and hip and decreased bone turnover in women who were experiencing early menopause.[35] Transdermal estrogen has been shown to decrease the risk of new vertebral fractures in women aged 47 to 75 years with established osteoporosis.[37] Estrogen therapy, therefore, is indicated in both the prevention and treatment of osteoporosis.[37]

Ongoing debate continues about the risk-benefit ratio of HT, mandating individualized assessment of the potential benefits to determine whether they outweigh the potential risks. In addition to increasing BMD, HT can also relieve hot flashes and atrophic vaginitis and improve sleep disorders and minor mood disturbances.[38] Other results from the WHI suggest that HT may reduce the risk of colorectal cancer.[33] Estrogen use also increases the risk of thromboembolism and gallstones. The clearly defined increased risk of endometrial cancer with unopposed estrogen therapy in women with an intact uterus is nullified by the concomitant use of progestin.[33] There is an increased risk of breast cancer diagnosis with prolonged HT use of greater than 4 to 5 years. The WHI also confirmed that combined estrogen/progestin use increased the risk of incident breast cancer.[6] Overall, there occurred no change in the number of deaths due to breast cancer in women who received HT in the WHI studies.[39]

The WHI is a large, prospective, randomized, controlled trial that set out to study 3 HT regimens: (1) conjugated equine estrogens (0.625 mg/d) in women who had a hysterectomy, (2) conjugated equine estrogens (0.625 mg/d) plus medroxyprogesterone acetate (2.5 mg/d), and (3) placebo. The primary end points were coronary artery disease (CAD) and invasive breast cancer. Recent controversy surrounding HT was spawned after the combined estrogen-progesterone arm of the WHI was stopped prematurely at approximately 5 years due to an increased "global risk index," which includes the risk of nonfatal myocardial infarction, stroke, pulmonary embolism, and breast cancer. However, no increase in overall mortality or overall cancer incidence occurred in the HT user. The estrogen-only arm vs placebo continues.[33]

Hormonal therapy is recommended for the prevention and/or management of osteoporosis in those who are also looking for concomitant perimenopausal symptom relief and in those who are within 5 years of menopause whose individual benefit-risk equation favors benefit over risk. The beneficial effects of HT on bone are lost when the drug treatment is discontinued. Consideration should be given to continuing HT indefinitely in older women if the benefits are deemed to outweigh the well-established risks because of the significant benefit of HT in preventing hip fractures in elderly women (80% reduction in risk in women older than 75 years of age).[40] Another potential benefit is reflected in studies that have suggested that HT for more than 10 years is associated with significant reductions in the risk of Alzheimer's dementia in older women.[41]

Selective estrogen receptor modulators

Selective estrogen receptor modulators are nonsteroidal mixed-estrogen agonists and antagonists. Two drugs belong to this class: raloxifene hydrochloride (Evista) and tamoxifen citrate. Both exhibit antagonist properties in the breast and partial estrogen agonist properties in trabecular bone (and cardiovascular tissue). Raloxifene is the only SERM approved for the prevention and treatment of osteoporosis in postmenopausal women. The impact on reduction in fracture risk has not been studied in tamoxifen. Raloxifene has been shown to reduce the risk of new vertebral fractures when used for 4 years by women with osteoporosis; studies show a reduction in vertebral fracture risk of 36%.[5] Fractures occurred in 10.1% of women who received placebo compared with 6.6% of those taking 60 mg/d of raloxifene and 5.4% of those taking 120 mg/d of raloxifene. At 60 mg, raloxifene reduced the vertebral fracture rate by 40% to 50% over 2 to 4 years; however, it did not reduce hip fractures as of the 4-year data report.[42]

Unlike tamoxifen, raloxifene has estrogen antagonist properties in the uterus and thus does not increase the risk of endometrial cancer.[5] The use of raloxifene does not appear to increase the risk of breast cancer and may actually reduce incidence, making raloxifene a helpful alternative in women who cannot take estrogen. Raloxifene has beneficial effects on serum lipids and decreases homocysteine levels.[43] The Raloxifene Use for the Heart (RUTH) Trial is under way to evaluate cardiovascular outcomes.[44,45]

The recommended daily dosage of raloxifene is 60 mg without regard to meal times. As with estrogen, the relative risk of venous thromboembolism is increased twofold to threefold with use of raloxifene.[15] Due to the increased incidence of vasomotor symptoms and leg cramps with use of SERMs, raloxifene may be limited to the later postmenopausal years.

Bisphosphonates

Newer and better tolerated oral bisphosphonates are available, which constitutes an important update in the treatment of osteoporosis. Risedronate sodium (Actonel) and alendronate sodium (Fosamax) are 2 oral agents in this class of drugs, which are approved for the prevention and treatment of postmenopausal and glucocorticoid-induced osteoporosis. Each has been proved to increase spine and hip BMD in a dose-dependent manner and to decrease fracture rate up to 50% or 60%. These drugs were associated with significant increases in BMD at all sites measured (lumbar spine, femoral neck, femoral trochanter, and midshaft radius). This was coupled with significant decreases in fracture rates.[46]

The exact mechanism by which bisphosphonates improve bone strength is not fully understood. Bisphosphonates increase BMD by preventing resorption of bone, but researchers suspect other mechanisms are involved. This is evidenced in results from a study of risedronate that showed an increase in BMD of only 3% to 4% vs placebo but a 50% to 60% reduction in fracture risk.[47]

In the placebo-controlled, randomized Fracture Intervention Trial, alendronate (5 to 10 mg/d) reduced the risk of a new vertebral fracture (the primary outcome of the trial) by 50% over 3 years in postmenopausal women with low BMD and a prior history of 1 vertebral fracture.[48] Relative risk of hip and wrist fracture, with alendronate compared with placebo, were 51% and 47%, respectively. Alendronate also reduced the number of days of "bed-disability" and days of limited activity caused by back pain.[49] In the Vertebral Efficacy With Risedronate Therapy (VERT) Trial, risedronate (5 mg/d) reduced incidence of new vertebral fractures by 41% in postmenopausal women with low BMD and a history of vertebral fracture.[47] Over 3 years, the relative risk of a new vertebral fracture in women younger than age 85 years was 0.59, and relative risk of a new nonvertebral fracture was 0.6. Bone mineral density at the lumbar spine increased 5.4%.[47] A separate trial looking at risedronate showed no decrease in the rate of hip fracture among women over age 80 years with 1 or more risk factors for falls, but not all participants had low BMD.[15] Most studies aimed at assessing the efficacy of bisphosphonates have been industry sponsored, thus the potential for bias.

The major adverse effects of bisphosphonates are gastrointestinal. Although several controlled trials have shown that the rate of gastrointestinal side effects was not significantly higher with alendronate therapy than with placebo, many of these excluded patients with a higher incidence of such disorders as a study entry disqualification.[50] Studies performed on risedronate did include patients with higher risks of gastrointestinal disorders and failed to show any increase incidence of such side effects.[51] Risedronate and alendronate begin to have notable effects on BMD within the first year of treatment.[48] The bisphosphonates have a prolonged half-life in bone, and therefore the effects on BMD tend to last long.[46,52]

The recommended doses of alendronate for prevention and treatment of osteoporosis in postmenopausal women are 5 mg/d or 35 mg once weekly for prevention and 10 mg/d or 70 mg once weekly for treatment. The recommended dose of risedronate is 5 mg/d or 35 mg once weekly for prevention and treatment. Once-weekly dosing with 7 times the daily dose of alendronate has demonstrated an increase in lumbar spine BMD at 12 months, making either dosing option equivalent.[53] Bisphosphonates are generally well tolerated, bone specific, and tend to have few drug interactions. The difficulty in administering them lies in their easily influenced and relatively poor absorption. Thus, it is important to tell patients that they must take these drugs with an 8-oz glass of water on an empty stomach and to remain upright for 30 minutes afterward. Once-weekly formulations were associated with fewer serious adverse effects in the upper gastrointestinal tract as well as a lower incidence of esophageal events compared with daily doses.[53] Although the once-weekly dosing has led to increased toleration and convenience, the associated cost remains equivalent and is approximately 3 times more expensive than HT.

Bisphosphonates are not approved for use in renal failure. The drug is cleared by the kidney, with the potential for resultant accumulation. Thus, use of biphosphates in the setting of substantial renal insufficiency (ie, creatinine clearance level 35 ml/min) cannot be recommended.[46] Safety of these drugs has not been determined in children or women of childbearing age, as bisphosphonates incorporate into the bony matrix and have prolonged effects. Bisphosphonates should be considered the first-line choice in women who cannot take estrogen therapy or are more than 5 years after menopause, in men with osteoporosis, and in the prevention and treatment of glucocorticoid-induced osteoporosis.

Although not yet approved by the Food and Drug Administration (FDA) as a treatment of postmenopausal osteoporosis, a 1-year randomized placebo-controlled trial found that intermittent administration of the intravenous bisphosphonate zoledronic acid (Zometa) increased spine and hip BMD and suppressed markers of bone turnover.[54] A new pharmaceutical-sponsored study called HORIZON (Health Outcomes and Reduced Incidence with Zoledronic Acid Once Yearly) is under way to further evaluate risk reduction of osteoporotic fractures with once yearly zoledronic acid in postmenopausal women and in men.

A few studies have looked at the potential benefits of combination therapy. One such study was a yearlong, randomized, controlled trial that found a greater increase in BMD, as well as a decrease in markers of bone turnover, with combined therapy using raloxifene and alendronate vs raloxifene alone. This study consisted of postmenopausal women with osteoporosis, and the end

points were additive and independent. However, fracture rates were not a direct end point.[55]

Parathyroid hormone

The injectable parathyroid hormone teriparatide (Forteo) is a recently FDA-approved anabolic agent of a different class from other antiresorptive therapies for osteoporosis. Parathyroid hormone stimulates both osteoblast-mediated bone formation and osteoclastic resorption. Continuous exposure to high levels of PTH, as occurs in primary hyperparathyroidism, stimulates bone catabolism over formation. When given subcutaneously and in intermittent low doses, bone formation is favored. Intermittent teriparatide has been shown in studies to increase BMD and decrease the risk of vertebral and nonvertebral fractures in postmenopausal women with at least one vertebral fracture. Although increases in BMD were seen in men as well, fracture data are pending the results of further studies. In patients with established osteoporosis, PTH has been shown to build mechanically strong new bone. The current recommended dose of 20 µg injected daily demonstrated a decreased risk of new vertebral fracture by 65% over 21 months in women with osteoporosis and a mean age of 70 years.[18,56,57] Teriparatide is currently FDA approved for treatment in women with osteoporosis at high risk of fracture, defined as those with a history of osteoporotic fracture, multiple risk factors for fracture, and/or failure to respond or intolerance to other therapies. The drug is also approved for the treatment of osteoporosis in men with primary or hypogonadal osteoporosis at high risk of fracture using the aforementioned criterion.

Potential side effects of PTH include transient hypercalcemia/calciuria, orthostatic hypotension, and leg cramps. No difference in dosing is required for patients with mild to moderate renal insufficiency (ie, creatinine clearance level 30–72 ml/min) or in patients with a history of congestive heart failure. The drug has not been studied in patients with chronic renal failure or substantial hepatic impairment. Initial studies were halted prematurely at 2 years instead of 3 years when concurrent rat studies developed dose-dependent increased rates of osteosarcoma. This led to current approval of only 2 years' duration of therapy. Longer term studies of PTH are under way to study more prolonged therapy. Currently at 30 months of 4 years of follow-up, no increased incidence of osteosarcoma was found. Contraindications to the use of PTH include inherent risk of osteosarcoma, Paget disease, pediatric and young adults with open epiphyses, and history of radiation therapy to the skeleton. The current cost of treatment is approximately $600 per month.[58]

Calcitonin-salmon

Calcitonin-salmon (Miacalcin) is a peptide hormone available in a nasal spray or injectable form that inhibits osteoclast formation and thereby reduces bone resorption.

The suggested intranasal dose (alternating nostrils daily) is 200 IU/d. In the Prevent Recurrence of Osteoporotic Fractures (PROOF) Study, calcitonin at a dose of 200 IU/d significantly reduced risk of vertebral fractures by 33% over 3 to 5 years in postmenopausal women with a history of fractures.[59] These results have been questioned, however, due to a high dropout rate, absence of dose response, and the lack of strong supporting data from BMD and bone markers. In addition, calcitonin did not reduce hip or other nonvertebral fracture rates and, compared with alendronate, was not as effective at increasing BMD of the lumbar spine.[60] Calcitonin remains FDA approved for treatment but not prevention of osteoporosis in women in the late postmenopausal phase. Use of calcitonin may have a mild analgesic effect in the treatment of compression fractures, although the mechanism is not well understood or established. Potential side effects of calcitonin include local nasal irritation, epistaxis, nausea, and flushing. Calcitonin is usually reserved for patients who cannot tolerate other agents.

Other pharmacotherapy

Phytoestrogens, predominantly as soy protein, have been used to treat menopausal symptoms. Few clinical trials, however, have evaluated effects of phytoestrogens on BMD and menopausal symptoms. Some studies have shown a benefit but were not dose dependent and were limited by their small sample size and short duration.[61] The safety of phytoestrogens is unclear in patients with contraindications to estrogen because of their weak estrogen-like effects.

Sodium fluoride is no longer recommended as a treatment option. Sodium fluoride does stimulate new bone formation via osteoblast activation but produces bone of unclear quality, and fracture rates are not reduced.

Certain HMG CoA reductase inhibitors (statins) may increase BMD by inducing expression of bone morphogenetic protein (BMP-2), although early research results are mixed.[3] One case-control study reported a 50% reduction in nonpathologic fractures in older women receiving statins for treatment of hypercholesterolemia.[62] Another case-control study did not demonstrate any reduction in the risk of fracture with statin drugs.[63] A prospective, randomized, controlled trial has yet to explore this reported association.

SURGICAL TREATMENT OF FRACTURES

In recent years, 2 procedures have been developed to relieve pain and restore function to patients with vertebral fracture: vertebroplasty and kyphoplasty. In vertebroplasty, the surgeon inserts a needle under fluoroscopic guidance and injects surgical cement into the compressed part of the vertebrae. Once the cement hardens, it supports the affected vertebrae and relieves pain in many patients.

Kyphoplasty is a newer procedure that may have fewer side effects than vertebroplasty. Kyphoplasty is similar to vertebroplasty except that, before the cement is injected, a balloon is inserted into the affected vertebrae and inflated. The balloon, which is then removed, creates a space for the cement to be injected in a controlled fashion, minimizing the risk of cement leakage out of the vertebrae.

REFERENCES

1. Consensus development conference: diagnosis, prophylaxis, and treatment of osteoporosis. *Am J Med.* 1993;94:646–650.

2. National Institutes of Health (NIH) Osteoporosis and Related Bone Diseases National Resource Center. Osteoporosis overview. Available at: www.osteo.org/osteo.html. Accessed November 20, 2002.

3. National Osteoporosis Foundation. Disease statistics: fast facts. Available at: www.nof.org/osteoporosis/stats.htm. Accessed November 20, 2002.

4. National Osteoporosis Foundation. America's bone health: the state of osteoporosis and low bone mass. Available at: www.nof.org/advocacy/prevalence. Accessed November 20, 2002.

5. NIH Consensus Development Conference. Osteoporosis prevention, diagnosis, and therapy. *JAMA.* 2001;285:785–795.

6. Stephen AB, Wallace WA. The management of osteoporosis. *J Bone Joint Surg Br.* 2001;83:316–323.

7. Fitzpatrick LA. Secondary causes of osteoporosis. *Mayo Clin Proc.* 2002;77:453–468.

8. American College of Rheumatology Ad Hoc Committee on Glucocorticoid-Induced Osteoporosis. Recommendations for the prevention and treatment of glucocorticoid-induced osteoporosis: 2001 update. *Arthritis Rheum.* 2001;44:1496–1503.

9. Bilezikian JP, Silverberg SJ. Clinical spectrum of primary hyperparathyroidism. *Rev Endocr Metab Disord.* 2000;1:237–245.

10. Geusens P, Hochberg MC, van der Voort DJ, et al. Performance of risk indices for identifying low bone density in postmenopausal women. *Mayo Clin Proc.* 2002;77:629–637.

11. Golden NH. Osteoporosis prevention: a pediatric challenge. *Arch Pediatr Adolesc Med.* 2000;154:542–543.

12. Cummings SR, Xu L, Chen X, Zhao X, Yu W, Ge Q. Bone mass, rates of osteoporotic fractures, and prevention of fractures: are there differences between China and Western countries? *Chin Med Sci J.* 1994;9:197–200.

13. Siris ES, Miller PD, Barrett-Connor E, et al. Identification and fracture outcomes of undiagnosed low bone mineral density in postmenopausal women: results from the

National Osteoporosis Risk Assessment. *JAMA.* 2001;286:2815–2822.

14. Wallach S, Cohen S, Reid DM, et al. Effects of risedronate treatment on bone density and vertebral fracture in patients on corticosteroid therapy. *Calcif Tissue Int.* 2000;67:277–285.

15. Nelson HD, Helfand M, Woolf SH, Allan JD. Screening for postmenopausal osteoporosis: a review of the evidence for the US Preventive Services Task Force. *Ann Intern Med.* 2002;137:529–543.

16. Miller P, Bonnick S, Johnston CJ, et al. The challenges of peripheral bone density testing. *J Clin Densitometry.* 1998;1:211–217.

17. Screening for osteoporosis in postmenopausal women: recommendations and rationale. *Ann Intern Med.* 2002;137:526–528.

18. National Osteoporosis Foundation. Physician's Guide to Prevention and Treatment of Osteoporosis, 2000. Available at: www.nof.org/physguide/. Accessed November 20, 2002.

19. Shaver K, et al. Kidney stones and calcium. *Prescriber's Letter,* March, 2002, p. 18. Available at: www.prescribersletter.com. Accessed November 20, 2002.

20. Chapuy MC, Arlot ME, Delmas PD, Meunier PJ. Effect of calcium and cholecalciferol treatment for three years on hip fractures in elderly women. *Br Med J.* 1994;308:1081–1082.

21. Gallagher JC, Goldgar D. Treatment of postmenopausal osteoporosis with high doses of synthetic calcitriol: a randomized controlled study. *Ann Intern Med.* 1990;113:649–655.

22. Cummings SR, Nevitt MC, Browner WS, et al. Risk factors for hip fracture in white women: Study of Osteoporotic Fractures Research Group. *N Engl J Med.* 1995;332:767–773.

23. Holbrook TL, Barrett-Connor E. A prospective study of alcohol consumption and bone mineral density. *BMJ.* 1993;306:1506–1509.

24. Rambaut PC, Goode AW. Skeletal changes during space flight. *Lancet.* 1985;2:1050–1052.

25. Kohrt WM, Snead DB, Slatopolsky E, Birge SJ Jr. Additive effects of weight-bearing exercise and estrogen on bone mineral density in older women. *J Bone Miner Res.* 1995;10:1303–1311.

26. The Writing Group for the Postmenopausal Estrogen/ Progestin Interventions (PEPI) trial. Effects of hormone therapy on bone mineral density: results from the Postmenopausal Estrogen/Progestin Interventions (PEPI) trial. *JAMA.* 1996;276:1389–1396.

27. Feskanich D, Willett W, Colditz G. Walking and leisure-time activity and risk of hip fracture in postmenopausal women. *JAMA.* 2002;288:2300–2306.

28. Kannus P, Parkkari J, Niemi S, et al. Prevention of hip fracture in elderly people with use of a hip protector. *N Engl J Med.* 2000;343:1506–1513.

29. Tannenbaum C, Clark J, Schwartzman K, et al. Yield of laboratory testing to identify secondary contributors to osteoporosis in otherwise healthy women. *J Clin Endocrinol Metab.* 2002;87:4431–4437.

30. Stall GM, Harris S, Sokoll LJ, Dawson-Hughes B. Accelerated bone loss in hypothyroid patients overtreated with L-thyroxine. *Ann Intern Med.* 1990;113:265–269.

31. Lips P. Epidemiology and predictors of fractures associated with osteoporosis. *Am J Med.* 1997;103(2A):3S–8S.

32. Hosking D, Chilvers CE, Christiansen C, et al, for the Early Postmenopausal Intervention Cohort Study Group. Prevention of bone loss with alendronate in postmenopausal women under 60 years of age. *N Engl J Med.* 1998;338:485–492.

33. Rossouw JE, Anderson GL, Prentice RL, et al. Risks and benefits of estrogen plus progestin in healthy postmenopausal women: principal results from the Women's Health Initiative randomized controlled trial. *JAMA.* 2002;288:321–333.

34. Recker RR, Davies KM, Dowd RM, Heaney RP. The effect of low-dose continuous estrogen and progesterone therapy with calcium and vitamin D on bone in elderly women: a randomized, controlled trial. *Ann Intern Med.* 1999;130:897–904.

35. Lindsay R, Gallagher JC, Kleerekoper M, Pickar JH. Effect of lower doses of conjugated equine estrogens with and without medroxyprogesterone acetate on bone in early postmenopausal women. *JAMA.* 2002;287:2668–2676.

36. Villareal DT, Binder EF, Williams DB, Schechtman KB, Yarasheski KE, Kohrt WM. Bone mineral density response to estrogen replacement in frail elderly women: a randomized controlled trial. *JAMA.* 2001;286:815–820.

37. Lufkin EG, Wahner HW, O'Fallon WM, et al. Treatment of postmenopausal osteoporosis with transdermal estrogen. *Ann Intern Med.* 1992;117:1–9.

38. Elder J, Thacker HL. Menopause. Available at: www.clevelandclinicmeded.com/diseasemanagement/ women/menopause/menopause.htm. Accessed November 20, 2002.

39. Batur P, Thacker HL, Moore HC. Discussing breast cancer and hormone replacement therapy with women. *Cleve Clin J Med.* 2002;69:838–848.

40. Cauley JA, Seeley DG, Ensrud K, Ettinger B, Black D, Cummings SR. Estrogen replacement therapy and fractures in older women: Study of Osteoporotic Fractures Research Group. *Ann Intern Med.* 1995;122:9–16.

41. Zandi PP, Carlson MC, Plassman BL, et al. Hormone replacement therapy and incidence of Alzheimer disease in older women: the Cache County Study. *JAMA.* 2002;288:2123–2129.

42. Delmas PD, Ensrud KE, Adachi JD, et al. Efficacy of raloxifene on vertebral fracture risk reduction in postmenopausal women with osteoporosis: four-year results from a randomized clinical trial. *J Clin Endocrinol Metab.* 2002;87:3609–3617.

43. Barrett-Connor E, Grady D, Sashegyi A, et al. Raloxifene and cardiovascular events in osteoporotic postmenopausal women: four-year results from the MORE (Multiple Outcomes of Raloxifene Evaluation) randomized trial. *JAMA.* 2002;287:847–857.

44. Mosca L. Rationale and overview of the Raloxifene Use for the Heart (RUTH) trial. *Ann N Y Acad Sci.* 2001;949:181–185.

45. Mosca L, Barrett-Connor E, Wenger NK, et al. Design and methods of the Raloxifene Use for The Heart (RUTH) study. *Am J Cardiol.* 2001;88:392–395.

46. Canalis E, Feld S, Miller P, et al. Osteoporosis and fracture prevention/reduction. *Med Crossfire.* 2002;3:1–15.

47. Harris ST, Watts NB, Genant HK, et al, for the Vertebral Efficacy With Risedronate Therapy (VERT) Study Group. Effects of risedronate treatment on vertebral and nonvertebral fractures in women with postmenopausal osteoporosis: a randomized controlled trial. *JAMA.* 1999;282:1344–1352.

48. Black DM, Thompson DE, Bauer DC, et al, for the Fracture Intervention Trial Research Group. Fracture risk reduction with alendronate in women with osteoporosis: the Fracture Intervention Trial. *J Clin Endocrinol Metab.* 2000;85:4118–4124.

49. Nevitt MC, Thompson DE, Black DM, et al, for the Fracture Intervention Trial Research Group. Effect of alendronate on limited-activity days and bed-disability days caused by back pain in postmenopausal women with existing vertebral fractures. *Arch Intern Med.* 2000;160:77–85.

50. Ettinger B, Pressman A, Schein J. Clinic visits and hospital admissions for care of acid-related upper gastrointestinal disorders in women using alendronate for osteoporosis. *Am J Manag Care.* 1998;4:1377–1382.

51. Taggart H, Bolognese MA, Lindsay R, et al. Upper gastrointestinal tract safety of risedronate: a pooled analysis of 9 clinical trials. *Mayo Clin Proc.* 2002;77:262–270.

52. Greenspan SL, Emkey RD, Bone HG, et al. Significant differential effects of alendronate, estrogen, or combination therapy on the rate of bone loss after discontinuation of treatment of postmenopausal osteoporosis: a randomized, double-blind, placebo-controlled trial. *Ann Intern Med.* 2002;137:875–883.

53. Schnitzer T, Bone HG, Crepaldi G, et al, for the Alendronate Once-Weekly Study Group. Therapeutic equivalence of alendronate 70 mg once-weekly and alendronate 10 mg daily in the treatment of osteoporosis. *Aging (Milano).* 2000;12:1–12.

54. Reid IR, Brown JP, Burckhardt P, et al. Intravenous zoledronic acid in postmenopausal women with low bone mineral density. *N Engl J Med.* 2002;346:653–661.

55. Johnell O, Scheele WH, Lu Y, Reginster JY, Need AG, Seeman E. Additive effects of raloxifene and alendronate on bone density and biochemical markers of bone remodeling in postmenopausal women with osteoporosis. *J Clin Endocrinol Metab.* 2002;87:985–992.

56. Neer RM, Arnaud CD, Zanchetta JR, et al. Effect of parathyroid hormone (1-34) on fractures and bone mineral density in postmenopausal women with osteoporosis. *N Engl J Med.* 2001;344:1434–1441.

57. Kuijpers G, Schneider B, Stadel B, Colman E. Recombinant human parathyroid hormone: preclinical data on rat osteosarcoma were not dismissed. *BMJ.* 2002;324:1218.

58. Forteo teriparatide (rDNA origin) injection: a prescriber's overview. Indianapolis, Ind: Eli Lilly and Co; 2002. PA 9241 FSAMP.

59. Chesnut CH, 3rd, Silverman S, Andriano K, et al, for the Prevent Recurrence of Osteoporotic Fractures Study Group. A randomized trial of nasal spray salmon calcitonin in postmenopausal women with established osteoporosis: the Prevent Recurrence of Osteoporotic Fractures study. *Am J Med.* 2000;109:267–276.

60. Downs RW Jr, Bell NH, Ettinger MP, et al. Comparison of alendronate and intranasal calcitonin for treatment of osteoporosis in postmenopausal women. *J Clin Endocrinol Metab.* 2000;85:1783–1788.

61. Tsourounis C. Clinical effects of phytoestrogens. *Clin Obstet Gynecol.* 2001;44:836–842.

62. Meier CR, Schlienger RG, Kraenzlin ME, Schlegel B, Jick H. HMG-CoA reductase inhibitors and the risk of fractures. *JAMA.* 2000;283:3205–3210.

63. van Staa TP, Wegman S, de Vries F, Leufkens B, Cooper C. Use of statins and risk of fractures. *JAMA.* 2001;285:1850–1855.

RESOURCES

National Institutes of Health Osteoporosis and Related Bone Diseases– National Resource Center.
Web site: www.osteo.org.

National Osteoporosis Foundation.
Web site: www.nof.org. (Information for physicians and patients regarding osteoporosis prevention, screening, and treatment.)

North American Menopause Society.
Web site: www.menopause.org. (Information for physicians, health care providers, and women on the topics of health and wellness, menopause, hormone therapy, and osteoporosis from nonprofit organization dedicated to women's health in midlife.)

Doctor's Guide to the Internet—OP Section:
www.docguide.com

Breast Cancer

Mark E. Mayer, MD

INTRODUCTION AND EPIDEMIOLOGY

The United States has one of the highest rates of breast cancer in the world. The US incidence rate was 85 cases per 100,000 people in 1980 and 117 cases per 100,000 in 1999. However, some of this high incidence is likely due to earlier case-finding and enhanced detection of ductal carcinoma in situ (DCIS).

Mortality from breast cancer in the United States has fallen since the early 1990s in both rate and in absolute terms. In 1991, the incidence was 175,000 new cases and there were 44,500 deaths. For 2002, it was estimated that there would be 205,000 breast cancer cases and 40,000 deaths due to breast cancer in the United States. The US death rate from breast cancer is approximately average among developed countries. The 5-year survival rate for all stages of breast cancer rose from 75% in 1974 to 1976 to 86% in 1992 to 1997.[1] As in most cancers, the survival rate correlates with the stage of the disease at diagnosis. In localized disease (negative lymph nodes, no skin or muscle invasion, and a lesion less than 3 cm), the 5-year survival is greater than 90%; with regional disease, it is approximately 70%; and with distant metastases, less than 20%. Unlike some malignancies, breast cancer can recur late; this reduces the significance of 5-year survival data.

RISK FACTORS

Known risk factors account for only 20% of breast cancer cases in younger patients and less than 30% in older patients.[2] The strongest risk factors (relative risk, >4) for the development of breast cancer include age over 65 years, prior invasive or in situ breast cancer, family history of 2 or more relatives with premenopausal or bilateral breast cancer, or atypical hyperplasia on prior breast biopsy. Lesser risk (relative risk, 2 to 4) is conferred by a family history of a first-degree relative with breast cancer, obesity, age at first full-term pregnancy greater than 30 years, nulliparity, or history of prior ovarian or endometrial cancer. A smaller increased risk

(relative risk, 1 to 2) is conferred by early menarche (age, <12 years) or late menopause (age, >55 years). In addition to obesity, several lifestyle factors are associated with a modest increased risk of breast cancer: weight gain, fat intake, inactivity, and alcohol consumption. Cigarette smoking may be weakly associated with breast cancer risk. The risk conferred by benign breast disease is greatest for those having atypical hyperplasia. If no proliferative changes are present, the relative risk of breast cancer is modest, between 1.4 and 1.9.

The Gail Model may be used to help calculate breast cancer risk from the patient's medical history: race, age, age at menarche, age at first live birth, number of first-degree relatives with breast cancer, number of previous breast biopsies, and prior biopsy showing atypical hyperplasia.[3] The Gail Model is based on major predictors of risk identified in the Breast Cancer Detection Demonstration Project. A computer disk for use of the Gail Model Risk Assessment Tool is available from the National Cancer Institute (see "Resources" at the end of the chapter). The Gail Model does not consider either breast cancer in second-degree relatives or age of onset of breast cancer in the affected relative. Consequently, the calculation may overestimate risk in women whose mothers or sisters had breast cancer at an elderly age and underestimate risk in women who have second- or third-degree relatives with breast cancer at early ages.

Breast cancer risk is increased even if the nearest relative with breast cancer is a third-degree relative.[4] Having multiple first-degree relatives with premenopausal breast cancer confers the highest risk, much of it associated with BRCA-1 or BRCA-2 gene mutations. Several models for assessing the risk of carrying a gene mutation have been proposed, to help guide decision making regarding when to recommend genetic testing.[5] Personal characteristics increasing likelihood of having the BRCA-1 or BRCA-2 gene include breast cancer at an early age, bilateral breast cancer, and both breast and ovarian cancer. Family history characteristics include breast cancer in male family members, multiple cases of breast cancer in the family, both breast and ovarian cancer in the family, 2 primary cancers in any family member, or Ashkenazi Jewish background. The cost of genetic testing for markers of breast cancer susceptibility ranges from $400 for limited testing, after a known marker is discovered in a family member, to $2800 for a full battery, with a woman being the "index case."

The risk of breast cancer due to postmenopausal hormone therapy (HT) is probably slightly increased. A large meta-analysis showed a relative risk of 1.35 for women who received HT for 5 years or longer but a reduction in risk after discontinuation of HT.[6] One recent large primary study (Iowa Women's Health Study) did not show an overall increased risk of breast cancer but did show an increase in some cancers with a "better prognosis."[7] The latest trial to assess this risk is the Women's Health Initiative. For women receiving estrogen plus progestin for a mean of 5.2 years, the relative risk of breast cancer was 1.26 compared with those taking a placebo.[8] The absolute risk was 1.95% for those receiving HT vs 1.53% for placebo, an absolute risk increase of 0.42% for a "number needed to harm" (NNH) of 238. There are no data showing increased mortality from breast cancer due to HT. Recently, data have emerged suggesting that HT given after breast cancer was diagnosed had no adverse impact on recurrence or mortality.[9] The overall consensus seems to be that there is some increased risk of breast cancer with HT, although this risk is probably modest, and there is no definite evidence of an increase in breast cancer mortality.

SCREENING AND DIAGNOSTIC METHODS

Clinical Breast Examination

The clinical breast examination (CBE) performed by a physician or health care professional should include inspection, done with the woman sitting with her hands on her hips, or with her hands on her head, pushing downward. The examiner looks for lumps, asymmetry, or skin dimpling. Careful, systematic palpation has been shown to increase the detection of breast lumps. Patient position, palpation of breast margins, and examination pattern and technique are important. The supine position is preferable for palpation because CBE requires flattening breast tissue against the patient's chest, and the distance from skin to chest wall is minimized with the patient supine. The patient's ipsilateral hand should be brought up to her head for examination of the lateral aspect of the breast; her elbow should be at shoulder level during examination of the medial part of the breast. The examination pattern should be systematic. It is important to include the area bordering the clavicle, and laterally toward the axilla, to ensure examination of all breast tissue.

During the examination, a rectangular area bordered by the clavicle, midsternum, midaxillary line, and "bra line" should be covered. The pattern of examination can be from outside to in (like spokes on a wheel) or in parallel,

vertical strips (the so-called lawnmower technique). The examiner should make circular motions at each step using the pads of the index, third, and fourth fingers (as if tracing the outer edge of a dime), with gradated pressure. Examination of the axillae for lymph nodes should follow examination of the breast. Examination along the chest wall is important. The position and size of any nodes should be recorded. The presence of lymphadenopathy should prompt referral to a breast surgeon, although the clinical significance of small (<1 cm) nodes is unclear.

The character of breast lumps is important. Characteristics that suggest cancer include a hard or gritty texture, immobility, an irregular border, and size greater than 2 cm. A new "dominant" mass, or a gritty or growing lump, deserves evaluation by a breast surgeon. Unfortunately, likelihood ratios that these signs indicate cancer are not large, except for the presence of fixed lesions and lump size greater than 2 cm (likelihood ratios of 2.4 and 1.9, respectively).[10]

Breast Self-examination

Monthly breast self-examination (BSE) has been frequently advocated and encouraged, but evidence for its effectiveness is weak. A case-control study nested within the Canadian National Breast Screening Study suggests that well-performed BSE may be effective. This study compared self-reported frequency of BSE with breast cancer mortality. Women who examined their breasts visually, used their finger pads for palpation, and used their 3 middle fingers had a lower breast cancer mortality.[11] Other studies, including a large randomized trial in China,[12] have failed to show a significant effect. The American Cancer Society (ACS) recommends including BSE in screening for breast cancer. The US Preventive Services Task Force (USPSTF) currently does not recommend BSE and notes that its use may increase the incidence of clinical assessments and biopsies. The National Cancer Institute (NCI) is silent on BSE, although it presents data from clinical trials, most of them showing no effect of BSE. The Canadian Task Force on Periodic Health Examination (CTF) recently revised its recommendations for BSE as a screening maneuver, noting that because there is some evidence of no benefit and good evidence of harm in BSE, it recommends that routine teaching of BSE be excluded from the periodic health examination of women.

Mammography

Mammography may be done as an adjunct to physical examination in the evaluation of breast lumps or as a screening tool in the absence of palpable lumps. Mammography is not generally useful in women under age 35 years who present with a lump of the breast.[13] Mammography is usually recommended as part of the evaluation in women older than 35 years who have a breast lump. Normal mammograms do not rule out breast cancer when a clinically suspicious lump is present. In such cases, mammography is a diagnostic adjunct to the surgeon and should *not* preclude referral. Mammographic findings that suggest cancer include increased density, irregular border, spiculation, and clustered irregular microcalcifications.

Whether and how to incorporate mammography in breast cancer screening programs are questions that have been debated vigorously. The ability of mammography to reduce morbidity and mortality has been contested, although the balance of evidence leans toward reduced breast cancer mortality using this screening modality. The presence of false-positives (and the prolonged anxiety these results engender) has been cited as a reason for the clinician to be circumspect when offering them. The possibility of false-negative results with mammography (more likely in younger women), and the false reassurance they give, is one of the strongest reasons to continue CBE as part of screening.

Previous estimates of mortality reduction derived from the screening trials varied from 26% for women aged 50 through 74 years to 18% (with follow-up of 10 to 18 years) for women who began getting screening mammograms in their 40s. More recent reanalysis by the USPSTF yielded an estimated mortality reduction of 16% for women of all ages covered in the screening trials.[14] It is apparent from mammographic registry data that the overall sensitivity of mammograms is approximately 81%, but sensitivity is less than 70% in women under age 40 years and improves with advancing age.[15] The overall positive predictive value (PPV) of mammography is surprisingly low, in the 3% to 4% range, which is comparable with the PPV of CBE. The PPV of mammography is better for women with a family history of breast cancer due to higher prior probability and improves with older age. The PPV is 7% in women in their 60s with a family history. Concern about lack of sensitivity of mammography refocuses our attention on the utility of CBE in screening.

The age at which to begin screening mammography is controversial. In addition to the debates over possible harm of false-positive and false-negative studies, there is concern about the numbers of women needed to be screened to prevent a death due to breast cancer. In the recent USPSTF summary, the "number needed to screen" (NNS) to prevent 1 breast cancer death ranged from 1224 (women of all ages) to 1792 (women aged 40 to 49 years).[14] The ACS and the USPSTF recommend starting screening mammography at age 40 years, although the USPSTF notes the problems with screening women in their 40s. The CTF recommends starting mammography at age 50 years. The NCI notes the controversies surrounding screening but maintains a recommendation to offer mammography every 1 or 2 years for women aged 40 to 70 years.

Ultrasonography

Ultrasonography does not have a role as a single or initial study in screening for breast cancer. However, it is useful for evaluating palpable lumps and in further defining mammographic abnormalities. It is especially useful in women younger than 35 years, when a "mass" is noted on screening mammography but is not palpable, when a patient declines aspiration of a nodule, and if a mass is too small or deep for aspiration.

The risk of cancer is low if a simple cyst is found on ultrasound. One study found no cancers is 223 cysts.[16] However, some experts recommend going directly to fine-needle aspiration if a cyst is found at the site of a palpable mass.[17]

Fine-needle Aspiration

Fine-needle aspiration can be performed to aspirate a palpable lump that is a suspected cyst. The practitioner inserts a 22- or 24-gauge needle into a cyst that has been stabilized with the other hand. If fluid without blood is obtained, it can be discarded. No cancers were found in nonbloody fluid from cysts in a large series.[18] A clinical recheck should be performed in 4 to 6 weeks; recurrence of the lump should prompt surgical referral. Cancer is found in approximately 1% of bloody aspirates. When no fluid is obtained, cells aspirated can be sent for cytologic evaluation (fine-needle aspiration biopsy).

Core Needle Biopsy

A larger needle (14- to 18-gauge) is used for core needle biopsy. This technique is used mostly for evaluating non-palpable breast masses (those found on mammography only). The procedure is performed with ultrasound or mammographic guidance. Agreement between results of core needle biopsy and those of surgical biopsy was 94% in several studies.[19]

Triple Diagnosis

The use of the physical examination, mammography, and fine-needle aspiration biopsy for diagnosing palpable lumps is referred to as "triple diagnosis." Sensitivity and specificity, both in the 99% range, are excellent with this approach.[20] If results of any of these 3 modalities suggest cancer, excisional biopsy is warranted.

Magnet Resonance Imaging

Magnetic resonance imaging (MRI) has been used to evaluate palpable masses, but its role in screening for breast cancer is not established. The PPV for an incidentally discovered solitary lesion on a magnetic resonance image of the breast in women who did not have prior breast cancer was less than 2%.[21] False-positive results are common. The role of MRI in breast imaging includes evaluating the integrity of silicone breast implants, assessing palpable masses after surgery or radiation therapy (it is useful in distinguishing a scar from cancer), and detecting breast cancer in patients with axillary nodal metastasis, when mammogram and ultrasound results are negative.

Ductal Lavage

Ductal lavage is a newer technology approved by the Food and Drug Administration (FDA) in which milk ducts of the nipple are cannulated and cells are obtained via saline lavage. Cytologic analysis is then applied to the cells to evaluate for atypia. Ductal lavage has been studied as a means to further evaluate high-risk women. Ductal lavage was performed in 383 women with either a history of breast cancer or a 5-year risk, using the Gail Model, of 1.7% or more; 299 (78%) of those women had samples adequate for cytologic interpretation.[22] Of the samples, 17% showed mild atypia, 6% showed marked atypia, and 1 showed malignancy. Ductal lavage has not been tested in a controlled screening trial but has been suggested as a means to stratify risk and to aid in decisions about chemoprevention or prophylactic mastectomy.

GENERAL SCREENING RECOMMENDATIONS

Several breast cancer screening guidelines have been outlined in North America. Table 30-1 outlines and compares screening guidelines for 4 major expert organizations or task forces. The American Cancer Society (ACS) recommendations as of January 2002 are that women begin

monthly BSE at age 20 years, have a CBE by a health care professional every 3 years between ages 20 and 39 years, and starting at age 40 have CBE and mammography annually.[23] National Cancer Institute recommendations were reaffirmed in January 2002, as follows: Women in their 40s should be screened every 1 to 2 years with mammography. Women aged 50 years and older should be screened every 1 to 2 years. Women who are at higher-than-average risk of breast cancer should seek expert medical advice about whether they should begin screening before age 40 and about the frequency of screening. Both the ACS and NCI have dropped recommendations for baseline screening mammography for women at age 35 years.

The USPSTF recommendations were updated in February 2002. They recommend screening mammography with or without CBE every 1 to 2 years for women aged 40 years and older and conclude that evidence is strongest for screening women aged 50 to 69 years. For women aged 40 to 49 years, evidence that screening mammography reduces mortality from breast cancer is weaker, and the absolute benefit is smaller than for older women. The USPSTF concludes that the evidence can be generalized to screening women aged 70 years and older if their life expectancy is not compromised by comorbid disease.[24]

The CTF recommends CBE and mammography every 1 or 2 years for women between 50 and 70 years of age as part of the periodic health examination. They note that current evidence of the effectiveness of screening mammography does not suggest the inclusion of mammography in, or its exclusion from, the periodic health examination of women aged 40 to 49 years at average risk of breast cancer.

TABLE 30-1

Recommendations for Breast Cancer Screening With Clinical Breast Examination (CBE) and Mammography (MGM)

Age, y	American Cancer Society	US Preventive Services Task Force	National Cancer Institute	Canadian Task Force on the Periodic Health Examination
20–39	CBE every 3 y ("no baseline" MGM)	No recommendations	No data for benefit, nor for performing baseline MGM	No recommendations
40–49	CBE and MGM yearly	MGM with or without CBE every 1–2 y	MGM every 1–2 y (screening data reviewed, value of CBE discussed, no formal CBE recommendation)	Recommend against screening (encourages discussion between patient and physician for high-risk patients)
50–69	CBE and MGM yearly	MGM with or without CBE every 1–2 y	MGM every 1–2 y with or without CBE	CBE and MGM during periodic health examination
≥70	Cessation of screening is not age related but due to comorbidity	MGM with or without CBE every 1–2 y, if life expectancy is not compromised by comorbidity	Screening may or may not be helpful	No recommendations

OUTCOMES OF SCREENING, CHEMOPREVENTION, AND TREATMENT

The age-adjusted breast cancer mortality has been declining about 2% per year since 1991 in the United States. A similar decrease has been noted in the United Kingdom. Breast cancer mortality has been decreasing even among women excluded from screening protocols by age.[25] Good evidence exists that adjuvant hormonal and cytotoxic treatment reduces mortality.[26,27] Recent controversy has occurred regarding the effectiveness of screening mammography. A previous meta-analysis of breast cancer screening trials yielded an estimated mortality reduction of 26% in screened women aged 50 to 74 years.[28] The most optimistic estimates of mortality reduction in women who began getting screening mammograms in their 40s is 16% to 18%. A greater proportion of screening mammograms are false-positive and false-negative among women in their 40s.[29,30]

Some recent analyses have raised questions about the degree of mortality reduction that is achieved with screening mammography. There have been 8 large trials of breast cancer screening that included mammography: The Health Insurance Plan/New York, NY; 2 Canadian National Breast Screening Studies (CNBSS-1 and CNBSS-2); Edinburgh, Scotland; Gothenburg, Stockholm; Malmö, Sweden; and the Swedish Two-County Trial. It was observed that, by 1999, breast cancer mortality had not significantly declined in Sweden, where some of the trials yielding more optimistic results had occurred and where screening protocols had been in place since 1985. Gotzsche and Olsen[31] excluded 5 of the 8 major trials, which they judged to have inadequate randomization; when they analyzed the remaining studies, the pooled relative risk of breast cancer mortality in women who underwent screening mammography was 1.04, suggesting no benefit for mammography. Whether major screening trials should be excluded from overall analysis has subsequently been the subject of much debate. A recent summary of the evidence for the USPSTF excluded only the Edinburgh trial (which the authors rated as poor quality because of significantly lower socioeconomic status and all-cause mortality in the control group, suggesting inadequate randomization).[14] The analysis by Humphrey et al[14] of 7 of the 8 trials of screening yielded an overall relative risk of breast cancer death of 0.84 (overall mortality reduction of 16% for women of all ages covered in 7 trials). Their estimates of NNS to prevent 1 breast cancer death were 1224 for women of all ages; and 1792 for women 40 to 49 years of age. The current consensus remains that screening mammography has a role in reducing mortality, but estimation of the magnitude of the effect has been tempered.

Debate has occurred regarding whether to include CBE in screening programs. Only 4 of the 8 randomized controlled trials of breast cancer screening (HIP/New York, the 2 Canadian trials, and the Edinburgh trial) included CBE; all 8 included mammography. No randomized trials of CBE as a sole screening modality have been performed. In the trials that included both CBE and mammography, training in CBE as well as mammography technology differed among the studies. Recognizing these differences, it is still apparent that there appears to be an incremental value of CBE beyond mammography. The range of breast cancers found by CBE but not by mammography was 3% to 45% in these 4 trials that included both screening tools; the average incremental value of CBE was 21%. The sensitivity of mammography for all ages as assessed via several large mammographic registries was 81%. The sensitivity is lower for women who are younger and increases with age of the women being screened.[15]

The ACS and the Canadian Task Force recommend CBE along with mammography (see Table 29-1). The USPSTF recommends mammography with or without CBE. The NCI recommends screening mammography and is silent on CBE. However, its discussion of breast cancer screening for health professionals covers the sensitivity, specificity, and PPV of CBE and compares it more favorably with mammography than in previous analyses.

An analysis of 752,081 CBEs performed between 1995 and 1998 as part of the National Breast and Cervical Cancer Early Detection Program found that 6.9% of CBE results were abnormal and that 3.8 invasive cancers and 1.2 cases of DCIS were detected per 1000 examinations. Sensitivity was 58.8%, specificity was 93.4%, and PPV was 4.3%; this compares favorably with the PPV of mammography.[32]

Chemoprevention of breast cancer is an area of intense interest in recent years. The National Surgical Adjuvant Breast and Bowel Project (NSABP) P-1 Breast Cancer Prevention Trial achieved a 49% reduction in the incidence of invasive breast disease in women at increased risk of breast cancer.[33] To be eligible for randomization, women were 60 years of age or older, or were aged 35 to 59 years with a 5-year predicted risk (by the Gail Model) of breast cancer of at least 1.66%, or had a history of lobular carcinoma in situ. These findings have stimulated further interest in risk assessment and identification of candidates for chemoprevention, as well as the ongoing Study of Raloxifene and Tamoxifen (STAR) trial to compare effectiveness of tamoxifen and raloxifene in chemoprevention. The greatest concern with tamoxifen is an elevated risk of thromboembolism. Currently, the criteria that were used in the NSABP P-1 trial are employed to help women assess their candidacy for chemoprevention. Efforts are under way to help define a subgroup more likely to benefit from chemoprevention. Parallel advances in understanding some of the genetic markers of very high risk (including BRCA-1 and BRCA-2) have had impact on decision making in addressing clinical dilemmas, including who should have genetic testing, whether newer techniques such as ductal lavage should be recommended, and whether to consider prophylactic mastectomy.

A retrospective study was performed to evaluate the impact of bilateral prophylactic mastectomy on subsequent breast cancer risk.[34] Most women had undergone subcutaneous rather than total mastectomy. The reduction in risk for women at moderate risk was 89% and for high-risk women was 90% to 94%. Information on BRCA-1 or BRCA-2 status was not known. Misclassification may have led to overestimation of the benefit. Bilateral prophylactic mastectomy should be considered in association with counseling regarding all the preventive options, which include tamoxifen chemoprevention.

FUTURE DIRECTIONS IN SCREENING AND PREVENTION

An ideal scenario from a public health perspective would be a reduction in breast cancer due to a concerted, multi-level population risk factor reduction. Although lifestyle factors individually confer lesser risks than some inherited factors do, the majority of women in whom breast cancer develops do not have a known genetic predisposition. Reduction in intake of dietary fat and alcohol, increase in physical activity, and reduction in weight could all have a positive effect on reducing the incidence of breast cancer.

Improved knowledge of the genetics of breast cancer should improve the ability to identify the subgroup of women at highest risk of breast cancer. Better data are needed on the role of ductal lavage in helping to further stratify risk. Hand in hand with better risk stratification is the need for better understanding of the risks and benefits of chemoprevention and of the role of prophylactic mastectomy. Inherent in this expanding knowledge is the responsibility to counsel patients about the evolving data on breast cancer prevention.

REFERENCES

1. Jemal A, Thomas A, Murray T, Thun M. Cancer statistics, 2002. *CA Cancer J Clin.* 2002;52:23–47.

2. Stoll BA. Quantifying the risk of breast cancer. *Eur J Surg Oncol.* 1991;17:36–41.

3. Gail MH, Brinton LA, Byar DP, et al. Projecting individualized probabilities of developing breast cancer for white females who are being examined annually. *J Natl Cancer Inst.* 1989;81:1879–1886.

4. Slattery ML, Kerber RA. A comprehensive evaluation of family history and breast cancer risk: the Utah population database. *JAMA.* 1993;270:1563–1568.

5. Ang P, Garber JE. Genetic susceptibility for breast cancer: risk assessment and counseling. *Semin Oncol.* 2001;28:419–433.

6. Collaborative Group on Hormonal Factors in Breast Cancer. Breast cancer and hormone replacement therapy: collaborative reanalysis of data from 51 epidemiologic studies in 52,705 women with breast cancer and 108,411 women without cancer. *Lancet.* 1997;350:1047–1059.

7. Gapstur SM, Morrow M, Sellers TA. Hormone replacement therapy and risk of breast cancer with a favorable histology: results of the Iowa Women's Health Study. *JAMA.* 1999;281:2091–2097.

8. Writing Group for the Women's Health Initiative Investigators. Risks and benefits of estrogen plus progestin in health postmenopausal women: principal results from the Women's Health Initiative Randomized Controlled Trial. *JAMA.* 2002;288:321–333.

9. O'Meara ES, Rossing MA, Daling JR, Elmore JG, Barlow WE, Weiss NS. Hormone replacement therapy after a diagnosis of breast cancer in relation to recurrence and mortality. *J Natl Cancer Inst.* 2001;93:754–762.

10. Barton MB, Harris R, Fletcher SW. Does this patient have breast cancer? The screening clinical breast examination: should it be done? How? *JAMA.* 1999;282:1270–1280.

11. Harvey BJ, Miller AB, Baines CJ, et al. Effect of breast self-examination techniques on the risk of death from breast cancer. *Can Med Assoc J.* 1997;157:1205–1212.

12. Thomas DB, Gao DL, Ray RM, et al. Randomized trial of breast self-examination in Shanghai: final results. *J Natl Cancer Inst.* 2002;94:1445–1457.

13. Hindle WH, Davis L, Wright D. Clinical value of mammography for symptomatic women 35 years of age and younger. *Am J Obstet Gynecol.* 1999;180(pt 1):1484–1490.

14. Humphrey LL, Helfand M, Chan BKS, Woolf SH. Breast cancer screening: a summary of the evidence for the U.S. Preventive Services Task Force. *Ann Intern Med.* 2002;137:347–360.

15. Kerlikowske K, Carney PA, Geller B, et al. Performance of screening mammography among women with and without a first-degree relative with breast cancer. *Ann Intern Med.* 2000;133:855–863.

16. Sickles EA, Filly RA, Callen PW. Benign breast lesions: ultrasound detection and diagnosis. *Radiology.* 1984;151:467–470.

17. Donegan WL. Evaluation of a palpable breast mass. *N Engl J Med.* 1992;3327:937–942.

18. Ciatto S, Cariaggi P, Bulgaresi P. The value of routine cytologic examination of breast cyst fluids. *Acta Cytol.* 1987;31:301–304.

19. Evans WP. Stereotactic core breast biopsy. In: Harris JR, Lippman ME, Morrow M, Hellman S, eds. *Diseases of the Breast.* Philadelphia, Pa: Lippincott-Raven Publishers; 1996:144–151.

20. Layfield LJ, Glasgow BJ, Cramer H. Fine-needle aspiration in the management of breast masses. *Pathol Annu.* 1989;24(pt 2):23–62.

21. Kuhl CK, Bieling HB, Gieseke J, et al. Healthy premenopausal breast parenchyma in dynamic contrast-enhanced MR imaging of the breast: normal contrast medium enhancement and cyclical-phase dependency. *Radiology.* 1997;203:137–144.

22. Dooley WC, Ljung BM, Veronesi U, et al. Ductal lavage for detection of cellular atypia in women at high risk for breast cancer. *J Natl Cancer Inst.* 2001;93:1624–1632.

23. Smith RA, Cokkinides V, Eschenbach AC, et al. American Cancer Society guidelines for the early detection of cancer. *CA Cancer J Clin.* 2002:52:8–22.

24. US Preventive Services Task Force. Screening for breast cancer: recommendations and rationale. *Ann Intern Med.* 2002;137:344–346.

25. Peto R, Boreham J, Clarke M, Davies C, Beral V. UK and USA breast cancer deaths down 25% in year 2000 at ages 20–69 years. *Lancet.* 2000;355:1822.

26. Early Breast Cancer Trialists' Collaborative Group. Tamoxifen for early breast cancer: an overview of the randomised trials. *Lancet.* 1998;351:1451–1467.

27. Early Breast Cancer Trialists' Collaborative Group. Polychemotherapy for early breast cancer: an overview of the randomised trials. *Lancet.* 1998;352:930–942.

28. Kerlikowske K, Grady D, Rubin S, Sandrock C, Ernster VL. Efficacy of screening mammography: a meta-analysis. *JAMA.* 1995;273:149–154.

29. Berry DA. Benefits and risks of screening mammography for women in their forties: a statistical appraisal. *J Natl Cancer Inst.* 1998;90:1431–1439.

30. Rajkumar SV, Hartmann LC. Screening mammography in women aged 40–49 years. *Medicine.* 1999;78:410-416.

31. Gotzsche PC, Olsen O. Is screening for breast cancer with mammography justifiable? *Lancet.* 2000;355:129–134.

32. Bobo JK, Lee NC, Thames SF. Findings from 752,081 clinical breast examinations reported to a national screening program from 1995 through 1998. *J Natl Cancer Inst.* 2000;92:971–976.

33. Fisher B, Costantino JP, Wickerham DL, et al. Tamoxifen for prevention of breast cancer: report of National Surgical Adjuvant Breast and Bowel Project P-1 study. *J Natl Cancer Inst.* 1998;90:1371–1388.

34. Hartmann LC, Schaid DJ, Woods JE, et al. Efficacy of bilateral prophylactic mastectomy in women with a family history of breast cancer. *N Engl J Med.* 1999;340:77–84.

RESOURCES

National Cancer Institute, 800 422-6237.

Web site: www.cancer.gov/cancerinformation/cancertype/breast. (Information about breast cancer; Gail Model Breast Cancer Risk Assessment Tool can be obtained by calling toll-free number.)

National Guideline Clearinghouse.

Web site: www.guidelines.gov. (Comparison of recommendations by organizations regarding screening.)

chapter 31

Gynecologic Cancers

Bobbie S. Gostout, MD

INTRODUCTION

Women are uniquely susceptible to the premalignant and malignant changes that affect the female reproductive system, including the uterus, fallopian tubes, ovaries, vagina, and vulva. Gynecologic cancers refer to a variety of neoplasms affecting girls and women throughout the life span. Prevention strategies are specific to the cancers that affect individual organs, but some themes are common to all. Early cancer detection can be lifesaving, and for many of the gynecologic cancers, early detection requires that women attend to and seek evaluation for subtle symptoms. Frequently, women with gynecologic cancers seek evaluation because of vaginal bleeding at unexpected times such as in a young girl before menarche, between periods in a woman of reproductive age, or unexpected bleeding after menopause. Pain is an uncommon sign of early cancer, and women are encouraged to seek preventive care and screening examinations so that changes can be detected before cancers become advanced to the point of causing pain.

Endometrial cancer is the most common gynecologic cancer, whereas cancer of the vagina is the rarest (Table 31-1). Ovarian cancer causes more deaths each year than any of the other gynecologic cancers. Gynecologic cancers have different etiologic associations, underlying biology, and pathophysiological mechanisms; therefore, it is not surprising that the risk factors, ages at onset, and protective measures are quite diverse. The various gynecologic cancers and their prevention strategies are described in this chapter.

OVARIAN AND FALLOPIAN TUBE CANCERS

Prevention of ovarian, fallopian tube, and primary peritoneal cancers will be considered together since these 3 cancers share many common features. Of the 3, ovarian cancer is by far the most common. The overall mortality rate of ovarian cancer is high, making this a feared disease among women who are familiar with this cancer. Because the fallopian tubes are extensions of the uterus, it is easy to imagine that cancers arising in them might resemble uterine cancers. However, they are more likely to mimic ovarian cancer in their appearance, pattern of spread, and response to treatment. Very little is known about the risk factors for fallopian tube cancer. What information is available will be pointed out in the discussion on ovarian cancer risk and prevention. Primary peritoneal cancer is a malignancy that arises from the abdominal or pelvic peritoneum. In early organogenesis, the ovaries arise as an outpouching of the peritoneal lining, and it is no doubt this embryologic connection that determines the shared characteristics between ovarian cancer and primary peritoneal cancer. Primary peritoneal cancer can create a confusing clinical picture of "ovarian cancer" arising in women who have had their ovaries removed.

Currently, an affordable and reliable test is not available for early detection of ovarian and related cancers. In realizing the limitations of early detection, the American Cancer Society recommends only a pelvic examination during a regular check-up. There is still much to learn about modifiable risk factors, and this is an area of active research. The following are known factors that raise or decrease the risk of ovarian cancer. These risk factors can be modified to varying degrees.

TABLE 31-1

Incidence and Mortality due to Gynecologic Cancers*

Cancer Site	Annual No. of Cases	Annual Deaths	Typical Age, y, of Affected Women
Uterus	38,300	6600	50–70
Ovary	23,400	14,000	50–80
Cervix	12,900	4400	40–55
Vagina	2100	600	60+
Vulva	3600	800	60+

*From the American Cancer Society. Cancer Facts and Figures, 2001.

Oral Contraceptives

Oral contraceptives have been shown to have a significant protective effect on ovarian cancer in several epidemiologic studies.[1,2] There are no randomized controlled studies demonstrating conclusive proof of causality of this association, but it is consistent across retrospective studies. Longer use of oral contraceptives provides greater protection. Cumulative years of use appear to be more important than consecutive years of use. The protective effect of oral contraceptives led to the theory that some aspect of ovulation triggers changes that lead to ovarian cancer, and interruption of incessant ovulation by any means should decrease ovarian cancer risk. This theory is supported by evidence of protection against ovarian cancer by other conditions or treatments that decrease total ovulations.

Additionally, a second mechanistic theory is emerging. Recent work has suggested a possible protective contribution at the molecular level from the progesterone component of oral contraceptives. Proponents of this theory observe that certain progesterones trigger apoptosis in some cells, so that ovarian cells that have suffered minor genetic damage will be targeted for death before further damage can accumulate and lead to the formation of a fully committed cancer cell.[3]

Parity

The incessant ovulation theory would lead one to predict that pregnancy might also be protective toward ovarian cancer, and indeed this has been shown to be true. As with oral contraceptives, evidence suggests that more interruption of ovulation is better.[4,5] Women who have had no pregnancies have twice the risk of ovarian cancer as that in the average population, and the adverse effect of nulliparity may be enhanced for women from high-risk families.[6]

Fertility Drugs

The increased risk of ovarian cancer for women who have never been pregnant might be related to the absence of pregnancy, but in recent years researchers have also questioned the possible role that infertility treatments might play in ovarian cancer risk. This topic is still controversial, however, and it is difficult to sort out which, if any, agents used in the treatment of infertility might have a role in ovarian cancer risk.[7] Overall, the effects are questionable enough that women desiring fertility should choose treatments on the basis of probable effectiveness for their specific fertility needs, rather than on the basis of possible ovarian cancer risk.

Hysterectomy and Tubal Ligation

Interestingly, tubal ligation and hysterectomy both have been shown to provide protection from ovarian cancer.[8,9]

This may seem a contradiction to the discussion above since both procedures limit the number of possible pregnancies, thereby limiting a woman's protective effect of pregnancy. One possible reason is the observed effect of hysterectomy and tubal ligation on reproductive life span. On average, menopause occurs 1 year earlier in women who have had a hysterectomy or tubal ligation. This change could be considered equivalent to 1 additional pregnancy.

Breast-feeding

The effect of breast-feeding on ovarian cancer risk is controversial. Some research suggests that exclusive and prolonged breast-feeding can decrease the risk of ovarian cancer. Studies that have been less selective in the definition of breast-feeding have shown less or no significant effect on ovarian cancer risk.[5]

Endometriosis

Endometriosis is a risk factor for ovarian cancer.[10,11] The impact of medical or surgical treatment on subsequent risk is uncertain. It is reasonable to assume that this increased risk is diminished after surgical and medical treatment of endometriosis, but this has never been tested in a prospective study.

Prophylactic Oophorectomy

Surgical removal of the ovaries clearly provides protection from ovarian cancer. It is important for women selecting this option to recall that primary peritoneal cancer can still occur in women after oophorectomy. There is a wide range of estimates for the incidence of primary peritoneal cancer in women who underwent oophorectomy for ovarian cancer protection. The risk is probably in the range of 2% to 3% for women from families with a high risk of ovarian cancer.[12] The frequency is undoubtedly lower for women from average-risk families, but no reliable numbers exist. In general, fallopian tubes are removed along with ovaries, although often this is not specifically mentioned to the patient. Therefore, most fallopian tube cancers will be prevented when ovaries are removed.

Talc

A series of retrospective studies suggest that use of talc-containing products might be associated with increased risk.[13] There is no clear consensus, however, and, at most, talc exposure may cause a small increase in risk.[14]

Hormone Replacement Therapy

Postmenopausal hormone replacement therapy (HRT) is under increased scrutiny. Some studies have suggested a link to ovarian cancer, but study designs leave room for question. There are not enough solid data on the relationship between HRT and ovarian cancer risk to influence the decision about taking HRT.

Genetics

A family history of ovarian cancer is not a modifiable risk factor, but for those women with a strong history of breast or ovarian cancer or both, careful consideration of hereditary risk is warranted. Syndromes with both breast and ovarian cancer risk, and also site-specific hereditary ovarian cancer have been described. Women affected by hereditary nonpolyposis colorectal cancer syndrome (HNPCC) are also at elevated risk of ovarian cancer.[15] The lifetime risk of ovarian cancer in patients with BRCA-1 mutations may be as high as 45%, while the risk in women with BRCA-2 mutations is estimated at approximately 20%. The risk of fallopian tube cancer is elevated in the presence of hereditary breast and ovarian cancer, but the total number of fallopian tube cancers in this cohort is relatively small. Genetic consultation should be considered for all suspicious pedigrees.

Until a reliable means of screening and early detection is available, women with more than 1 first-degree or 1 first-degree plus 1 second-degree family member affected by ovarian cancer should be offered prophylactic oophorectomy when childbearing is complete. Options include laparoscopic removal of both fallopian tubes and ovaries vs hysterectomy with removal of tubes and ovaries. Prophylactic oophorectomy has the added advantage of decreasing a high-risk woman's odds of developing breast cancer, perhaps by as much as 50%.[16] Another option is protection through use of oral contraceptives. Ten years of oral contraceptive use is estimated to provide an 80% risk reduction in high-risk women.[17] However, women in this category should be appropriately cautious about oral contraceptive use because of the possible adverse influence on breast cancer risk.

Ovarian Germ Cell Tumors

Rarely, the ovaries are involved by malignant germ cell tumors or ovarian stromal cell tumors. These tumors affect young women more often than does epithelial ovarian cancer, but women of all ages can be affected. Germ cell and stromal cells tumors may produce hormonal abnormalities with clinical manifestations of excess estrogen or androgen, interruption of periods, or a pelvic mass. Risk factors for these tumors are mostly unknown, although germ cell tumors are more common in young women with genetic syndromes in which a Y chromosome is present. XY gonadal dysgenesis should be considered a diagnostic possibility when a young woman does not begin menstruation by age 15 years. Chromosome analysis should be considered as part of the evaluation of delayed menarche, and girls with Y chromosome abnormalities should be referred to a gynecologic oncologist for consultation. Prophylactic removal of the dysgenetic gonads is usually recommended, although the optimal age may depend on the specific syndrome.

UTERINE CANCER

The term *uterine cancer* is often used to denote cancer of the uterine lining. This type of cancer is more precisely called endometrial cancer to distinguish this common cancer from cancer of the uterine cervix and from unusual malignancies arising in the muscle wall of the uterus. Endometrial cancer is the most common of the gynecologic cancers. Traditionally this cancer has been associated with the best chance for survival of all the gynecologic cancers, partly because the cancer commonly triggers the symptom of abnormal vaginal bleeding, providing an opportunity for early diagnosis. However, over the past 15 years the death rate of endometrial cancer has more than doubled. The reason for this worrisome trend is unknown.

Estrogen Excess

Usually, the occurrence of endometrial cancer is the result of a relative or absolute excess of estrogen. In the United States, the majority of estrogen excess is due to obesity. During the premenopausal years, excess adipose tissue causes changes in the hormone balance that are associated with insulin resistance and suppression of ovulation. During the postmenopausal years, fat cells continue to produce the weak estrogen, estrone, causing long-term low-level stimulation of the endometrium.

Estrogen excess may also occur as a result of medication use. Estrogen-containing medications are used to manage conditions such as hot flashes and sleep disturbances of menopause, osteoporosis, and urogenital atrophy. The preventive role of estrogens for cardiovascular conditions, including heart attacks and strokes, has come into question since the release of data from the Women's Health Initiative study.[18] When estrogens were first introduced for the treatment of menopausal symptoms, the cancer-causing effect of estrogens alone was demonstrated. From this unintended experiment, the concept of balanced estrogen plus progesterone treatment was adopted and remains the standard treatment today whenever the uterus is in place and estrogens are indicated. Whether in the form of daily combined estrogen plus progesterone treatment as in oral contraceptives or daily vs cyclic estrogen plus progesterone hormone replacement regimens, combining estrogens with progesterones effectively mitigates the endometrial cancer-promoting action of estrogen alone.

Other common medications that affect uterine estrogen activity are listed in Table 31-2. When endometrial

Medications That Affect Uterine Estrogen Activity

Drug Class	Medication	Effects
Nonsteroidal antiestrogen	Tamoxifen	Antiestrogen for breast tissue, weak estrogen for endometrium, uterine cancer relative risk 2.5
Selective estrogen receptor modulator (SERM)	Raloxifene	Antiestrogen for breast tissue, no significant effect on the endometrium, uterine cancer relative risk 1.0
Nonsteroidal aromatase inhibitor	Anastrozole	≥70% systemic reduction in circulating estrogen
Intravaginal estrogens	Conjugated estrogen cream, estradiol cream	Weak systemic effect; increased absorption and therefore potential for increased systemic effect in women with vaginal atrophy

stimulation is possible as a result of medications such as tamoxifen or vaginal estrogen creams, physicians should counsel patients about risks and caution women to report any vaginal spotting or bleeding. Ultrasound surveillance of endometrial thickness may be useful for women receiving long-term therapy with vaginal estrogen cream. However, ultrasound is of questionable value in women receiving tamoxifen therapy, where cystic atrophy frequently results in the appearance of a thickened endometrial stripe.[19,20]

In therapeutic use, estrogen plus progesterone is standard therapy, but when estrogen exposure is natural, the need to supplement progesterone may not be as obvious. The primary clinical symptom of polycystic ovary syndrome (PCO) is infrequent menses, with or without symptoms of androgen excess. Infertility or subfertility is common. Ovulation induction is the recommended treatment for women desiring pregnancy. However, women who do not have regular menses and do not desire fertility should consider the possibility of using oral contraceptives or cyclic progesterone to guard against endometrial hyperplasia and endometrial cancer. Cyclic progesterone supplementation or oral contraceptives should be prescribed for women with menstrual intervals of 3 months or longer, or 4 or fewer menses per year. If the menstrual history is unclear, endometrial biopsy or ultrasound should be used as a screen for endometrial hyperplasia to determine the need for progesterone supplementation.[21]

Recently, consumers have been provided with information about the health benefits of natural estrogens from plant sources. These phytoestrogens have been touted as one reason for the reported low incidence of menopausal symptoms in women consuming an Asian diet. Interestingly, Asian women have a risk of uterine cancer 40 times lower than that of US women, suggesting that soy phytoestrogens do not produce substantial endometrial stimulation. One possible explanation is that phytoestrogens are weak estrogens—too weak to cause an increase in cancer incidence.

Endometrial Cancer Without Estrogen Excess

It is clear that excess or unbalanced estrogen stimulation can result in endometrial cancer. But what of the women who develop endometrial cancer in the absence of excess estrogens? Current theory divides endometrial cancer into 2 categories, type 1 and type 2 endometrial cancer, based on the early description published by Bokhman.[22] The discussion above pertains to type 1 cancers. The causes of type 2 endometrial cancers for women with no history of estrogen excess are largely unknown. Cancers arising in women without estrogen excess tend to be more unpredictable in their clinical course. Genetic predisposition contributes to a fraction of these cases. In women affected with HNPCC, endometrial cancer is the second most common malignancy, with lifetime risk approximating 20%.[23] Prophylactic hysterectomy with bilateral salpingo-oophorectomy should be offered to women affected with HNPCC when childbearing is complete. Annual screening with endometrial biopsy can be offered to women who do not want a hysterectomy, although it must be acknowledged that the procedure is uncomfortable and the benefits of such screening have not been tested in clinical trials.

Nonendometrial Uterine Cancers

Approximately 3% of uterine malignancies arise from the muscle wall of the uterus or from the stromal tissue underlying the glands. This group of malignancies includes leiomyosarcoma, endometrial stromal sarcoma, and uterine carcinosarcoma (also called malignant mixed mullerian tumor). These uncommon malignancies appear to be increasing in frequency and are more deadly than uterine endometrial carcinoma. Most sarcomas arise in individuals with no known predisposing conditions. However, prior pelvic radiation increases a woman's risk of sarcomas and rare, predisposing genetic conditions have been recognized. Recently, an association between the use of tamoxifen and uterine sarcomas has been reported.[24,25] Fortunately, sarcomas remain rare even in tamoxifen-treated women.

Given these risk factors, what can a woman do to reduce her risk of uterine cancer? Women should be advised to maintain a healthy weight through balanced eating and exercise. During the menstruating years, it is important to maintain menstrual regularity, if necessary through the use of medication. Oral contraceptives offer significant protection against endometrial cancer after as little as 1 year of use.[26] Current standards support the use of progesterone medication in addition to estrogens in postmenopausal women who have not had a hysterectomy if they choose to use HRT. There are well-documented benefits from the use of tamoxifen in women who have had breast cancer or are at risk of breast cancer, and the risk of uterine cancers and sarcomas does not negate the overall advantages gained by appropriate use of this drug. However, women who are receiving or have received tamoxifen should be especially alert for signs of abnormal uterine bleeding, as follows:

1. bleeding between menstrual periods
2. bleeding after intercourse
3. menses lasting longer than 7 days, especially if that is a change
4. menstrual bleeding requiring change in protection more than once every 2 hours
5. any vaginal bleeding after menopause, except regular bleeding induced by cyclic HRT

If abnormal uterine bleeding becomes a problem, women over age 35 years, regardless of risk factors, should receive careful evaluation, including an endometrial biopsy.

CERVICAL CANCER

The etiology, epidemiology, and preventive measures for cancers of the uterine cervix are distinct from those associated with cancer of the endometrium or muscular uterine wall. Historically, cervical cancer ranked as the leading cause of cancer death in women. Fortunately, in the United States the number of deaths due to cervical cancer has decreased dramatically, although the virus that causes cervical cancer is at least as prevalent today as it was 50 years ago and there is still no effective treatment of the virus. In 1928 Dr George Nicholas Papanicolaou first reported on the potential for detecting cervical cancer at a treatable stage through the use of cervical cytology. The Papanicolaou (Pap) test did not come into common use until the 1950s, but today it is recognized as one of the most effective cancer screening and prevention tools ever developed. Of note is that the efficacy of the Pap test has never been proved in a randomized, controlled trial. However, temporal trends and other indirect evidence strongly support its value.

The human papillomaviruses (HPV) that cause more than 90% of cervical cancers are members of a large family of viruses with an array of hosts and a spectrum of disease manifestations. More than 200 HPV types have been at least partially characterized. The HPV types that are fully characterized are assigned a number. A new type is identified if an HPV virus is found to have less than 90% homology with any known type. Certain HPV types, such as types 6 and 11, are associated with genital warts and mild Pap test abnormalities. Other types, especially types 16 and 18, are associated with more severe Pap test abnormalities and cervical cancer. Still other types cause common skin warts and plantar warts. We know that the HPV types that cause common warts and plantar warts are found in the environment and can be transferred from person to person. It is believed that this transfer does not require direct contact.

In contrast, there is evidence that cervical infection with HPV does require intimate contact and that transmission through contact other than sexual intercourse is unusual. It is not known whether men or women can come in contact with HPV through nonsexual contact and subsequently transfer the virus to the susceptible cervix of the female through sexual intercourse. It is known that HPV infection is by far the most common sexually transmitted disease (STD) and that somehow this infection has been transmitted to an estimated 75% of sexually active women. If HPV is transmitted only sexually, then this virus has somehow managed to spread through the community of sexually active adults in a more aggressive manner than herpes, the acquired immunodeficiency syndrome (AIDS), chlamydia, or any other STD. Fortunately, most men and women have no clinical sequelae from HPV exposure. A study of young women demonstrated that after exposure to HPV, 52% of women cleared the virus without clinical sequelae. An additional 37% intermittently had the same virus type detectable on their cervix, and 8% consistently tested positive for the same virus over 13 to 40 months of observation.[27] The 2-year incidence of moderate to severe cervical dysplasia after a positive HPV test has been estimated at 28%,[28] and the risk of dysplasia is dramatically elevated in women with persistence of the same virus type over 2 years.[29]

Host factors are thought to influence the likelihood that a woman will acquire a clinically significant cervical infection with HPV. Age at exposure is thought to be a prominent host factor. Women who report first coitus during their early teen years have a higher chance of cervical cancer and dysplasia developing, although some argue that this increase is due to the overall increase in the number of sexual partners in women reporting early age at first coitus.[30] Conditions associated with suppressed immune function increases the chance that exposure to the virus will result in dysplasia and cancer. Infection with AIDS and transplant drugs are potent immune suppressors that increase the virulence of HPV infection. However, these factors are responsible for only a small fraction of cervical cancer cases. Far more commonly, cigarette smoking has a mild immunosuppressive effect that appears to play a very significant role in promoting cervical cancer. In addition to immunosuppression, tobacco use may contribute to cervical cancer risk through a variety of different mechanisms. The net effect is a twofold to threefold elevated risk of cervical cancer in women who smoke.[31]

Beyond host factors, an important consideration in determining whether a woman will develop cervical cancer is which of the multiple HPV types she is exposed to. The likelihood of being exposed to the high-risk types increases with increasing number of sexual partners, such that women with a lifetime history of 8 or more sexual partners have an 18% to 59% chance, depending on age, of harboring high-risk HPV types.[32]

Prevention Through Screening

The messages in the preceding paragraphs might leave readers with the fatalistic notion that HPV exposure is an almost inevitable consequence of sexual activity. Except for lifelong mutually monogamous couples, this might be true. However, HPV exposure is not synonymous with cervical cancer, especially for women who undergo regular screening with a Pap test. Most Pap test abnormalities are a consequence of HPV infection, but fortunately with time or treatment, most dysplasia resolves.

In 2003, the American Cancer Society revised their cervical cancer screening recommendations.[33] The new

recommendations include descriptions of optimal use of the sample collection techniques for the newer liquid-based Pap test. Just 6 months after these recommendations were released, the US Food and Drug Administration (FDA) approved the application of the Hybrid Capture II test for HPV to be used for cervical cancer screening. These 2 changes are rapidly being incorporated into clinical practice. New guidelines for Pap test screening are briefly summarized in Table 31-3. The addition of direct testing for HPV as part of cervical cancer screening for women over 30 years of age means that women and their doctors will no longer have to guess at individual risk categories by reviewing sexual history risk factors. Instead, women can be directly tested for the presence or absence of the virus types that are known to cause cervical cancer. With direct testing for HPV, women with low-risk sexual histories can be appropriately alerted to continue Pap test screening if they are found to be carriers of cancer-causing HPV types, thereby reducing the risk of dangerous complacency. Conversely, women with histories of higher risk behavior might be reassured to find that they do not harbor cancer-causing virus types, so that maximal screening effort can be directed to those women at highest risk. All women will benefit by the new screening methods that make the direct association between HPV, cervical dysplasia, and cervical cancer more apparent.

Recommendations for follow-up of abnormal Pap test results have also recently been revised.[34] As a result of recent research and collaborative thought, many providers test for high-risk HPV types to triage indeterminate or atypical squamous cells of undetermined significance

T A B L E   31-3

American Cancer Society Cervical Cancer Screening Guidelines, 2003*

Screening Parameter	Screening Guideline
When to begin screening	Approximately 3 y after onset of vaginal intercourse, no later than 21 y of age
When to discontinue screening	At age ≥70 y if a woman has had ≥3 documented, consecutive, technically satisfactory normal Pap test results and no abnormal test results within 10 y. Continue screening 70+-year-old women with a history of cervical cancer, DES exposure, women who test positive for high-risk HPV types, or women who are immunocompromised.
Screening intervals	Screen annually with conventional smears or every 2 y with liquid-based Pap test.
Screening women aged ≥30 y	If a woman has had 3 consecutive, technically satisfactory, normal smears, then screen every 2–3 y after age 30 y unless she has had no exposure to DES or is immunocompromised.
HPV testing for women aged ≥30 y	As alternative to cervical cytology alone, cervical cancer screening may be performed every 3 y using cytology combined with test for high-risk HPV DNA.
After hysterectomy	If complete hysterectomy is performed for benign reasons (CIN two thirds is not benign), screening is no longer indicated. If a woman has had subtotal hysterectomy, DES exposure, or cervical cancer, she should continue to be screened.

*Pap indicates Papanicolaou; DES, diethylstilbestrol; HPV, human papilloma virus; and CIN, cervical intraepithelial neoplasia. From Smith et al.[33]

(ASCUS) Pap test results. New guidelines reflect a refocusing of effort to identify and treat high-grade dysplasia, while emphasizing the avoidance of overtreatment of low-grade dysplasia. The importance of thoughtful assessment of glandular abnormalities is also emphasized.

Vaccines for Prevention

Development of an HPV vaccine is an area of active research with promising early results. In a recently reported clinical trial, a viruslike particle HPV 16 vaccine provided remarkable protection from acquisition of a long-term infection with HPV 16.[35] Since HPV 16 is the most common virus type associated with cancer, accounting for an estimated 50% of cervical cancers in the United States, protection from this one virus type alone could have a huge impact on the worldwide incidence of cervical cancer. Importantly, vaccine therapy appears promising for prevention if administered before exposure to HPV. Vaccine therapy for established HPV infection, precancer, or invasive cancer does not appear as promising.

VAGINAL AND VULVAR CANCER

Vaginal and vulvar cancers are the least common gynecologic cancers. In many cases, the causes of these cancers are unknown. Certain conditions that cause long-term vulvar irritation are associated with increased risk of vulvar cancer. Clear cell cancer is an aggressive form of vaginal cancer strongly associated with exposure to diethylstilbestrol (DES) during early embryo formation.[36] During the 1950s, DES was prescribed for pregnant women with the intent of preventing miscarriage. Two decades later, the cancer-promoting effects that this seemingly innocuous treatment had on female offspring were finally recognized. Women who have a history of DES exposure require careful physical examination and Pap test screening of not only the uterine cervix but the entire vagina. The lessons of the DES story serve as a reminder of the importance of avoiding all unnecessary medications during pregnancy.

An increasingly common cause of vaginal and vulvar cancer is HPV. While HPV causes more than 90% of cervical cancers, the same virus is also associated with vaginal and vulvar precancer and cancer. Some women with HPV experience its effects at all 3 sites: cervical, vaginal, and vulvar. Because of the possibility that HPV might infect vaginal tissues, women who undergo hysterectomy for cervical cancer or precancer should continue to have Pap tests of the vagina after hysterectomy. The same risk factors and preventive aspects that were discussed for cervical cancer apply to HPV-induced cancer of the vagina and vulva. It is potentially beneficial to limit exposures to different sexual partners, avoid firsthand and secondhand tobacco smoke, use condoms, and avoid behaviors associated with increased risk of HIV infection and AIDS. Vulvar and vaginal dysplasia can be a particular problem for women receiving immune suppressive medications after kidney or bone marrow transplantation, highlighting the importance of gynecologic examinations for this group.

Studies suggest that HPV is found in approximately one half of vaginal and vulvar cancers.[37,38] Cancers associated with HPV typically occur in a background of vulvar or vaginal dysplasia. The cause of atrophic vulvar dystropy or lichen sclerosis is unknown; however, this condition is also associated with an increased risk of vulvar cancer. It is not known whether treatment of the vulvar dystrophy, usually with high-potency topical steroids, alters the subsequent risk of vulvar cancer.

As with the other gynecologic cancers, women should be aware of the symptoms of vulvar cancer so that they can seek proper evaluation and care. It most often presents as a plaquelike thickened area, or sometimes as a skin or mucosal ulcer that will not heal. Pigment changes are common, including a pale or red appearance. Vaginal and vulvar melanomas account for less than 2% of melanomas in women and present as black lesions much like those seen on other body surfaces.[39] Vaginal cancer is often asymptomatic unless a woman or her partner notices a vaginal plaque, a mass, or unexpected vaginal bleeding. In general, all vaginal and vulvar lesions, whether palpable or visible, require biopsy to determine the presence or absence of precancerous or malignant cells. Too often, a series of creams are prescribed over the course of several months before a biopsy is finally obtained and reveals the true diagnosis.

SUMMARY

Patients and physicians have access to measures that can reduce the risk of developing or dying of gynecologic cancers. The most important measures for prevention and early detection of gynecologic cancers include the following:

1. Perform Pap test screening according to guidelines appropriate for age and risk category for cervical cancer. All women who have had vaginal intercourse are at some level of risk.

2. In the appropriate clinical situation, consider the use of oral contraceptives for their cancer protection in addition to the contraceptive benefits. If pills are a reasonable option for a woman, consider accumulating 10 years of use through the reproductive years.

3. Counsel patients to eat a balanced diet high in cancer-fighting nutrients and to avoid obesity.

4. Educate patients on the symptoms of gynecologic cancer to improve the chance for early diagnosis.

REFERENCES

1. Bosetti C, Negri E, Trichopoulos D, et al. Long-term effects of oral contraceptives on ovarian cancer risk. *Int J Cancer.* 2002;102:262–265.

2. Riman T, Dickman PW, Nilsson S, et al. Risk factors for invasive epithelial ovarian cancer: results from a Swedish case-control study. *Am J Epidemiol.* 2002;156:363–373.

3. Bu SZ, Yin DL, Ren XH, et al. Progesterone induces apoptosis and up-regulation of p53 expression in human ovarian carcinoma cell lines. *Cancer.* 1997;79:1944–1950.

4. Chiaffarino F, Parazzini F, Negri E, et al. Time since last birth and the risk of ovarian cancer. *Gynecol Oncol.* 2001;81:233–236.

5. Purdie DM, Siskind V, Bain CJ, Webb PM, Green AC. Reproduction-related risk factors for mucinous and nonmucinous epithelial ovarian cancer. *Am J Epidemiol.* 2001;153:860–864.

6. Titus-Ernstoff L, Perez K, Cramer DW, Harlow GL, Baron JA, Greenberg ER. Menstrual and reproductive factors in relation to ovarian cancer risk. *Br J Cancer.* 2001;84:714–721.

7. Vachon CM, Mink PJ, Janney CA, et al. Association of parity and ovarian cancer risk by family history of breast or ovarian cancer in a population-based study of postmenopausal women. *Epidemiology.* 2002;13:66–71.

8. Mosgaard BJ, Lidegaard O, Kjaer SK, Schou G, Andersen AN. Infertility, fertility drugs, and invasive ovarian cancer: a case-control study. *Fertil Steril.* 1997;67:1005–1012.

9. Hankinson SE, Hunter DJ, Colditz GA, et al. Tubal ligation, hysterectomy, and risk of ovarian cancer: a prospective study. *JAMA.* 1993;270:2813–2818.

10. Green A, Purdie D, Bain C, et al, for Survey of Women's Health Study Group. Tubal sterilization, hysterectomy and decreased risk of ovarian cancer. *Int J Cancer.* 1997;71:948–951.

11. Yoshikawa H, Jimbo H, Okada S, et al. Prevalence of endometriosis in ovarian cancer. *Gynecol Obstet Invest.* 2000;50(suppl 1):11–17.

12. Zanetta GM, Webb MJ, Li H, Keeney GL. Hyperestrogenism: a relevant risk factor for the development of cancer from endometriosis. *Gynecol Oncol.* 2000;79:18–22.

13. Eisen A, Rebbeck TR, Wood WC, Weber BL. Prophylactic surgery in women with a hereditary predisposition to breast and ovarian cancer. *J Clin Oncol.* 2000;18:1980–1995.

14. Cramer DW, Liberman RF, Titus-Ernstoff L, et al. Genital talc exposure and risk of ovarian cancer. *Int J Cancer.* 1999;81:351–356.

15. Wong C, Hempling RE, Piver MS, Natarajan N, Mettlen CJ. Perineal talc exposure and subsequent epithelial ovarian cancer: a case-control study. *Obstet Gynecol.* 1999;93:372–376.

16. Vasen HFA, Wijnen JT, Menko FH, et al. Cancer risk in families with hereditary nonpolyposis colorectal cancer diagnosed by mutation analysis. *Gastroenterology.* 1996;110:1020–1027.

17. Rebbeck TR, Levin AM, Eisen A, et al. Breast cancer risk after bilateral prophylactic oophorectomy in BRCA1 mutation carriers. *J Natl Cancer Inst.* 1999;91:1475–1479.

18. Piver MS. Hereditary ovarian cancer: lessons from the first twenty years of the Gilda Radner familial ovarian cancer registry. *Gynecol Oncol.* 2002;85:9–17.

19. Writing Group for the Women's Health Initiative Investigators. Risks and benefits of estrogen plus progestin in healthy postmenopausal women: principal results from the Women's Health Initiative randomized controlled trial. *JAMA.* 2002;288:321–333.

20. Suh-Burgmann EJ, Goodman A. Surveillance for endometrial cancer in women receiving tamoxifen. *Ann Intern Med.* 1999;131:127–135.

21. Giorda G, Crivellari D, Veronesi A, et al. Comparison of ultrasonography, hysteroscopy, and biopsy in the diagnosis of endometrial lesions in postmenopausal tamoxifen-treated patients. *Acta Obstet Gynecol Scand.* 2002;81:975–980.

22. Cheung AP. Ultrasound and menstrual history in predicting endometrial hyperplasia in polycystic ovary syndrome. *Obstet Gynecol.* 2001;98:325–331.

23. Bokhman JV. Two pathogenetic types of endometrial carcinoma. *Gynecol Oncol.* 1983;15:10–17.

24. Watson P, Lynch HT. Extracolonic cancer in hereditary nonpolyposis colorectal cancer. *Cancer.* 1993;71:677–685.

25. Wickerham DL, Fisher B, Wolmark N, et al. Association of tamoxifen and uterine sarcoma. *J Clin Oncol.* 2002;20:2758–2760.

26. Bouchardy C, Verkooijen HM, Fioretta G, Sappino AP, Vlastos G. Increased risk of malignant mullerian tumor of the uterus among women with breast cancer treated by tamoxifen. *J Clin Oncol.* 2002;20:4403.

27. Gwinn ML. Oral contraceptives and breast, endometrial, and ovarian cancers: the Cancer and Steroid Hormone Study Group, Atlanta, Georgia. *J Obstet Gynaecol.* 1985;5(suppl 2):S83–S87.

28. Moscicki AB, Palefsky J, Smith G, Siboshski S, Schoolnik G. Variability of human papillomavirus DNA testing in a longitudinal cohort of young women. *Obstet Gynecol.* 1993;82:578–585.

29. Koutsky LA, Holmes KK, Critchlow CW, et al. A cohort study of the risk of cervical intraepithelial neoplasia grade 2 or 3 in relation to papillomavirus infection. *N Engl J Med.* 1992;32:1272–1278.

30. Kjaer SK, van den Brule AJC, Paull G, et al. Type specific persistence of high risk human papillomavirus (HPV) as indicator of high grade cervical squamous intraepithelial lesions in young women: population based prospective follow up study. *BMJ.* 2002;325:572–576.

31. Brinton LA, Hamman RF, Huggins GR, et al. Sexual and reproductive risk factors for invasive squamous cell cervical cancer. *J Natl Cancer Inst.* 1987;79:23–30.

32. Castle PE, Wacholder S, Lorincz AT, et al. A prospective study of high-grade cervical neoplasia risk among human papillomavirus-infected women. *J Natl Cancer Inst.* 2002;94:1406–1414.

33. Peyton CL, Gravitt PE, Hunt WC, et al. Determinants of genital human papillomavirus detection in a US population. *J Infect Dis.* 2001;183:1554–1564.

34. Smith RA, Cokkinides V, Eyre HJ, for American Cancer Society. American Cancer Society guidelines for the early detection of cancer, 2003. *CA Cancer J Clin.* 2003;53:27–43.

35. Wright TC, Cox JT, Massad LS, Twiggs, LB, Wilkinson EJ. 2001 consensus guidelines for the management of women with cervical cytological abnormalities. *JAMA.* 2002;287:2120–2129.

36. Koutsky LA, Ault KA, Wheeler CM, et al. A controlled trial of a human papillomavirus type 16 vaccine. *N Engl J Med.* 2002;347:1645–1651.

37. Merino MJ. Vaginal cancer: the role of infectious and environmental factors. *Am J Obstet Gynecol.* 1991;165:1255–1262.

38. Monk BJ, Burger RA, Lin F, Parham G, Vasilev SA, Wilczynski SP. Prognostic significance of human papillomavirus DNA in vulvar carcinoma. *Obstet Gynecol.* 1995;85:709–715.

39. Ikenberg H, Runge M, Goppinger A, Pfleiderer A. Human papillomavirus DNA in invasive carcinoma of the vagina. *Obstet Gynecol.* 1990;76:432–438.

chapter 32

The Adult Male

Adele Fowler, MD, and Alan M. Weiss, MD, MBA

INTRODUCTION

The past 30 years have been marked by a major refocusing of health research and policies on women. Although these laudable efforts have successfully garnered research and attention on a sex whose health issues were historically often ignored, they have also revealed a great disparity in men's health. Men's life expectancy remains lower than that of women, and men have a higher mortality rate for all 15 leading causes of death.[1] The inequality is wider for men of less affluent backgrounds and in some minority groups. In the United States, white men live nearly 6 years less than white women do (73.9 vs 79.8 years), whereas black men live 8 years less than black women (66.1 vs 74.3).[2]

Cardiovascular disease remains the most common cause of death in men. One in 4 men will die of a heart attack. One in 5 men will die prematurely before age 75 years due to disease of the heart and circulatory system.[3] Furthermore, half of sudden coronary deaths in men occur in patients without a prior history of heart disease. Contributing to these problems is the fact that hypertension and high cholesterol levels are more common in men. Twenty-eight percent of men have high cholesterol levels.[4] Because men are less likely to see a physician on a regular basis, they are also less likely to have these issues addressed. Furthermore, only 31% of men are physically active enough to give them protection against coronary artery disease (CAD).[4]

Congestive heart failure (CHF) remains the most common cause of hospital admission in the United States. Given the higher rate of cardiovascular disease in men, CHF disproportionately affects them. It is estimated that 30% of men over the age of 65 years have hypertension, which can cause CHF. Unfortunately, it is undiagnosed in nearly one third. Studies have also shown that, even in men with the diagnosis, congestive heart failure is untreated or undertreated in up to one third.[5]

An increasing number of men, just like women, are obese. According to the National Health and Nutrition Examination Survey (NHANES) data, the prevalence of adult obesity (body mass index ≥30) has increased from 23% to 30% in the United States over the past decade.[6] This problem disproportionately affects certain minority groups. Among adolescent Hispanic boys, for example, obesity increased from 14.1% in 1994 to 27.5% in 2000.[7] Since obesity is itself a significant risk factor for hypertension, high cholesterol levels, diabetes, and strokes,[8] the epidemic may worsen male mortality. One recent study seems to confirm this idea and concluded that the years of life lost due to obesity is 13 for white men and 20 for black men. These values compare to 8 years of life lost for white women and 5 for black women.[9]

Men often exhibit increased risk-taking and aggressive behaviors. These behaviors may help explain why the most common causes of death in men younger than 40 years are accidents and homicide.[10] Similarly, these same attitudes contribute to unhealthy lifestyles with a high prevalence of smoking and drug and alcohol abuse in men. These behaviors place men at greater risk of disease. Psychosocial disorders, including alcohol and substance abuse, depression, and domestic violence, play a large role in men's health.[11] Alcoholism is a male-dominated issue with considerable social implications. Excessive alcohol intake is more common in men of lower education and socioeconomic status. Men drink more than women do. Two thirds of Americans with alcohol abuse or alcohol dependence disorders are men according to the 2001 National Household Survey on Drug Abuse.[12] Thirty-seven percent of men drink more than the recommended amount of alcohol per day,[4] and men make up 81% of binge drinkers.[13] Moreover, excess alcohol intake plays a role in 50% of deaths due to car accidents.

Suicide continues to be a major concern and appears to have an increasing incidence. Men are well known for attempting suicide through more violent means and consequently being more successful. The incidence of suicide is increasing among young men.[14] The rate of suicide together with accidents is now 4 times higher in teenaged boys than girls. A man's lifetime risk of suicide is twice that of women.[15] Since 45% of people committing suicide had contact with primary care physicians within 1 month of committing suicide,[16] there is a substantial opportunity for physicians to address this problem.

Men's cancer survival rate is lower than women's, possibly because of later presentations.[17] Furthermore, men more frequently contract cancer than women do. Worldwide colon cancer rates are almost double those in women, and lung cancer rates are nearly 5 times higher in men.[18] Lung cancer remains the most common cancer-related death in men. Contributing to the cancer issue is the fact that compared with women only half as many men have cancer-related check-ups. An exception, however, is colon cancer screening; men are more likely than women to undergo routine screening via flexible sigmoidoscopy or colonoscopy (34.2% vs 30.3%).[19] Nonetheless, men are still more likely than women to die of colon cancer.

Men underuse primary care health services.[20] They are less likely than women to seek help for acute medical problems.[21] To explain men's health care avoidance, a panel of physicians suggested 3 contributing factors. First, men get most of their support for health concerns from their female partners, who often force them to seek medical care, a notion supported by the mortality of divorced men being double that of women.[22] Second, perceived vulnerability, fear, and denial of illness force men to pursue help for specific problems rather than for more general health concerns. Third, both personal and systemic barriers prevent men from seeking help. The personal barriers are deeply rooted in society's view of masculinity that encourages a sense of immunity and immortality, and a belief system that relinquishing control and seeking help is unacceptable. Systemically, lack of time and access, having to state a reason for the visit, and lack of a male care provider were also mentioned as barriers preventing men from pursuing routine health care.[21]

Men's health cannot be separated from their socially constructed roles and the culturally shaped views of masculinity. Societal expectations of men may make them less able to recognize physical and emotional distress. The male stereotype of risk-taking and aggressive behaviors is incompatible with being ill and showing weakness. Signs of weakness, particularly regarding health, are not compatible with men's social status. Men often see themselves as invulnerable. These psychosocial aspects of men's health become more obvious as men retire from the work force. Retirement means the loss not only of the economic rewards but also the social and psychological ones. These issues may contribute to depression, anxiety, and suicide, which are increasingly common as men age. In some cultures, the traditional male role of producer and economic supplier lead to devaluation at older ages and retirement. With their traditional role of provider gone and failing health shattering their notions of invulnerability, men often grow increasingly depressed as they age.

HORMONAL CHANGES OF MALE AGING

Background

Women have an inevitable end of their reproductive cycle with ovarian failure. There is increasing evidence that some men go through similar hormonal changes as they age. Unlike women, however, these hormonal changes are often subtle and gradual and are not present in all men. The most common hormone attributed to these male hormonal changes, often called male menopause, is testosterone. The healthy adult male has 2 sources of androgens, testosterone secreted by the Leydig cells of the testes and androstenedione produced by the adrenal cortex. Most of testosterone (98%) is bound to proteins in the plasma, leaving only a small amount of free hormone. Approximately 40% of testosterone is bound to sex hormone–binding globulin (SHBG), with the rest bound to albumin and other proteins. Testosterone production is regulated by gonadotropin-releasing hormone (GnRH) and luteinizing hormone (LH) in a negative feedback system. The enzyme 5-α reductase metabolizes the hormone to dihydrotestosterone (DHT) within the testes, and aromatase converts it to estradiol, usually in the peripheral tissues.

In healthy men, there is a slow, continuous, age-associated decrease in testosterone levels.[23] There are wide variations in the prevalence of the deficiency. It affects about 7% of men younger than 60 years, and 20% of those older than 60.[24] Free testosterone is affected more than total testosterone due to the age-associated increase in SHBG. At age 75 years, the mean total testosterone in the morning is about two thirds the mean at ages 20 to 30. The free level is only 40% of the mean levels at the same age. Testosterone levels follow a circadian rhythm in men, with higher levels in the morning than the evening. This diurnal variation is also disrupted in elderly men.

The loss of testosterone has 3 general causes. First, the number and volume of Leydig cells in the testicles decreases with age at about 1% per year after the age of 50 years.[24] Second, aging leads to a loss of the LH pulse amplitude as well as a decreased response of LH to GnRH. Centrally, there is also an increased gonadotropic sensitivity to testosterone, increasing the negative feedback control arch. Third, increases in SHBG lead to a further decrease in free testosterone. Increased SHBG may be the result of increased adiposity, which in turn increases estradiol and leads to more SHBG. Abdominal obesity is itself associated with a decrease in testosterone, possibly because adipose tissue metabolizes testosterone to estradiol. Testosterone administration decreases abdominal fat and increases lean body mass.[25]

Other factors also play a role in the levels of testosterone in men, including genetics, alcohol (which is known to suppress testosterone likely by its toxic effect on the testicles), decreased blood flow to the testicles, and smoking.[26] Obesity itself may play both a causative and effectual role in decreasing testosterone levels. Abdominal fat mass is inversely correlated with free testosterone independent of age. The increased fat mass may lead to an increase in aromatase, causing even more testosterone to be converted to estradiol. Obesity also may decrease testosterone levels by increasing SHBG by itself. Furthermore, morbid obesity leads to an additional decrease in free testosterone for reasons that remain unclear.[27]

The prevalence of cardiovascular disease increases in men as they age and may correlate with the decrease in testosterone levels. High-density lipoprotein cholesterol (HDL-C) is positively correlated with testosterone levels and negatively correlated with total cholesterol levels.[28] Testosterone also has direct effects on endothelin, prostacyclin, and fibrinogen, which may partially explain the inverse correlation between testosterone levels and CAD.[29]

The major adrenal androgen, dehydroepiandrosterone sulfate (DHEAS), also declines with aging in both men and women. The hormone reaches its maximum serum value in the third decade and declines by about 10% per decade. The mean serum value at age 70 years of age reaches only 20% of the young adult levels. Elderly men with higher DHEAS levels appear to be leaner and more fit, but it is unclear if this observation is caused by the hormone or by other disease processes. Further controversy exists as to whether low DHEAS levels increase the risk of cardiovascular disease and whether supplements can help.[30]

Changes in levels of both growth hormone and insulin-like growth factor can also be responsible for the symptoms of the male menopause. Growth hormone production declines by 14% per decade after puberty.[31] The production of insulin-like growth factor, which is dependent on growth hormone secretion, decreases correspondingly. The combined decreases lead to changes in lean muscle mass, bone density, hair distribution, and obesity. It has been shown that administration of growth hormone reverses some of these changes and can improve mood as well.[32]

Melatonin is secreted by the pineal gland in a carefully controlled process governed by both circadian rhythms and by hypoglycemia. Light and temperature also play a role in its secretion. Melatonin secretion decreases in both sexes with age, and its loss may have an effect on gonadal function.[33] Similarly, it has been shown that melatonin secretion is also altered by hypotestosteronism.[34] There currently is no consensus that melatonin supplementation can positively affect this issue.

As the US population continues to age, more men reach the age of being affected by symptoms attributable to male menopause, and thus the diagnosis and treatment of this syndrome become increasingly important. The syndrome is now widely recognized and is known by many different names, including andropause, viropause, androgen decline in the aging male (ADAM), partial endocrine deficiency syndrome (PEDAM), male climacteria, adult hypogonadism, and progressive decline in androgen function.

Symptoms

The male menopause involves physical, psychological, and intellectual changes. These symptoms are varied, usually subtle, and often can be explained by many other disease processes. Furthermore, assessing which symptoms are effects of normal aging vs those of hypogonadism is often difficult. Hypogonadal men may have decreases in muscle mass and strength, loss of body hair, and an increase in visceral fat, leading especially to truncal obesity. A decrease in hematopoiesis can lead to anemia. Changes in libido and sexual activity may occur and may be accompanied by erectile dysfunction (ED). Cognitive function may also decline and be manifested by change in memory and difficulty concentrating.[35] Accompanying all of these symptoms may be fatigue and mood changes, including depression and anger. There seems to be a relation between testosterone levels and age-associated osteopenia, although this is somewhat controversial.[23] Bone mineral density and bone mass both can decrease, leading to an increased risk of osteoporosis. The risk of hip fractures is twice as great in elderly men with hypogonadism.[36]

Diagnosis and Testing

The diagnosis of androgen deficiency in men requires both symptoms and confirmatory laboratory tests. Unfortunately, androgen requirements for elderly men are currently still unknown. Further complicating the issue is the fact that testosterone receptor concentration and sensitivity to testosterone change in men as they age, making it difficult to assess supplemental requirements. Values less than 2 standard deviations below the value of healthy young males are usually thought to confirm the diagnosis. The screening test for androgen deficiency is an early morning serum total testosterone level, with values less than 10.4 nmol/L (300 ng/dL) often considered suggestive of the diagnosis of hypogonadism. Once a low level is found, it is appropriate to rule out other causes of a low testosterone level and to obtain a free testosterone level.

Prevention and Management

Prevention advice to be offered to men concerned about declining testosterone level should include cessation of smoking, avoidance of excessive alcohol intake, maintenance of an appropriate healthy weight, and regular exercise. The initiation of testosterone therapy should be made on a case-by-case basis. Patients should be advised that little consensus exists not only on the diagnosis of the male menopause but also on which therapies to use and on the dose of each therapy.

Testosterone has been implicated in the development of benign prostatic hypertrophy, also called benign prostatic hyperplasia (BPH). For that reason, androgen replacement may potentially induce BPH or worsen related symptoms. Although there is consensus that testosterone replacement does not increase the risk of prostate cancer, prostate cancer is an absolute contraindication to testosterone replacement.[37]

Concerns have been expressed about the effect of testosterone on lipid profiles and atherosclerosis. Testosterone has been shown to decrease HDL-C levels, which may thereby increase the risk of cardiovascular disease. A meta-analysis of intramuscular testosterone therapy limited to patients treated for an average of only 6 months failed, however, to show that replacement had significant effect on cholesterol profiles compared with placebo.[38] The effect of testosterone on CAD also remains controversial. Some studies have shown serum testosterone levels to be lower in elderly men with CAD than in age-matched controls. Whereas this result does not implicate testosterone deficiency as the cause of CAD, studies have shown that testosterone administration increases both coronary and cerebral circulation as well as decreases symptoms associated with peripheral vascular disease.[37]

Androgens stimulate erythropoiesis, and replacement therapy has been used in the past to treat patients with anemia of chronic disease. Anemia is corrected in about 50% of patients receiving androgen therapy.[28] Polycythemia can result from androgen therapy in up to 24% of treated patients.[39] This problem increases the risk of heart failure and stroke. While polycythemia can be a risk factor for the development of sleep apnea, controversy exists as to whether testosterone itself plays a role. There is some evidence that sleep apnea may be associated with a dysfunction of the pituitary-gonadal axis, including a low testosterone level.[40] At the same time, several reports have linked the administration of testosterone to sleep apnea.[41] Other potential side effects of testosterone supplementation are acne; gynecomastia; testicular atrophy, leading to a decrease in spermatogenesis and sperm counts; flushing; edema; mood changes, including excitation, aggressive behavior, sleeplessness, anxiety, and depression; headaches; nausea and gastrointestinal (GI) tract irritation; epididymitis; priapism; bladder irritability; cholestatic hepatitis; and hepatic necrosis.

Long-acting testosterone esters are available, but they require painful intramuscular injections weekly or every few weeks and lack a diurnal variation common in younger men. A more physiological approach involves using gels or patches on a daily basis. Testosterone is absorbed through the skin, and the level peaks several hours after administration and declines thereafter. Short-acting formulations of testosterone include testosterone aqueous and testosterone propionate, each administered by the intramuscular route. Scrotal patches provide a formulation advantage since genital skin is the only skin on the body across which sufficient testosterone can be absorbed without chemical enhancement. The patches are applied to the scrotal skin once a day. They are worn continuously except when bathing. Scrotal shaving needs to occur on a regular basis to enhance absorption as well as adhesion of the patch. Absorption can be further enhanced by warming the patch with a hair dryer immediately after application as well as by wearing jockey-style underwear. The serum testosterone peaks 3 to 5 hours after application of the scrotal patch. Nonscrotal patches are applied to a clean, dry area on the skin of the arm, back, or upper buttocks. Each of the 2 approved patches delivers 5 mg of testosterone in a 24-hour period. The testosterone levels peak 6 to 8 hours after its application. Some patches may cause skin irritation and/or a rash, which can be treated with a steroid cream or by switching to another form of treatment. Testosterone gels should be applied daily, preferably in the morning. Dry, clean skin of the shoulders, upper arms, or abdomen should be used. The entire contents of the gel packet should be used in each application. After application, the patient should allow the gel to dry and avoid contact with other people during that time.

BENIGN PROSTATIC HYPERTROPHY

Background

Benign prostatic hyperplasia becomes increasingly problematic as men age. Approximately 50% of men over age 50 years report symptoms. The incidence rises by nearly 10% per decade so that nearly 90% of men over 80 are affected.[42] Although prostate cancer has a 1 in 10 lifetime risk, there is histologic evidence that BPH will develop in all men if they live long enough. At the same time, progression from histologic to symptomatic BPH will occur in only 30% to 50% of men throughout their lifetimes. Symptomatic BPH and prostate cancer can coexist; prostate cancer is found is 10% to 15% of men undergoing prostatectomy for BPH.[43] Benign prostatic hyperplasia can have a substantial mortality burden. The most common causes of deaths are renal failure, urologic infections, sepsis, and complications from surgery.[44] Both medical and surgical treatments have improved considerably, leading to a much lower mortality.

While a number of risk factors have been identified for the development of BPH, the 2 most widely recognized are age and functioning testes. Some studies have suggested a genetic predisposition as well as racial differences. Heritable forms of the disease are more common in men under the age of 60 years who undergo prostatectomy.

Up to 50% of that population may be affected by an autosomal dominant form of BPH that increases the risk to first-degree relatives fourfold.

The pathogenesis of BPH remains controversial and is likely multifactorial. It is generally accepted that the male sex hormone dehydrotestosterone stimulates tissue growth in aging men. For that reason, functioning testicles are required for prostate growth. Castrated men do not experience BPH, demonstrating the endocrinologic control of prostate growth. Paradoxically, serum androgens decrease as men age. It is also believed, since estrogen also increases in elderly men, that that hormone may indirectly encourage prostatic cell growth. For reasons that remain unclear, the dominant growth of the prostate in BPH is periurethral. The growth is often nodular and affects both the glandular and stromal elements of the gland.[45]

Symptoms

The symptoms of BPH can be categorized as either obstructive or irritative. Both types of symptoms can coexist. The obstructive symptoms are the result of the enlarged gland blocking urination; they consist of a weak stream of urine, hesitancy, incomplete bladder emptying, and a need to strain to urinate. The irritative symptoms arise from increased tone in the prostate and consist of urinary urgency, frequency, and dribbling as well as nocturia. The most age-dependent syndrome is nocturia. Benign prostatic hyperplasia can also lead to occasional urinary retention, renal insufficiency, and either microscopic or gross hematuria. Another way to categorize the symptoms of BPH is being either static or dynamic. The static component is related to the pure mechanical obstruction provided by the increased prostatic mass impinging on the urethra. The dynamic component is related to the α-adrenergic tone in the prostate, prostatic capsule, and bladder neck. This latter component reflects the smooth muscle tone in the prostate gland. Categorizing the symptoms in this fashion helps in the consideration of treatment options.

Diagnosis and Screening

The diagnosis of BPH is usually clinical based on symptoms followed by digital rectal examination, urinalysis to exclude infections, measurement of serum creatinine, and perhaps a prostate-specific antigen (PSA) test. It is important to exclude nonurologic factors causing symptoms. Certain medications, especially over-the-counter allergy and cold medicines, can impair bladder contractility and increase outlet obstruction. The use of diuretics at night also can simulate the nocturnal symptoms of BPH. Diabetes and resultant glycosuria causing nocturia can mimic symptoms of BPH.

The PSA test is often used as an adjunct in the diagnosis of BPH. This test roughly approximates the size of the prostate gland.[46] According to the Baltimore Longitudinal Aging Study, serum PSA is also a strong predictor of growth of the prostate, with higher values indicative of higher future growth.[47] In the 4-year, placebo-controlled Proscar Long-Term Efficacy and Safety (PLESS) trial, prostate volume and PSA were strong predictors of future episodes of acute urinary retention as well as the need for BPH-related surgery in placebo-treated patients with BPH.[48]

One way to both diagnose BPH and judge the effects of treatments is to use the International Prostate Symptom Score. This 7-question questionnaire was adapted from the American Urological Association (AUA) Symptom Index (Table 32-1) and has become the standardized, validated tool for the evaluation of BPH. A total score can range from 0 to 35.[49] Values of 0 to 7 are considered to be mild prostatism; 8 to 18, moderate prostatism; and 19 to 35, severe prostatism. The risk of acute urinary retention in men with severe symptoms is about 2.5% per year.

Management and Prevention

A number of treatment options exist for BPH, which include lifestyle modifications, medical devices and surgical therapies, medications, and herbal preparations. The use of each therapy depends on the severity of symptoms. Most urologists prefer a watchful waiting approach for patients with mild symptoms (AUA score of 0 to 7). Moderate symptoms (AUA score of 8 to 19) are often initially treated with α-blockers, although finasteride and transurethral prostatic resection can be used if treatment with α-blockers fails. Treatment of severe symptoms (AUA score, 20 to 35) often depends on the size of the prostate. Surgical intervention is performed for larger prostates (greater than 40 cc), although medical therapies are often tried as well.[50]

Lifestyle modifications can be very effective in treating the symptoms of BPH. Since nocturia is often one of the more troublesome symptoms, reducing liquid consumption in the evening is particularly useful. Both caffeinated beverages and alcoholic beverages can cause a diuresis, exacerbating the symptoms of BPH, and therefore should be avoided particularly in the afternoon and evening. Patients should also be encouraged to void just before going to sleep.

While the etiology of BPH remains controversial, there is increasing evidence that diet and exercise may prevent some of the symptoms of BPH. One observational study of men in the Physician's Health Study showed an inverse correlation of physical activity with BPH.[51] Men who walked 2 or 3 hours per week had a 25% lower risk of BPH developing. It appears that moderate physical activity level over long periods reduces sympathetic nervous system activity at rest and therefore lowers prostatic glandular tone.

Phytochemicals, substances found most often in soybeans and many fruits, may have an inhibitory effect on

T A B L E   32-1

American Urological Association (AUA) Symptom Index

1. Over the past month or so, how often have you had a sensation of not emptying your bladder completely after you finished urinating?	*For questions 1–6, score as follows:* 0—Not at all 1—Less than 1 in 5
2. Over the past month or so, how often have you had to urinate again less than 2 hours after you finished urinating?	2—Less than half the time 3—About half the time 4—More than half the time 5—Almost always
3. Over the past month or so, how often have you found you stopped and started again several times when you urinated?	
4. Over the past month or so, how often have you found it difficult to postpone urination?	
5. Over the past month or so, how often have you had a weak urinary stream?	*For question 7, score as follows:* 0—None
6. Over the past month or so, how often have you had to push or strain to begin urination?	1—1 time 2—2 times 3—3 times
7. Over the past month, how many times did you most typically get up to urinate from the time you went to bed at night until you got up in the morning?	4—4 times 5—5 or more times

Printed by permission of the AUA.

5α-reductase, the enzyme required to make DHT. Ingestion of large amounts of these compounds may explain why Asian men who eat more soy and vegetables are less likely to have BPH develop.[52] Isoflavonoids and flavonoids, which are also found in fruits and vegetables, have a mild estrogenic effect. They may act as a competitive inhibitor of the body's own estrogen receptors in the prostate, thereby decreasing the symptoms of BPH. A study in Greece seems to confirm this observation, finding that men who eat more fruit appear less likely to have BPH develop.[53]

The medication finasteride (Proscar) produces a modest improvement in urinary symptoms, likely by reducing the size of the gland. Finasteride inhibits the enzyme 5α-reductase in the testicles. This enzyme acts to convert testosterone to DHT, the hormone that stimulates growth of the prostate. Treatment over 6 to12 months leads to reduction in prostatic volume averaging 20%. With finasteride treatment, AUA scores improved by 26%, and peak urinary flow rates improved by approximately 23%. The benefit of finasteride was greatest in men with larger prostates.[54]

Finasteride is prescribed in a dosage of 5 mg/d. No titration of doses is required. Because 6 to 12 months are needed to judge its effectiveness, a prolonged trial may be required. Finasteride is generally well tolerated and has an excellent toxicity profile. Side effects may include impotence, decrease in libido, and decrease in ejaculation volume and are more common during the first year of use. Finasteride reduces PSA values by about 50%, so this laboratory value requires careful interpretation in treated patients.[55] Studies have shown that finasteride may pre-

vent urinary retention as well as a need for surgical intervention, particularly in men with higher PSA levels and a larger initial prostate size.[55,56]

The prostate gland contains both α-1 and α-2 receptors, with the α-1 receptors being more prevalent. Hyperplastic prostatic tissue may actually contain a higher density of the receptors. The α-blockers relax the smooth-muscle aspect of prostatic tissues, affecting the dynamic glandular symptoms. These medications, therefore, are generally considered to be more effective at improving symptoms than are 5-α reductase inhibitors, and they act more quickly.

α-Blockers include the following:

- Nonselective drugs (eg, phenoxybenzamine, thymoxamine)

- Short-acting α-1 selective drugs (eg, alfuzosin, indoramin, prazosin)

- Long-acting α-1 selective drugs (eg, doxazosin, tamsulosin, terazosin)

Few direct comparisons of the α-blockers have been performed. They are generally similar in efficacy. Prostate symptom scores can be expected to improve by 30% to 40%, and urinary flow rates may improve as well. A number of the α-blockers require dose titration to achieve efficacy. The most important side effects of the α-blockers are orthostatic hypotension and dizziness, which are less common in the selective agents. Abnormal ejaculation is associated with both types of medications. Tamsulosin has a low potential for causing hypotension. Terazosin can cause dizziness, generalized weakness, rhinitis, and postural hypotension.

Saw palmetto (*Serenoa repens* or *Sabal serrulata*) has become a popular herbal product for treatment of BPH. Its efficacy may be linked to its ability to decrease the estrogen receptors in prostate cells, thereby inhibiting the hormone's growth-promoting effect. Saw palmetto may also have anti-inflammatory effects as well as possibly decreasing SHBG. A review of 18 randomized, controlled clinical trials involving 2939 men confirms the herb's efficacy in decreasing urinary symptoms and increasing urine flow. It improved urinary tract symptoms by 28%, nocturia by 25%, peak urine flow by 24% and residual urine volume by 43%. In general, saw palmetto has fewer side effects compared with finasteride.[57] The side effects are usually mild and can include headache, nausea, and dizziness.

Other over-the-counter preparations used to treat BPH include *Pygeum africanum,* developed from the African evergreen and for which there is some evidence suggesting it can reduce prostate inflammation, and vitamin E. Vitamin E is an essential, fat-soluble vitamin that has not been studied for effectiveness in the treatment or prevention of BPH.

Nearly 400,000 prostatectomies are performed annually in the United States, and 200,000 of them are performed for relief of BPH symptoms alone.[51] Most procedures are performed transurethrally, unless the prostate is exceptionally large, in which case an open procedure is preferred. Prostatectomy tends to be very effective; one study reports an 85% improvement after a transurethral resection of the prostate (TURP). Surgical interventions should be considered in men with moderate to severe symptoms who are unresponsive to medical therapies. Surgery should also be advocated for patients with recurrent urinary tract infections or recurrent or persistent gross hematuria. A history of bladder stones, renal insufficiency, or refractory urinary retention also may require surgery. Some 20% to 25% of patients with TURP have unsatisfactory outcomes. Side effects include retrograde ejaculation in 70% to 75% of patients, impotence in 5% to 10%, postoperative urinary tract infections in 5% to 10%, and urinary incontinence in 2% to 4%.[58]

Other procedures for treatment of BPH include transurethral incision of the prostate, urethral stents, microwave therapy, laser prostatectomy, balloon dilation, focused high-intensity transrectal ultrasound, and transurethral needle ablation.

ERECTILE DYSFUNCTION

Background

Erectile dysfunction is defined as the persistent inability to attain or maintain a penile erection sufficient for sexual intercourse.[59] The term has replaced *impotence,* as it is believed to more accurately define the problem. Erectile dysfunction can greatly affect quality of life, relationships, and self-esteem. Recent estimates indicate that approximately 30 million men in the United States are affected by some degree of ED. The Massachusetts Male Aging Study (MMAS), a community-based survey of 1200 men, found 52% of men between the ages of 40 and 70 years reported some degree of ED.[60] The incidence of ED appears higher for men with diabetes, heart disease, and hypertension. The risk was 4 times higher in men aged 60 to 69 years than for those aged 40 to 49.

The ability to attain and maintain an erection depends on psychological, neurological, vascular, and hormonal factors. Impairment of any of these factors can affect the quality of erection. The penis consists of 3 parallel cylinders of tissue, the 2 corpora cavernosa and the centrally located corpus spongiosum, which surrounds the urethra. The corpora cavernosa act as an interconnected space that fills with blood, resulting in erection. The penis has both autonomic and somatic innervation. The parasympathetic innervation comes from the sacral spinal cord, while sympathetic innervation comes from the lower thoracic and upper lumbar segments of the spinal cord. Somatic innervation is via the pudendal nerve. With direct sexual stimulation, nerve impulses cause the release of neurotransmitters from nerve terminals and relaxing factors, including nitric oxide. This results in increased blood flow to erectile tissue. Erections can also be initiated centrally in response to sensory stimuli—visual, olfactory, or auditory. With stimulus, either central or direct, nerve impulses result in the release of neurotransmitters from nerve terminals and relaxing factors, including nitric oxide. Nitric oxide activates guanylate cyclase, which results in the production of cyclic guanosine monophosphate (cGMP). This leads to a smooth-muscle relaxation through a complex series of reactions, and the result is increased blood flow.

Any disorder that affects blood flow or somatosensory or autonomic innervation to the penis can result in some ED. Psychological disorders, such as anxiety or depression, can cause some ED by interfering with concentration and awareness of one's senses. The causes of ED can be broadly categorized into organic and psychological. Organic causes can be further divided into vascular, neurologic, and hormonal. In 80% of cases, ED is thought to have an organic cause.[61]

The most common medical conditions associated with ED are those that interfere with arterial blood flow, and ED can actually be a presenting symptom of underlying vascular disease. Also, factors such as hypertension, low HDL-C, and heart disease have been found to be associated with an increased risk of ED. In the MMAS, the probability of complete impotence was 39% in those with treated heart disease and 15% in those with treated hypertension compared with 9.6% in the entire sample. The probability of ED varies inversely with the level of HDL-C. Cigarette smoking compounds the association of ED with conditions including treated hypertension and treated heart disease.

Diabetic men have a threefold increased risk of ED over nondiabetics.[60] Increased risk in this population is associated with obesity, elevated glycosylated hemoglobin (Hb A_{1C}), smoking, and duration of diabetes.[62] This increased risk of ED comes from many factors associated with the disease, including damage to vascular supply to the penile tissue, and somatic and autonomic nerve damage. Especially sensitive is the parasympathetic nerve supply to erectile tissue, which is vulnerable due to its long physical length. Furthermore, many of these patients may be treated with medications that have been implicated in ED, including antihypertensive agents, diuretics, and tricyclic antidepressants.

In the setting of ED, a careful medication history, including over-the-counter agents, is important. Onset of symptoms may correlate with new medications. Drugs may be responsible for up to 25% of cases of ED. Drugs used to treat hypertension and psychiatric disorders are those most often implicated.

Evaluation

Evidence suggests that patients want to discuss sexual function with their physician but are reluctant to bring it up and are relieved when their doctor raises the topic.[63] A written questionnaire, such as the International Index of Erectile Dysfunction, can help facilitate communication and evaluation of this issue. This questionnaire contains 5 questions on specific aspects of sexual functioning. It is important to differentiate ED from loss of libido or ejaculatory problems. The patient should be questioned on the frequency and quality of erections and also whether he has spontaneous and morning erections. Maintenance of these spontaneous erections, with difficulty attaining or maintaining erection during sex points to a psychogenic cause. Patients should be questioned about all medications, including over-the-counter and herbal products. It is also important to ask about social habits, including tobacco, alcohol, and illicit drug use, and prior psychiatric illness. The physician should also inquire about any history of back or perineal trauma and genitourinary surgery or neurosurgery. Other pertinent history includes that of diabetes, hypertension, or heart disease.

Physical examination is targeted to assess blood pressure, arterial circulation, neurologic function, and hormonal state. The anal reflex can be evaluated by lightly touching the perianal skin and watching for contraction of the external anal sphincter. The bulbocavernosus reflex can be tested by inserting a finger into the rectum and eliciting anal sphincter contraction by squeezing the glans penis. The genital examination should include evaluation for undescended testicles, hypospadias, and phimosis. Gynecomastia and facial and body hair distribution should be noted for any signs of testosterone deficiency. Laboratory diagnostic testing includes studies for diabetes, thyroid abnormalities, hyperlipidemia, and testosterone deficiency.

Treatment

Sildenafil citrate (Viagra) was approved in 1998 for use in ED and brought the management of this problem into the primary care provider's office. Sildenafil is a selective inhibitor of phosphodiesterase type 5 (PDE5), the enzyme responsible for degradation of cGMP in the corpora cavernosa. Sexual stimulus leads to the release of nitric oxide, which stimulates the production of cGMP. This results in smooth-muscle relaxation, allowing increased penile blood flow and erection.[64] By inhibiting degradation of cGMP, more is available for further augmentation of this process. Sildenafil has been studied in over 3000 men in more than 20 clinical trials. These studies, which included subjects with organic, psychogenic, and mixed ED, have shown sexual satisfaction to be significantly higher with sildenafil than placebo.[65,66]

Sildenafil reaches maximum serum concentration approximately 1 hour after ingestion. The usual starting dose is 50 mg, which may be increased to 100 mg or decreased to 25 mg depending on effectiveness and side effects. Although most patients respond within 2 or 3 attempts at their optimum dose, some take more than 6 attempts before success is achieved. Patients should therefore be encouraged to try the medication a few times before concluding it to be ineffective.[67] This drug should be taken no more than once per day. The only absolute contraindication to sildenafil is nitrate therapy because of the risk of severe hypotension in patients receiving both medications.[64]

Other treatments of ED include alprostadil, yohimbine, and the vacuum tumescence device. Alprostadil, a synthetic prostaglandin that relaxes arterial smooth muscle in the corpora cavernosa, is administered transurethrally (MUSE) or by intercavernosal injection. Yohimbine, an α-adrenergic antagonist agent produced from the bark of yohimbe trees, has been found in men with ED to be better than placebo, particularly in nonorganic ED.[68] Surgical implantation of a penile prosthesis is used when more conservative therapies fail or in men who have sustained severe corporal injury or neurologic damage.

VASECTOMY

Vasectomy is a common surgical procedure used for contraception, which involves cutting and usually occluding the vas deferens. Approximately 42 to 60 million men, or 5% of couples, worldwide use vasectomy for contraception.[69] The vas can be occluded by various techniques, including ligation or cautery. Varying lengths of the vas can be removed and varying amounts of fascia can be interposed between the cut ends. The procedure is usually done in the office with the patient under local anesthesia.

The failure rate for vasectomy is generally less than 1%.[70] Early failure is thought to be due to unprotected intercourse shortly after the procedure, before all sperm are cleared from the reproductive tract. Overall, 95% of men will be azoospermic after approximately 23 ejaculations, and patients should be advised to use alternative contraception until then.[70] Semen should be examined a few weeks after vasectomy to ensure reduced numbers of sperm, all of which should be immotile. Late failure occurs after proof of successful vasectomy when motile sperm reappear in the ejaculate and is usually detected after a pregnancy has occurred. Failure after technical success means that either recanalization has occurred, duplication of the vas deferens is present, or the wrong structure was ligated.[71] Early complications of vasectomy include bleeding, hematoma, and infection. The incidence of these complications varies inversely with the surgical technique and with the number of procedures performed annually by the physician. Sperm granuloma is a usually painless, inflammatory reaction to extravasated sperm at the vasectomy site. Pain may occur in 2% to 3% of vasectomies, usually 2 to 3 weeks after the procedure.[72] The most common but still rare late complication of vasectomy is chronic pain, usually attributed to congestive epididymitis. Pain may last weeks to months and is usually treated with pain relievers and antibiotics.

Several studies have evaluated the potential relationship of vasectomy and prostate cancer. In 1993, the National Institutes of Health (NIH) convened an expert panel to evaluate the evidence and make recommendations. The panel concluded that medical evidence did not support such an association.[73] In 1998, a systematic review of 14 studies published between 1985 and 1996 was undertaken and also concluded no causal association between vasectomy and prostate cancer.[74] A 2002 population-based, case-control study of 923 men with prostate cancer showed no association between prostate cancer and vasectomy.[69] Questions have also been raised regarding testicular cancer and vasectomy. The 2 largest studies to date found no elevated risk of testicular cancer in men with vasectomy.[75,76]

A common question raised by patients considering vasectomy is the potential for reversal. The success rate as measured by pregnancy is between 30% and 60%.[70] The reversal procedure involves reanastomosis of the vas deferens. The success of the procedure depends on the original method of occlusion and how much of the vas was removed. Studies also show that success rates decline with time since vasectomy. In a 1991 study of 1469 men undergoing vasectomy reversal, pregnancy was achieved in 76% of those with less than a 3-year interval since their vasectomy. This success rate declined to 30% in those who had their vasectomy more than 15 years previously.[77] Overall, vasectomy appears to be a safe and reliable method of contraception.

PROSTATITIS

Prostatitis is a major health care problem with a prevalence rate of 5% to 8.8%, resulting in 2 million office visits per year.[78] Prostatitis can be a source of substantial morbidity because of the potential for chronic symptoms. The NIH International Prostatitis Collaborative Network

evaluated the literature and clinical practice and has developed a classification of prostatitis syndromes.[79] The classification consists of 4 categories:

1. Acute bacterial prostatitis
2. Chronic bacterial prostatitis
3. Chronic prostatitis/pelvic pain syndrome
   a. Inflammatory
   b. Noninflammatory
4. Asymptomatic inflammatory prostatitis

Management for each of these varies but often includes antibiotics, usually the quinolones and trimethoprim sulfamethoxazole. Prostate massage is also used, but not in the setting of suspected acute bacterial prostatitis because of the possibility of inducing bacteremia.[80]

The theory behind prostate massage is that living and/or dead bacteria may be blocking the prostatic ducts and preventing clearing of infection.[81] Other treatment modalities used for prostatitis have included α-blockers, anti-inflammatory drugs, allopurinol, thermotherapy, and psychotherapy. Evidence for the efficacy of these modalities is lacking, and further research is needed. Surgery does not play an important role in the treatment of chronic prostatitis. It is used in certain cases such as bladder neck obstruction and infected prostatic calculi.

OSTEOPOROSIS

Osteoporosis should not be thought of only as a women's health issue. Approximately 1.5 million men over the age of 65 years in the United States have osteoporosis.[82] The lifetime risk of hip fracture in men is 6%.[83] The incidence of hip fracture in men reaches the same level as that of women at an age approximately 5 years older. For example, 80-year-old men have the same fracture risk as 75-year-old women.[84] The morbidity and mortality of hip fracture in men are substantial. The estimated 1-year mortality after hip fracture in men is about 30% compared with 17% in women.[85] In one study of men with hip fracture, more than 50% needed institutionalized care after the fracture and 79% of those who survived 1 year still resided in nursing homes or intermediate care centers, or were attended by home care.[86]

The key to reducing osteoporotic fractures in men lies both in prevention and in identifying those men at high risk of osteoporosis. A number of important risk factors have been identified, many of which are the same as those in women. Both alcohol and tobacco use are associated with diminished bone density in men. Current smokers have lower bone density than former smokers or men who never smoked[87-89] and a higher risk of fracture.[90] Heavy alcohol consumption is associated with lower bone density[89,91] and possibly with higher fracture risk.[92] Sex hormones appear to play a large role in bone health in men. Hypogonadism, both primary and secondary, is a well-characterized risk factor for osteoporosis in men.[93]

Testosterone therapy can be beneficial to bone density in men with hypogonadism.[94] Men of low weight or BMI and sedentary lifestyle are more likely to lose bone density.[95] Other risk factors for low bone density and/or fractures in men are endogenous and exogenous corticosteroids, long-term anticonvulsant therapy, untreated hyperthyroidism, excess thyroid hormone replacement, disorders of calcium metabolism, nutritional disorders, and gastrointestinal diseases that result in calcium malabsorption. Bone density measurement should be performed in men with any of these risks and also in elderly men with a low-trauma fracture or evidence of osteopenia on plain radiograph. However, a strict definition for osteoporosis for men based on bone density is still lacking.

Treatment of osteoporosis in men includes calcium and vitamin D supplementation as well as counseling about smoking and excessive alcohol use, regular weight-bearing exercise, and fall prevention. Bisphosphonates have been shown to effectively increase bone density in osteoporotic men and, therefore, should be considered in men with established osteoporosis.[96]

REFERENCES

1. Mathers CD, Sadana R, Salomon JA, Murray CJ, Lopez AD. Healthy life expectancy in 191 countries, 1999. *Lancet.* 2001; 357:1685–1691.

2. Centers for Disease Control and Prevention. *Ntl Vital Stat Rep.* 2002;50.

3. Barton A. Men's health: a cause for concern. *Nurs Stand.* Nov. 22, 2000:47–52, 54–55.

4. Kannel WB, McGee DL, Schatzkin A. An epidemiological perspective of sudden death; 26-year follow-up in the Framingham Study. *Drugs.* 1984;28(Suppl 1):1–16.

5. WHO Study Group. *Epidemiology and Prevention of Cardiovascular Disease in Elderly People.* Geneva, Switzerland: World Health Organization; 1995.

6. National Center for Health Statistics. National Health and Nutrition Examination Survey, 1999–2000 findings: prevalence of overweight and obesity among adults, United States, 1999–2000. Available at: www.cdc.gov/nchs/products/pubs/pubd/hestats/obese/obse99.htm#Table%202. Accessed June 5, 2003.

7. Flegal KM, Caroll MD, Ogden CL, Johnson CL. Prevalence and trends in obesity among US adults, 1999–2000. *JAMA.* 2002;288:1723–1727.

8. Kurth T. Body mass index and the risk of stroke in men. *Arch Intern Med.* 2002;162:2557–2571.

9. Fontaine K, Redden DT, Wang C, Westfall AO, Allison DB. Years of life lost due to obesity. *JAMA.* 2003;289:187–193.

10. Centers for Disease Control and Prevention. *Ntl Vital Stat Rep.* 2001;49.

11. Epperly T. Health issues in men: Part II. common psychosocial disorders. *Am Fam Physician.* 2000;62:117–124.

12. Substance Abuse and Mental Health Services Administration. National Household Survey on Drug Abuse. Rockville, Md: US Dept of Health and Human Services; 2001. Available at: www.samhsa.gov/oas/nhsda/2k1nhsda/vol1/chapter7.

13. Naimi T. Binge drinking among US adults. *JAMA.* 2003;289:70–75.

14. Singh GK, Siahpush M. Increasing rural-urban gradients in US suicide mortality, 1970–1997. *Am J Public Health.* 2002;92:1161–1167.

15. Griffiths S. Men's health: unhealthy lifestyles and an unwillingness to seek medical help. *Br Med J.* 1996;312:69–70.

16. Luoma JB, Martin CE, Pearson JL. Contact with mental health and primary care providers before suicide: a review of the evidence. *Am J Psychiatry.* 2002;159:909–916.

17. Rafuse J. Men's attitudes about seeking health care may put them at risk, conference told. *Calif Med Assoc J.* 1993;149:329–330.

18. International Society for Men's Health. World Congress on Men's Health Web site. Available at: http://www.wcmh.info. Accessed June 5, 2003.

19. Smith R. American Cancer Society guidelines for the early detection of cancer. *CA Cancer J Clin.* 2002;52:19.

20. Bradlow J. *Patterns of Referral.* Oxford, England: University of Oxford Health Services Research Unit; 1992.

21. Tudiver F. Why don't men seek help? Family physicians' perspective on help-seeking behavior in men. *J Fam Pract.* 1999;48:47–52.

22. Kposowa AJ. Marital status and suicide in the National Longitudinal Mortality Study. *J Epidemiol Community Health.* 2000;54:254–261.

23. Vermeulen A. Androgen replacement therapy in the aging male: a critical evaluation. *J Clin Endocrinol Metab.* 2001;86:2380–2390.

24. Vermeulen A. Ageing of the hypothalamo-pituitary axis in men. *Hum Res.* 1995;43:35.

25. Marin P. Assimilation and mobilization of triglycerides in subcutaneous abdominal and femoral adipose tissue in vivo in men: effects of androgen. *J Clin Endocrinol Metab.* 1995;80:239–243.

26. McVary KT, Carrier S, Wessells H, for Subcommittee on Smoking and Erectile Dysfunction Socioeconomic Committee, Sexual Medicine Society of North America. Smoking and erectile dysfunction: evidence based analysis. *J Urol.* 2001;166:1624–1632.

27. Vermeulen A. Influence of some biological indices on the sex hormone binding globulin and androgens in aging and obese men. *J Clin Endocrinol Metab.* 1997;81:1821–1827.

28. Snyder PJ. Effects of testosterone treatment on body composition and muscle strength in men over 65 years of age. *J Clin Endocrinol Metab.* 1999;84:2647–2653.

29. Phillips G. The association between hypotestosteronemia and coronary heart disease in men. *Arterioscl Thromb.* 1994;14:701–706.

30. Larkin M. DHEA: will science confirm the headlines? *Lancet.* 1998;352:208.

31. Veldhuis J. Elements in the pathophysiology of diminished growth hormone secretion in aging humans. *Endocrine.* 1997;7:41.

32. Baum H. Effect of physiological growth hormone therapy on cognition and quality of life in patients with adult-onset GH deficiency. *J Clin Endocrinol Metab.* 1998;83:3184.

33. Liu R, Zhou JN, van Heerikhuize J, Hofman MA, Swaab DF. Decreased melatonin levels in postmortem cerebrospinal fluid in relation to aging, Alzheimer's disease and apolipoprotein E-epsilon4/4 genotype. *J Clin Encrinol Metab.* 1999;84:323–327.

34. Leibenluft E. Effects of leuprolide-induced hypogonadism and testosterone replacement on sleep, melatonin and prolactin secretion in men. *J Clin Endocrinol Metab.* 1997;82:3203.

35. Barrett-Connor E. Bio-available testosterone and depressive mood in older men: the Rancho-Bernano Study. *J Clin Endocrinol Metab.* 1999;84:573–577.

36. Jackson JA. Testosterone deficiency as a risk factor for hip fractures in men: a case control study. *Am J Med Sci.* 1992;204:4–8.

37. Basaria S. Hypogonadism and androgen replacement therapy in elderly men. *Am J Med.* 2000;110:563–572.

38. Whisel EA. Intramuscular testosterone esters and plasma lipids in hypogonadal men: a meta-analysis. *Am J Med.* 2001;111:261–269.

39. Hajjar RR. Outcomes of long term testosterone replacement in older hypogonadal males: a retrospective analysis. *J Clin Endocrinol Metab.* 1997;82:3793–3896.

40. Luboshitzky R, Aviv A, Hefetz A, et al. Decreased pituitary-gonadal secretion in men with obstructive sleep apnea. *J Clin Endocrinol Metab.* 2002;87:3394–3398.

41. Cistulli PA, Grunstein RR, Sullivan CE. Effect of testosterone administration on upper airway collapsibility during sleep. *Am J Resp Crit Care Med.* 1994;149:530–532.

42. Berry S. The development of human benign prostatic hyperplasia with age. *J Urol.* 1984;132:474.

43. Barry M. A 73-year-old man with symptomatic benign prostatic hyperplasia. *JAMA.* 1997;278:2178–2184.

44. Boyle P. Decrease in mortality from benign prostatic hyperplasia: a major unheralded health triumph. *J Urol.* 1996;155:176–180.

45. Grayhack J. The pathogenesis of benign prostatic hyperplasia: a proposed hypothesis and critical evaluation. *J Urol.* 1998;160:2375–2380.

46. Polascik TJ, Oesterling JE, Partin AW. Prostate specific antigen: a decade of discovery—what we have learned and where we are going. *J Urol.* 1999;162:293–306.

47. Wright EJ, Fang J, Metter EJ, et al. Prostate specific antigen predicts the long-term risk of prostate enlargement: results from the Baltimore Longitudinal Study of Aging. *J Urol.* 2002;167:2484–2487; discussion 2487–2488.

48. Roehrborn CG, McConnell JD, Lieber M, et al. Serum prostate specific antigen concentration is a powerful predictor of acute urinary retention and need for surgery in men with clinical benign prostatic hyperplasia. *Urology.* 1999;53:473.

49. Barry M. The American Urological Association symptom index for benign prostatic hyperplasia. *J Urol.* 1992;148:1549.

50. Gee WF, Holtgrewe HL. 1997 American Urological Association Gallup survey: changes in diagnosis and management of prostate cancer and benign prostatic hyperplasia, and other practice trends from 1994 to 1997. *J Urol.* 1998;160:1804–1807.

51. Platz E. Physical activity and benign prostatic hyperplasia. *Arch Intern Med.* 1998;158:2349–2356.

52. Thomas J. Diet, micronutrients and the prostate gland. *Nutr Rev.* 57:95.

53. Lagiou P, Wuu J, Trichopoulou A, Hsieh CC, Adami HO, Trichopoulos D. Diet and benign prostatic hypertrophy: a study in Greece. *Urology.* 1999;54:284–290.

54. Abrams P, Schafer W, for Finasteride Urodynamics Study Group. Improvement of pressure flow parameters with finasteride is greater in men with large prostates. *J Urol.* 1999;161:1513–1517.

55. McConnell J. The effect of finasteride on the risk of acute urinary retention and the need for surgical treatment among men with benign prostatic hyperplasia. *N Engl J Med.* 1998;338:557–563.

56. Anderson J. Finasteride significantly reduces acute urinary retention and need for surgery in patients with symptomatic benign prostatic hyperplasia. *Urology.* 2000;56:610–616.

57. Wilt T, Ishani A, Stark G, MacDonald R, Lau J, Mulrow C. Saw palmetto extracts for treatment of benign prostatic hyperplasia: a systemic review. *JAMA.* 1998;280:1604–1609.

58. Mebust WK. Transurethral prostatectomy: practice aspects of the dominant operation in American urology. *J Urol.* 1989;141:248–253.

59. National Institutes of Health Consensus Development Panel on Impotence. *JAMA.* 1993;270:83–90.

60. Feldman HA, Goldstein I, Hatzichristou DG, Krane RJ, McKinlay JB. Impotence and its medical and psychosocial correlates: results of the Massachusetts male aging study. *J Urol.* 1994;151:54–61.

61. Dewire DM. Evaluation and treatment of erectile dysfunction. *Am Fam Physician.* 1996;53:2101–2107.

62. Klein R, Klein BE, Lee KE, Moss SE, Cruickshanks KJ. Prevalence of self-reported erectile dysfunction in people with long-term IDDM. *Diabetes Care.* 1996;19:135–141.

63. Ende J, Rockwell S, Glasgow M. The sexual history in general medicine practice. *Arch Intern Med.* 1984;144:558–561.

64. Lue TF. Drug therapy: erectile dysfunction. *N Engl J Med.* 2000;342:1802–1813.

65. Goldstein I, Lue TF, Padma-Nathan H, Rosen RC, Steers WD, Wicker PA. Oral sildenafil in the treatment of erectile dysfunction. *N Engl J Med.* 1998;338:1397–1404.

66. Padma-Nathan H, Steers WD, Wicker PA. Efficacy and safety of oral sildenafil in the treatment of erectile dysfunction: a double-blind, placebo-controlled study of 329 patients. *Int J Clin Pract.* 1998;52:375–380.

67. Levine LA. Diagnosis and treatment of erectile dysfunction. *Am J Med.* 2000;109:3S–13S.

68. Ernst E, Pittler MH. Yohimbine for erectile dysfunction: a systematic review and meta-analysis of randomized clinical trials. *J Urol.* 1998;159:433–436.

69. Cox B, Sneyd MJ, Paul C, Delahunt B, Skegg DCG. Vasectomy and risk of prostate cancer. *JAMA.* 2002;287:3110–3115.

70. Schwingl PJ, Guess HA. Safety and effectiveness of vasectomy. *Fertil Steril.* 2000;73:923–936.

71. Peterson HB, Huber DH, Belker AM. Vasectomy: an appraisal for the obstetrician-gynecologist. *Obstet Gynecol.* 1990;76:568–572.

72. Kendrick JS, Gonzales B, Huber DH, Grubb GS, Rubin GL. Complications of vasectomies in the United States. *J Fam Pract.* 1987;25:245–248.

73. Healy B. From the National Institutes of Health. Does vasectomy cause prostate cancer? *JAMA.* 1993;269:2620.

74. Bernal-Delgado E, Latour-Perez J, Pradas-Arnal F, Gomez-Lopez LI. The association between vasectomy and prostate cancer: a systematic review of the literature. *Fertil Steril.* 1998;70:191–200.

75. Moller H, Knudsen LB, Lynge E. Risk of testicular cancer after vasectomy: cohort study of over 73,000 men. *Br Med J.* 1994;309:295–299.

76. United Kingdom Testicular Cancer Group. Aetiology of testicular cancer: association with congenital abnormalities, age at puberty, infertility, and exercise. *Br Med J.* 1994;308:1393–1399.

77. Belker AM, Thomas AJ Jr, Fuchs EF, Konnak JW, Sharlip ID. Result of 1,469 microsurgical vasectomy reversals by the Vasovasostomy Study Group. *J Urol.* 1991;145:505–511.

78. Anderson RU. Management of chronic prostatitis-chronic pelvic pain syndrome. *Urol Clin N Am.* 2002;29:235–239.

79. Krieger JN, Nyberg L, Nickel JC. NIH consensus definition and classification of prostatitis. *JAMA.* 1999;282:236–237.

80. Naber KG, Weidner W. Chronic prostatitis: an infectious disease? *J Antimicrob Chemother.* 2000;46:157–161.

81. Nickel JC. Effective office management of chronic prostatitis. *Urol Clin N Am.* 1998;25:677–684.

82. Siddiqui NA, Shetty KR, Duthie EH Jr. Osteoporosis in older men: discovering when and how to treat. *Geriatrics.* 1999;54:20–22, 27–28.

83. Kaufman JM, Johnell O, Abadie E, et al. Background for studies on the treatment of male osteoporosis: state of the art. *Ann Rheum Dis.* 2000;59:765–772.

84. De Laet C, van Hour BA, Burger H, Hofman A, Pols HAP. Bone density and risk of hip fracture in men and women: cross sectional analysis. *Br Med J.* 1997;315:221–225.

85. Forsen L, Sogaard AJ, Meyer HE, Edna T, Kopjar B. Survival after hip fracture: short and long-term excess mortality according to age and gender. *Osteoporosis Int.* 1999;10:73–78.

86. Poor G, Atkinson EJ, Lewallen DG, O'Fallon WM, Melton LJ. Age-related hip fractures in men: clinical spectrum and short-term outcomes. *Osteoporosis Int.* 1995;5:419–426.

87. Egger P, Duggleby S, Hobbs R, Fall C, Cooper C. Cigarette smoking and bone mineral density in the elderly. *J Epidemiol Community Health.* 1996;50:47–50.

88. Kiel DP, Zhang Y, Hannan MT, Anderson JJ, Baron JA, Felson DT. The effect of smoking at different life stages on bone mineral density in elderly men and women. *Osteoporosis Int.* 1996;6:240–248.

89. Slemenda CW, Christian JC, Teed T, Reister TK, Williams CJ, Johnston CC. Long-term bone loss in men: effects of genetic and environmental factors. *Ann Intern Med.* 1992;117:286–291.

90. Scane AC, Francis RM, Sutcliffe AM, et al. Case-control study of the pathogenesis and sequelae of symptomatic vertebral fractures in men. *Osteoporosis Int.* 1999;9:91–97.

91. Felson DT, Kiel DP, Anderson JJ, Kannel WB. Alcohol consumption and hip fractures: the Framingham Study. *Am J Epidemiol.* 1988;128:1102–1110.

92. Hoidrup S, Gronbaek M, Gottschau A, Lauritzen JB, Schroll M. Alcohol intake, beverage preference, and risk of hip fracture in men and women: Copenhagen Centre for prospective population studies. *Am J Epidemiol.* 1999;149:993–1001.

93. Kelepouris N, Harper KD, Gannon F, Kaplan FS, Haddad JG. Severe osteoporosis in men. *Ann Intern Med.* 1995;123:452–460.

94. Katznelson L, Finkelstein JS, Schoenfeld DA, et al. Increase in bone density and lean body mass during testosterone administration in men with acquired hypogonadism. *J Clin Endocrinol Metab.* 1996;81:4358.

95. Hannan MT, Felson DT, Dawson-Hughes B, et al. Risk factors for longitudinal bone loss in elderly men and women: the Framingham Osteoporosis Study. *J Bone Min Res.* 2000;15:710–720.

96. Ringe JD, Faber H, Dorst A. Alendronate treatment of established primary osteoporosis in men: results of a 2-year prospective study. *J Enocrin Metab.* 2001;86(11):5252–5255.

chapter 33

Prostate Cancer

Eric A. Klein, MD

INTRODUCTION

Prostate cancer has been the most common visceral malignancy in US men since 1984.[1] The American Cancer Society estimates more than 220,000 new cases of prostate cancer to occur in the United States in 2003.[1] Recently the National Cancer Institute reported a reduction in overall cancer mortality between 1990 and 1997, including a decrease of approximately 6% in prostate cancer mortality.[2] Tarone et al[3] have also reported that the mortality rate for prostate cancer in US whites has declined to a level lower than that observed before the introduction of prostate-specific antigen (PSA)–based screening in 1987. These improvements in mortality have been variously ascribed to screening, improvements in therapeutic modalities, earlier and more aggressive therapy, and more appropriate application of hormone manipulation. However, there remain marked disparities in prostate cancer incidence and mortality among various ethnic groups in the United States and around the world. These observations highlight the relatively poor state of knowledge regarding genetic, environmental, nutritional, and biologic variables important to this disease.[3,4] Additionally, most men who develop metastatic disease are still destined to die of prostate cancer. Between 1989 and 1998, more than 334,000 men in the United States have died of this disease.[5]

For some cancers, early intervention after the detection of occult or preinvasive disease has been demonstrated to be beneficial with respect to reduced morbidity and mortality compared with treatment of clinically evident disease. For various reasons, an effective primary prevention strategy (lifestyle or dietary change, or intervention with a nontoxic agent) is preferable to screening. However, for most cancers (including prostate cancer), prevention and early detection should be viewed as complementary strategies—prevention to reduce the prevalence of a given cancer, and early detection and therapy to maximize the chance for cure when prevention has failed.[6]

Screening for prostate cancer remains controversial because of the lack of randomized controlled trials demonstrating a reduction in mortality in screened populations. However, recent studies documenting a declining rate of mortality due to prostate cancer in the United States and observed trends in PSA-induced clinical and pathological stage migration provide inferential evidence that screening is beneficial. Recognizing these trends, the US Preventive Services Task Force recently upgraded its position on screening for prostate cancer from one of indicating evidence of harm and recommending *against* screening to one indicating that there is insufficient evidence to recommend for or against screening. In justifying this change, the task force concluded that there is "good evidence that PSA screening can detect early-stage prostate cancer but mixed and inconclusive evidence that early detection improves health outcomes"[7] (Table 33-1). To the contrary, the American Cancer Society[8] and the American Urological Association[9] (Table 33-1) recommend that "prostate-specific antigen (PSA) testing and digital rectal examination (DRE) should be offered annually, beginning at age 50 years, to men who have at least a 10-year life expectancy. Men at high risk should begin testing at age 45 years. Information should be provided to men regarding potential risks and benefits of early detection and treatment of prostate cancer."

For disease screening to be effective, the target disease must be an important health problem with a definable epidemiology, natural history, and latent period; the screening test should be simple, safe, and have agreed-on cutoffs with a standard policy for further diagnostic evaluation in those with a positive result; and treatment should be effective, with evidence that early treatment leads to better outcomes than does late treatment.[10] Evidence supporting a role for screening for prostate cancer for each of these areas follows.

EPIDEMIOLOGY AND RISK FACTORS

Prostate cancer is the most frequently occurring visceral cancer in the industrialized world, with an estimated

TABLE 33-1

Screening Recommendations for Prostate Cancer

Organization and Source	Policy Statement
US Preventive Services Task Force[7]	The evidence is insufficient to recommend for or against routine screening for prostate cancer using PSA testing or DRE.
	Rationale: There is good evidence that PSA screening can detect early-stage prostate cancer but mixed and inconclusive evidence that early detection improves health outcomes. Screening is associated with important harms, including frequent false-positive results and unnecessary anxiety, biopsies, and potential complications of treatment of some cancers that may never have affected a patient's health. Task force concludes that evidence is insufficient to determine whether benefits outweigh risks for a screened population.
American Cancer Society[8]	Both PSA testing and DRE should be offered annually, beginning at age 50 years, to men who have at least a 10-year life expectancy. Men at high risk (eg, African Americans and men who have a first-degree relative diagnosed with prostate cancer at a young age) should begin testing at age 45 years. Men at even higher risk, due to multiple first-degree relatives (father, brother, or son) affected at an early age, could begin testing at age 40. Depending on the results of this initial test, no further testing might be needed until age 45.
	For all men aged 40 and older, information should be provided regarding potential risks and benefits of early detection and treatment of prostate cancer.
	Men who ask their doctor to make the screening decision on their behalf should be tested. Discouraging testing is not appropriate. Also, not offering testing is not appropriate. Testing for prostate cancer in asymptomatic men can detect tumors at a more favorable stage (anatomical extent of disease). There has been a reduction in mortality due to prostate cancer, but it has not been established that this is a direct result of screening.
	An abnormal PSA test result has been defined as a value >4.0 ng/mL. Some elevations in PSA may be due to benign conditions of the prostate.
	The DRE of the prostate should be performed by health care workers skilled in recognizing subtle prostate abnormalities, including those of symmetry and consistency, as well as more classic findings of marked induration or nodules. Compared with PSA, DRE is less effective in detecting prostate carcinoma.
American Urological Association[9]	Both PSA screening and DRE should be offered annually, beginning at age 50 years, to men who have a life expectancy of at least 10 years. Men at high risk should begin testing at age 45. Information should be provided to patients before testing about benefits and limitations of testing, specifically, testing for early prostate cancer detection and treatment. Men who ask the clinician to make the testing decision on their behalf should be tested. A clinical policy of not offering testing, or discouraging testing in men who request early prostate cancer detection tests, is inappropriate.
	High-risk groups include men of African descent (specifically, sub-Saharan African descent) and men with a first-degree relative diagnosed at a young age. Risk increases with the number of first-degree relatives affected by prostate cancer. Work group recommended that these men begin testing for early detection of prostate cancer at age 45 years. Among men of African descent, age-specific risk increases steadily beginning at age 45. Men at appreciably higher risk of prostate cancer due to multiple first-degree relatives who were diagnosed with prostate cancer at an early age could begin testing at age 40. However, if PSA is <1.0 ng/mL, no additional testing is needed until age 45. If PSA is >1.0 ng/dL but <2.5 ng/dL, annual testing is recommended. If PSA is ≥2.5 ng/dL, further evaluation with biopsy should be considered. Men at high risk also should be informed about benefits, limitations, and uncertainties associated with testing for early prostate cancer detection.

PSA indicates prostate-specific antigen; DRE, digital rectal examination.

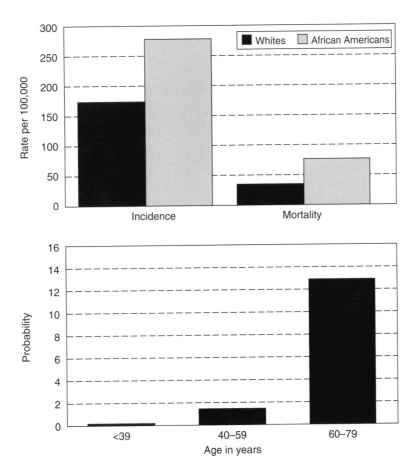

FIGURE 33-1

Race- and age-related risk of prostate cancer. Data from Jemal et al.[1]

220,900 new cases and 28,900 deaths estimated in the United States in 2003.[1] More than 100,000 men with prostate cancer are treated with curative intent in the United States yearly.

The epidemiology of prostate cancer is well defined. The main risk factors include living in an industrialized Western nation, age, race, and family history. Although the incidence of prostate cancer is low in the Far East, many studies have documented an increased incidence in second- and later-generation migrants to industrialized nations.[11,12] This increase in risk has been ascribed to both dietary and environmental factors. The probability of prostate cancer developing increases with age, with probabilities of 1 in 19,299 for those younger than 39 years, 1 in 45 for those aged 40 to 59, and 1 in 7 for men aged 60 to 79.[1] The estimated lifetime risk of developing prostate cancer is 1 in 6, although clinically evident disease is rare before age 50 years. African American men have a 1.6 times higher likelihood of prostate cancer developing and a 3 times higher likelihood of dying of prostate cancer than whites (Fig 33-1).[1]

TABLE 33-2

Family History and Risk of Prostate Cancer

Family History	Relative Risk	Absolute Risk (%)
None	1	8
Father or brother	2	15
Father or brother affected <60 y	3	20
Father and brother	4	30
Hereditary prostate cancer	5	35–45

Men with a family history of prostate cancer are twice as likely to be affected, and relative risk increases according to the number of affected family members, their degree of relatedness, and the age at which they were affected (Table 33-2). Hereditary prostate cancer, caused by inheritance of 1 or more autosomal dominant susceptibility genes, accounts for 5% to 10% of all prostate cancers.[13,14] Hereditary cancers are more common in those affected at an early age and may account for up to one half of cases in men affected before age 55 years.[15] Missense mutations in at least 1 prostate cancer susceptibility gene are also important in sporadic prostate cancers.[16]

NATURAL HISTORY

Although not all premalignant or invasive cancers progress to clinically significant disease, important steps in the molecular progression of prostate cancer have been defined. There is an impressive amount of epidemiologic, histologic, immunohistochemical, and gene expression data suggesting that many prostate cancers begin as a premalignant lesion called high-grade prostatic intraepithelial neoplasia (PIN, a lesion conceptually similar to carcinoma in situ in other organs) and then progress to invasive cancer.[17] Progression along this molecular pathway is fueled by oxidative stress leading to mutations, clonal expansion, genetic instability, and clinically evident cancer. Autopsy evidence suggests that PIN is present in 5% to 10% of men in their 20s and 30s and increases with age in parallel to age-related increases in invasive cancers.[18] Like carcinoma, PIN tends to be multifocal and is most often found in the peripheral zone of the prostate.[19] High-grade PIN demonstrates a number of genetic and molecular changes including alterations in DNA ploidy, chromosomal abnormalities, loss of heterozygosity, suppression of apoptosis, hypermethylation of DNA, and increased cell proliferation markers that are similar to those of prostate cancer or lie intermediate between benign and malignant prostate. The prevalence of high-grade PIN ranges from 25% to 43% in benign prostates at autopsy to 63% to 94% in prostates that harbor carcinomas.[20] The prevalence and extent of PIN tend to increase with age, with the peak prevalence approximately 5 to 10 years before that of prostate cancer.[21,22] In addition, PIN is more prevalent in African Americans than whites. Furthermore, the finding of high-grade PIN portends an increased risk of the patient having prostatic carcinoma.[23] Along with the known long natural history of progressive prostate cancer, these observations clearly define a latent period during which an effective screening test can identify localized and potentially curable disease. The identification of the molecular steps involved in progression from premalignant to invasive to clinically apparent disease also provides a framework for the development of effective chemoprevention strategies.

PROSTATE-SPECIFIC ANTIGEN AND SCREENING

Prostate-specific antigen is an androgen-regulated serine protease of the tissue kallikrein family of proteases.

Prostate-specific antigen is produced by both benign and malignant prostatic epithelium and is a major component of the proteins in semen, where it functions to cleave seminogelins in the seminal coagulum. Prostate-specific antigen is secreted into the prostatic ducts as an inactive precursor (proPSA) that is activated by the enzyme hK2.[24] Most PSA that enters the serum is bound by protease inhibitors (primarily alpha-1-antichymotrypsin) to form complexed PSA (cPSA), but a small fraction circulates in free form (free PSA or fPSA). In men with cancer, higher levels of total PSA (cPSA + fPSA) and cPSA are found in the serum, making it a useful test for detection and staging. The main limitation of the use of PSA as a screening tool is poor specificity, with substantial overlap of "abnormal" values in men with early-stage prostate cancer and those with benign prostatic hyperplasia (BPH). Measurement of free vs total PSA can increase specificity for prostate cancer, limiting the number of negative biopsy results obtained in screened men. The utility of monoclonal antibodies for proPSA and other PSA isoforms in improving specificity is currently under investigation.[24]

Results of several large-scale screening trials have established that the optimal cutoff of total PSA for triggering a prostate biopsy is 4 ng/mL, based on 95% sensitivity.[25,26] Using an extended transrectal biopsy technique, approximately 35% to 40% of men with a total PSA between 4 and 10 ng/mL and a normal DRE result will have cancer at biopsy.[27] However, recent observations suggest that a PSA between 2.5 and 4 ng/mL is associated with a cancer detection rate of 20%, and there is a growing consensus among urologists that younger men (below age 50 years) and those at high risk of prostate cancer (African Americans and those with a family history) should undergo biopsy when the PSA reaches 2.5 ng/mL or greater.[28] Many studies have demonstrated that PSA-detected cancers are clinically significant, as defined by tumor volume greater than 0.5 mL and Gleason grade.[25,26,28]

Prostate-specific antigen–based screening has been responsible for a marked stage migration in newly diagnosed prostate cancers. In the pre-PSA era, when prostate cancer was diagnosed by DRE or symptoms, the proportion of clinically organ-confined tumors was one half that discovered in the PSA era.[29] Multiple longitudinal and cross-sectional studies have confirmed that PSA testing increases the lead time for diagnosis of prostate cancer and results in the discovery of prostate cancer earlier in the natural history of the disease. For example, in a prospective evaluation of banked serum from the Physicians' Health Study, PSA was determined to have high sensitivity for detecting aggressive disease, with a lead time of 5.5 years.[30] The same study documented that the relative risk of prostate cancer is increased even with PSA levels below 4 ng/mL. Compared with men with PSA levels less than 1 ng/mL, those with PSA levels between

1.01 and 1.50 ng/mL had a 2.2 times greater relative risk of cancer, and those with PSA levels between 2.01 and 3.00 had a more than fivefold increased risk.

Prostate-specific antigen–based screening has also induced a profound downward migration in clinical stage among newly diagnosed prostate cancers. The National Prostate Cancer Detection Project demonstrated a reduction in locally advanced and metastatic tumors to under 5% of all newly diagnosed cancers in 2999 men undergoing serial screening with PSA, DRE, and transrectal ultrasound during a 5-year interval, compared with a combined incidence of 41% for these stages in the American College of Surgeons' 1982 survey.[31,32] Other studies comparing changes in both clinical and pathological staging in the pre-PSA vs the PSA era have demonstrated a doubling of the proportion of organ-confined tumors during the latter era. Thompson et al[33] reported that only 33% of men in the pre-PSA era with DRE-detected cancers had pathologically organ-confined disease, and Catalona et al[25] found more pathologically organ-confined tumors in men undergoing initial and serial PSA-based screening compared with those detected by DRE alone. A similar high rate of organ-confined disease was observed in a study of 6630 men undergoing surgery for PSA-detected cancers.[26] Other studies have shown that serum PSA correlates directly with advancing clinical and pathological stage.[34]

Prognosis after radical prostatectomy is closely linked to pathological findings, including Gleason grade, margin status, and the presence of extracapsular extension (ECE). Those with organ-confined disease (ie, no ECE and negative tumor margins) have the best chance for cure. Prostate-specific antigen screening has resulted in a decrease in Gleason score 8–10 tumors, an increase in Gleason score 5–7 tumors, and a marked reduction in rates of positive margins and ECE. In a recent study of trends of pathological findings in prostatectomy specimens in men with PSA-detected cancers, a statistically significant twofold decline in the rate of ECE was observed during the first 10 years after PSA was introduced.[29] The observed decline in ECE was seen for all clinical stages, preoperative serum PSA levels, and Gleason grades at biopsy. The results suggest that in addition to previously reported effects on migration to earlier clinical stage disease, PSA screening also causes an important downward pathological stage migration, resulting in more favorable pathological parameters for each clinical stage. This finding has resulted in higher cure rates in men with tumors diagnosed later in the PSA era, likely the result of repeated screening. In another recent report, the likelihood of organ-confined disease was shown to be related to age and PSA level at the time of diagnosis, suggesting that the best chance for cure is in younger men who have the lowest PSA values.[35]

In summary, despite a relative lack of specificity, PSA-based screening detects clinically significant cancers with an average lead time of more than 5 years and has resulted in a substantial downward clinical and pathological migration to early-stage, more curable disease.

TREATMENT OF PROSTATE CANCER

Localized prostate cancer is curable by several treatment modalities, including surgery (radical prostatectomy), external beam radiotherapy, or interstitial brachytherapy. Of the 13 most prevalent visceral cancers, prostate cancer is the only site where 100% 5-year survival is observed for both localized and regional disease.[1] Many studies document 10-year biochemical disease-free relapse rates of 93% to 97% for men with clinical T1 and T2 tumors treated by radical prostatectomy.[36-39] Modern radiotherapy series using various forms of dose escalation also report excellent disease control at shorter intervals.[40] Even patients whose cancer relapses after radical prostatectomy have an excellent chance of living 10 or more years.[41,42]

The most powerful evidence for the effectiveness of treatment of prostate cancer comes from a recently reported randomized trial of observation vs radical prostatectomy.[43] In this trial, 695 men with localized cancer were randomized to radical prostatectomy vs observation. With a median follow-up of 6.2 years, men treated by radical prostatectomy had a 37% reduction in the risk of bony metastases developing and a 50% reduction in the risk of dying of prostate cancer compared with the observation group. Although there was no difference in overall mortality between the 2 groups, the higher rate of bony metastases in the observation group suggests that with additional follow-up mortality rates will be higher in this group because (1) bone metastases precede death due to prostate cancer in most patients and (2) virtually all patients with bone metastases die of their disease. A common criticism of screening for prostate cancer is that the treatment-associated side effects of therapy have a negative impact on quality of life (QOL), and that observation is a way of maintaining QOL. In a companion study to the randomized trial, however, no difference in overall QOL measures were found when comparing the 2 groups, although there were significant differences in the symptoms that affected QOL in each group.[44] Not surprisingly, the progression of cancer in the untreated group resulted in significant reduction in the patients' QOL during the study period. Although only about 10% of the men in these studies had cancers detected by PSA alone, the findings give strong support to the contention that untreated prostate cancer progresses and kills more men than those undergoing potentially curative therapy, without sacrificing overall QOL. An updated analysis of the study results is planned in 2005.

Although some may still question the effectiveness of therapy for prostate cancer, there is no question that therapy is more effective for early-stage than late-stage disease. Evidence to support this assertion comes from biochemical failure rates after radical prostatectomy or radiation therapy based on disease extent at the time of treatment. In every series reported in the PSA era, those individuals with earlier-stage disease, as defined by lower pretreatment PSA, earlier clinical T stage, and lower biopsy grade, fare better than those with features of more advanced disease.[36-39,45] These findings are mirrored when investigators examine outcomes based on pathological disease extent.[36-39,45] The improved outcomes observed with more favorable pathological stages, coupled with the previously discussed observations that PSA screening results in a significant shift toward more favorable pathological stages, clearly suggest that PSA screening is likely to result in an improved cure. This contention is supported by analyses indicating that men treated in more recent years have a more favorable outcome.[45]

The favorable results in treating early-stage prostate cancer are in sharp contrast to outcomes in men with distant or metastatic disease. The 100% 5-year survival achieved for localized and regional disease contrasts markedly with the 34% 5-year survival seen for distant disease, as reported by the American Cancer Society.[1] Furthermore, virtually all men who have progression to androgen-independent disease die of prostate cancer. The evidence that treatment of early-stage disease is more effective than late-stage disease is overwhelmingly clear.

TRENDS IN PROSTATE CANCER INCIDENCE AND MORTALITY

Recent data from the American Cancer Society Surveillance, Epidemiology, and End Results (SEER) program of the National Cancer Institute highlight a rise, fall, and new baseline incidence rates for prostate cancer after the introduction of PSA screening in the late 1980s. These data parallel exactly what would be predicted if screening were effective: a marked increase in incidence rates immediately after introduction of PSA screening (as previously occult disease is identified), a subsequent decline as occult cancers are culled from the population, and ultimately establishment of a new baseline rate higher than before PSA screening was introduced, representing the improved sensitivity of the screening test. Before the introduction of PSA screening, the baseline incidence of prostate cancer increased by 2.7% per year between 1973 and 1988. The incidence increased by 16.2% per year between 1988 and 1992, just after the introduction of PSA screening, and declined by 11.7% per year from 1992–1995. A new baseline was established, with the incidence rate increasing by 1.4% per year between 1995 and 1999.

Furthermore, the mortality rate for prostate cancer has been falling since 1991. A recent report documents several other important trends in prostate cancer mortality.[46] First,

the age-adjusted prostate cancer mortality rates for men aged 50 to 84 years dropped below the rate observed in 1986; this occurred in 1995 for white men and in 1997 for African Americans and still persists. Second, for white men aged 50 to 79 years, the 1998 and 1999 rates were the lowest observed since 1950. Third, incidence-based mortality rates by disease stage revealed that the recent declines were due to declines in distant disease mortality. Moreover, the decrease in distant disease mortality was due to a decline in distant disease incidence and not to improved survival of patients with distant disease. Whereas the decreases in mortality due to prostate cancer in the last decade may not be solely attributable to screening, the observations are consistent with the notion that increased detection of prostate cancer by screening before it becomes metastatic will lower mortality. Other factors that may have contributed to declines in mortality include both more aggressive and earlier use of curative therapy.

In summary, there is substantial evidence that screening for prostate cancer results in the diagnosis of clinically significant disease early in its natural history, when it is most curable; that therapy for screen-detected cancers is effective and does not result in decreased overall QOL; and that the trends in prostate cancer incidence and mortality are consistent with a beneficial effect of screening. Current screening guidelines endorsed by the American Urological Association and the American Cancer Society are outlined in Table 33-1.

CHEMOPREVENTION

Chemoprevention of prostate cancer is based on an understanding of the underlying molecular events that lead to neoplastic growth, resulting in opportunities for both primary and secondary prevention. A number of hypotheses regarding the pathogenesis of prostate cancer have led to several large clinical trials with oral agents meant to prevent the development of this cancer. The use of nontraditional dietary supplements is widespread among men with prostate cancer and those who perceive themselves to be at risk. The willingness to use such agents provides a ripe opportunity for their use in well-controlled clinical trials to determine if they are as effective as generally perceived.

Hormonal Prevention

The basis for hormonal prevention of prostate cancer relies on the observation that only 2 requirements exist for the development of prostate cancer: aging and the lifetime presence of androgens. The requirement for androgens in the development of prostate cancer is based on observations from clinical studies of individuals afflicted with androgen insensitivity or deficiency syndromes. As these individuals were followed up into adulthood, it was

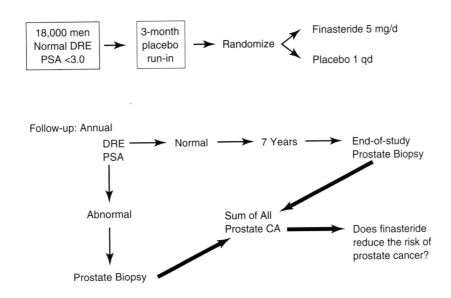

FIGURE 33-2
Design of the Prostate Cancer Prevention Trial. DRE indicates digital rectal examination; PSA, prostate-specific antigen; qd, every day; and CA, cancer.

recognized that they had rudimentary prostates with an undetectable level of PSA. Prostate biopsy revealed no epithelium and follow-up has identified no cases of either BPH or prostate cancer.[47,48] Many other epidemiologic and preclinical observations support the hypothesis that androgens are required for the development of prostate cancer.[49-53]

The recognition that the androgenic milieu of the prostate was important in the development of prostate cancer led to the first wide-scale effort at prostate cancer prevention, the Prostate Cancer Prevention Trial (PCPT), Southwest Oncology Group (SWOG-9217) with finasteride (Fig 33-2). Finasteride is a testosterone analogue that competitively inhibits the enzyme 5α-reductase (type 2) that converts testosterone to dihydrotestosterone (DHT) in the prostate and causes a profound reduction in circulating and cellular DHT. Finasteride inhibits growth of prostate cancer cells in vitro and is an active preventive agent in certain animal models of prostate carcinogenesis. The PCPT is an ongoing phase III, double-blind, placebo-controlled, randomized trial to determine the efficacy of finasteride in the reduction of the period prevalence of prostate cancer. In addition to determining if finasteride prevents prostate cancer, PCPT will also yield a wealth of information on the effectiveness of PSA screening and on the natural history of BPH.

A second large-scale industry-sponsored trial called REDUCE will examine the effect of another 5α-reductase inhibitor, dutasteride, on its ability to prevent biopsy-proven cancer at 2 and 4 years of follow-up in men with an elevated PSA and normal initial biopsy result. Dutasteride inhibits both isoforms (types 1 and 2) of 5α-reductase.

Antioxidants

Selenium

Selenium (Se) is an essential trace element occurring in both organic and inorganic forms. The organic form is found predominantly in grains, fish, meat, poultry, eggs, and diary products and enters the food chain via plant consumption. There is marked geographic variability of Se in food related to local soil content. In addition to dietary sources, Se is widely available in over-the-counter supplements and multivitamins, typically in doses of 20 μg for inorganic forms and 50 to 200 μg of organic Se in the form of selenized yeast, or selenomethionine.

Selenium is widely distributed in body tissues and is an important constituent of antioxidant enzymes. Many epidemiologic observations support the proposition that Se acts to protect against the development of some cancers, and there is compelling experimental evidence that Se induces cell cycle arrest and stimulates apoptosis.[54] Several placebo-controlled, randomized trials in humans have further supported Se as an anticancer agent. In the most important trial, Clark et al[55] randomized subjects with a prior history of skin cancer to receive 200 μg/d of elemental Se in the form of selenized yeast or placebo. With an average follow-up of 4.5 years, there were no differences in rates of skin cancer. However, further analysis found that prostate cancer incidence was reduced by two-thirds among those in the Se supplemented group. A recent update of the trial by Clark et al added an additional 25 months of follow-up to the study cohort to reach a mean of 7.45 years.[56] Reanalysis of the effect of Se supplementation continues to show a marked reduction on the incidence of prostate cancer. As in the initial analysis, the

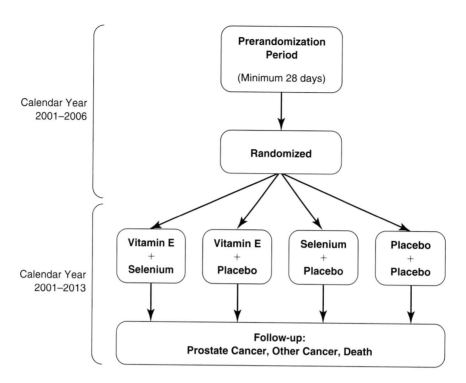

FIGURE 33-3

Design of Selenium and Vitamin E Cancer Prevention Trial (SELECT).

effect was strongest for those with a PSA level less than 4 ng/mL and those with the lowest serum Se levels at study entry. These observations give strong scientific support to ongoing clinical trials testing the ability of Se to prevent prostate cancer.

Vitamin E

Vitamin E is a family of naturally occurring, essential, fat-soluble vitamin compounds. Vitamin E functions as the major lipid-soluble antioxidant in cell membranes; it is a chain-breaking, free radical scavenger and inhibits lipid peroxidation, specifically biologic activity relevant to carcinogen-induced DNA damage.[57] The most active form of vitamin E is α-tocopherol; it is also among the most abundant and is widely distributed in nature and the predominant form in human tissues.[58] Studies suggest that vitamin E can inhibit the growth of certain human cancer cell lines, including prostate cancer.[59]

One large-scale, randomized, placebo-controlled trial, the Alpha-Tocopherol, Beta-Carotene Cancer Prevention Trial (ATBC), supports the role of vitamin E in the prevention of prostate cancer. The ATBC was a randomized, double-blind, placebo-controlled trial of α-tocopherol (50 mg synthetic *dl*-α-tocopheryl acetate daily) and beta carotene (20 mg/d alone or in combination with α-tocopherol) among 29,133 male smokers who were 50 to 69 years old at entry into the study.[60,61] During the median follow-up period of 6.1 years, there were 246 new cases and 64 deaths of prostate cancer. Among those

assigned to the α-tocopherol arm (n = 14,564), there were 99 incident prostate cancers compared with 147 cases among those assigned to the non-α-tocopherol arm (n = 14,569). This represented a statistically significant 32% reduction in prostate cancer incidence. The observed preventive effect appeared stronger in clinically evident cases, in which the incidence was decreased 40% in subjects receiving α-tocopherol. Data for prostate cancer mortality, although based on fewer events, suggested a similarly strong effect of 41% lower mortality. Although the incidence of prostate cancer was only a secondary endpoint in this trial, these findings suggest a potentially substantial benefit of α-tocopherol in reducing the risk of prostate cancer.

Selenium and Vitamin E Cancer Prevention Trial (SELECT)

Based on the epidemiologic, preclinical, and clinical evidence that selenium and vitamin E may prevent prostate cancer, the National Cancer Institute has organized and launched the Selenium and Vitamin E Cancer Prevention Trial. This double-blind, placebo-controlled, 2 × 2 factorial study (Fig 33-3) of selenium and vitamin E alone and in combination was performed in 32,400 healthy men with a DRE result not suggestive of cancer and a serum PSA level less than or equal to 4 ng/mL. Study duration will be 12 years, with a 5-year uniform accrual period and a minimum of 7 years and maximum of 12 years of intervention depending on the time of randomization.

The study supplements are 200 μg of *l*-selenomethionine, 400 mg of racemic α-tocopheryl, and an optional multivitamin containing no selenium or vitamin E. The primary endpoint for the trial is the clinical incidence of prostate cancer, as determined by a recommended routine clinical diagnostic workup, including yearly DRE and serum PSA level. Secondary endpoints will include prostate cancer-free survival, all-cause mortality, and the incidence and mortality of other cancers and diseases (lung and colorectal cancers and cardiovascular disease) potentially affected by the long-term use of selenium and vitamin E. Other trial objectives will include periodic QOL assessments, assessment of serum micronutrient levels and prostate cancer risk, and studies of the evaluation of biological and genetic markers with the risk of prostate cancer.

Dietary Supplements

Soy and isoflavones

Marked disparities in the worldwide incidence of prostate cancer has led to speculation that dietary influences may be important in tumor development. For example, legumes play an important role in the traditional diets of Eastern countries where prostate cancer incidence is low, but only a minor role in the West where the incidence is highest worldwide.[62] Legumes are low in fat and rich in protein, dietary fiber, and a variety of micronutrients and phytochemicals.[62] Soybeans are unique among the legumes because they are a concentrated source of isoflavones, which have weak estrogenic activity. Genistein, the predominant isoflavone in soy, also appears to have an influence on signal transduction. Epidemiologic observations dating to the early 1990s on the inverse relationship of soy intake and incidence of prostate cancer have stimulated research is this arena.

Many studies have demonstrated a consistent and statistically significant anticancer effect of soy-based diets compared with controls in various animal models of prostate cancer. Epidemiologic evidence also supports the role of soy as an anticancer agent. Severson and colleagues[63] found that consumption of tofu was associated with a markedly reduced but not quite statistically significant risk of prostate cancer in those who consumed tofu 5 times per week compared with those who ate it just once per week. Japanese men excrete high levels of isoflavones in the urine, and those urinary levels correlated with intake of soybean products.[64] In a follow-up study, the same investigators compared plasma levels of 4 isoflavonoids in 14 Japanese and 14 Finnish men. The mean plasma total isoflavonoid levels were 7 to 110 times higher in the Japanese men, and genistein occurred in the highest concentration.[65] These observations sparked much interest because Finnish men have one of the highest worldwide mortality rates for prostate cancer. A larger study by Hebert et al[66] investigated predictive variables for prostate cancer mortality in data from 59 countries.

Prostate cancer mortality was inversely associated with estimated consumption of cereals, nuts and oilseed, and fish. In the 42 countries for which data were available, soy products were found to be protective with an effect size per kilocalorie at least 4 times as large as that of any other dietary factor.[66] No large-scale clinical trials using soy or soy-based products as preventive or therapeutic agents in prostate cancer have been reported.

Lycopene

Lycopene is a red-orange carotenoid found primarily in tomatoes and tomato-derived products, including tomato sauce, tomato paste, and ketchup, and in other red fruits and vegetables, including pink grapefruit, apricots, watermelon, and guava. Lycopene is a highly unsaturated acyclic isomer of beta carotene, is the predominant carotenoid in human plasma, and possesses potent antioxidant activity.[67] Lycopene is concentrated in liver, adrenal, and testis and is the predominant carotenoid in human prostate. The most important anticancer activity of lycopene may be its antioxidant capacity, which is the strongest among all carotenoid species.[68]

In a review of the epidemiologic evidence for all cancers, Giovannucci and Clinton[69] summarized 72 studies and concluded that 57 studies showed a reduced risk of cancer in individuals with highest tomato intake. Summarizing the data specific to prostate cancer, they concluded that high dietary intake of tomatoes or lycopene was associated with a 30% to 40% reduction in prostate cancer risk in 6 studies, 3 studies showed a similar risk reduction but the differences were not statistically significant, and 7 did not support an association.[70] Among a cohort of 47,365 men in the Health Professionals Follow-up Study, 2481 incident prostate cancer cases were observed between 1986 and 1998.[71] High lycopene intake was associated with a statistically significant risk of prostate cancer of 16%, and high intake of tomato sauce was associated with a 23% risk reduction. The observations held even when controlling for potential confounders, including overall fruit and vegetable intake, Mediterranean diet, prevalence of PSA screening, and ethnicity.

Two non–placebo-controlled, prospective clinical trials that examined the effect of lycopene on known prostate cancer have been reported.[71,72] In the first trial, 26 men with clinically localized prostate cancer scheduled for radical prostatectomy were randomized to receive either 15 mg of lycopene orally twice a day for 3 weeks or no lycopene preoperatively. Statistically significant reductions in serum PSA level (18% drop vs 14% increase) and in the rate of positive margins (from 72% to 17%) were observed in the lycopene group, with no differences seen in various biological endpoints. In the second trial, 32 patients with localized disease scheduled for radical prostatectomy ate pasta dishes with tomato sauce for 3 weeks (equally 30 mg of lycopene per day) before surgery. Serum and prostate lycopene concentrations were statistically significantly increased in the intervention group. Compared with preintervention levels, both leukocyte and prostate oxidative DNA damage were also significantly reduced after intervention. A small but statistically significant reduction in serum PSA level also was observed (from 10.9 ng/mL to 8.7 ng/mL). Together these clinical trials support the hypothesis that lycopene is active against prostate cancer. Additional larger studies with appropriate controls are indicated.

Vitamin D

Consistent with a role for vitamin D in the prevention of prostate cancer is the fact that prostate cancer is more common in northern countries as compared with those closer to the equator. Prostate cancer mortality rates in the United States are inversely proportional to sunlight exposure (ultraviolet radiation), which is necessary for the synthesis of vitamin D.[73] Low serum $1,25(OH)_2D_3$ levels are associated with increased risk of prostate cancer, and insufficient levels of vitamin D allow progression to clinical disease.[74] There is a significant relation between low serum vitamin D levels and risk of palpable and anaplastic tumors in men over the age of 57 years. Among younger men (<52 years) low serum vitamin D entailed a higher risk of nonlocalized cancers. High calcium intake, leading to a lowering of serum concentration of vitamin D, may increase risk of prostate cancer, and this relation may underlie associations between dairy products and prostate cancer. High consumption of dairy products in a case-control study was associated with a 50% increased risk of prostate cancer.[75]

Vitamin D currently is being studied in clinical trials in men with various stages of prostate cancer. In one study, 7 patients with prostate cancer that recurred after radiation therapy or radical prostatectomy underwent 6 to 15 months of therapy. The rate of rise of serum PSA level significantly decreased in all 7 of the individuals, providing preliminary evidence that calcitriol effectively prolongs tumor doubling time in selected cases. Differentiation therapy with vitamin D analogues have a reduced toxicity profile and have the potential for preventing or slowing cancer progression.

Cyclooxygenase-2 Inhibitors, Nonsteroidal Anti-inflammatory Drugs, and Aspirin

A growing body of evidence suggests that anti-inflammatory medications may have a chemoprotective effect on a variety of neoplasms. Aspirin, nonsteroidal anti-inflammatory drugs (NSAIDs), and, more recently, cyclooxygenase-2 inhibitors all have been variously reported to be associated with a lower risk of prostate cancer. Expression of cyclooxygenase inhibitors (COX-1 and 2) appears to be higher in the prostate gland than in any other organ, making them attractive targets.[76] A population-based case-control study from New Zealand compared 317 patients with newly diagnosed disease, 192 patients with advanced disease, and 480 age-matched controls.[77] After adjusting for dietary fat and socioeconomic status, a trend toward a reduced risk of advanced prostate cancer was found in men who used NSAIDs on a regular basis. Similar findings were encountered for aspirin. In a longitudinal study of 1362 men, Roberts and colleagues[78] found that 4% of 569 NSAID users were subsequently found to have prostate cancer compared to 9% of men who were not NSAID users.[75] The Baltimore Longitudinal Study of Aging has been analyzed for the effect of NSAIDS on prostate cancer by Pearson and colleagues.[79] They found that aspirin use was associated with a relative risk of 0.85 and that NSAIDs were associated with an even lower risk. With each additional year of NSAID exposure, there was a 6% further risk reduction for prostate cancer.

A large-scale, population-based, industry-sponsored trial of a COX-2 inhibitor in men at risk of prostate cancer is currently being designed. The trial will randomize 8000 men to placebo vs 25 μg rofecoxil per day for 6 years, and the primary endpoint will be the incidence of prostate cancer in each arm.

REFERENCES

1. Jemal A, Murray T, Samuels A, Ghafoor A, Ward E, Thun MJ. Cancer statistics, 2003. *CA Cancer J Clin.* 2003;53:5–26.

2. Ries LAG, Eisner MP, Kosary CL, et al, eds. *SEER Cancer Statistics Review, 1973–1997.* Bethesda, Md: National Cancer Institute; 2000.

3. Tarone RE, Chu KC, Brawley OW. Implications of stage-specific survival rates in assessing recent declines in prostate cancer mortality rates. *Epidemiology.* 2000;11:167–170.

4. Hsing AW, Tsao L, Devesa SS. International trends and patterns of prostate cancer incidence and mortality. *Int J Cancer.* 2000;85:60–67.

5. *US Mortality Public Use Data Tapes 1989–1998.* Atlanta, Ga: National Center for Health Statistics, Centers for Disease Control and Prevention; 2000.

6. Ford LG, Minasian LM, McCaskill-Stevens W, et al. Prevention and early detection clinical trials: opportunities for primary care providers and their patients. *CA Cancer J Clin.* 2003:53:82–101.

7. US Preventive Services Task Force. Screening: prostate cancer. Agency for Healthcare Research and Quality Web site. 2002. Available at: www.ahrq.gov/clinic/uspstf/uspsprca.htm. Accessed July 18, 2003.

8. American Cancer Society. ACS cancer detection guidelines. 2003. Available at: www.cancer.org/docroot/PED/content/PED_2_3X_ACS_Cancer_Detection_Guidelines_36.asp?sitearea=PED. Accessed July 18, 2003.

9. American Urological Association. Policy statements: early detection of prostate cancer. November 2002. Available at: www.auanet.org/aboutaua/policy_statements/services.cfm#detection. Accessed July 18, 2003.

10. Frankel S, Smith GD, Donovan J, Neal D. Screening for prostate cancer. *Lancet.* 2003;361:1122–1128.

11. Shimizu H, Ross RK, Bernstein L, Yatani R, Henderson BE, Mack TM. Cancers of the prostate and breast among Japanese and white immigrants in Los Angeles County. *Br J Cancer.* 1991;63:963–966.

12. Muir CS, Nectoux J, Staszewski J. The epidemiology of prostatic cancer: geographical distribution and time-trends. *Acta Oncol.* 1991;30:133–140.

13. Bratt O. Hereditary prostate cancer. *Br J Urol Int.* 2000;85:588–598.

14. Carpten J, Nupponen N, Isaacs S, et al. Germline mutations in the ribonuclease L gene in families showing linkage with HPC1. *Nat Genet.* 2002;30:181.

15. Bratt O, Kristofferson U, Lundgren R, Olsson H. Familial and hereditary prostate cancer in southern Sweden: a population-based case-control study. *Eur J Cancer.* 1999;35:272–277.

16. Casey G, Neville PJ, Plummer SJ, et al. RNASEL Arg462Gln variant is implicated in up to 13% of prostate cancer cases. *Nat Genet.* 2002;32:581–583.

17. DeMarzo AM, Nelson WG, Isaacs WB, Epstein JI. Pathological and molecular aspects of prostate cancer. *Lancet.* 2003;361:955–964.

18. Sakr WA, Grignon DJ, Crissman JD, et al. High grade prostatic intraepithelial neoplasia (HGPIN) and prostatic adenocarcinoma between the ages of 20–69: an autopsy study of 249 cases. *In Vivo.* 1994;8:439–443.

19. Qian J, Wollan P, Bostwick DG. The extent and multicentricity of high-grade prostatic intraepithelial neoplasia in clinically localized prostatic adenocarcinoma. *Hum Pathol.* 1997;28:143–148.

20. Sakr WA, Billis A, Ekman P, Wilt T, Bostwick DG. Epidemiology of high-grade prostatic intraepithelial neoplasia. *Scand J Urol Nephrol.* 2000;205(suppl):11–18.

21. Sakr WA, Haas GP, Cassin BJ, Pontes JE, Crissman JD. Frequency of prostatic intraepithelial neoplasia and invasive carcinoma in young males. *J Urol.* 1993;150:379–385.

22. Sakr WA, Grignon DJ, Haas GP. Pathology of premalignant lesions and carcinoma of the prostate in African-American men. *Semin Urol Oncol.* 1998;16:214–220.

23. Epstein JI, Potter SR. The pathological interpretation and significance of prostate needle biopsy findings: implications and current controversies. *J Urol.* 2001;166:402–410.

24. Balk SP, Ko Y-J, Bubley GJ. Biology of prostate-specific antigen. *J Clin Oncol.* 2003;21:383–391.

25. Catalona WJ, Smith DS, Ratliff TL, et al. Detection of organ confined prostate cancer is increased through prostate-specific antigen-based screening. *JAMA.* 1993;270:948–954.

26. Catalona WJ, Richie JP, Ahmann FR, et al. Comparison of digital rectal examination and serum prostate specific antigen in the early detection of prostate cancer: results of a multicenter trial in 6630 men. *J Urol.* 1994;151:1283–1290.

27. Potter SR, Horninger W, Tinzl M, et al. Age, prostate specific antigen, and digital rectal examination as determinants of the probability of having prostate cancer. *Urology.* 2001;57:100–110.

28. Catalona WJ, Smith DS, Ornstein DK. Prostate cancer detection in men with serum PSA concentrations of 2.6 to 4.0 ng/mL and benign prostate examination: enhancement of specificity with free PSA measurements. *JAMA.* 1997;277:1452–1455.

29. Jhaveri FM, Klein EA, Kupelian PA, Zippe C, Levin HS. Declining rates of extracapsular extension in radical prostatectomy: evidence for continued stage migration. *J Clin Oncol.* 1999;17:3167–3172.

30. Gann PH, Hennekens CH, Stampfer MJ. A prospective evaluation of plasma prostate-specific antigen for detection of prostatic cancer. *JAMA.* 1995;273:289–294.

31. Murphy GP, Natarajan N, Pontes JE, et al. The national survey of prostate cancer in the United States by the American College of Surgeons. *J Urol.* 1982;127:928–934.

32. Mettlin C, Murphy GP, Babaian RJ, et al, for Investigators of the American Cancer Society National Prostate Cancer Detection Project. The results of a five-year early prostate cancer detection intervention. *Cancer.* 1996;77:150–159.

33. Thompson IM, Ernst JJ, Gangai MP, et al. Adenocarcinoma of the prostate: results of routine urological screening. *J Urol.*1984;l32:690–694.

34. Partin AW, Yoo JK, Carter HB, et al. The use of prostate-specific antigen, clinical stage and Gleason score to predict pathological stage in men with localized prostate cancer. *J Urol.* 1993;150:110–114.

35. Aleman MA, Klein EA, Kupelian PA, et al. Age and PSA predict the likelihood of organ-confined disease in men presenting with PSA <10 ng/ml: implications for screening. *Urology.* 2003;62:70–74.

36. Clark PE, Levin HS, Kupelian PA, Reddy C, Zippe CD, Klein EA. Intermediate-term outcome with radical prostatectomy for localized prostate cancer: The Cleveland Clinic experience. *Prostate J.* 2001;3:118–125.

37. Eastham JA, Scardino PT. Radical Prostatectomy for clinical stage T1 and T2 prostate cancer. In: Vogelzang NJ, Scardino PT, Shipley WU, Coffey DS, eds. *Comprehensive Textbook of Genitourinary Oncology.* 2nd ed. Philadelphia, Pa: Lippincott, Williams & Wilkins; 1999:722–738.

38. Walsh PC, Partin AW, Epstein JI. Cancer control and quality of life following anatomical radical retropubic prostatectomy: results at 10 years. *J Urol.* 1994;152:1831.

39. Catalona WJ, Ramos CG, Carvalhal GF. Contemporary results of anatomic radical prostatectomy. *CA Cancer J Clin.* 1999;49:282.

40. Kupelian PA, Mohan DS, Lyons JA, Klein EA, Reddy CA. Higher than standard radiation doses (≥72 Gy) with or without androgen deprivation in the treatment of localized prostate cancer. *Int J Rad Oncol Biol Phys.* 2000;46:567–574.

41. Jhaveri FM, Zippe CD, Klein EA, Kupelian PA. Biochemical failure does not predict overall survival after radical prostatectomy for localized prostate cancer: 10 year results. *Urology.* 1999;54:884–890.

42. Pound CR, Partin AW, Eisenberger MA, Chan DW, Pearson JD, Walsh PC. Natural history of progression after PSA elevation following radical prostatectomy. *JAMA.* 1999;281:1591–1597.

43. Holmberg L, Bill-Axelson A, Helgesen F, et al. A randomized trial comparing radical prostatectomy with watchful waiting in early prostate cancer. *N Engl J Med.* 2002;347:781–789.

44. Steineck G, Helgesen F, Adolfsson J, et al. Quality of life after radical prostatectomy or watchful waiting. *N Engl J Med.* 2002;347:790–795.

45. Kupelian PA, Elshaikh M, Reddy CA, Zippe CD, Klein EA. Comparison of the efficacy of local therapies for localized prostate cancer in the PSA era: a large single institution experience with radical prostatectomy and external beam radiotherapy. *J Clin Oncol.* 2002;20:3376–3385.

46. Chu KC, Tarone RE, Freeman HP. Trends in prostate cancer mortality among black men and white men in the United States. *Cancer.* 2003;97:1507–1516.

47. Imperato-McGinley J, Peterson RE, Gautier T, Sturla E. Androgens and the evolution of male-gender identify among male pseudohermaphrodites with 5-alpha reductase deficiency. *N Engl J Med.* 1979;300:1233–1237.

48. Imperato-McGinely J, Gautier T, Zirinsky K, et al. Prostate visualization studies in males homozygous and heterozygous for 5-alpha reductase deficiency. *J Clin Endocrinol Metab.* 1992;75:1022–1026.

49. Ross RK, Bernstein L, Lobo RA, et al. 5-alpha reductase activity and risk of prostate cancer among Japanese and US white and black males. *Lancet.* 1992;339:887–889.

50. Henderson BE, Bernstein L, Ross RK, et al. The early in utero estrogen and testosterone environment of blacks and whites: potential effects on male offspring. *Br J Cancer.* 1988;57:216–218.

51. Rebbeck TR, Jaffe JM, Walk AH, et al. Modification of clinical presentation of prostate tumors by a novel genetic variant in CYP3A4. *J Ntl Cancer Inst.* 1998;90:1225–1229.

52. Sartor O. Molecular factors in the assessment of prostate cancer risk. In: Resnick MI, Thompson IM, eds. *Advanced Therapy of Prostate Disease.* Hamilton, Ontario: BC Decker Inc; 2000:44–49.

53. Henderson BE, Ross RK, Pike MC, et al. Endogenous hormones as a major factor in human cancer. *Cancer Res.* 1982;42:3232–3239.

54. Klein EA. Selenium: epidemiology and basic science. *J Urol.* In press.

55. Clark LC, Combs GF, Turnbull BW, et al. Effects of Se supplementation for cancer prevention in patients with carcinoma of the skin. *JAMA.* 1996;276:1957–1963.

56. Duffield-Lillico AJ, Dalkin BL, Reid ME, et al. Se supplementation, baseline plasma Se status, and incidence of prostate cancer: an analysis of the complete treatment period of the nutritional prevention of cancer study group. *Br J Urol Intl.* 2003; 91:608–612.

57. Burton GW, Ingold KU. Autoxidation of biological molecules: I. The antioxidant activity of vitamin E and related chain-breaking phenolic antioxidants in vitro. *J Am Chem Soc.* 1981;103:6472.

58. Pappas AM. Vitamin E: Tocopherols and tocotrienols. In: Pappas AM, ed. *Antioxidant Status, Diet, Nutrition, and Health.* Boca Raton, Fla: CRC; 1998; chap 2.

59. Israel K, Sanders BG, Kline K. RRR-alpha-tocopheryl succinate inhibits the proliferation of human prostatic tumor cells with defective cell cycle/differentiation pathways. *Nutr Cancer.* 1995;24:161–169.

60. ATBC Cancer Prevention Study Group. The effect of vitamin E and beta carotene on the incidence of lung cancer and other cancers in male smokers. *N Engl J Med.* 1994;330:1029–1035.

61. Heinonen OP, Albanes D, Huttunen JK, et al. Prostate cancer and supplementation with alpha-tocopherol and beta-carotene: incidence and mortality in a controlled trial. *J Ntl Cancer Inst.* 1998;90:440–446.

62. Messina MJ. Legumes and soybeans: overview of their nutritional profiles and health effects. *Am J Clin Nutr.* 1999;70(suppl):439S–450S.

63. Severson KJ, Nomura AMY, Grove JS, Stemmermann GN. A prospective study of demographics, diet, and prostate cancer among men of Japanese ancestry in Hawaii. *Cancer Res.* 1989;49:1857–1860.

64. Adlercreutz H, Honjo H, Higashi A, et al. Urinary excretion of lignans and isoflavonoid phytoestrogens in Japanese men and women consuming a traditional Japanese diet. *Am J Clin Nutr.* 1991;54:1093–1100.

65. Adlercreutz H, Markkanen H, Watanabe S. Plasma concentrations of phyto-oestrogens in Japanese men. *Lancet.* 1993;342:1209–1210.

66. Hebert JR, Hurley TG, Olendzki BC, Teas J, Ma Y, Hampl JS. Nutritional and socioeconomic factors in relation to prostate cancer mortality: a cross-national study. *J Natl Cancer Inst.* 1998;90:1637–1647.

67. Agarwal S, Rao AV. Tomato lycopene and its role in human health and chronic diseases. *Can Med Assoc J.* 2000;163:739–744.

68. Sies H, Stahl W. Vitamins E and C, β-carotene, and other carotenoids as antioxidants. *Am J Clin Nutr.* 1995;62(suppl 6):1315S–1321S.

69. Giovannucci E, Clinton SK. Tomatoes, lycopene, and cancer: review of the epidemiologic literature. *J Natl Cancer Inst.* 1999;91:317–331.

70. Giovannucci E, Rimm EB, Liu Y, Stampfer MJ, Willet WC. A prospective study of tomato products, lycopene, and prostate cancer risk. *J Natl Cancer Inst.* 2002;94:391–398.

71. Kucuk O, Sarkar FH, Sakr W, et al. Phase II randomized clinical trial of lycopene supplementation before radical prostatectomy. *Cancer Epidemiol Biomarkers Prev.* 2001;861–868.

72. Chen L, Stacewicz-Sapuntzakis M, Duncan C, et al. Oxidative DNA damage in prostate cancer patients consuming tomato sauce-based entrees as a whole-food intervention. *J Natl Cancer Inst.* 2001;93:1872–1879.

73. Hanchette CL, Schwartz GG. Geographic patterns of prostate cancer mortality: evidence for protective effect of ultraviolet radiation. *Cancer.* 1992;70:2861–2869.

74. Schwartz GG, Hulka BS. Is vitamin D deficiency a risk factor for prostate cancer? *Anticancer Res.* 1990;10:1307–1311.

75. Giovannucci E. Dietary influences of 1,25(OH)$_2$ vitamin D in relation to prostate cancer: a hypothesis. *Cancer Causes Control.* 1998;9:567–582.

76. O'Neill GP, Ford-Hutchinson AW. Expression of mRNA for cyclooxygenase-1 and cyclooxygnease-2 in human tissues. *FEBS Lett.* 1993;330:156–160.

77. Norrish AE, Jackson RT, McRae CU. Non-steroidal anti-inflammatory drugs and prostate cancer progression. *Intl J Cancer.* 1998;77:511–515.

78. Roberts RA, Jacobson DJ, Lieber MM. Prostate cancer and non-steroidal anti-inflammatory drugs: a protective association. *J Urol.* 2001;165:62.

79. Pearson JD, Watson DJ, Corrada MM, et al. A prospective cohort study of nonsteroidal anti-inflammatory drugs and risk of prostate cancer: Baltimore Longitudinal Study of Aging. *J Urol.* 2001;165:63.

PART 7

Racial and Ethnic Considerations in Clinical Prevention

chapter 34

Hispanics

Raul J. Seballos, MD

INTRODUCTION

In Census 2000, the US government considered race and Hispanic origin to be separate and distinct.[1] Hispanics are persons of Cuban, Mexican, Puerto Rican, South or Central American, or other Spanish culture of origin, regardless of race. Thus, Hispanic Americans may be of any race. Statistics from Census 2000 revealed Hispanics to represent 12.5% of the US population, or about 35 million persons. The Hispanic population is the fasting growing minority group in the United States and has increased by nearly 60% in the past decade compared with an increase of 13.2% of the total US population. The Census Bureau projects that by 2035 approximately 75 million Hispanics, comprising 20% of the population, will be living in the United States.[2]

SOCIODEMOGRAPHICS

The Census Bureau in 2002 updated its data on Hispanics, which revealed that 66.9% of Hispanics were Mexican Americans, 14.3% Central and South Americans, 8.6% Puerto Ricans, 3.7% Cuban Americans, and 6.5% other Hispanic origins[3] (Fig 34-1). In 2000, three fourths of the Hispanic population lived in the West and South, with half of all Hispanics living in California and Texas.

Hispanics tend to be younger than the remainder of the US population.[3] The median age of all Hispanics is 25.9 years, nearly 10 years younger than the median age of the entire US population. Of the Hispanic subgroups, Cuban Americans tend to be older and Mexican Americans, younger.

As of 2002, 40% of Hispanics were foreign-born,[3] with half of those entering the United States between 1990 and 2002. Hispanics tend to live in larger family households, demonstrated by more than 25% living in households of 5 or more people, compared with 10.8% of non-Hispanic white families.[3] Hispanics are more likely than non-Hispanic whites never to have been married and less likely to graduate from high school. Hispanics are also more likely to have less than a ninth grade education than non-Hispanic whites (27.0% vs 4.0%), and were less likely to hold a bachelor's degree (11% vs 29.4%).

Hispanics are more likely than non-Hispanic whites to be unemployed, more likely to work in service occupations, and less likely to hold managerial or professional positions. Full-time year-round Hispanic workers earn less than do non-Hispanic white counterparts. Hispanics are more likely to live in poverty, with slightly more than 21% living below poverty level. While Hispanic children represent 17.7% of all children in the United States, they comprise nearly one third of all children living in poverty.

HEALTH PROFILES

Just as the Hispanic population is a heterogeneous group, variability exists in their health profiles. Distinction of Hispanic groups may vary by study. Accurate reporting of race and ethnicity may limit statistics from surveys, such as the National Center for Health Statistics. The National Health and Nutrition Examination

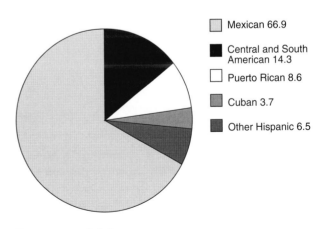

FIGURE 34-1

US Hispanics (percent) by origin in 2002. Data from US Census Bureau.[3]

Survey III in 1988 to 1994 (NHANES III) provides more comprehensive Hispanic-specific information, which helps to recognize patterns of susceptibility among Hispanic subgroups. For example, Puerto Ricans are more likely to have asthma, human immunodeficiency virus (HIV)/acquired immunodeficiency syndrome (AIDS), and infant mortality, and Mexican Americans are more likely to have diabetes. Being younger than the non-Hispanic white US population, Hispanics in general are less likely to report a chronic health condition.[4] By age 50 years, however, Hispanics appear to report chronic diseases at rates similar to all US adults aged 50 and older.

CARDIOVASCULAR DISEASE AND STROKE

Cardiovascular Disease

Cardiovascular disease (CVD) is a common cause of death among Hispanics. More than 25% of Mexican American men and women have CVD.[5] Death rates due to CVD, however, are lower in the Hispanic population. In 2000, for every 100,000 persons in the United States, 187 people died of coronary heart disease whereas the same age-adjusted rate for Hispanics was 138.[6] In a study based on death certificates, Swenson and colleagues[7] also reported lower CVD mortality among Hispanics compared with non-Hispanic whites.

Stroke

As in CVD, death rates due to stroke are less in the Hispanic population than in the overall US population. The stroke death rates between Hispanics and non-Hispanic whites were similar under age 65 but slightly less for Hispanics over age 65.[8] Puerto Ricans have the highest age-adjusted death rate for stroke in both men and women. Frey and colleagues,[9] in a hospital-based study, found that Hispanics have a higher proportion of hemorrhagic stroke in the younger age group.

Risk Factors for Atherosclerosis

Hypertension

Among Hispanics aged 20 to 74 years, 24.2% of men and 2.4% of women have hypertension.[5] Unfortunately, only half of hypertensive Hispanics know they have hypertension, and only one fourth of those have their blood pressure under control.[10] Hispanic women have higher rates of awareness, treatment, and control of their blood pressure than do Hispanic men.[11] Puerto Ricans are more likely than any Hispanic subgroup to have hypertension.[12]

Smoking

Smoking is a known risk factor for CVD, stroke, and lung cancer. Lower smoking rates may contribute to the lower cardiovascular and stroke mortality found in Hispanics.[13] The National Health Interview Survey data show smoking rates of 20.4% in Hispanic adults, compared with 25.3% in non-Hispanic whites, 26.7% in African Americans, and 34.1% in American Indians and Alaskan Natives.[14] Hispanic men were twice as likely than Hispanic women to smoke. One third of Hispanic high school students (grades 9 through 12) were current smokers.[15] Fortunately, cigarette smoking among Hispanic high school students plateaued between 1997 and 1999. Use of other forms of tobacco such as cigars is also common. One in 5 Hispanic male high school students smokes cigars, slightly less than in non-Hispanic whites but more than in African American male high school students.[15]

Diabetes mellitus

The risk of diabetes mellitus (DM) is greater for the Hispanic population than for non-Hispanic whites. Hispanics also tend to have poorer glycemic control among minority groups with diabetes.[16] The risk of DM for Hispanics—particularly Mexican Americans and Puerto Ricans—and African Americans is 2 times greater than for non-Hispanic whites.[8] After controlling for socioeconomic status, Sacco and colleagues[17] reported diabetes prevalence of 41% among Hispanics vs 26% for non-Hispanic whites. Diabetes in the Mexican American subgroup is particularly problematic. Among Mexican Americans older than age 20 years, 8.1% of men and 11.4% of women have physician-diagnosed DM. Another 5.8% of men and 3.9% of women have undiagnosed DM and an additional 12.1% of men and 6.7% of women have impaired fasting glucose levels. Nearly one fourth of Mexican Americans and Puerto Ricans older than age 65 years have DM.[12]

Obesity

Obesity, defined as body mass index at or above 30 kg/m^2, is less prevalent in Hispanics than in African Americans but greater than in non-Hispanic whites. In the pediatric population, Dwyer and colleagues[18] reported a greater prevalence of obesity among Hispanics and African Americans in both sexes compared with non-Hispanic whites. Interestingly, parental income and education does not seem to be associated with childhood obesity in Hispanics, as appears to be the case in non-Hispanic whites.[19]

Lipids

Lipid patterns in Hispanics are similar to those found in African Americans and non-Hispanic whites. There are slight differences. Hispanics are slightly less likely to have low-density lipoprotein cholesterol (LDL-C) levels greater than 3.36 mmol/L (130 mg/dL) compared with non-Hispanic whites and African Americans. Also, Mexican American women are more likely than African American and non-Hispanic white women to have high-density lipoprotein cholesterol (HDL-C) levels less than 0.91 mmol/L (35 mg/dL). Mexican American men are more likely than African American men and less likely than non-Hispanic white men to have HDL-C levels lower than 0.91 mmol/L (35 mg/dL).

CANCER

Cancer is the second leading cause of death among Hispanic adults. In 1998, lung cancer was the leading cause of cancer death in Hispanic men, with an age-adjusted rate of 28.6 per 100,000 population.[20] Among Hispanic women, breast cancer is the leading cause of cancer death, with an age-adjusted rate of 14.2 per 100,000 population, less than in non-Hispanic white and African American women. Death rates due to cancers of the lung, colon, prostate, and breast have declined in the past decade among Hispanics. Changes in the death rate for lung cancer reflect the decline in smoking during 1965 to 1985.[21] Other decreases likely reflect increased screening and more effective cancer treatment.

The Centers for Disease Control and Prevention (CDC) reported in a press release on March 19, 2003, that Hispanic women who live in border counties along the US–Mexican border, were less likely than non-Hispanic women to undergo screening for breast and cervical cancers.[22] Access to health care preventive services in the border regions and lower socioeconomic status, particularly for Hispanic women living in border states, may partly account for lower cancer screening rates. The Collaborative Research Unit at the former Cook County (Ill) Hospital reported that when equivalent insurance and a regular source of care were available, Hispanic patients received cancer screening procedures at the same rate as non-Hispanics.[23] This led the authors to conclude that availability of insurance coverage and continuity of care may be more important than cultural factors.[23] The CDC is funding the National Breast and Cervical Cancer Early Detection Program to offer cancer screening to low-income women, including new immigrants.

HUMAN IMMUNODEFICIENCY VIRUS

In 1999, the age-adjusted death rate due to HIV in Hispanics was 3 times higher than in non-Hispanic whites but 3 times less than in African Americans.[12] In the Hispanic subgroup, Puerto Ricans were more likely to die of HIV complications and AIDS, particularly in the states of New York and New Jersey. As with other minority groups, HIV infection is associated with intravenous drug use and men having sex with men.[24] Hispanics are less likely to cite written information and more likely to cite radio as sources for HIV information. Hispanic parents are also less likely to discuss HIV and AIDS with their children.[24]

TUBERCULOSIS

Between 1986 and 1995, the number of cases of tuberculosis (TB) increased 61% among foreign-born immigrants.[25] One in 5 foreign-born immigrants are born in Mexico. Using DNA fingerprinting of TB isolates in northern Manhattan in New York from 1990 to 1999, Geng and colleagues[26] reported TB to be more likely caused by reactivation of latent infection among foreign-born persons, rather than by recent transmission, which was the more common mode in US-born persons. A 400% increase in TB occurred among children living in San Diego County (Calif) from 1985 to 1993. In a retrospective review of medical records, the largest increase was noted in children younger than age 5 years.[27] Three fourths of these children were born in the United States. However, nearly two thirds had a foreign-born parent, and nearly half of these children visited Mexico. Most of these children were also from non–English-speaking households. Of note, 27.5% exhibited drug resistance to one of the first-line antituberculous medications. The authors concluded that TB infection in children was most likely due to transmission either outside the United States or within the United States via household contacts with foreign-born parents from highly endemic countries such as Mexico.

Successful screening and treatment of TB, particularly latent TB, can be achieved. The Johns Hopkins School of Nursing demonstrated a successful program of screening and treating Hispanic immigrants by partnering with a local health department's pulmonary clinic.[28]

HOMICIDE AND SUICIDE

In 1999, homicides among Hispanics were 3 times more likely than in non-Hispanic whites but less than half that of African Americans.[12] Of the Hispanic subgroups, Puerto Ricans were more likely to die of homicide. Factors such as lower socioeconomic status, residence in urban areas with higher rates of violent crimes, substance abuse, and delay in emergency treatment to indigent patients contribute to higher homicide rates.[24]

Cuban Americans and Puerto Rican men, especially foreign-born, have higher rates of suicide than non-Hispanic whites and African Americans. Underdiagnosed depression caused by cultural and language barriers, and political uncertainty with loss of access to their homeland, particularly with Cuban-born immigrants, may contribute to higher rates of suicide.

BARRIERS TO HEALTH CARE

Lack of personal health insurance, low socioeconomic status, and language and cultural isolation, all serve as barriers to health care and contribute to poor health outcomes for Hispanics.[29] Hispanics under age 65 years are more than twice as likely to be uninsured than are non-Hispanic whites.[12] More than one third of Hispanics do not have private health insurance, Medicare, or Medicaid coverage. According to The Commonwealth Fund 2001 Health Care Quality Survey, the number of uninsured Hispanics has dramatically increased from 7.0 million in 1990 to 11.2 million in 2000.[30] Mexican Americans and immigrants from Central and South America were most likely of the Hispanic subgroups not to have insurance. Nearly 75% of Hispanics who have lived in the United States less than 5 years are uninsured. Hispanics are more likely to be unemployed, more likely to work in service occupations, and more likely to live in poverty than non-Hispanic whites.

Hispanic patients who speak English are more likely to seek regular medical care than those who speak only Spanish.[31] Hispanics who primarily speak Spanish report poorer health status, are less likely to have a regular primary care physician, and more likely to lack health insurance.[30] Sixty-one percent of primarily Spanish-speaking Hispanic adults aged 18 to 64 years are uninsured all or part of the year. Primarily Spanish-speaking Hispanics are more likely to use community health clinics for their health care, compared with primarily English-speaking Hispanics, African Americans, and non-Hispanic whites.[30] In addition to poorer health status, primarily Spanish-speaking Hispanics are less likely to visit a physician, have more difficulty understanding prescription instructions, and have greater difficulty understanding instructions from physician's office.

SUMMARY

Because the Hispanic population is a heterogeneous group, variability in its health profiles also exists. Distinction of Hispanic groups also varies by study. Reporting of disease prevalence by race and ethnicity may be inaccurate and underestimated within the Hispanic subgroups. Although Hispanics are younger compared to the US population, they are less likely to report a chronic health condition.[4] However, over a third reported having at least one chronic disease and are more likely to report a poorer health status. Low socioeconomic status, lower educational attainment levels, lack of personal health insurance, language and cultural barriers, all contribute to access to health care leading to poorer health outcomes. Programs to curb smoking and obesity are needed among children, teenagers, and adult Hispanic Americans. Additional health screening programs are needed, such as the CDC's National Breast and Cervical Cancer Early Detection Program, that offer cancer screening to low-income women. Further research should also focus on the Central and South American Hispanic subgroup, illegal immigrants, and others not surveyed because of language and cultural barriers. Once we include as many Hispanic Americans in the health database, we can better understand the health care issues faced by this fastest growing minority group.

REFERENCES

1. US Bureau of the Census. US Census 2000. Washington, DC: US Bureau of the Census; 2000. Available at: www.census.gov. Accessed October 1, 2003.

2. Overview of race and Hispanic origin: Census 2000 brief. Washington, DC: US Bureau of the Census; 2001. Available at: www.census.gov/prod/2001pubs/c2kbr01–3.pdf. Accessed October 1, 2003.

3. Ramirez RR, de la Cruz GP. The Hispanic population in the United States: March 2002. *Current Population Reports.* Washington DC: US Census Bureau; 2002. P-20-545.

4. Doty M, Ives BL. Quality of healthcare for Hispanic populations: findings from The Commonwealth Fund 2001 Health Care Quality Survey. March 2002. Available at: www.cmwf.org/programs/minority/doty_hispanic_fs_526.pdf. Accessed October 1, 2003.

5. American Heart Association. *Heart Facts 2003: Latino/Hispanic Americans.* Available at: www.americanheart.org/downloadable/heart/1046366143509HFLHFS.pdf.

6. *National Vital Statistics Report.* September 16, 2002. Available at: www.cdc.gov/nchs. Accessed October 1, 2003.

7. Swenson CJ, Trepka MJ, Rewers MJ, Scarbro S, Hiatt WR, Hamman RF. Cardiovascular disease mortality in Hispanics and non-Hispanic whites. *Am J Epidemiol.* 2002;156:919–928.

8. Guillum RF. Epidemiology of stroke in Hispanic Americans. *Stroke.* 1995;26:1707–1712.

9. Frey JL, Jahnke HK, Bulfinch EW. Difference in stroke between white, Hispanic, and Native American patients: Barrow Neurological Institute Stroke database. *Stroke.* 1998;29:29–33.

10. Cangiano JL. Hypertension in Hispanic Americans. *Clev Clin J Med.* 1994;61:345–350.

11. Crespo CJ, Loria CM, Burt VL. Hypertension and other cardiovascular disease risk factors among Mexican American, Asian Americans, and Puerto Ricans from the Hispanic Health and Nutrition Examination Survey. *Public Health Rep.* 1996;111(suppl 2):7–10.

12. *A Demographic and Health Snapshot of the U.S. Hispanic/Latino Population: 2002 National Hispanic Health Leadership Summit.* Atlanta, Ga: Centers for Disease Control and Prevention; 2002. Available at: www.cdc.gov/NCHS/data/hpdata2010/chcsummit.pdf. Accessed October 1, 2003.

13. Bruno A. Are there differences in vascular disease between ethnic and racial groups? *Stroke.* 1998;29:29–33.

14. Centers for Disease Control and Prevention. Cigarette smoking among adults: United States, 1997. *MMWR Morb Mortal Wkly Rep.* 1999;48:993–996.

15. Centers for Disease Control and Prevention. Youth risk behavior surveillance: United States, 1999. *MMWR Morb Mortal Wkly Rep.* 2000;49:No.SS–5.

16. Summerson JH, Konen JC, Dignan MB. Race-related differences in metabolic control among adults with diabetes. *South Med J.* 1992;85:953–956.

17. Sacco RL, Kargman DE, Zamanillo MC. Race-ethnic differences in stroke risk factors among hospitalized patients with cerebral infarction: the Northern Manhattan Stroke Study. *Neurology.* 1995;45:659–663.

18. Dwyer JT, Stone EJ, Yang M, Webber LS, Must A, Feldman HA, Nader PR, Perry CL, Parcel GS. Prevalence of marked overweight and obesity in multiethnic pediatric population: findings from the Child and Adolescent Trial for Cardiovascular Health (CATCH) Study. *J Am Diet Assoc.* 2000;100:1149–1156.

19. Crawford PB, Story M, Wang MC, et al. Ethnic issues in the epidemiology of childhood obesity. *Pediatr Clin North Am.* 2001;48:855–878.

20. Centers for Disease Control and Prevention. Recent trends in mortality rates for four major cancers by sex, and race/ethnicity: United States, 1990–1998. *MMWR Morb Mortal Wkly Rep.* 2002;51:49–53.

21. Wingo PA, Ries LAG, Giovino GA, et al. Annual report to the nation on the status of cancer, 1973–1996, with a special section on lung cancer and tobacco smoking. *J Natl Cancer Inst.* 1999;91:675–690.

22. Centers for Disease Control and Prevention Office of Communication. Hispanic women in border states less likely to receive screening for breast and cervical cancers [press release]. March 19, 2003. Available at: www.cdc.gov/od/oc/media/pressrel/r030319.htm. Accessed October 1, 2003.

23. Jacobs EA, Lauderdale DS. Receipt of cancer screening procedures among Hispanics and non-Hispanic health maintenance organization members. *Cancer.* 2001;91(suppl):257–261.

24. Bassford T. Special health problems of Hispanics in the United States. In: Matzen RN, Lang R, Mayshark C, eds. *Clinical Preventive Medicine.* St Louis, Mo: Mosby; 1993:677–688.

25. Characteristics of foreign-born Hispanic patients with tuberculosis: eight U.S. counties bordering Mexico, 1995. *MMWR Morb Mortal Wkly Rep.* 1996;45:1032–1036.

26. Geng E, Kreisworth B, Driver C, et al. Changes in transmission of tuberculosis in New York City from 1990 to 1999. *N Engl J Med.* 2002;346:1453–1458.

27. Kenyon TA, Driver C, Haas E, et al. Immigrants and tuberculosis among children in the United States-Mexico border, County of San Diego, California. *Pediatrics.* 1999;104:8.

28. D'Lugoff MI, Jone W, Kub J, et al. Tuberculosis screening in an at-risk immigrant Hispanic population in Baltimore city: an academic health center/local health department partnership. *J Cultural Diversity.* 2002;9:79–85.

29. *The Heath Care Challenge: Acknowledging Disparity, Confronting Discrimination, and Ensuring Equality.* Washington, DC: A report of the US Commission on Civil Rights; September 1999.

30. The Commonwealth Fund. 2001 Health Care Quality Survey. Available at: www.cmwf.org/programs/minority/doty_hispanicchartpack_684.pdf. Accessed October 1, 2003.

31. American Medical Association Council on Scientific Affairs. Council report: Hispanic health in the United States. *JAMA.* 1991;265:248–252.

RESOURCES

Overview of Race and Hispanic Origin. Available at: www.census.gov/prod/2001pubs/c2kbr01-3.pdf

A demographic and health snapshot of the U.S. Hispanic/Latino population. 2002 National Hispanic Health Leadership Summit. Available at: www.cdc.gov/NCHS/data/hpdata2010/chcsummit.pdf

The Commonwealth Fund. Health Care Quality Survey. Available at: www.cmwf.org/programs/minority/doty_hispanicchartpack_684.pdf

chapter 35

African Americans

Oluranti Aladesanmi, MD, MPH, and Carol E. Blixen, PhD, RN

INTRODUCTION

Disparities in the burden of death and illness experienced by African Americans compared with the general US population are well documented, and they persist and, in many areas, continue to increase.[1] African Americans today live substantially shorter lives than do whites; die more frequently of cancer, heart disease, stroke, and diabetes; and see their infants die at nearly twice the rate of white infants, partly as a result of their unique and tragic historical experience in America.[2] In 1999, African Americans had an age-adjusted death rate due to heart disease that was 30% higher than in whites and were 30% more likely to die of cancer than were whites.

To address these overwhelming disparities, the Clinton administration led the Initiative to Eliminate Racial and Ethnic Disparities in Health by the year 2010.[3] In addition, the US Congress in 1999 requested an Institute of Medicine (IOM) study to assess disparities in the kinds and quality of health care received by racial and ethnic minorities and patients who are not minorities. The March 2002 IOM report, *Unequal Treatment: Confronting Racial and Ethnic Disparities in Healthcare,* concluded that the sources of these disparities are multiple, complex, and rooted in historic and contemporary inequities.[4] Additionally, the report concluded that many sources, including health care systems, health care providers, patients, and utilization managers, are potential causes of health disparities and that bias, stereotyping, prejudice, and the clinical uncertainty of clinicians may contribute to the problem. It also found that the rates that minority patients refuse procedures and treatments are generally small and do not fully explain health care disparities. The IOM recommendations include the following:

1. Increase the awareness of the public and health care providers about the extent of these differences.

2. Enact legal, regulatory, and policy interventions.

3. Initiate specific health system interventions such as promoting the consistency and equity of care through the use of evidence-based guidelines, structuring payment systems to ensure an adequate supply of services to minority patients, limiting provider incentives that may promote disparities, and enhancing patient-provider communication and trust by providing financial incentives for practices that reduce barriers and encourage evidence-based practice.

THE AFRICAN AMERICAN/ BLACK POPULATION IN THE UNITED STATES

According to US Census 2000, 36.4 million, or 12.9% of the US population, were reported on April 1, 2000, to be black or African American. The question on race in the 2000 census was changed and respondents were given the option of selecting one or more race categories to indicate their racial identities. 34.7 million people, or 12.3%, reported being solely black, and an additional 1.8 million people reported black and at least one other race. Within this group, the most common combinations were "Black and White," "Black and Some Other Race," "Black and American Indian and Alaska Native," and "Black and White and American Indian and Alaska Native." Census 2000 also asked separate questions on race and Hispanic or Latino origin. Hispanics who reported their race as black, either alone or in combination with one or more other races, are included in the numbers for blacks.[5]

MAJOR HEALTH PROBLEMS

The top 10 causes of mortality of African Americans in 2000 are listed in Table 35-1. Despite overall declines in mortality, racial and ethnic disparities in mortality persist.[6] Although many conditions contribute to socioeconomic and racial disparities in mortality, a few conditions account for most of these disparities. Smoking-related diseases such as ischemic heart disease and lung cancer are more prevalent in persons with fewer years of education, and hypertension, human immunodeficiency virus (HIV), diabetes mellitus, and trauma are more

T A B L E 35-1

Leading Causes of Death Among African Americans in the United States, 2000*

Cause of Death	Rank	% of Deaths
Heart disease	1	27.0
Malignant neoplasms	2	21.7
Cerebrovascular disease	3	6.7
Accidents (unintentional injuries)	4	4.3
Diabetes mellitus	5	4.2
Assault (homicide)	6	2.8
Human immunodeficiency virus disease	7	2.7
Chronic lower respiratory tract diseases	8	2.7
Nephritis, nephrotic syndrome, and nephrosis	9	2.4
Influenza and pneumonia	10	2.1

*From Anderson RN. Deaths: Leading causes for 2000. *Natl Vital Stat Rep.* 2002;50:1–85.

prevalent in African Americans than in other races. Therefore, targeting ischemic heart disease and lung cancer would be most useful in reducing the disparities in mortality attributable to educational status, whereas targeting hypertension, HIV, trauma, and diabetes would have the greatest effect on racial disparities in mortality.[7]

Cardiovascular Disease and Stroke

Cardiovascular disease (CVD) remains the leading cause of death in blacks in the United States.[8] The increased morbidity and mortality of CVD in African Americans have been validated in population-based studies, which have defined the role of hypertension in the disparities in prevalence and death of CVD, stroke, and end-stage renal disease (ESRD) between African Americans and whites.[9] Compared with whites, African Americans have an earlier age at onset of CVD, stroke, and ESRD; a greater prevalence of congestive heart failure; poorer survival rates after myocardial infarction (MI) and stroke; higher overall CVD-associated mortality rates; greater levels of hypertension-related cardiac ischemia; and a higher incidence of cardiac arrest and sudden cardiac death.[10-13] African American women have the highest prevalence of CVD, followed by African American men, white women, and white men.[14] African American women have a 60% greater prevalence of MI and stroke than do white women, whereas African American men have a somewhat lower prevalence of MI compared with white men.[14,15] Recent declines in death rates due to coronary heart disease have been more significant in whites than in minority populations in the United States.[16]

Stroke is the third leading cause of death among African Americans. Prevalence of stroke is highest in African American women. African Americans between the ages of 35 and 54 years have a risk of stroke 4 times that of white Americans; African Americans aged 55 to 64 years have a threefold risk; and those between ages 65 and 74 years have almost twice the risk.[14,15]

Diabetes

Approximately 13% of all African Americans have diabetes, and are twice as likely to have diabetes as white Americans of similar age.[17] Compared with diabetic white Americans, African Americans with diabetes are more likely to have diabetic complications and to experience greater disability from these complications, and are 27% more likely to die.[17] African American women aged 45 to 64 years have a 2.4 times greater relative risk of diabetes than white women do, as well as a high prevalence of concomitant hypertension with type 2 diabetes.[18] The Atherosclerosis Risk in Communities Study found African American men to have an approximately 60% increased risk of concomitant type 2 diabetes and hypertension compared with white men.[19] These observations indicate that the presence of the comorbid conditions of diabetes and hypertension affords an especially increased risk of CVD, stroke, and ESRD in African Americans.[9,18]

Hypertension

The prevalence of hypertension is estimated to be 25% in the overall adult US population compared with 37% for African Americans.[14] The excess risk of hypertension and CVD in African Americans is more strongly linked to being born and living in the United States than with African ancestry.[9] This is supported by the results of a cross-sectional study showing that the prevalence of hypertension was 14% in rural Nigerians and 26% in Jamaicans of African descent.[20] Currently, racial differences in response to drugs have not yet been sufficiently disentangled from social and cultural influences to provide a sound basis for clinical decision making.[9,21] Recent studies such as the Antihypertensive and Lipid-Lowering Treatment to Prevent Heart Attack Trial (ALLHAT) and the African American Study of Kidney Disease and Hypertension Study Group (AASK) allow the evaluation of the effects of hypertension treatment on groups, such as blacks, who were underrepresented in or excluded from previous clinical trials.[22,23] All antihypertensive drug classes offer blood pressure–lowering efficacy in African Americans. Ethnicity alone does not predict response to antihypertensive therapy, and there is no rationale to use race as a reason to avoid certain classes of agents.[21] The expectancy among medical professionals that blood pressure can and should be adequately controlled in African American patients must be strengthened.

Obesity

African American adults have substantially higher rates of obesity than do white Americans.[24,25] Additionally, African Americans have a greater tendency to develop upper-body obesity, which has been found to increase risk of diabetes. Although African Americans have higher rates of obesity, researchers do not believe that obesity alone accounts for their higher prevalence of diabetes. Even when compared with white Americans with the same levels of obesity, age, and socioeconomic status, African Americans still have higher rates of diabetes. Other factors, yet to be understood, appear to be responsible.[26]

Cancer

The survival rate in African American patients for most cancers, including the 4 major types (colorectal, lung and bronchus, female breast, and prostate), is poorer than that in white patients, although survival rates have improved in recent years for both groups.[27] The observed racial or ethnic differences in relative risks of cancer death may relate to differences in access to optimal treatments that reduce cancer mortality rates. Low socioeconomic status, lack of health insurance, and low literacy can also delay diagnosis and reduce access to optimal therapies.[28-31]

From 1992 to 1998, African American men were almost twice as likely to have a diagnosis of prostate cancer compared with white men. Although incidence rates for African American men declined 4.0% per year for these years, white men experienced a 5.7% decline per year for the same period.[32,33] African American men were twice as likely to die of prostate cancer in comparison with white men between 1992 and 1998. Reasons proposed for higher incidence and death rates due to prostate cancer among African American men include biologically more aggressive cancer, younger age at presentation,[34-38] genetic factors,[39-41] higher testosterone level,[42,43] and adverse pathological factors after radical prostatectomy.[44] Socioeconomic factors such as income, education, nutrition, and screening also have been cited as factors contributing to the more aggressive and advanced stage of prostate cancer in African American men.[45-47]

Breast cancer is an important cause of mortality in African American women. Studies have shown lower breast cancer survival rates for African American women compared with white women when controlled for prognostic factors, such as age, tumor stage, menopausal status,[48] socioeconomic status,[49-51] Medicaid or Medicare status,[49] tumor size,[48-50] histologic grade,[50] lymph node

status,[48] or hormone receptor status.[48] From 1988 to 1997, despite minor differences in their reported mammography screening rates in 1998, localized breast cancer was diagnosed in a smaller percentage of African American patients compared with non-Hispanic whites, and African Americans had a higher adjusted risk of breast cancer death.[52] These findings may partly account for breast cancer mortality rates being higher in African American women than in white women in whom the disease was diagnosed during 1990 to 1996.[53,54] The mammography screening benefits in African American women may have not yet been realized because decreases in breast cancer mortality rates due to screening lag behind increases in mammography utilization.[52] In addition, as many as 30% to 50% of minority women with abnormal mammography findings do not receive timely follow-up.[55-57] Other potential explanations include the low use of repeated screening, higher prevalence of obesity, and, possibly, breast density and other biologic factors that contribute to younger age at diagnosis.[58]

African Americans bear a disproportionate share of the mortality burden from colon cancer in the United States.[59] Although mortality rates are declining overall, they began to decline earlier and more rapidly in whites vs African Americans during the past 2 decades.[60] The group disparities in colorectal cancer mortality are partly attributable to differences in risk factors; however, variations in health care practices, primarily early detection and treatment, are also potential contributing causes.

HIV Infection

The impact of HIV and acquired immunodeficiency syndrome (AIDS) in the African American community has been devastating.[61] Representing only 12% to 13% of the total US population, African Americans make up almost 38% of all AIDS cases reported in the United States.[61] The proportional distribution of AIDS cases among racial and ethnic groups has shifted since the beginning of the epidemic, decreasing among whites over time and increasing among blacks and Hispanics. In 2000, AIDS was reported to affect more African Americans than any other racial or ethnic group. Almost two thirds (63%) of all women reported having AIDS were African American, and African American children made up almost two thirds (65%) of all reported pediatric AIDS cases.

Among African American men reported with AIDS, men having sex with men represent 37% of cases and injection drug use 34%. Heterosexual exposure accounts for 8% of cumulative cases. Among African American women reported to have AIDS, injectable drug use has accounted for 41% of all AIDS case reports since the epidemic began, with another 38% due to heterosexual contact. According to the Centers for Disease Control and Prevention (CDC), factors contributing to this problem include continued health disparities between economic classes, challenges related to controlling substance abuse, and the role of substance abuse within the epidemic of HIV and other sexually transmitted diseases. Fewer than half as many black patients as white patients attempt to obtain experimental HIV medications, suggesting that less awareness and more widespread negative attitudes about research exist in minority communities.[62]

Sickle Cell Anemia

Sickle cell anemia is the most common inherited blood disorder in the United States, affecting about 72,000 Americans, or 1 in 500 African Americans. Characterized by episodes of pain, chronic hemolytic anemia, and severe infections, this disorder usually begins in early childhood. An autosomal recessive condition, sickle cell anemia is caused by a point mutation in the hemoglobin beta gene *(HBB)* found on chromosome 11p15.4. The carrier frequency of *HBB* varies significantly around the world, with high rates associated with zones of high malaria incidence, as carriers appear somewhat protected against malaria. Approximately 8% of the African American population are carriers.

Adult patients are managed by preventive health maintenance, early recognition and treatment of complications, continuous assessment of social status, psychological assessment and support, and continuing patient education. Initial evaluation should include assessment of the patient's and family's understanding of the disease. Educational activities should focus on correcting deficits in knowledge about more common complications.

Asthma

African Americans account for a disproportionately high 23.7% of asthma-related deaths in the United States. Asthma prevalence rates show similar disparities, and the reason is unknown.[63] Not only are asthma rates higher in African Americans compared with whites, there are racial differences in use of health services for patients with asthma. African American patients with asthma are more likely to seek emergency care and less likely to visit primary care providers for asthma than are whites with asthma.[64] The researchers note that more asthma education programs specifically targeted for low-income African Americans are needed to improve use of asthma-related health care.

Sarcoidosis

Sarcoidosis is a multiorgan granulomatous disease of unknown cause that usually affects adults between 20 and 40 years of age. The prevalence of sarcoidosis is more

than 8 times greater in African Americans than whites. Although sarcoidosis is not a common cause of death, in 1998 the mortality rate due to sarcoidosis was 12 times greater for African Americans than for whites.[65] The primary care physician plays an important and necessary role in providing comprehensive care, evaluating the extent of organ and system involvement, and coordinating specialty consultations and services.[66]

Glaucoma

Glaucoma is the second leading cause of blindness in the United States, the greatest cause of preventable blindness, and the leading cause of blindness among African Americans. Glaucoma is 6 to 8 times more common in African Americans than Caucasians. African Americans aged 45 to 65 years are 14 to 17 times more likely to become blind from glaucoma than are whites with glaucoma in the same age group. Other high-risk groups include people over 60 years old, those with a family history of glaucoma, diabetic individuals, and people who are severely nearsighted. A recent survey found that 16.1% of African Americans were unfamiliar with glaucoma.[67] The American Academy of Ophthalmology recommends a comprehensive eye examination for every patient over age 40 years, to be performed every 1 to 4 years, and an eye examination every 2 to 4 years for blacks aged 20 to 39 years.[68]

Tobacco use

Cigarette smoking remains the most important contributor to preventable morbidity and mortality in the United States.[69] African Americans living in the inner city have a smoking rate as high as 45%, whereas the general population's smoking rate is 25%.[70] Despite African Americans being likely to attempt to quit smoking more times in any given year compared with whites, the success rate for smoking cessation is 34% lower for blacks than for whites.[71,72] Studies show that the higher number of quit attempts would likely result in sustained abstinence if improved smoking cessation modalities for African Americans were developed and disseminated.[73,74] Smoking patterns in African Americans are different from those of whites.[74] African Americans smoke fewer cigarettes per day (15 vs 25 for whites), prefer mentholated and higher tar or nicotine cigarettes,[75] and are more likely to smoke within 10 minutes of awakening.[74] Researchers have found that African Americans metabolize nicotine slower and have higher serum cotinine levels per cigarette smoked than do whites.[76,77] These factors merit consideration in organization of smoking cessation programs and in treating individual patients for smoking cessation.

Alcohol Abuse

Alcohol consumption patterns and resultant health effects differ between African American and white populations. For example, data collected from the National Health and Nutrition Examination Survey (NHANES) and the NHANES Epidemiologic Followup Study (NHEFS) showed an absence of a protective effect at lower volumes of consumption in a large sample of African Americans after a long period of longitudinal follow-up.[78] Given that the protective effect of the J-shaped mortality curve was seen in the same study for white respondents, the absence of this effect in the African Americans was striking. The NHANES study also confirmed earlier findings that African Americans drink less often but in larger amounts than do whites—a biologically less protective pattern. In addition, in some subgroups, such as those that are socioeconomically disadvantaged, special kinds of drinks (eg, malt liquor) that come in large serving sizes prevail.[79] The larger containers and higher alcohol content of these beverages marketed to African Americans may therefore underestimate the heavy quantities consumed by ethnic minorities. These factors help to explain in part the higher risks of liver cirrhosis among African American and Hispanic populations compared with whites. Preventive interventions for alcohol use in the African American population often focus on reducing the *average* volume of drinking. Assessing and addressing drinking *patterns* in this population may lead to improved outcomes.

Violence

Homicide is the second leading cause of death for persons 15 to 24 years of age and is the leading cause of death for African American youth in this age group, according to national statistics.[80-82] Guns are a factor in most youth homicides. In 1999, 81% of homicide victims aged 15 to 24 years were killed with firearms.[82]

Violence prevention strategies incorporate social-cognitive training for children and adolescents, parent training, nurse home visits to high-risk young parents, and mentoring programs for young people.[83]

BARRIERS TO HEALTH CARE

Socioeconomic and Cultural Barriers

Causes of disparities in health status have consistently been attributed to such variables as socioeconomic status (especially income, lack of education, and unemployment), lifestyle choices and behavioral risks, occupational and environmental hazards, inferior housing, poor nutrition, and different cultural beliefs about health and illness.

Another factor is lack of minority access to health care, particularly the lack of either public or private health insurance, which has persisted despite the introduction and expansion of programs such as Medicare and Medicaid.[84,85] Efforts to reduce or eliminate disparities in health care must consider the complex relationship between the social, cultural, and economic factors that form the matrix of the lives of African Americans.

The Health Behavior Model hypothesizes that characteristics of the external environment, the health care delivery system, and personal features of the population influence health maintenance behaviors.[86,87] The model organizes personal population characteristics (ie, individual-level predictors) into 3 categories: predisposing, need, and enabling factors. Predisposing factors, which precede current illness, reflect differences in the propensity for specific behaviors and are conceptualized as the sociocultural element of the model. They include sociodemographic factors, health attitudes, and beliefs. Before deciding to pursue treatment or adhere to treatment recommendations, individuals must perceive a need (ie, a condition warranting intervention or behavior change). The enabling component incorporates circumstances that hinder or facilitate access to formal services.

Culture may be defined as the sharing of modes of behavior and outlook within a community.[88,89] The traditional European cultural perspective, proposed as being appropriate for African Americans, is divergent from the African cultural perspective. Whereas Europeans focus on individuality, uniqueness, and difference, African culture prioritizes "groupness," sameness, and commonality. European values of competition, independence, and "survival of the fittest" contrast with the values of collective responsibility, interdependence, and tribal survival found in African culture. African Americans display their need for "groupness" by relying more on informal resource networks than do members of the white community.[90,91] Multigenerational households frequently are found in African American communities. Living, being close with, and reliance on grandparents, aunts and uncles, cousins, and other close relatives may be seen as another demonstration of the "groupness" that is an essential component of this culture. Therefore, a health care intervention for African Americans framed in the context of "groupness" will be more likely to succeed.

Because African Americans depend on extended kin and neighbors for advice and support, they may underuse the health care system. Instead of seeking care, African Americans may be more likely to trivialize or ignore symptoms of disease and may be more likely to exhibit an external locus of control orientation.[90,91] An orientation in the present time, which is culturally reinforced,[90] also may interfere with African Americans attaining optimal health care outcomes.

Bailey[92] described the following pattern of health care–seeking behavior among African Americans:

- Individual waits for days or weeks after symptoms of illness appear
- Allows body to heal itself (prayer or alternative strategies)
- Modifies daily activities (reduces work and stress)
- Seeks advice from family member, close friend, church leader, and traditional healer
- Eventually goes to emergency department, health clinic, or family doctor

The above pattern of delay translates into greater disease progression and ultimately greater intensity of treatment and cost—both to the individual and to society.

Mistrust of the Health Care System

It has been shown that African American patients are more likely to reject treatment recommendations.[93,94] These findings may be attributable to the long history of distrust of the medical profession, negative experiences in the clinical encounter, a perception that their doctor is not invested in their care, and a propensity for rumor generation among African Americans, which exists to encode persistent and pervasive anxieties. These anxieties or "legends and rumors" serve a role in African American culture[95]; they flourish where "official" news is perceived as untrustworthy. Common urban legends believed by African Americans can be traced back to the 16th century, to the earliest contacts between white European explorers and black sub-Saharan Africans, and to the post-Reconstruction period in the South.[95] The general theme of these legends and rumors involves threats to the well-being of the community and/or physical dangers to the bodies of African Americans.

The so-called "Tuskegee study" initiated by the US Public Health Service in 1932 on 600 indigent African American males in Macon County, Alabama, touched off a wave of controversy and indignation 30 years later.[96-99] The purpose of this now-famous study was to examine the course of untreated syphilis. Acknowledgment that this project was carried out has instilled a deep mistrust among African Americans toward the health care system and has validated the notion that they are viewed as potential targets for medical experimentation.[98] A recent survey of 1056 African American church members in 5 cities that evaluated the widespread misconception that AIDS is a plot to wipe out African Americans found 35% of respondents believing AIDS was a genocidal plot, 30% "unsure," and 44% believing the government was not telling the truth about AIDS.[100] The collective knowledge and consciousness of African Americans understandably includes mistrust of the health care system; ongoing disparities in health care outcomes have been taken as

evidence that reconfirms these suspicions.[101] Although there is historical justification, this mistrust serves to perpetuate and widen the racial disparities in health care outcomes; it also interferes with many African Americans achieving the goals of disease management, while continuing to fuel the trends for disproportionately high morbidity and mortality in certain diseases.

Cultural Competency

Culturally competent health care includes knowledge about diverse patient groups and understanding the ways that different beliefs of patients, families, and health care professionals influence the patient's health-related behavior and treatment outcomes. Culturally competent health care allows health care professionals to assess, consider, and plan for the biological, cultural, psychosocial, and spiritual aspects of patient care. However, the provision of culturally appropriate and competent health care can be a complex and difficult task. Variation within certain races or cultural or ethnic groups adds to the complexity of delivering culturally competent health care. Among African Americans, major cultural differences exist between urban and rural dwellers, native-born individuals and immigrants from the Caribbean and elsewhere, and Christians and Muslims.

Cultural competency training aims to increase cultural awareness, knowledge, and skills with a potential for behavior change (both clinical and administrative). Cross-cultural education is one of the strategies needed to address disparities in health care. Other strategies include interpreter services, recruitment and retention strategies aimed at increasing minority providers, use of minority community health workers, and including family and community members in the care of minority patients.[102]

SUMMARY

The knowledge of disparities in the health care and health status of African Americans and an understanding of health-related attitudes, perceptions, and behaviors are crucial in the provision of primary care services to this population.

Health care providers and administrators need to seek solutions in clinical, research, and educational settings to address these disparities.

REFERENCES

1. Williams DR. Race, socioeconomic status, and health: the added effects of racism and discrimination. *Ann N Y Acad Sci.* 1999;896:173–188.

2. Blendon RJ. Foreword. In: Byrd WM, Clayton LA. *An American Health Dilemma.* Vol 1. *A Medical History of African Americans and the Problem of Race: Beginnings to 1900.* New York, NY: Routledge; 2000.

3. Office of Minority Health. Available at: www.omhrc.gov. Accessed January 6, 2003.

4. Smedley BD, Stith AY, Nelson AR, eds. *Unequal Treatment: Confronting Racial and Ethnic Disparities in Health Care.* Washington, DC: National Academy Press; 2002.

5. McKinnon J. *The Black Population: 2000. Census 2000 Brief.* US Census Bureau, Census 2000 Redistricting Data (Public Law 94-171) Summary File, Table PL1. Washington, DC: US Government Printing Office; 2000.

6. Hoyert DL, Arias E, Smith BL, Murphy SL, Kochanek KD. Deaths: final data for 1999 [serial online]. *Natl Vital Stat Rep.* September 21, 2001. Available at: www.cdc.gov/nchs/data/nvsr/nvsr49/nvsr49_08.pdf. Accessed January 7, 2003.

7. Wong MD, Shapiro MF, Boscardin WJ, Ettner SL. Contribution of major diseases to disparities in mortality. *N Engl J Med.* 2002;347:1585–1592.

8. Office of Minority Health. Available at: www.omhrc.gov. Accessed January 6, 2003.

9. Sowers JR, Ferdinand KC, Bakris GL, Douglas JG. Hypertension-related disease in African Americans: factors underlying disparities in illness and its outcome. *Postgrad Med.* 2002;112:24–34.

10. Brancati FL, Kao WH, Folsom AR, et al. Incident type 2 diabetes mellitus in African American and white adults: the Atherosclerosis Risk in Communities Study. *JAMA.* 2000;283:2253–2259.

11. Gillum RF, Mussolino ME, Madans JH. Coronary heart disease risk factors and attributable risks in African-American women and men: NHANES I epidemiologic follow-up study. *Am J Public Health.* 1998;88:913–917.

12. Goldstein LB, Adams R, Becker K, et al. Primary prevention of ischemic stroke: a statement for healthcare from the Stroke Council of the American Heart Association. *Circulation.* 2001;103:163–182.

13. Becker LB, Han BH, Meyer PM, et al. Racial differences in the incidence of cardiac arrest and subsequent survival: the CPR Chicago Project. *N Engl J Med.* 1993;329:600–606.

14. American Heart Association. *2000 Heart and Stroke Statistical Update.* Dallas, Tex: American Heart Association; 2001.

15. Goldstein LB, Adams R, Becker K, et al. Primary prevention of ischemic stroke: a statement for healthcare from the Stroke Council of the American Heart Association. *Circulation.* 2001;103:163–182.

16. Sempos C, Cooper R, Kovar MG, McMillen M. Divergence of the recent trends in coronary mortality for the four major race-sex groups in the United States. *Am J Public Health.* 1988;78:1422–1427.

17. National Diabetes Information Clearinghouse. National diabetes statistics [fact sheet]. NIH publication 02-3892. Available at: www.niddk.nih.gov/health/diabetes/pubs/dmstats/dmstats.htm. Accessed January 18, 2003.

18. Sowers JR, Epstein M, Frohlich E. Diabetes, hypertension, and cardiovascular disease: an update. *Hypertension.* 2001;37:1053–1059.

19. Brancati FL, Kao WH, Folsom AR, et al. Incident type 2 diabetes mellitus in African American and white adults: the Atherosclerosis Risk in Communities Study. *JAMA.* 2000;283:2253–2259.

20. Cooper R, Rotimi C. Hypertension in blacks. *Am J Hypertens.* 1997;10:804–812.

21. Jamerson K, DeQuattro V. The impact of ethnicity on response to antihypertensive therapy. *Am J Med.* 1996;101(3A):22S–32S.

22. ALLHAT (Antihypertensive and Lipid-Lowering Treatment to Prevent Heart Attack Trial): quick reference for health care providers. Available at: www.nhlbi.nih.gov/health/allhat/qckref.htm. Accessed February 1, 2003.

23. Wright JT Jr, Bakris G, Greene T, et al, for the African American Study of Kidney Disease and Hypertension Study Group. Effect of blood pressure lowering and anti-hypertensive drug class on progression of hypertensive kidney disease: results from the AASK trial *JAMA.* 2002;288:2421–2431.

24. Kuzmarski RJ, Flegal KM, Campbell SM, Johnson CL. Increasing prevalence of overweight among US adults: the National Health and Nutrition Examination Surveys, 1960 to 1991. *JAMA.* 1994;272:205–211.

25. Troiano RP, Flegal KM, Kuczmarski RJ, Campbell SM, Johnson CL. Overweight prevalence and trends for children and adolescents. *Arch Pediatr Adolesc Med.* 1995;149:1085–1091.

26. National Diabetes Information Clearinghouse. Diabetes in African Americans [fact sheet]. Available at: www.niddk.nih.gov/health/diabetes/pubs/afam/afam.htm. Accessed January 18, 2003. NIH Publication No. 02–3266.

27. Ries LAG, Eisner MP, Kosary CL, et al. *SEER Cancer Statistics Review, 1973–1997.* Bethesda, Md: National Cancer Institute; 2000.

28. Ayanian JZ, Kohler BA, Abe T, Epstein AM. The relation between health insurance coverage and clinical outcomes among women with breast cancer. *N Engl J Med.* 1993;329:326–331.

29. McWhorter WP, Mayer WJ. Black/white differences in type of initial breast cancer treatment and implications for survival. *Am J Public Health.* 1987;77:1515–1517.

30. Bennett CL, Ferreira MR, Davis TC, Kaplan J, Weinberger M, Kuzel T. Relation between literacy, race, and stage of presentation among low-income patients with prostate cancer. *J Clin Oncol.* 1998;16:3101–3104.

31. Lannin DR, Mathews HF, Mitchell J, Swanson MS, Swanson FH, Edwards MS. Influence of socioeconomic and cultural factors on racial differences in late-stage presentation of breast cancer. *JAMA.* 1998;279:1801–1807.

32. American Cancer Society. Prostate cancer in minorities. Cancer Facts and Figures in 2001. Available at: www.cancer.org/eprise/main/docroot/stt/stt_0. Accessed January 15, 2003.

33. Howe HL, Wingo PA, Ries AG, et al. Annual report to the nation on the status of cancer (1973 through 1998), featuring cancers with recent increasing trends. *J Natl Cancer Inst.* 2001;93:824–841.

34. Moul JW, Sesterhenn IA, Connelly RR, et al. Prostate-specific antigen values at the time of prostate cancer diagnosis in African-American men. JAMA. 1995;274:1277–1281.

35. Moul JW, Connelly RR, Mooneyhan RM, et al. Racial differences in tumor volume and prostate specific antigen among radical prostatectomy patients. *J Urol.* 1999;162:394–397.

36. Ibrahim GK, Coetzee LJ, Paulson DF. Outcomes of surgical therapy for clinically localized prostatic carcinoma adenocarcinoma: Caucasians and Afro-Americans. *J Urol.* 1995;153:504a.

37. Powell IJ, Banerjee M, Novallo M, et al. Prostate cancer biochemical recurrence stage for stage is more frequent among African-American than white men with locally advanced but not organ-confined disease. *Urology.* 2000;55:246–251.

38. Pettaway CA, Troncoso P, Ramirez EI, et al. Prostate-specific antigen and pathological features of prostate cancer in black and white patients: a comparative study based on radical prostatectomy specimens. *J Urol.* 1998;160:437–442.

39. Sartor O, Zheng Q, Eastham JA. Androgen receptor gene CAG repeat length varies in a race-specific fashion in men without prostate cancer. *Urology.* 1999;53:378–380.

40. Giovannucci E, Stampfer MJ, Krithivas K, et al. The CAG repeat within the androgen receptor gene and its relationship to prostate cancer. *Proc Natl Acad Sci USA* 1997;94:3320–3323.

41. Reichardt JK, Makridakis N, Ross RK, et al. Genetic variability of the human SRD5A2 gene: implications for prostate cancer risk. *Cancer Res.* 1995;55:3973–3975.

42. Kubricht WS, Williams BJ, Whatley T, et al. Serum testosterone levels in African-American and white men undergoing prostate biopsy. *Urology.* 1999;54:1035–1038.

43. Ross R, Bernstein L, Judd H, et al. Serum testosterone levels in healthy young black and white men. *J Natl Cancer Inst.* 1986;76:45–48.

44. Freedland SJ, Dorey F, Aronson WJ. Multivariate analysis of race and adverse pathologic findings after radical prostatectomy. *Urology.* 2000;56:807–811.

45. Vijayakumar S, Weichselbaum R, Vaida F, et al. Prostate-specific antigen levels in African-American correlate with insurance status as an indicator of socioeconomic status. *Cancer J Sci Am.* 1996;2:225–233.

46. Dale W, Vijayakumar S, Lawlor E, et al. Prostate cancer, race, and socioeconomic status: inadequate adjustment for social factors in assessing racial differences. *Prostate.* 1996;29:271–281.

47. Vijayakumar S, Winter K, Sause W, et al. Prostate specific antigen levels are higher in African-American than in white patients in a multicenter registration study: results of RTOG 94-12. *Int J Radiat Oncol Biol Phys.* 1998;40:17–25.

48. Lyman GH, Kuderer NM, Lyman SL, Cox CE, Reintgen D, Baekey P. Importance of race on breast cancer survival. *Ann Surg Oncol.* 1997;4:80–87.

49. Simon MS, Severson RK. Racial differences in survival of female breast cancer in the Detroit metropolitan area. *Cancer.* 1996;77:308–314.

50. Simon MS, Severson RK. Racial differences in breast cancer survival: the interaction of socioeconomic status and tumor biology. *Am J Obstet Gynecol.* 1997;176:S233–S239.

51. Greenwald HP, Polissar NL, Dayal HH. Race, socioeconomic status and survival in three female cancers. *Ethn Health.* 1996;1:65–75.

52. Clegg LX, Li FP, Hankey BF, Chu K, Edwards BK. Cancer survival among US whites and minorities: a SEER (Surveillance, Epidemiology, and End Results) Program population-based study. *Arch Intern Med.* 2002;162:1985–1993.

53. Ries LAG, Kosary CL, Hankey BF, Miller BA, Clegg LX, Edwards BK. *SEER Cancer Statistics Review, 1973–1996.* Bethesda, Md: National Cancer Institute; 1999.

54. National Center for Health Statistics. *Health, United States, 1998 With Socioeconomic Status and Health Chartbook.* Hyattsville, Md: National Center for Health Statistics; 1998.

55. Mandelblatt J, Traxler M, Lakin P, Kanetsky PL, Thomas L, Chauhan P. Breast and cervical cancer screening of poor, elderly, black women: clinical results and implications. *Am J Prev Med.* 1993;9:133–138.

56. Wells BL, Horm JW. Stage at diagnosis in breast cancer: race and socioeconomic factors. *Am J Public Health.* 1992;82:1383–1385.

57. Gregorio D, Cummings K, Michalek A. Stage of disease, and survival among white and black women with breast cancer. *Am J Public Health.* 1983;73:590–593.

58. Jones BA, Patterson EA, Calvocoressi L. Mammography screening in African American women: evaluating the research. *Cancer.* 2003;97(suppl):258–272.

59. Ries LAG, Wingo PA, Miller DS, et al. The annual report to the nation on the status of cancer, 1973–1997, with a special section on colorectal cancer. *Cancer.* 2000;88:2398–2424.

60. Greenlee RT, Hill-Harmon MB, Murray T, et al. Cancer statistics, 2001. *CA Cancer J Clin.* 2001;51:15–36.

61. Centers for Disease Control and Prevention, National Center for HIV, STD, and TB Prevention. HIV/AIDS among African Americans: key facts. Available at: www.cdc.gov/ hiv/pubs/facts/afam.htm. Accessed January 19, 2003.

62. Gifford AL, Cunningham WE, Heslin KC, et al. The HIV Cost and Services Utilization Study Consortium: participation in research and access to experimental treatments by HIV-infected patients. *N Engl J Med.* 2002;346:1373–1382.

63. American Lung Association. Minority lung disease data: asthma. Available at: www.lungusa.org/pub/minority/ asthma. Accessed January 20, 2003.

64. Blixen CE, Havstad S, Tilley BC, Zoratti E. A comparison of asthma-related healthcare use between African-Americans and Caucasians belonging to a health maintenance organization (HMO). *J Asthma.* 1999;36:195–204.

65. American Lung Association. African Americans and Lung Disease. Available at: www.lungusa.org/diseases/ africanlung_factsheet.html. Accessed January 20, 2003.

66. Young RC Jr, Rachal RE, Nelson-Knuckles B, Arthur CN, Nevels HV. Primary care paradigm for management of sarcoidosis, Part 1. *J Natl Med Assoc.* 1997;89:181–190.

67. Glaucoma Research Foundation. Glaucoma facts. Available at: www.glaucoma.org/learn/facts.html. Accessed January 20, 2003.

68. American Academy of Ophthalmology. Preferred practice pattern; comprehensive adult medical eye evaluation. San Francisco, Calif: American Academy of Ophthalmology; 1992. Available at: www.aao.org/aao/education/library/ ppp.cfm. Accessed April 22, 2003.

69. Centers for Disease Control and Prevention. Smoking-attributable mortality and years of potential life lost—United States, 1984. *MMWR Morb Mortal Wkly Rep.* 1997;46:444–451.

70. Resnicow K, Futterman R, Weston RE, et al. Smoking prevalence in Harlem, New York. *Am J Health Promot.* 1996;10:343–346.

71. Giovino GA, Schooley MW, Zhu BP, et al. Surveillance for selected tobacco-use behaviors—United States, 1900–1994. *MMWR Morb Mortal Wkly Rep.* 1994;43:1–43.

72. Fiore MC, Novotny TE, Pierce JP, Hatziandreu EJ, Patel KM, Davis RM. Trends in cigarette smoking in the US—the changing influence of gender and race. *JAMA.* 1989;261:49–55.

73. Hahn LP, Folsom AR, Sprafka JM, Norsted SW. Cigarette smoking and cessation behaviors among urban blacks and whites. *Public Health Rep.* 1990;105:290–295.

74. Royce JM, Hymowitz N, Corbett K, Hartwell TD, Orlandi MA, for the COMMIT Research Group. Smoking cessation factors among African Americans and whites. *Am J Public Health.* 1993;83:220–226.

75. Kabat GC, Morabia A, Wynder EL. Comparison of smoking habits of blacks and whites in a case-control study. *Am J Public Health.* 1991;81:1483–1486.

76. Caraballo RS, Giovino GA, Pechacek TF, et al. Racial and ethnic differences in serum cotinine levels of adult cigarette smokers: Third National Health and Nutrition Examination Survey, 1988–1991. *JAMA.* 1998;280:135–139.

77. Perez-Stable EJ, Herrera B, Jacob III P, Benowitz NL. Nicotine metabolism and intake in black and white smokers. *JAMA.* 1998;280:152–156.

78. National Center for Health Statistics. National Health and Nutrition Examination Survey (NHANES) I Epidemiologic Followup Study. Available at: www.cdc.gov/nchs/ about/major/nhefs/nhefs.htm. Accessed January 21, 2003.

79. Sempos CT, Greenfield TK. Patterns of alcohol consumption among African Americans are more deadly. Available at: www.eurekalert.org/pub_releases/2003–01/ ace-poa010603.php. Accessed January 21, 2003.

80. National Center for Health Statistics (NCHS). NCHS National Vital Statistics System. Available at: www.cdc.gov/ nchs/nvss.htm. Accessed January 21, 2003.

81. US Census Bureau. Census 2000. Washington, DC: US Census Bureau; 2000. Available at: www.census.gov/ main/www/cen2000.html. Accessed January 21, 2003.

82. Centers for Disease Control and Prevention. WISQARS (Web-based Injury Statistics Query and Reporting System) Atlanta, Ga: National Center for Injury Prevention and Control, Centers for Disease Control and Prevention; 2001. Available at: www.cdc.gov/ncipc/wisqars. Accessed January 21, 2003.

83. National Center for Injury Prevention and Control. Youth Violence in the United States. Fact Sheet. Available at: www.cdc.gov/ncipc/dvp/youth/newfacts.htm. Accessed January 21, 2003.

84. Blendon RJ, Aiken LH, Freeman JE, Corey CR. Access to medical care for black and white Americans: a matter of continuing concern. *JAMA.* 1989;261:278–281.

85. Weinick RM, Zuvekas SH, Cohen JW. Racial and ethnic differences in access to and use of health care services, 1977 to 1996. *Med Care Res Rev.* 2000;57(suppl 1):36–54.

86. Andersen R, Newman J. Societal and individual determinants of medical care utilization in the US. *Milbank Mem Fund Q.* 1973;51:95–124.

87. Andersen R. Revisiting the behavioral model and access to medical care: Does it matter? *J Health Soc Behav.* 1995;36:1–10.

88. Stoller E, Gibson RC. *Worlds of Difference: Inequality and the Aging Experience.* 3rd ed. Newbury Park, Calif: Pine Forge Press; 2000.

89. Coultas DB, Gong H, Grad R, et al. Respiratory diseases in minorities in the United States. *Am J Respir Crit Care Med.* 1994;149:S93–S131.

90. Mitchell RE, Barbarin OA, Hurley DJ. Problem solving, resource utilization, and community involvement in a black and a white community. *Am J Community Psych.* 1981;9:233–246.

91. Wilson WJ. *When Work Disappears: The World of the New Urban Poor.* New York, NY: Alfred A. Knopf; 1996.

92. Bailey EJ. Sociocultural factors and health care seeking behavior among black Americans. *J Natl Med Assoc.* 1987;79:389–392.

93. Ayanian JZ, Clearly PD, Weissman JS, Epstein AM. The effect of patients' preferences on racial differences in access to renal transplantation. *N Engl J Med.* 1999b;341:1661–1669.

94. Hannan EL, van Ryn M, Burke J, et al. Access to coronary artery bypass surgery by race/ethnicity and gender among patients who are appropriate for surgery. *Soc Sci Med.* 1999;50:813–828.

95. Turner PA. *I Heard It Through the Grapevine.* Berkeley, Calif: University of California Press; 1993.

96. Gamble VN. Under the shadow of Tuskegee: African Americans and health care. *Am J Public Health.* 1997; 87:1773–1778.

97. Siminoff LA, Saunders-Sturm CM. African American reluctance to donate: beliefs and attitudes about organ donation and implications for policy. *Kennedy Inst Ethics J.* 2000;10:59–74.

98. The Tuskegee study's legacy. *Philadelphia Inquirer.* August 15, 1993:A1, A5.

99. Fry GM. *Night Riders in Black Folk History.* Chapel Hill, NC: University of North Carolina Press; 2001.

100. Corbie-Smith G, Thomas SB, Williams MV, Moody-Ayers S. Attitudes and beliefs of African Americans toward participation in medical research. *J Gen Intern Med.* 1999;14:537–546.

101. Dula A. African American suspicion of the healthcare system is justified: What do we do about it? *Cambridge Q J Healthcare Ethics.* 1994;3:347–357.

102. Fraser I. Can cultural competency reduce racial and ethnic disparities? A review and conceptual model: implementation of sound cultural competency techniques in health services is an important step in reducing racial disparities. *Medical Care Res Rev.* 2002;57.

RESOURCES

For Clinicians

Institute of Medicine. Unequal treatment: confronting racial and ethnic disparities in health care. Web site: www.iom.edu/iom/iomhome.nsf/Pages/Report+Summaries.

National Academy of Sciences. Examining unequal treatment in American health care. Web site: www4.nationalacademies.org/onpi/webextra.nsf/web/minority.

National Heart, Lung, and Blood Institute. The management of sickle cell disease. July 12, 2002. Web site: www.nhlbi.nih.gov/health/prof/blood/sickle/index.htm.

Office of Minority Health. Web site: www.omhrc.gov.

Patient Care [online]. Caring for diverse populations. May 15, 2000. Web site: www.patientcareonline.com.

Postgraduate Medicine. Symposium on hypertension in African Americans. October 2002. Vol 112. Web site: www.postgradmed.com.

For Patients

MEDLINEplus.
   Web site: www.nlm.nih.gov/medlineplus/ medlineplus.html. (Health information and interactive tutorials.)
National Heart, Lung, and Blood Institute.
   Web site: www.nhlbi.nih.gov/health/index.htm. (Health information about cardiovascular diseases, asthma and lung diseases, and sickle cell anemia and blood disorders.); Your guide to lowering high blood pressure.
   Web site: www.nhlbi.nih.gov/hbp.

chapter 36

European Americans

Stephen P. Hayden, MD

INTRODUCTION

This chapter will review variations in the prevalence of selected conditions in the European population and compare these, when appropriate, to the existing general North American population. European immigration to the United States has fallen somewhat and is now a much smaller proportion of overall immigration than in the past (Fig 36-1). The children of European immigrants are likely to share many of the same cultural traits as well as genetic makeup.

The European population is far from homogeneous, and therefore cannot be characterized as a single group.

This chapter divides Europe when appropriate into northern, southern, and central and eastern Europe, since the medical literature demonstrates various differences between these geographical groupings. Northern Europe includes the countries of Belgium, Denmark, Finland, Holland, Germany, Iceland, Ireland, Liechtenstein, Luxembourg, Norway, Sweden, Switzerland, and the United Kingdom. Southern Europe is composed of Albania, Andorra, Croatia, Cyprus, France, Greece, Italy, Macedonia, Malta, Monaco, Portugal, San Marino, Slovenia, Spain, and Yugoslavia. In central and eastern Europe are Armenia, Azerbaijan, Austria, Bulgaria, Belarus, Czech Republic, Estonia, Georgia, Hungary, Latvia, Lithuania,

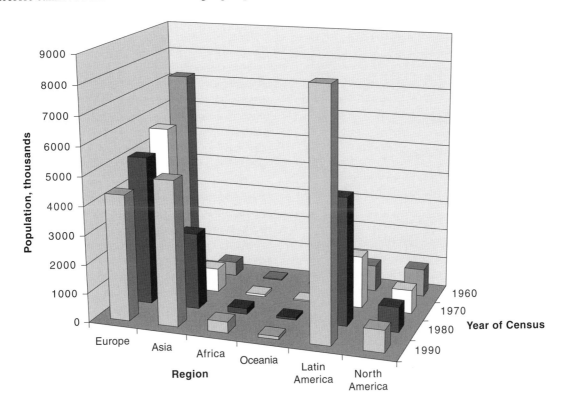

FIGURE 36-1

Region of birth of foreign-born population of United States, 1960–1990. From US Census Bureau; 1999.

Moldavia, Poland, Romania, Russia, Slovak Republic, and Ukraine.

Migration is currently considered to be a major political and health problem in parts of Europe, with relatively large numbers of asylum seekers and economic migrants seeking new lives or opportunities in the developed countries. Citizens of European Union (EU) member countries may obtain employment in any other EU country, which has increased legal migration in the EU. Some individual countries have relatively large populations of native-born persons of non-European extraction. These factors may change the propensity to certain diseases in these countries over time both in Europe as a whole and when different regions are compared.

The European population in some countries, mostly in the northern and western parts of Europe, has experienced many of the same changes and trends as have the North American people. Indeed, some of the longest life expectancies anywhere in the world are to be found in Europe, but now there are trends of increasing obesity and diabetes, which may threaten the major gains in length of life due to increases in coronary artery disease and stroke. The trends in mortality due to major diseases in Europe have shown steady and substantial declines in overall mortality in 20 major European countries.[1] In western European countries, there has been a decline in mortality due to coronary heart disease (CHD), cerebrovascular disease, and cancer. In eastern Europe, females show a modest improvement, and males show worsening mortality, which are thought to be the result of nutrition, environmental factors, alcohol and tobacco use, and delayed treatment of hypertension; there is also a high rate of homicides and suicide.

DISEASE PREVALENCE

Cardiovascular Disease

Blood pressure generally is higher in men than women, and a considerable variation exists between countries and within countries in data collected as part of the World Health Organization (WHO) MONICA project. Compared with Stanford, United States, and Halifax, Canada, the prevalence of elevated blood pressure is generally higher in Europe, with notable exceptions in Spain, southern France, Belgium, Denmark, and Iceland. The people in eastern European countries appear to have higher blood pressures on average.[2] Mortality rates for CHD and all circulatory diseases are comparable in North America and northern and southern Europe. The mortality rates for cerebrovascular disease are higher in Europe in general. In eastern Europe, the rates are strikingly higher than the other European regions and North America.[3]

Pulmonary Disease

Mortality due to pulmonary disease is broadly comparable, although slightly lower in southern Europe and in Canada than in northern and eastern Europe and the United States. However, mortality due to obstructive lung disease appears strikingly higher in eastern Europe.[3] There are very large variations in asthma prevalence between countries, with the highest rates of symptoms in the United Kingdom and Ireland, as well as in Australia and New Zealand. Lower rates were noted in several eastern European countries and in Greece. North America also had rates close to the highest European rates.[4] In the former East Germany, rates have increased in the 8 years after unification.[5] There are differences between the prevalence of sarcoidosis between European countries. Scandinavia has the highest rates and rates are also high among Irish females living in London.[6] There has long been suspicion that an infectious or environmental agent is responsible, and that genetic determinants have a role, but proof is lacking.[7]

Digestive Disease

Statistics from the WHO indicate that in northern Europe and North America mortality due to digestive disease and mortality from liver disease and cirrhosis are comparable. These rates are somewhat higher in southern Europe and strikingly higher in eastern Europe.[3]

Much of the recent literature has focused on the role of *Helicobacter pylori* infection in peptic ulcer disease. Numerous articles from Europe have demonstrated that overcrowding, poor living conditions, immigration from a high-prevalence area, and lower socioeconomic class are associated with higher rates of this infection. In Siberia very high rates have been found. In Italy, lower rates are found in the north than in the south and in the Italian islands.[8-10] Gastroesophageal reflux disease has a similar prevalence in developed countries in Europe and in North America but is lower in developing countries.[11]

Crohn disease and ulcerative colitis have a higher incidence and prevalence in northern Europe and North America than in southern Europe.[12] Celiac disease is most common in persons of European origin with a strong genetic component, related to the HLA-DQ alpha beta heterodimeric, and a second locus in the major histocompatibility complex.[13] Italian studies have shown significant iron deficiency among children with celiac disease detected by screening.[14]

Hepatic, Gallbladder, and Renal Disease

Gallstone prevalence increases with age in a number of European and North American studies. The prevalence appears to be similar in western Europe and in the overall

North American population, typically under 10% in men and between 10% and 20% in women.[15]

The reported prevalence of primary biliary cirrhosis has increased in Europe, but this may be a result of improved awareness and diagnosis.[16] In Europe, 28% of hepatic cancer cases have been attributed to chronic hepatitis B viral infection and 21% to hepatitis C viral infection. Intermediate incidence rates of hepatic cancer are found in southern, eastern, and western Europe, Central America, western Asia, and northern Africa. Low rates are found among men in northern Europe, America, Canada, south central Asia, Australia, and New Zealand. These compare to high rates found in southeastern Asia, Japan, Africa, and the Pacific Islands.[17]

Rates of liver cancer in the United States have increased by 70% over the past 2 decades, and there are similar trends in Europe.[18] In addition to hepatitis B and C virus infection, factors such as aflatoxin exposure in diets, cigarette smoking, alcohol consumption, and oral contraceptives may explain the residual variation between and in countries.[19]

The probability of developing renal stone disease is higher in North America (13%) than in Europe (5% to 9%). Stones in the upper tract seem associated with greater affluence.[20]

Neurologic Disease

Creutzfeldt-Jakob disease has been described in sporadic and iatrogenic forms, and is associated with eating food. Persons who have lived in the United Kingdom for certain periods of time are proscribed from donating blood, as a result of this epidemic, which is still unfolding and whose magnitude is unknown. As a worst-case scenario, it has been estimated that many thousands of cases may yet develop as a result of eating contaminated beef.[21] As a result, the American Red Cross does not accept blood donations from persons who have lived 3 months or more since 1980 or received a blood transfusion in any of the following countries: England, Scotland, Wales, Northern Ireland, Isle of Man, Falkland Islands, Gibraltar, and the Channel Islands. The same applies to those who have lived 6 months or more in any part of Europe or have received bovine insulin from a European source.[22]

Prevalence rates for multiple sclerosis are high in northern Europe in a north-south gradient, particularly in persons of Scandinavian ancestry.[23] There appears to be a familial recurrence rate of 15%, highest for siblings, especially monozygotic twins, whereas for adoptees, the risk is similar to that in the general population. Hopefully, current or new genetic techniques will further illuminate the genetics of this disease.[24]

Parkinson's disease and parkinsonism increase with age, but no differences exist between different parts of Europe, except for lower rates in France.[25]

Hemoglobinopathies

Whereas hemoglobinopathies were chiefly problems of Mediterranean countries in the past, they are now endemic in Europe and North America, through the effects of migration on the gene pool. Prevention efforts for these conditions have been 80% to 100% successful in some endemic Mediterranean countries.[26]

Hormonal and Nutritional Disorders

Prevalence for diabetes in individual countries varies significantly. Reported rates are lower for eastern European countries, but others are generally similar to the US and Canadian statistics.[27]

An increased incidence of thyroid disease (Hashimoto disease, thyroid adenoma, and thyroid cancer, particularly papillary microcarcinoma) diagnosed on thyroid surgery records was noted in a study of the Kiev region for the 4 years before and 8 years after the Chernobyl nuclear accident.[28] The United Nations has prepared a detailed report on the effects of the Chernobyl accident.[29] Among other findings, a total of 7.1 million people were affected, and there are still 4.5 million people living in the contaminated territories of Ukraine, Russia, and Belarus. This report confirms the increased rates of thyroid cancer in those exposed in childhood. The psychosocial effects have been high, especially among persons who moved from the contaminated areas.

Obesity rates are rising both in developed and developing countries.[30] In only Finland and the United Kingdom are obesity rates comparable to the high rates of the United States at dates close to the most recent National Health and Nutrition Examination Survey (NHANES) period. Childhood obesity is more common in southern and eastern Europe, but there is considerable variation.[31]

Rheumatic Disease

A gradient for incidence of polymyalgia rheumatica exists from the south to the north of Europe.[32] Primary osteoarthritis of the hip is 3% to 6% in the white population, and hip replacements are rare in those of Asian origin, and low in the black and Hispanic populations. Family studies show increased risk of osteoarthritis of the hip in relatives of an index patient in Sweden, Britain, and the United States.[33]

Infectious Disease

The WHO statistics on tuberculosis (TB) are extensive. Few countries have lower rates of TB than in North America. In many countries, the rates remain alarmingly high and are increasing. The countries of the former Yugoslavia have had high TB rates, and among more

Western countries, Portugal had the highest rate. The incidence of drug-resistant TB is rising, especially in eastern Europe.[34] An outbreak of multiple drug-resistant TB (MDR-TB) in persons infected with the human immunodeficiency virus (HIV) was reported in Italy, associated strongly with hospital exposure to MDR-TB or previous use of anti-TB drugs.[35] The percentage of HIV-infected adults aged 15 to 49 years are similar across the European and North American populations.[36]

Northern Europe compares broadly with North America in hepatitis B carrier status. Many areas of southern and eastern Europe have higher rates. However, these rates are not as high as in the Far East and sub-Saharan Africa.[37]

Since the 1980s, most of Europe has seen a decline in gonorrhea except for some Baltic countries in the 1990s and among men who have sex with men. There is increased gonorrhea drug resistance to penicillin and tetracycline and also to fluoroquinolones, through importation from Southeast Asia.[38] Human papillomavirus infection is increasing over time in western Europe, paralleling other sexually transmitted diseases.[39] Lyme borreliosis occurs throughout Europe, and is more prevalent in the East.[40]

Cancer

The all-cause cancer mortality is comparable in North America and northern and southern Europe but is distinctly higher in eastern Europe. The main difference in cancer mortality is due to the gradient in gastric cancer from North America to northern, southern, and eastern Europe. Other cancer mortality is comparable, except respiratory cancers have a higher mortality rate in North America than in Europe. Smoking remains a major contributor to cancer mortality.[41]

Breast cancer mortality is higher in the northern part of Europe than the south. Whether this is the result of genetic or environmental factors is uncertain.[3] In eastern European countries, mortality due to cervical and uterine cancer is appreciably higher than in most of western Europe.[42]

A higher incidence of ovarian cancer mortality exists in northern Europe than in North America; however, only 5% to 10% of cancers are familial.[43] Prostate cancer mortality is higher in northern Europe.[3] Norway has the highest in the Nordic countries and among the highest in the world.[44]

In Europe the highest lung cancer mortality rates in men are in Hungary, the Czech Republic, and Russian Federation, followed by the other eastern European countries, which also showed high rates of tobacco- and alcohol-related cancers. The highest European lung cancer rates for women are in Scotland and Denmark; rates are similar to those in the United States.[45] Smoking rates are higher in Europe in general than in North America. Current US smoking rates are about 25% for adults, whereas in the EU countries the rate is 30% to 31%. Among younger men, especially in eastern Europe, head and neck cancer rates have been rising, mostly related to tobacco and alcohol use and perhaps to nutritional deficiencies and human papillomavirus.[46] In England and Wales, there has been an overall reduction in oral cancer during the last century but an increase among younger men during the last 30 years, perhaps as a result of alcohol consumption.[47]

Higher rates for gastric cancer mortality exist in eastern and central Europe than in the rest of Europe. Gastric cancer rates have been declining worldwide, perhaps as a result of improved lifestyle, food storage, and lower infection rates.[48] In Finland, there has been a decline in gastritis as well as gastric carcinoma with time, together with a decline in *H pylori* infection rates in childhood, suggesting that *H pylori* infection may be playing a part.[49] In Europe, the highest mortality rates due to colorectal cancer were in the Czech Republic and Hungary.[45]

Melanoma incidence has risen for the last 3 decades. In Europe the highest rates are in Scandinavia and in the Mediterranean countries. Overall rates are generally lower than those in the United States.[50]

External causes of mortality and morbidity

Statistics from the WHO show that in eastern Europe and the United States external causes of death including homicide were higher than in Canada and other regions of Europe. Suicide was more than twice as frequent in eastern than in southern Europe.

Environmental pollution may be a major problem, particularly in eastern European countries, although it is not known how much this contributes to morbidity such as cancer. Drinking water standards in many areas are inadequately monitored. Many people drink water from unmonitored wells, which may have high levels of pesticides, nitrates, arsenic, and fluoride.[51] In men, occupational exposures are considered to account for 13% to 18% of lung cancers, 2% to 10% of bladder cancers, and 2% to 8% of laryngeal cancers, with much lower rates in women.[52]

The cancer burden of eastern European countries is substantial, and mortality has increased, perhaps related to environmental exposure and lifestyle.[53]

Cancer screening and immunization practices

Cancer screening may be of particular importance for those who move from Europe to North America. Breast and cervical cancer screening is widespread in developed countries, and women are likely to have been enrolled in screening programs.[54] Screening for other cancers may be less common. For instance, colon cancer screening is not yet employed by the UK National Health Service, but a pilot program for fecal occult blood testing is under way. Prostate cancer screening remains an area of uncertainty. Although there is no UK National Health Service screening program, information is available through the

National Health Service and other sources.[55] Gastric cancer screening is not currently carried out on a large scale in Europe or North America as it is in Japan, but there is some interest in using screening for *H pylori* and eradication to reduce the incidence.[56]

Detailed information is available from the WHO on immunization rates worldwide.[57] General recommendations for Europe have been developed.[58] In Europe, including the former Soviet Union, no cases of poliovirus have been reported since November 1998. This is very promising and has led to a change in immunization policy in many European countries. Where live attenuated oral poliovirus vaccine (OPV) has been used predominantly, vaccine-associated paralytic poliomyelitis—although very rare—occurs more frequently than wild-type virus infection. Consequently, immunization with OPV has been replaced by injectable inactivated poliovirus vaccine.[59]

By the end of 2002, 41 of the 51 countries of the WHO European Region were implementing universal hepatitis B immunization.[60] Universal measles immunization policies are in place in Europe. However, outbreaks still occur as a result of failure to immunize.[61]

SUMMARY

European populations have environmental exposures and inherited factors that differentiate their risks for some conditions. Although Europe does not supply as high a proportion of total immigration to the United States as in the past, persons of European origin still form a substantial number of persons living in the United States and Canada. Table 36-1 provides a summary of the patterns of medical conditions in regions of Europe and differences between Europe and North America.

T A B L E 36-1

Conditions of High Frequency in Europe

Condition	Region of High Frequency	Comment
Down syndrome	Ireland	Termination not permitted
Hypertension	Most of Europe, and more in eastern Europe	
Coronary artery and cerebrovascular disease	Most of Europe; mortality appears much higher in eastern Europe	
Chronic obstructive lung disease	Eastern Europe	
Asthma	United Kingdom and Ireland	North America comparable to United Kingdom and Ireland
Sarcoidosis	Scandinavia	
Digestive diseases	Eastern Europe	
Liver cancer	Higher in eastern, southern, and western Europe than northern Europe and United States	
Inflammatory bowel disease	Northern Europe and northern United States	
Creutzfeldt-Jakob disease	United Kingdom at risk of emerging epidemic	
Multiple sclerosis	Northern Europe, especially Scandinavian ancestry	
Diabetes	Higher in western and southern than eastern Europe	
Thyroid cancer	Areas affected by Chernobyl accident (Ukraine, Belarus, Russia)	Highest numbers in persons exposed in childhood
Obesity	United Kingdom and Finland are comparable to United States	
Polymyalgia rheumatica	Scandinavia	
Tuberculosis	Eastern and parts of southern Europe	Drug-resistant TB higher in eastern Europe
Hepatitis B	Southern and eastern Europe	
Cancer mortality	Eastern Europe	Also all-cause mortality higher in eastern Europe
Gastric cancer	Eastern and southern Europe	
Breast cancer	Northern Europe	
Uterine cancer	Eastern Europe	Improved screening programs needed
Prostate cancer	Northern Europe, especially Norway	
Lung cancer	Hungary, Czech Republic, and Russian Federation	Females highest in Scotland and Denmark
Aerodigestive tract cancer	Southern Europe, rising in eastern Europe and younger UK men	
Gastric cancer	Eastern Europe	Declining worldwide
Colon cancer	Hungary and Czech Republic	
Melanoma	Scandinavia and Mediterranean	Higher in United States and Australia
Smoking	Europe higher than North America	
Illness and death due to external causes	Eastern Europe and North America are comparable	

REFERENCES

1. La Vecchia C, Levi F, Lucchini F, Negri E. Trends in mortality from major diseases in Europe, 1980–1993. *Eur J Epidemiol.* 1998;14:1–8.

2. WHO MONICA Project database. British Heart Foundation Statistics Web site; 2002. Available at: www.heartstats.org. Accessed June 2003.

3. *1997–1999 World Health Statistics Annual.* Geneva, Switzerland: World Health Organization; 1999.

4. Worldwide variation in prevalence of symptoms of asthma, allergic rhinoconjunctivitis, and atopic eczema: ISAAC. The International Study of Asthma and Allergies in Childhood (ISAAC) Steering Committee. *Lancet.* 1998;351:1225–1232.

5. Matricardi PM. Prevalence of atopy and asthma in eastern versus western Europe: why the difference? *Ann Allergy Asthma Immunol.* 2001;87(suppl 3):24–27.

6. Crystal RG. In: Braunwald E, Fauci AS, Issebacher KG, et al, eds. *Harrison's Online.* Available at: http://harrisons.accessmedicine.com/. Accessed June 12, 2003.

7. Newman LS, Rose CS, Maier LA. Sarcoidosis 139. *N Engl J Med.* 1997;336:1224–1234.

8. Moayyedi P, Axon AT, Feltbower R, et al. Relation of adult lifestyle and socioeconomic factors to the prevalence of *Helicobacter pylori* infection. *Int J Epidemiol.* 2002;31:624–631.

9. Reshetnikov OV, Haiva VM, Granberg C, Kurilovich SA, Babin VP. Seroprevalence of *Helicobacter pylori* infection in Siberia. *Helicobacter.* 2001;6:331–336.

10. Stroffolini T, Rosmini F, Ferrigno L, Fortini M, D'Amelio R, Matricardi PM. Prevalence of *Helicobacter pylori* infection in a cohort of Italian military students. *Epidemiol Infect.* 1998;120:151–155.

11. Sonnenberg A, El-Serag HB. Clinical epidemiology and natural history of gastroesophageal reflux disease. *Yale J Biol Med.* 1999;72:81–92.

12. Shivananda S, Lennard-Jones J, Logan R, et al. Incidence of inflammatory bowel disease across Europe: is there a difference between north and south? Results of the European Collaborative Study on Inflammatory Bowel Disease (EC-IBD). *Gut.* 1996;39:690–697.

13. Pena AS, Wijmenga C. Genetic factors underlying gluten-sensitive enteropathy. *Curr Allergy Asthma Rep.* 2001;1:526–533.

14. Schuppan D, Esslinger B, Dieterich W. Pathomechanisms in celiac disease. *Int Arch Allergy Immunol.* 2003;132:98–108.

15. Wang HH, Afdhal NH, Gendler SJ, Wang DQ. Targeted disruption of the murine mucin gene 1 decreases susceptibility to cholesterol gallstone formation. *J Lipid Res.* 2004;1.

16. Myszor M, James OF. The epidemiology of primary biliary cirrhosis in north-east England: an increasingly common disease? *Q J Med.* 1990;75:377–385.

17. Bosch FX, Ribes J. Epidemiology of liver cancer in Europe. *Can J Gastroenterol.* 2000;14:621–630.

18. Yu MC, Yuan JM, Govindarajan S, Ross RK. Epidemiology of hepatocellular carcinoma. *Can J Gastroenterol.* 2000;14:703–709.

19. Bosch FX, Ribes J, Borras J. Epidemiology of primary liver cancer. *Semin Liver Dis.* 1999;19:271–285.

20. Ramello A, Vitale C, Marangella M. Epidemiology of nephrolithiasis. *J Nephrology.* 2000;13(suppl 3):S45–S50.

21. Pedersen NS, Smith E. Prion diseases: epidemiology in man. *Apmis.* 2002;110:14–22.

22. Blood Donation Eligibility Guidelines. Available at: www.redcross.org.

23. Hogancamp WE, Rodriguez M, Weinshenker BG. The epidemiology of multiple sclerosis. *Mayo Clin Proc.* 1997;72:871–878.

24. Compston A. The genetic epidemiology of multiple sclerosis. *Philos Trans Roy Soc Lond Biol.* 1999;354:1623–1634.

25. de Rijk MC, Tzourio C, Breteler MM, et al. Prevalence of parkinsonism and Parkinson's disease in Europe: the EUROPARKINSON Collaborative Study: European Community Concerted Action on the Epidemiology of Parkinson's disease. *J Neurol Neurosurg Psychiatr.* 1997;62:10–15.

26. Angastiniotis M, Modell B. Global epidemiology of hemoglobin disorders. *Ann N Y Acad Sci.* 1998;850:251–269.

27. Amos AF, McCarty DJ, Zimmet P. The rising global burden of diabetes and its complications: estimates and projections to the year 2010. *Diabet Med.* 1997;14(suppl 5):S1–S85.

28. Avetisian IL, Gulchiy NV, Demidiuk AP, Stashuk AV. Thyroid pathology in residents of the Kiev region, Ukraine, during pre- and post-Chernobyl periods. *J Environ Pathol Toxicol Oncol.* 1996;15:233–237.

29. *A Report Commissioned by UNDP and UNICEF With the support of UN-OCHA and WHO: The Human Consequences of the Chernobyl Nuclear Accident: A Strategy for Recovery.* January 25, 2002.

30. Saw SM, Rajan U. The epidemiology of obesity: a review. *Ann Acad Med Singapore.* 1997;26:489–493.

31. Livingstone B. Epidemiology of childhood obesity in Europe. *Eur J Pediatr.* 2000;159(suppl 1):S14–S34.

32. Cimmino MA, Zaccaria A. Epidemiology of polymyalgia rheumatica. *Clin Exp Rheumatol.* 2000;18(suppl 20):S9–S11.

33. Hoaglund FT, Steinbach LS. Primary osteoarthritis of the hip: etiology and epidemiology. *J Am Acad Orthop Surg.* 2001;9:320–327.

34. Rusch-Gerdes S. Epidemiology of resistant tuberculosis in Europe. *Infection.* 1999;27(suppl 2):S17–S18.

35. Angarano G, Carbonara S, Costa D, Gori A, for Italian Drug-Resistant Tuberculosis Study Group. Drug-resistant tuberculosis in human immunodeficiency virus infected persons in Italy. *Int J Tuberc Lung Dis.* 1998;2:303–311.

36. *Report on the Global HIV/AIDS Epidemic 2002.* Geneva, Switzerland: World Health Organization; 2002.

37. WHO Department of Vaccines and Biologicals. *Introduction of Hepatitis B Vaccine into Childhood Immunization Services.* Geneva, Switzerland: World Health Organization; 2001.

38. van Duynhoven YT. The epidemiology of Neisseria gonorrhoeae in Europe. *Microbes Infection.* 1999;1:455–464.

39. Dillner J, Meijer CJ, von Krogh G, Horenblas S. Epidemiology of human papillomavirus infection. *Scand J Urol Nephrol Suppl.* 2000;205:194–200.

40. O'Connell S, Granstrom M, Gray JS, Stanek G. Epidemiology of European Lyme borreliosis. *Zentralbl Bakteriol.* 1998;287:229–240.

41. Levi F, Lucchini F, Negri E, La Vecchia C. Worldwide patterns of cancer mortality, 1990–1994. *Eur J Cancer Prev.* 1999;8:381–400.

42. Levi F, Lucchini F, Negri E, Franceschi S, la Vecchia C. Cervical cancer mortality in young women in Europe: patterns and trends. *Eur J Cancer.* 2000;36:2266–2271.

43. Holschneider CH, Berek JS. Ovarian cancer: epidemiology, biology, and prognostic factors. *Semin Surg Oncol.* 2000;19:3–10.

44. Harvei S. *Tidsskr Nor Laegeforen.* 1999;119:3589–3594.

45. Levi F, Lucchini F, Negri E, Boyle P, La Vecchia C. Cancer mortality in Europe, 1990–1994, and an overview of trends from 1955 to 1994. *Eur J Cancer.* 1999;35:1477–1516.

46. La Vecchia C, Franceschi S, Bosetti C, Levi F, Talamini R, Negri E. Time since stopping smoking and the risk of oral and pharyngeal cancers. *J Natl Cancer Inst.* 1999;91:726–728.

47. Hindle I, Downer MC, Moles DR, Speight PM. Is alcohol responsible for more intra-oral cancer? *Oral Oncol.* 2000;36:328–333.

48. Corella D, Guillen M. Dietary habits and epidemiology of gastric carcinoma. *Hepatogastroenterology.* 2001;48:1537–1543.

49. Sipponen P. *Helicobacter pylori* gastritis—epidemiology. *J Gastroenterol.* 1997;32:273–277.

50. Garbe C, Blum A. Epidemiology of cutaneous melanoma in Germany and worldwide. *Skin Pharmacol Appl Skin Physiol.* 2001;14:280–290.

51. Jedrychowski W, Maugeri U, Bianchi I. Environmental pollution in central and eastern European countries: a basis for cancer epidemiology. *Rev Environ Health.* 1997;12:1–23.

52. Boffetta P, Kogevinas M. Introduction: epidemiologic research and prevention of occupational cancer in Europe. *Environ Health Perspect.* 1999;107(suppl 2):229–231.

53. Dobrossy L. Cancer mortality in central-eastern Europe: facts behind the figures. *Lancet Oncol.* 2002;3:374–381.

54. UK National Health Service. *Breast Screening Programme Annual Review.* 2002; 2003.

55. *The Prostate Cancer Risk Management Programme.*

56. Davies R, Crabbe D, Roderick P, Goddard JR, Raftery J, Patel P. A simulation to evaluate screening for *Helicobacter pylori* infection in the prevention of peptic ulcers and gastric cancers. *Health Care Manage Sci.* 2002;5:249–258.

57. WHO Vaccine Preventable Diseases Monitoring System. *2002 Global Summary.* Geneva, Switzerland: World Health Organization; 2002.

58. Helwig H, Mertsola J, Harvey D, Nicolopoulos D, Schaack JC, Sedlak W, for Confederation of European Specialists in Paediatrics (CESP). Childhood immunisation in the European Union. *Eur J Pediatr.* 1998;157:676–680.

59. Heininger U. Eradication of poliomyelitis: where do we stand in Europe? *Arch Dis Child.* 2001;84:124.

60. Van Damme P, Vorsters A. Hepatitis B control in Europe by universal vaccination programmes: the situation in 2001. *J Med Virol.* 2002;67:433–439.

61. Hanratty B, Holt T, Duffell E, et al. UK measles outbreak in non-immune anthroposophic communities: the implications for the elimination of measles from Europe. *Epidemiol Infect.* 2000;125:377–383.

chapter 37

Asians and Pacific Islanders

Xian Wen Jin, MD, PhD, FACP, and Carol E. Blixen, PhD, RN

INTRODUCTION

The United States represents the most culturally diverse nation in the world. Whereas in 1990 ethnically diverse individuals represented 25% of the total US population, by the year 2010 they will comprise 60% of our population.[1] Asian Americans and Pacific Islanders (hereafter called Asian/Pacific Islanders) are the fastest growing ethnic minorities in the United States. It is estimated that by 2010 there will be more than 17 million Asian/Pacific Islanders in this country.[2]

According to the 2000 census, the US population on April 1, 2000, was 281.4 million. Of the total respondents, 11.9 million, or 4.2%, reported being Asian. This number included 10.2 million people (3.6%) who reported only Asian and 1.7 million people (0.6%) who reported Asian as well as one or more other races. Because Census 2000 asked separate questions on race and Hispanic or Latino origin, Hispanics who reported their race as Asian, either alone or in combination with 1 or more races, are included in the numbers for Asians. More than half (51%) of the Asian American population lived in just 3 states: California (4.2 million), New York (1.2 million), and Hawaii (0.7 million).

The term *Asian* is misleading in that this title refers to a great number of cultural groups and at least 25 linguistic groups (Table 37-1). However, in Census 2000, Chinese were the largest Asian group in the United States, with 2.7 million people reporting Chinese alone or in combination with 1 or more other races or Asian groups. Filipinos (2.4 million) and Asian Indians (1.7 million) were the next 2 largest identified Asian groups.[3]

The rapid growth and diversity of Asian/Pacific Islanders in the United States will certainly result in more encounters with this population in the primary care setting. However, little is known about the sociocultural issues and health beliefs and practices related to their care. Lack of awareness or misunderstanding of these issues as well as the special health care problems found in this population present a unique challenge for physicians and other health care providers in providing culturally

competent health care to this population. The increasing focus by both consumers and payers on providing culturally competent health care requires that primary care physicians become knowledgeable about the health care issues facing this fastest growing minority population.

American Asian patients are a group of heterogeneous individuals with multicultural and multilingual backgrounds. More commonly encountered Asian patients come from areas of East Asia (ie, China, Japan, and Korea) and from Southeast Asia (ie, India, Vietnam, Cambodia, and Thailand), although widely divergent cultures exist within and among these populations.

This chapter will review diseases that are more common in Asians, conditions with unique clinical significance, and issues that influence preventive care in this population.

DISEASES THAT ARE MORE COMMON IN ASIANS

Lactose Intolerance

Lactose intolerance is found in as many as 75% to 100% of Chinese, Japanese, and Koreans. Studies of Chinese

TABLE 37-1

Asian Ethnic Groups in the United States

Asian		Pacific Islanders
Asian Indian	Japanese	Fijian
Bangladeshi	Korean	Northern Mariana Islander
Burmese	Laotian	Palauan
Cambodian	Malaysian	Tahitian
Chinese	Okinawan	Tongan
Filipino	Pakistani	
Guamanian	Samoan	
Hawaiian	Sri Lankan	
Hmong	Thai	
Indonesian	Vietnamese	

children receiving a physiological dose of lactose (0.5 g/kg) showed that all 3-years-olds were able to digest lactose. By 4 to 6 years of age, lactose intolerance was found in 12% to 14%; by 7 years of age, in 43%; and by 13 to 14 years of age, in 74%.[4] In evaluating an Asian patient who presents with subacute or chronic watery diarrhea, the physician should first rule out any infectious causes based on a careful medical history, physical examination, and stool cultures. Then a lactose-free diet should be tried before an extensive diagnostic workup is initiated. Especially if the patient has recently immigrated to the United States, increases in dairy product intake may make the diarrhea worse.

Tuberculosis

In the United States, half of all cases of tuberculosis (TB) occur in foreign-born persons who represent only 10% of the total population. Tuberculosis is more common in Asian Americans compared with other ethnic groups. The incidence of TB is estimated to be 8.7 times higher in Asian/Pacific Islanders than that in US whites.[5] Most cases of TB in foreign-born Asians develop within the first 2 years after arrival in the United States.[6] Many countries in Asia still use bacille-Calmette-Guérin (BCG) vaccination as part of their TB control program, especially for infants. Initially, BCG vaccine was derived from a strain of *Mycobacterium bovis* and was attenuated through years of serial passage in culture.[7] A positive reaction to the tuberculin skin test may result due to BCG immunization. This phenomenon complicates the clinical decisions about prophylactic therapy for BCG-vaccinated Asian patients who have a positive skin test result, as there is no reliable method of distinguishing tuberculin reactions caused by BCG from those caused by natural infection. According to the Centers for Disease Control and Prevention (CDC), a positive reaction to tuberculin in a person with a history of BCG vaccination is more likely to be due to infection with tuberculosis if: (1) the induration is large, (2) the person was vaccinated a long time ago, (3) the person recently came into contact with someone with TB, (4) there is a family history of TB, (5) the person comes from an area where TB is common, and (6) chest X-ray findings show evidence of previous TB. Recent recommendations from the American Thoracic Society and the CDC advocate testing patients at increased risk of TB. If a recent Asian immigrant (<5 years) has a purified protein derivative (PPD) skin induration of 10 mm or larger, he or she should be considered to have a positive test. If the skin induration measures 5 mm or greater in an Asian patient who had recent contact with someone having active TB, the patient is considered to have a latent TB infection.[8] Therefore, an Asian immigrant who comes from a country where TB is common and who has a positive PPD skin test should undergo chest radiography to rule out active pulmonary TB infection and be considered for preventive therapy with isoniazid after active disease has been ruled out.[9,10]

Hepatitis B

Hepatitis B is much more common in Asians than in the general US population. About 8% to 22% of Asians may carry hepatitis B, whereas the carrier rate in the US general population is only 0.2% to 0.9%.[11,12] Consequently, primary hepatocellular carcinoma among Asians is also increased in the US general population. In California alone, Asians were 5 times more likely to have liver cancer develop and 4 times more likely to die of the disease than were whites.[13] It is prudent for the practitioner to obtain hepatitis B serologic findings before vaccinating Asian immigrants since they may already have protective hepatitis B antibodies due to prior exposure.

Parasitic Diseases

Several parasitic diseases, such as malaria, schistosomiasis, and tapeworm, are more common in Asians. Today malaria remains an overwhelming problem in India and Southeast Asia. Immigrants or Asian patients who have recently visited Southeast Asia may carry malaria to the United States.[14] Cyclic fevers in these patients should prompt the physician to include malaria in the differential diagnosis. A thin or thick peripheral blood smear for microscopic examination of malarial parasites is the diagnostic test of choice.

Patients from Southeast Asia and the Philippines may harbor *Schistosoma japonicum.*[15] Symptoms of this disease may develop after a prolonged latent period. Intermittent diarrhea or dysentery, enlargement of liver and spleen, and portal hypertension are the most common symptoms and signs of chronic schistosomiasis.[16] In the right clinical setting, a fecal sample or liver biopsy specimen should be submitted for identification of schistosome eggs.

Fish tapeworm (*Diphyllobothrium latum*) infection is more common in Japanese and Chinese from the Guangdong province of southern China because of consumption of sushi prepared from raw freshwater fish, and rice soup made with raw fish.[17] Clinical presentation may include salt craving, diarrhea, and intermittent abdominal discomfort. Prolonged infection of *D latum* may lead to megaloblastic anemia caused by vitamin B_{12} deficiency due to parasite-mediated dissociation of vitamin B_{12} and intrinsic factors. A careful history regarding raw fish ingestion, examination of the stool for fish tapeworm eggs, and contrast studies of the intestine may lead to the definitive diagnosis.

Nasopharyngeal Carcinoma

Nasopharyngeal carcinoma is rare in the general population but remarkably common in Cantonese Chinese, likely because of a high incidence of Epstein-Barr virus infection in the region.[18,19] An otolaryngology referral is essential in evaluating a Chinese patient with epistaxis or cervical adenopathy to rule out a nasopharyngeal lesion before lymph node biopsy is performed. The biopsy site will not heal during subsequent radiation therapy for nasopharyngeal carcinoma.

Invasive Cervical Carcinoma

Cervical carcinoma is relatively uncommon in the US general population, but it remains the second leading cause of death due to cancer in women worldwide, with approximately 500,000 deaths annually.[20] The incidence of invasive cervical carcinoma is high in Southeast Asia, where screening programs are scarce and the prevalence of risk factors is high.[21,22] Cervical cancer is prevalent among Asians and is generally diagnosed at later stages in Japanese, Chinese, Vietnamese, Filipino, and Korean women than in their white counterparts.[23] Primarily, this is because of lack of screening with the Papanicolaou test in this population. The "Pap" test screening rate in Cambodian American women is lower than in any other racial or ethnic group in the United States.[24]

Takayasu's Arteritis

Takayasu's arteritis is an inflammatory and stenotic disease of medium- and large-sized arteries characterized by a strong predilection for the aortic arch and its branches. The disease is most prevalent in young females of Asian descent.[25] Clinically, patients can present with generalized symptoms, such as malaise, fever, night sweats, arthralgias, weight loss, and localized symptoms such as pain over involved vessels and absence of pulses.[26,27] The diagnosis of Takayasu's arteritis should be strongly suspected in a young Asian female who has a decrease or absence of peripheral pulses, discrepancies in blood pressure, and arterial bruits.

Human Immunodeficiency Virus Infection

Currently, human immunodeficiency virus (HIV) is not common in Asians; however, the number of new cases in Asian countries is accelerating rapidly. The magnitude of the epidemic is projected to exceed that of sub-Sahara Africa in the early part of the 21st century. According to the Joint United Nations Programme on HIV/AIDS (UNAIDS), more than 20 million people in India alone could be infected with the acquired immunodeficiency virus (AIDS) by 2010.[28] The estimated number of cases in China is still relatively small; however, the potential exists for a major explosion of the epidemic in that nation of more than 1 billion people. India and China could have 40 million HIV-positive people by the end of this decade—the same number the entire world has today.

This poses risks to epidemiologic trends among Asian/Pacific Islanders. Although the US immigration policy of HIV testing will screen out those with the virus and viral antibodies, those with a false-negative test will be missed. Furthermore, many Asians travel to their homeland to visit relatives and are at risk if they engage in risky sexual behavior with infected individuals. Therefore, in the right clinical setting, a diagnostic test for HIV should be included in the evaluation of Asian patients with recent travel to endemic Asian countries such as India, Thailand, and China.

CONDITIONS WITH UNIQUE ASPECTS

Sensitivity to Medications

Chinese patients may have increased sensitivity to β-blockers.[29] In clinical practice, these patients may require only a very low dosage of a β-blocker to treat hypertension or congestive heart failure while avoiding side effects. Studies have shown that the effective weight-standardized neuroleptic dose for Asian American patients is significantly lower than that for their white counterparts. Likewise, the weight-standardized dose associated with the development of extrapyramidal symptoms was much lower for Asian Americans than for whites.[30]

Mental Health

Mental health problems among Asian patients may be masked by a negative cultural attitude that prevents many Asians from seeking professional care.[31] Studies have shown that Asians are more vulnerable to mental disorders than are whites.[32] The nature of mental illnesses in Asian immigrants is strongly affected by several factors, including the circumstances that motivated them to leave their countries, the expectations for starting a new life in the United States, and the adjustment experience they have had. Refugees forced to leave their native country because of civil war or political persecution may bring with them memories of torture and atrocities and may suffer from post-traumatic stress disorder and intrusive, frightening thoughts. Sleep disturbances are therefore common.[31] Mental illness is perceived as out-of-control behavior and a sign of weakness in most traditional Asian cultures. The primary care physician, in assessing for psychological disorders, should inquire about the circumstances surrounding the patient's decision to leave his or her native country, with the understanding that it may be difficult for the person to recall painful memories.

In contrast to the psychological factors involved with refugees, major depression in educated, professional immigrants is much more difficult to recognize. This group of Asian immigrants tends to include US-educated professionals with fewer language barriers and higher education levels, who are usually perceived as successful by society.[32] However, they also face culture shock, separation from family, and unsatisfactory employment. Frequently, these patients present to primary care physicians with multiple physical complaints, and diagnostic tests often reveal no organic cause. Primary care providers should search for clues beneath the surface as the cultural expectation of self-control is strengthened by the perspective that direct expression of strong feeling is rude and disgraceful.

ISSUES THAT INFLUENCE CARE

Language Barriers

The conversation between patient and primary care physician is probably the most fundamental part of medical practice. Many Asian-born patients have some difficulties in English proficiency, and medical terminology is even more challenging for them. Therefore, making appointments, stating reasons for the visit, registering, nurse triage, and following instructions may present considerable difficulties for these patients. Studies have shown that Vietnamese men who could not speak English well were less likely to obtain stool hemoccult tests,[33] and Chinese patients with limited English fluency were less likely to obtain serum cholesterol screening.[34] Language barriers can lead to unnecessary diagnostic testing as a result of inaccurate history information given or lost in the translation.

An executive order issued in 2000 and policy guidance from the US Department of Health and Human Services mandate that health care providers who accept federal funds, such as Medicare or Medicaid, must provide language assistance at no cost to any patient with limited English proficiency.[35] However, most physicians in the United States are probably not sufficiently bilingual to practice medicine in a language other than English. Professional interpreters are rarely available in the health care community. Consequently, patients and physicians rely on their own language skills, family or friends, or ad hoc interpreters (bilingual strangers from the waiting room or employees). Family, friends, and ad hoc interpreters may add, omit, substitute, or edit while translating. These services may be problematic in terms of patient confidentiality. Nonetheless, good interpreter services are still possible despite these problems. The local Asian community can be a helpful resource, by providing a number of individuals with a broad spectrum of language skills. Church missionaries who have been assigned to Asian countries usually have satisfactory language skills. In addition, translating for Asian Pacific Islanders provides an opportunity for missionaries to maintain language proficiency. Physicians and nurses fluent in an

Asian language also generally make excellent interpreters because of familiarity with the language and the cultural dimensions of the patient's illness. Volunteer interpreter service should be highly encouraged if locally available, since many hospitals are struggling to comply with federal rules regarding medical interpreters.

Other simple interventions can be helpful for Asian patients with limited English proficiency.[36,37] Examples include:

- Bilingual signs to assist patients making appointments, filling prescriptions, and obtaining laboratory testing.
- A bilingual list of common phrases, medical terms, and questions for both staff and patients.
- The AT&T language line, a 24-hour telephone interpreter service, available in all major languages (1-800-874-9426); there is a charge for this service.

Health Literacy

One fourth of the US population is estimated to be functionally illiterate.[38] Furthermore, an individual's functional health literacy—the ability to read and comprehend prescription directions, appointment slips, and other essential health-related materials required to successfully function as a patient—may be much worse than his or her general literacy. A large-scale study of functional health literacy revealed that one third of English-speaking patients at 2 public hospitals could not read or understand basic health-related materials. Twenty-six percent of patients in the study could not understand information on an appointment slip.[39] The functional health literacy of Asian/Pacific Islanders is virtually unknown. Compounding the problem of functional health illiteracy in these populations is the added dimension of heterogeneous ethnicity and language. To provide culturally appropriate health education programs and deliver culturally competent care for Asian/Pacific Islanders, it may be important to develop a language-specific test to assess the level of functional health literacy in this population.[40]

Socioeconomic Status

Contrary to the stereotype that US Asians are a homogeneous, high-achieving "model minority," they are actually bimodal in aspects of socioeconomic status. According to the March 2000 current population survey of the US Census Bureau, Asians and Pacific Islanders were more likely than non-Hispanic whites to have earned a college degree but were also more likely to have less than a ninth grade education. While one third of Asian and Pacific Islander families had incomes of $75,000 or more, one fifth reported incomes of less than $25,000 and were almost twice as likely as non-Hispanic white families to be in poverty.[41] Thus, Asian/Pacific Islanders demonstrate the same social and economic vulnerability as other minority groups in this country have experienced.

Socioeconomic status has a major impact on the health care of patients in general, and Asian patients are no exception. Impoverished Asian immigrants usually have low-income jobs with long working hours and no health insurance. Consequently, they often do not seek medical care, especially for disease prevention, unless they have acute symptoms. A study in California revealed that 23% of uninsured Chinese over age 40 years never had their blood pressure checked compared with only 6% of insured Chinese.[34] Poverty has also been associated with failure to have a screening mammogram. In a study of Vietnamese immigrants, being married and poverty status, rather than traditional health beliefs and practices, were the most consistent predictors of health care access. Furthermore, having some form of health insurance or having a regular doctor were the strongest predictors of use of preventive health care services.[42] Patients who are poor are usually reluctant to seek medical attention, even when they are ill, because of potential loss of work time and inability to pay medical bills. In addition, an unknown number of Asian immigrants reside in the United States illegally. This subgroup is more vulnerable and may refuse to seek medical help for fear of being reported to federal authorities and deported.

Socioeconomic barriers are more complex to address than language barriers. Some Asian patients with low socioeconomic status may have the cultural belief that seeking public assistance is shameful. Encouraging immigrant Asian patients to comply with treatment of tuberculosis or sexually transmitted diseases is important because of the impact on public health. It is often helpful to involve social workers in making patients aware of available social services. On the other hand, the assumption that all Asian immigrants are poor or that they have been receiving suboptimal medical service in their native countries is inaccurate, as this group is very heterogeneous.[31] Although lack of health insurance is an important barrier to seeking care, evidence exists of disparities in quality of care among persons who are insured and among persons with the same type of insurance or in the same health plan.[43] Interventions aimed at reducing disparities among minority populations should examine all aspects of socioeconomic status as well as each minority group's health beliefs and practices.

Health Beliefs and Practices

A person's beliefs about health are influenced by his or her culture, social background, experience of health and illness, and exposure to health promotion. These, in turn, may influence the use of preventive health services and compliance with disease management efforts.

Balance and harmony: yin and yang

Chinese Taoist philosophy is the foundation of most traditional Asian medical theories and practices. Traditional Chinese medicine is grounded not in biochemistry or pathology but in concepts of balance and harmony between yin and yang, the "5 elements" (wood, fire, earth, metal, and water), the "6 pathogenic factors" (cold, wind, dryness, heat, dampness, and fire), the "7 emotions" (joy, anger, anxiety, obsession, sadness, horror, and fear), and the "way of life" (diet, sexual activity, physical activity, etc). An excess or deficiency in these areas can cause imbalance—"illness" according to traditional Chinese medical theory. An imbalance can also be caused by too much or too little food, drink, sex, work, or exercise.[44] It is also believed that good health requires the life force or vital energy that Chinese call *qi* (pronounced "chee") to flow smoothly through the body along 14 major channels or meridians.[45]

Asian patients who hold these culturally rooted health beliefs may exhibit health behaviors that influence preventive screening, diagnostic testing, and treatment. For example, Asian American patients may be reluctant to have blood tests for cholesterol or glucose determination since they may believe that blood is a nonrenewable vital energy and that blood loss may lead to weakness. A patient may resist a magnetic resonance imaging (MRI) test for fear that the magnetic force may cause imbalance between yin and yang or the 5 elements. Finally, a patient with a febrile illness may present with persistent high fever. This person may have not been taking an antipyretic and believes that the fever is caused by cold or wind (one of the "6 pathogenic factors"), which is necessary to overcome the illness, and that the medication may cause worsening of the disease by reducing fever.

The issue of culturally related health beliefs is even more complex because of the heterogeneity of the ethnic and cultural backgrounds of Asian immigrants. It is virtually impossible for physicians to understand the health beliefs of each distinct group of Asian patients. A simple and very helpful approach in overcoming cross-cultural barriers is to ask the patient for his or her perception of the illness. This approach avoids assumptions of the patient's ethnic heritage and level of acculturation, and acknowledges the differences between a patient's culturally rooted health beliefs and biomedical culture.[46]

Herbal medicine

Herbal medicine is an increasingly common form of alternative therapy in the United States. A 1997 survey estimated that 12.1% of US adults had used an herbal medicine in the previous 12 months vs 2.5% in 1990.[47] Among Asian/Pacific Islanders, the percentage of people using herbal remedies is estimated even higher than the general population, although the exact number is unknown. Contrary to popular myth, herbal remedies can pose serious health risks, since some herbs contain pharmacologically active substances that can have adverse effects and interact with prescription drugs. Only a small fraction of the thousands of herbs used worldwide has been studied vigorously in randomized, controlled clinical trials.[48] Ginkgo or Ginkgo biloba, a Chinese plant that is the oldest living tree species on earth, has been used in China for centuries to treat dementia, peripheral vascular diseases, and tinnitus.[49] Asian ginseng root or ginseng is believed to help the body build resistance to stress, improve immunity, and enhance sexual function.[50] For these reasons, ginseng remains one of the most popular herbs among Asian patients. Toxicity or side effects such as central nervous system stimulation and a rise in blood pressure have been reported.[51] Patients ingesting excessive amounts of ginseng may present with headache, insomnia, and palpitations. Ginseng also may decrease the diuretic effect of furosemide.[52] Therefore, patients with congestive heart failure receiving diuretics or with tachyarrhythmia should avoid consuming ginseng.

Acupuncture

Acupuncture has been an important therapy in East Asian medicine since the first century BC.[53] Many Asian/Pacific Islanders seek acupuncture therapy before seeing primary care physicians and may continue to use acupuncture and Western medical care simultaneously. Asian patients believe acupuncture can correct disruptions of a person's harmony and can moisten, dry, cool, warm, augment, deplete, redirect, reorganize, and unblock a person's internal weather patterns. Of all East Asian complementary medical treatments, acupuncture enjoys the most credibility in the medical community.[54] In 1997, the National Institutes of Health Consensus Development Panel on Acupuncture reviewed the available evidence from almost 500 randomized clinical trials since the early 1970s and concluded: "There is clear evidence that needle acupuncture is efficacious for adult postoperative and chemotherapy nausea and vomiting and probably for nausea of pregnancy. Much of the research focuses on various pain problems. There is evidence of efficacy for postoperative dental pain. There are reasonable studies (although sometimes only single studies) showing relief of pain with acupuncture on diverse pain conditions."[55]

Furthermore, a substantial body of data exists showing acupuncture in the laboratory having measurable and replicable physiological effects that can offer plausible mechanisms for the clinical effects. Extensive neurophysiological research has shown that acupuncture analgesia may be initiated by stimulation of high-threshold, small-diameter nerves in the muscles. These nerves are able to send messages to the spinal cord, brain stem, and hypothalamic (arenate) neurons, which, in turn,

trigger endogenous opioid mechanisms. These responses include changes in plasma or corticospinal fluid levels of endogenous opioids (endorphins) or stress-related hormones (adrenocorticotropic hormones).[56]

Functional magnetic resonance imaging also is beginning to demonstrate that acupuncture has regionally specific, quantifiable effects on relevant structures of the human brain. One study found that a specific acupuncture point on the foot traditionally related to vision activated an occipital visual cortex that was the same area activated by light stimulation of the eye.[57] For patients with chronic musculoskeletal pain, intractable nausea, vomiting during pregnancy or chemotherapy, or migraine headaches intolerant to medication, acupuncture may offer an effective alternative therapeutic modality.

Other traditional Eastern Asian therapies

Asian/Pacific Islanders may also use other traditional Eastern Asian therapies in addition to herbal remedies and acupuncture. For example, "coin rubbing" is one of the commonly used traditional healing techniques in East Asia. The basis of this technique is a belief that ecchymosis induced by rubbing the skin in certain patterns with an object, such as a metal coin, will release toxins that cause illness and will relieve congestion, thus allowing energy qi to flow smoothly.[31] Lack of knowledge of this traditional Asian healing technique may lead physicians to suspect physical abuse. The distribution of ecchymoses produced is often symmetrical and linear (Fig 37-1).

Another common traditional remedy is intake of mo-her (black tree fungus). Mo-her is one of the main ingredients of a popular Chinese restaurant dish—Mooshu pork. This remedy is often taken to enhance circulation. Mo-her may have anticoagulation effects and cause bleeding in patients receiving warfarin.[58] In a patient receiving warfarin whose prothrombin time continues to be elevated above the therapeutic level despite adjustment in dose, a detailed history specifically regarding mo-her intake should be sought.

SUMMARY

In many ways, caring for the Asian patient is no different than caring for any other patient in diagnosing the disease, eliciting the patient's ideas about his or her illness, and negotiating a treatment plan. However, Asian patients encountered in the primary care setting are a group of heterogeneous individuals with multicultural, multiethnic, and multilingual backgrounds. Caring for patients with a different culture, language, religion, socioeconomic status, and health beliefs is a major challenge for health care providers and health care systems. The cultural and ethnic backgrounds of patients can shape their views of illness and well-being. Meeting the health needs of minority populations requires a cultural awareness of the diversity and commonality in peoples' health beliefs and practices.

Useful guidelines to address these issues in the care of Asian patients include the following:

1. Use a translator when possible if language barriers exist. Take a creative approach when a professional translator is not available.

2. Be aware of a patient's socioeconomic status and involve a social worker early on.

3. Avoid making assumptions about the patient's ethnic heritage and level of acculturation. When in doubt, ask the patient about his or her comfort with a particular plan.

4. Respect and acknowledge the differences in culture.

5. Learn about your patient's culture through research and conversing with colleagues from other cultural backgrounds.

6. Cultivate openness toward, and tolerance of, different values and beliefs, and be aware of your own inherent cultural biases.

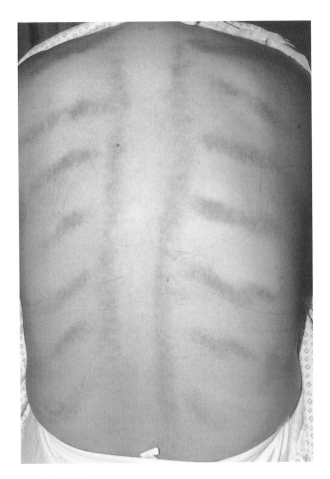

F I G U R E 37–1

Ecchymosis produced by coin rubbing, a traditional Asian healing technique.

REFERENCES

1. Francese P. America at mid-decade. *Am Demographic.* 1995;17:2–31.

2. Yu ES, Liu WT. US National Health Data on Asian Americans and Pacific Islanders: a research agenda for the 1990s. *Am J Public Health.* 1992;82:1645–1652.

3. Barnes J, Bennett C. The Asian Population: 2000. Census 2000 Brief. US Census Bureau, Census 2000 Redistricting Data (Public Law 94-171) Summary File, Table PL1. Washington, DC: US Government Printing Office; 2002.

4. Ting CW, Hwang B, Wu TC. Developmental changes of lactose malabsorption in normal Chinese children: a study using breath hydrogen test with a physiological dose of lactose. *J Pediatr Gastroenterol Nutr.* 1988;7:848–851.

5. Tuberculosis among Asian/Pacific Islanders: US, 1985. *MMWR. Morb Mortal Wkly Rep.* 1987;36:331–334.

6. Tuberculosis cases and case rates per 100,000 population by origin: United States, 1991–2001. Atlanta, Ga: Centers for Disease Control and Prevention. Available at: www.cdc.gov/nchstp/tb/surv/surv2001/pdf/tabpost4.pdf. Accessed December 5, 2002.

7. Luelmo F. BCG vaccination. *Am Rev Respir Dis.* March 1982;125(pt 2):70–72.

8. American Thoracic Society and the Centers for Disease Control and Prevention. Targeted tuberculin testing and treatment of latent tuberculosis infection. *Am J Respir Crit Care Med.* 2000;161:5221–5247.

9. Greenberg PD, Lax KG, Schechter CB. Tuberculosis in house staff: a decision analysis comparing the tuberculin screening strategy with the BCG vaccination. *Am Rev Respir Dis.* 1991;143:490–495.

10. Snider DE Jr. Bacille Calmette-Guerin vaccinations and tuberculin skin tests. *JAMA.* 1985;253:3438–3439.

11. Engebretsen B, Knight A, Shah R. Hepatitis B in Southeast Asian refugees in Iowa. *Iowa Med.* 1984;74:105–108.

12. McQuillan GM, Townsend TR, Fields HA, Carroll M, Leahy M, Polk BF. Seroepidemiology of hepatitis B virus infection in the United States: 1976 to 1980. *Am J Med.* 1989;87(3A):5S–10S.

13. Perkins C, Morris C, Wright W. *Cancer Incidence and Mortality in California by Race/Ethnicity.* Sacramento, Calif: California Department of Health Services, Cancer Surveillance Section; 1996.

14. Krogstad D. Plasmodium species (malaria). In: Mandell G, Bennett J, Dolin R, eds. *Principles and Practice of Infectious Diseases.* 15th ed. New York, NY: Churchill-Livingstone Inc; 2000:2817–2831.

15. Markel SF, LoVerde PT, Britt EM. Prolonged latent schistosomiasis. *JAMA.* 1978;240:1746–1747.

16. Mahmoud A. Trematodes (schistosomiasis) and other flukes. In: Mandell G, Bennett J, Dolin R, eds. *Principles and Practice of Infectious Diseases.* 15th ed. New York, NY: Churchill-Livingstone Inc; 2000.

17. Ebe T, Matsumura M, Mori T, et al. Eight cases of diphyllobothriasis *Kansenshogaku Zasshi.* 1990;64:328–334.

18. Yu MC, Ho JH, Ross RK, Henderson BE. Nasopharyngeal carcinoma in Chinese: salted fish or inhaled smoke? *Prev Med.* 1981;10:15–24.

19. Raab-Traub N, Hood R, Yang CS, Henry B II, Pagano JS. Epstein-Barr virus transcription in nasopharyngeal carcinoma. *J Virol.* 1983;48:580–590.

20. Wright TC, Ferenczy A, Kuman RJ. Carcinoma and other tumors of the cervix. In: Kurman RJ, ed. *Pathology of the Female Genital Tract.* 4th ed. New York, NY: Springer-Verlag; 1994:279–326.

21. Cannistra SA, Niloff JM. Cancer of the uterine cervix. *N Engl J Med.* 1996;334:1030–1038.

22. Jin XW, Cash J, Kennedy AW. Human papillomavirus typing and the reduction of cervical cancer risk. *Cleve Clin J Med.* 1999;66:533–539.

23. Flaskerud JH, Kim S. Health problems of Asian and Latino immigrants. *Nurs Clin North Am.* 1999;34:359–380.

24. Carey Jackson J, Taylor VM, Chitnarong K, et al. Development of a cervical cancer control intervention program for Cambodian American women. *J Community Health.* 2000;25:359–375.

25. Hashimoto H. Takayasu's arteritis and giant cell (temporal or cranial) arteritis. *Intern Med.* 2000;39:4–5.

26. Feng YX, Jin XW. Diagnosis and treatment of polyarteritis. *Zhonghua Wai Ke Za Zhi.* 1985;23:138–140, 189.

27. Kerr GS, Hallahan CW, Giordano J, et al. Takayasu arteritis. *Ann Intern Med.* 1994;120:919–929.

28. Joint United Nations Programme on HIV/AIDS (UNAIDS). *Report on the global HIVAIDS epidemic.* Geneva, Switzerland: World Health Organization; June 2000.

29. Wood AJ, Zhou HH. Ethnic differences in drug disposition and responsiveness. *Clin Pharmacokinet.* 1991;20:350–373.

30. Lin KM, Finder E. Neuroleptic dosage for Asians. *Am J Psychiatry.* 1983;140:490–491.

31. Jin XW, Slomka J, Blixen CE. Cultural and clinical issues in the care of Asian patients. *Cleve Clin J Med.* 2002;69:50–61.

32. Browne C, Fong R, Mokuau N. The mental health of Asian and Pacific Island elders: implications for research and mental health administration. *J Ment Health Adm.* 1994;21:52–59.

33. McPhee SJ, Jenkins CNH, Hung S, Nguyen KP, Ha NT, Fordham DC. Behavioral risk factor survey of Vietnamese: California, 1991. *MMWR. Morb Mortal Wkly Rep.* 1991;41:69–72.

34. Chen A, Lew R, Thai V, Ko KL, Okahara L, Hirota S, et al. Behavioral risk factor survey of Chinese: California, 1989. *MMWR. Morb Mortal Wkly Rep.* 1992;41:269–270.

35. Hawryluk M. Lost in the translation. *Am Med News.* 2002;45:5–6.

36. Woloshin S, Bickell NA, Schwartz LM, Gany F, Welch HG. Language barriers in medicine in the United States. *JAMA.* 1995;273:724–728.

37. Putsch RW III. Cross-cultural communication: the special case of interpreters in health care. *JAMA.* 1985;254:3344–3348.

38. Kirsch I, Jungeblut, Jenkins L, Kolstad A. *A First Look at the Findings of the National Adult Literacy Survey.* Washington, DC: National Center for Education Statistics, US Department of Education; 1993.

39. Williams MV, Parker RM, Baker DW, et al. Inadequate functional health literacy among patients at two public hospitals. *JAMA.* 1995;274:1677–1682.

40. Baker DW, Williams MV, Parker RM, Gazmararian J, Narss J. Development of a brief test to measure functional health literacy. *Patient Education Counseling.* 1999;38:33–42.

41. Current population survey. Washington, DC: US Census Bureau, Racial Statistics Branch, Population Division; March 2000.

42. Jenkins C, Le T, McPhee SJ, Stewart S, Ha NT. Health care access and preventive care among Vietnamese: do traditional practices pose barriers? *Soc Sci & Med.* 1996;43(7):1049–1056.

43. Nerenz D, Bonham V, Green-Weir R, Joseph C, Gunter M. Eliminating racial/ethnic disparities in health care: can health plans generate reports? *Health Aff.* 2002;21:259–263.

44. Hsu H. *Chinese Herb Medicine and Therapy.* Rev ed. Los Angeles, Calif: Oriental Healing Arts Institute, 1994.

45. Eisenberg D. *Encounters with Qi: Exploring Chinese Medicine.* New York, NY: WW Norton; 1985.

46. Kleinman A, Eisenberg L, Good B. Culture, illness, and care: clinical lessons from anthropologic and cross-cultural research. *Ann Intern Med.* 1978;88:251–258.

47. Eisenberg DM, Davis RB, Ettner SL, et al. Trends in alternative medicine use in the United States, 1990–1997: results of a follow-up national survey. *JAMA.* 1998;280:1569–1575.

48. De Smet PA. Herbal remedies. *N Engl J Med.* 2002;347:2046–2056.

49. Blumenthal M. *The Complete German Commission E Monographs: Therapeutic Guide to Herbal Medicines.* Austin, Tex: American Botanical Council; 1998.

50. Vogler BK, Pittler MH, Ernst E. The efficacy of ginseng: a systematic review of randomised clinical trials. *Eur J Clin Pharmacol.* 1999;55:567–575.

51. Hammond TG, Whitworth JA. Adverse reactions to ginseng. *Med J Aust.* 1981;1:492.

52. Becker BN, Greene J, Evanson J, Chidsey G, Stone WJ. Ginseng-induced diuretic resistance. *JAMA.* 1996;276:606–607.

53. Kaptchuk TJ. Acupuncture: theory, efficacy, and practice. *Ann Intern Med.* 2002;136:374–383.

54. Astin JA, Marie A, Pelletier KR, Hansen E, Haskell WL. A review of the incorporation of complementary and alternative medicine by mainstream physicians. *Arch Intern Med.* 1998;158:2303–2310.

55. NIH Consensus Conference. Acupuncture. *JAMA.* 1998;280:1518–1524.

56. Pomeranz B, Stux G. *Scientific Bases of Acupuncture.* New York, NY: Springer-Verlag; 1989.

57. Cho ZH, Chung SC, Jones JP, et al. New findings of the correlation between acupoints and corresponding brain cortices using functional MRI. *Proc Natl Acad Sci USA.* 1998;95:2670–2673.

58. Fitzgerald F, Ainsworth M, Bach H, Humphrey HJ, Lubin MF, Schuster BL. Cross-cultural medicine. *Medical Knowledge Self-Assessment Program.* Philadelphia, Pa: American College of Physicians; 1995:140–142.

59. Chen A, Ng P, Sam P, et al. Special health problems of Asians and Pacific Islanders. In: Matzen RN, Lang RS eds, *Clinical Preventive Medicine.* St. Louis, Mo: Mosby–Year Book, Inc; 1993:739–761.

RESOURCES

Association of Asian Pacific Community Health Organizations (AAPCHO), 439 23rd St, Oakland, CA 94612. Web site: www.AAPCHO.org.

Asian American Health Forum, 450 Sutter St, Suite 600, San Francisco, CA 94108. Web site: www.APIAHF.org.

Oriental Healing Arts Institute, 1945 Palo Verde Ave, Suite 208, Long Beach, CA 90815.

chapter 38

Persons of Mideast Origin

Anita D. Misra-Hebert, MD

INTRODUCTION

When treating ethnic patients, the clinician should become familiar with not only diseases that are prevalent in those ethnic groups but also the approach to health and illness that may be unique to cultural context. As the US population becomes more diverse, the clinician's ability to optimally care for patients from different cultural backgrounds will be determined by a combination of ethnicity-specific medical knowledge and cross-cultural communication skills. Knowledge of the unique health issues of patients of Mideast origin and implications of specific cultural norms may serve to enhance doctor-patient communication and thus the provision of health care within this population.

Countries that make up the Middle East, according to the Centers for Disease Control and Prevention, are Bahrain, Cyprus, Iran, Iraq, Israel, Jordan, Kuwait, Lebanon, Oman, Qatar, Saudi Arabia, Syrian Arab Republic, Turkey, United Arab Emirates, and Yemen.[1] The World Book definition, with the addition of Egypt and Sudan, includes 17 countries.[2] Most people in the Middle East are of Arab ancestry, followed in number by those of Iranian or Turkish origin, with other smaller ethnic groups, such as Kurds, Copts, Greeks, Armenians, and black African groups.[2] In terms of religion, greater than 90% of the population are Muslim, approximately 7% are Christian, and 1% are Jewish.[2]

MEDICAL ISSUES

Much of the information in this section is derived from epidemiologic studies of small groups of patients from various regions in the Middle East, but it may serve as a reference for specific disease processes to be considered in the medical evaluation of this diverse population.

Red Blood Cell Disorders

Thalassemias, sickle cell disease, and glucose 6-phosphate dehydrogenase deficiency are common in the Middle East.[3,4] β-Thalassemia, especially β-thalassemia trait, is seen frequently in the Middle East, while α-thalassemia with symptoms is rare in persons from the Middle East.[4] Consanguineous marriage is not uncommon among Middle Eastern cultures,[5] and it has been suggested that consanguinity is responsible for the increased incidence of β-thalassemia in these populations.[6] Hemoglobin H disease, seen in Saudi Arabia, is caused by dysfunctional α-globin genes and presents as a chronic hemolytic anemia.[4]

Sickle cell disease is seen with some frequency in the Middle East, specifically in the Arabian peninsula.[4] Interestingly, those Arabic patients with homozygous hemoglobin S disease seem to have milder disease than do patients with African hemoglobin S disease, possibly due to elevated levels of hemoglobin F noted in Arabic patients.[4,7,8]

Glucose 6-phosphate dehydrogenase deficiency is prevalent in many Middle Eastern countries, which is of particular relevance in treating Mideastern patients because ingestion of fava beans, a common food in the Middle Eastern diet, and certain prescription drugs may precipitate a hemolytic crisis.[4,9] Obtaining a baseline complete blood cell count as part of preventive screening for persons of Mideast origin is appropriate. Clinical and laboratory findings that may suggest an underlying red blood cell disorder are listed in Table 38-1.

Familial Mediterranean Fever

Familial Mediterranean fever is an autosomal recessive disease, which affects patients of non-Ashkenazi Jewish origin and of Armenian, Turkish, and Middle Eastern Arab origin.[10] This disease is characterized by acute episodes of fever, with abdominal pain and peritonitis, pleurisy, and arthritis.[10,11] Although most patients with familial Mediterranean fever will present with the disease in childhood, presentation can rarely occur in later years. A physician should consider this diagnosis when caring for patients of Mideast origin.[12]

Creutzfeldt-Jakob Disease

Creutzfeldt-Jakob disease has been found to be prevalent in Libyan-born Jews in Israel, with a large number of

TABLE 38-1

Clinical and Laboratory Findings That May Indicate
Underlying Red Blood Cell Disorder*

Anemia

Polycythemia

Microcytosis

Macrocytosis

Target cells or basophilic stippling

Evidence of hemolysis

  Elevated levels of lactate dehydrogenase, indirect
    bilirubin, and aspartate aminotransferase

  Decreased haptoglobin

  Hemoglobinuria or hemosiderinuria

  Bilirubin cholelithiasis

Hematuria or isosthenuria

Splenomegaly and/or hyposplenism

  Howell-Jolly bodies on peripheral blood test

Paradoxical or implausible glycosylated hemoglobin
  measurements

Growth retardation

Unexplained vaso-occlusive episodes

  Bone pain or avascular necrosis

  Colicky abdominal pain

  Priapism

  Retinal infarction and vitreous hemorrhage

  Digital ischemia and dactylitis

*Adapted with permission from Steensma DP, Hoyer JD,
Fairbanks VF.[4]

familial cases and the implication of genetic factors.[3,13,14]
This disease should be considered in the appropriate clinical setting.

Infectious Diseases

Schistosomiasis is prevalent in the Middle East, especially
in Egypt.[15] Chronic pulmonary infection or infection of
the gastrointestinal tract, liver, or bladder may occur
without severe symptoms of acute infection.[15] Infection
with *Schistosoma haematobium* has been associated with
bladder cancer, with a higher frequency of bladder cancer
noted in Africa and the Middle East than in North
America and Europe.[3,16]

Risk of malaria is present in Iran, Iraq, Oman, Saudi
Arabia, the Syrian Arab Republic, Turkey, the United
Arab Emirates, and Yemen.[2] Dengue and plague also are
seen in the Middle East. These infectious diseases should
be considered in the care of patients of Mideast origin
who have recently either immigrated to the United States
or returned from a visit to the region and who present
with appropriate symptoms.

Sarcoidosis

A study of sarcoidosis in 20 Arab patients showed clinical
features similar to presentation of the disease in Western
patients. Notable differences, however, in this small
sample included frequent initial presentation with
chest infection, and rare ocular and central nervous
system involvement.[3,17]

Asthma

The prevalence of asthma in the Middle East likely reflects
the role of environmental factors and specific allergens in
the region.[18] A relationship with asthma and parasitic disease has been proposed.[18] The prevalence of asthma among
high school students in Israel has been found to be approximately 9%.[3,19] A high prevalence of smoking, along with
increased number of cigarettes smoked compared with
smokers in the United States, was reported in Arab American immigrants to the United States in the early 1990s.[20]

Inflammatory Bowel Disease

An increased incidence of inflammatory bowel disease
(IBD) has been reported in Jewish patients. A study of
ulcerative colitis in northern Israel between 1967 and 1986
showed an average annual incidence of 2.23 per 100,000
persons, with the highest average annual incidence in
Israeli-born Jews.[3,21] The reported incidence of Crohn's
disease ranged from 0.5 to 1.8 per 100,000 persons in
Israel in the 1970s,[22] with both genetic and environmental
factors implicated.[23] A study of IBD from 1977 to 1979
found higher incidence rates among Jewish persons in
Baltimore, Maryland, for all types of IBD and for both
ulcerative colitis and Crohn's disease separately.[22]

Renal Stones

Renal stones are common in Arab patients.[16] However,
diet and environmental factors are more commonly
linked to stone formation than genetic predisposition.
Renal stones are seen more frequently in patients with
a high intake of animal protein, whereas bladder
stones are more common in the setting of protein-
energy malnutrition.[3,16]

CULTURAL COMPETENCE IN HEALTH CARE

Although knowledge of specific medical conditions likely
to be encountered in patients of Mideast origin is important, having a familiarity with cultural norms of patients
from this region cannot be overemphasized. *Cultural
competence* refers to the ability of health care providers
to effectively communicate with persons of backgrounds

different from their own. As defined by the American Medical Association, culturally competent physicians are able to provide patient-centered care by adjusting their attitudes and behaviors to the needs and desires of different patients, and by accounting for the impact of emotional, cultural, social, and psychological issues on the main biomedical ailment.[24] Effective communication between clinician and patient will lead to optimal health care delivery and likely greater patient adherence to recommendations. If communication barriers are encountered and culturally competent care is not provided, this may negatively affect health care delivery and thus the overall health of specific ethnic groups. In attempts to review general themes regarding any cultural group, the dangers of stereotyping do need to be acknowledged, as factors such as socioeconomic status, educational level, occupation, and family values and belief systems may contribute as much to cultural norms as does ethnicity.[25]

The following factors may contribute to a patient's ethnic identity:[26]

■ Generation
■ Length of time in host country
■ Language spoken
■ Social network
■ Educational background
■ Economic status
■ City vs rural residence in native country
■ Motivation for acculturation

When acculturation is high, one may find little effect of ethnicity on the patient's cultural identity.

Overall, preventive care is not emphasized in Middle Eastern cultures.[26,27] To explain why health prevention may not be given great emphasis, one must consider the concept of fatalism, or the sense of an external (vs internal) locus of control, which dominates the belief systems in many non-Western cultures.[28] A person of Mideast origin not accustomed to belief systems of the mainstream United States may be more likely to believe that his or her health is predetermined by external forces, such as a higher power. If external forces determine one's health outcomes, the importance of health prevention decreases. This same thinking also may apply to end-of-life decision making; maintaining hope until the end may be viewed as a sign of faith in God, whereas preparing for death may be thought to hasten the process.[26] Regarding treatment options for disease, many patients from the Middle East may adhere to practices of nontraditional healing, or complementary medicine. As stated by Boyle,[26] the "wearing of amulets, meditation, use of herbal teas, eating fresh and complimentary foods, are all thought to negate illness and hasten recovery." This is not to imply that the physician's "traditional" recommended treatments would not be followed, but that an open discussion of the patient's

practices and health belief system would help build a collaborative relationship.

Lipson and Meleis,[27] in their review of health care issues in Middle Eastern patients, state, "An approach that combines expertise and authority with personal warmth more likely encourages trust than would a stiff professional facade." Although pertinent to patients across all cultures, this statement serves to highlight important issues among Middle Eastern patients—issues of status and personal relationships. Expertise and authority are highly respected in the Middle Eastern culture. Boyle[26] states, "[A] premium value is affixed to social status in the Middle East, hence, requesting the person with the most prominent title—the department head, the best surgeon, or the nurse in charge—to intervene on the patient's behalf, is the norm, not the exception." However, personal warmth is also important, perhaps stemming from the importance placed on close relationships, beginning with family relationships, in the culture. Salimbene,[29] in her discussion of culturally sensitive health care for patients from the Middle East, notes that "trust is established only when a personal relationship between caregiver and patients and their families is formed." The need for close relationships may also be reflected in differing concepts of personal space in the Middle East. The appropriate conversational distance in the Middle East is 0.6 m, whereas for Americans, it is 1.5 m.[27] This differing definition of personal space may initially cause some discomfort for the physician not accustomed to working with patients from this region.

The closeness of family ties in the Middle East extends into health care. The family of patients of Middle Eastern origin is often equally involved in medical decision making. One of Salimbene's[29] recommendations for establishing good relationships with Middle Eastern patients is to "include the family, especially older male relatives, in the medical decision-making process." This statement also underscores the patriarchal nature of the Middle Eastern culture and the importance of gender in the evaluation and treatment of Middle Eastern patients. It is always advisable, if possible, to allow the Middle Eastern patient the opportunity to choose a same-sex provider and interpreter, when needed. Female patients of Mideast origin will more likely feel comfortable with a female physician.

Barriers exist in the preventive care of Arab women. This is demonstrated in a statement from an Arab client regarding women's health issues noted by Kulwicki et al,[18] in their study of health services for the Arab American community: "It's like *ayb* (shame) to talk about this." The 1995 Michigan Behavioral Risk Factor Survey showed that Arab women in Detroit, Michigan, performed breast self-examinations less frequently than did white women, 39.6% vs 56.8%, respectively, and underwent Papanicolaou tests less often, 59.9% vs 78.5%, respectively.[20] The prevalence of domestic violence in Arab American women appears similar to that in the rest of the US population, but barriers for use of domestic violence services may be greater among Arab women.[20] The decreased use of screening practices in women of Arab origin may be a reflection of cultural attitudes toward health prevention or may also relate to health care access in this population. Cultural competence of health care providers, attention to same-sex pairing of provider and patient, and creating an appropriate comfort level to allow discussion of preventive recommendations are important to overcoming preventive health barriers in this female population.

RECOMMENDATIONS FOR HEALTH PREVENTION

Specific recommendations for health prevention in patients of Mideast origin are outlined in Table 38-2. A framework for providing culturally competent care also is provided.

SUMMARY

The Middle East is composed of a heterogeneous population from many countries. Although the largest percentage of people of Mideast origin are Muslim Arabs, and much of the literature regarding cultural issues in this population refers to customs of this group, it is important to realize that individual differences and level of acculturation may be much more important in determining cultural attitudes than ethnicity alone. Treating each patient as an individual, and with respect, along with a background of general knowledge about specific diseases and cultural norms prevalent in persons of Mideast origin, will go far to ensure optimal health care delivery to this diverse group of patients.

TABLE 38-2

Issues in Health Prevention in Persons of Mideast Origin*

Issue	Recommendation
Medical Issues	
RBC disorders	Perform CBC count
Tobacco use	Perform usual screening; refer to smoking cessation program
Women's health	Thoroughly discuss age-appropriate preventive screening
Differential diagnosis	In appropriate clinical scenario, consider diagnosis of familial Mediterranean fever, schistosomiasis, malaria, dengue, plague, IBD, renal stones, and Creutzfeldt-Jakob disease
Cultural Competence Issues	
Attitudes toward preventive care	Assess overall attitudes toward preventive care
Gender	Acknowledge gender as a possible communication barrier; offer opportunity for sex-matched provider and interpreter
Complementary medicine	Inquire about complementary medicine practices
Family	Acknowledge role of family in health care decisions
Personal space	Acknowledge differing concepts of personal space
Personal relationship	Respect expectation for a more "personal" relationship between patient and doctor
Status	Acknowledge importance placed on status

*RBC indicates red blood cells; CBC, complete blood cell; and IBD, inflammatory bowel disease.

REFERENCES

1. National Center for Infectious Diseases. Health information for travelers to the Middle East. *Travelers' Health*. Available at: www.cdc.gov/travel/mideast.htm. Accessed March 26, 2003.

2. Le Gall D, Le Gall M. Middle East. *World Book Online Americas Edition*. Available at: www.worldbookonline.com. Accessed December 2002.

3. Hayden SP. Special health problems of European Americans, including peoples of the Mediterranean Basin. In: Matzen RN, Lang RS eds. *Clinical Preventive Medicine*. St Louis, Mo: Mosby-Yearbook Inc; 1993:715–728.

4. Steensma DP, Hoyer JD, Fairbanks VF. Hereditary red blood cell disorders in Middle Eastern patients. *Mayo Clin Proc*. 2001;76:285–293.

5. Hoodfar E, Tebi AS. Genetic referrals of Middle Eastern origin in a western city: inbreeding and disease profile. *J Med Genet*. 1996;33:212–215.

6. Kamel K. Hemoglobin variants in the Middle East. In: Winter WP, ed. *Hemoglobin Variants in Human Populations*. Vol 2. Boca Raton, Fla: CRC Press; 1987:45–64.

7. Wood WG, Pembrey ME, Serjeant GR, Perrine RP, Weatherall DJ. Hb F synthesis in sickle cell anaemia: a comparison of Saudi Arab cases with those of African origin. *Br J Haematol*. 1980;45:431–445.

8. Kamel K. Heterogeneity of sickle cell anemia in Arabs: review of cases with various amounts of fetal haemoglobin. *J Med Genet*. 1979;16:428–430.

9. Gelpi AP. Glucose 6-phosphate dehydrogenase deficiency in Saudi Arabia: a survey. *Blood*. 1965;25:486–493.

10. Pras E, Aksentijevich I, Gruberg L, et al. Mapping of a gene causing familial Mediterranean fever to the short arm of chromosome 16. *N Engl J Med*. 1992;326:1509–1513.

11. Wright DG. Familial Mediterranean fever. In: Bennett JC, Plum F, eds. *Cecil Textbook of Medicine*. Vol 1. Philadelphia, Pa: WB Saunders Co; 1996:907–908.

12. Orbach H, Ben-Chetrit E. Familial Mediterranean fever: a review and update. *Minerva Medica*. 2001;92:421–430.

13. Zilber N, Kahana E, Abraham M. The Libyan Creutzfeldt-Jakob disease focus in Israel: an epidemiologic evaluation. *Neurology*. 1991;41:1385–1389.

14. Korczyn AD. Creutzfeldt-Jakob disease among Libyan Jews. *Eur J Epidemiol*. 1991;7:490–493.

15. National Center for Infectious Diseases. Schistosomiasis [Travelers' Health]. Available at: www.cdc.gov/travel/diseases/schisto.htm. Accessed March 28, 2003.

16. Challah S, Wing AJ. The epidemiology of genito-urinary disease. In: Holland WW, Detels R, and Knox G, eds. *The Oxford Textbook of Public Health*. Oxford, England: Oxford University Press; 1984:181–202.

17. Diab SM, Karnik AM, Ouda BA, et al. Sarcoidosis in Arabs: the clinical profile of 20 patients and review of the literature. *Sarcoidosis*. 1991;8:56–62.

18. Glazer I. Epidemiology of asthma in the Middle East. *Ann Allergy*. 1988;61:312–314.

19. Brook U. The prevalence of bronchial asthma among high school pupils in Holon (Israel). *J Trop Pediatr*. 1991;37:176–178.

20. Kulwicki AD, Miller J, Schim SM. Collaborative partnership for culture care: enhancing health services for the Arab community. *J Transcultural Nurs*. 2000;11:31–39.

21. Niv Y, Torten D, Tamir A, et al. Incidence and prevalence of ulcerative colitis in the Upper Galilee, Northern Israel, 1967–1986. *Am J Gastroenterol*. 1990;85:1580–1583.

22. Calkins BM, Mendeloff AI. Epidemiology of inflammatory bowel disease. *Epidemiol Rev*. 1986;8:60–91.

23. Fireman Z, Grossman A, Lilos P, et al. Epidemiology of Crohn's disease in the Jewish population of central Israel, 1970–1980. *Am J Gastroenterol*. 1989;84:255–258.

24. American Medical Association. *Report of the Council on Medical Education: Enhancing the Cultural Competence of Physicians*. CME Report 5-A-98. Available at: www.ama-assn.org/meetings/public/annual98/reports/cme/cmerpt5.htm. Accessed March 28, 2003.

25. Misra-Hebert AD. Physician cultural competence: cross-cultural communication improves care. *Cleve Clin J Med*. 2003; 70(4):289–303.

26. Boyle DM. Cultural awareness: the cultural context of dying from cancer. *Int J Palliat Nurs*. 1998;4:70–83.

27. Lipson JG, Meleis AI. Issues in health care of Middle Eastern patients. *West J Med*. 1983;139:854–861.

28. Gardenswartz L, Rowe A. *Managing Diversity in Health Care*. San Francisco, Calif: Jossey-Bass Inc; 1998.

29. Salimbene S. *What Language Does Your Patient Hurt In? A Practical Guide To Culturally Competent Patient Care*. Amherst, Mass: Diversity Resources; 2000.

chapter 39

American Indian and Alaska Native People

David R. Baines, MD, J. Anthony Kendrick, MS, and Michael H. Trujillo, MD, MPH, MS

EPIDEMIOLOGY, BACKGROUND, AND RISK FACTORS

American Indians and Alaska Natives are the original inhabitants of North America, or the first "Americans." However, they are the smallest of the US population groups and one of the most diverse. There are more than 560 federally recognized tribes.[1] Each is a sovereign nation with a government-to-government relationship with the federal government. They are nations within a nation, and each has its own language, traditions, heritage, and culture. For the purpose of this chapter, the term *Native American* refers to American Indians and Alaska Natives (AI/AN) and does not include Native Hawaiians. Although technically Native Americans, Native Hawaiians generally are considered within the population group of Asian/Pacific Islanders, as outlined in the US Constitution, Article 1, Section 8. They do, however, have similar health problems and much of what is said about AI/ANs can be

extended to Native Hawaiians. Alaska has 3 distinct racial aborigines. These are American Indian (Athabascan, Tlingit, Tsimshian, and Haida nations), Inuit (formerly known as Eskimo), and Alutiiq (formerly known as Aleut).

There are 2.6 million American Indians and Alaska Natives identified in the 2000 US census. Another 1.6 million reported being American Indian and Alaska Native in combination with 1 or more other races.[2] Approximately one-third live on reservations or historic federal trust lands, and about one-half live in urban areas. Those remaining live on rural nontrust lands[3] (Fig 39-1).

The Indian Health Service (IHS), an agency of the Public Health Service of the US Department of Health and Human Services, provides health care for members of the federally recognized tribes, or approximately 1.6 million AI/AN people. Those remaining receive care, as do all Americans, including the 1.6 million federally recognized Indians in other federal, state, or county programs for which they are eligible or in the private sector. The

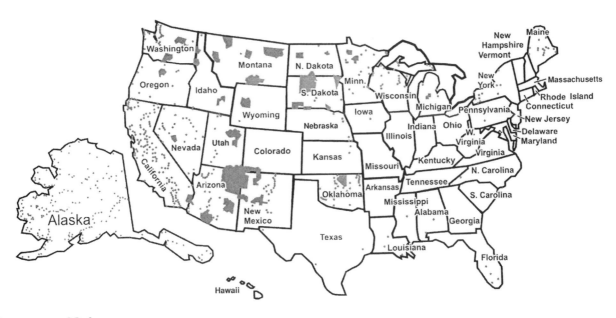

FIGURE 39-1

American Indian and Alaska Native tribal reservations and communities.

T A B L E   39-1

American Indian and Alaska Native Socioeconomic Profile

	American Indian	US All Races
High school graduate	71%	90%
College graduate	11%	15.5%
Average age	28.7	35.3
Health per-capita expenditure	$1,384*	$5,427
Without health insurance	27.1%	14.5%
Annual income	$32,000	$43,000
Poverty	24.5%	11.6%
Unemployment rate		5.8%
Home ownership	55%	67.5%
Homes without safe water	11.7%	2.1%
Homes with phones	70%	95%
Persons per household	3.09	2.59
Family size	3.58	3.14

*Expenditures by the Indian Health Service.

Source information:

(1) US Census Bureau, Current Population Survey 2000, 2001, and 2002 Annual Demographic Supplements.

(2) Indian Health Service, Federal Employee Health Benefit Program Disparity Index, Key Findings by FY 2001 page. Available at: http://www.ihs.gov/NonMedicalPrograms/Lnf/IHCIF2002/IHCIF%20ILLUST%202002.pdf

lack of health coverage for AI/ANs is 42% compared with 14% for non-Hispanic whites.[4]

The annual appropriation for the IHS is insufficient to meet the health needs of all Indian people, which is estimated to be at least 40% greater than appropriation levels.[5] Within its limited resources, the IHS has ongoing programs to address all preventable causes of death in this population. It does not have health facilities in all eligible locations because of financial, personnel, and geographical limitations as well as limited patient workload sufficient for justification. The result is that within "Indian Country" access to medical services involves overcoming transportation issues, such as distance, weather, lack of road access during certain times of the year, and limited medical vehicles and aircraft.[6] To address the unmet health needs in Indian Country, the IHS, tribal, and urban Indian health programs increasingly collaborate with other federal programs such as the Centers for Disease Control and Prevention (CDC), the National Institutes of Health; and the IHS also benefits from the grants and contracts programs administered by the Substance Abuse and Mental Health Services Administration, the Health Resources Services Administration, and the Center for Medicare and Medicaid Services.[7] Collaborations also include alliances with other health organizations, academic medical centers, and philanthropic foundations. Still, there remains a tremendous unmet health need.

SOCIOECONOMICS

Native American family income is well below the national average ($32,116 compared with $45,514 for non-Hispanic whites), and 24.5% live in poverty compared with 11.6% for United States all races (Table 39-1).[8,9] Unemployment is over twice the national average and can exceed 70% in some communities. Only 71% of Native Americans graduate from high school (vs 90% for United States all races), only 11% have a college degree (vs 15.5% for United States all races), and they have the lowest educational attainment of all the minority groups. The average size for a Native American family is 3.58 members, which is the largest for any minority or nonminority group.[10]

The Native American population is relatively young. The median age is 7.3 years younger than the national average. This is due to a high birth rate and the fact that 32% of deaths occur before age 45 years, compared with 9% for the group United States all races.[10,11]

DEMOGRAPHICS

The 10 leading causes of death for American Indians in reservation states in 1996 are shown in Fig 39-2.[12] Death rates due to injuries, liver disease, diabetes, and suicide are significantly higher than for non-Hispanic whites. Other

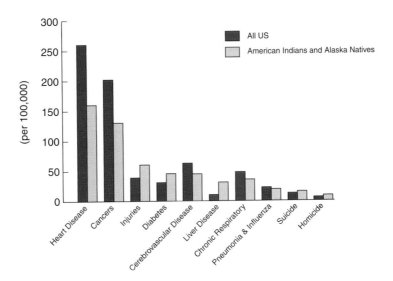

F I G U R E 39-2

Top 10 leading causes of American Indian and Alaska Native deaths.

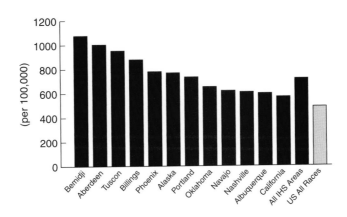

F I G U R E 39-3

Age-adjusted death (all causes) rates (per 100,000 population) for American Indians and Alaska Natives 1996–1998.

conditions more prevalent in the AI/AN population include infant mortality, nephritis, septicemia, and tuberculosis. There are regional differences for these problems (Fig 39-3). These differences have not been broken down by race (eg, Indian vs Inuit), and there has been little effort to determine the etiology of most of these differences.

CARDIOVASCULAR DISEASE

Cardiovascular disease (CVD) is now the leading cause of death in American Indians.[13,14] Early medical literature indicates that ischemic heart disease in this population was rare.[15-18] In 1979 Sievers[19] noted increasing rates of myocardial infarction, and others have recently noted that as well.[20-22] As advances were made in other areas, such as infant mortality and infectious disease, and as the Native American population aged and adopted Western lifestyles, heart disease has become the leading cause of

mortality, and the rate continues to rise.[21,22] Rates very from one area to another. The highest rates are seen in the IHS Bemidji Area (covering the states of Minnesota, Wisconsin, and Michigan) and the IHS Aberdeen Area (covering the states of North Dakota, South Dakota, Nebraska, and Iowa).

Risk Factors

Cardiovascular disease is decreasing in the general population but continues to be on the rise in the American Indian population. The Strong Heart Study (SHS), funded by the National Heart, Lung, and Blood Institute of the National Institutes of Health, was started in 1988 to study CVD and CVD risk factors in 13 tribes in 3 geographic areas.[23,24] It is currently in its fourth phase and has provided a great deal of important information. The SHS has documented that AI/AN are not protected from CVD as

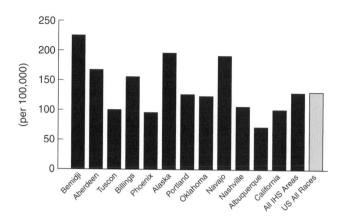

FIGURE 39-4

Age-adjusted malignant neoplasm death rates (per 100,000 population) for American Indians and Alaska Natives 1996–1998.

previously believed and that diabetes and renal disease are the strongest risk factors for CVD in the AI/AN population. The SHS has increased awareness of CVD in AI/AN communities and, as a result, has led to more interventions for primary and secondary CVD prevention programs—programs that are justified by the findings of the SHS over the past 15 years.

Cholesterol

Several studies in American Indians have shown that a high low-density lipoprotein cholesterol (LDL-C) level is the strongest independent lipid abnormality, followed by a low high-density lipoprotein cholesterol (HDL-C) level.[25-28] Lipoprotein(a) was not an independent risk factor in this population.[28] The mean HDL-C level has been decreasing in both men and women. Slight improvements in LDL-C were seen in men; however, women continued to show a slight decrease.[29]

Hypertension

Hypertension was noted to be almost nonexistent in early studies of the AI/AN population.[30-32] More recently, numerous studies have shown an increasing prevalence of hypertension in Indians.[33-35] Hypertension has been found in all populations to be associated with obesity, and those with impaired glucose or diabetes have higher rates of hypertension.[36-38] Because obesity and smoking are linked to multiple morbidities, they will be discussed later in this chapter.

CANCER

Cancer is the second leading cause of death. Similar to CVD, it was previously noted to be rare but is now increasing in this population.[39-41] After a diagnosis of cancer, AI/AN have the poorest 5-year survival rates of any population.[42] Cancer rates vary by area (Figs 39-4 through 39-9). The most common cancers are similar to those found in the general population, but several cancers

that are rare in the general population are more prevalent in some AI/AN populations. Cancer of the gallbladder is more prevalent in the Southwest, and cancer of the liver is more prevalent in Alaska.[43] A high incidence of hepatitis B infection in Alaska Natives is the primary reason for this high prevalence of liver cancer. High rates of smoking play a significant role in lung cancer. Cancer of the cervix is also noted to be more common in Native Americans compared with all US races.[44] Access to culturally sensitive care and lack of knowledge about cancer and cancer screening have been found to be significant factors for the underutilization of cancer screening.[45] Also, limited access to early detection and a population-wide fatalism[46] have resulted in historically low cancer survival rates.[47]

INJURIES

Unintentional injuries are the third leading cause of death. Motor vehicle accidents are the most common cause of unintentional injury and the leading cause of death in Native Americans under 45 years.[48] Low seat belt use and alcohol are the major risk factors. Rural Native Americans are at greater risk because of higher speeds and more distant medical care.[49,50] Other types of injuries vary greatly by area. Drownings are highest in Alaska, and fire- and burn-related deaths are very high in the Northern plains.[51] Native American children have the highest rates of injury morbidity and mortality of any ethnic group in the United States, and rates are almost double compared with all races of children in the United States.[52] If unintentional and intentional injuries were combined, they would be the leading cause of death and the largest cause of years of potential life lost in this population.[53,54]

DIABETES

Once rare,[18,55] type 2 diabetes has grown to epidemic levels and is now the fourth leading cause of death for AI/AN.[56-59] Diabetes ranks as the third leading cause of death in Native Americans aged 55 to 64 years and is 3.6 times higher than

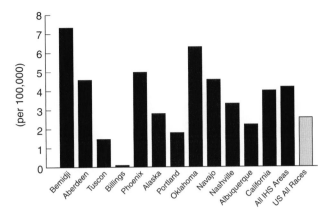

FIGURE 39-5

Age-adjusted cervical cancer death rates (per 100,000 population) for American Indians and Alaska Natives 1996–1998.

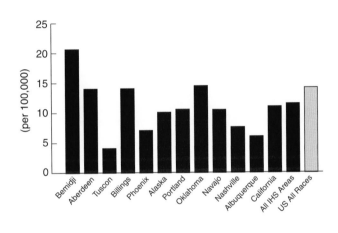

FIGURE 39-6

Age-adjusted prostate cancer death rates (per 100,000 population) for American Indians and Alaska Natives 1996–1998.

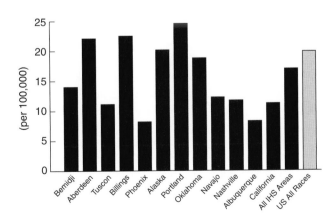

FIGURE 39-7

Age-adjusted breast cancer death rates (per 100,000 population) for American Indians and Alaska Natives 1996–1998.

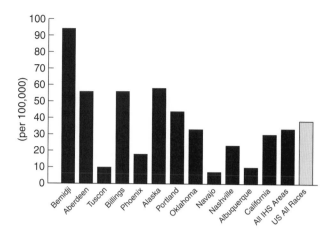

FIGURE 39-8

Age-adjusted lung cancer death rates (per 100,000 population) for American Indians and Alaska Natives 1996–1998.

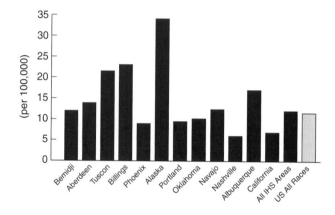

FIGURE 39-9

Age-adjusted colon-rectal cancer (per 100,000 population) for American Indians and Alaska Natives 1996–1998.

the rate for United States all races.[48] The Strong Heart Study found that diabetes prevalence varied among regions. Arizona had the highest prevalence (69%), followed by Oklahoma (39%) and North and South Dakota (38%) in the study population aged 45 to 74 years.[60] Factors shown to increase the risk of diabetes are increasing age, obesity, degree of Indian heritage, and family history of diabetes.[60] Diabetes is associated with hypertension and CVD,[24] stroke,[58] retinopathy,[61] nephropathy,[62] lower extremity amputation,[63] periodontal disease,[61] and risk of infection.[61] Gestational diabetes is found in 2% to 5% of all pregnancies in the United States but is found in 3.4% to 14.5% in Native Americans.[61] This is a great concern, as gestational diabetes is a major cause of congenital anomalies, malformations, and perinatal death.[64] In almost one third of women who had gestational diabetes, diabetes will develop within 8 years of their pregnancy.[61] Of more concern is that longitudinal studies have shown that infants born to gestational diabetic mothers were 9 times more likely to have diabetes develop by 19 years of age and 32 times more likely by 24 years of age, compared with children in the same population born to mothers who did not have gesta-

tional diabetes.[65] This is troublesome because the younger children are when diabetes develops, the younger they will be when complications develop (ie, increased disease burden). It has yet to be determined if better control of diabetes during pregnancy will prevent or delay the subsequent development of diabetes in the offspring of those pregnancies.[66] The marked rise in the incidence of diabetes has been attributed to obesity secondary to increasingly sedentary lifestyles and high-fat, high-calorie diets.[67,68]

Diabetes is also a contributing factor for kidney disease. Increases in the rate of kidney disease, nephritis, and kidney failure have been noted in every age group in the United States.[69] The increased incidence in the AI/AN population is 4 times higher than that for non-Hispanic whites.[70] Contributing factors include diabetes and high blood pressure, which account for up to 65% of cases.[71] The link between end-stage renal disease and diabetes appears to be strong. In the 10-year period between 1991 and 2000, the prevalence of end-stage renal disease per million population that was attributed to diabetes increased from 78 to 145. The prevalence of diabetes

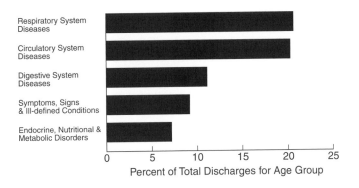

FIGURE 39-10

Leading causes of hospitalization: ages 65+ for IHS and tribal direct and contract hospitals, provisional fiscal year 1997.

in the AI/AN population appears to correlate with the increase of reported end-stage renal disease for the same 10-year period, increasing from 548 per million in 1991 to 716 per million in 2000.[72]

STROKE

There is little information on cerebrovascular disease for AI/AN.[73,74] They have been reported to have a lower incidence of stroke compared with Hispanics and non-Hispanic whites.[75] Stroke is the fifth leading cause of death for Native Americans. It was reported that compared with Hispanics and non-Hispanic whites, stroke-related deaths in Indians were more likely to have diabetes and heavy alcohol use as risk factors,[73] to be coded as subarachnoid hemorrhage,[74] and to be lacunar.[75] Even though strokes were more likely to be coded as a hemorrhage, hemorrhage as a percent of all strokes was lowest among Indians (27%) compared with non-Hispanic whites (37%) and Hispanics (48%).[73] Much more research needs to be done in this area.

LIVER DISEASE

Cirrhosis is a major problem in Native American communities. Although the age-adjusted alcoholism death rate decreased 35% between 1980 and 1993, it is still 5 times the rate for all races in the United States.[48] Chronic liver disease is the second leading cause of death in the 25- to 44-year-old Native American age group and overall is the sixth leading cause of death.[48] Alcoholism accounts for much of chronic liver disease, but hepatitis C is also a culprit, especially in urban AI/AN populations.

CHRONIC RESPIRATORY DISEASE, PNEUMONIA, AND INFLUENZA

Native Americans are particularly susceptible to respiratory tract diseases,[48,76] especially the elders (Fig 39-10).[77] Some consider the susceptibility to be associated with the relatively low adherence to influenza and pneumococcal immunization guidelines by health care providers and the

low level of use of preventive services by minority adults.[78] Other studies suggest that, similar to some Third World countries, those living in remote and isolated locations rely on biomass fuel sources that create high levels of particulate and pollution and, thus, increase the risk of lung diseases, such as emphysema, bronchitis, asthma, and pneumonia. For example, smoke from wood-burning fires interferes with normal lung development in infants and young children.[79] Heating using a wood-burning stove is also associated with symptoms of respiratory illness in young children.[80] Two studies (1988 and 1993) of Navajo households using biomass fuel in enclosed metal heating or cooking stoves with chimneys showed a lower mortality rate for American Indian children compared with children in developing countries.[81] However, the rate was still 6 times that of non-Hispanic white children. In addition, smoking among American Indian and Alaska Native youth predisposes to increased respiratory disease as they age.

Chronic respiratory disease is the seventh leading cause of death for American Indians and Alaska Natives. Influenza and invasive pneumococcal disease are the leading causes of respiratory tract disease and overall it is the eighth leading cause of death. Tuberculosis remains an issue, especially in Alaska Natives, occurring at a rate 6 times that of all US races.[82]

SUICIDE

The suicide rate is 50% higher in Indians compared with all US races and is especially a problem in the 15- to 44-year age group.[14,83] It is the seventh leading cause of death in the AI/AN population. Tribes with higher levels of social integration (eg, clans) and tribes that retain more traditional beliefs (are less acculturated into mainstream society) have lower rates of suicide. Conversely, tribes with higher acculturation have higher rates of suicide.[83,84] Profiles of suicide victims indicate they came from unstable families with substantial alcohol and drug abuse, and other self-destructive behaviors. Physical and sexual abuse are also more common among those who attempt or complete suicide.

A large number commit suicide while incarcerated or intoxicated.[83] As with unintentional injuries, alcohol is a significant factor in both suicide and homicide.

HOMICIDE

The age-adjusted homicide rate for AI/AN has decreased 37% since the 1970s.[82] Despite this, the homicide rate is 33% higher than that for all US races and is 2.2 times higher compared with non-Hispanic whites.[12] The age-specific death rate for homicide is higher for males in all age groups except for male infants less than 1 year old or men over 85 years. It is most prominent in the 15- to 44-year age group.

INTERVENTION PROGRAMS AND STRATEGIES

All of the top 10 causes of death have preventable risk factors. Although no estimation of cost savings is known, substantial savings would certainly occur if risk factors were brought to a level equivalent to those for all Americans. This is the federal goal outlined in Healthy People 2010—to eliminate health disparities between all of America's population groups.[13] Many deaths in American Indians are attributable to several risk factors:

- tobacco use
- alcohol abuse
- obesity or sedentary lifestyle
- low socioeconomic status
- limited access to care

Tobacco

Traditionally, tobacco has major religious and cultural importance. Indians believe that tobacco is a sacred substance given to the tribes by the Creator for ceremonial purposes. Recreational use of tobacco began after contact with Europeans.[85] Tobacco use varies by region, with the North Central plains having the highest prevalence and the Southwest the lowest. The number of cigarettes smoked per day is also lower in the Southwest.[86,87] In many regions of the United States, current smoking rates among Indians can approach 70%. Use is consistently higher than in the non-Indian population, but number of cigarettes per day is lower.[88-90] A high incidence of smokeless tobacco use has been noted in Alaska, even among females.[88] Although tobacco use has generally been shown to be a risk factor for heart disease,[21,25] surprisingly, smoking has not consistently been shown to be an independent risk factor for CVD in this population. This is most likely due to the low number of cigarettes smoked per day in some populations. Smoking has been consistently shown to be a significant

risk factor for lung and other cancers, chronic lung disease, and susceptibility to pneumonia. Maternal smoking during pregnancy and having a current smoker in the household significantly increases the risk of sudden infant death syndrome (SIDS). As mentioned in the next section, SIDS also is linked to maternal alcohol use.[91] The IHS and a number of tribes have programs available to communities and providers to teach patients about the risks of SIDS and, as is typical, the need exceeds the resources.

Tobacco use is very high among Native American adolescents. Having a family member who smokes, experiencing a death or loss, and experiencing other stressful life events are linked to increased risk of tobacco use in adolescents. Being connected to their traditional culture increases Indian youths' ceremonial use of tobacco and decreases their risk of recreational tobacco use. Good family and tribal support and being academically oriented lowers the risk of tobacco abuse.[92] Studies consistently show tobacco use starts early; therefore, intervention should be targeted at youths before they enter the eighth grade.[15,34,87] Programs to address poverty, racism, and social isolation are needed and should be supported at the tribal or community level as well as the state and federal levels.

Alcohol Abuse

Alcohol plays a significant role in 4 of the top 10 causes of death (unintentional injury, liver disease, suicide, and homicide). In addition, alcohol increases infant mortality and morbidity in the form of fetal alcohol syndrome/fetal alcohol effect and SIDS. Alcohol and substance abuse have been attributed to transgenerational trauma or historical grief (ie, loss of culture), depression, poverty, and exposure to destructive life forces.[93-95] Comorbid mental health diseases are often present.[96] Dealing with the historical grief and the comorbid psychiatric conditions in an appropriate cultural manner has proved more successful than using traditional Western approaches alone.[93,94,97] A school-based prevention program showed lower rates of smokeless tobacco, alcohol, and marijuana use in the intervention arm of the study, with cigarette use left unaffected.[98] This demonstrates that a school-based curriculum can be effective in preventing alcoholism.

Obesity

Obesity was rare in the AI/AN population before 1940.[99-102] Since then, studies have shown that obesity is increasing at an alarming rate in this population and is especially a problem in children.[103] The prevalence of obesity has been documented to be twice that of the general population.[104-106] Sedentary lifestyles and westernization of diet are the culprits of this epidemic.[97]

Because obesity is a potent risk factor for diabetes, which is, in turn, a potent risk factor for CVD, most lifestyle intervention programs have used body mass index (BMI), glucose intolerance, and diabetes as end points. Positive results in primary[107] and secondary[20] prevention have been demonstrated with lifestyle modification. The Diabetes Program Research Group studied diabetes prevention in a high-risk population using lifestyle changes vs drug therapy with metformin. There was a 58% reduction in the incidence of diabetes in the lifestyle modification arm and a 31% reduction in the metformin arm of the study.[108] These same lifestyle changes have been shown to reduce the risk of obesity in school-aged children as well.[100,109]

Physical activity decreases as children age. Female adolescents are generally less active than their male counterparts and establish their adult physical activity levels earlier.[87]

Successful intervention programs received support from community members and leaders, brought in extra resources, used members of the community in most or all phases of the study, and provided a culturally appropriate message to bring people back to the healthy ways their people had traditionally followed.

Low Socioeconomic Status

Education; job opportunities; and a strong, safe, culturally appropriate environment can provide a base to develop self-esteem. Unfortunately, this is the exception rather than the rule in many AI/AN communities. Low self-esteem leads to many psychological and behavioral problems. This population is one of the poorest, least educated, and most unemployed groups in the United States.[110] Suicide, homicide, depression, substance abuse, tobacco abuse, SIDS and other infant mortality, and unintentional injury have been linked to low socioeconomic status.[111]

Traditionally, the family and tribal community (extended family) first taught the children to respect themselves (ie, they are important and have gifts given to them by the Creator). Next, they were taught to respect others and, when older, they were taught to respect their surroundings or environment according to the beliefs and culture of their individual tribe. This was done through traditional stories passed on by the elders. The loss of the traditional culture and teaching system has been widespread. This was exacerbated by mandatory federal and church-run boarding schools where Indian children were forcibly removed from their families and acculturated and educated.[112] This disruption of the culture continues to have a strong negative influence in the Indian population. Many communities are trying to bring back the traditional ways, but much has been lost. Providing strong psychological and social services and using traditional healers and elders in treatment and prevention protocols can be beneficial, especially during times of heavy stress. This has been shown to be particularly effective in suicide prevention.[80]

Limited Access to Care

The IHS, as well as many rural and inner city locations where Native Americans reside, has limited workforce and financial resources. Tribal programs and the IHS have had difficulty in filling many of its primary care positions, and many remote locations are understaffed. The IHS has used physician extenders such as community health representatives (CHR), nurse practitioners, physician assistants, pharmacists, and temporary providers to help alleviate some of the problem.[113] In addition, a triage method using nurses has been successful in alleviating some of the excess patient load. This has led to better acute and preventive care.[114]

Many populations live in remote locations and smaller communities may have only a CHR. Telemedicine has greatly improved care to these remote sites. Further development of this system is important to continue to address access to care for this population. As mentioned earlier, funding for the IHS, tribal, and urban Indian health programs does not meet the personal and public health needs of AI/AN. Per capita spending on AI/AN patients is less than half that of the general US population.[115]

In addition to disparities in health status, access to health services, and funding, there is also racial disparity in health care. Former Secretary of Health and Human Services Louis Sullivan said that "there is clear demonstrable, undeniable evidence of discrimination and racism in our healthcare system." Discrimination, the differential treatment of people based on their race or ethnicity, can determine the quality of care at the individual and institutional level.[115] Studies also show that even when controlling for variable factors, such as age, insurance status, medical conditions, and symptom expression, racial and ethnic populations receive lower quality of services and are less likely to receive routine medical procedures than is the non-Hispanic white population.[116,117]

Many groups have put forward ideas to try to address the various disparities that many people, including Native Americans, in this country face in accessing and receiving health services. Ideas frequently mentioned include increasing the percentage in the workforce who are primary care providers, increasing the number of minority providers and researchers, and mandating cultural sensitivity training in medical education curriculum.[113]

Targeted Efforts

Cardiovascular disease

The Intertribal Heart Project, funded jointly by the IHS and the CDC, was started in 1992 and looked at CVD and its risk factors. As a result of that study, community-based heart disease prevention programs were implemented in 3 Native American communities in Minnesota and Wisconsin, where heart disease mortality is very high.[22]

The Native American Cardiology Program was developed in 1993 as a collaboration between the IHS Navajo, Phoenix, and Tucson areas (covering the states of Arizona, Utah, and Nevada and portions of New Mexico) and is based at the University of Arizona. Its mission is to coordinate treatment, education, and prevention of CVD in American Indian patients in the Southwest. It is a unique collaboration of resources that also does research on CVD and its risk factors and that develops and implements prevention strategies for CVD.[118]

Cancer

The Native American Cancer Survivors Network, spearheaded by the Native American Cancer Research Center in Pine, Colo, was started in 1999. It has had a major positive impact on the social support as well as the fatalism about cancer that is common in this population.[119]

The Mayo Cancer Center has a national resource for individuals, communities, and providers called the Native Cancer Information Resource Center and Learning Exchange (CIRCLE). Native CIRCLE has 5 goals.[120] First, it maintains and distributes culturally appropriate materials designed for community cancer education, recruitment of AI/AN subjects into clinical trials for the benefit of Indian people, and cancer prevention and intervention programs. Second, it provides information on current and prior cancer prevention and control research among AI/AN populations. Third, it maintains information on resources relevant to cancer prevention and control such as a speaker's bureau, support groups, tribal resolutions, grant cycle information, and foundation resources for pilot projects. Fourth, it maintains an interactive Internet site for immediate dissemination of new data and resources. Fifth, it conducts an active dialog with AI/AN organizations, advocacy groups, and extramural investigators.

Injuries

The IHS Injury Prevention Program promotes community-based interventions to reduce severe injuries in Indian Country. Using data and community input, the program staff designs programs to train members of the community as injury prevention specialists. The community injury prevention specialist then designs programs targeting the most common types of injuries in the individual communities. Started in the mid 1980s, the program has had a major impact in decreasing injury-related morbidity and mortality.[51]

The IHS tribal and urban clinics have an infant and child restraint program, which provides these important devices without charge. This program has significantly decreased the rates of injuries in the infant and child population.[121]

Other Prevention Efforts

The IHS, tribal and urban Indian clinics have aggressive immunization programs for influenza and pneumococcal disease. The AI/AN population is especially vulnerable to these diseases, and this effort needs to be adopted by private, county, state, and federal health programs that serve AI/AN patients.[122]

Multiple studies have shown the benefits of breast-feeding for the health of infants and mothers. Benefits increase with the duration of breast-feeding after the birth of the child. Reductions in gastrointestinal and respiratory tract infections have been noted in infants who are breast-fed.[123] A study on the Navajo reservation showed that a breast-feeding promotion program significantly increased breast-feeding rates (16.4% to 54.6%) and decreased the percent of children having pneumonia by 32.2% and gastroenteritis by 14.6%.[111] Based on these and other data, breast-feeding should be more aggressively promoted.

Counseling and Compliance

When responding to the health concerns of Native American patients, it is important for the health care provider to understand the patients' beliefs regarding health, disease, and healing. This allows for more effective communication and a better chance for a positive outcome.[124] Indian patients claim that many non-Indian providers cannot communicate well, are difficult to work with, and do not stay long enough to learn about Indian culture and traditions. Providers complain that American Indian patients cannot communicate well, are difficult to work with, exclude themselves from their community activities, and are not motivated enough to care for themselves. These beliefs make for poor doctor-patient relationships. Many providers, particularly those contracted by the IHS and tribal programs to augment their professional staff on a temporary basis, do not get adequate cultural training for working with this population. These relationships can be improved by increasing the understanding and sensitivity of providers to relevant aspects of Native American culture as well as increasing the understanding of tribal members concerning the potential for a newcomer in a community to feel isolated and lacking in cultural sensitivity.

Health in Native culture is not the absence of disease, but rather harmony with oneself (mind, body, and spirit), others, and the surroundings or environment. When harmony is lost, illness is allowed to enter. The culture of many tribes considers spirituality or religion as inseparable from health and wellness. Traditional Indian healers use a spiritual means to diagnose and heal, based on the unique beliefs of the tribe. Traditional healers are viewed as healing from the inside (of the body) because they spiritually correct what is out of harmony. Therefore, they treat the cause of the illness. Western medicine is viewed by many Indian cultures as using a physical means to diagnose and treat. It is viewed as healing from the outside (of the body), and it treats the symptoms (headaches, dyspepsia). Both methods are viewed as compatible and are not considered competitive. They have the same goal—a healthy patient. Studies have shown that compliance with medical treatment is influenced by many factors, and one of them is their relevance to an individual's belief system.[125] Through a better understanding, encounters between Native American patients and providers can be more effective and satisfying.

Both reservation-based and urban Native Americans use traditional healers, and these healers should be kept in mind as a possible consultant to whom to refer Native American patients. Traditional healers are frequently underutilized and can be a major resource for treating the AI/AN patient. Traditional healers often are reluctant to work with non-Indians until they get to know them; however, just indicating to the individual or that person's family that he or she may wish to consider contacting a traditional healer may be the only referral that is necessary. Traditional healing is a very personal matter between the individual and the healer and cannot be prescribed as a referral would be in a typical Western model of health treatment. In some IHS locations, there is a history of a collaborative approach to healing and sometimes a traditional healer will refer an individual to the local health clinic to treat symptoms first. In turn, a provider will recommend a patient consider contacting a traditional healer. Some hospitals and clinics even have areas for the traditional healers to work. Through better understanding, this may become the rule rather than the exception in Indian communities.

The Association of American Indian Physicians (see "Resources" at the end of this chapter) has an American Indian cross-cultural training workshop that has had excellent success in training medical and nursing students, residents, nurses, physicians, and researchers who provide care for Native American patients. The workshop uses Native physicians and traditional healers who discuss traditional Indian beliefs, cultural norms, and specific case histories. For further information on Indian culture, see Suggested Readings under "Resources."

REFERENCES

1. Indian Health Service. Year 2003 profile. January 2003. Available at: www.info.ihs.gov/Infrastructure/Infrastructure6.pdf. Accessed March 20, 2003.

2. Centers for Disease Control and Prevention. Table 3, American Indian or Alaska Native resident population by state and Hispanic origin: United States 2000. Atlanta, Ga: Centers for Disease Control and Prevention; March 2003. Available at: ftp://ftp.cdc.gov/pub/Health_Statistics/NCHS/datasets/nvss/bridgepop/table3.xls. Accessed March 20, 2003.

3. US Dept of Health and Human Services. *Trends in Indian Health 1997*. Rockville, Md: US Dept of Health and Human Services, Public Health Service, Indian Health Service; 1997.

4. Indian Health Service. *Disparities in health insurance coverage for American Indians and Alaska Natives*. May 2002. Available at: http://info.ihs.gov/Resources/Resource5.pdf. Accessed March 22, 2003.

5. Indian Health Service. LNF Workgroup Report—Level of Need Funded Cost Model, May 1999. Available at: www.ihs.gov/nonmedicalprograms/lnf/Dld_files/p1sum.pdf. Accessed March 21, 2003.

6. US Dept of Health and Human Services. *Healthy People 2010: Understanding and Improving Health*. 2nd ed. Washington, DC: US Government Printing Office; November 2000.

7. Grim C. IHS plans a healthy future. *US Med.* January 2003.

8. US Bureau of the Census. *Current Population Survey 2000, 2001, and 2002,* annual demographic supplements. Washington, DC: US Bureau of the Census; 2000–2002.

9. Indian Health Service, Federal Employee Health Benefit Program Disparity Index, Key Findings for FY 2001. Available at: www.ihs.gov/NonMedicalPrograms/Lnf/IHCIF2002/IHCIF%20ILLUST%202002.pdf. Accessed January 31, 2003.

10. US Dept of Commerce. *U.S. Census 2000.* Suitland, Md: US Dept of Commerce, Economics and Statistics Administration, US Census Bureau; 2001.

11. US Dept of Health and Human Services. *Trends in Indian Health 1994*. Rockville, Md: US Dept of Health and Human Services, Public Health Service, Indian Health Service; 1994.

12. US Dept of Health and Human Services. *Health, United States, 2002, With Chart Book on Trends in the Health of Americans.* Hyattsville, Md: US Dept of Health and Human Services, Centers for Disease Control and Prevention; 2002.

13. US Dept of Health and Human Services. *Health, United States, 1998, With Socioeconomic Status and Health Chart Book.* Hyattsville, Md: US Dept of Health and Human Services, Centers for Disease Control and Prevention; 1998.

14. US Dept of Health and Human Services. *Regional Differences in Indian Health, 1998–1999*. Rockville, Md: US Dept of Health and Human Services, Public Health Service, Indian Health Service, Office of Public Health; 2000.

15. Gilbert J. Absence of coronary thrombosis in Navajo Indians. *Calif Med.* 1955;82:114–115.

16. Kunitz SJ. *Disease Change and the Role of Medicine: The Navajo Experience.* Berkeley, Calif: University of California Press; 1983.

17. Leo TF. Cardiovascular surgery in a population of Arizona Indians. *Circulation.* 1958;18:748.

18. Salisbury CF. Disease incidence among the Navajos. *Southwest Med.* 1937;21:230–233.

19. Sievers ML, Fisher JF. Increasing rate of acute myocardial infarction in Southwestern American Indians. *Arizona Med.* 1979;36:739–742.

20. Gilliland SS, Zane SP, Perez GE, Carter JS. Strong in body and spirit: lifestyle intervention for Native American adults with diabetes in New Mexico. *Diabetes Care.* 2002;25:78–83.

21. Howard VF. Rising tide of cardiovascular diseases in American Indians: the Strong Heart Study. *Circulation.* 1999;99:2389–2395.

22. Sewell JL. The increasing incidence of coronary artery disease and cardiovascular risk factors among a Southwest Native American tribe: the White Mountain Apache Heart Study. *Arch Intern Med.* 2002;162:1368–1372.

23. Welty TK. The Strong Heart Study: a study of cardiovascular disease and its risk factors in American Indians. *IHS Provider.* 1992;17:32–33.

24. Welty TK. Cardiovascular disease risk factors among American Indians: the Strong Heart Study. *Am J Epidemiol.* 1995;142:269–287.

25. Howard BV. Coronary heart disease prevalence and its relation to risk factors in American Indians: the Strong Heart Study. *Epidemiology.* 1995:142:254–268.

26. Howard BV. LDL cholesterol as a strong predictor of coronary heart disease in diabetic individuals with insulin resistance and low LDL: the Strong Heart Study. *Arteriosclerosis, Thrombosis, and Vascular Biology.* 2000;20:830–835.

27. Hu D. Accuracy of lipoprotein lipid and apportions in predicting heart disease in diabetic American Indians: the Strong Heart Study. *Ann Epidemiol.* 2002;12:79–85.

28. Wang W, Hu D, Yen JL, et al. Lipoprotein (a) in American Indians is low and not independently associated with cardiovascular disease: the Strong Heart Study. *Ann Epidemiol.* 2002;12:107–117.

29. Welty TK. Changes in cardiovascular risk factors among American Indians: the Strong Heart Study. *Ann Epidemiol.* 2002;12:97–106.

30. Clifford NJ. Coronary heart disease and hypertension in the White Mountain Apache Tribe. *Circulation.* 1963;28:926–931.

31. Fulmer H. Coronary heart disease among the Navajo Indians. *Arch Intern Med.* 1963;59:740–764.

32. Sievers ML. Historical overview of hypertension among American Indians and Alaska Natives. *Ariz Med.* 1977;34:607–610.

33. Destrehan F, Coulehan JL, Want MK. Blood pressure survey on the Navajo Indian reservation. *Am J Epidemiol.* 1979;109:335–345.

34. Howard BV. Blood pressure in 13 American Indian communities: the Strong Heart Study. *Public Health Rep.* 1996;36(suppl 12):47–48.

35. Young TK. Prevalence and correlates of hypertension in a subarctic Indian population. *Prev Med.* 1991;20:474–485.

36. Howard BV. Hypertension in adult American Indians: the Strong Heart Study. *Hypertension.* 1996;28:256–264.

37. Saad MF. Insulin and hypertension: relationship to obesity and glucose intolerance in Pima Indians. *Diabetes.* 1990;39:1430–1435.

38. Strotz CR. Hypertension in Papago Indians. *Circulation.* 1973;48:1299–1303.

39. Burhansstipanov L, Hampton JW, Tenny MJ. American Indian and Alaska Native cancer data issues. *Am Indian Culture Res J.* 1999;23:217–241.

40. Cobb N, Paisano RE. Patterns of cancer mortality among Native Americans. *Cancer.* 1998;83:2377–2383.

41. Valway S, Kileen M, Paisano R, et al. *Cancer Mortality Among Native Americans in the United States: Regional Differences in Indian Health, 1984–1988 and Trends Over Time.* Rockville, Md: US Dept of Health and Human Services, Public Health Service, Indian Health Service; 1992.

42. Horn JW. Cancer incidence, mortality, and survival among racial and ethnic minority groups in the United States. In: Schottenfeld D, Fraumeni JF Jr, eds. *Cancer Epidemiology and Prevention.* New York, NY: Oxford University Press; 1996.

43. Boss LP, Lanier AP, Dohan PH, et al. Cancers of the gallbladder and biliary tract in Alaska Natives. *J Natl Cancer Inst.* 1982;69:1005–1007.

44. US Dept of Health and Human Services. *Regional Differences in Indian Health, 2000–2001.* Rockville, Md: US Dept of Health and Human Services, Public Health Service, Indian Health Service, Office of Public Health; 2002.

45. Risendal B. Pap smear screening among urban southwestern American Indian women. *Prev Med.* 1999;29:510–518.

46. Hanno WK, Weisbrod JA, Ericson K, eds. *Psychosocial and Behavioral Aspects of Medicine.* Baltimore, Md: Williams & Wilkins; 2003.

47. Joe J. Cancer in American Indian Women. In: Glanz K, ed. *Cancer in Women of Color Monograph.* Bethesda, Md: US Dept of Health and Human Services, National Institutes of Health, National Cancer Institute; January 2003.

48. US Dept of Health and Human Services. *Trends in Indian Health 1996.* Rockville, Md: US Dept of Health and Human Services, Public Health Service, Indian Health Service, Office of Public Health; 1997.

49. Grossman DC, Kriger JW, Sugarman JR, Forquera RA. Health status of urban American Indians and Alaska Natives: a population-based study. *JAMA.* March 16, 1994;271(11):845–850.

50. Grossman DC. Motor vehicle crash—injury risk factors among American Indians. *Accident Analysis and Prev.* 1977;29(3):313–319.

51. Smith RJ, Dellapena AJ, Berger LR. Training injury control practitioners: the Indian Health Service model. *Unintentional Injuries Child.* Spring/Summer 2000;10(1):175–188.

52. Chilton L. The prevention of unintentional injury among American Indian and Alaska Native children: a subject review. *Pediatrics.* 1999;104:1397–1399.

53. Gallaher MM, Fleming DW, Berger LR, et al. Pedestrian and hypothermia deaths among native Americans in New Mexico. *JAMA.* 1992;267:1345–1348.

54. US Dept of Health and Human Services. *Indian Health Focus: Injuries 1998–1999.* Rockville, Md: US Dept of Health and Human Services, Public Health Service, Indian Health Service, Office of Public Health; 1999.

55. Joslin EP. The universality of diabetes: a survey of diabetic morbidity in Arizona. *JAMA.* 1940;115:2033–2038.

56. Burrows, NR, Geiss LS, Engelgau MM, Acton KJ. Prevalence of diabetes among Native Americans and Alaska Natives, 1990–1997: an increasing burden. *Diabetes Care.* 2000;23:1786–1790.

57. Mokdad AH, Bowman BA, Englegau MM, Vinicor F. Diabetes trends among American Indians and Alaska Natives: 1990–1998. *Diabetes Care.* 2001;24:1508–1509.

58. Schraer CD, Adler AI, Mayer AM, Halderson KR, Trimble BA. Diabetes complications and mortality among Alaska Natives: 8 years of observation. *Diabetes Care.* 1997;20:314–321.

59. Will J. Diabetes trends in the U.S.: 1990–1998. *Diabetes Care.* 2000;23:1278–1283.

60. Lee ET. Diabetes and impaired glucose tolerance in 3 American Indian populations ages 45–74 years: the Strong Heart Study. *Diabetes Care.* 1995;18:599–610.

61. Ghodes D. Diabetes in North American Indians and Alaska Natives. In: National Diabetes Data Group. *Diabetes in America.* 2nd ed. Bethesda, Md: National Institutes of Health; 1995:683–701. NIH Publication 95–1468.

62. Carter JS, Pugh JA, Monterrosa A. Non-insulin-dependent diabetes mellitus in minorities in the United States. *Ann Intern Med.* 1996;125:221–232.

63. Rith-Najarian SJ, Stolusky T, Ghodes DM. Identifying diabetic patients at high risk for lower-extremity amputation in a primary health care setting: evaluation of simple screening criteria. *Diabetes Care.* 1992;15:1386–1389.

64. Aberg A, Westbom L, Kallen B. Congenital malformations among infants whose mothers had gestational diabetes or preexisting diabetes. *Early Hum Dev.* 2001;61:85–95.

65. Pettitt DJ, Aleck KA, Baird HR, Carraher MJ, Bennett PH, Knowler WC. Congenital susceptibility to NIDDM: role of intrauterine environment. *Diabetes* 1988;37:622–628.

66. Pettit DJ, Knowler WC. Long-term effects of the intrauterine environment, birth weight, and breast-feeding in Pima Indians. *Diabetes Care.* 1998;21(suppl 2):B138–B141.

67. Knowler WC, Pettitt DJ, Savage PJ, Bennett PH. Diabetes incidence in Pima Indians: contributions of obesity and parental diabetes. *Am J Epidemiol.* 1981;113:144–156.

68. Lillioja S, Bogardus C. Obesity and insulin resistance: lessons learned from the Pima Indians. *Diabetes Metab Rev.* 1988;4:517–540.

69. US Dept of Health and Human Services. *Healthy People 2010.* Washington, DC: US Dept of Health and Human Services; January 2000.

70. US Dept of Health and Human Services. *Baseline Report: Strategic Development and Planning Meeting.* Bethesda, Md: National Institutes of Health, National Institute of Diabetes and Digestive and Kidney Diseases; June 2001.

71. US Dept of Health and Human Services. The National Women's Health Information Center Web site. Available at: www.4woman.gov/faq/diabetes.htm. Accessed March 27, 2003.

72. US Dept of Health and Human Services. *U.S. Renal Data System 2002 Annual Data Report: Atlas of End-Stage Renal Disease in the United States.* Bethesda, Md: National Institutes of Health, National Institute of Diabetes and Digestive and Kidney Diseases; 2002.

73. Frey JL, Jahnke HK, Bulfinch EW. Differences in stroke between white, Hispanic, and Native American patients: the Barrow Neurological Institute Stroke database. *Stroke* 1988;29:29–33.

74. Gillum RF. The epidemiology of stroke in Native Americans. *Stroke.* 1995;26:514–521.

75. Kattapong VJ, Becker TM. Ethnic differences in mortality from cerebrovascular disease among New Mexico's Hispanics, Native Americans, and non-Hispanic whites, 1958 through 1987. *Ethnic Dis.* 1993;3:75–82.

76. Rhoades ER. The major respiratory diseases of American Indians. *Am Rev Respir Dis.* 1990;141:595–600.

77. John R. *American Indian and Alaska Native Elders: An Assessment of Their Current Status and Provision of Services.* Rockville, Md: Indian Health Service, Office of Health Programs; 1995.

78. Buchwald D, Sheffield J, Furman R, Hartman S, Dudden M, Manson S. Influenza and penumococcal vaccination among Native American elders in a primary care practice. *Arch Intern Med.* 2000;160:1443–1448.

79. Air Quality Program. *Health Effects of Wood Smoke.* Olympia, Wash: Washington State Dept of Ecology; March 1997.

80. Honicky RE, Osborne JS III, Akpom CA. Symptoms of respiratory illness in young children and the use of wood-burning stoves for indoor heating. *Pediatrics.* 1985;75:587–593.

81. Smith KR, Samet JM, Romieu I, Bruce N. Indoor air pollution in developing countries and acute lower respiratory infections in children. *Thorax.* 2000;55:518–532.

82. US Dept of Health and Human Services. *Trends in Indian Health 1998–1999.* Rockville, Md: US Dept of Health and Human Services, Public Health Service, Indian Health Service; 1999.

83. May PA. Suicide and self-destruction among American Indian youths. *Am Indian Alaska Native Ment Health Res.* 1987;1:52–69.

84. Middlebrook DL, LeMaster PL, Beals J, Novins DK, Manson SM. Suicide prevention in American Indian and Alaskan Native communities: a cultural review of programs. *Suicide Life-Threatening Behav.* 2001;31(suppl):132–149.

85. Gillum RF, Gillum BS, Smith N. Cardiovascular risk factors among urban American Indians: blood pressure, serum lipids, smoking, diabetes, health knowledge, and behavior. *Am Heart J.* 1984;107:765–776.

86. Kimball EH, Goldberg HI, Oberle MW. The prevalence of selected risk factors for chronic disease among American Indians in Washington State. *Public Health Rep.* 1996;111:264–271.

87. Nelson DE, Moon RW, Holtzman D, Smith P, Siegel PZ. Patterns of health risk behaviors for chronic disease: a comparison between adolescent and adult American Indians living on or near reservations in Montana. *J Adolesc Health.* 1997;21:25–32.

88. Kaplan SD, Lanier AP, Merritt RK, Siegel PZ. Prevalence of tobacco use among Alaska Natives: a review. *Prev Med.* 1997;26:460–465.

89. LeMaster PL, Connell CM, Mitchell CM, Manson SM. Tobacco use among American Indian adolescents: protective and risk factors. *J Adolesc Health.* 2002;30:426–432.

90. Welty TK, Tanaka ES, Leonard B. Indian Health Service facilities become smoke-free. *MMWR Morb Mortal Wkly Rep.* 1987;36:348–350.

91. Randall LL, Welty TK, Iyasu, S, Willinger M. *I Will Never Forget My Child: Results of the Aberdeen Area Infant Mortality Study.* Rockville, Md: US Dept of Health and Human Services, Public Health Service, Indian Health Service; 1998.

92. US Dept of Health and Human Services. *Tobacco Use Among U.S. Racial/Ethnic Minority Groups—African Americans, American Indians and Alaska Natives, Asian Americans and Pacific Islanders, and Hispanics: A Report of the Surgeon General.* Atlanta, Ga: US Dept of Health and Human Services, Centers for Disease Control and Prevention, National Center for Chronic Disease Prevention and Health Promotion, Office on Smoking and Health; 1998.

93. Braveheart M, DeBruyn LM. The American Indian Holocaust: healing historical unresolved grief. *Am Indian Alaska Native Ment Health Res J Natl Center.* 1998;8:60–82.

94. Gray N. American Indian and Alaska Native substance abuse: co-morbidity and cultural issues. *Am Indian Alaska Native Ment Health Res J Natl Center.* 2001;10:67–84.

95. Walters KL, Simoni JM. Reconceptualizing Native women's health: an 'indigenist' stress-coping model. *Am J Public Health.* 2002;92:520–524.

96. Westermeyer J. Alcoholism and comorbid psychiatric disorders among American Indians. *Am Indian Alaska Native Ment Health Res J Natl Center.* 2001;10:27–50.

97. Walters KL. Substance use among American Indians and Alaska Natives: incorporating culture in an 'indigenist' stress-coping paradigm. *Public Health Rep.* 2002;177(suppl):S104–S117.

98. Schinke SP, Tepavac L, Cole KC. Preventing substance use among Native American youth: three-year results. *Addictive Behav.* 2000;25:387–397.

99. Broussard BA, Johnson A, Himes JH, et al. Prevalence of obesity in American Indians and Alaska Natives. *Am J Clin Nutr.* 1991;53:1535–1542.

100. Cook VV, Hurley JS. Prevention of type 2 diabetes in childhood. *Clin Pediatr.* 1998;37:123–129.

101. Davis CE, Hunsberger S, Murray DM, et al. Design and statistical analysis for the Pathways Study. *Am J Clin Nutr.* 1999;69(suppl):760S–763S.

102. Jackson MY. Nutrition in American Indians and Alaska Natives. *Am J Clin Nutr.* 1991;53:1535–1542.

103. Acton KJ, Burrows NR, Moore K, Querec L, Geiss LS, Engelgau MM. Trends in diabetes prevalence among American Indian and Alaska Native children, adolescents, and young adults [published erratum appears in *Am J Public Health.* 2002;92(11):1709]. *Am J Public Health.* 2002;92(9):1485–1490.

104. Centers for Disease Control and Prevention. *Intertribal Heart Project: Results from the Cardiovascular Health Survey.* Atlanta, Ga: Centers for Disease Control and Prevention; 1996.

105. Harwell TS, Ghodes D, Moore K, McDowall JM, Smilie JG. Cardiovascular disease and risk factors in Montana American Indians and non-Indians. *Am J Prev Med.* 2001;20:196–201.

106. Sugarman J, Percy C. Prevalence of diabetes in a Navajo Indian community. *Am J Public Health.* 1989;79:511–513.

107. Tuomilehto J, Lindstrom J, Eriksson JG, et al. Prevention of Type 2 diabetes mellitus by changes in lifestyle among subjects with impaired glucose tolerance. *N Engl J Med.* 2001;344:1343–1350.

108. Diabetes Prevention Program Research Group. Reduction in the incidence of type 2 diabetes with lifestyle intervention or metformin. *N Engl J Med.* 2002;393–403.

109. Broussard BA, Sugarman JR, Bachman-Carter K, et al. Toward comprehensive obesity prevention programs in Native American communities. *Obes Res.* 1995;3:289S–2897S.

110. Keppel KG, Pearcy JN, Wagener DK. Trends in racial and ethnic-specific rates for the health status indicators: United States, 1990–1998. *Healthy People Statistical Notes, No. 23.* Hyattsville, Md: National Center for Health Statistics; January 2002.

111. May PA. The health status of Indian children: problems and prevention in early life [monograph]. *Am Indian Alaska Native Ment Health Res.* 1988;1:244–289 (ADAI jl).

112. Marr C. Assimilation through education: Indian boarding schools in the Pacific Northwest [essay]. 2003.

113. Johnson KG. Strategies for prevention using allied health professionals. *Prev Med.* 1977;6:386–390.

114. Shorr G. Improving outpatient care with concurrent visit planning: a case for industrial strength triage. Rockville, Md: US Dept of Health and Human Services, Indian Health Service, Division of Health Systems Development; 2003. Unpublished draft.

115. Baines DR. Obstacles to equality: Issues for purchaser and provider. *Ethnicity and Health.* 1999;4(3):182–210.

116. Smedley BD, Stith AY, Nelson AR, eds. *Unequal Treatment: Confronting Racial and Ethnic Disparities in Health Care (2002).* Washington, DC. National Academies Press: 2003.

117. Schneider EC, Zaslavsky AM, Epstein AM. Racial disparities in the quality of care for enrollees in medicare managed care. *JAMA.* 2002:287(10):1288–1294.

118. Indian Health Service. The Native American Cardiology Program page. Available at: www.ihs.gov/MedicalPrograms/Cardiology/index.cfm. Accessed March 24, 2003.

119. Burhansstipanov L, Gilbert A, LaMarca K, Kreb LU. An innovative path to improving cancer care in Indian country. *Public Health Rep.* 2001; 116(5):424–433.

120. Mayo Foundation for Medical Education and Research. The Native CIRCLE page. Available at: www.mayo.edu/nativecircle/. Accessed March 24, 2003.

121. Indian Health Service. The Injury Prevention Program page. Available at: www.ihs.gov/MedicalPrograms/InjuryPrevention/index.cfm. Accessed March 24, 2003.

122. Indian Health Service. The American Indian and Alaska Native Immunizations Child Health page. Available at: www.ihs.gov/medicalprograms/MCH/C/CHIMO l.cfm. Accessed January 2, 2004.

123. Kramer MS, Chalmers B, Hodnett ED, et al. Promotion of breastfeeding intervention trial (PROBIT): A cluster-randomized trial in the Republic of Belarus. In: Koletzko B, Michaelsen KF, Hernell O, eds. *Short and Long Term Effects of Breast Feeding on Child Health.* New York: Kluwer Academic/Plenum Publishers; 2000;327–345.

124. US Dept of Health and Human Services. Mental Health: culture, race, ethnicity. In supplement to: *Mental Health: A Report of the Surgeon General 1999.* Rockville, Md; 2001.

125. Consortium of Social Science Associations. *Not What the Doctor Ordered—Challenges Individuals Face in Adhering to Medical Advice and Treatment, Congressional Briefing. Executive Summary* [Web site]. April 1999. Available at: www.cossa.org/docbrief.html. Accessed January 2, 2004.

RESOURCES

Suggested Readings

Aitken LP, Haller EW. *Two Cultures Meet: Pathways for American Indians to Medicine.* Duluth, Minn: University of Minnesota—Duluth; 1990.

Axtell H, Aragon M. *A Little Bit of Wisdom: Conversations With a Nez Perce Elder.* Lewiston, Idaho: Confluence Press; 1997.

Coulehan JL. Navajo Indian medicine: implication for healing. *J Fam Pract.* 1980;10:55–61.

Halfe LB. The circle: death and dying from a Native perspective. *J Palliative Care.* 1989;5:37–41.

Hammerschlag CA. *The Dancing Healers: A Doctor's Journey of Healing With Native Americans.* San Francisco, Calif: Harper & Row; 1988.

Kunitz SJ. Traditional Navajo health beliefs and practices. In: *Disease Change and the Role of Medicine: The Navajo Experience.* Berkeley, Calif: University of California Press; 1983:118–145.

Rhoades ER. *American Indian Health: Innovations in Health Care, Promotion, and Policy.* Baltimore, Md: The Johns Hopkins University Press; 2000.

Organizations and Programs

Association of American Indian Physicians, 1235 Sovereign Row, Suite 103, Oklahoma City, OK 73108.

Injury Prevention Program, Indian Health Service, Reyes Building, Suite 610, Rockville, MD 20852-1627.

Native American Cancer Research Corporation, 3022 S Nova Road, Pine, CO 80470-7830.

Native American Cardiology Program, University of Arizona, 1501 N Campbell Ave, PO Box 245037, Tucson, AZ 85724-5046.

Native CIRCLE, Department of Oncology, Mayo Clinic, 200 First St SW, Rochester, MN 55905.

PART 8

Genetics

chapter 40

The Human Genome—Present State of the Art

David B. Schowalter, MD, PhD

INTRODUCTION

The importance of the Human Genome Project to the preventive care of patients remains unclear. In 1999, *Time* magazine published a special issue on the future of medicine, in which it reported on a public opinion poll regarding predictive genetic testing. Around the same time, the American Medical Association performed a similar poll. Both polls found the same results: Most people would like to know, through genetic testing, what harmful diseases they may suffer from later in life. Yet, there are many issues to be addressed before the use of genetic information is a routine occurrence in clinical preventive practice.

The predictions regarding the future of medicine after the completion of the Human Genome Project are many.[1] For a typical family, the impact on various members may differ. For a woman, the growing understanding of the molecular basis for familial breast cancer serves as one example. Breast cancer is common in that approximately 8% of women will develop it in their lifetime. Although it is clear that various environmental factors can alter a woman's risk of breast cancer, no single risk factor seems to be more potent than a disease-causing mutation in either the BRCA-1 or BRCA-2 gene, which is associated with nearly a tenfold increase in risk. For women identified as having this mutation, an array of therapeutic options need to be discussed, including prophylactic surgeries and increased surveillance aimed at identifying disease at a curable stage.

For our children, the hope of predictive genetics is foreseen as large genetic panels that will be performed early in life to identify which common diseases may affect an individual later in life. This identification process would facilitate the development of a patient-specific, proactive health care plan tailored to the patient's needs. Perhaps medical therapies could be initiated to prevent a disease process entirely. For a number of years, states have mandated screening of infants for particular metabolic conditions in which early dietary or other intervention could avoid an undesirable outcome.

More recently, some states, such as Wisconsin, have extended this to include DNA screening for mutations that are responsible for one of the more common autosomal recessive conditions found in people of Northern European ancestry—cystic fibrosis (CF). A curative therapy for this disease does not currently exist, but aggressive medical management has greatly helped prolong a high quality of life for many people with CF. It is thus felt that the identification of newborns with this condition would provide them with similar aggressive medical management at an even earlier age, with the hope of improving development and quality of life. With the completion of the Human Genome Project in April 2003, it is anticipated that there will be an expansion in the number of these types of screening tests, not only for rare genetic diseases but also more common diseases as well.

Many people believe that the initial benefits from the completion of the Human Genome Project will come in the area of pharmacogenetics. *Pharmacogenetics* is defined as the study of pharmacologic responses and their modification by hereditary influences. All family members could reap the rewards for more appropriate and safer use of medications. Adverse drug reactions, estimated to be the fourth to sixth leading cause of death,[2] have been an important national issue. Efforts to eliminate most of these adverse reactions would be welcomed by all. Given the characterization of an individual's particular drug absorption, metabolism, and processing systems, medications may be used that display the highest efficacy and least likelihood for a life-threatening adverse reaction.

An example of this is the gene for thiopurine methyltransferase (TPMT), an enzyme involved in the phase 2 metabolism of 6-mercaptopurine (6-MP) and azathioprine. Particular alterations in this gene have been identified, which result in a wide variability among individual clearance of these medications. Although most of the population has a high rate of metabolism, approximately 1 in 20 people may have 2 copies of the gene, which functions less efficiently. Administration of 6-MP in standard doses to an individual with 2 copies of the lower functioning TPMT gene could result in toxic and life-threatening serum levels of the medication. Clarification of an individual's genotype before starting chemotherapy with 6-MP for childhood acute leukemia allows for adjustment of doses and better cure rates.[3]

The future use of genetic testing to help care for our patients in a more personalized fashion is a worthy and, in some sense, an already realized outcome of the Human Genome Project. The completion of the Human Genome Project is expected to lead to a rapid expansion in the number of predictive genetic tests that are available for use in clinical practice. To better understand the basis for this revolution and its limitations, we first need to understand the genome and how it functions.

THE GENOME

In this section, a brief review of several basic genetic concepts is presented to help readers better understand some of the issues associated with genetic testing. A number of outstanding books are available for readers to pursue the details of molecular biology and genomics.[4,5] *Genetics* is the study of heredity and variation in all living things. *Medical genetics* is the study of human genetic variation that is relevant to the practice of medicine. *Genomics* is the study of the *genome,* the genetic material that makes up a species, its organization, and its function.

The human genome sequence is now completed according to the National Institutes of Health genome Web site.[6] The product of the Human Genome Project is the sequence of the human haploid genome that is estimated to be approximately 3 billion nucleotides or base pairs (bp) in length. Nucleotides are composed of a ribose sugar, a phosphate group, and a purine or pyrimidine base attached to the sugar group. The nucleotides not only are responsible for the structure of DNA but also encode all the molecules required to make a human. The 4 different types of nucleotides that compose DNA are adenine, guanine, thymine, and cytosine and are abbreviated A, G, T, and C, respectively. The alternating sugar and phosphate molecules are covalently attached and form the backbone for each half of the DNA structure. The bases face the interior of the molecule and pair together with weaker hydrogen bonds in a particular way: A with T and G with C. It was Watson and Crick[7] in 1953 who used the available X-ray crystal data to propose the double helix as the structure for the DNA molecule.

Figure 40-1 shows a portion of the human genome from the short arm of chromosome 11, which contains the gene for hemoglobin-β. This portion and the approximately 2 million other fragments that together make up the human genome are the result of the Human Genome Project. If the regions of DNA that encode the hemoglobin-β protein were not underlined, it would be quite difficult to find them by inspection. It is the ability of human cell machinery to identify the necessary regions

of DNA to make a particular cell function that is outlined in the central dogma of molecular biology.

THE CENTRAL DOGMA

If each cell of the human body contains the same DNA in the nucleus, what is the basis for the difference among all the cells that make it up? The answer lies in the combination of genes expressed and proteins produced, which provide a cell with the tools needed to perform a particular function. For example, a skin cell produces many different types of collagen that, together with other connective tissue molecules, provides the barrier we need from the environment around us. A liver cell does not produce the same amount or type of collagen but does produce many different enzymes important in the processing of many different compounds into forms that can be used for energy production or energy storage. The collection of expressed mRNA molecules that encode a particular set of proteins serves to give a cell a particular function. The collection of RNA molecules found in a particular cell type is referred to as the *transcriptome.* Similarly, the collection of proteins produced in a particular cell is referred to as the *proteome.* Given the many tissues that make up a human, there are many different transcriptomes and proteomes. The study of these varied transcriptomes and proteomes is known as *transcriptomics* and *proteomics,* respectively.

Comparison of expression profiles from 2 different tissues using high-density array technologies, which can assess the levels of thousands of different genes at a time, is a growing approach used to identify therapeutic targets for many diseases. With the completion of the Human Genome Project, the identification of the gene expression profiles for all tissues will likely follow. This will lead to the identification of tissue-specific gene regulators, important targets for new therapeutics, and markers that can help classify diseases.

The central dogma of molecular biology outlines the fundamental processes for protein production. RNA molecules are first transcribed from the nuclear DNA and then processed and transported to the cytoplasm from the nucleus of the cell. In the cytoplasm, the messenger RNA (mRNA) is translated into a protein by the ribosome complex. The area of the genome that encodes a particular cellular function is called a *gene.* Some genes for specialized RNA molecules are less than 100 nucleotides in length, while others span more than 1 million bp. Current estimates suggest that the human genome encodes around 30,000 genes. The "average" gene is 27,000 bp in length.

In Fig 40-2 is a schematic diagram of the central dogma, which outlines the production of 1 protein from a gene. RNA polymerase is the nuclear protein that recognizes a particular stretch of DNA and transcribes the DNA sequence into a single RNA message. The specific region of a gene that is recognized by the RNA polymerase is

```
   1 ccctgtggag ccacaccta gggttggcca atctactccc aggagcaggg agggcaggag
  61 ccagggctgg gcataaaagt cagggcagag ccatctattg cttacatttg cttctgacac
 121 aactgtgttc actagcaacc tcaaacagac acc[atg]gtgc acctgactcc tgaggagaag
 181 tctgccgtta ctgccctgtg gggcaaggtg aacgtggatg aagttggtgg tgaggccctg
 241 ggcaggttgg tatcaaggtt acaagacagg tttaaggaga ccaatagaaa ctgggcatgt
 301 ggagacagag aagactcttg ggtttctgat aggcactgac tctctctgcc tattggtcta
 361 ttttcccacc cttaggctgc tggtggtcta cccttggacc cagaggttct ttgagtcctt
 421 tgggatctg tccactcctg atgctgttat gggcaaccct aaggtgaagg ctcatggcaa
 481 gaaagtgctc ggtgccttta gtgatggcct ggctcacctg gacaacctca agggcacctt
 541 tgccacactg agtgagctgc actgtgacaa gctgcacgtg gatcctgaga acttcagggt
 601 gagtctatgg gacccttgat gttttctttc cccttctttt ctatggttaa gttcatgtca
 661 taggaagggg agaagtaaca gggtacagtt tagaatggga aacagacgaa tgattgcatc
 721 agtgtggaag tctcaggatc gtttttagttt cttttatttg ctgttcataa caattgtttt
 781 cttttgttta attcttgctt tctttttttt tcttctccgc aatttttact attatactta
 841 atgccttaac attgtgtata acaaaaggaa atatctctga gatacattaa gtaacttaaa
 901 aaaaaacttt acacagtctg cctagtacat tactatttgg aatatatgtg tgcttatttg
 961 catattcata atctccctac tttattttct tttattttta attgatacat aatcattata
1021 catatttatg ggttaaagtg taatgtttta atatgtgtac acatattgac caaatcaggg
1081 taattttgca tttgtaattt taaaaaatgc tttcttcttt taatatactt ttttgtttat
1141 cttatttcta atactttccc taatctcttt ctttcagggc aataatgata caatgtatca
1201 tgcctctttg caccattcta aagaataaca gtgataattt ctgggttaag gcaatagcaa
1261 tatttctgca tataaatatt tctgcatata aattgtaact gatgtaagag gtttcatatt
1321 gctaatagca gctacaatcc agctaccatt ctgcttttat tttatggttg ggataaggct
1381 ggattattct gagtccaagc taggcccttt tgctaatcat gttcatacct cttatcttcc
1441 tcccacagct cctgggcaac gtgctggtct gtgtgctggc ccatcacttt ggcaaagaat
1501 tcaccccacc agtgcaggct gcctatcaga aagtggtggc tggtgtggct aatgccctgg
1561 cccacaagta tcac[taa]gct cgctttcttg ctgtccaatt tctattaaag gttcctttgt
1621 tccctaagtc caactactaa actggggggat attatgaagg gccttgagca tctggattct
1681 gcctaataaa aaacatttat tttcattgca atgatgtatt taaattattt ctgaatattt
1741 tactaaaaag ggaatgtggg aggtcagtgc atttaaaaca taaagaaatg atgagctgtt
1801 caaaccttgg gaaaatacac tatatcttaa actccatgaa agaaggtgag gctgcaacca
1861 gctaatgcac attggcaaca gcccctgatg cctatgcctt attcatccct cagaaaagga
1921 ttcttgtaga ggcttgattt gcaggttaaa gttttgctat gctgtatttt acattactta
1981 ttgttttagc tgtcctcatg aatgtctttt cactacccat ttgcttatcc tgcatctctc
2041 tcagccttga ct
```

F I G U R E 40-1

Shown is DNA sequence from the short arm of chromosome 11 that encodes the human hemoglobin beta gene that represents 0.00006% of the total human genome. The three sequence sections are the three coding regions (exons) of the gene. The "atg" start site of translation and "taa" stop signal for translation are boxed. The other segments are important in "splicing out" the segments between the exons known as introns.

called the *promoter.* Promoters have some features that are common to other promoters, as well as many unique features. Intricate cell "signals" can interact with the promoter region to alter the expression of a gene, including enhancers, silencers, and numerous regulatory proteins.

After the transcription of the RNA in the nucleus, the transcript is then processed into an mRNA molecule by the removal of all intervening (intronic) sequences and transport to the cytoplasm. In the cytoplasm, the ribosome complex recognizes a portion of the mRNA as the translation start site. The particular order of incorporation of the 20 different amino acids is translated from the mRNA using a code of 3 nucleotides for each amino acid. This triplet code is recognized by a specific transfer RNA (tRNA) molecule that has a specific amino acid attached to it. In a stepwise fashion, the translation of the mRNA continues until a stop codon (particular triplet sequence) is encountered. Once a protein is completely synthesized, there are a number of post-translational modifications that may or may not occur. The first stretch of amino acids is often also a leader signal, which directs the protein to a particular subcellular location.

The derivative studies of transcriptomics and proteomics will be important ongoing programs well beyond the Human Genome Project. Unlike genomics, the information from these studies will most likely be tissue specific and will help with disease diagnosis, but will be less helpful in the prediction of diseases that patients may develop.

GENETIC VARIATION: DETECTION AND DISEASE

All of us display a remarkable degree of variation in the way we appear, our response to medications, and the

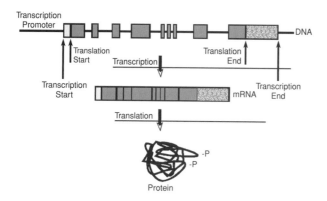

FIGURE 40-2

Shown is a "typical" human gene and the two steps of the central dogma, transcription and translation. The black boxes represent the nine exons of the gene separated by 8 introns of varying length. The left and right grey regions represent the 5 prime and 3 prime untranslated regions of the RNA molecules, respectively. Just ahead of the transcription start is the promoter region of the gene, which is important in initiating the transcription of RNA for this gene. The molecule below the upper open arrow represents the processed mRNA molecule in the cytoplasm where translation can take place to produce the particular protein. -P represents two phosphorylated sites of the protein, one example of post-translational modifications.

diseases we acquire. It is estimated that in every 300 to 500 nucleotides, we have a variance from the "normal" or predominant DNA sequence. Thus, approximately 10 million alterations may exist in the 3 billion bp of human DNA. Given that less than 1% of DNA actually encodes the proteins necessary for life, most of these changes may not alter protein structure or expression. All genetic variation originates from a process known as mutation, which means change in DNA sequence. These alterations can occur in somatic cells or in germline cells. Somatic cell mutation accumulation over time is thought to be an important mechanism leading to the formation of cancer. Mutations in human germlines (eggs or sperm) are transmitted mutations from one generation to the next and can be either silent or the basis of disease. The differentiation of disease-causing mutations from harmless sequence alterations is an important process that needs to be understood before meaningful predictions can be made from DNA alterations identified by genomic testing.

Some of the earliest recognized genomic alterations were variations in chromosome number and content. The ability to visualize chromosomes isolated and stained from white blood cells has progressed over the last 30 years. Figure 40-3 shows a white blood cell karyotype from a girl with Down syndrome showing the 2 X chromosomes and the extra chromosome 21. The inclusion of an extra chromosome 18 or 13 may also result in the birth of a child with distinctive features of a particular syn-

drome such as Edward or Patau syndrome. The deletion of regions of particular chromosomes such as 22q, 17p, and 5p results in other well-described medical conditions known as, respectively, velocardiofacial syndrome (or DiGeorge syndrome), William syndrome, and cri du chat syndrome. Tremendous strides in the ability to identify submicroscopic DNA alterations has occurred with the use of fluorescent-labeled DNA probes that have a binding specificity for 1 region of DNA in fluorescent in situ hybridization (FISH) studies. Using FISH techniques, we can rapidly identify submicroscopic DNA alterations. For example, the use of FISH probes specific for the telomeres (ends) of each chromosome has allowed us to identify alterations that are responsible for developmental delays in up to 5% of children who previously did not have a known cause of their developmental delays.

With the development of the tools to directly analyze DNA using polymerase chain reaction and DNA sequencing, it has become clear that there are many genomic variations in human DNA. Traditionally, the molecular consequences of a single nucleotide alteration have been classified according to the effect it has on gene expression. If the changed nucleotide alters the sequence such that a different amino acid is incorporated into a growing polypeptide, several outcomes are possible. Often, the amino acid substitution is "tolerated" by a protein, but other times it can completely inactivate the function of a protein. In addition, a single nucleotide change in a promoter region of a gene could result in diminished transcription and loss of gene expression from 1 allele. Single nucleotide changes in other noncoding regions can also decrease the stability of an mRNA transcript or the efficiency of its translation. The redundancy of the genetic code does allow for some genomic alterations to be "tolerated" in that the new recognition codon might also code for the same amino acid. Finally, a sequence alteration could create an internal ribosomal stop codon that would result in the production of a shortened protein product that may not function appropriately. All these possible outcomes from a single nucleotide alteration present a daunting task in developing an understanding of the effect that the millions of known single nucleotide polymorphisms contained in human genomes have on our health.

SNP are a subset of single nucleotide alterations that have been identified in people. This implies that all the serious single nucleotide alterations that are not compatible with life are not included in the millions of SNP, which are listed as part of the SNP consortium. Many different technologies, beyond the scope of this discussion, are being developed in hopes of bringing the ability to identify a particular SNP with clinical significance to the physician. The ability to assay thousands of SNP in a single test is used in the research community and will likely be available to the medical community soon—that

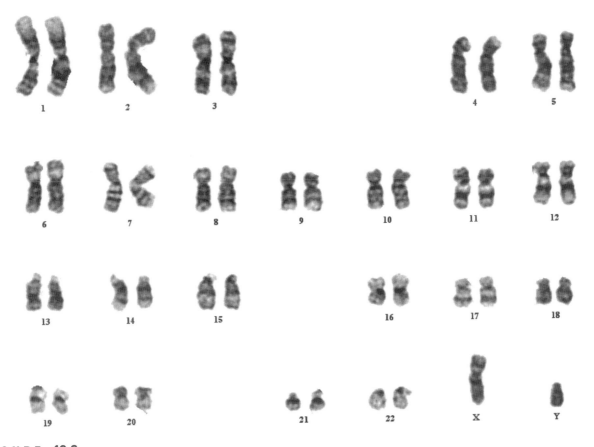

FIGURE 40-3

White blood cell karyotype from girl with Down syndrome.

is, as soon as we can accurately predict the outcomes that a particular SNP may have for patients.

In addition to single nucleotide alterations, insertion and deletion of nucleotides is another mechanism for DNA alteration. In reviewing chromosome alterations, mobile DNA elements known as *transposons* have been identified in the noncoding DNA from many species, including humans. The function of these mobile elements is somewhat unclear, but they obviously played an important role in the evolutionary process. Currently, the use of these mobile elements is being evaluated as a tool for use in gene therapy systems to correct the loss of gene function.[8]

Finally, *minisatellites* and *microsatellites* are regions of the DNA in which the same sequence of DNA is repeated over and over again in tandem. The function of these sequence alterations is often unknown. The utility of these alterations has been the ability to mark genomic regions and follow their inheritance through a family. Using a particular statistical process known as linkage analysis, the region or regions of the genome shared by only the people with a particular condition from a collection of families can be identified. Further analysis of these shared regions can lead to the identification of candidate genes, which are then evaluated for specific causative mutations in people

with the disease. This process originally took many years in that extensive sequencing of a particular region of the genome had to be done first. With the Human Genome Project completed this will no longer be necessary and disease gene identification should be more accelerated.

PUTTING IT ALL INTO PRACTICE

The power of genomic testing is clear. For some diseases, genetic tests are already a part of clinical practice in the verification of a suspected clinical diagnosis. In this situation, a paucity of pretest counseling is usually the norm, in that a discussion regarding the suspected disease process has already occurred, including the risks to others in the family. The use of genetic testing to predict diseases a person might develop in the future has received much media coverage and is currently available for a number of conditions. The use of these predictive tests has been a part of medical genetic practice for a number of years and has led to the identification of several important issues in the application of these tests.

One important issue in accurate predictive testing is knowing that the test result can identify the disease in the family, as outlined in the following clinical case study.

CASE STUDY

A young woman has come to your office for presymptomatic testing of Huntington Disease (HD), a degenerative neurologic disorder involving chorea, dementia, and psychiatric disease. The particular gene alteration for HD is well described, and testing is very sensitive and specific. The diagnosis for this disease was made in your patient's paternal uncle at a reputable medical institution and was confirmed on brain autopsy. Your patient's father and older brother died of a similar disease involving a severe movement disorder and dementia with the exception that the patient's brother had vision loss early in the disease course. The patient had heard through the news media that HD gene testing was clinically available and wanted to have this test performed to clarify her life plan, given her 50% risk of inheriting this autosomal dominant disease from her father.

After an extensive genetic counseling session, she agreed to hold off on testing until a DNA sample could be obtained from banked tissue from her affected brother. Testing of this DNA showed that he did not have HD. Additional testing of the DNA from the same brother identified a spinocerebellar ataxia (SCA7) gene alteration. If the patient's older brother had not been tested, a negative (normal) HD test result for your patient would have provided a false sense of comfort, because the disease in the patient's immediate family was not HD. This clinical case demonstrates the concept of genetic heterogeneity; a single phenotype is the result of alterations in different genes. Clearly, one needs to be sure of the genetic basis for the disease in the family for accurate predictive genetic testing.

Genetic heterogeneity is not only seen for rare neurologic diseases as discussed in the case study, but even more so in common diseases such as hypertension and cancer. Most common diseases are multifactorial in nature, in that multiple genes and environmental exposures can contribute to the development of a disease in a person. As mentioned earlier, predictive testing to clarify a person's risk of breast and ovarian cancer, a current clinical practice, demonstrates the use of predictive testing for a common multifactorial disease. This brings up another important issue. Many women (and men) would like to know if they are at an increased risk of cancer if they have a mother, maternal aunt, and sibling with breast or ovarian cancer, or both. If testing is performed on this at-risk family member first, a positive, or abnormal, test result (identification of a disease-causing alteration) does indicate that this person is at a significantly increased risk of the development of breast or ovarian cancer. Counseling regarding risk to other family members and for prophylactic measures can be instituted. Unfortunately, if the test result is negative, or normal (a disease-causing alteration

was not identified), there is again a false sense of security in that we do not know for sure the cause of the disease in the rest of the family. For this reason, in many cases, it is important to try to test an affected individual first to ascertain if the test can identify the basis for the disease in the family. If the genetic alteration of the disease in the family is known through previous testing, then "at risk" family members with negative test results can be reassured that their risk of disease (in this case breast or ovarian cancer) is reduced to that of the general population.

It is not uncommon to hear from patients in this clinical situation that they were unaware that storing DNA (DNA banking) is clinically available. Given the good probability that many more tests for common diseases will be developed over the next 5 to 10 years, it would be reasonable to talk to almost all patients about the possibility of DNA banking. The amount and quality of stored DNA is important. The small amounts of DNA that can be isolated from a cheek swab or toothbrush will most likely not be sufficient to perform the necessary testing for common disease prediction but can be helpful for identification purposes using informative microsatellite studies. In the back of various popular journals, there are offers for banking DNA and enclosing it in glass jewelry. Unfortunately, these small samples may not be of sufficient amount or quality for use in predictive genetic testing.

Additional factors hinder the ability to accurately predict the clinical outcome of a particular genetic change. One important issue in this regard is disease penetrance. Hemochromatosis is an iron storage disorder that is caused by several common alterations in the HFE gene. After this discovery, discussions of population screening started because regular phlebotomy can greatly alter the disease course and prevent many of the late complications (ie, liver failure) and it was believed that the majority of people with the most common mutations would develop the condition. Recent studies in large populations have determined that actually less than half of the people with the most common HFE gene alterations eventually get the disease. Given this low level of disease penetrance, discussion of population screening stopped due to the inability to accurately predict which persons with the identified gene alteration would progress to development of the disease. Over time, the other genes that influence the development of hemochromatosis will also be identified and may make this type of predictive genetic testing possible. Many additional studies that test large populations for particular genetic alterations and correlate these findings with clinical disease will facilitate a more rapid development of meaningful genetic tests.

The issue of testing in minors is an important topic to briefly discuss. The author has seen several families referred to medical genetics for counseling because factor V Leiden mutations were identified in some of their children. Often, the parent had recurrent thrombosis and in further evaluations to identify a cause was found to have a factor V mutation. With the knowledge that each child is at a 50% risk of inheriting this mutation from a parent, testing of all children was performed. Although an argument can be made that, before offering young women birth control, it would be important to know if they had this genetic predisposition for thrombosis, predictive testing for adult-onset disease generally is deferred until the child reaches adult age. Predictive testing is offered when interventions are known to be of benefit to the child. One example of this is the identification of children with gene alterations that predispose to multiple endocrine neoplasia type 2 (MEN2B) in which life-saving thyroidectomies need to be performed in very young children.

Finally, pretest counseling needs to include a discussion of all possible test results, especially the possibility of results of unclear significance. The risk to other family members needs to be addressed, as well as a review of the psychosocial impact the test results may have on the patient, and the patient's employer and insurance carrier. It is clear from extensive use of predictive genetic testing in the practice of medical genetics that much benefit to families with both common and rare diseases has resulted from the information. The rapid expansion of test availability is going to challenge us to continue to use this information in a way that is helpful and not harmful for patients.

SUMMARY

The future impact that the Human Genome Project and its derivative sciences will have on patients is going to be enormous. As more and more genetic tests become available, their use as predictive tests will continue to expand.

The following list summarizes the major issues emphasized in this chapter and gives tips for genetic testing:

- If a patient does not have disease signs or symptoms, allow extra time for predictive test counseling, including familial implications and impact on self, insurability, and employment.
- Always discuss the implications of all possible test results, including that some identified alterations may be of unclear significance.
- If unable to provide appropriate pretest counseling, consider a referral to a medical genetics specialist.
- Presymptomatic testing in minors is usually deferred until the child is an adult unless life-saving interventions are necessary.
- Remember to test an affected member first (if possible) so as to ascertain that the family disease is identified with the test.
- Positive (abnormal) test results do not accurately predict disease course in many cases (ie, variable penetrance and modifier genes).
- Consider talking to your patients about DNA banking to provide a resource for their children and grandchildren.
- A negative (normal) test result does not always mean the patient is not at risk of the disease; it means the patient is at the population risk of the condition.

With thoughtful use of genetic testing, you will provide your patients with much-sought-after information that will change their lives and potentially allow you to tailor a much more personalized preventive medicine program in a more cost-effective manner.

REFERENCES

1. Collins FS. Shattuck lecture—medical and societal consequences of the Human Genome Project. *N Engl J Med.* 1999;341:28–37.

2. Lazarou J, Pomeranz BH, Corey PN. Incidence of adverse drug reactions in hospitalized patients: a meta-analysis of prospective studies. *JAMA.* 1998;279:1200–1205.

3. Weinshilboum RM, Otterness DM, Szumlanski CL. Methylation pharmacogenetics: catechol O-methyltransferase, thiopurine methyltransferase, and histamine N-methyltransferase. *Annu Rev Pharmacol Toxicol.* 1999;39:19–52.

4. Thompson MW, McInnes RR, Willard HR. *Thompson & Thompson Genetics in Medicine.* 5th ed. Philadelphia, Pa: WB Saunders Co; 1996.

5. Gelehrter TD, Collins FS, Ginsburg D. *Principles of Medical Genetics.* 2nd ed. Baltimore, Md: Williams & Wilkins; 1998.

6. National Center for Biotechnology Information, National Library of Medicine, National Institutes of Health. Genome sequencing. Available at: www.ncbi.nlm.nih.gov/genome/seq/HsHome.shtml. Accessed August 28, 2003.

7. Watson JD, Crick FHC. Molecular structure of nucleic acids. *Nature.* 1953;171:737–738.

8. Yant SR, Ehrhardt A, Mikkelsen JG, et al. Transposition from a gutless adenotransposition vector stabilizes transgene expression in vivo. *Nature Biotechnol.* 2002;20:999–1005.

RESOURCES

Gelehrter TD, Collins FS, Ginsburg D. *Principles of Medical Genetics.* 2nd ed. Baltimore, Md: Williams and Wilkins; 1998.

Jorde LB, Corey JC, Bamshad MJ, White RL. *Medical Genetics.* St. Louis, Mo: Mosby; 2003.

Thompson MW, McInnes RR, Willard HF. *Thompson & Thompson Genetics in Medicine.* 6th ed. Philadelphia, Pa: Saunders; 2001.

National Center for Biotechnology Information. Available at: www.ncbi.nlm.nih.gov/About/index.html.

chapter 41

Integrating Genetic History into Preventive Care

Howard M. Saal, MD

INTRODUCTION

As most physicians learned during medical training, the key to making a diagnosis is at least 80% dependent on information gained in the medical history. Individual and family medical histories take on greater importance in the diagnosis and management of genetic disorders. With the advances in genomics, the genetic links to common disease have become increasingly evident. There has been a remarkable increase in the identification of conditions for which there is a known genetic predisposition in the absence of signs and symptoms. These include many hereditary cancers, hypertension, renal disease, bleeding disorders, and neurodegenerative disorders. Of the 10 leading causes of death in the United States (Table 41-1), genetic factors play a role in most of them except for, perhaps, unintentional injury and pneumonia/influenza. Even for these disorders, one can identify potential genetic issues such as alcoholism, depression, and bipolar illness for unintentional injury, and neurodegenerative disorders for pneumonia and influenza (eg, living in a chronic care facility). It is clear that genetic factors play an important role in the development of common diseases by influencing etiology, natural history, and response to therapy.

There are often subtle clues in the medical history, which, when identified, play important roles in leading to the appropriate diagnosis. Such data include pregnancy loss, fertility, ethnicity, race, age at death, response to specific medications, and learning problems. Similar information is also available from the family history.

There are many single gene disorders that are important causes of disease. Individually, these genetic disorders are infrequent, but when combined they cause a formidable number of disease conditions. On the other hand, common diseases are defined as being present in greater than 1 in 1000 individuals in the population.[1] Most research into common diseases in the past has focused on identification of environmental factors, including diet, tobacco use, activity levels, alcohol, and infectious agents. Because of the Human Genome Project, a great deal of attention has been given to the interaction of genetic and environmental factors as causes of morbidity and mortality. It is becoming more apparent that many common diseases are multifactorial (ie, caused by the interaction of several genes and environmental factors). Information about genes that predispose to certain disorders related to environmental factors is emerging. For many individuals much information about disease predisposition exists in the medical and family history and is readily available as long as the right questions are asked and appropriate data are obtained.

With increasing identification of heredity as an important factor in the etiology of disease, the model of medical management will have to undergo certain changes. Because hereditary factors have been characterized that identify a predisposition to disease and morbid conditions, physicians will have to focus less on disease and acute management and more on prevention and counseling.

TABLE 41-1

Ten Leading Causes of Death in the United States in 2001*

Causes	No. (%) of Deaths
Heart disease	700,142 (29.0)
Cancer	553,768 (22.9)
Stroke	163,538 (6.8)
Chronic lower respiratory tract disease	123,013 (5.1)
Accidents	101,537 (4.2)
Diabetes	71,372 (3.0)
Pneumonia/influenza	62,034 (2.6)
Alzheimer disease	53,852 (2.2)
Nephritis, nephritic syndrome, and nephrosis	39,480 (1.6)
Septicemia	32,238 (1.3)

*From Centers for Disease Control and Prevention, National Center for Health Statistics, Web site. Available at: www.cdc.gov/nchs. Accessed 12/14/03.

Also, the focus on the individual patient in the traditional medical model will have to change to encompass the family as we incorporate more genetic information.

DEFINITIONS AND BACKGROUND

It is estimated that the human genome contains 30,000 genes.[2] More than 1000 genes have been implicated in disease processes,[3] and clinical and research testing is available for almost 1000 genetic disorders.[4] It is likely that not all 30,000 genes will be found to be associated with human disease, since the functions of many of these genes is so fundamental to normal development that mutations will likely result in early miscarriage or failure to implant.

All genes are paired, except for those on the sex chromosomes in males, with males having only 1 X and 1 Y chromosome and, therefore, only 1 copy of the genes on the X and Y chromosomes. Females have 2 copies of the X chromosome. *Genotype* refers to the entire genetic information of an organism or individual. It can also refer to the specific genetic information at a single gene locus. *Phenotype* refers to an organism's specific clinical features, as influenced by the genotype.

As noted previously, most individuals with genetic disorders have a multifactorial disorder, such that morbidity or disease is caused by the interaction of several genes with environmental factors. However, thousands of single gene disorders have been recognized. A *single gene* disorder refers to a disorder that is caused by mutations at a single gene locus. Information for these disorders can be accessed through Online Mendelian Inheritance in Man.[3]

Autosomal dominant disorders are the most common single gene disorders. These conditions occur when an individual inherits a gene for a disorder from a parent. An individual who has an autosomal dominant condition has a 50% chance of having a child with the same genetic condition with each pregnancy. A family history will show that there are affected individuals with a specified disorder in consecutive generations. Male-to-male transmission of genetic disorders confirms that a disorder is autosomal dominant and not X-linked dominant, since males cannot transmit their X chromosome to their sons. It is common to have an autosomal dominant disorder without a family history. This is because many autosomal dominant disorders have a high mutation rate. For example, neurofibromatosis type 1 is a common autosomal disorder with an incidence of 1 in 3000 live births. In approximately 50% of cases, there is no family history.[5] Those individuals with no family history have a new mutation of the neurofibromin gene that causes neurofibromatosis type 1. Similarly, approximately 50% of individuals with Marfan syndrome have new mutations.

Autosomal dominant disorders often affect more than 1 organ system or may have more than 1 physical presentation, a phenomenon called *pleiotropy*. An example of this would be Marfan syndrome, in which an individual may present with ocular findings (eg, myopia, dislocated lenses), cardiovascular findings (mitral valve prolapse, aortic root dilatation), or skeletal findings (arachnodactyly, scoliosis).[6] Autosomal dominant disorders also demonstrate *variable expressivity*. For example, some individuals with tuberous sclerosis complex may present with brain hamartomas, seizures, enamel pits, hypopigmented patches, and shagreen patches, whereas other individuals with the same disorder may present only with hypopigmented patches or other minor manifestations.[7] *Penetrance* is the percentage of individuals with a certain genotype who show any signs or symptoms of the specific disorder. The penetrance of a BRCA-1 and BRCA-2 gene mutation causing either breast cancer or ovarian cancer or both is 50% to 85%.[8,9] Therefore, 20% to 40% of individuals with BRCA-1 or BRCA-2 gene mutations will not have breast or ovarian (or related) cancers develop and will be nonpenetrant carriers.

Autosomal recessive disorders occur less frequently than do autosomal dominant disorders. Since all autosomal genes are paired, if there are mutations of both members of a pair of genes at a single locus, that individual will have an autosomal recessive disorder. This implies that an individual who has a mutation of only 1 of the paired genes is phenotypically normal, and this individual is termed a *carrier*. When 2 carriers for a mutation at the same locus have children, their risk of having an affected child with an autosomal recessive condition is 1 in 4 (25%) for each pregnancy.

X-linked disorders are those conditions for which the causative gene is located on the X chromosome. Most X-linked disorders, such as hemophilia and Duchenne muscular dystrophy are X-linked recessive. Carrier females are expected to have a normal phenotype since they have 2 X chromosomes and, therefore, 1 normal gene and 1 mutated gene. Affected males, on the other hand, have only 1 X chromosome and are unable to make any normal gene product. Some disorders are X-linked dominant, and both males and females are affected. An example of an X-linked dominant disorder is amelogenesis imperfecta, in which affected individuals do not make normal tooth enamel. The clue to X-linked dominant inheritance is that there is no male-to-male transmission, and all daughters of affected males are affected.

Sex-limited disorders are those conditions that are not X-linked; rather, they are autosomal dominant or autosomal recessive disorders that are more likely seen in 1 sex because of an underlying phenotype related to sex. For example, hereditary hemochromatosis is an autosomal recessive disorder that tends to affect men much more frequently than females, mainly because females menstruate and decrease their iron load on a regular basis.

Genetic heterogeneity refers to the fact that a similar phenotype can be seen in 2 unrelated individuals and can be caused by a different gene in each. An example of genetic heterogeneity is Usher syndrome. This autosomal recessive disorder causes both sensorineural deafness and a pigmentary retinopathy that leads to blindness. At least 6 different genes (gene loci) have been identified that can cause this disorder.[10] One lesson learned from genetic heterogeneity is that a normal genetic test result for a specific disorder may be valid, but this does not exclude the diagnosis and other family members may still be at risk. Often, further testing is indicated, but unfortunately testing for all genetic disorders is not available. This implies that a thorough medical history, family history, and physical examination remain essential in the management of individuals who are at risk of common or rare genetic disorders.

Genetic anticipation is a phenomenon in which earlier onset or more severe phenotypes or both are seen in successive generations.[11] This is most common in autosomal dominant and X-linked disorders. Anticipation is most often associated with disorders in which genetic changes in zygotes are possible, usually related to conditions mediated by expansion of trinucleotide repeats.

FAMILY HISTORY

Genetic disorders may present at any point in life. For this reason, it is often helpful to know an individual's predisposition to a specific disorder. Although screening and diagnostic tests are available for a wide array of disorders, such tests may be more specific and sensitive when performed in individuals who are at high risk. The family history and pedigree are powerful tools for identifying familial genetic disorders and individuals within a family who are at risk of these disorders. In addition, by having knowledge of inheritance patterns, it is possible to determine individuals in a pedigree who are not at risk of a specific disorder. An example of this would be a man whose maternal uncle has hemophilia A (factor VIII deficiency). Clearly, if this man is unaffected, neither he nor his children would be at risk of having this disorder.

The pedigree is extremely useful for identifying inheritance patterns. In a pedigree, males are signified by squares and females, by circles. Pregnancies are designated by diamonds, and miscarriages are designated by small triangles. An arrow is used to designate the proband (patient). The object is to obtain at least 3, and hopefully 4, generations of family history. It is most important to identify health issues in closely related individuals, especially parents, siblings, aunts, uncles, and grandparents. Health and medical information about more distantly related individuals may also be helpful, particularly when a practitioner suspects autosomal dominant disorders or, in the case of consanguinity, rare conditions.

By understanding inheritance patterns, one can identify risks for certain conditions as well as risks for recurrence. As noted, in autosomal dominant conditions one will see

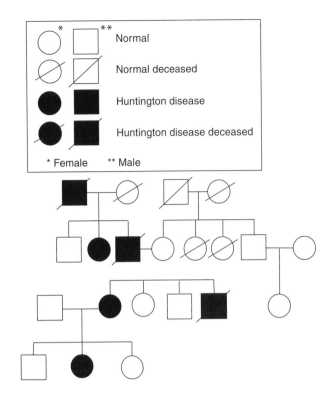

FIGURE 41-1

A pedigree of a family with Huntington disease. Note that there are several consecutive generations affected and male-to-male transmission, consistent with autosomal dominant inheritance.

consecutively affected generations within a family and male-to-male transmission (Fig 41-1). In newly affected individuals with an autosomal dominant condition, a single affected individual will be present in the pedigree (Fig 41-2). Usually, autosomal recessive disorders are seen in a single generation and limited to siblings. Autosomal recessive disorders are seen more frequently in the case of consanguinity, when related individuals have children. They have more genes in common (including genes with pathologic mutations) because they share common ancestors (Fig 41-3).

Autosomal recessive disorders are also more common in the case of genetic isolates, often because of geographic or cultural isolation (Table 41-2). For example, the incidence of congenital adrenal hyperplasia (21-hydroxylase deficiency) is very high in the Inuit population.[12] Some autosomal recessive conditions are relatively common, such as cystic fibrosis in whites and sickle cell anemia in Africans and African Americans. In some of these conditions, despite the morbidity associated with the homozygous state, evolution has conferred disease protection on heterozygotes (carriers of a single mutant gene). Sickle cell anemia and thalassemia heterozygotes have some protection against contracting malaria.[13,14]

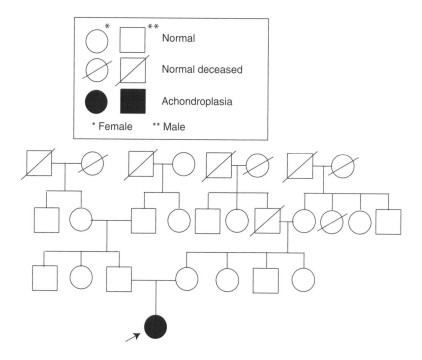

A pedigree of a family with a single affected child with achondroplasia. Although one cannot interpret the inheritance pattern from this pedigree, achondroplasia is a well-documented autosomal dominantly inherited disorder and, therefore, this child has a new mutation for this disorder. Knowledge of the diagnosis and inheritance pattern will be very helpful when counseling the parents about recurrence risks.

Some autosomal recessive disorders are so common that they actually may appear in successive generations, giving the appearance of being autosomal dominant. This type of inheritance is called pseudodominant inheritance. For example, the carrier frequency of hereditary hemochromatosis is approximately 1 in 11, with 1 in 200 to 1 in 400 whites in the general population being affected. The onset of this disorder is more frequent in men between the ages of 40 and 60 years. Therefore, it would not be a rare event for an affected male or female to have an affected child, since the likelihood that their spouse would be a gene carrier is close to 10%.

As has been reviewed, most X-linked disorders are recessively inherited and, therefore, affect predominantly males. Because female gene carriers are usually unaffected or minimally affected, they are often not identified unless there is a family history of the condition (Fig 41-4). X-linked recessive disorders may give the appearance of skipping generations, since there may not be an affected male in a generation, despite the presence of carrier females.

In addition to identifying specific disorders and disease entities in a pedigree, a comprehensive family history can help with identification of other patterns of anomalies and family conditions. A strong family history of infertility or recurrent pregnancy loss may indicate a familial balanced chromosome translocation or possibly uterine anomalies.

A family history of mental retardation in multiple members may indicate balanced and unbalanced chromosome anomalies or perhaps a hereditary mental retardation condition, particularly fragile X syndrome, which is an X-linked disorder with variable expression that can affect both males and females.

Documentation of stillbirths and infant death is important because of the risks for chromosome anomalies as well as the risks for rare genetic disorders. If a specific diagnosis for the infant death or stillbirth can be identified, this information is very useful for counseling regarding recurrence risks, identifying possible health maintenance issues, and often for reassurance for the family.

The pedigree should always include information about consanguinity and racial and ethnic background of the patient and family. There are many conditions with a greater incidence in particular populations (Table 41-1). The incidence of sickle cell disease is 1 in 500 in African Americans.[15] The carrier frequency for Tay-Sachs is 1 in 25 for both Ashkenazi (eastern European) Jews and French Canadians.[16] Because of the degree of consanguinity seen in Amish and Mennonite populations, the incidence of maple syrup urine disease and chondroecto-dermal dysplasia is much higher among these groups than in the general population.[17,18]

Not all conditions that show an increased racial or ethnic predisposition are autosomal recessive. Glucose-6-

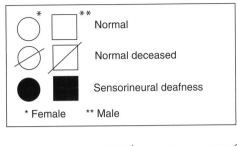

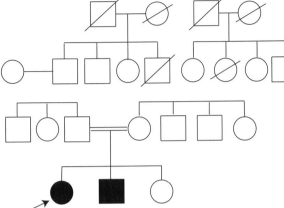

F I G U R E   41-3

A pedigree demonstrating two siblings with sensorineural deafness. From the pedigree, one can infer that this is an autosomal recessive disorder. This is supported by the fact that only two individuals (siblings) are affected in a single generation and the parents are unaffected. This is not an X-linked recessive disorder, since a female is affected. Also supportive of autosomal recessive inheritance is the fact that the parents are first cousins (their fathers are brothers). The consanguinity is denoted by a double line connecting the parents.

phosphate dehydrogenase deficiency (favism), seen in higher frequency in individuals of Mediterranean and African ancestry, is an X-linked recessive disorder.[19] The autosomal dominant genes that predispose to breast and ovarian cancer, BRCA-1 and BRCA-2, are known to have specific mutations that are seen in high frequency in individuals of Ashkenazi Jewish ancestry.[20]

REPRODUCTIVE HISTORY

Individual and familial reproductive history can be very helpful in determining risks for recurrent pregnancy loss, stillbirths, and children with birth defects. In approximately 5% of couples with 2 or more pregnancy losses, one of the members of the couple will have a balanced reciprocal chromosome translocation.[21] Approximately 1 in 500 individuals has a balanced chromosome translocation.[22]

Primary amenorrhea is uncommon. In adolescent females, Turner syndrome is a commonly identified cause. A chromosome study will disclose the presence

of a single X chromosome, or a single normal X chromosome with either a deleted X or Y chromosome or some other rearrangement of the X chromosome. Androgen insensitivity syndromes are very uncommon disorders, in which the phenotype is female with normal-appearing external genitalia, but testes are present, the uterus and müllerian structures are absent, and there is a blind-ending vagina. The karyotype is 46,XY, that of a male. However, there is no androgen influence, resulting in no development of a penis, a scrotum, or male secondary sexual characteristics at puberty. This is a genetically heterogeneous disorder with multiple genes identified.

Male infertility may also have numerous causes. A common disorder encountered in infertility clinics is Klinefelter syndrome, males with a karyotype of 47,XXY. Many men with this disorder are healthy with few medical issues, but typically have azoospermia or oligospermia. Congenital bilateral absence of the vas deferens is seen in 2% to 5% of males seen in infertility clinics.[23] The most common cause of this disorder is having at least 1 mutation for the cystic fibrosis gene, which is responsible for 75% of cases.[23] Pregnancy can be accomplished with assisted reproductive techniques. However, there is an increased risk of having a child with cystic fibrosis, since the partner has up to a 4% chance of being a carrier of the cystic fibrosis gene.

CANCER SYNDROMES AND PREDISPOSITION

Many genes predispose to the development of malignancies. Some are associated with known syndromes, of which cancer is but one manifestation, and some are associated primarily with neoplasias (Table 41-3).

Breast cancer will strike 1 in 9 women at some time in their lives. Most cases are sporadic; however, approximately 5% of cases will be found in women who have a genetic predisposition to cancer.[8] Genetic risk factors for hereditary breast and ovarian cancer syndrome include:[9,24]

- Breast and ovarian cancer in the same individual
- Two or more family members under 50 years of age with breast cancer or ovarian cancer at any age
- Male breast cancer
- One or more family members under age 50 years with breast cancer and Ashkenazi Jewish ancestry
- Ovarian cancer with Ashkenazi Jewish ancestry
- Known BRCA-1 or BRCA-2 gene mutation in the family

The best known genetic risk factors are the autosomal dominant BRCA-1 and BRCA-2 genes. Women who have a mutation of either BRCA-1 or BRCA-2 have a cumulative risk of up to 85% for the development of breast

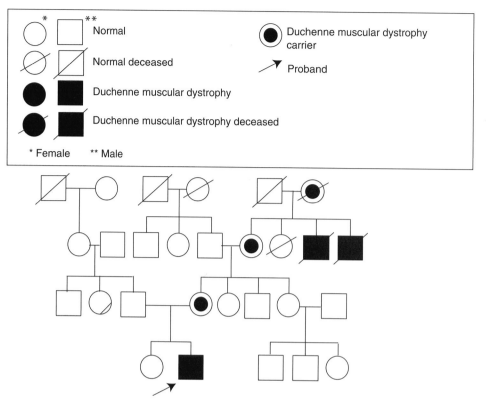

FIGURE 41-4

A pedigree of a family with Duchenne muscular dystrophy. This is an X-linked recessive disorder for which each male has a 50% risk for inheriting the gene from an unaffected female carrier. From this pedigree, it appears that this condition can "skip" generations; however, it is clear that each affected woman has a 25% risk to have an affected son with each pregnancy.

cancer by 70 years, although it is often seen in pre-menopausal women.[24] Moreover, the risk of ovarian cancer developing by age 70 is up to 40%.[8,24] The risk of prostate cancer in male carriers may be 3 times greater than baseline, with up to 8% getting this form of cancer by age 70 years.[25] The incidence of breast cancer in a male is a potential indicator of BRCA-1 or BRCA-2 mutation, especially in the presence of a family history of breast cancer or ovarian cancer or both, or Ashkenazi Jewish ancestry.[20] Other cancers occurring with increased frequency include colon and pancreatic cancer and malignant melanoma (with BRCA-2).

Colorectal cancers comprise approximately 15% of all malignancies, and approximately 5% of them are associated with a hereditary predisposition.[26] In the past, most attention has focused on familial adenomatous polyposis (FAP) (Table 41-3). Although an uncommon genetic condition, the penetrance is very high and there is greatly increased morbidity and mortality in individuals who are not appropriately identified and managed. A family history is considered "positive" when multiple individuals are affected in consecutive generations with an autosomal dominant inheritance pattern. Laboratory testing for mutations of the adenomatous polyposis (APC) gene is

clinically available.[27] Nonclassic presentations of this condition also exist. Other types of malignancies have also been identified with APC tumors (Table 41-3). A family history of these tumors and a young age at diagnosis of colon cancer should alert one to the possibility of FAP in the family. There is a specific mutation of the APC gene that is seen in Ashkenazi Jews. This mutation does not cause classic FAP, and neither does it have as high a penetrance as other mutations of this gene. This mutation is associated with a 10% to 20% risk of colorectal cancer, and 6% of individuals of Ashkenazi Jewish ancestry are carriers of this mutation.[28]

Hereditary nonpolyposis colorectal cancer (HNPCC) accounts for almost all genetically predisposed colorectal cancers.[29] Risk factors for HNPCC include the following:[9,27,29]

- Individuals who fulfill Amsterdam criteria (≥3 relatives with colorectal cancer, one of whom is a first-degree relative of the other 2; ≥2 affected generations; 1 or more affected individuals diagnosed before age 50 years)
- Individuals with 2 HNPCC-related cancers (see Table 41-3)

TABLE 41-2

Racial and Genetic Risk Factors*

Racial or Ethnic Group	Genetic Disorder	Inheritance	Gene	Gene Location
African American	Sickle cell disease	AR	β-globin	11
	Glucose-6-phosphate dehydrogenase deficiency	XR	Glucose-6-phosphate dehydrogenase	Xq28
Ashkenazi Jewish	Tay-Sachs disease	AR	Hexosaminidase A	15q22-q25
	Canavan disease	AR	Aspartoacylase	17pter-17p13
	Bloom syndrome	AR	Helicase	15q26
	Gaucher disease	AR	Acid β-glucosidase	1q21
	Niemann-Pick disease type A	AR	Sphingomyelinase	11p15
	Cystic fibrosis	AR	Cystic fibrosis transmembrane conductance regulator (CFTR)	7q31.2
	Breast/ovarian cancer (BRCA-1/BRCA-2)	AD	BRCA-1 BRCA-2	17q11 13q
	Familial dysautonomia	AR	IKBKAP	9q31-q33
	Sensorineural deafness	AR	Connexin 26	
	Mucolipidosis type IV	AR	Neuraminidase	19p13.3-13.2
Mediterranean (Italian, Greek, North African)	β-thalassemia	AR	β-globin	11
	Glucose-6-phosphate dehydrogenase deficiency	XR	Glucose-6-phosphate dehydrogenase	Xq28
French Canadian	Tyrosinemia	AR	Fumarylacetoacetate hydrolase	15q23-q25
	Tay-Sachs disease	AR	Hexosaminidase A	15q23-q24
Amish/Mennonite	Maple syrup urine disease	AR	Branched-chain keto acid dehydrogenase	19q13-q12
	Chondroectodermal dysplasia (Ellis-van Creveld syndrome)	AR	EVC	4p16
Finnish	Hereditary nephrosis	AR	Nephrin	19q13.1
Southeast Asian	α-thalassemia	AR	α-globin	16p13
Inuit	Congenital adrenal hyperplasia	AR	21-hydroxylase	6p21.3
Northern European/ white	Cystic fibrosis	AR	Cystic fibrosis transmembrane conductance regulator (CFTR)	7q31.2
Portuguese	Machado-Joseph disease	AD	MJD	14q24.3-q31
Puerto Rican	Hermansky-Pudlak syndrome	AR	HPS1	10q23.1-q23.2

*AR indicates autosomal recessive; XR, X-linked recessive; and AD, autosomal dominant. From McKusick VA.[3]

TABLE 41-3

Genetic Causes of Cancer Predisposition*

Syndrome	Types of Neoplasia	Inheritance	Gene and Chromosome Location	Clinical Testing
Familial adenomatous polyposis	Colorectal carcinoma, periampullary carcinoma, gastric adenocarcinoma, small-intestine carcinoid, desmoid tumor, medulloblastoma, astrocytoma, hepatoblastoma, fibrosarcoma	AD	APC gene 5q21-q22	Gene sequencing, protein truncation studies
Hereditary nonpolyposis colorectal cancer (HNPCC)	Colorectal carcinoma, uterine leiomyosarcoma, transitional cell carcinoma of bladder, renal cell carcinoma, gastric carcinoma, biliary carcinoma, endometrial carcinoma, ovarian cancer	AD	At least 13 genes identified, including: hMSH2 2p21-p22 hMLH1 3p21.3 hPMS1 2q31-33 hPMS2 7p22 hMSH6 2p16	Gene sequencing of hMSH2 and hMLH1, commercial testing of other genes not available
Hereditary breast and ovarian cancer	Breast cancer, ovarian cancer, melanoma (BRCA2), pancreatic cancer, papillary serous carcinoma of peritoneum	AD	BRCA-1 17q21 BRCA-2 13q12.3	Gene sequencing of BRCA-1 and BRCA-2
Li-Fraumeni syndrome	Rhabdomyosarcoma, soft-tissue sarcoma, breast cancer, brain tumors, osteosarcoma, leukemia, adrenocortical carcinoma, lymphocytic or histiocytic lymphoma, lung adenocarcinoma, melanoma, gonadal germ cell tumors, prostate carcinoma, pancreatic carcinoma	AD	p53 17p13.1 CHEK2 22q12.1	Gene sequencing of p53
Multiple endocrine neoplasia type 1 (MEN1)	Pancreatic islet cell adenoma, parathyroid adenoma, pituitary adenoma, adrenocortical adenoma, prolactinoma, glucagonoma, insulinoma, vasointestinal peptide tumor, gastrinoma subcutaneous lipoma	AD	Menin gene 11q.13	Gene sequencing of menin gene
Multiple endocrine neoplasia type 2 (MEN2)	Pheochromocytoma, medullary thyroid carcinoma, parathyroid adenoma	AD	RET proto-oncogene 10q11.2	Gene sequencing of RET gene
Von Hippel-Lindau syndrome	Pheochromocytoma, cerebellar hemangioblastoma, hypernephroma, renal cell carcinoma, pancreatic cancer, paraganglioma, adenocarcinoma of ampulla of Vater, retinal angioma	AD	VHL gene 3p26-3p25	Gene sequencing of VHL gene
Peutz-Jeghers syndrome	Gastrointestinal carcinoma, breast cancer, thyroid cancer, lung cancer, pancreatic cancer, uterine cancer, Sertoli cell testicular tumors, ovarian sex cord tumors	AD	STK 11 19p13.3 (serine/threonine kinase gene)	Gene sequencing of STK 11

Syndrome	Types of Neoplasia	Inheritance	Gene and Chromosome Location	Clinical Testing
Cowden syndrome	Oral papillomas, cerebellar gangliocytoma, breast cancer, ovarian carcinoma, cervical carcinoma, uterine adenocarcinoma, follicular cell thyroid cancer, bladder carcinoma, colon adenocarcinoma, meningioma	AD	PTEN 10q23.31	Gene sequencing of PTEN
Neurofibromatosis-1 (NF-1)	Neurofibroma, optic pathway glioma, meningioma, neurofibrosarcoma, rhabdomyosarcoma, pheochromocytoma, astrocytoma	AD	Neurofibromin 17q11.2	Gene linkage analysis
Neurofibromatosis-2 (NF-2)	Vestibular schwannoma, neurinoma, meningioma, schwannoma	AD	Merlin 22q12.2	Mutation analysis and mutation scanning of merlin gene
Nevoid basal cell carcinoma (Gorlin syndrome)	Basal cell carcinoma, hamartomatous stomach polyps, ovarian carcinoma, medulloblastoma, lymphomesenteric cysts	AD	PTCH 9p22.2	Linkage analysis and sequencing of PTCH gene

*AD indicates autosomal dominant. From McKusick VA.[3]

- Colorectal cancer and a first-degree relative with HNPCC-related cancer or adenoma, at least one of the cancers diagnosed before age 50 years
- HNPCC-related cancer in 2 first-degree relatives regardless of age
- Individuals with early-onset colorectal or endometrial cancer regardless of family history

Although the term *nonpolyposis* is used, individuals who have a mutation for HNPCC will generally have a small number of polyps, not the thousands of polyps seen in FAP. In addition, polyps are likely to be present in the ascending colon, making the diagnosis dependent on colonoscopy.[29] A family history of colorectal cancer, especially under the age of 50 years, should lead to further inquiry and possible diagnostic testing for HNPCC. A problem with testing for HNPCC is that there are 13 genes identified that cause this disorder. However, 3 genes are primarily implicated: MLH1 and MSH2, which account for 90% of mutations, and MSH6. Clinical molecular testing is available for these 3 genes. A person with a family history suggestive of HNPCC who tests negative for the condition may still have a gene mutation. Therefore, that person must be followed up as if he or

she has the condition, as should family members at risk. Carriers of HNPCC mutations have a high risk of other tumors, especially endometrial, ovarian, and bladder cancers. This underscores the importance of identifying HNPCC-affected families. Mutation carriers and at-risk individuals should be aggressively monitored.

Although thyroid malignancies may have multiple causes, most of which are not related to predisposing genetic factors, medullary thyroid carcinoma (MTC) has been shown to be associated with mutations of the RET proto-oncogene.[30] It has been shown that 25% of all MTCs are seen in individuals with a RET proto-oncogene mutation. Also, MTC is seen as a clinical component of the multiple endocrine neoplasia type 2 (MEN2). In addition to MTC, individuals with MEN2 are also at risk of pheochromocytomas and parathyroid adenomas. Of interest is that other mutations of the RET proto-oncogenes can cause familial Hirschsprung disease with no apparent increased risk of malignancies.[31] Individuals with familial MTC and MEN2 are at high risk of thyroid cancer. If RET proto-oncogene mutations are identified in an individual with a family history of MTC or MEN2 or both, it is recommended that a thyroidectomy be performed.[32]

COMMON DISEASES AND MULTIFACTORIAL INHERITANCE

When obtaining a family history, it becomes clear that many conditions that are common in a family do not necessarily follow a mendelian pattern of inheritance. Examples include type 1 and type 2 diabetes mellitus, coronary artery disease, rheumatoid arthritis, hypertension, and Alzheimer disease, all of which are multifactorial disorders.

As the term *multifactorial* implies, there are several factors involved in the etiology of these disorders, including genes and nongenetic factors related to environment and lifestyle. Genetic factors clearly play a role, since individuals who have a multifactorial disorder are more likely to have a first-degree relative with the same condition compared with the general population. A predisposing gene or genes that alter genetic background (ie, polygenic or oligogenic inheritance) is termed an epigenetic phenomenon. In some racial or ethnic populations, there may be an increased incidence of specific multifactorial disorders. In the Pima Indians of the Southwest, the prevalence of type 2 diabetes is very high: 50% as compared with 10% of whites and 12% of other Native Americans.[33,34]

The severity of a multifactorial disorder may also give some indication with regard to recurrence risks. With isolated cleft lip and cleft palate, the incidence in the general white population is approximately 1 in 700 live births.[35] The recurrence risk after having a child with unilateral cleft lip is 3%, whereas the recurrence risk after having a child with bilateral cleft lip and cleft palate rises to 5%. Similarly, the more affected individuals there are in a family, the greater the recurrence risk. The incidence of spina bifida is 1 in 2000 live births in the United States.[36] If a couple has 1 child with spina bifida, their chance for having another child with this disorder is increased to 3% or greater. With 2 affected children, the recurrence risk increases to 10% or more.[36]

Multifactorial disorders comprise a large number of conditions that influence morbidity and mortality in the general population. Unfortunately, one cannot perform genetic testing for most of these disorders, although other screening tests exist for conditions such as hypercholesterolemia and hypertension. For the most part, it becomes important to identify these conditions in the family history to appropriately inform patients regarding changes in lifestyle and the need to avoid exposures to potentially harmful substances. In addition, more frequent medical screening should be performed, with the goal of early identification and treatment to avoid morbidity.

AGE AT ONSET OF GENETIC DISORDERS

The age at onset of a condition may give clues as to the severity and inheritance of a disorder. In the case of genetic anticipation, trinucleotide repeats may be inserted in the gene responsible for the disorder during oogenesis or spermatogenesis. Larger trinucleotide expansions will result in earlier onset of signs and symptoms. This has been well documented for Huntington disease, myotonic dystrophy, and several other neurogenetic disorders.

Generally, type 1 diabetes is diagnosed during childhood and type 2 diabetes in later adulthood (although ages at diagnoses for both of these conditions appear to be changing). Two forms of diabetes are genetically heterogeneous and have a milder clinical course. Maturity-onset diabetes of youth (MODY) type 1 is a mild form of juvenile-onset diabetes. This is an autosomal dominant condition and maps to the HNF4 gene on chromosome 20q12-q13.1.[37] The more common MODY type 2, also autosomal dominant, is a relatively mild early-adult-onset diabetes, which is caused by mutations of the glucokinase gene on chromosome 7p15-p13.[37]

Alzheimer disease is another multifactorial condition, for which too little genetic data exist. Approximately 25% of cases are familial, including early-onset and late-onset, and the remaining 75% of cases are sporadic with late-onset.[38] The late-onset familial Alzheimer disease is a complex disorder that involves what appear to be several susceptibility genes for which testing has not proved particularly helpful. Early-onset Alzheimer disease accounts for only 2% of all cases of Alzheimer disease. Three genes have been identified: presenilin 1, presenilin 2, and β-amyloid precursor protein. Clinical testing is available for presenilin 1 and presenilin 2.[39,40]

SUMMARY

As our technology advances and we are able to test for more genetic disorders and susceptibility to many multifactorial disorders, we must become more sensitive to the impact of this information on the individual patient and the family unit. It must be emphasized that before ordering genetic testing for a suspected hereditary disorder, the physician should be aware of the inheritance pattern, natural history of the disorder, distribution of the disorder in the family, and family members who are at risk of the disorder. Personal genetic information has the potential to radically change health care and improve the quality of life for millions. However, this information is very sensitive. In addition to positive uses, there is great potential for misuse of the same information, particularly because it affects not only the individual patient but also the entire family. Results of genetic testing have the potential to be ambiguous or result in unexpected information, including that related to nonpaternity issues. For this reason, genetic testing is ideally accompanied by genetic counseling in which these issues can be discussed with the patient *before* ordering tests.

Medical genetics is both a high-tech and a low-tech specialty. Valuable information can be obtained from simple procedures, including a careful medical and family history. These data are essential for genetic testing and subsequent management of patients.

REFERENCES

1. King RA, Rotter JI, Motulsky AG. Approach to genetic basis of common disease. In: King RA, Rotter JI, Motulsky AG, eds. *The Genetic Basis of Common Diseases.* New York, NY: Oxford University Press; 2002:3–17.

2. Claverie J-M. GENE NUMBER What If There Are Only 30,000 Human Genes? *Science.* 2001;291:1255–1257.

3. McKusick VA. OMIM, Online Mendelian Inheritance in Man. Baltimore, Md: Johns Hopkins University; 2003. Available at: www.ncbi.nlm.nih.gov/omim. Accessed August 18, 2003.

4. Pagon R. GeneTests. Available at: www.genetests.org. Accessed August 18, 2003.

5. DeBella K, Szudek J, Friedman JM. Use of the National Institutes of Health criteria for diagnosis of neurofibromatosis 1 in children. *Pediatrics.* 2000;105:608–614.

6. Dietz HC, Pyeritz RE. Marfan syndrome and related disorders. In: Scriver CR, Beaudet AL, Sly WS, Valle D, eds. *The Metabolic and Molecular Basis of Inherited Disease.* New York, NY: McGraw-Hill; 2001:5287–5311.

7. Northrup H, Wheless JW, Bertin TK, Lewis RA. Variability of expression in tuberous sclerosis. *J Med Genet.* 1993;30:41–43.

8. Culver JB, Hull J, Levy-Lahad E, Daly M, Burke W. Breast cancer genetics: an overview. *GeneReviews.* 2000. Available at: www.geneclinics.org. Accessed May 3, 2003.

9. Eng C, Hampel H. Genetic testing for cancer predisposition. *Annu Rev Med.* 2000;58(2):371–400.

10. Gregory-Evansa K, Bhattacharyaa SS. Genetic blindness: current concepts in the pathogenesis of human outer retinal dystrophies. *Trends Genetics.* 1998;14:103–108.

11. Lindblad K, Schalling M. Expanded repeat sequences and disease. *Semin Neurol.* 1999;19:289–299.

12. Pang S, Murphey W, Levine LS, et al. A pilot newborn screening for congenital adrenal hyperplasia in Alaska. *J Clin Endocrinol Metab.* 1982;55:413–420.

13. Aidoom M, Terlouwb DJ, Kolczaka MS, et al. Protective effects of the sickle cell gene against malaria morbidity and mortality. *Lancet.* 2002;359:1311–1312.

14. Smith TG, Ayi K, Serghides L, Mcallister CD, Kain KC. Innate immunity to malaria caused by *Plasmodium falciparum. Clin Invest Med.* 2002;25:262–272.

15. Flint J, Harding RM, Boyce AJ, Clegg JB. The population genetics of the haemoglobinopathies. *Baillieres Clin Hematol.* 1998;11:1–50.

16. Kaback M, Lim-Steele J, Dabholkar D, Brown D, Levy N, Zeiger K, for International TSD (Tay-Sachs Disease) Data Collection Network. Tay-Sachs disease—carrier screening, prenatal diagnosis, and the molecular era: an international perspective, 1970 to 1993. *JAMA.* 1993;270:2307–2315.

17. Zhang B, Zhao Y, Harris RA, Crabb DW. Molecular defects in the E1 alpha subunit of the branched-chain alpha-ketoacid dehydrogenase complex that cause maple syrup urine disease. *Mol Biol Med.* 1991;8:39–47.

18. McKusick VA. Ellis-van Creveld syndrome and the Amish. *Nat Genetics.* 2000;24:203–204.

19. Weber WW. Populations and genetic polymorphisms. *Mol Diagn.* 1999;4:299–307.

20. Levy-Lahad E, Catane R, Eisenberg S, et al. Founder BRCA1 and BRCA2 mutations in Ashkenazi Jews in Israel: frequency and differential penetrance in ovarian cancer and in breast-ovarian cancer families. *Am J Hum Genet.* 1997;60:1059–1067.

21. Bourrouillou G, Colombies P, Dastugue N. Chromosome studies in 2136 couples with spontaneous abortions. *Hum Genet.* 1986;74:399–401.

22. Hamerton JL, Canning N, Ray M, Smith S. A cytogenetic survey of 14,069 newborn infants: I. Incidence of chromosome abnormalities. *Clin Genetics.* 1975;8:223–243.

23. Weiske WH, Salzler N, Schroeder-Printzen I, Weidner W. Clinical findings in congenital absence of the vasa deferentia. *Andrologia.* 2000;32:13–18.

24. Wooster R, Weber BL. Breast and ovarian cancer. *N Engl J Med.* 2003;348:2339–2347.

25. Johannsson O, Loman N, Moller T, Kristoffersson U, Borg A, Olsson H. Incidence of malignant tumours in relatives of BRCA1 and BRCA2 germline mutation carriers. *Eur J Cancer.* 1999;35:1248–1257.

26. Cohen AM, Minsky BD, Schilsky RL. Cancer of the colon. In: DeVita VTJ, Hellman S, Rosenberg SA, eds. *Cancer: Principles and Practice of Oncology.* Philadelphia, Pa: Lippincott-Raven; 1997:1144–1197.

27. Lynch HT, de la Chapelle A. Hereditary colorectal cancer. *N Engl J Med.* 2003;348:919–932.

28. Gryfe R, Di Nicola N, Lal G, Gallinger S, Redston M. Inherited colorectal polyposis and cancer risk of the APC I1307K polymorphism. *Am J Hum Genetics.* 1999;64:378–384.

29. Hampel H, Peltomaki P. Hereditary colorectal cancer: risk assessment and management. *Clin Genetics.* 2000;58:89–97.

30. Bachelot A, Lombardo F, Baudin E, Bidart JM, Schlumberger M. Inheritable forms of medullary thyroid carcinoma. *Biochimie.* 2002;84:61–66.

31. Parisi MA, Kapur RP. Genetics of Hirschsprung disease. *Curr Opin Pediatr.* 2000;12:610–617.

32. Conte-Devolx B, Schuffenecker I, Niccoli P, et al, for French Study Group on Calcitonin-Secreting Tumors (GETC). Multiple endocrine neoplasia type 2: management of patients and subjects at risk. *Horm Res.* 1997;47:221–226.

33. Knowler WC, Saad MF, Pettitt DJ, Nelson RG, Bennett PH. Determinants of diabetes mellitus in the Pima Indians. *Diabetes Care.* 1993;16:216–227.

34. Pettitt DJ, Nelson RG, Saad MF, Bennett PH, Knowler WC. Diabetes and obesity in the offspring of Pima Indian women with diabetes during pregnancy. *Diabetes Care.* 1993;16:310–314.

35. Saal HM. Classification and description of nonsyndromic oral clefts. In: Wyszynski DF, ed. *Cleft Lip and Palate: From Origin to Treatment.* New York, NY: Oxford University Press; 2002:47–52.

36. Northrup H, Volcik KA. Spina bifida and other neural tube defects. *Curr Probl Pediatr.* 2000;30:313–332.

37. Fajans SS, Bell GI, Polonsky KS. Molecular mechanisms and clinical pathophysiology of maturity-onset diabetes of the young. *N Engl J Med.* 2001;345:971–980.

38. Cummings JL, Vinters HV, Cole GM, Khachaturian ZS. Alzheimer's disease: etiologies, pathophysiology, cognitive reserve, and treatment opportunities. *Neurology.* 1998;51:S2–S17; discussion S65–S67.

39. St George-Hyslop PH, Haines JL, Polinsky RJ, et al. Molecular genetics of familial Alzheimer's disease. *Can J Neurol Sci.* 1989;16:465–467.

40. Levy-Lahad E, Bird TD. Genetic factors in Alzheimer's disease: a review of recent advances. *Ann Neurol.* 1996;40:829–840.

RESOURCES

Gardner RJM, Sutherland GR. *Chromosome Anomalies and Genetic Counseling.* New York, NY: Oxford University Press; 1996:478.

King RA, Rotter JI, Motulsky AG. Approach to genetic basis of common disease. In: King RA, Rotter JI, Motulsky AG, eds. *The Genetic Basis of Common Diseases.* New York, NY: Oxford University Press; 2002:3–17.

McKusick VA. OMIM, Online Mendelian Inheritance in Man. Baltimore, Md: Johns Hopkins University; 2003. Web site: www.ncbi.nlm.nih.gov/omim.

National Library of Medicine, National Center for Biotechnology Information. Web site: www.NCBI.nlm.nih.gov/genome/guide/human/ (A publicly funded genetics information resource with links to multiple Web sites with comprehensive information regarding human genetics.)

National Institutes of Health, Office of Rare Diseases. Bethesda, Md: National Institutes of Health; 2003. Web site: http://rarediseases.info.nih.gov.

Nussbaum RL, McInnes RR, Willard HF, Thomson MW. *Thompson and Thompson Genetics in Medicine.* Philadelphia, Pa: WB Saunders; 2001.

Pagon R. GeneTests. Web site: www.genetests.org. (A publicly funded medical genetics information resource for physicians, other healthcare providers, and researchers, available free.)

Rimoin DL, Connor M, Pyeritz RE, Korf BR, Emery AE. *Emery and Rimoin's Principles and Practice of Medical Genetics.* New York, NY: Churchill Livingstone; 2002:4936.

US Dept of Energy, Office of Science. Human Genome Project information. Washington, DC: US Dept of Energy; 2003. Web site: www.ornl.gov/TechResources/Human_Genome/home.html.

chapter 42

Health and Genetic Risk Assessment Instruments

Robin G. Molella, MD, MPH

INTRODUCTION

Two main reasons exist to quantify individual or population health risk. Such an assessment can inform clinical decision making or health policy formation, and it can be used to facilitate behavior change. In their most basic form, health risk assessment (HRA) tools are mathematical models of the probability that an individual with given risk factors will develop a disease or die in a given time frame. The models are constructed from epidemiologic data. The usefulness of these HRA tools is therefore limited by (1) the quality of the parameters entered by the individual, (2) the quality or validity of the source data, (3) the quality or validity of the model to predict interaction of the risk factors, and (4) the methods used to present the output of the tool.

The most widely used HRAs have focused primarily on health behaviors and rudimentary biometrics, such as height, weight, blood pressure, pulse, and lipids. Data are obtained by survey, which may be self-administered or administered by a trained technician. The instruments may be hand scored or computer scored. The advancement of personal computing technology and the Internet has made these tools widely available in various formats.[1]

With the explosion of data created by the sequencing of the human genome, genetic information will be increasingly included in HRA tools. A change toward assessing genetic data to estimate risk adds an invasive character to HRAs not present before and creates ethical, legal, and social concerns not present in standard HRAs.[2] As our knowledge of the genome increases, so will the number of HRAs using the information. These will be available for use by clinicians, health promotion professionals, and the lay public. Experts in preventive medicine and related specialties will be called on to judge these tools for their validity, relevance, and usefulness.

The term *HRAs* will be used to represent all tools intended to estimate health risks for either clinical decision making or behavior change.

HEALTH HAZARD APPRAISAL APPROACH

Epidemiology is focused on the study of populations and population risks. Any given individual is subject to a series of risks, which relate to heredity, behavior, and exposures, and to the interaction of these features. In the late 1950s, with increasing knowledge gained from prospective trials and the desire to intervene in the course of disease prospectively, preventive medicine and public health professionals wanted to use epidemiologic data to quantify an individual's health risk. The leader of this approach was Lewis C. Robbins. In 1957, Dr Robbins became the first chief of cancer control for the US Public Health Service.[3] In that role, he worked with others to focus on the value of prevention as part of the periodic health examination and was instrumental in lobbying for the creation of risk tables showing the probability of death initially over 1 year but later changed to over 10 years.[4] These tables, called Geller tables because they were compiled by Harvey Geller of the cancer control program, formed the basis of the first HRAs.

The approach was simple. The devices were hand scored and intended to be used to inform the physician and patient of the risk reduction that could be achieved by a particular health prevention strategy. A baseline mortality risk stratified for age, sex, and race was assigned for each of the top causes of mortality, and a multiplier was assigned for each identified risk factor. The patient's estimated 10-year mortality was then recalculated. A factor was assigned for each risk reduction strategy and the risk was recalculated. The difference between the risk with and without prevention was obtained, allowing the calculation of a percent advantage for each strategy. This approach allowed the clinician, as part of a periodic health examination, to quantitate individual patient risks and the risk reduction associated with one or a series of interventions.[5] The approach was sound, but the state of the art at inception was limited. The original risk tables assumed that the risks were independent. In addition, Drs Sadusk and Robbins[3] wrote of the early work, "An important part of the methodology of health hazard appraisal to be established in the future will be the scientific validity of the factors for changing health hazards. It is here that the epidemiologist must meet the challenge and produce better data."

The first known book about the HRA, *How to Practice Prospective Medicine,* was written by Robbins and Hall[5] in 1970 and published by Methodist Hospital in Indianapolis, Ind, where much of the early development of the HRA took place. In the mid-1970s, the Centers for Disease Control and Prevention (CDC) developed its own HRA, which was widely used. In 1974, the Society of Prospective Medicine was formed, with a primary focus on HRAs. By 1987, it was estimated that between 5 million and 15 million people had completed an HRA.[6]

MODERN HRAs

Over the past 30 years, the use of the HRA has become a standard health promotion practice, although, for the most part, Robbins' vision of the HRA as an integral part of the periodic health examination has yet to be fully recognized.[7] Modern HRAs make full use of the statistical, mathematical, and epidemiologic methods as they are developed. Although the first HRAs assumed independence of risk factors and were self-scored, modern HRAs can use multivariate analysis and branching logic.

In formulating an HRA, one must first consider the outcome of interest. In Sadusk and Robbins' initial formulation, this was 10-year mortality from the leading causes of death. However, HRAs need not focus on the leading causes of death but may quantify the risk of a condition developing or mortality from a rare disease. Depending on the group of interest, HRAs may focus on diverse outcomes, such as the risk of nursing home admission, having a low-birth-weight child, or the development of low back pain.[8] An HRA intended to be used in an occupational setting for health promotion purposes will focus on leading causes of death and leading health indicators. An HRA intended to be used in the clinical setting for decision making may focus on specific outcomes.

With the release of Adult Treatment Panel III (ATPIII) guidelines for treatment of cholesterol, the method of quantifying risk to make clinical decisions has become mainstream.[9] The guidelines use risk tables from the Framingham Heart Study to estimate 10-year mortality to determine the patient's need for medication. Although this risk may be estimated, it can also be calculated using an online risk calculator.[10] Risk calculation tools for the risk of breast cancer help women understand their risks and make informed choices about prevention strategies.[11] These tools are widely available through their adaptation as interactive Internet applications.[12]

It has become convention not to include an outcome in an HRA unless there is at least one risk indicator that may lead to an intervention to decrease risk. However, initial HRAs gave risk estimates for causes of death that were not modifiable.[3,5] In some cases, it may be useful to know the risk to put various outcomes in perspective. This debate will become more important as more genetic information is used in HRAs.

Selection of risk indicators depends on the value of the indicator in predicting risk. Multiple questions may need to be asked to assess risk. For example, the risk reduction attributable to cervical cancer screening depends not only on when the last screen was performed but also on the number of sexual partners, whether condoms are used, if there was a previous abnormal Papanicolaou test result, or if there was a diagnosis of human papillomavirus or other sexually transmitted disease. Most HRAs designed for use outside the clinical setting do not include extensive physiologic measurements or detailed past health history or clinical measurements. This is generally because many people do not know or cannot remember these values.[13] In addition, there is always a question of how reliable self-reported values are. Finally, when these instruments are used outside the clinical environment, there is a natural sensitivity to privacy issues. This is especially true with Internet-based instruments if the instruments can be linked to a single individual.[1]

The HRA questionnaire must be carefully designed, and the questions intended to assess risk must be validated, as in any survey. It is always best to ask questions in the same format as they were asked in the original epidemiologic research. Generally, shorter instruments are more likely to be completed and, depending on the intent of the risk assessment, may be adequate. Lengthy questionnaires may be desirable in a comprehensive setting or when the instrument is administered by allied health personnel rather than self-administered. Use of incentives may be helpful in encouraging participation.[14] Health literacy issues are important, as are cultural issues.[15] Literacy is an especially important issue in self-administered instruments; technology can help somewhat, with the use of video streaming and other interactive technologies. Telephonic systems also can be employed and can easily be offered in a variety of languages. It is important to recognize that technologic interfaces such as telephonic systems, touch screens, keyboards, or mouse interfaces may be variably accepted by different groups.[5,16]

Just as the HRA must define the outcome of interest, that is, mortality, morbidity, or disability, the HRA must define the period in question; for example, 10-year risk of myocardial infarction or a lifetime risk of breast cancer. Risk for an individual is then estimated by applying the results of groups or families with similar characteristics. In this way, epidemiologic data are translated by the use of algorithms and mathematical models into risks for a specific individual. Although the principle is simple, a critical eye is required to assess the quality of a given instrument. The risk estimate is only as good as the data from which it was derived. Any flaws in the original investigation are transmitted to the HRA. In addition, flaws can be introduced by assumptions made in constructing the model. A single risk indicator, smoking, might be linked to multiple diseases. Moreover, risk indicators are often not independent. Smoking and elevated cholesterol may have a dependent relationship with regard to the risk of death due to stroke, and that may be a different dependent relationship than with death from myocardial infarction. Or, perhaps smoking is not a risk factor for myocardial infarction if cholesterol is not elevated.[17] For many of these relationships, data are simply not available.

Epidemiologic study designs vary in their value in measuring risk. Prospective cohort studies give an estimate of absolute risk. A cohort of outcome-free individuals is sorted by a risk indicator and then observed to determine the number of individuals who develop the outcome over time. The *absolute risk* is the number of people with the risk indicator who develop the disease divided by the total number of people in the study with the risk indicator. By dividing the absolute risk of those with the factor by the absolute risk of those without the factor, a *relative risk* can be estimated. It may also be the case that the relative risk is estimated by dividing the absolute risk of those with the factor by the population average risk. Prospective studies are costly and not useful for rare outcomes because they would require following a very large sample over a long period to observe a statistically significant relationship. For rare outcomes, one often relies on the case-control study design. In this instance, individuals with the outcome of interest are selected and compared with controls. The odds of cases having the risk factor are compared with the odds of controls having the risk factor. This approach gives an estimate of relative risk.

One can use biostatistical methods to estimate absolute risk if one knows the prevalence of the risk factor in the population and the incidence of disease. Family studies can provide estimates of the probability that, with age, an unaffected individual will become affected given that another specific family member (sibling, parent, grandparent, etc) is affected. Once the risk estimation for a given risk indicator is determined, that risk indicator must be used to adjust the baseline risk of the individual. Multivariate techniques can be used to directly estimate absolute risk and can account for interaction among risk factors. Again, any method employed in epidemiology and biostatistics can be used in an HRA, but all of the potential flaws of the technique are transferred to the HRA.

Scoring is often by computer but may be by hand as in the original Robbins/Hall HRA. Self-scoring is not ideal unless the process is rather simple. Similar to literacy skill, computation skill varies among subjects and errors in the scoring decrease the accuracy of the HRA.[18]

If the value of the HRA is affected by the structure of the survey instrument and the methods of risk estimation, the output of the HRA is equally important. Here, just as in prior portions of the HRA process, the output must be tailored to its intended population and use. An HRA for health promotion intended to be used with individuals who have limited literacy might do best to present risk information in the form of graphics.

Relative risks may be presented, but they are not useful for comparing across diseases and may provide a false sense of security if one is at average risk of a common disorder. Absolute risks allow for ranking of outcomes. *Achievable risk* is calculated by substituting the patient's modifiable high-risk behaviors with low-risk behaviors, as in Sadusk and Robbins'[3] original concept. Risks may be conveyed without using numerical values. Terms such as *high risk, moderate risk,* or *low risk* may be used. A comparison of an individual's risk with the average risk at various ages for that person's sex and race allows one to find the age, sex, and race risk closest to the individual's own risk. That age then becomes the "risk age" or "health age" of the individual. A similar strategy for conveying global risk is to predict life expectancy. Changes in life expectancy can then be adjusted depending on the changes in behavior an individual considers.

An HRA output is intended to facilitate action. In the clinical setting, the clinician who has determined the need to utilize the instrument should have plans for how to use the output, eg, whether to use a 3-hydroxy-3-methylglutaryl coenzyme A (HMG CoA) reductase inhibitor based on the Framingham study 10-year mortality. When an HRA is used for health promotion, the output must be linked to specific risk reduction recommendations. Information obtained during the survey can be used to tailor the information. For example, stage of change[19,20] or self efficacy[21-23] for each risk indicator can be recorded and feedback given so that the most prominent message relates to the behavior change the individual is most ready to make, or so that messages are stage related. Recommendations for risk reduction should have demonstrated effectiveness in reducing risk.

USES OF HRA

Many uses of the HRA have already been alluded to earlier in this chapter. HRAs can be focused on specific diseases and used to facilitate clinical decision making, or they can be more global and focus on the major causes of death, as was intended by Robbins, Hall, and Sadusk. The HRA is a tool for adapting what is known about risk factors for disease into an instrument that can quantitate risk estimates for individuals. In this way, the HRA can serve as a core for health promotion activities at health clubs, in community settings such as churches and grocery stores, and in occupational settings. When aggregate population risk is the focus instead of individuals, the data can be used to formulate health policies and population-based health programs. It can also be used to assess outcomes of interventions. Because HRAs can be packaged with other facets of wellness programming, commercial firms have become involved, which has increased the availability and variety of HRAs.

CRITICISMS OF HRA

Despite their frequent use, HRAs are not without their critics. Criticism may relate to the validity of the risk estimate, concerns about the output, or questions about effectiveness. The effectiveness question is an interesting one because HRAs have been created to be a risk estimation tool or risk calculator. They are not really interventions intended on their own to reduce risk. There are challenges in evaluating approaches that rely solely on the provision of health education.[24-26] Certainly, recent advances in our understanding of behavior change would suggest that a clear understanding of the risks of a behavior is essential before lasting behavior change is possible.[20-24]

Validity is always a concern, as noted previously. There may be data collection errors, the risk factor measured in the HRA may not be equivalent to the reference factor evaluated in the original research, the risk estimate from the epidemiologic study may not be generalizable, or the original study may have methodological errors that compromise the results. There may be flaws in the HRA algorithm. There may be difficulties with test-retest reliability, especially with regard to self-reported biometric values such as blood pressure, weight, and lipids.[27] There have been concerns that individuals will answer in ways that make them appear in a more positive light.

Studies have evaluated the validity of HRA risk estimates. In this type of research, the predictions are compared with actual outcomes in prospective trials. The tendency has been for the HRA to overestimate risk.[28] Although predicted and actual results do correlate, estimated risks must be viewed with some degree of caution. Clearly, the value of risk estimation will improve as further research is done in this area. Finally, the presentation of the outcome involves other disciplines, including behavioral psychology and health communication. The effectiveness of the strategy of health risk estimation is reliant on the ability to translate that risk into a message that is meaningful for the individual.[12]

USE OF GENETIC INFORMATION IN HEALTH RISK APPRAISAL

Family history information as a risk of disease has been included in health risk appraisals since they were originally conceived.[3] Traditionally, family history has been less enthusiastically included than other risk indicators in HRAs for a variety of reasons. Family members may have been subjected to environmental and behavioral risks that may not be a factor in the individual in question. A genetic trait, which exists in a family and confers risk of disease, may not have been passed to a given individual. Knowledge of the absence or presence of that genetic trait may alter risk dramatically. Use of family history of disease information may also be subject to recall bias. Family history information changes over time, meaning that as new illnesses and conditions occur, the risk must be recalculated. There has also been resistance to including family history of disease information because it is traditionally viewed as unmodifiable. However, estimating family history of disease risk is a subject of renewed interest with the increase in genomic information.[29] To understand why, one needs to understand some of the issues associated with using genetic testing to estimate risk.

In theory, genetic information represents a much more precise approach to estimating risk than is family history of disease. Each individual's genetic makeup is uniquely his or her own. There may come a time when a simple blood test will allow a physician to inform patients, perhaps at infancy, of all potential risks posed by their particular genetic makeup.[30] The physician may be able to calculate the likelihood of various outcomes related to behaviors or choices the individual might make, and then make recommendations on how to maximize health and avoid adverse consequences. Although we have made tremendous strides in our knowledge of the human genome, we are not yet at a point where we can provide this information. An analysis of the 2042 published articles in the epidemiologic literature on human genes in 2001 revealed that most reported on only the population prevalence of gene variants or simple gene-disease associations (82.0%), while 14.5% integrated the study of interactions (gene-gene and gene-environment) and only 3.5% dealt with evaluation of genetic tests.[31]

The use of genetic tests, similar to the use of other risk indicators, is reliant on the quality of the epidemiologic information that summarizes the relationships between genotype, environment, and outcome. For the bulk of chronic diseases, the pathogenesis is not from a single gene (causal gene) but rather from a series of less consequential genetic changes (susceptibility genes). These susceptibility genes, when present in the same individual or combined with certain environmental conditions, lead to disease. The magnitude of interaction might vary with age. For example, smoking may have a more significant risk in a particular genotype at a young age. Another example is that for some time it was postulated that smoking might be a less significant risk factor if low-density lipoprotein cholesterol (LDL-C) levels were low. A recent study has not borne this out,[13] but these examples illustrate the level of detailed epidemiologic data necessary, given the possible permutations of the genome, to use genotype to assess risk.

To be useful in estimating risk, genetic test information must be analytically valid, clinically valid, and have clinical utility.[32] *Analytic validity* refers to the ability of the test to identify the genetic characteristic of interest (ie, the test's sensitivity and specificity). Different methods may be used to reach the same diagnosis, and the sensitivity and specificity of those methods can have an impact on other inferences made about the epidemiology of disease.[32] *Clinical validity* is the positive or negative predictive value of a test. This is often uncertain for new genetic tests, which may have been based on studies in limited or biased populations.[33] The BRCA1 and BRCA2 genes were originally studied in high-risk families.[34] A woman who tests positive for one of these genes has an approximately 85% lifetime risk of breast cancer. However, when one looks at less selected populations, the risk associated with the mutation falls to between 36% and 56%.[35-39] *Clinical utility* refers to the likelihood that the test will lead to an improved health outcome. The issues of concern are whether effective interventions exist for people who test positive for a gene, as well as the social and emotional consequences for people with both "positive" (abnormal) and "negative" (normal) results.[40-43]

In addition to issues regarding validity and utility, genetic tests also have ethical, legal, and social implications. There are concerns about access to testing and treatment, and their cost. Concerns exist about insurance or employment discrimination, which are difficult to study. There are concerns on the potential long-term psychologic harm that may be caused by testing, or perhaps medical harm if knowledge of risk or perhaps the false security of a negative test result causes a change in behavior that is harmful. Holtzman's[44] concerns from 1989, suggesting that there is a great need to "proceed with caution" in applying genetic testing in human populations, still hold today despite the growth in the number of available genetic tests and in our knowledge of the human genome. He noted that society's use of genetics had led to human rights abuses in the past. Additionally, he pointed out that the commercialization of genetics testing may lead to development of some commercially profitable tests, but not others. He noted that indiscriminate testing could occur without an understanding of the limits of the test or an ability to interpret the results. Finally, he pointed out that our ability to detect susceptibility genes would outstrip our ability to provide effective intervention. These 4 issues continue to have an impact on our ability to use genetic testing information in risk estimation.

It will likely be a decade or more before adequate information regarding genetic risk indicators will be available for many of the leading causes of morbidity and mortality.[45] Therefore, there has been a renewed interest in measures of risk based on a family history of disease.[46] Having a family history of a common chronic disease has been associated with relative risks that range from 2 to 5 times that of the general population.[47] More specific estimates can be made by accounting for the risk indicators of the family and the relationship of the affected family member to the subject (more weight for those more closely related). Testing for the reliability of the information obtained (analytic validity) has demonstrated generally positive results.[48,49] But not all studies have been positive, and the issues seem to be related to the specific diseases in question as well as the social and economic setting where the study was done.[50,51] Once again, the power of the family history as a disease tool (ie, the clinical utility) is dependent on the epidemiologic data. As with genetic testing, great uncertainty still exists as to what is the impact of quantifying the family history of disease risk. Some studies have shown that knowledge of increased risk may increase the likelihood of adherence to preventive interventions.[52,53] However, it is possible that some individuals will respond adversely to the knowledge and view their family history as fatalistic.

FUTURE OF RISK ESTIMATION TOOLS

As our knowledge of the risk indicators of disease grows, regardless of whether those risk indicators are behavioral, environmental, family history, or genetic, there will be increasing pressure to quantitate those risks for individuals and groups, and report them in such a way that the information results in the prevention of morbidity and mortality. There is likely to be an increase in the availability of disease-specific and global risk estimation tools. These tools will continue to be of variable quality and available in multiple settings. The ready availability of these tools to the public will increase the need for clinicians who understand these tools and can interpret the results.

The rising burden of chronic disease demands renewed efforts at modifying risk factors,[15] and the HRA can serve as the initial step toward identifying the risks and guiding individuals and groups to the best resources to support change. The original intent of the HRA was to empower the physician and patient to make rational prevention decisions based on quantitative risk measurements. The pressures of medical economics, explosive growth in medical information, and the importance of obtaining informed consent before beginning medical interventions makes the risk assessment approach more valuable in the clinical setting than, perhaps, it has ever been.

REFERENCES

1. Roseman J, et al. A computerized system to assess risk of disease specific morbidity and mortality utilizing immunogenetic marker information. In: *Proceedings of the 25th Annual Meeting of the Society of Prospective Medicine.* Indianapolis, Ind: Society of Prospective Medicine; 1990:205–212.

2. Vineis P. Ethical issues in genetic screening for cancer. *Ann Oncol.* 1997;8:945–949.

3. Sadusk JF, Robbins LC. Proposal for health-hazard appraisal in comprehensive care. *JAMA.* 1968;203:1108–1112.

4. Geller H, Steele F. Updating tables of probability of dying within the next 10 years. In: *Proceedings of the 13th Annual Meeting of the Society of Prospective Medicine.* Bethesda, Md: Society of Prospective Medicine; 1978.

5. Robbins LC, Hall JH. *How to Practice Prospective Medicine.* Indianapolis, Ind: Methodist Hospital of Indiana; 1970.

6. Roseman JM, Acton RT, Bamberg R. Health and genetic risk assessment instruments. In: Matzen RN, Lang RS, eds. *Clinical Preventive Medicine.* St Louis, Mo: Mosby; 1993.

7. Fletcher DJ, Smith GL. Health risk appraisal: helping patients predict and prevent health problems. *Postgrad Med.* 1986;80:69–82.

8. DeFriese GH, Fielding JE. Health risk appraisal in the 1990's: opportunities, challenges, and expectations. *Annu Rev Public Health.* 1990;11:401–418.

9. The Third Report of the National Cholesterol Education Program (NCEP) Expert Panel on Detection, Evaluation, and Treatment of High Blood Cholesterol in Adults. Available at: www.nhlbi.nih.gov/guidelines/chol/atp3full.pdf. Accessed January 31, 2003.

10. National Cholesterol Education Program. Risk assessment tool for estimating 10-year risk of developing hard CHD (myocardial infarction and coronary death). Available at: www.hin.nhlbi.nih.gov/atpiii/calculator.asp?usertype=prof. Accessed January /31, 2003.

11. Euhus DM. Understanding mathematical models for breast cancer risk assessment and counseling. *Breast J.* 2001;7:224–232.

12. Available at: www.brca.nci.nih.gov. Accessed January 9, 2003.

13. Sacks JJ, Krusat WM, Newman J. Reliability of the health hazard appraisal. *Am J Public Health.* 1980;70:730–732.

14. Jeffrey RW, Forster JL, Baxter JE, French SA, Kelder SH. An empirical evaluation of the effectiveness of tangible incentives in increasing participation and behavior change in a worksite health promotion program. *Am J Health Promotion.* 1993;8:98–100.

15. US Dept of Health and Human Services. *Healthy People 2010.* 2nd ed. *With Understanding and Improving Health and Objectives for Improving Health.* Vol 1. Washington, DC: US Government Printing Office; November 2000.

16. Eng TR, Gustafson TH, eds. *Wired for Health and Well-Being: The Emergence of Interactive Health Communication.* Washington, DC: Science Panel on Interactive Communication and Health, US Dept of Health and Human Services; 1999.

17. Blanco-Cedres L, Daviglus ML, Garside DB, et al. Relation of cigarette smoking to 25-year mortality in middle-aged men with low baseline serum cholesterol. *Am J Epidemiol.* 2002;155:354–360.

18. Smith KW, McKinlay SM, McKinlay JB. The reliability of health risk appraisals for coronary heart disease: results from a randomized field trial. *Am J Public Health.* 1991;81:466–470.

19. DiClemente CC, Prochaska JO. Toward a comprehensive transtheoretical model of change. In: Miller, Heather, eds. *Treating Addictive Behaviors.* 2nd ed. New York, NY: Plenum Press; 1998.

20. Prochaska JO, Velicer WF. The transtheoretical model of health behavior change. *Am J Health Promotion.* 1997;12:39–50.

21. Bandura A. *Self-Efficacy: the Exercise of Control.* New York, NY: WH Freeman & Co; 1997.

22. Bandura A. *Social Learning Theory.* Englewood Cliffs, NJ: Prentice Hall; 1977.

23. Bandura A. Self-efficacy mechanism in human agency. *Am Psychol.* 1982;37:122–142.

24. Breslow L. A policy assessment of preventive health practice. *Prev Med.* 1977;6:242–251.

25. Cohen CI, Cohen EJ. Health education: panacea, pernicious or pointless? *N Engl J Med.* 13:718–720.

26. Green LW. Determining the impact and effectiveness of health education as it relates to federal policy. *Health Educ Monogr.* 1978;6:28–66.

27. Alexy BJ. Health risk appraisal: reliability demonstrated. In: Miller LA, ed. *Proceedings of the 19th Annual Meeting of the Society of Prospective Medicine.* Bethesda, Md: Society of Prospective Medicine Publishers; 1984.

28. Fletcher DJ, Smith GL. Health-risk appraisal: helping patients predict and prevent health problems. *Postgrad Med.* 1986;80:69–82.

29. Scheuner MT, Wang S, Raffel LJ, et al. Family history: a comprehensive genetic risk assessment method for the chronic conditions of adulthood. *Am J Med Genet.* 1997;71:315–324.

30. Collins FS. Shattuck Lecture: medical and societal consequences of the Human Genome Project. *N Engl J Med.* 1999;341:28–37.

31. Khoury MJ. Commentary: epidemiology and the continuum from genetic research to genetic testing. *Am J Epidemiol.* 2002;156:297–299.

32. Little J, Bradley L, Bray MS, et al. Reporting, appraising, and integrating data on genotype prevalence and gene-disease associations. *Am J Epidemiol.* 2002;156:300–310.

33. Burke W, et al. Genetic test evaluation: information needs of clinicians, policy makers and the public. *Am J Epidemiol.* 2002;156:311–318.

34. Ford D, Easton DF, Bishop DT, et al. Risks of cancer in BRCA1-mutation carriers: Breast Cancer Linkage Consortium. *Lancet.* 1994;343:692–695.

35. Fodor FH, Weston A, Bleiweiss IJ, et al. Frequency and carrier risk associated with common BRCA1 and BRCA2 mutations in Ashkenazi Jewish breast cancer patients. *Am J Hum Genet.* 1998;63:45–51.

36. Struewing JP, Hartge P, Wacholder S, et al. The risk of cancer associated with specific mutations of BRCA1 and BRCA2 among Ashkenazi Jews. *N Engl J Med.* 1997;336:1401–1408.

37. Thorlacius S, Struwing JP, Hartge PP, et al. Population-based study of risk of breast cancer in carriers of BRCA2 mutation. *Lancet.* 1998;352:1337–1339.

38. Hopper JL, Southey MC, Dite GS, et al. Population-based estimate of the average age-specific cumulative risk of breast cancer for a defined set of protein truncating mutations in BRCA1 and BRCA2. Australian Breast Cancer Family Study. *Cancer Epidemiol Biomarkers Prev.* 1999:8:741–747.

39. Burke W, Press NA, Pinsky LE. BRCA1 and BRCA2: a small part of the puzzle. *J Natl Cancer Inst.* 1999;91:904–905.

40. Prospero L, Seminsky M, Honeyford J, et al. Psychosocial issues following a positive result of genetic testing for BRCA1 and BRCA2 mutations: findings from a focus group and a needs-assessment survey. *Can Med Assoc J.* 2001;164:1005–1009.

41. Akan-Collan K, Mecklin J, et al. Predictive genetic testing for hereditary non-polyposis colorectal cancer: uptake and long term satisfaction. *Int J Cancer.* 2000;89:44–50.

42. Murphy AE. Dealing with the uncertainty of developing a cancer. *Eur J Cancer Care.* 1999;8:233–237.

43. Kupila A, Muona P, Simell T, et al. Feasibility of genetic and immunological prediction of Type 1 diabetes in a population based cohort. *Diabetologia.* 2001;44:290–297.

44. Holtzman NA. *Proceed With Caution: Predicting Genetic Risks in the Recombinant DNA Era.* Baltimore, Md: The Johns Hopkins University Press; 1989.

45. Yoon PW, Chen B, Faucett A, et al. The public health impact of genetic tests at the end of the 20th century. *Genet Med.* 2001;3:405–410.

46. Yoon PW, Scheuner MT, et al. Can family history be used as a tool for public health and preventive medicine? *Genet Med.* 2002;4:304–310.

47. King RA, Rotter JI, Motulsky AG, eds. *The Genetic Basis of Common Diseases.* New York, NY: Oxford University Press; 1992.

48. Hunt SC, Williams RR, Barlow GK. A comparison of positive family history definitions for defining risk of future disease. *J Chronic Dis.* 1986;39:809–821.

49. Kahn LB, Marshall JA, Baxter J, Shetterly SM, Hamman RF. Accuracy of reported family history of diabetes mellitus: results from San Luis Valley Diabetes Study. *Diabetes Care.* 1990;13:796–798.

50. Napier JA, Metzner MA, Johnson BC. Limitations of morbidity and mortality data obtained from family histories: a report from the Tecumseh Community Health Study. *Am J Public Health.* 1972;62:30–35.

51. Go R, et al. Analyses of HLA linkage in white families with multiple cases of seropositive rheumatoid arthritis. *Arthritis Rheum.* 1987;30:1115–1123.

52. Murabito JM, Evans JC, Larson MG, et al. Family breast cancer history and mammography. *Am J Epidemiol.* 2001;154:916–923.

53. Codori AM, Peterson GM, Miglioretti DL, Boyd P. Health beliefs and endoscopic screening for colorectal cancer: potential for cancer prevention. *Prev Med.* 2001;33:128–136.

chapter 43

Genetic Impact on Disease Risk

Brad T. Tinkle, MD, PhD, and Howard M. Saal, MD

INTRODUCTION

Diseases due to a single gene defect are rare. The vast majority of adult-onset diseases are considered "complex." Complex disease refers to multifactorial etiology in which the products of more than 1 gene interact with the environment and are influenced by development, growth, maturation, and aging to produce a disease.

As the roles of genes are uncovered, it is clear that complex diseases have a large number of genetic components. A review of the Online Mendelian Inheritance in Man (OMIM) database shows that more than 500 single genes have been shown to predispose to cancer, more than 400 for heart disease, approximately 300 for diabetes and thyroid disease, and 100 to 150 for dementia and arthritis.[1] It is thought that the more genes an individual has that predispose to a particular disorder, the greater the likelihood that the disorder will develop in that person. This is known as the threshold model. For example, 4% of people have an activated protein C resistance due to the factor V Leiden mutation. However, if 2 predisposing clotting disorders coexist, the likelihood of a venous thrombotic event rises to nearly 25%. This chapter will review the role genetics plays in important complex diseases in adults.

OPHTHALMOLOGY

Macular Degeneration

Age-related macular degeneration (AMD) is a leading cause of blindness. A large fraction of AMD is likely caused by genetic factors, but they remain largely unidentified.[2] Several genes have been found that are associated with macular dystrophy, including a juvenile-onset form of macular degeneration, which accounts for up to 7% of all human retinal degenerative diseases.[3] The diagnosis can be made by functional studies, associated findings, and a family history.

Cataracts

Cataracts are seen in multiple genetic syndromes, including more than 200 listed in OMIM. Presenile cataracts as defined as onset before the age of 50 years. They are more associated with diabetes, trauma, and treatment with phenytoin or steroids, and are seen in several rare genetic conditions. In neurofibromatosis type 2 (NF2), 70% to 80% of patients will have cataracts, often developing before adulthood.[4] Fortunately, less than 20% will have substantial visual impairment due to their cataracts. Patients with presenile cataracts should be evaluated for signs of NF2. Galactosemia is due to the deficiency of the enzymes galactose-uridyl transferase (type 1) and galactokinase (type 2). Homozygotes typically have cataracts in childhood, but presenile cataracts can also be seen in heterozygotes. Therefore, first-degree relatives of patients with galactosemia are at exceptionally increased risk of presenile cataracts, and heightened attention should be given to any visual disturbance.[5]

Retinitis Pigmentosa

Retinitis pigmentosa (RP) is a retinal degeneration that leads to night blindness, loss of peripheral vision, and retinal pigment deposition, and may eventually cause total loss of vision. Retinitis pigmentosa is both clinically and genetically heterogeneous. It can be seen in a number of genetic syndromes or as a single trait. More than 50 genetic loci have been implicated in RP.[6] The most common form of syndromic RP, Usher syndrome, is associated with progressive hearing loss. Regardless of the cause, individuals with a family history need to be closely monitored. Anyone presenting with RP should be closely evaluated for other features of the syndrome, especially hearing loss.

T A B L E   43-1

Disorders due to Dynamic Mutations of Specific Nucleotide Repeats*

Disease Name	Clinical Description	Inheritance	Type of Repeat	No. of Repeats Normal	No. of Repeats Pathologic
Bipolar disorder	Mania/hypomania; depression	AD	(CTG)		>40
Dentatorubral-pallidoluysian atrophy (DRPLA)	Cerebellar ataxia; chorea; myoclonus; seizures; dementia; mean age at onset, 30 y	AD	(CAG)	3–36	49–88
Episodic ataxia type 2	Allelic to SCA6; onset in childhood	AD	(CAG)	<18	>19
Fragile X syndrome	Mental retardation; characteristic facies; macro-orchidism	XLD	(CGG)	6–40	>200
FraXE mental retardation	Mild mental retardation	XLR	(CCG)	6–35	>200
FraXF	Possible developmental delay	XL	(CGG)	6–38	>300
Fra16A	Congenital malformations; infertility	AD	(CCG)		
Friedreich ataxia	Gait and limb ataxia; hyporeflexia; cardiomyopathy	AR	(GAA)	5–34	66–1700
Haw River syndrome	Allelic to DRPLA; seizures; extensive demyelinization; basal ganglia calcifications; neuroaxonal dystrophy	AD	(CAG)		
Huntington disease	Involuntary choreiform movements; personality changes; dementia; cognitive decline; depression	AD	(CAG)	6–35	36–121
Kennedy disease (spinal and bulbar muscular atrophy)	Slowly progressive adult-onset spinobulbar muscular atrophy; fasciculations; androgen insensitivity	XLR	(CAG)	9–36	38–62
Male infertility with testicular failure	Hypospermatogenesis	XLD	(CAG)	8–27	17–33
Progressive myoclonic epilepsy (Unverricht-Lundborg disease)	Seizures; ataxia; onset 6–13 y	AR	(CCCCGC CCCGCG)	1–3	>17
Myotonic dystrophy, type I	Distal muscle weakness; myotonia; cataracts; arrhythmias	AD	(CTG)	5–36	57–5000

Continued

NEUROLOGY AND NEURODEGENERATIVE DISORDERS

Neurologic disorders, which include neurodegenerative and neuropsychiatric conditions, are among some of the more unusual genetic syndromes. Families with many of these disorders, in particular the ataxias, show clinical anticipation, as seen by an earlier age at onset and usually an increase in severity in successive generations. Many of these syndromes that show clinical anticipation have been demonstrated to have dynamic mutations (Table 43-1). Nearly all of the syndromes are seen as having an expansion of trinucleotide repeats that affect gene expression or function.

Alzheimer Disease

Most dementias are sporadic, but some families show varying degrees of genetic predisposition.[7] Alzheimer disease (AD) is the most common of these in the general population older than 65 years of age. The disease can occur before age 65 years as early-onset AD, which has a clear autosomal dominant inheritance pattern. At least 3 genes are known: β-amyloid precursor protein, presenilin 1, and presenilin 2. Presenilin 1 is the most common and most severe form of early-onset AD and has its onset in the fifth decade. Presenilin 2 is far more variable, with a later onset. These mutations account for approximately 5% of patients with AD but are nearly completely penetrant.

One of the contributing factors to late-onset AD aside from age is the apolipoprotein E (apoE) genotype. Those individuals with none of the apoE4 alleles have been found

TABLE 43-1

Disorders due to Dynamic Mutations of Specific Nucleotide Repeats*—*Concluded*

Disease Name	Clinical Description	Inheritance	Type of Repeat	No. of Repeats Normal	Pathologic
Myotonic dystrophy, type II	Distal muscle weakness; myotonia; cataracts; arrhythmias	AD	(CCTG)		75–11,000
Oculopharyngeal muscular dystrophy	Progressive dysphagia; ptosis; proximal limb weakness	AD/AR	(GCG)	6	7–13
Spinocerebellar ataxia, type 1	Progressive ataxia; optic atrophy; peripheral neuropathy; chorea; onset in third or fourth decade of life	AD	(CAG)	6–38	39–83
Spinocerebellar ataxia, type 2	Progressive ataxia; dementia; peripheral neuropathy; dysphagia; onset in third or fourth decade	AD	(CAG)	14–31	32–400
Spinocerebellar ataxia, type 3 (Machado-Joseph disease)	Progressive ataxia; sensory loss; amyotrophic fasciculations; dystonia; ophthalmoplegia	AD	(CAG)	12–42	55–86
Spinocerebellar ataxia, type 6 (SCA6)	Very slowly progressive ataxia; nystagmus	AD	(CAG)	4–19	20–33
Spinocerebellar ataxia, type 7	Gait ataxia; vision loss; chorea; mean age at onset, 32 y	AD	(CAG)	4–35	37–300
Spinocerebellar ataxia, type 8	Progressive ataxia; hyperreflexia	AD	(CTG)	16–37	100–320
Spinocerebellar ataxia, type 10	Progressive ataxia; seizures; cerebellar atrophy	AD	(ATTCT)	10–22	800–4500
Spinocerebellar ataxia, type 12	Progressive cerebellar ataxia; tremor; cerebellar and cortical atrophy	AD	(CAG)	6–45	55–78
Spinocerebellar ataxia, type 17	Gait ataxia; dementia; dystonia	AD	(CAG)	25–42	43–63
Synpolydactyly	Syndactyly; polydactyly of third or fourth finger	AD	(GCG)	15	22–25

*Italic indicates disorders with controversial linkage to repeat expansion mutations but that may exhibit genetic anticipation; AD, autosomal dominant; AR, autosomal recessive; XL, X-linked; XLD, X-linked dominant; and XLR, X-linked recessive.

to have a 9% lifetime risk of AD, whereas those with 2 copies have a 25% to 50% lifetime risk.[8] Testing for apoE alleles has been erroneously used to predict the likelihood of developing AD and in confirmation of a suspected diagnosis. A more appropriate view is that the apoE4 allele in single- or double-dosage forms raises the risk of AD by twofold to fivefold and fivefold to tenfold, respectively. This allele is, therefore, a risk factor but not predictive or confirmatory of AD. Its use in diagnosis should be limited to adjunctive evidence and not confirmation.

Ataxia

The ataxias are a group of heterogeneous disorders characterized by slowly progressive gait disturbances and may involve poor coordination of the hands and speech as well. Most forms of genetic ataxias involve a sporadic occurrence. The remaining proportion has one of multiple genetic syndromes. The spinocerebellar ataxias are genetically heterogeneous but involve nucleotide repeat sequences (Table 43-1). Because of the clinical overlap, persons with ataxia and a family history suggestive of an autosomal dominant ataxia need to be differentiated by molecular diagnosis, which is clinically available, for 8 forms of spinocerebellar ataxia.[9]

Some of the autosomal recessive ataxias include Friedreich ataxia (Table 43-1) and ataxia-telangiectasia. Ataxia-telangiectasia presents before the age of 4 years. Both parents are heterozygotes, as are two thirds of the unaffected siblings. Persons heterozygous for ataxia-telangiectasia are known to have a cancer rate as much as 4 times higher than that in the general population, especially for breast cancer. Genetic counseling is recommended for all first-degree relatives of the affected person. Carrier testing is not routinely offered unless the specific mutation of the proband is identified. Therefore, the clinician must have increased vigilance for cancer in those at risk of being heterozygotes.

Huntington Disease

Huntington disease (HD) is an autosomal dominant disorder with progressive motor disability involving both involuntary and voluntary movement, cognitive decline, and personality changes. Symptoms usually begin at around age 40 years but can occasionally show clinical anticipation in successive generations. Once early symptoms have begun in those with a family history of the disease, depression occurs in 9% to 44% and the incidence of suicide is 0.5% to 12.7%. Death usually occurs about 15 years after disease onset. Huntington disease is caused by a mutation in the gene Huntington located on chromosome 4 as a repeat expansion of the CAG trinucleotide. This is available as a clinical test (Table 43-1). Many children of those affected with HD prefer not to have genetic testing. Because of the high rate of depression and suicide, counseling *before* genetic testing is a must, and a psychologic evaluation is required. Those at risk need to undergo continued counseling and be observed for signs of depression.

Tuberous Sclerosis

Tuberous sclerosis (TSC) is an autosomal dominant condition that affects multiple organ systems and occurs in 1 of every 5800 births.[10] It is caused by defects in 1 of 2 genes, *TSC1* and *TSC2*. Patients with TSC have a multitude of findings, and some features present only in adulthood. The characteristic features of TSC are infantile spasms, seizures, cortical tubers, subependymal nodules, cardiac rhabdomyomas, shagreen patches, and hypopigmented macules. Of the cases identified, 70% arise from new mutations. However, it is not uncommon to find a parent with the dermatologic findings who reports good health but is unknowingly at future risk.

Adult patients with TSC are at risk of facial angiofibromas, ungual fibromas, giant cell astrocytomas, pulmonary lymphangiomyomatosis, renal angiomyolipomas, and polycystic renal disease. The facial angiofibromas and ungual fibromas have low malignant potential and are more a cosmetic concern. Subependymal giant cell astrocytomas and nodules are infrequently malignant (6% to 14%), but growth may cause increased intracranial pressure. Renal angiomyolipomas occur in about 70% of cases and are benign, but continued growth carries a substantial risk of spontaneous, life-threatening bleeding. In addition, as the angiomyolipomas continue to grow, they replace normal renal parenchyma, resulting in hypertension and renal insufficiency and may even lead to end-stage renal disease. These lesions must be followed closely with renal ultrasound every 1 to 3 years and preferably by someone experienced in TSC, as these lesions may require embolization or nephrectomy.[11] Polycystic renal disease occurs in about one fifth of patients, specifically those having a deletion of TSC2 and the contiguous gene, APKD1. Pulmonary lymphangiomyomatosis occurs almost exclusively in women and may present in early to midadulthood with sudden onset of dyspnea. Therefore, patients with TSC who may have some or no involvement during childhood are at risk of future complications as adults and must be monitored appropriately. Relatives of patients with TSC should also undergo evaluation, as some individuals who have had no clinical consequences as children may go on to have life-threatening complications as adults.

Neurofibromatosis

Neurofibromatosis type 1 (NF1) is an autosomal dominant condition that affects 1 in 3000 people in the United States.[12] Its clinical manifestations include café au lait spots, neurofibromas, axillary or inguinal freckling, optic gliomas, Lisch nodules, and tibial dysplasia. Many of these features are readily seen in or before adolescence. The dermatofibromas continue to grow throughout the patient's lifetime, with a particular increase in growth rate during puberty and pregnancy. These lesions are rarely malignant but are worrisome for their cosmetic appearance for most patients. Plexiform fibromas are congenital but may not be visible initially. These continue to grow, and they envelop the nerve and sometimes the surrounding tissue. Growth may be disfiguring and may lead to neurologic involvement, including paresthesias and pain. Patients also carry a 10% lifetime risk of malignant nerve sheath tumors.[13] Partial removal is palliative and should be done by an experienced surgeon.

Patients are also at an increased risk of high blood pressure, which may be essential hypertension but vasculopathy is also seen. Neurofibromatosis type 1 vasculopathy may present as stenosis of any artery, but renal, aortic, and carotid artery stenoses have the highest morbidity. Overall, the lifespan of someone with NF1 is reduced by approximately 15 years due to vasculopathy and malignancy.[12]

Patients with NF1 also have higher complaints of neuropsychiatric issues. Nearly half complain of headache. These headaches do not respond to migraine treatment regimens but respond better to chronic pain management. A seizure disorder is seen in 5% to 10% of patients and responds to the usual antiepileptic drugs. These patients also have a higher incidence of mental retardation (8% to 10%), and half have learning disabilities.[14] Any adult patients with NF1 need to be carefully monitored for neuropsychiatric symptoms, seizures, and brain tumors as well as for behavioral and affective disorders. Although diagnostic testing for NF1 is available, clinical diagnostic criteria are well characterized, sensitive, and quite specific.[15] Relatives of patients should be screened clinically for signs of NF1, as some may have only skin lesions but remain undiagnosed.

Myotonic Dystrophy

Myotonic dystrophy is an autosomal dominant disorder characterized by skeletal muscle myotonia, progressive myopathy, and abnormalities in the heart, brain, and endocrine system.[16] This can be phenotypically variable and show clinical anticipation (Table 43-1). Expansion of the number of repeats to more than 1000 presents as infantile hypotonia, mental retardation, and respiratory deficits. It is recommended that patients with myotonic dystrophy have yearly electrocardiographic or Holter monitoring, be followed up by an ophthalmologist for evaluation of cataracts, and have an annual endocrine evaluation consisting of fasting serum glucose and thyrotropin levels. Virtually all people with myotonic dystrophy have a parent with it. Due to genetic anticipation, some parents may have less severe forms, such as mild or classical myotonic dystrophy. Once an affected family is identified, all first-degree relatives should be offered testing.

PULMONOLOGY

Emphysema is associated with genetic disorders of connective tissue such as Marfan syndrome and Ehlers-Danlos syndrome, as well as α_1-antitrypsin deficiency (AAT). An autosomal recessive disorder, AAT has a prevalence of 1 in 3000 in the United States. In homozygous-deficient infants, neonatal cholestasis progressing to cirrhosis of the liver may develop in early childhood. Approximately 20% of adults will show cirrhosis. Heterozygous individuals have an increased risk of liver disease, connective tissue disease, inflammatory eye disorders, glomerulonephritis, and panacinar emphysema. Confirmation of AAT can be made by the reduction of α_1-antitrypsin activity levels or by identification of α_1-antitrypsin isoenzymes by electrophoresis. Heterozygotes should be strongly advised against chronic smoke exposure to avoid increasing the risk of emphysema.

CARDIOLOGY

Heart disease is a complex disease and one of the leading causes of death. There are many known risk factors, including heritable traits such as low-density lipoprotein cholesterol (LDL-C), high-density lipoprotein cholesterol (HDL-C), homocysteine, and triglyceride levels as well as dysrhythmias and cardiomyopathies. Overall, there are more than 400 single genes that can contribute to heart disease and many more genes that can cause other disorders that predispose an individual to the development of heart disease. It is difficult to imagine using genetic testing in most individuals to predict a predisposition to heart disease given its complexity. However, certain diseases predisposing to heart disease are more amenable to identification and early intervention.

Hypertension

Essential hypertension accounts for 90% to 95% of all cases of hypertension. It occurs in approximately 25% of the general population and is more common among African Americans. Heritability is estimated to be about 50%. Hypertension is a complex disease with many environmental factors, and more than 100 genes have been proposed to affect blood pressure. Several genes have been implicated as important contributing factors, including an M235T variant of the angiotensinogen gene that has been associated with HTN in 70% of African-Americans. Further delineation of the genetic causes and the pathophysiology may influence the medical management of HTN.

Venous Thrombosis

Venous thromboses are associated with Virchow's triad: stasis, vascular injury, and hypercoagulability. Hypercoagulability may be caused by medications, cancer, pregnancy, or a genetic defect. Briefly, protein C, protein S, and antithrombin deficiency are disorders of coagulation factor inhibitors. These deficiencies are associated with the first occurrence of venous thrombosis before the age of 60 years. Activated protein C due to factor V Leiden, prothrombin gene mutations, and to dysfibrinogenemia cause an increase in the functional levels of coagulation proteins and are associated with venous thrombosis after the age of 60 years. Hyperhomocysteinemia is also associated with venous thrombosis as well as arterial disease. Anyone with a family history of deep-vein thrombosis (DVT) should be advised to avoid prolonged stasis. With the first episode of DVT, it may be prudent to screen for known congenital predisposing factors.

Hypertrophic Cardiomyopathy

Hypertrophic cardiomyopathy (HCM) is a disease of contractile sarcomeric apparatus. Mutations in 11 sarcomeric proteins to date have been identified that predispose to HCM. Mutations in the β-myosin heavy chain, myosin binding protein-C, and cardiac troponin T account for nearly two thirds of all cases of HCM. These defects impair myocyte function leading to increased stress, which, in turn, induces cardiac hypertrophy, interstitial fibrosis, and myocyte disarray.

GASTROENTEROLOGY

Hereditary hemochromatosis (HH), an autosomal recessive disorder of iron metabolism, is one of the most common single-gene disorders, affecting nearly 1 million people in the United States. Eighty-five percent to 90% of HH is caused by a mutation in the HFE gene, and 1 in 20 people of Northern European ancestry is a carrier for one of the mutations. Those carrying 2 mutations are at risk of diabetes, hepatic cirrhosis, liver cancer, heart failure, and hypogonadism due to iron overload. These complications can be avoided and in some cases reversed by the removal of iron with phlebotomy. There are only a few mutations known of HFE, and C282Y (a cysteine is substituted for a tyrosine reside at amino acid 282) accounts for nearly all cases of HH either in the homozygous (C282Y/C282Y) or compound heterozygous (C282Y/H63D) state. Because the disease process is amenable to identification and prevention, genetic testing is an attractive option. Massive population screening has been proposed, but findings from a multitude of studies have questioned the penetrance of carrying 2 mutations. Thus, detection of the C282Y mutation, either in homozygous or compound heterozygous forms, may label a person with hemochromatosis, but that person may never have a clinical presentation. For those at risk, screening with serum percent transferrin saturation and ferritin is more disease specific and sensitive. Transferrin saturation above 45% identifies 98% of individuals with a genetic defect in the HFE gene. Those at risk may benefit from a reduction in excess iron intake by limiting foods rich in iron, abstinence of alcohol, and avoidance of supplements containing iron or vitamin C.

NEPHROLOGY

Autosomal dominant polycystic kidney disease (ADPKD) is characterized by progressive cyst development leading to enlarged, polycystic kidneys. This disease has a variable presentation, genetic heterogeneity involving 2 genes (PKD1 and PKD2), has nearly 100% penetrance by age 80 years, and accounts for nearly 10% of all end-stage renal disease. Typically, ADPKD presents between the ages of 15 and 30 years. Slowly progressive renal failure becomes evident usually by the fourth decade of life and results in end-stage renal disease in approximately 50% by 60 years of age.[17] Cysts also can be found in extrarenal organs, such as the liver, pancreas, seminal vesicles, and arachnoid membrane.

Polycystic liver disease is the most common extrarenal manifestation of ADPKD, with 75% having hepatic cysts after the sixth decade.[18] These hepatic cysts are usually asymptomatic. However, the cysts can rupture, hemorrhage, or become infected. They may also cause extrinsic compression of the hepatic veins, the inferior vena cava, and the bile duct. Mitral valve prolapse has been demonstrated in up to 25% of patients. Intracranial aneurysms occur in approximately 10% of individuals with ADPKD. Patients with ADPKD and a family history of intracranial aneurysms are at increased risk of intracranial aneurysm compared with those who do not have a family history (22% vs 6%).[19]

Autosomal dominant polycystic kidney disease is diagnosed by the presence and number of renal cysts, based on age.[17] Patients who have a family member with ADPKD and who meet the age-related criteria can be definitively diagnosed. Molecular testing may be used for those with renal and extrarenal cysts not yet meeting the age-related criteria. A family history of ADPKD can be suspected in first-degree relatives having extrarenal manifestations such as hernias, aneurysms, mitral valve prolapse, and hypertension. First-degree relatives of a patient with ADPKD should be offered counseling, renal ultrasound examinations, and molecular testing.

REPRODUCTIVE HEALTH

Infertility affects about 5% of the male population. Most causes are unknown. However, genetic causes of male infertility are being investigated. To date, some of the genetic causes include Klinefelter syndrome, congenital bilateral absence of vas deferens (CBAVD), Y-chromosome microdeletions, and androgen receptor mutations (Table 43-1).

Klinefelter syndrome is the most common sex chromosome abnormality and is the most common cause for male hypogonadism and infertility. Typically, males present in late adolescence or adulthood with a eunuchoid appearance, gynecomastia, micro-orchidism, or infertility. Sexual drive is reduced and can be treated by testosterone supplementation. Although infertility is the rule, advances in reproductive technology have allowed some patients to become fathers using intracytoplasmic sperm injection.

Congenital bilateral absence of vas deferens resulting in azoospermia may be seen in cystic fibrosis as the result of 2 mutations in the CFTR gene. It is also seen in the presence of 1 or 2 5T tract alleles with or without the presence of a known CFTR mutation. Because CBAVD does not alter testicular development or spermatogenesis, individuals with CBAVD are candidates for assisted reproductive technologies.

ENDOCRINOLOGY

Diabetes

Type 1 diabetes mellitus (DM) is a multifactorial disease with a strong genetic component. Fifty percent of monozygotic twins will have concordance. However, less than 10% of first-degree relatives are known to be affected. There is a strong linkage to the genetic loci containing antigens HLA-

DR3, HLA-DR4, and HLA-DQ, which supports the proposal that type 1 DM is an autoimmune disorder.

Type 2 DM is a complex disease and accounts for most cases of diabetes, with approximately 5% of all Americans affected and a prevalence as high as 12% in African Americans, Hispanics, and Native Americans. It has a concordance rate in identical twins of 90%, suggesting a strong genetic predisposition. Furthermore, siblings of a person with type 2 DM have up to a 40% chance of type 2 DM themselves, and children of a person with type 2 DM have about a 33% risk.

The presence of type 2 DM presenting in childhood is known as maturity onset of diabetes in the young (MODY). A milder form, MODY is genetically heterogeneous with at least 3 forms, all of which are autosomal dominant. Despite the milder elevations of plasma glucose, these patients are still at risk of the same diabetic complications.

Polycystic Ovary Syndrome

Polycystic ovary syndrome (PCOS) is a common endocrine disorder in women of reproductive age, especially adolescents. The disorder is characterized by hyperandrogenism, menstrual irregularities, central obesity, and hyperinsulinemia. This syndrome is associated with an increased risk of infertility, type 2 DM, dyslipidemia, cardiovascular disease, and endometrial cancer. The genetic basis of PCOS is largely unknown, but there is a strong familial component. There are several candidate genes leading to susceptibility, including insulin minisatellite located 596 base pairs (bp) upstream of the insulin promoter, CYP11A (cholesterol side chain cleavage) gene, and a polymorphic variant in the insulin receptor gene.[20] Treatment with metformin during pregnancy reduces the rate of spontaneous abortions and gestational diabetes, and is not associated with any adverse affects on birth weight, developmental achievement at 6 months of age, or birth defects.[21]

Pendred Syndrome

Pendred syndrome involves severe to profound congenital sensorineural hearing loss and related abnormality of the bony labyrinth. It is an autosomal recessive condition, so patients are unlikely to have a family history. All patients with Pendred syndrome should be monitored for a euthymic goiter, which presents in nearly 75% of patients.[22]

MUSCULOSKELETAL DISORDERS

Marfan Syndrome

Marfan syndrome is a systemic disorder of connective tissue with a high degree of clinical variability and a prevalence of 1 in 3000 to 5000. Patients with Marfan syndrome may present in the neonatal period throughout adulthood. Clinical manifestations involve the ocular, skeletal, and cardiovascular systems (Table 43-2). Cardiovascular manifestations, which are the major sources of morbidity and mortality, include dilation of the aorta with a predisposition for aortic tear and rupture, mitral valve prolapse with or without regurgitation, tricuspid valve prolapse, and enlargement of the proximal pulmonary artery. With proper management, the life expectancy for someone with Marfan syndrome approximates that of the general population.

The diagnosis of Marfan syndrome is based on clinical manifestations. The family history may be remarkable for disproportionate tallness for family, retinal detachment, recurrent hernias, spontaneous pneumothorax, or sudden death due to aortic dissection. Any individual with suspected Marfan syndrome and a family history of aortic dissection is especially at increased risk of aortic dissection. For women with Marfan syndrome, pregnancy can be complicated by further progression of aortic dilation. These women should be counseled before conception and evaluated appropriately during pregnancy. Any first-degree relative of those suspected of having Marfan syndrome warrants detailed physical, ophthalmologic, orthopedic, and cardiac evaluation in addition to genetic counseling.

Ehlers-Danlos Syndrome

There are several types of Ehlers-Danlos syndrome (Table 43-2). In general, these types demonstrate joint laxity, hyperextensibility of skin, and poor wound healing with widened atrophic scars. Adults with Ehlers-Danlos syndrome have a much higher incidence of aortic root dilation and possible rupture or dissection.[23] They may also have chronic joint pain and develop joint dislocations, as well as degenerative joint disease due to their joint hypermobility.

RHEUMATOLOGY

Rheumatoid Arthritis

Rheumatoid arthritis is a chronic systemic inflammatory disease that afflicts 0.1% to 2% of the general population. Genetic linkage has been found with certain HLA haplotypes. The lifetime risk of those homozygous for an HLA-DRB1 allele was found to be 41% to 48%.

Systemic Lupus Erythematosus

Systemic lupus erythematosus (SLE) is a multisystem inflammatory disorder with a prevalence of 1 per 2500 people in the United States and a female-to-male ratio of 9:1.[24] It is of unknown etiology; however, epidemiologic evidence supports a strong genetic component with an overall tenfold greater risk than expected of SLE in

TABLE 43-2

Syndromes With Primary Musculoskeletal Involvement*

Syndrome	Inheritance	Gene Involved	Features
Ehlers-Danlos syndrome			
Classical type	AD	COL5A1, COL5A2	Skin hyperextensibility; widened atrophic scars; joint hypermobility
Hypermobile type	AD	Unknown	Smooth, velvety skin or skin hyperextensibility; joint hypermobility
Vascular type	AD	COL3A1	Thin, almost translucent skin; arterial fragility; easy bruisability; characteristic facies
Marfan syndrome	AD	FBN1, FBN2	Aortic root dilation; ectopia lentis; retinal detachment; pectus excavatum/carinatum scoliosis; lumbosacral dural ectasia
Congenital contractural arachnodactyly	AD	FBN2	Contractural arachnodactyly; kyphoscoliosis; valvular defects
MASS** phenotype	AD	FBN1	Myopia; mitral valve prolapse; mild aortic dilatation; striae; skeletal (marfanoid)
Homocystinuria	AR	CBS, NTHFR	Ectopia lentis; marfanoid habitus; hypercoagulability
Stickler syndrome	AD	COL2A1, COL11A1, COL11A2	High myopia; retinal detachment; deafness; micrognathia; cleft palate; arthropathy

*AD indicates autosomal dominant; AR, autosomal recessive.

**MASS indicates mitral value prolapse, mild aortic dilatation, skeletal and skin involvement.

monozygotic twins.[25] Multiple genetic loci have been linked to SLE but are without clinical significance at this time.

PSYCHIATRY

Schizophrenia

Schizophrenia is a complex, multifactorial disease with a worldwide prevalence of approximately 1%. Although multifactorial, it has a strong heritability component. Concordance among monozygotic twins is 40% to 90%. Additionally, based on epidemiologic evidence, a child of a couple who each has schizophrenia has a lifetime risk of the disease of 15% to 55%.

Finding a major genetic contribution has remained elusive. However, at least 7 loci have been found with significant linkage. It is clear from previous studies that a single locus in a given family can be a strong familial predisposing factor. For example, catechol O-methyltransferase (COMT) is an enzyme that degrades catecholamines. The COMT haplotype was found to highly correspond to the development of schizophrenia in an Ashkenazi Jewish population.[26] The COMT gene also resides on chromosome 22q11 and is commonly deleted in the contiguous gene deletion syndrome, velocardiofacial syndrome. Approximately 20% to 30% of patients with velocardiofacial syndrome have been found to have schizophrenia.[27]

Bipolar Disorder

Bipolar disorder, also known as manic-depressive psychosis, involves alternating episodes of mania (type 1) or hypomania (type 2) with depression. Concordance for monozygotic twins is 57% and for dizygotic is 14%. Pedigree analysis suggests that bipolar disorder undergoes clinical anticipation with successive generations (Table 43-1). However, candidate genes with trinucleotide repeats have not consistently been associated with the occurrence of bipolar disorder.

ONCOLOGY

Breast Cancer

Five percent to 10% of breast cancer is related to a single gene defect. Breast cancer with an underlying single gene defect may present as early-onset or bilateral disease or both. Patients may have multiple affected relatives with breast cancer or higher incidences of ovarian, colorectal, pancreatic, and prostate cancer, as well as melanoma.

The most common single gene defects for breast cancer are BRCA-1 and BRAC-2. Both genes encode tumor suppressors. Inheritance of just one copy of either gene increases a woman's lifetime risk of breast cancer to 50% to 85% compared with 12% in the general population. Any patient with breast cancer or a family history of breast cancer with early onset or bilateral disease should be offered counseling and testing for BRCA-1 or BRCA-2. If a patient is found to carry one of the BRCA-1 and 2 mutations, further counseling and prophylactic mastectomy should be offered. Prophylactic mastectomy has been found to significantly reduce a woman's chance of breast cancer.[28] Alternatively, patients may elect chemoprevention with tamoxifen, which may reduce the occurrence of a second primary breast cancer by as much as 50% to 75%.[29] Once diagnosed with breast cancer, BRCA-1 and -2 carriers need intensive follow-up not only for the initial primary lesion but also because these patients have a 10% to 20% risk of a second breast cancer and higher incidences of other cancers.

BRCA-1 and -2 carriers also have a significant risk of ovarian cancer, with a lifetime prevalence of 20% to 40% compared with 1% in the general population. Patients who are found to be carriers of BRCA-1 and -2 mutations should be counseled and offered prophylactic oophorectomy. Removal of both ovaries reduces the risk of ovarian cancer by 95%.[29] This is not 100% effective, as some ovarian cells remain in the peritoneum along the tracts of the developmental descent of the gonads.

Colorectal Cancer

Familial adenomatous polyposis (FAP) accounts for less than 1% of all colorectal cancers. Patients with FAP present with polyps in their teens and continue to have tens, hundreds, or even thousands of polyps in their lifetime. Each polyp has a malignant potential. It is estimated that the lifetime incidence of colorectal cancer is nearly 100%. Most individuals inherit the adenomatous polyposis (APC) mutation from 1 parent and, therefore, have a known family history. Family history may also be remarkable for associated features such as gastric polyps, dental anomalies, desmoid tumors, and osteomas. The incidence rates of other cancers in the family may also be increased.[30]

Familial adenomatous polyposis should be suspected in anyone presenting with polyps at a young age or with multiple polyps. It can be clinically diagnosed when someone has more than 100 polyps or has fewer than 100 polyps but has a first-degree relative with FAP. Confirmation can be obtained by molecular testing, which detects approximately 95% of cases. Any first-degree relative should be counseled and offered colonoscopy and molecular genetic testing.[31] Any individual with a known APC mutation should be evaluated routinely by colonoscopy and offered colectomy when adenomatous polyps begin to develop, which often occurs in the second or third decade of life.

Hereditary nonpolyposis colorectal cancer (HNPCC) is an autosomal dominant trait that accounts for 3% to 5% of all colorectal cancers. The lifetime risk of CRC is approximately 80% compared with a general population risk of 2%. Also, HNPCC increases the risk of endometrial cancer to a lifetime risk of 40% to 60% vs a population risk of 1.5% for women. Aggressive surveillance with colonoscopy reduces the mortality associated with HNPCC. Subtotal colectomy should be considered for those at risk and has been shown to reduce the occurrence of a second colorectal cancer. Women carrying HNPCC mutations should consider total hysterectomy with bilateral salpingo-oophorectomy for prevention of endometrial and ovarian cancer.

Prostate Cancer

Prostate cancer occurs in as many as 1 in 8 American men during their lifetime and is the second leading cause of cancer deaths among men in the United States.[32] Nearly all of these cases are sporadic; however, familial clustering has been demonstrated in up to 10%.[33] Screening for prostate cancer has been debated for its efficacy, and studies are under way to evaluate this. However, it may be useful to identify those individuals at higher risk. High-risk families can be identified if they meet the Hopkins criteria,[34] which include:

1. 3 or more first-degree relatives with prostate cancer
2. 3 or more generations from either the maternal or paternal side with prostate cancer
3. a cluster of 2 relatives affected before the age of 55 years

Segregation analyses of familial prostate cancer suggests the existence of multiple, highly penetrant, susceptibility alleles. Although multiple genetic loci have been linked to prostate cancer susceptibility, only a few genes have been identified. Recently, it was found that CAG repeats in the androgen receptor (AR) gene inversely correlate with disease susceptibility (Table 43-1).[35] The expanded repeat sequences in AR are thought to reduce expression of the gene product. This corresponds to the observation of the lower incidence among Asians, who have a higher number of repeats in the AR gene, and also the higher incidence of prostate cancer among African Americans, who have a lower number of CAG repeats. This increased susceptibility is likely due to a shift in the age at onset seen in those individuals with the fewest CAG repeats in the AR gene.[36]

There is a higher incidence of prostate cancer among families with heritable breast cancer. In a study of 263 men with prostate cancer before the age of 55 years, 2.3% had mutations in the breast-ovarian cancer susceptibility gene BRCA-2.[37] It was also found that males of first-degree relatives who had breast cancer carrying a BRCA-2 mutation had a relative risk of 7.3 for development of prostate cancer before age 65 years.[38] Similar results were also found in known BRCA-1 mutation carriers, with a relative risk of 1.8 before the age of 65.[39] It is unknown whether these individuals at higher risk would have better health outcomes if screening measures were started earlier than 50 years of age.

Melanoma

Multiple risk factors for melanoma are well known and include the number of melanocytic nevi, propensity to sunburn, number of sunburn episodes during youth, and presence of dysplastic nevi. Additionally, it is noted that there is a familial tendency that may be related to freckling tendency, lighter skin tones, and red hair color. Familial cutaneous malignant melanoma, also known as dysplastic nevus syndrome, usually has an earlier age at onset, has a smaller diameter of the lesion, and carries an increased risk of multiple primary tumors. Patients usually have 10 to 100 moles on their upper torso and limbs. Germline mutations in CDKN2A and CDK4 have been found in more than half of families. Melanoma may also be seen associated with other family cancer syndromes, including Li-Fraumeni and breast/ovarian cancer involving BRCA-2 mutations. Anyone with known risk factors, especially a family history of melanoma, should be instructed to observe any moles for dysplastic changes and should be seen on an annual basis.

Multiple Endocrine Neoplasia

Multiple endocrine neoplasia type 2 (MEN2) is an autosomal dominant disorder and is classified into 3 subtypes: MEN2A, familial medullary thyroid carcinoma (FMTC), and MEN2B. All carry the risk of the development of medullary thyroid carcinoma (MTC). Both MEN2A and MEN2B carry a 50% risk of pheochromocytoma. The MEN2A subtype is associated with parathyroid adenoma or hyperplasia, whereas MEN2B is distinguished by a marfanoid habitus, neuromas of the lips and tongue, and ganglioneuromas of the gastrointestinal tract. All subtypes are due to mutations in the RET oncogene. Mutations have a specific genotype-phenotype correlation for the different subtypes.

Most patients present with MTC from 5 to 25 years of age with biochemical disease or a painful neck mass or both. If presentation occurs with neck pain or a mass, more than 50% of these patients already have metastatic disease.[40] Some will present with hypertension related to a pheochromocytoma. Once a person is identified with MEN2, careful screening for a pheochromocytoma is needed, which may be bilateral. Malignant transformation occurs in about 4%. However, death can occur due to anesthesia-induced hypertensive crisis. In MEN2B, these patients present shortly after birth with mucosal neuromas. Once identified, thyroidectomy usually is done at about 1 year of age due to the occurrence of earlier and more severe onset of MTC in MEN2B.

Family history is usually remarkable for a parent or sibling with MTC, if not MEN2. A personal history of Hirschsprung disease is seen in some, as this may also be caused by mutations in the RET gene. Those with a suspected family history or relatives of a known patient should undergo genetic testing at less than 5 years of age

for MEN2A and FMTC, and at less than 1 year for MEN2B. Genetic testing detects greater than 90% of RET mutations associated with MEN2. Prophylactic thyroidectomy is recommended as early as ages 3 to 5 years for MEN2A and FMTC, and at 1 year of age for MEN2B. Thyroidectomy usually is accompanied by parathyroid autotransplantation. Screening for a pheochromocytoma should be done before thyroidectomy to avoid perioperative crises. Patients should continue to have biochemical screening for a pheochromocytoma annually. Those individuals at risk but not identified by genetic testing should undergo annual calcitonin stimulation testing in addition to biochemical pheochromocytoma screening.

Li-Fraumeni Syndrome

Li-Fraumeni syndrome is an autosomal dominant cancer predisposition syndrome. Affected patients are at a considerably increased risk of multiple primary cancers involving the colon, brain, breast, adrenal cortex, and pancreas in addition to soft-tissue sarcoma, leukemia, osteosarcoma, and melanoma. Greater than 50% have identifiable disease-causing mutations in the tumor suppressor gene, TP53.[41] Those without TP53 gene mutations may have mutations in the CHEK2 gene. The cancer risk in Li-Fraumeni syndrome is 50% by age 40 years and 90% by age 60. A second primary tumor develops in 15% of those with the syndrome in their lifetime.

Other Cancers

Molecular testing should be offered to anyone having a sarcoma, brain tumor, breast cancer, or adrenocortical tumor before the age of 36 years and at least 1 first-degree relative with cancer younger than 46 years, anyone with a relative having multiple primary tumors at any age, or anyone with multiple primary tumors with the initial one occurring before 36 years. Recommended surveillance includes breast cancer monitoring, urinalysis, and annual abdominal ultrasound examination. Breast cancer monitoring includes semiannual clinical breast examination and annual mammography. Due to the potential radiosensitivity of cells with a germline p53 mutation, some advocate annual breast ultrasounds or magnetic resonance imaging (MRI) instead of mammography.[42]

TRANSITIONAL CARE

Many genetic syndromes present and are traditionally managed in the pediatric population. Current management of many such syndromes has increased life expectancy and hopefully quality of life. For example, people with cystic fibrosis who previously had a life expectancy in their teens are now living into their late 20s and even 30s. Although many pediatric subspecialists are capable of continuing the patient's care related to their underlying disorder, these patients have other age-related medical and emotional needs. Patients are encouraged in adolescence to start asserting independence and medical decision making. As young adults, these same individuals have vocational, financial, and psychosocial concerns. Additionally, they are also susceptible to the same illnesses and age-related disorders as in the general population. As adults, these patients are best served by an adult primary care physician with continued subspecialty supervision. Transitional care should be considered in adolescence, which involves empowering the patient and establishing the patient-physician relationship of an adult provider. Transition can be done over a long period such as years but should be mapped out carefully with the patient and family.

Down Syndrome

Down syndrome is the most common genetic cause of mental retardation occurring in about 1 in 600 to 700 newborns. The genetic defect involves the presence of a third copy of at least part of chromosome 21, with 95% having a pure trisomy 21. Clinical features include characteristic facial features, hypotonia, congenital heart defects, gastrointestinal anomalies, and mild to moderate mental retardation. There is also an approximately 1% chance of leukemia, which usually presents in childhood. With age, these individuals have increasing challenges for education and social needs. It is not uncommon to have behavior disorders and depression secondary to poor socialization. Most remain dependent but can gain productive skills and self-confidence through vocational training. In the third and fourth decades of life, there is a much higher incidence of AD, and nearly all have histopathologic features at autopsy.

Fragile X Syndrome

Fragile X syndrome is the most common form of inherited mental retardation. It is caused by the expanded repeat of the trinucleotide (CGG) in the fragile X mental retardation gene 1 (Table 43-1). Those with 50 to 200 repeats were once thought of as silent carriers but have now been recognized as having milder involvement. The classic physical appearance includes an elongated face, large prominent ears, prognathism, and macro-orchidism. They also have connective tissue dysplasia giving them joint hyperextensibility and making them more prone to dislocations, scoliosis, flat feet, and degenerative joint disease. Approximately half of adult patients with fragile X syndrome also have mitral valve prolapse and hypertension, and appropriate anticipatory management is indicated. Women who are permutation carriers have an approximately 25% risk of premature menopause as early as their 20s.[43]

Adults with fragile X syndrome have difficulty transitioning. The mental retardation varies greatly but is usually moderate to severe. Hyperactivity and impulsivity are common problems in childhood but may be less severe in adolescence and adulthood. Anxiety disorders, especially social anxiety, are very common among both males and females with fragile X. Males with an anxiety disorder may be more prone to aggressive or violent behavior. Obsessive-compulsive disorder and psychosis are also more common. Transition becomes more difficult in attempting to train these individuals to be a productive part of society, given their mental capacity and neuropsychological behaviors. Fortunately, patients with fragile X typically respond to the standard pharmacologic management of these disorders.

Velocardiofacial (DiGeorge) Syndrome

Velocardiofacial syndrome, also known as DiGeorge syndrome, is a highly variable disorder that is due to a microdeletion of chromosome 22q11.2. Those affected may have characteristic facies, cleft palate, conotruncal cardiac lesions, and renal anomalies. These patients commonly have mild developmental delays most notably in speech, learning disabilities, and hypernasal speech. In adolescence, those affected exhibit social immaturity, phobias, and other psychiatric illnesses. Young adults with velocardiofacial syndrome are at approximately 20% risk of bipolar disorder or schizophrenia.[27]

Williams Syndrome

Williams syndrome is a microdeletion disorder that involves the elastin gene located on chromosome 7q11.23. Affected persons have a constellation of features, including dysmorphic facies, short stature, idiopathic hypercalcemia, joint laxity, supravalvular stenosis, developmental delays, and peculiar personality traits. The facial characteristics coarsen into adulthood. They typically have a gaunt appearance, prominent supraorbital brow, broad nasal tip, and wide mouths with full lips. The elastin defect can cause a generalized arterial stenosis but its most common feature is the supravalvular aortic stenosis, encountered in 75% of cases.[44] Supravalvular aortic stenosis and pulmonic artery stenosis may cause cardiac hypertrophy and may result in congestive heart failure, and renal artery stenosis may cause hypertension. Hypertension can be adequately treated with β-blockade in most cases. In severe forms of stenosis, surgical repair of the aorta or other arteries may be necessary. Most patients with Williams syndrome have mild mental retardation and remarkable auditory rote memory and language skills, but they perform poorly in visual spatial tasks. Vocational training needs to begin in adolescence through early adulthood. Health supervision guidelines are available.[45]

Prader-Willi Syndrome

Prader-Willi syndrome is characterized by hypotonia, obesity, mental retardation, hypogonadism, and characteristic behaviors. It is the result of a microdeletion of the long arm of chromosome 15. It is the most common genetic cause of obesity, with an overall incidence of 1 in 15,000. Adults usually remain mildly hypotonic, obese, mildly mentally retarded, hypogonadic, and infertile. In early childhood, these patients exhibit hyperphagia and lack of satiety. They may gorge themselves on food without vomiting and eat garbage, spoiled foods, and frozen foods, as well as pet foods. They may hoard food and actively steal food or money to buy food. Other behaviors manifesting in childhood or adulthood include aggressiveness, lying, stealing, obsessive-compulsive tendencies, and stubbornness. Complications of obesity are the major cause of morbidity and mortality in these patients, including sleep apnea, type 2 DM, and hypertension. Management includes strict routines and making unavailable all foods other than those on their nutritional plan.

SUMMARY

With the advancement of the Human Genome Initiative, the field of genetics has moved from one gene: one phenotype in many "classic" genetic diseases to understanding how the gene products function on a molecular level. Gene expression is influenced by other genes and environmental factors such as nutritional components, smoking, or obesity among many. The information that is being acquired about our genes and their products is exploding, but we are far from understanding all of the myriad of factors that interact on the molecular level to affect the function of a particular gene product. What is becoming clear is that certain environmental factors have a larger contribution to the phenotype of a complex trait if that person has a genetic predisposition. For example, a gene may have an allelic variant that reduces its expression by 30%, which in itself is not sufficient to cause disease. However, when one is exposed to the proper environmental factor(s), usually on a chronic basis, this combination leads to a disease state. The future of genetics in clinical practice will include the ability to identify those people who are genetically susceptible to a given disease, counsel them to avoid the known environmental triggers, and monitor those patients carefully for the signs and symptoms of those diseases.

REFERENCES

1. Khoury MJ, Burke W, Thomson EJ. Genetics and public health: a framework for the integration of human genetics into public health practice. In: Khoury MJ, Burke W, Thomson EJ, eds. *Genetics and Public Health in the 21st Century: Using Genetic Information to Improve Health and Prevent Disease.* New York, NY: Oxford University Press; 2000.

2. Stone EM, Sheffield VC, Hageman GS. Molecular genetics of age-related macular degeneration. *Hum Mol Genetics.* 2001;10:2285–2292.

3. Musarella MA. Molecular genetics of macular degeneration. *Doc Ophthalmol.* 2001;102:165–177.

4. Bouzas EA, Perry DM, Eldridge R, et al. Visual impairment in patients with neurofibromatosis 2. *Neurology.* 1993;43:622–623.

5. Endres W. Inherited metabolic diseases affecting the carrier. *J Inherit Metab Dis.* 1997;20:9–20.

6. Saleem RA, Walter MA. The complexities of ocular genetics. *Clin Genetics.* 2002;61:79–88.

7. Schott JM, Fox NC, Rossor MN. Genetics of the dementias. *J Neurol Neurosurg Psychiatry.* 2002;73(suppl 2):II27–31.

8. Breitner JC, Wyse BW, Anthony JC, et al. APOE-epsilon4 count predicts age when prevalence of AD increases, then declines: the Cache County Study. *Neurology.* 1999;53:321–331.

9. Bird TD. Hereditary ataxia overview. *GeneReviews.* Available at: www.geneclinics.org. Accessed July 23, 2003.

10. Osborne JP, Fryer A, Webb D. Epidemiology of tuberous sclerosis. *Ann N Y Acad Sci.* 1991;615:125–127.

11. van Baal JG, Smits NJ, Keeman JN, Lindhout D, Verhoef S. The evolution of renal angiomyolipomas in patients with tuberous sclerosis. *J Urol.* 1994;152:35–38.

12. Rasmussen SA, Yang Q, Friedman JM. Mortality in neurofibromatosis 1: an analysis using U.S. death certificates. *Am J Hum Genetics.* 2001;68:1110–1118.

13. Evans DG, Baser ME, McGaughran J, Sharif S, Howard E, Moran A. Malignant peripheral nerve sheath tumours in neurofibromatosis 1. *J Med Genetics.* 2002;39:311–314.

14. North KN, Riccardi V, Samango-Sprouse C, et al. Cognitive function and academic performance in neurofibromatosis 1: consensus statement from the NF1 Cognitive Disorders Task Force. *Neurology.* 1997;48:1121–1127.

15. Gutmann DH, Aylsworth A, Carey JC, et al. The diagnostic evaluation and multidisciplinary management of neurofibromatosis 1 and neurofibromatosis 2. *JAMA.* 1997;278:51–57.

16. Harper PS. Myotonic dystrophy and other autosomal dominant muscular dystrophies. In: Scriver CR, Beaudet AL, Sly Ws, Valle D, eds. *The Metabolic and Molecular Basis of Inherited Disease.* New York, NY: McGraw-Hill; 1995:4227–4251.

17. Ravine D, Gibson RN, Walker RG, Sheffield LJ, Kincaid-Smith P, Danks DM. Evaluation of ultrasonographic diagnostic criteria for autosomal dominant polycystic kidney disease 1. *Lancet.* 1994;343:824–827.

18. Torres V. Polycystic liver disease. In Watson MT, Torres VE, eds. *Polycystic Kidney Disease.* Oxford, England: Oxford Medical Publications; 1996.

19. Harris PC, Torres V. Autosomal dominant polycystic kidney disease. *GeneReviews.* 2001. Available at: www.geneclinics.org. Accessed July 23, 2003.

20. Waterworth DM, Bennett ST, Gharani N, et al. Linkage and association of insulin gene VNTR regulatory polymorphism with polycystic ovary syndrome. *Lancet.* 1997;349:986–990.

21. Glueck CJ, Wang P, Goldenberg N, Sieve-Smith L. Pregnancy outcomes among women with polycystic ovary syndrome treated with metformin. *Hum Reprod.* 2002;17:2858–2864.

22. Smith RJH, Van Camp G. Pendred syndrome. *GeneReviews.* 2002. Available at: www.geneclinics.org. Accessed July 23, 2003.

23. Wenstrup RJ, Meyer RA, Lyle JS, et al. Prevalence of aortic root dilation in the Ehlers-Danlos syndrome. *Genet Med.* 2002;4:112–117.

24. Hochberg MC. The epidemiology of systemic lupus erythematosus. In: Wallace DJ, Hahn BJ, eds. *Dubois' Lupus Erythematosus.* Baltimore, Md: Williams & Wilkins; 1997.

25. Deapen D, Escalante A, Weinrib L, et al. A revised estimate of twin concordance in systemic lupus erythematosus. *Arthritis Rheum.* 1992;35:311–318.

26. Shifman S, Bronstein M, Sternfeld M, et al. A highly significant association between a COMT haplotype and schizophrenia. *Am J Hum Genet.* 2002;71:1296–1302.

27. Murphy KC, Jones LA, Owen MJ. High rates of schizophrenia in adults with velo-cardio-facial syndrome. *Arch Gen Psychiatry.* 1999;56:940–945.

28. Meijers-Heijboer H, van Geel B, van Putten WL, et al. Breast cancer after prophylactic bilateral mastectomy in women with a BRCA1 or BRCA2 mutation. *N Engl J Med.* 2001;345:159–164.

29. Narod SA, Brunet JS, Ghadirian P, et al. Tamoxifen and risk of contralateral breast cancer in BRCA1 and BRCA2 mutation carriers: a case-control study. *Lancet.* 2000;356:1876–1881.

30. Solomon C, Burt RW. Familial adenomatous polyposis. *GeneReviews.* 2002. Available at: www.geneclinics.org. Accessed July 23, 2003.

31. Heiskanen I, Luostarinen T, Jarvinen HJ. Impact of screening examinations on survival in familial adenomatous polyposis. *Scand J Gastroenterol.* 2000;35:1284–1287.

32. Reis LAG, Kosary CL, Hankey BF, Miller BA, Clegg L, Edward BK, eds. *SEER Cancer Statistics Review, 1973–96.* Bethesda, Md: National Cancer Institute; 1999.

33. Eeles RA, for UK Familial Prostate Cancer Study Collaborators. Genetic predisposition to prostate cancer. *Prostate Cancer Prostatic Dis.* 1999;2:9–15.

34. Carter BS, Bova GS, Beaty TH, et al. Hereditary prostate cancer: epidemiologic and clinical features. *J Urol.* 1993;150:797–802.

35. Nelson KA, Witte JS. Androgen receptor CAG repeats and prostate cancer. *Am J Epidemiol.* 2002;155:883–890.

36. Hardy DO, Scher HI, Bogenreider T, et al. Androgen receptor CAG repeat lengths in advanced prostate cancer: correlation with age of onset. *J Clin Endocrinol Metab.* 1996;81:4400–4405.

37. Edwards SM, Kote-Jarai Z, Meitz J, et al. Two percent of men with early-onset prostate cancer harbor germline mutations in the BRCA2 gene. *Am J Hum Genetics.* 2003;72:1–12.

38. Breast Cancer Linkage Consortium. Cancer risks in BRCA2 mutations carriers. *J Natl Cancer Inst.* 1999;91:1310–1316.

39. Thompson D, Easton DF, for Breast Cancer Linkage Consortium. Cancer incidences in BRCA1 mutation carriers. *J Natl Cancer Inst.* 2002;94:1358–1365.

40. Robbins J, Merino MJ, Boice JD Jr, et al. Thyroid cancer: a lethal endocrine neoplasm. *Ann Intern Med.* 1991;115:133–147.

41. Nichols KE, Malkin D, Garber JE, Fraumeni JF Jr, Li FP. Germ-line p53 mutations predispose to a wide spectrum of early-onset cancers. *Cancer Epidemiol Biomarkers Prev.* 2001;10:83–87.

42. Eng C, Hampel H, de la Chapelle A. Genetic testing for cancer predisposition. *Annu Rev Med.* 2000;52:371–400.

43. Allingham-Hawkins DJ, Babul-Hirji R, Chitayat D, et al. Fragile X permutation is a significant risk factor for premature ovarian failure: the International Collaborative POF in Fragile X study—preliminary data. *Am J Med Genetics.* 1999;83:322–325.

44. Morris CA, Demsey SA, Leonard CO, Dilts C, Blackburn BL. The natural history of Williams syndrome: physical characteristics. *J Pediatr.* 1988;113:318–326.

45. American Academy of Pediatrics Committee on Genetics. Health care supervision for children with Williams syndrome. *Pediatrics.* 2001;107:1192–1204.

RESOURCES

Genetic Alliance. Web site: www.geneticalliance.org. (An international coalition composed of millions of individuals with genetic conditions and more than 600 advocacy, research, and health care organizations that represent their interests.)

Online Mendelian Inheritance in Man (OMIM). Web site: www.ncbi.nlm.nih.gov/OMIM. (A catalog database of genetic conditions and their genes.)

PART 9

Cardiovascular Risk Prevention

Cardiovascular Risk Assessment and Reduction

Julie C. Huang, MD, and Dennis L. Sprecher, MD

INTRODUCTION

Cardiovascular disease (CVD) has been and remains the most prevalent disease and most potent killer of the population of the Western world. Although death rates have declined markedly in the past 40 years with advances in the understanding of its epidemiology, physiology, and pharmacology,[1] CVD continues to be the number one cause of disability, death, and expense to society. In the United States alone, approximately 1 million deaths per year are attributed to CVD.[2]

Cardiovascular disease is commonly divided into 3 major areas: (1) coronary heart disease (CHD), including myocardial infarction (MI), angina pectoris, and congestive heart failure/ischemic cardiomyopathy; (2) cerebrovascular disease, including stroke and transient ischemic attack; and (3) peripheral vascular disease (PVD), manifested by claudication or limb loss. The focus on CHD assessment reflects its prevalence of approximately one half of all CVD.[2]

The challenge to physicians through the years has been to identify those patients at danger for the development of CVD and to modify their risk, as well as to slow progression of disease in those already afflicted. The Framingham Heart Study, begun in 1948, was the first large-scale prospective epidemiologic study to address the growing epidemic, and it continues to this day. It accumulated data showing the presence of risk factors, spurring public health initiatives against cigarette smoking in the 1960s, hypertension in the 1970s, and dyslipidemia in the 1980s. Along with other studies, the Framingham Heart Study showed a strong impact on development of CVD due to diabetes mellitus, physical inactivity, obesity, menopause, and psychosocial factors. The Framingham Heart Study also identified novel risk factors, such as homocysteine and apolipoprotein E isoforms, whose significance is still under investigation.

A risk factor is the existence of a characteristic, whether genetic or behavioral, modifiable or not, that is associated with an increased risk of developing a disease. A "true" risk factor predates the disease and is therefore presumed to be associated with causality, although the elucidation of the mechanism may lag behind the discovery of the factor by many years. Most risk factors contain a gradation of risk, with the likelihood of developing disease existing in proportion to the degree of derangement; that is, a higher level of low-density lipoprotein cholesterol (LDL-C) connotes higher risk. In most instances, a decrease in the risk factor level corresponds with a decrease in risk. Therefore, an assessment of risk is accompanied by several goals: identification, modification, and decrease of total risk of disease.

Commonly accepted cardiovascular risk factors can be divided into those that can be modified and those that cannot. Nonmodifiable risk factors include the following[3]:

- Age
- Sex
- Family history

Modifiable risk factors include[3]:

- Cigarette smoking
- Hypertension
- Obesity
- Physical inactivity
- Diabetes mellitus/glucose intolerance
- Dyslipidemias

Table 44-1 provides a proposed list of serologic cardiovascular risk factors based on modification.[3]

AGE AND SEX

Age remains one of the strongest predictors of cardiovascular risk, morbidity, and mortality.[4-7] The accumulation of additional risk factors with advancing age may be inevitable in some patients; hypertension develops with decreasing arteriolar compliance, and physical inactivity and obesity increase in the setting of accompanying comorbidities. Epidemiologic data show that the risk of CHD rises dramatically in men over the age of 45 years

T A B L E   44-1

Proposed Cardiovascular Risk Factors Based on Modification*

Proatherogenic
  Homocysteine
  Lipoprotein particle oxidation
  Hyperinsulinemia
  Lipoprotein particle subspecies
  Apolipoprotein E isoforms
  Cholesteryl ester transferase protein
Prothrombinogenic
  Plasminogen
  Fibrinogen
  Factor VII
  Plasminogen activator inhibitor 1
  Lipoprotein(a)
Antiatherogenic
  Apolipoprotein A-1
  Lecithin–cholesterol acyltransferase
  Low-density lipoprotein receptor
  Very-low-density lipoprotein receptor
  Apolipoprotein E (depending on isoform)
  Interleukins 4 and 10
Transforming growth factor-β
Proinflammatory
  High-sensitivity C-reactive protein
  Intercellular adhesion molecule 1
  Interleukin 6
  Tumor necrosis factor-α

*Partial listing from Hoeg JM.[3]

and in women over the age of 55 years compared with the rise observed during the younger years.

In addition, there is a marked discrepancy in cardiovascular risk between the sexes. Whereas during the early to middle adulthood years (ages 21 to 60 years), women (particularly whites) enjoy considerable protection from heart disease, compared with men (perhaps a twofold to threefold contrast), this differential disappears in later years.[8,9] There remains, however, an approximate 10-year difference in overall mortality rates between men and women.[8] Nearly half of this earlier disparity in disease rates (30% in the group above 55 years old) is thought to be associated with known risk entities, specifically the high-density lipoprotein cholesterol (HDL-C)/total cholesterol ratio and cigarette use.[8]

FAMILY HISTORY

While family history and genetic heritage play a role in determining susceptibility to various cardiovascular risk factors such as dyslipidemia and diabetes, family history is also an independent risk factor for CVD.

A 12-year prospective study of more than 15,000 individuals in Finland showed that acute MI is associated with a family history of premature CHD (fatal or nonfatal MI or angina before the age of 60 years) in either parent. The risk ratio was 1.61 in men and 1.85 in women, with a slight decrease after adjustment for smoking, cholesterol, hypertension, diabetes, and obesity. The relative risk associated with family history was higher for early MI (less than age 55 years) vs later MI (at or greater than age 55 years) in the study population, especially in women (relative risk [RR] 2.87 vs 1.49).[10] Prospective data from the Physicians' Health Study and the Women's Health Study (female US health professionals enrolled in 1992) confirmed these findings and showed that in both men and women, having a maternal history of MI had a higher relative risk of CVD than having a paternal history. In addition, while an early history of parental MI conferred higher risk, the effect of family history was continued even to maternal ages 70 to 79 years in men and maternal age 60 years or older in women.[11]

Many studies are ongoing to discover the genetic determinants of CVD that may be contributing to the importance of family history as a risk factor.

CIGARETTE SMOKING

Cigarette smoking is the single most preventable cause of premature death in the United States. The American Heart Association estimates that it accounts for more than 400,000 deaths annually.[12] It is a powerful risk factor for CVD and is associated with increased rates of MI, sudden death, stroke, and PVD, as well as lung and other cancers and acute and chronic pulmonary disease. The dangers of cigarettes have been widely publicized, and the prevalence of adult smokers in the United States has fallen from approximately 42% in 1965 to 23% in 2000.[13] This figure, however, still represents more than 45 million smokers, and estimates exist of over 1 billion smokers worldwide.[14]

On average, the risk of MI is doubled with cigarette smoking and is related to quantity, duration, and whether smoke is inhaled.[15-17] Women appear to be more sensitive than men to current smoking as a CHD risk factor, with a relative risk in women of 3.3 and in men of 1.9 compared with people who have never smoked, according to a 12-year follow-up of the Finnmark study.[18] Low serum cholesterol levels do not confer a protective effect on CVD risk in smokers.[19] However, alcohol consumption, as reputed in the general population to be beneficial in moderate doses,[20] does have a protective effect in this group.[21,22]

In individuals who already have CHD and continue to smoke, the RR of mortality was 1.7 compared with those who quit smoking, as shown in a subgroup of the

Coronary Artery Surgery Study (CASS) registry.[23] Persistent smokers also have an increased risk of all-cause mortality (RR 1.68), cardiac death (RR 1.75), and need for revascularization (RR 1.41) after coronary artery bypass graft (CABG) surgery compared with those who quit smoking for at least 1 year.[24] In patients who underwent percutaneous coronary revascularization, persistent smokers have a greater relative risk of death (RR, 1.76) or Q-wave MI (RR, 2.08) compared with nonsmokers, as well as a greater risk of death compared with those who quit smoking (RR, 1.44).[25] The incidences of recurrent heart failure, MI, and death are significantly higher in smokers with left ventricular dysfunction compared with ex-smokers and nonsmokers.[26]

Cigarette smoking is also an independent risk factor for stroke, with the relative risk being twice that in heavy smokers (>40 cigarettes per day) compared with light smokers (<10 cigarettes per day) in the Framingham Heart Study cohort. Similarly to CHD risk, the risk of stroke decreases markedly by 2 years after smoking cessation, and the risk approaches that of nonsmokers 5 years after cessation.[27]

Passive smoking, or "second-hand smoke," also presents substantial cardiovascular risk. The large prospective Cancer Prevention Study II showed an approximately 20% higher rate of CHD mortality in persons who never smoked but were exposed to environmental tobacco smoke compared with those who were not exposed.[28] Cigar smokers generally have a lower exposure to smoke than cigarette smokers due to lesser quantity smoked and less inhalation; however, cigar smokers also had an increased relative risk of 1.27 for CHD compared with nonsmokers.[29]

Studies and observations support a concerted effort by health care professionals to encourage smoking cessation. The risk of CVD decreases soon after quitting smoking and continues to fall with time.[30] In men under the age of 55 years with their first MI, one study showed the risk of CHD in smokers who had quit decreased by half within 1 year, and approached that of persons who have never smoked within about 2 years.[31]

The mechanisms by which cigarette smoking are linked to CVD are incompletely understood; several possible factors have been implicated. Smoking is known to activate the sympathetic nervous system, causing increased heart rate, blood pressure, and vasomotor tone. Free radicals in smoke cause oxidation of LDL-C, resulting in highly atherogenic particles. It is also associated with lowered HDL-C levels,[32] increased triglycerides levels, and insulin resistance.

Methods of smoking cessation include nicotine replacement, antidepressant drugs, and behavioral therapy (see Chapter 11) but are rarely successful unless the smoker is highly motivated to quit. Physician intervention

TABLE 44-2

Classification of Blood Pressure*

Blood Pressure, mm Hg		
Classification	**Systolic**	**Diastolic**
Optimal blood pressure	<120	< 80
Normal blood pressure	120–129	80–84
High-normal blood pressure	130–139	85–89
Hypertension		
Stage 1	140–159	90–99
Stage 2	160–179	100–109
Stage 3	≥180	≥110

*From the Joint National Committee.[33]

in the form of simple advice or counseling may help improve the rate of quitting.

HYPERTENSION

Hypertension is an accepted and well-established risk factor for CVD, including CHD, ischemic and hemorrhagic stroke, congestive heart failure, and sudden cardiac death. Many large epidemiologic trials have shown a strong correlation between degree of hypertension and cardiovascular mortality, as well as demonstrated a reduction in risk with blood pressure control, both through lifestyle modification and pharmacologic means. The classification of blood pressure given in Table 44-2 was devised by the Joint National Committee.[33]

A large segment of the population, young and old, suffers from hypertension, placing a large burden of potential CVD on this risk factor. Based on data from the National Health and Nutrition Examination Survey (NHANES III) phase 1 (1988–1991), the prevalence of hypertension in the US adult population was approximately 24%, affecting more than 43 million persons. The age-adjusted prevalence in the non-Hispanic black, non-Hispanic white, and Mexican American populations was 32.4%, 23.3%, and 22.6%, respectively.[34] The risk of developing hypertension rises with advancing age. In the Framingham Heart Study, hypertension incidence per 2-year period increased with age in men from 3.3% at ages 30 to 39 years to 6.2% at ages 70 to 79 years; in women, hypertension incidence increased from 1.5% at ages 30 to 39 years to 8.6% at ages 70 to 79.[35] On average, there is an individual 20 mm Hg systolic and 10 mm Hg diastolic increase in blood pressure between ages 30 and 65 years.[36] The residual lifetime risk of developing stage 1 or higher hypertension (140/90 mm Hg or greater) in nonhypertensive 55- and 65-year-old subjects in the Framingham cohort was 90%, indicating a profound public health burden.[37]

The association between blood pressure and CVD has been demonstrated in many large trials. The Seven Countries Study showed a relative risk of death of 1.28 for every 10 mm Hg rise in systolic or 5 mm Hg rise in diastolic blood pressure.[38] The Framingham Heart Study showed a fourfold risk of ischemic stroke in hypertensives compared with normotensives.[39] The Chicago Heart Association Detection Project in Industry study followed up more than 10,000 young adult men: over a 25-year follow-up, risk-adjusted hazard ratios for 1 standard deviation higher systolic and diastolic blood pressures were 1.26 and 1.17, respectively. Estimated life expectancy was shortened by 2.2 and 4.1 years in subjects with high-normal blood pressure and stage 1 hypertension.[40]

Systolic blood pressure, contrary to earlier hypotheses regarding the pathophysiology of hypertension's cardiovascular risk, is as important, and in the elderly may be more important, than diastolic blood pressure as a determinant of risk.[41,42] Between ages 50 and 60 years, diastolic blood pressure often starts to fall.[43] Isolated systolic hypertension (systolic blood pressure ≥160 mm Hg when diastolic blood pressure <95 mm Hg) is especially prevalent in the elderly, and by itself has a significant association with CVD. [44,45] Pulse pressure (the difference between the systolic and diastolic blood pressures) also serves as a predictor of mortality and adverse outcomes, perhaps as a function of the fall in diastolic blood pressure and decreased arterial compliance with aging. In the Framingham Study, a 10-mm Hg increment in pulse pressure was associated with a CHD hazard ratio of 1.23.[46] Similar findings were reported in the SHEP (Systolic Hypertension in the Elderly Program), Syst-Eur (European drug intervention study of subjects greater than 60 years of age with isolated systolic hypertension), and the Multiple Risk Factor Intervention Trial.

Blood pressure represents a continuous, graded risk factor, and the threshold above which cardiovascular risk begins to rise is believed to be approximately 115/75 mm Hg.[47] Even in patients with high-normal blood pressure (130 - 139 over 85 to 89 mm Hg based on JNCVI), the adjusted hazard ratio for cardiovascular disease over 10 years was 1.6 in men and 2.5 in women compared with optimal blood pressure.[48] The decision to treat and the intensity of treatment should be determined by global risk stratification and presence of end-organ damage.

DYSLIPIDEMIA

Total Cholesterol and LDL-C

The importance of cholesterol and lipids in the development of atherosclerosis and CHD has been well established, initially based on Framingham data[49,50] and confirmed in many subsequent epidemiologic studies. Both serum total cholesterol and LDL-C have a direct relationship with the risk of developing CHD, and

TABLE 44-3

Classification of Cholesterol Levels*

Cholesterol, mmol/L (mg/dL)	Classification
LDL-C	
<2.59 (<100)	Optimal
2.59–3.33 (100–129)	Near optimal/above optimal
3.36–4.11 (130–159)	Borderline high
4.14–4.89 (160–189)	High
≥4.91(≥190)	Very high
Total cholesterol	
<5.17 (<200)	Desirable
5.17–6.18 (200–239)	Borderline high
≥6.21 (≥240)	High
HDL-C	
<1.03 (<40)	Low
≥1.55 (≥60)	High

*LDL-C indicates low-density lipoprotein cholesterol; HDL-C, high-density lipoprotein cholesterol. From the National Cholesterol Education Program Panel.[51]

evidence that supports their lowering as a strategy for primary and secondary prevention is particularly robust.

Table 44-3 provides a classification of cholesterol levels from the National Cholesterol Education Program (NCEP).[51]

The Seven Countries Study in 1980 showed a strong association between a higher level of total cholesterol with a higher rate of CHD, a correlation of relative risk that was echoed among different European populations.[52] However, through differences in diet and lifestyle, the absolute risks between countries differed greatly.[53] The Multiple Risk Factor Intervention Trial[54] evaluated more than 350,000 middle-aged American men to establish a continuous, graded relationship between serum cholesterol and CHD death rate, with almost half of CHD deaths attributed to cholesterol levels greater than 180 mg/dL. Other data have shown that a similar relationship exists for LDL-C.

Small dense LDL is emerging as another risk factor for CHD and is frequently associated with elevated triglycerides levels and lowered HDL-C levels. A subtype of LDL-C (LDL phenotype B), small dense LDL appears to be more atherogenic than regular LDL, perhaps because of its prolonged residence time in plasma and its increased rate of oxidation.[55]

High-Density Lipoprotein Cholesterol

Plasma HDL-C levels correlate inversely with the degree of CHD risk.[56] In men and particularly in women, an elevated HDL-C appears to have an atheroprotective effect, lowering CHD risk even in subjects in the highest quartile of total cholesterol levels in a 12-year follow-up of the Framingham Heart Study. In the setting of normal total cholesterol levels (<200 mg/dL), there was an increase in CHD when HDL-C levels were low.[57] Numerous studies now suggest that the changes in HDL-C with treatment, primarily fibrates but also potentially statins and niacin, correlate with disease outcomes.[58]

The exact mechanism of HDL-C metabolism and its cardioprotective effect are not fully understood. Reverse cholesterol transport, in which HDL operates as a vehicle to transport lipid from vascular membranes through triglyceride metabolic pathways back to the liver,[59] as well as HDL-C's antioxidant properties may be the relevant contributions to cardiovascular protection. Furthermore, HDL-C values may be representative of fatty acid metabolism or the inflammatory state, as HDL has been viewed as an acute-phase reactant.

Triglycerides

The role of triglycerides in cardiovascular risk has been controversial, although recent guidelines have provided some clarification of the importance of triglycerides in the setting of the metabolic syndrome. Classification of serum triglycerides levels is provided in Table 44-4. Whereas most studies showed an increased risk of CHD in subjects with elevated serum triglycerides levels, the Lipid Research Clinics Follow-up Study showed no significant independent association.[60] In contrast, in the Copenhagen Male Study, among approximately 2900 middle-aged men followed up over 8 years, there was a relative risk of 1.5 and 2.2 of developing CHD in the middle and highest third of triglycerides levels, an association that was independent of HDL-C and LDL-C levels.[61] A probable confounding factor in establishing the correlation between triglycerides and CHD risk is the well-reported inverse correlation between triglycerides and HDL-C levels as well as the heterogeneity of triglyceride-rich lipoproteins, the smaller, denser particles believed to be more atherogenic.[62]

Apolipoproteins

An excess of lipoprotein(a), or Lp(a), a modified form of LDL that bears a structural similarity to plasminogen, has been associated with an increased risk of CHD. The prospective study PROCAM (prospective cardiovascular Munster) study, an observational study of employees in Munster, Germany following subjects recruited between ages 35 and 65 years, followed up 788 males for 10 years and found that those with Lp(a) levels 20 mg/dL and above had a risk of a major adverse cardiac event of 2.7 times greater than those with lower levels.[63] The risk was more pronounced in subjects with low HDL-C levels and hypertension.[63] The atherogenic effect of Lp(a) is thought to be mediated through high-affinity binding with macrophages

TABLE 44-4

Classification of Serum Triglycerides

Classification	Triglycerides, mmol/L (mg/dL)
Normal	<1.69 (<150)
Borderline high	1.69–2.25 (150–199)
High	2.26–5.63 (200–499)
Very high	≥5.65 (≥500)

and subsequent foam cell formation, as well as through interference with plasminogen activation and fibrinolysis.[64]

Defects in the protein portion of lipoproteins, the apolipoproteins, can lead to abnormal lipid metabolism and are also associated with an increased risk of CHD. For example, apolipoprotein B-100 mutation is associated with significantly increased serum cholesterol levels as well as increased risk of CVD.[65] Low levels of apolipoprotein A-I, high levels of apolipoprotein B, and the ratio of apolipoprotein B to apolipoprotein A-I were found to be highly predictive of cardiovascular risk in the AMORIS study.[66] Baseline apolipoprotein B and apolipoprotein B/apolipoprotein A-I ratio values were independent risk factors in the Air Force/Texas Coronary Atherosclerosis Prevention Study (AFCAPS/TexCAPS; primarily healthy men and women in the military service).[67] Screening for these conditions is recommended in patients who present with premature coronary disease.

Treatment

Recommendations for treatment of the dyslipidemias have most recently been made by the NCEP in the Adult Treatment Panel III (ATP III).[51] The guidelines focus on primary prevention of CHD in patients with multiple risk factors, adding more intensive treatment than recommended in earlier versions of ATP, as well as recommending a high level of attention to secondary prevention. As defined in ATP III, major risk factors (not including cholesterol levels) include: (1) cigarette smoking, (2) hypertension (blood pressure ≥140/90 mm Hg or patient receiving antihypertensive medications), (3) low HDL-C (<1.03 mmol/L [<40 mg/dL]), (4) family history of premature CHD (male first-degree relative <55 years or female first-degree relative <65 years), and (5) age (men, ≥45 years, women, ≥55 years). Of note, HDL-C greater than or equal to 1.55 mmol/L (≥60 mg/dL) is a "negative" risk factor. Risk equivalents for CHD include: other forms of atherosclerotic disease, including peripheral arterial disease, abdominal aortic aneurysm, and symptomatic carotid artery disease; diabetes mellitus; and multiple risk factors that confer a 10-year risk of CHD greater than 20%, as estimated by Framingham risk scores.

Heart Disease Risk Categories and LDL-C Goals*

Risk Category	LDL-C Goal	Initiation of TLC	Drug Therapy
CHD or CHD risk equivalent	<2.59 (<100)	≥2.59 (≥100)	≥3.36 (≥130)
2+ risk factors	<3.36 (<130)	≥3.36 (≥130)	≥3.36 (≥130) (10-year risk 10%–20%) ≥4.14 (≥160) (10-year risk <10%)
0–1 risk factor	<4.14 (<160)	≥4.14 (≥160)	≥4.91 (≥190)

*LDL-C indicates low-density lipoprotein cholesterol; TLC, therapeutic lifestyle changes; CHD, coronary heart disease. Values are in millimoles per liter (and milligrams per deciliter). From the National Cholesterol Education Program Panel.[51]

The assessment of risk factors and risk equivalents places patients in risk categories that guide the goals for LDL-C levels (Table 44-5). For instance, the highest risk category is composed of patients with existing CHD or CHD risk equivalents, including diabetes, for which an intensive prevention strategy and the lowest LDL-C goal (<2.59 mmol/L [<100 mg/dL]) is recommended. Therapeutic lifestyle changes (TLC) include decreasing dietary intake of cholesterol and saturated fats, increasing physical activity, and controlling weight and are the cornerstone of the population-wide approach for primary prevention. The decision to institute a more intensive strategy, namely drug therapy, in higher-risk patients is based on clinical studies showing benefit of LDL-C lowering on CHD risk in primary and secondary prevention. Table 44-6 provides a summary of commonly used lipid-lowering medications.

The most commonly cited primary prevention trials include the West of Scotland Coronary Prevention Study (WOSCOPS) and the AFCAPS/TexCAPS. In WOSCOPS, 6595 men with hypercholesterolemia (average cholesterol level, 7.03 mmol/L [272 mg/dL]; LDL-C, >4.0 mmol/L [>155 mg/dL]) and no prior evidence of CHD were randomized to receive either pravastatin or placebo. After a nearly 5-year follow-up, there was a 31% reduction in nonfatal MI or CHD death and a 22% reduction in all-cause mortality in the pravastatin group.[68] To study patients with average cholesterol levels, the AFCAPS/TexCAPS randomized 6605 subjects with average levels of total cholesterol of 5.72 mmol/L (221 mg/dL); LDL-C, 3.88 mmol/L (150 mg/dL); HDL-C, 0.93 mmol/L (36 mg/dL) for men and 1.03 mmol/L (40 mg/dL) for women to receive either lovastatin or placebo. After an approximately 5-year follow-up, the lovastatin group demonstrated a relative risk reduction of 37% for first acute major coronary event, 40% for MI, and 33% for coronary revascularization procedures compared with placebo.[69]

Secondary prevention trials also cite convincing data for lowering cholesterol. Patients with hypercholesterolemia (total cholesterol levels, 5.48 to 7.99 mmol/L

[212 to 309 mg/dL]) and known CHD were randomized to simvastatin or placebo in the Scandinavian Simvastatin Survival Study (4S). Over the 5.4-year follow-up, there was a 30% relative reduction in the risk of death, 34% reduction in risk of major coronary events, and 37% reduction in risk of undergoing myocardial revascularization in the simvastatin group.[70] The Cholesterol and Recurrent Events (CARE) Trial examined patients after MI with "average" total cholesterol and LDL-C levels and compared the incidence of MI or coronary death during therapy in patients receiving pravastatin or placebo. Again, there was a significant decrease in the primary endpoint in the patients receiving drug therapy with pravastatin.[71]

Most recently, the Heart Protection Study provided additional convincing evidence for LDL-C lowering, irrespective of baseline cholesterol levels. In a study of 20,536 individuals with known CAD, PVD, or diabetes who were randomized to groups receiving simvastatin (40 mg) or placebo, all-cause mortality was decreased from 14.7% to 12.9% in the treated group. This difference included the subgroup of patients with total cholesterol levels below 4.99 mmol/L (<193 mg/dL) and LDL-C levels below 3.0 mmol/L (<116 mg/dL).[72]

Other targets of therapy include low HDL-C and elevated triglycerides levels. In the Veterans Affairs HDL Intervention Trial (VA-HIT), 2531 patients with CHD and low HDL-C levels (≤1.03 mmol/L [40 mg/dL]) were randomized to receive gemfibrozil or placebo. At 5-year follow-up, the gemfibrozil group had a significant decrease in the combined primary endpoint of nonfatal MI and cardiac death compared with placebo (17.3% vs 21.7%). Interestingly, the HDL-C levels in the treatment arm rose by only 6%, while levels of triglycerides were lowered by 31%; total cholesterol levels decreased by 4%, and LDL-C was unaffected. The increase in serum HDL-C levels and potentially the fall in triglycerides levels partially predicted the observed risk reduction with gemfibrozil treatment.[73,74] Guidelines from ATP III recommend initial nonpharmacologic therapy such as weight loss and exercise in those with low HDL-C levels,

TABLE 44-6

Lipid-Lowering Therapies

Drug Class	Examples	Mechanism	TC	LDL-C	HDL-C	TG	Side Effects/Interactions
HMG-CoA reductase inhibitors	Lovastatin, pravastatin, simvastatin, atorvastatin, rosuvastatin	↓Hepatic cholesterol synthesis, upregulation of LDL receptors	↓↓	↓↓	↔,↑	↔,↓	Myopathy, transaminase elevations (especially in combination with fibrates)
Bile acid sequestrants	Cholestyramine, colestipol, colesevelam	↓ Enterohepatic circulation of bile acids, upregulation of LDL receptors	↓	↓	↔,↑	↑	GI upset, ↓ absorption of fat-soluble drugs and vitamins
Fibrates	Gemfibrozil, fenofibrate, bezafibrate	↑ Peripheral lipolysis, ↓ hepatic TG production	↓	↓,↔ ↑	↑↑	↓↓	GI upset, myopathy, transaminase elevations (especially in combination with statins)
Nicotinic acid	Extended-release niacin	↓ Hepatic production of VLDL and apolipoprotein B	↓	↓	↑↑	↓↓	Flushing, itching, hepatotoxicity, hyperglycemia, hyperuricemia
Cholesterol uptake inhibitors	Ezetimibe	Blocks cholesterol absorption at intestinal brush border	↓	↓	↑	↓	GI upset, arthralgias

*TC indicates total cholesterol; LDL-C, low-density lipoprotein cholesterol; HDL-C, high-density lipoprotein cholesterol; TG, triglycerides; HMG-CoA, 3-hydroxy-3-methylglutaryl coenzyme A; ↑, increased; ↓, decreased; ↔, no significant change on the average; GI, gastrointestinal tract; and VLDL, very-low-density lipoprotein. From the National Cholesterol Education Program (NCEP) Expert Panel.[51]

and the addition of nicotinic acid or a fibrate if lifestyle changes are ineffective. The approach to lowering serum triglycerides is similar, with the primary goal of therapy being to achieve targets for LDL-C.[51]

DIABETES MELLITUS

From the earliest days of the Framingham Heart Study, diabetes mellitus was recognized to be an important cardiovascular risk factor, conferring a twofold to threefold increased risk.[75,76] Both microvascular and macrovascular complications of diabetes lead to a high degree of morbidity and mortality. Thus, identification of patients with diabetes as targets of primary and secondary prevention is of paramount importance.

Diabetic men followed up in the Multiple Risk Factor Intervention Trial demonstrated a higher absolute and adjusted mortality than did nondiabetic men at 12-year follow-up. Even in nonsmokers with optimized blood

pressure and serum cholesterol levels, diabetic patients had a relative risk of cardiovascular death of 5.1 compared with those without diabetes. The presence of additional risk factors such as smoking, hypertension, and hyperlipidemia resulted in a higher excess cardiovascular risk compared with the same risk factors in nondiabetic men.[77] Similar findings were reported in a large cohort of female nurses.[78]

Although tight glycemic control has been shown to decrease the microvascular complications associated with diabetes mellitus, such as retinopathy, nephropathy, and neuropathy, there are conflicting data regarding the effect on macrovascular complications. The United Kingdom Prospective Diabetes Study (UKPDS) did not find a significant difference in the incidence of macrovascular complications among individuals with type 2 diabetes treated with intensive blood glucose control (either a sulfonylurea or insulin) vs conventional therapy (diet).[79] A subgroup analysis, however, did show a 14% relative risk reduction in MI associated with each 1% reduction in hemoglobin A_{1C}.[80] Metformin administered to obese diabetic patients reduced the composite vascular event rate by 30%.[81] In the Diabetes Control and Complications Trial (DCCT) comparing intensive with conventional blood glucose control in type 1 diabetes, there was a trend, although not significant, toward fewer macrovascular events after a 6.5-year follow-up. Mean levels of total cholesterol, LDL-C, and triglycerides were significantly reduced in the intensive therapy group, suggesting that glycemic control may at least be helpful in reducing the risk factors of diabetic patients.[82]

The pathophysiology of CVD in diabetic individuals is multifactorial and incompletely understood. Dyslipidemias, including elevated total cholesterol, LDL-C, and triglycerides levels and reduced HDL-C levels, are common in this population, as is hypertension. Endothelial dysfunction, increased oxidative stress, changes in coagulation factors and platelets, causing a hypercoagulable state, and the effects of hyperinsulinemia also contribute to increased risk.

METABOLIC SYNDROME

Linked to diabetes and insulin resistance is the metabolic syndrome, also termed syndrome X, a constellation of risk factors that together constitute a higher aggregate risk of CHD. The diagnosis of the metabolic syndrome is made when 3 of the risk determinants shown below are present.[51]

Abdominal obesity	
Men	Waist circumference >102 cm (>40 in)
Women	Waist circumference >88.9 cm (>35 in)
Triglycerides	≥3.88 mmol/L (≥150 mg/dL)
HDL-C	
Men	<1.03 mmol/L (<40 mg/dL)
Women	<1.29 mmol/L (<50 mg/dL)
Blood pressure	≥130/≥85 mm Hg
Fasting glucose	≥2.84 mmol/L (≥110 mg/dL)

By a cross-sectional health survey, the prevalence of the metabolic syndrome in the United States was 22%, corresponding to approximately 47 million Americans.[83] A prospective study of 1209 Finnish men without previous CVD or diabetes showed that those with the metabolic syndrome, as defined by the NCEP, had an adjusted relative risk of CHD mortality of 2.9 compared with those without the metabolic syndrome.[84]

Treatment of the metabolic syndrome, as directed by the ATP III, involves targeting the underlying causes by instituting TLC to decrease weight and increase physical activity. Other cardiovascular risk factors such as hyper-

tension and elevated serum triglycerides and decreased HDL-C levels also require therapy if they persist despite lifestyle changes.[51] Ongoing studies are evaluating the role of the thiazolidinedione class of insulin-sensitizing agents in improving insulin resistance and perhaps decreasing adverse cardiovascular effects.[85]

OBESITY

The prevalence of overweight and obesity has become an international epidemic, one that may "threaten global well-being" as it begins to overtake malnutrition and infectious diseases in public health importance in many countries.[86] In the United States, data from the NHANES III obtained from 1988 to 1994 suggested that over half the adult American population (63% of men; 55% of women) is overweight (body mass index, or BMI, 25 to 29.9 kg/m^2) or obese (BMI of 30 kg/m^2 or greater).[87] In a 2001 survey, the prevalence of a BMI 30 kg/m^2 or greater was 20.9% and of BMI 40 kg/m^2 or above was 2.3%.[88] In children and adolescents aged 6 to 19 years, 15% are considered overweight in being at or greater than 95th percentile of sex-specific BMI for age-growth charts.[89]

Obesity is associated with the development of many other cardiovascular risk factors, including hypertension, diabetes and glucose intolerance, and dyslipidemias, but is also itself an independent risk factor for CVD.[90] In the Nurses' Health Study, there was a gradation of risk based on increasing BMI; women with a BMI 32 kg/m^2 or more who had never smoked had a relative risk of 4.1 for death due to CVD compared with women with a BMI <19 kg/m^2.[91] Within the same cohort, the BMI at 18 years of age and at midlife were associated with development of hypertension: weight gain of 5 to 9.9 kg was associated with a relative risk of 1.74; a gain of 25 kg or more, with a relative risk of 5.21. Conversely, long-term weight loss resulted in a significantly lower risk of hypertension.[92]

PHYSICAL INACTIVITY

The advances of modern technology, while bringing about massive socioeconomic changes and, happily, convenience into human lives, have eliminated much of the need for hard physical labor. Our society has become increasingly sedentary and has experienced an attendant rise in CVD. The Centers for Disease Control and Prevention (CDC) estimate that only 15% of adult Americans get regular vigorous physical activity; 60% of Americans are not regularly active, and 25% are not active at all.[93] Multiple studies have shown an association between physical inactivity, poor fitness, and cardiovascular and all-cause mortality, with sedentary individuals experiencing approximately double the risk of active individuals.[94-96]

Intensity of exercise is inversely associated with cardiovascular risk. In a study of more than 72,000 female nurses, the age-adjusted relative risk of coronary events was 0.77, 0.65, 0.54, and 0.46 for increasing quintiles of energy expenditure.[97] An increase in physical activity decreases cardiovascular risk even if no weight loss is achieved, perhaps through improvements in the lipid profile.[98] The CDC currently recommends at least 30 minutes of moderate exercise or 15 to 20 minutes of strenuous exercise per day.[93,99] The American Heart Association recommends 30 to 60 minutes of exercise 3 to 6 times per week.[100] Perhaps more exercise overall is better than less; however, it is clear that any exercise is better than none.

INFLAMMATORY AND THROMBOTIC MARKERS

More recently in the investigation of the pathogenesis of CVD, the idea that atherosclerosis is an inflammatory disease has evolved. Acute-phase reactants such as C-reactive protein (CRP) and serum amyloid A lack diagnostic specificity. Nonetheless, they have proved useful in identifying patients who may be at higher risk of development of manifest CVD and therefore who will benefit from an intensified regimen of risk factor modification.

C-Reactive Protein

C-reactive protein has been rigorously investigated and shown to be a strong independent risk predictor of CVD. In apparently healthy men and women, the serum CRP concentration predicts long-term mortality as well as risk of MI, stroke, PVD, and sudden cardiac death.[101-106] In a sample of subjects from the Physicians' Health Study, those in the highest quartile of CRP levels had a relative risk of 2.9 for MI and 1.9 for ischemic stroke; this risk was significantly decreased by the use of aspirin.[102]

Concurrently, CRP levels appear to correlate with the presence, both in number and severity, of other risk factors, including age, smoking, cholesterol, BMI, blood pressure, Lp(a), apolipoprotein B, fibrinogen, and homocysteine; these correlations suggest a possible role for CRP as a marker of preclinical disease.[107] In a study of nearly 28,000 apparently healthy American women, elevated CRP levels appeared to be more predictive of first cardiovascular event than were LDL-C levels. Other evidence suggests that evaluation of CRP in conjunction with other risk factors provides more predictive power for CVD than any one of the factors alone.[108]

Management of elevated CRP levels remains problematic; there are currently no therapies targeted specifically to CRP, nor is there any evidence that lowering CRP in and of itself lowers cardiovascular risk. More studies are needed and are ongoing to investigate the relationship between CRP, inflammation, and cardiovascular risk. Meanwhile, many investigators have suggested that CRP be part of the standard lipid screening to improve global risk assessment.[101]

Homocysteine

Homocysteine, an intermediary in methionine and cysteine amino acid metabolism, has also been associated with CVD as an independent risk factor. The Physicians' Health Study identified men with MI as having higher homocysteine levels than did matched controls; there was a relative adjusted risk of 3.4 for MI between those with the highest 5% and lowest 90% of values.[109] A meta-analysis evaluating the effects of the MTHFR 677C→T polymorphism, which result in elevated levels of plasma homocysteine and were correlated with CHD, suggests a more causal link than previously thought.[110]

Microalbuminuria

Microalbuminuria is known to be a marker of microvascular as well as macrovascular disease in diabetes, but has also been found to be an independent cardiovascular risk factor in the nondiabetic population. In the Heart Outcomes Prevention Evaluation (HOPE) Trial, increased urinary albumin concentration was associated with an adjusted relative risk of cardiovascular events or death of 1.97 in persons without diabetes and 1.61 in diabetic patients.[111]

Abnormal coagulation factors and platelet function also have been found to be associated with the development of atherosclerosis. These derangements are found especially in conjunction with diabetes. Elevated levels of plasminogen activator inhibitor 1 (PAI-1) and fibrinogen[112,113]; decreased levels of antithrombin III, protein C, and protein S[114]; increased levels of von Willebrand factor and factor VIII[115]; and increased platelet adhesion and aggregation[116] all exist.

Other markers of inflammation, such as white blood cell count, interleukin 6 (IL-6), myeloperoxidase (MPO), and matrix metalloproteinase 9 (MMP-9), along with CRP, are being studied to uncover possible roles in atherosclerosis.

CARDIOVASCULAR RISK SCORING

With epidemiologic data collected from the Framingham Heart Study, a scoring system has been devised to help assess individual cardiovascular risk. Incorporating age, total cholesterol or LDL-C levels, HDL-C levels, blood pressure, diabetes, and smoking, a point score is generated to give an estimate of 10-year CHD risk[117] (Fig 44-1). The European Society of Cardiology has also created a tool for stratification of patients into high, intermediate, or low risk of CHD. This scheme differs from the Framingham score in that it does not incorporate HDL-C into the calculation of risk[118,119] (Fig 44-2). Both tools provide a useful means of assessing cardiovascular risk and thereby guiding the strategy of prevention and intervention for an individual.

Estimate of 10-Year Risk for Men
(Framingham Point Scores)

Age	Points
20–34	−9
35–39	−4
40–44	0
45–49	3
50–54	6
55–59	8
60–64	10
65–69	11
70–74	12
75–79	13

Total cholesterol (mg/dl)	Points Age: 20–39	40–49	50–59	60–69	70–79
<160	0	0	0	0	0
160–199	4	3	2	1	0
200–239	7	5	3	1	0
240–279	9	6	4	2	1
≥280	11	8	5	3	1

	Points Age: 20–39	40–49	50–59	60–69	70–79
Nonsmoker	0	0	0	0	0
Smoker	8	5	3	1	1

HDL (mg/dl)	Points
≥60	−1
50–59	0
40–49	1
<40	2

Systolic BP (mm Hg)	Points If untreated	If treated
<120	0	0
120–129	0	1
130–139	1	2
140–159	1	2
≥160	2	3

Point total	10-year risk %
<0	<1
0	1
1	1
2	1
3	1
4	1
5	2
6	2
7	3
8	4
9	5
10	6
11	8
12	10
13	12
14	16
15	20
16	25
≥17	≥30

10-year risk ___%

Estimate of 10-Year Risk for Women
(Framingham Point Scores)

Age	Points
20–34	−7
35–39	−3
40–44	0
45–49	3
50–54	6
55–59	8
60–64	10
65–69	12
70–74	14
75–79	16

Total cholesterol (mg/dl)	Points Age: 20–39	40–49	50–59	60–69	70–79
<160	0	0	0	0	0
160–199	4	3	2	1	1
200–239	8	6	4	2	1
240–279	11	8	5	3	2
≥280	13	10	7	4	2

	Points Age: 20–39	40–49	50–59	60–69	70–79
Nonsmoker	0	0	0	0	0
Smoker	9	7	4	2	1

HDL (mg/dl)	Points
≥60	−1
50–59	0
40–49	1
<40	2

Systolic BP (mm Hg)	Points If untreated	If treated
<120	0	0
120–129	1	3
130–139	2	4
140–159	3	5
≥160	4	6

Point total	10-year risk %
<9	<1
9	1
10	1
11	1
12	1
13	2
14	2
15	3
16	4
17	5
18	6
19	8
20	11
21	14
22	17
23	22
24	27
≥25	≥30

10-year risk ___%

FIGURE 44-1

Framingham risk tables for estimating 10-year risk of coronary heart disease.[51] Cholesterol levels are given in milligrams per deciliter. To convert to the Systeme International (SI) unit of micromoles per liter, multiply by 0.02586.

Coronary Risk Chart

Primary Prevention of Coronary Heart Disease

MEN

Risk of Coronary Heart Disease

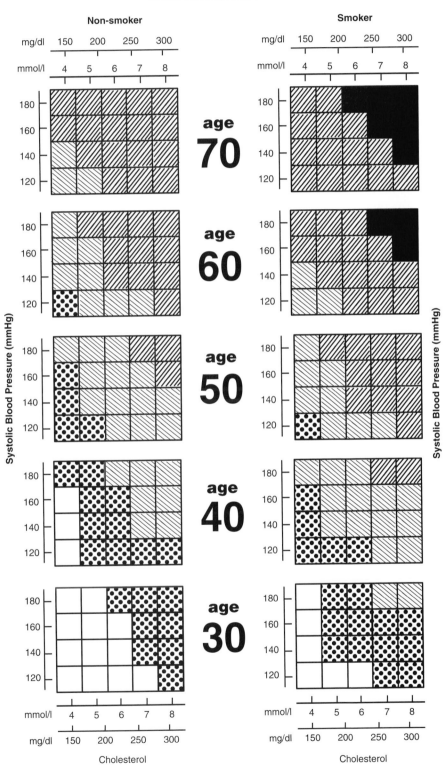

10-Year Risk Level	
Very high	over 40 %
High	20 % to 40 %
Moderate	10 % to 20 %
Mild	5 % to 10 %
Low	under 5 %

FIGURE 44-2

European Society of Cardiology Risk Model for estimating 10-year risk of coronary heart disease.[118]

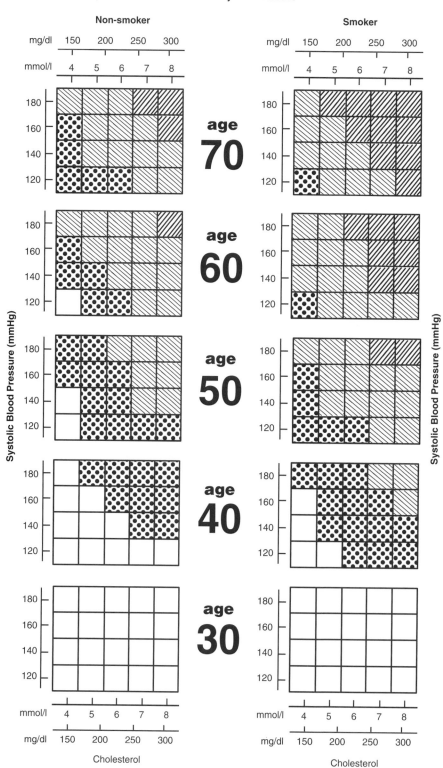

Coronary Risk Chart

Primary Prevention of Coronary Heart Disease

WOMEN

Risk of Coronary Heart Disease

10-Year Risk Level

Very high	■	over 40 %
High	▨	20 % to 40 %
Moderate	▨	10 % to 20 %
Mild	▨	5 % to 10 %
Low	□	under 5 %

F I G U R E   44-2

(continued)

DIET AND NUTRITION

Dietary patterns are an important contributor to the risk profile of certain susceptible individuals. Studies of Japanese immigrants to the United States in whom CHD subsequently developed in significantly higher numbers than in their nonimmigrant counterparts provided strong early evidence for the potentially detrimental effects of a Western diet and lifestyle.[120]

Saturated fat intake is the primary determinant of serum LDL-C levels,[121] while *trans* fatty acids can increase LDL-C and reduce HDL-C levels.[122] In the Nurses' Health Study, each increase of 5% of saturated fat intake, compared with an equivalent energy intake from carbohydrates, was associated with a 17% increase in the risk of coronary disease. The relative risk for a 2% increment in energy intake from *trans* unsaturated fats was 1.93.[123] Current dietary guidelines recommend a saturated fat intake less than 10% of energy and dietary cholesterol less than 300 mg/d.[124]

On the other hand, foods rich in omega-3 fatty acids, such as docosahexaenoic acid (DHA) and eicosapentaenoic acid (EPA) from fatty fish and α-linolenic acid from vegetable oils, which are more common in the Mediterranean diet, appear to confer a cardioprotective effect as seen in the Lyon Diet Heart Study[125] and the GISSI-Prevenzione Trial.[126] Similarly, there is an inverse relationship between fiber intake in the form of fruits, vegetables, and cereals and the risk of CHD, although these data are less convincing when adjusted for other cardiovascular risk factors.[127] Currently, there is insufficient evidence to recommend the use of antioxidant supplements such as vitamin E, vitamin C, and beta carotene; however, the American Heart Association does advocate a balanced diet with an emphasis on antioxidant-rich foods.[128]

PHARMACOLOGIC THERAPY

Strategies for decreasing global risk may involve lifestyle and pharmacologic therapies (eg, antihypertensive medications or lipid-lowering therapies) that address each individual risk factor. However, some pharmaceuticals may have a more general role in risk reduction.

Aspirin is known to have both antiplatelet and anti-inflammatory properties, making it a valuable tool in the armamentarium against CHD. There is ample evidence for the importance of aspirin in secondary prevention, but there are currently no set guidelines for initiation of aspirin in the primary prevention setting. Most experts agree that a decision be made based on an assessment of the individual patient's absolute risk. Figures 44-1 and 44-2 outline scoring to estimate CHD risk. Aspirin therapy should be initiated in patients with an annual risk of coronary events by a Framingham score of 1.5% or greater and no contraindications to aspirin (ie, allergy,

bleeding diathesis, platelet disorders, active peptic ulcer disease). Patients with annual risk of 0.6% or less derive little benefit in proportion to bleeding risk; in those with intermediate CHD risk (0.7% to 1.4% per year), patient preference and other comorbidities such as diabetes or hypertension must be taken into account.[129]

It is currently unclear if vitamin or folate therapy is useful in reducing cardiovascular risk, specifically in patients with elevated levels of plasma homocysteine. Current recommendations are to encourage meeting recommended daily allowances (RDAs) through intake of a well-balanced diet. In high-risk patients with plasma homocysteine levels greater than or equal to 10.0 μmol/L, supplementation with 0.4 mg of folic acid, 2 mg of vitamin B_6, and 6 μg of vitamin B_{12} is advised.[130]

Although women experience a great increase in their risk of CVD after menopause, studies to show an improvement in that risk by estrogen or hormone replacement therapy have not been successful. There was no difference in the outcome of nonfatal MI or coronary death in postmenopausal women with a history of CHD taking either estrogen/progesterone or placebo after 4.1 years of follow-up in the Heart and Estrogen/Progestin Replacement Study (HERS).[131] The Women's Health Initiative (WHI), a study of hormone replacement therapy for primary prevention, was terminated early after preliminary results showed an increased risk of breast cancer and total CVD in subjects receiving hormone therapy.[132] Current recommendations do not endorse the initiation of hormone replacement therapy for either secondary or primary prevention of CHD.[133]

STRATEGIES FOR RISK ASSESSMENT AND SCREENING

Current American Heart Association guidelines suggest that risk factor screening begin in adults starting at age 20 years, including assessment of family history, smoking status, diet, alcohol intake, physical activity, and measurements of blood pressure, heart rate, BMI, and waist circumference taken every 2 years. Baseline fasting lipid profile and blood glucose levels should also be measured and rechecked at least every 5 years or every 2 years if risk factors are present. At age 40 years and older or in those with 2 or more risk factors, a global assessment of 10-year CHD risk using the multiple risk score should be performed every 5 years (or more frequently if risk factors change), and a subsequent course mapped accordingly.[134] Meanwhile, routine assessment of higher risk individuals may include CRP level, lipoprotein subtypes, homocysteine level, and inflammatory and thrombotic markers; however, many of these screening tests remain for research purposes only, and the value of their modulation (or the ability to do so) is as yet unrealized.

SUMMARY

Inherent in the pursuit of risk assessment is the desire to affect risk reduction. In this respect, many strides have been made through the application of epidemiologic data to public health initiatives such as blood pressure and cholesterol screening and antismoking campaigns. Such initiatives have resulted in the remarkable decline in cardiovascular mortality over the past 40 years. The future is by no means secure, however. The continued rise in obesity and physical inactivity, with attendant increases in diabetes mellitus and the metabolic syndrome, ensure the need for continued vigilance and effective primary and secondary prevention strategies. "Primordial prevention" or health promotion to the public may even prevent the onset of risk factors in the first place.[135]

In the future, our ability to more accurately assess cardiovascular risk will undoubtedly be improved with the advent of new laboratory tests, such as inflammatory markers; diagnostic testing such as ultrasound and computed tomography; and genetic screening. Further research to translate new screening techniques into strategies for prevention will also be needed.

REFERENCES

1. Sytkowski PA, Kannel WB, D'Agostino BR. Changes in risk factors and the decline in mortality from cardiovascular disease: the Framingham Heart Study. *N Engl J Med.* 1990;322:635–641.

2. Minino AM, et al. Deaths: final data for 2000. *Natl Vital Stat Rep.* 2002;50:1–119.

3. Hoeg JM. Evaluating coronary heart disease risk: tiles in the mosaic. *JAMA.* 1997;227:1387–1390.

4. Gordon T, et al. Predicting coronary heart disease in middle-aged and older persons: the Framington study. *JAMA.* 1977;238:497–499.

5. Schildkraut JM, et al. Coronary risk associated with age and sex of parental heart disease in the Framingham Study. *Am J Cardiol.* 1989;64:555–559.

6. Kannel WB, Gordon T. Evaluation of cardiovascular risk in the elderly: the Framingham study. *Bull N Y Acad Med.* 1978;54:573–591.

7. D'Agostino RB, et al. Trends in CHD and risk factors at age 55–64 in the Framingham Study. *Int J Epidemiol.* 1989;18:S67–S72.

8. Jousilahti P, et al. Sex, age, cardiovascular risk factors, and coronary heart disease: a prospective follow-up study of 14,786 middle-aged men and women in Finland. *Circulation.* 1999;99:1165–1172.

9. Lerner DJ, Kannel WB. Patterns of coronary heart disease morbidity and mortality in the sexes: a 26-year follow-up of the Framingham population. *Am Heart J.* 1986;111:383–390.

10. Jousilahti P, et al. Parental history of premature coronary heart disease: an independent risk factor of myocardial infarction. *J Clin Epidemiol.* 1996;49:497–503.

11. Sesso HD, et al. Maternal and paternal history of myocardial infarction and risk of cardiovascular disease in men and women. *Circulation.* 2001;104:393–398.

12. Ockene IS, Miller NH, for American Heart Association Task Force on Risk Reduction. Cigarette smoking, cardiovascular disease, and stroke: a statement for healthcare professionals from the American Heart Association. *Circulation.* 1997;96:3243–3247.

13. Smith SS, Fiore MC. The epidemiology of tobacco use, dependence, and cessation in the United States. *Primary Care.* 1999;26:433–461.

14. Jha P, et al. Estimates of global and regional smoking prevalence in 1995, by age and sex. *Am J Public Health.* 2002;92:1002–1006.

15. Cook DG, et al. Giving up smoking and the risk of heart attacks: a report from the British Regional Heart Study. *Lancet.* 1986;2:1376–1380.

16. Kaufman DW, et al. Nicotine and carbon monoxide content of cigarette smoke and the risk of myocardial infarction in young men. *N Engl J Med.* 1983;308:409–413.

17. Prescott E, et al. Smoking and risk of myocardial infarction in women and men: longitudinal population study. *BMJ.* 1998;316:1043–1047.

18. Njolstad I, Arnesen E, Lund-Larsen PG. Smoking, serum lipids, blood pressure, and sex differences in myocardial infarction: a 12-year follow-up of the Finnmark Study. *Circulation.* 1996;93:450–456.

19. Jee SH, et al. Smoking and atherosclerotic cardiovascular disease in men with low levels of serum cholesterol: the Korea Medical Insurance Corporation Study. *JAMA.* 1999;282:2149–2155.

20. Rimm EB, et al. Prospective study of alcohol consumption and risk of coronary disease in men. *Lancet.* 1991;338:464–468.

21. Manttari M, et al. Alcohol and coronary heart disease: the roles of HDL-cholesterol and smoking. *J Intern Med.* 1997;241:157–163.

22. Foody JM, et al. A propensity analysis of cigarette smoking and mortality with consideration of the effects of alcohol. *Am J Cardiol.* 2001;87:706–711.

23. Hermanson B, et al. Beneficial six-year outcome of smoking cessation in older men and women with coronary artery disease: results from the CASS registry. *N Engl J Med.* 1988;319:1365–1369.

24. van Domburg RT, et al. Smoking cessation reduces mortality after coronary artery bypass surgery: a 20-year follow-up study. *J Am Coll Cardiol.* 2000;36:878–883.

25. Hasdai D, et al. Effect of smoking status on the long-term outcome after successful percutaneous coronary revascularization. *N Engl J Med.* 1997;336:755–761.

26. Suskin N, et al. Relationship of current and past smoking to mortality and morbidity in patients with left ventricular dysfunction. *J Am Coll Cardiol.* 2001;37:1677–1682.

27. Wolf PA, et al. Cigarette smoking as a risk factor for stroke: the Framingham Study. *JAMA.* 1988;259:1025–1029.

28. Steenland K, et al. Environmental tobacco smoke and coronary heart disease in the American Cancer Society CPS-II cohort. *Circulation.* 1996;94:622–628.

29. Iribarren C, et al. Effect of cigar smoking on the risk of cardiovascular disease, chronic obstructive pulmonary disease, and cancer in men. *N Engl J Med.* 1999;340:1773–1780.

30. The Surgeon General's 1990 Report on the Health Benefits of Smoking Cessation: executive summary. *MMWR Morb Mortal Wkly Rep.* 1990;39(RR-12):i–xv, 1–12.

31. Rosenberg L, et al. The risk of myocardial infarction after quitting smoking in men under 55 years of age. *N Engl J Med.* 1985;313:1511–1514.

32. Criqui MH, et al. Cigarette smoking and plasma high-density lipoprotein cholesterol: the Lipid Research Clinics Program Prevalence Study. *Circulation.* 1980;62:IV70–76.

33. The sixth report of the Joint National Committee on prevention, detection, evaluation, and treatment of high blood pressure. *Arch Intern Med.* 1997;157:2413–2446.

34. Burt VL, et al. Prevalence of hypertension in the US adult population: results from the Third National Health and Nutrition Examination Survey, 1988–1991. *Hypertension.* 1995;25:305–313.

35. Dannenberg AL, Garrison RJ, Kannel WB. Incidence of hypertension in the Framingham Study. *Am J Public Health.* 1988;78:676–679.

36. Kannel WB. Blood pressure as a cardiovascular risk factor: prevention and treatment. *JAMA.* 1996;275:1571–1576.

37. Vasan RS, et al. Residual lifetime risk for developing hypertension in middle-aged women and men: the Framingham Heart Study. *JAMA.* 2002;287:1003–1010.

38. van den Hoogen PC, Feskens AJ, Nagelkerke NJ, Menotti A, Nissinen A, Kromhout D, for Seven Countries Study Research Group. The relation between blood pressure and mortality due to coronary heart disease among men in different parts of the world. *N Engl J Med.* 2000;342:1–8.

39. Kannel WB, et al. Epidemiologic assessment of the role of blood pressure in stroke: the Framingham Study, 1970. *JAMA.* 1996;276:1269–1278.

40. Miura K, et al. Relationship of blood pressure to 25-year mortality due to coronary heart disease, cardiovascular diseases, and all causes in young adult men: the Chicago Heart Association Detection Project in Industry. *Arch Intern Med.* 2001;161:1501–1508.

41. Kannel WB, Gordon T, Schwartz MJ. Systolic versus diastolic blood pressure and risk of coronary heart disease: the Framingham study. *Am J Cardiol.* 1971;27:335–346.

42. Stamler J, Stamler R, Neaton JD. Blood pressure, systolic and diastolic, and cardiovascular risks: US population data. *Arch Intern Med.* 1993;153:598–615.

43. Franklin SS, et al. Hemodynamic patterns of age-related changes in blood pressure: the Framingham Heart Study. *Circulation.* 1997;96:308–315.

44. Wilking SV, et al. Determinants of isolated systolic hypertension. *JAMA.* 1988;260:3451–3455.

45. Kannel WB, Dawber TR, McGee DL. Perspectives on systolic hypertension: the Framingham study. *Circulation.* 1980;61:1179–1182.

46. Franklin SS, et al. Is pulse pressure useful in predicting risk for coronary heart disease? The Framingham Heart Study. *Circulation.* 1999;100:354–360.

47. Lewington S, et al. Age-specific relevance of usual blood pressure to vascular mortality: a meta-analysis of individual data for one million adults in 61 prospective studies. *Lancet.* 2002;360:1903–1913.

48. Vasan RS, et al. Impact of high-normal blood pressure on the risk of cardiovascular disease. *N Engl J Med.* 2001;345:1291–1297.

49. Kannel WB, Castelli WP, Gordon T. Cholesterol in the prediction of atherosclerotic disease: new perspectives based on the Framingham study. *Ann Intern Med.* 1979;90:85–91.

50. Kannel WB, et al. Serum cholesterol, lipoproteins, and the risk of coronary heart disease: the Framingham study. *Ann Intern Med.* 1971;74:1–12.

51. Third Report of the National Cholesterol Education Program (NCEP) Expert Panel on Detection, Evaluation, and Treatment of High Blood Cholesterol in Adults (Adult Treatment Panel III): final report. *Circulation.* 2002;106:3143–3421.

52. Keys A. Wine, garlic, and CHD in seven countries. *Lancet.* 1980;1:145–146.

53. Kromhout D. Serum cholesterol in cross-cultural perspective: the Seven Countries Study. *Acta Cardiol.* 1999;54:155–158.

54. Stamler J, Wentworth D, Neaton JD. Prevalence and prognostic significance of hypercholesterolemia in men with hypertension: prospective data on the primary screenees of the Multiple Risk Factor Intervention Trial. *Am J Med.* 1986;80:33–39.

55. Kwiterovich PO Jr. Clinical relevance of the biochemical, metabolic, and genetic factors that influence low-density lipoprotein heterogeneity. *Am J Cardiol.* 2002;90:30i–47i.

56. Gordon T, et al. High density lipoprotein as a protective factor against coronary heart disease: The Framingham Study. *Am J Med.* 1977;62:707–714.

57. Abbott RD, et al. High density lipoprotein cholesterol, total cholesterol screening, and myocardial infarction: the Framingham Study. *Arteriosclerosis.* 1988;8:207–211.

58. Sprecher DL, Watkins TR, Behar S, Brown WV, Rubins HB, Schaefer EJ. Importance of high-density lipoprotein cholesterol and triglyceride levels in coronary heart disease. *Am J Cardiol.* 2003;91:575–580.

59. Kashyap ML. Mechanistic studies of high-density lipoproteins. *Am J Cardiol.* 1998;82:42U–48U; discussion 85U–86U.

60. Criqui MH, et al. Plasma triglyceride level and mortality from coronary heart disease. *N Engl J Med.* 1993;328:1220–1225.

61. Jeppesen J, et al. Triglyceride concentration and ischemic heart disease: an eight-year follow-up in the Copenhagen Male Study. *Circulation.* 1998;97:1029–1036.

62. Gotto AM Jr. Triglyceride as a risk factor for coronary artery disease. *Am J Cardiol.* 1998;82:22Q–25Q.

63. von Eckardstein A, et al. Lipoprotein(a) further increases the risk of coronary events in men with high global cardiovascular risk. *J Am Coll Cardiol.* 2001;37:434–439.

64. Loscalzo J, et al. Lipoprotein(a), fibrin binding, and plasminogen activation. *Arteriosclerosis.* 1990;10:240–245.

65. Tybjaerg-Hansen A, et al. Association of mutations in the apolipoprotein B gene with hypercholesterolemia and the risk of ischemic heart disease. *N Engl J Med.* 1998;338:1577–1584.

66. Walldius G, et al. High apolipoprotein B, low apolipoprotein A-I, and improvement in the prediction of fatal myocardial infarction (AMORIS study): a prospective study. *Lancet.* 2001;358:2026–2033.

67. Gotto AM Jr, et al. Relation between baseline and on-treatment lipid parameters and first acute major coronary events in the Air Force/Texas Coronary Atherosclerosis Prevention Study (AFCAPS/TexCAPS). *Circulation.* 2000;101:477–484.

68. Shepherd J, et al, for West of Scotland Coronary Prevention Study Group. Prevention of coronary heart disease with pravastatin in men with hypercholesterolemia. *N Engl J Med.* 1995;333:1301–1307.

69. Downs JR, et al. Primary prevention of acute coronary events with lovastatin in men and women with average cholesterol levels: results of AFCAPS/TexCAPS (Air Force/Texas Coronary Atherosclerosis Prevention Study). *JAMA.* 1998;279:1615–1622.

70. Randomised trial of cholesterol lowering in 4444 patients with coronary heart disease: the Scandinavian Simvastatin Survival Study (4S). *Lancet.* 1994; 344:1383–1389.

71. Sacks FM, et al, Cholesterol and Recurrent Events Trial investigators. The effect of pravastatin on coronary events after myocardial infarction in patients with average cholesterol levels. *N Engl J Med.* 1996;335:1001–1009.

72. MRC/BHF Heart Protection Study of cholesterol lowering with simvastatin in 20,536 high-risk individuals: a randomised placebo-controlled trial. *Lancet.* 2002;360:7–22.

73. Rubins HB, et al, for Veterans Affairs High-Density Lipoprotein Cholesterol Intervention Trial Study Group. Gemfibrozil for the secondary prevention of coronary heart disease in men with low levels of high-density lipoprotein cholesterol. *N Engl J Med.* 1999;341:410–418.

74. Robins SJ, et al. Relation of gemfibrozil treatment and lipid levels with major coronary events: VA-HIT: a randomized controlled trial. *JAMA.* 2001;285:1585–1591.

75. Kannel WB, McGee DL. Diabetes and cardiovascular risk factors: the Framingham study. *Circulation.* 1979;59:8–13.

76. Kannel WB, McGee DL. Diabetes and cardiovascular disease: the Framingham study. *JAMA.* 1979;241:2035–2038.

77. Stamler J, et al. Diabetes, other risk factors, and 12-yr cardiovascular mortality for men screened in the Multiple Risk Factor Intervention Trial. *Diabetes Care.* 1993;16:434–444.

78. Manson JE, et al. A prospective study of maturity-onset diabetes mellitus and risk of coronary heart disease and stroke in women. *Arch Intern Med.* 1991;151:1141–1147.

79. UK Prospective Diabetes Study (UKPDS) Group. Intensive blood-glucose control with sulphonylureas or insulin compared with conventional treatment and risk of complications in patients with type 2 diabetes (UKPDS 33). *Lancet.* 1998;352:837–853.

80. Stratton IM, et al. Association of glycaemia with macrovascular and microvascular complications of type 2 diabetes (UKPDS 35): prospective observational study. *BMJ.* 2000;321:405–412.

81. UK Prospective Diabetes Study (UKPDS) Group Effect of intensive blood-glucose control with metformin on complications in overweight patients with type 2 diabetes (UKPDS 34). *Lancet.* 1998;352:854–865.

82. Effect of intensive diabetes management on macrovascular events and risk factors in the Diabetes Control and Complications Trial. *Am J Cardiol.* 1995;75:894–903.

83. Ford ES, Giles WH, Dietz WH. Prevalence of the metabolic syndrome among US adults: findings from the third National Health and Nutrition Examination Survey. *JAMA.* 2002;287:356–359.

84. Lakka HM, et al. The metabolic syndrome and total and cardiovascular disease mortality in middle-aged men. *JAMA.* 2002;288:2709–2716.

85. Raji A, Plutzky J. Insulin resistance, diabetes, and atherosclerosis: thiazolidinediones as therapeutic interventions. *Curr Cardiol Rep.* 2002;4:514–521.

86. Kopelman PG. Obesity as a medical problem. *Nature.* 2000;404:635–643.

87. Must A, et al. The disease burden associated with overweight and obesity. *JAMA*. 1999;282:1523–1529.

88. Mokdad AH, et al. Prevalence of obesity, diabetes, and obesity-related health risk factors, 2001. *JAMA*. 2003;289:76–79.

89. Ogden CL, et al. Prevalence and trends in overweight among US children and adolescents, 1999–2000. *JAMA*. 2002;288:1728–1732.

90. Hubert HB, et al. Obesity as an independent risk factor for cardiovascular disease: a 26-year follow-up of participants in the Framingham Heart Study. *Circulation*. 1983;67:968–977.

91. Manson JE, et al. Body weight and mortality among women. *N Engl J Med*. 1995;333:677–685.

92. Huang Z, et al. Body weight, weight change, and risk for hypertension in women. *Ann Intern Med*. 1998;128:81–88.

93. *Physical Activity and Health: A Report of the Surgeon General*. Washington, DC: US Dept of Health and Human Services, Centers for Disease Control and Prevention, National Center for Chronic Disease Prevention and Health Promotion, The President's Council on Physical Fitness and Sports; 1996.

94. Powell KE, et al. Physical activity and the incidence of coronary heart disease. *Annu Rev Public Health*. 1987;8:253–287.

95. Morris JN, et al. Exercise in leisure time: coronary attack and death rates. *Br Heart J*. 1990;63:325–334.

96. Blair SN, et al. Physical fitness and all-cause mortality: a prospective study of healthy men and women. *JAMA*. 1989;262:2395–2401.

97. Manson JE, et al. A prospective study of walking as compared with vigorous exercise in the prevention of coronary heart disease in women. *N Engl J Med*. 1999;341:650–658.

98. Kraus WE, et al. Effects of the amount and intensity of exercise on plasma lipoproteins. *N Engl J Med*. 2002;347:1483–1492.

99. Pate RR, et al. Physical activity and public health: a recommendation from the Centers for Disease Control and Prevention and the American College of Sports Medicine. *JAMA*. 1995;273:402–407.

100. Fletcher GF, et al. Statement on exercise: benefits and recommendations for physical activity programs for all Americans: a statement for health professionals by the Committee on Exercise and Cardiac Rehabilitation of the Council on Clinical Cardiology, American Heart Association. *Circulation*. 1996;94:857–862.

101. Ridker PM. High-sensitivity C-reactive protein: potential adjunct for global risk assessment in the primary prevention of cardiovascular disease. *Circulation*. 2001;103:1813–1818.

102. Ridker PM, et al. Inflammation, aspirin, and the risk of cardiovascular disease in apparently healthy men. *N Engl J Med*. 1997;336:973–979.

103. Ridker PM, et al. Prospective study of C-reactive protein and the risk of future cardiovascular events among apparently healthy women. *Circulation*. 1998;98:731–733.

104. Ridker PM, et al. Plasma concentration of C-reactive protein and risk of developing peripheral vascular disease. *Circulation*. 1998;97:425–428.

105. Koenig W, et al. C-reactive protein, a sensitive marker of inflammation, predicts future risk of coronary heart disease in initially healthy middle-aged men: results from the MONICA (Monitoring Trends and Determinants in Cardiovascular Disease) Augsburg Cohort Study, 1984 to 1992. *Circulation*. 1999;99:237–242.

106. Albert CM, et al. Prospective study of C-reactive protein, homocysteine, and plasma lipid levels as predictors of sudden cardiac death. *Circulation*. 2002;105:2595–2599.

107. Rohde LE, Hennekens CH, Ridker PM. Survey of C-reactive protein and cardiovascular risk factors in apparently healthy men. *Am J Cardiol*. 1999;84:1018–1022.

108. Ridker PM, Rifai N, Rose L, Buring JE, Cook NR. Comparison of C-reactive protein and low-density lipoprotein cholesterol levels in the prediction of first cardiovascular events. *N Engl J Med*. 2002;347:1557–1565.

109. Stampfer MJ, et al. A prospective study of plasma homocyst(e)ine and risk of myocardial infarction in US physicians. *JAMA*. 1992;268:877–881.

110. Klerk M, et al. MTHFR 677C—>T polymorphism and risk of coronary heart disease: a meta- analysis. *JAMA*. 2002;288:2023–2031.

111. Gerstein HC, et al. Albuminuria and risk of cardiovascular events, death, and heart failure in diabetic and nondiabetic individuals. *JAMA*. 2001;286:421–426.

112. Landin K, Tengborn L, Smith U. Elevated fibrinogen and plasminogen activator inhibitor (PAI-1) in hypertension are related to metabolic risk factors for cardiovascular disease. *J Intern Med*. 1990;227:273–278.

113. Gray RP, Yudkin JS, Patterson DL. Plasminogen activator inhibitor: a risk factor for myocardial infarction in diabetic patients. *Br Heart J*. 1993;69:228–232.

114. Hughes A, et al. Diabetes, a hypercoagulable state? Hemostatic variables in newly diagnosed type 2 diabetic patients. *Acta Haematol*. 1983;69:254–259.

115. Conlan MG, et al. Associations of factor VIII and von Willebrand factor with age, race, sex, and risk factors for atherosclerosis: the Atherosclerosis Risk in Communities (ARIC) Study. *Thromb Haemost*. 1993;70:380–385.

116. Winocour PD. Platelet abnormalities in diabetes mellitus. *Diabetes*. 1992;41(suppl 2):26–31.

117. Wilson PW, et al. Prediction of coronary heart disease using risk factor categories. *Circulation.* 1998;97:1837–1847.

118. Prevention of coronary heart disease in clinical practice: recommendations of the Second Joint Task Force of European and Other Societies on Coronary Prevention. *Eur Heart J.* 1998;19:1434–1503.

119. Wood D, et al. Prevention of coronary heart disease in clinical practice: summary of recommendations of the Second Joint Task Force of European and Other Societies on Coronary Prevention. *J Hypertens.* 1998;16:1407–1414.

120. Robertson TL, et al. Epidemiologic studies of coronary heart disease and stroke in Japanese men living in Japan, Hawaii and California: incidence of myocardial infarction and death from coronary heart disease. *Am J Cardiol.* 1977;39:239–243.

121. Hegsted DM, et al. Dietary fat and serum lipids: an evaluation of the experimental data. *Am J Clin Nutr.* 1993;57:875–883.

122. Judd JT, et al. Dietary trans fatty acids: effects on plasma lipids and lipoproteins of healthy men and women. *Am J Clin Nutr.* 1994. 59:861–868.

123. Hu FB, et al. Dietary fat intake and the risk of coronary heart disease in women. *N Engl J Med.* 1997;337:1491–1499.

124. Krauss RM, et al. AHA Dietary Guidelines: revision 2000: a statement for healthcare professionals from the Nutrition Committee of the American Heart Association. *Circulation.* 2000;102:2284–2299.

125. de Lorgeril M, et al. Mediterranean diet, traditional risk factors, and the rate of cardiovascular complications after myocardial infarction: final report of the Lyon Diet Heart Study. *Circulation.* 1999;99:779–785.

126. Dietary supplementation with n-3 polyunsaturated fatty acids and vitamin E after myocardial infarction: results of the GISSI-Prevenzione trial: Gruppo Italiano per lo Studio della Sopravvivenza nell'Infarto miocardico. *Lancet.* 1999;354:447–455.

127. Rimm EB, et al. Vegetable, fruit, and cereal fiber intake and risk of coronary heart disease among men. *JAMA.* 1996;275:447–451.

128. Tribble DL, for American Heart Association Science Advisory. Antioxidant consumption and risk of coronary heart disease: emphasis on vitamin C, vitamin E, and beta-carotene: a statement for healthcare professionals from the American Heart Association. *Circulation.* 1999;99:591–595.

129. Lauer MS. Clinical practice: aspirin for primary prevention of coronary events. *N Engl J Med.* 2002;346:1468–1474.

130. Malinow MR, Bostom AG, Krauss RM. Homocyst(e)ine, diet, and cardiovascular diseases: a statement for healthcare professionals from the Nutrition Committee, American Heart Association. *Circulation.* 1999;99:178–182.

131. Hulley S, et al, for Heart and Estrogen/progestin Replacement Study (HERS) Research Group. Randomized trial of estrogen plus progestin for secondary prevention of coronary heart disease in postmenopausal women. *JAMA.* 1998;280:605–613.

132. Rossouw JE, et al. Risks and benefits of estrogen plus progestin in healthy postmenopausal women: principal results from the Women's Health Initiative randomized controlled trial. *JAMA.* 2002;288:321–333.

133. Mosca L, et al. Hormone replacement therapy and cardiovascular disease: a statement for healthcare professionals from the American Heart Association. *Circulation.* 2001;104:499–503.

134. Pearson TA, et al, for American Heart Association Science Advisory and Coordinating Committee. AHA guidelines for primary prevention of cardiovascular disease and stroke: 2002 update: consensus panel guide to comprehensive risk reduction for adult patients without coronary or other atherosclerotic vascular diseases. *Circulation.* 2002;106:388–391.

135. Pearson TA, et al. American Heart Association guide for improving cardiovascular health at the community level: a statement for public health practitioners, healthcare providers, and health policy makers from the American Heart Association Expert Panel on Population and Prevention Science. *Circulation.* 2003;107:645–651.

RESOURCES

American College of Cardiology.
Web site: www.acc.org.

American Heart Association.
Web site: www.americanheart.org.

American Stroke Association.
Web site: www.strokeassociation.org.

National Heart, Lung, and Blood Institute.
Web site: www.nhlbi.nih.gov.
(Includes information about National Cholesterol Education Program and Framingham Heart Study Risk Assessment Tool.)

chapter 45

Screening for Asymptomatic Coronary Artery Disease

Anjli Maroo, MD, and Michael B. Rocco, MD

INTRODUCTION

Major advances in the prevention and treatment of coronary heart disease (CHD) over the past 3 decades have led to a marked decline in mortality due to cardiovascular disease.[1] Nevertheless, CHD remains the leading cause of death in both men and women in the United States.[2] It is estimated that 39.4% of total deaths in the United States in 2000 were due to all causes of cardiovascular disease. One in 5 deaths, or 186.9 deaths per 100,000 people, was due to CHD. This sobering statistic translates into a death due to CHD every 60 seconds.[3]

Coronary heart disease has a tremendous impact on the elderly segment of the population. The average age on presentation with a first heart attack is 65.8 years for men and 70.4 years for women; 84% of people who die of CHD are aged 65 years or older. The lifetime risk of CHD after age 40 years is 49% for men and 32% for women. As our population ages, the prevalence of CHD is expected to increase. Moreover, the prevalence of CHD is increasing worldwide,[4] with an accompanying increase in global mortality and economic burden ($129.9 billion in direct and indirect costs in the United States alone).[3] Therefore, methods for early detection and treatment of CHD, even before symptoms emerge, are of paramount importance in improving these statistics.

Traditionally, treatment strategies for CHD have focused on patients with clinically apparent disease, manifested by prior myocardial infarction (MI), angina, or congestive heart failure. These patients are a high-risk population that faces an increased subsequent risk of MI, recurrent angina, heart failure, stroke, and death. However, many patients with underlying, and sometimes severe, CHD remain asymptomatic for long periods. Coronary stenoses sufficiently severe to compromise coronary blood flow may produce only intermittent symptoms or no symptoms at all. Ambulatory monitoring for ischemia in patients with known CAD has demonstrated that up to 86% of ischemic episodes are not associated with symptoms.[5] Alarmingly, the first manifestation of disease may be sudden cardiac death or fatal MI. It is estimated that MI is the first manifestation of coronary disease in 50% of men and 63% of women[3] and that sudden cardiac death is the presenting cardiac event in 15% of patients with CHD.[6] The prevalence of unrecognized ischemia in individuals with CHD is difficult to assess but has been estimated to be 2% to 4% of the general population and up to 10% of individuals with 2 or more major risk factors for CHD.[7]

In addition, a large segment of the population suffers from subclinical and nonobstructive coronary disease that is not associated with symptoms and often cannot be detected with commonly used functional studies, such as stress testing. A subset of these individuals may be at increased risk of adverse cardiac events. Pathophysiological data suggest that subclinical coronary stenoses (less than 50%) may be responsible for up to 68% of MIs.[8] Necropsy and intravascular ultrasound (IVUS) studies have clearly demonstrated that coronary artery disease (CAD) is widespread and present as early as the second decade of life and increases in frequency with aging.[9,10] Identification of these largely asymptomatic individuals to allow initiation of early preventive strategies is essential to reduce future adverse events.

Consequently, there has been increasing interest in early detection of both clinically silent obstructive disease and potentially vulnerable subclinical CHD in the overtly healthy and asymptomatic population. Strategies for screening asymptomatic individuals include the following: (1) identification of clinically silent, obstructive coronary lesions that may benefit from pharmacologic and/or revascularization procedures and (2) identification of nonobstructive, diffuse atherosclerosis that would warrant a more aggressive preventive strategy.

SCREENING GUIDELINES

An effective screening test must fulfill several criteria before widespread application. It must enable diagnosis of disease at an earlier stage to allow introduction of therapies that are likely to reduce morbidity and mortality associated with that disease. Therefore, there must be a reliable testing method for identification of latent disease and an acceptable therapeutic option proved to reduce adverse outcomes. Based on our current understanding of the pathophysiology of coronary atherosclerosis, CHD meets the criteria of a disease with a prolonged latent period that may benefit from early screening and treatment. Treatment of hypertension and dyslipidemia, therapy with angiotensin-converting enzyme (ACE) inhibitors, and antiplatelet therapy has benefited both patients with clinically overt CAD and high-risk subgroups without overt disease; thus, these interventions may decrease morbidity and mortality in patients with preclinical asymptomatic CAD if instituted early and in the appropriate populations.[11-15] However, are appropriate screening tools available? Many testing modalities are available to assess coronary atherosclerosis at various stages of development, including stress testing, perfusion imaging, coronary calcium scoring, and markers of vascular inflammation, plaque vulnerability, and diffuse atherosclerotic disease. The appropriateness of the widespread application of these screening tests in the general population is currently controversial. Although early detection and treatment of CHD is desirable, the accuracy of traditional screening tests is markedly diminished in individuals with a low pretest probability of disease. Thus, the benefits of early detection must be weighed against the consequences of false-positive and false-negative test results.

The objective then is to identify the subset of the asymptomatic population at increased risk and therefore the most likely to benefit from early detection and treatment. The initial evaluation of presymptomatic individuals involves screening for known risk factors for CHD and stratifying patients according to levels of risk. Simple risk stratification can be accomplished with routinely obtained history, physical findings, and laboratory test results. Major risk factors for CHD have been identified in large epidemiologic studies, such as the Framingham Heart Study, and are outlined in guidelines by the National Cholesterol Education Program Adult Treatment Panel III (NCEP/ATP III)[16]:

- Low-density lipoprotein cholesterol (LDL-C) greater than or equal to 3.37 mmol/L (130 mg/dL)

- Age 45 years or older in men and 55 years or older in women

- Family history of premature CHD (MI or sudden cardiac death before age 55 years in any first-degree male relative or before age 65 years in any first-degree female relative)

- Current cigarette smoking

- Hypertension (≥140/90 mm Hg on repeated examinations or while receiving antihypertensive medication)

- Low high-density lipoprotein cholesterol, or HDL-C (≤1.03 mmol/L [40 mg/dL]) a high HDL-C (≥1.55 mmol/L [60 mg/dL]) decreases risk for CHD.

The NCEP/ATP III guidelines summarize an easy-to-use risk score, constructed from risk models identified in the Framingham Heart Study.[17] Based on this simple calculation, individuals can be grouped into risk categories for decision making regarding further testing and treatment. Populations with a 10-year risk of MI or cardiac death of less than 10% are in a low-risk group; between 10% and 20% in an intermediate-risk group; and greater than 20% in a high-risk group.

The presence of diabetes or the metabolic syndrome also identifies a high-risk group that may benefit from early screening and institution of prevention strategies. Diabetes, without previously diagnosed CAD, is associated with the same mortality rate as seen in individuals without diabetes who have already experienced a first MI.[18] It is estimated that 75% to 80% of diabetic mortality is due to cardiovascular events, three fourths of which is due to CHD. Asymptomatic diabetic patients have an increased likelihood of CHD in the presence of one of the following additional factors: age older than 35 years, type 2 diabetes longer than 10 years' duration, type 1 diabetes longer than 15 years' duration, any major cardiac risk factor, microvascular disease (proliferative retinopathy, nephropathy, microalbinuria), peripheral vascular disease, or autonomic neuropathy. Thus, according to NCEP/ATP III guidelines[16] and the American Diabetic Association, diabetes should be considered a CAD equivalent, and lipid and blood pressure management should be equivalent to that in individuals with established CHD. The metabolic syndrome may be defined clinically by the presence of 3 or more of the following: waist circumference greater than 101.6 cm (40 in) in men and more than 88.9 cm (35 in) in women, hypertension (≥130/85 mm Hg), fasting serum triglycerides level of 150 mg/dL or greater, fasting HDL-C level under 40 mg/dL in men and less than 50 mg/dL in women, and fasting glucose level of 110 mg/dL or higher.[16] Observational studies have demonstrated a gradation of increasing cardiovascular risk with increasing glucose intolerance, insulin resistance, and hyperinsulinemia (hallmarks of the metabolic syndrome).[19]

Despite the high prevalence of CHD, its risk factors, and associated morbidity and mortality, the US Preventive Services Task Force 1996 Guidelines concluded that there is insufficient evidence to recommend routine screening of middle-aged men and women for asymptomatic CHD with resting electrocardiography (ECG), ambulatory ECG, or exercise ECG. Routine screening of individuals with a low-risk of CHD was not recommended. Similarly, routine screening of children, adolescents, or young adults during routine health visits was not recommended.

Over the past several years, however, the American College of Cardiology (ACC) and the American Heart Association (AHA) have published joint guidelines for

TABLE 45-1

ACC/AHA 2002 Guidelines for Screening Asymptomatic Individuals Without Known CAD Using Exercise ECG Testing*

Class	Definition of Class	Who Should Be Screened
I	Conditions for which there is evidence and/or general agreement that a procedure or treatment is useful and effective	None
IIa	Conditions for which the weight of evidence or opinion favors usefulness or efficacy	Asymptomatic persons with DM who plan to start vigorous exercise
IIb	Conditions for which usefulness or efficacy is less well established by evidence or opinion	Persons with multiple CHD risk factors[†] as a guide to risk-reduction therapy. Asymptomatic men >45 years old or women >55 years old who: 1. Plan to start vigorous exercise 2. Have an occupation in which impairment may affect public safety 3. Have a high risk of CHD due to comorbid illnesses
III	Conditions for which evidence and/or general agreement suggests that the procedure or treatment is not useful or effective and, in some cases, may be harmful	Routine screening of asymptomatic men and women

*ACC/AHA indicates American College of Cardiology/American Heart Association; CAD, coronary artery disease; ECG, electrocardiogram; DM, diabetes mellitus; and CHD, coronary heart disease. Data from Ritchie et al.[22]

[†]Multiple risk factors include total cholesterol >240 mg/dL, systolic blood pressure >140 mm Hg, diastolic blood pressure >90 mm Hg, smoking, diabetes, family history of heart attack, or sudden cardiac death in a first-degree relative younger than 60 years old.

the use of exercise ECG testing (Table 45-1),[20,21] nuclear perfusion imaging,[22] calcium scoring,[23] and inflammatory markers[24] in the management of patients with CAD. Routine screening of asymptomatic men or women generally is not recommended. The guidelines do recommend selective use of screening tests, based on clinical risk assessment and stratification. For example, although diabetic patients have higher cardiovascular risk, generalized screening of all asymptomatic diabetic individuals with exercise ECG stress testing (ETT) for detection of ischemia has not been advocated. However, diabetic patients who are about to embark on an exercise program or who participate in regular vigorous exercise may be screened to detect the presence of severe asymptomatic ischemia. Abnormal results of ETT screening should be followed by confirmatory perfusion studies or echocardiography; further abnormal test results with a poor prognostic index should prompt consideration of cardiac catheterization. The diabetic patient's high-risk status should prompt aggressive measures to try to stabilize underlying atherosclerosis and to prevent adverse events. In diabetic persons and other individuals at increased risk, several tests are available for the detection of asymptomatic obstructive or nonobstructive CHD. Preliminary studies suggest that the measurement of more novel disease and risk markers may help to better separate intermediate-risk patients into groups that may benefit from early and more intensive risk factor modification.

TRADITIONAL SCREENING TESTS FOR OBSTRUCTIVE ISCHEMIC CHD

Exercise Stress Testing

The ETT is the most commonly used tool for evaluation of individuals with known or suspected CHD. It may be used to diagnose severe obstructive atherosclerotic coronary disease and to assess long-term prognosis. It is relatively easy to perform, safe, and inexpensive and can provide several levels of prognostic information based on exercise capacity, hemodynamic and clinical responses, and electrocardiographic changes. The most commonly used definition of an abnormal ECG response is greater than or equal to 1 mm of horizontal or downsloping ST-segment depression or elevation for at least 60 to 80 milliseconds after the end of the QRS complex.[20] The addition of other clinical variables, such as symptoms and exercise duration, can further increase the diagnostic accuracy for detecting severe CHD and the prognostic value of the ETT. An abnormal Duke exercise treadmill score [Exercise Time − 5 × (Amount of ST-Segment Deviation in millimeters) − 4 × Exercise Angina Index (which equals 0 if there is no exercise angina, 1 if exercise angina occurs, and 2 if the test is stopped due to angina)] identifies patients with high average annual cardiovascular mortality.[25] Two variables with significant prognostic value are chronotropic incompetence, defined as failure to achieve 80% to 85% age-predicted maximal heart rate during peak exercise, and low chronotropic index, defined as a change of less than or equal to 12 beats per minute from peak heart rate to heart rate measured 2 minutes later. Abnormality in either measure is associated with an increase in all-cause mortality.[26,27]

The reported sensitivity, specificity, and positive predictive value of ETT for the diagnosis of obstructive CHD varies widely; meta-analyses that included symptomatic patients but excluded patients with a prior MI report a sensitivity of 67% and a specificity of 72%.[20] Diagnostic accuracy is diminished in the presence of baseline ECG abnormalities. They include:

- Digoxin effect
- Left ventricular hypertrophy with repolarization abnormalities
- Resting ST-segment depression
- Left bundle branch block
- Right bundle branch block
- Ventricular pacemaker

Most studies of test performance have been performed on patients with symptoms and known or suspected CHD. Unfortunately, a true estimate of the diagnostic accuracy of exercise testing in *asymptomatic* individuals has never been defined, mainly due to the inability to obtain angiographic correlation that is free from referral bias. According to bayesian analysis, the positive predictive value of exercise ECG testing in this population is markedly attenuated, due to the low pretest probability of disease. This fact, as well as a higher likelihood of false-positive testing outcomes, limits the usefulness of the test as a mass screening tool for the identification of asymptomatic ischemia in the low-risk population. General population screening for CHD with exercise testing is not recommended because severe CHD in most asymptomatic individuals is rare and because false-positive test results may lead to unwarranted anxiety and unnecessary invasive follow-up testing, with its associated morbidity. However, exercise testing has important prognostic value in asymptomatic patients with multiple risk factors. Exercise stress testing is recommended for these individuals before initiation of an exercise program and for individuals with jobs whose poor cardiovascular health might place others at risk, such as airline pilots or bus drivers.

As stated earlier, the diabetic population represents a group at particularly high risk of cardiovascular morbidity and mortality. Detection of asymptomatic ischemia on ambulatory ECG monitoring has been shown to be predictive of multivessel coronary disease, increased adverse clinical outcomes, and poor survival, particularly in individuals with longstanding diabetes mellitus. The prevalence of silent ischemia in diabetic persons approaches 10% to 15%, which is significantly higher than in their nondiabetic counterparts. Due to the higher pretest probability of disease, the yield of diagnostic screening tests may be higher in this population. The ETT is the most commonly used screening tool for detecting asymptomatic ischemia in diabetic individuals. Abnormal ETT results should be subsequently confirmed by radionuclide or echocardiographic imaging, to reduce false-positive test results. Current ACC/AHA guidelines recommend screening for CHD with ETT in diabetic individuals who are about to embark on a moderate to vigorous exercise program. Extending this recommendation to screen the diabetic patient with 2 or more additional risk factors should be considered.

Resting ECG

The resting ECG may reveal baseline abnormalities, such as ST depression, T-wave inversions, abnormal Q waves, left ventricular hypertrophy, or left bundle branch block. These findings have been shown to be predictive of a twofold to threefold increased risk of cardiovascular mortality.[28,29] However, the positive and negative predictive value of the resting ECG is poor. One third to one half of patients with angiographically normal coronary arteries have resting ECG abnormalities.[30] Conversely, 29% of individuals with angiographically proven CAD in the Coronary Artery Surgery Study had normal resting ECG findings.[31] Moreover, the baseline resting ECG of patients presenting with acute coronary syndromes often has normal findings. Thus, although the resting ECG is a simple, relatively inexpensive test, it is not a useful single screening tool for the diagnosis of CHD. However, in individuals at higher risk of CHD, resting ECG abnormalities consistent with ischemia, silent MI, or left ventricular hypertrophy may prompt further structural and functional assessment with echocardiography or stress testing. In addition, when screening is indicated, the resting ECG may be useful in selecting the most appropriate type of stress test protocol.

Ambulatory ECG Monitoring

Ambulatory ECG (Holter) monitoring is another method of testing for asymptomatic ischemia. Holter monitoring of the ST segment allows long-term assessment of ischemic events while the patient is engaged in usual daily activities. Indications for testing have been outlined in guidelines published by the ACC/AHA (Table 45-2). Diagnostic criteria for ischemia on Holter monitoring include flat or down-sloping ST depression of at least 1 mm, with a gradual onset and offset, which lasts at least 1 minute. Diagnostic accuracy is attenuated by the same baseline ECG abnormalities as in ETT, described in the "Exercise Stress Testing" section. Ischemic ST-segment depression on Holter monitoring has been shown to correlate with ischemia on myocardial perfusion imaging in patients with known CHD, although it may not accurately reflect the site or extent of perfusion defects detected by nuclear imaging. Most studies employing

TABLE   45-2

ACC/AHA 1999 Guidelines for Use of Ambulatory ECG for Monitoring of Myocardial Ischemia*

Class	Definition of Class	Who Should Be Screened
I	Conditions for which there is evidence and/or general agreement that a procedure or treatment is useful and effective	None
IIa	Conditions for which the weight of evidence or opinion favors usefulness or efficacy	Patients with suspected variant angina
IIb	Conditions for which usefulness or efficacy is less well established by evidence or opinion	Evaluation of patients with chest pain who cannot exercise Preoperative evaluation for vascular surgery of patients who cannot exercise Patients with known CAD and atypical chest pain syndrome
III	Conditions for which evidence and/or general agreement suggests that the procedure or treatment is not useful or effective and, in some cases, may be harmful	Routine screening of asymptomatic men and women Initial evaluation of patients with chest pain who are able to exercise

*ACC/AHA indicates American College of Cardiology/American Heart Association; CAD, coronary artery disease; ECG, electrocardiogram; DM, diabetes mellitus; and CHD, coronary heart disease. Data from Knutsen et al.[28]

ambulatory Holter monitoring have been undertaken in patients with known CAD and/or abnormal results of stress tests. The detection of asymptomatic ischemia in this subgroup has been shown to offer important additional prognostic information. However, in a study of patients with angiographically proven CAD and abnormal stress test results, only 57% had 1 or more episodes of ST-segment depression during 48 hours of monitoring, raising questions about the sensitivity of the test for detection of obstructive coronary disease.[5] Moreover, there is currently no evidence that ambulatory ECG monitoring provides reliable information concerning ischemia or prognosis in asymptomatic subjects without known CHD.[32] Therefore, Holter monitoring is not recommended for population screening. Although ambulatory monitoring may be used for screening in high-risk patients unable to exercise (class IIb recommendation), pharmacologic stress testing with adenosine, dipyridamole, or dobutamine is the testing modality of choice, as it offers greater sensitivity, reproducibility, and accuracy.

Myocardial Perfusion Imaging and Stress Echocardiography

Nuclear imaging may be used in conjunction with exercise testing or pharmacologic stress testing for the detection of ischemia, most commonly when there are abnormalities in the baseline ECG or as a confirmatory measure after an abnormal ETT result. Frequently used isotopes include thallium 201, technetium 99m sestamibi, or technetium 99m tetrofosmin. The sensitivity of myocardial perfusion imaging is superior to ETT alone and approaches 80% to 90% without loss of specificity. However, much like conventional ETT, the post-test accuracy of nuclear imaging modalities is affected by the pretest likelihood of disease,

and in low-risk populations the false-positive rate can be as high as 20% or even 30%. Other causes of false-positive test results specific to perfusion imaging include motion artifacts, regional photon attenuation (diaphragmatic attenuation, breast artifact, obesity), conduction abnormalities (left bundle branch block, ventricular pacing), hypertension, and cardiomyopathies (infiltrative, hypertrophic, dilated). In addition to attenuated diagnostic accuracy in low-risk populations, high cost makes nuclear imaging an impractical screening tool. This testing should be reserved for screening individuals with intermediate to high risk who also have baseline resting ECG abnormalities or other attributes that obscure the interpretation of the exercise ECG. Nuclear imaging also may be used as a confirmatory test in individuals with an abnormal result of a screening exercise ECG test. Asymptomatic individuals with a markedly abnormal result of an exercise ECG test (eg, ≥2 mm ST-segment depression) and a normal result on a perfusion scan are at low risk of future CHD events and can be managed with close follow-up and aggressive risk factor modification. In contrast, asymptomatic individuals with a markedly abnormal result of a perfusion scan have a high likelihood of disease and should be considered for further invasive testing. Stress echocardiography with exercise or with dobutamine infusion is gaining wider acceptance with advances in imaging harmonics, digital ECG gating of imaging, and use of contrast medium to enhance definition of the endocardial borders. Sensitivity and specificity are comparable to that seen with nuclear imaging and can be performed at a lower cost.

Recently, stress technetium 99m sestamibi myocardial perfusion single-photon emission computed tomography (SPECT) has been used to screen asymptomatic diabetic individuals for silent ischemia.[33] An abnormal result of a SPECT scan was associated with a significantly increased risk of future MI or cardiac death, while a normal scan result was associated with a low risk of future cardiac events. Other recent studies suggest that dobutamine stress echocardiography in patients with asymptomatic diabetes with at least 3 other risk factors has similar predictive value but fewer false-negative results compared with ETT or nuclear stress testing.[34] Nevertheless, use of SPECT or stress echocardiography as a primary screening tool has not been demonstrated to be cost-effective and is not recommended as a first-line screening strategy in the asymptomatic population with normal resting ECG findings.

Positron Emission Tomography

Positron emission tomography (PET) can be used to assess myocardial blood flow and flow reserve, regional perfusion, and metabolic activity. Positron emission tomography is a sensitive test for detection of myocardial ischemia and assessment of its severity. Once the diagnosis of CAD is established, PET also may be used to differentiate scar tissue from viable tissue via measurement of myocardial glucose utilization. Although PET has an established role in the assessment of symptomatic patients and of patients with known coronary disease and left ventricular dysfunction, PET is not a cost-effective screening modality to be used for widespread screening of asymptomatic individuals.

NOVEL NONINVASIVE IMAGING AND MARKERS FOR DETECTION OF SUBCLINICAL OR NONOBSTRUCTIVE CHD

Electron Beam Computed Tomography

Electron beam computed tomography (EBCT) and ultrafast computed tomography (CT) are new technologies used to detect and quantitate calcium deposits in the coronary arteries. Electron beam computed tomography allows rapid scanning times, with 30 to 40 adjacent axial scans obtained in 1 or 2 breath-holding sequences. The effect of cardiac motion is minimized by rapid ECG-triggered image acquisition. The total test time is approximately 15 minutes. Radiation exposure is equivalent to a standard CT scan of the chest. The average cost of an EBCT is approximately $400, but most insurance plans do not cover EBCT. This type of imaging allows measurement of coronary calcium area and density. The coronary calcium score is composed of an X-ray attenuation coefficient, measured in Hounsfield units (H), and the total area of coronary calcium deposits. The coronary calcium score serves as a semiquantitative measure of coronary plaque burden, which must be adjusted for age and sex.

Coronary artery calcification occurs during the process of atherosclerotic plaque formation and is absent in normal vessels. A weak correlation exists between the degree of coronary artery calcification and the exact location or size of atherosclerotic plaque.[35] However, plaque calcification does not predict plaque vulnerability, as unstable plaques are frequently not calcified.[36] Nevertheless, recent studies indicate a good correlation between disease activity (previously healed ruptured plaques are more likely to calcify) and extent of overall plaque burden.

The current role of EBCT for screening asymptomatic individuals for CHD is controversial. The prevalence of coronary calcium in asymptomatic adults is high and varies by age and sex, ranging from 21% and 11%, respectively, in men and women aged 30 to 40 years to 94% and 89%, respectively, in men and women aged 70 to 80 years.[37,38] The reported pooled sensitivity and specificity for predicting the angiographic presence of CAD by EBCT from 16 reports (n = 3683) is 91% and 49%, respectively.[33] This high sensitivity and low specificity may be a function of referral bias for angiographic studies. Electron beam computed tomography is not as well validated with respect to diagnostic or prognostic accuracy as traditional diagnostic tests for CHD, such as ETT, exercise perfusion imaging, exercise echocardiography, and pharmacologic stress testing. Because of this and its low specificity, EBCT has not demonstrated superior diagnostic capacity for detection of substantial flow-limiting coronary stenoses compared with traditional diagnostic tests.

Preliminary data from small studies indicate that EBCT calcium scores may be useful in predicting CHD risk. Various studies suggest that the presence of coronary calcification is associated with a 4-fold to 10-fold increase in risk of future cardiovascular events. Calcium scores higher than 1000 H are associated with significantly increased risk even in the elderly. Scores greater than 400 H may also identify a high-risk subgroup, particularly at younger ages. However, prediction of hard end points such as cardiac death or MI has not been consistently demonstrated in currently available study results, and it is unclear whether EBCT offers incremental predictive value over traditional risk models, such as the Framingham risk score.[23] While there is general agreement that the presence of coronary calcium predicts cardiovascular risk, the precise predictive value of calcium scoring for cardiac events remains uncertain. The ACC and AHA do not recommend EBCT for general screening.

There are emerging roles for the use of EBCT in subpopulations for assessment of CHD risk. For example, it is estimated that the Framingham risk score identifies only 60% to 70% of cardiovascular events. In addition, a broad segment of the screened population (estimated at 30% to 50%) is characterized as intermediate risk by this method. Therefore, newer modalities are desirable to improve our ability to better predict outcomes in this large intermediate-risk group. These individuals may not qualify for pharmacologic interventions, such as lipid-lowering agents and antiplatelet therapies, under current guidelines. Although EBCT may not offer major advantages over more traditional tests for the detection of severe obstructive coronary disease, it may provide insight into the total burden of coronary atherosclerosis and help identify the subset of intermediate-risk individuals who are likely to benefit from early, more aggressive pharmacologic risk factor modification. This may be particularly true in young individuals with a strong family history of CHD for whom the heavily age-weighted Framingham risk score may underestimate the degree of risk. A recent study indicated that chronologic age adjusted by the quantity of calcification was a better predictor of death in multivariate models, including standard risk factors.[39] Studies addressing the role of EBCT and other noninvasive testing in the evaluation of patients at intermediate risk of CHD by traditional risk models are under way. Abnormal markers of subclinical disease in intermediate-risk individuals may help improve patient motivation to modify lifestyle measures, such as diet and exercise regimens, and to accept the use of medications for risk factor reduction.

Another potential future role for EBCT is as a tool for monitoring progression, stabilization, or regression of coronary artery lesions during pharmacologic interventions, such as lipid-lowering therapy. Meaningful comparison of serial EBCT scans relies on a high level of reproducibility between the calcium scores derived from each scan. Variability among repeated scans appears to be at least 30% in most studies, although it decreases with higher amounts of calcium deposits. Introduction of a new calcium volume score that quantifies the actual volume of plaque and better defined gating techniques have allowed improvement in test-retest reproducibility compared with the traditional Agatston calcium score.[40] Preliminary non-controlled studies have demonstrated that EBCT can be used to monitor the effect of 3-hydroxy-3-methylglutaryl coenzyme A (HMG-CoA) reductase inhibitor therapy on coronary plaque burden.[41] Until more data are available in which newer techniques are used prospectively, serial EBCT testing is not suggested for routine use.

Magnetic Resonance Coronary Angiography

Magnetic resonance coronary angiography (MRCA) is an exciting research tool under development for noninvasive imaging of the coronary arteries. It has the potential to yield information about plaque size and composition, specifically identifying lesions vulnerable to rupture. However, at present, the small size of the coronary arteries, their tortuosity, and the effects of cardiac motion limit the resolution and diagnostic accuracy of MRCA.[42] The sensitivity and specificity of MRCA in a low-risk population have not been established. Cardiac computed tomography is another imaging technique that is being developed for the noninvasive assessment of CAD. Contrast-enhanced multidetector computed tomography, also known as multisection CT, is capable of identifying coronary and graft stenoses.[43] Further research is needed to determine whether MRCA or CT angiography will become suitable noninvasive substitutes for coronary angiography or appropriate screening tools for the detection of subclinical, vulnerable plaques. At present, these investigational tools do not have a role in general population screening but hold substantial promise for the future.

Noncardiac Noninvasive Tests of Systemic Atherosclerosis

A strong association has been shown to exist between other systemic forms of atherosclerosis such as carotid, aortic, and peripheral vascular disease and CAD presence and risk. Therefore, noninvasive tools for identifying systemic atherosclerosis may identify individuals with a high likelihood of subclinical CAD. Two modalities, in particular, are well-established screening tools for systemic atherosclerosis: the ankle-brachial index (ABI) for assessing peripheral vascular disease and B-mode ultrasonography for measurement of carotid intimal medial thickness (IMT). Whereas carotid IMT measurements require more experienced ultrasonographers and interpreters and the precise carotid location for optimal screening is disputed, the ABI is a simple, inexpensive test that can be performed easily in the office. Both tests are highly predictive of future CHD events and mortality,[44,45] and both tests provide additional information about cardiovascular risk above and beyond traditional risk assessment. The NCEP ATP III panel has classified carotid, peripheral, and/or aortic disease as CHD risk equivalents (even in the absence of known CAD), suitable for aggressive lowering of LDL-C level and CHD risk factor modification. Tests such as the IMT and ABI can be applied to asymptomatic patients in a cost-effective manner and may be used to implement early pharmacologic intervention in patients with intermediate-risk profiles.

Novel Serum Markers

Serum markers such as lipoprotein(a), fibrinogen, lipoprotein particle size, and homocysteine have been shown to offer independent prognostic information and have been offered as means to further modify assessment of risk (NCEP ATP III).[11] Recently, several serum markers of inflammation have been identified that predict increased cardiovascular risk, including high-sensitivity C-reactive protein (hsCRP), interleukins (IL-6), white blood cell (WBC) count, other cytokines, and soluble adhesion molecules. The hsCRP has been evaluated in multiple, large, prospective, population-based studies and appears to be the best candidate for more widespread use based on cost, precision, standardization, and ease of use. Most studies have shown a dose-response relationship between the level of hsCRP and the risk of CHD. Meta-analyses comparing individuals in the upper tertile of hsCRP with those in the lower tertile have found a relative odds ratio of 2.0 or greater (confidence interval 1.6 to 2.5) for major coronary events.[46,47] In addition, hsCRP has been shown to be an independent risk factor for CHD and yields additive predictive information above traditional cardiovascular risk scores in patients with unstable angina, MI, stroke, and peripheral arterial disease. However, not all established risk factors were controlled for in all prospective studies, and the true independent predictive value of new cardiovascular events in the asymptomatic population has not been well established.

The AHA recently evaluated hsCRP as a novel test for the identification of asymptomatic individuals who might benefit from aggressive primary prevention measures.[24] At present, the use of hsCRP for widespread screening of the general adult population is not recommended, and serial measurements of hsCRP to assess the response to pharmacologic risk factor reduction are not currently suggested. The hsCRP may be used as an adjunct to standard risk factor assessment in individuals deemed at intermediate risk to help modify the risk level, to guide use of earlier and more intensive primary prevention measures,

and to aid in motivating patients to improve lifestyle behaviors and comply with treatment recommendations. A recent report of the ongoing Women's Health Study suggests that a combined evaluation of hsCRP and LDL-C may be a superior method of risk detection.[48]

The guidelines suggest that hsCRP should be measured with the patient either fasting or not fasting, on 2 occasions at least 2 weeks apart, in the absence of any other metabolic or inflammatory syndromes. Values less than 1.0 mg/L define a low-risk group; values between 1 and 3 mg/L, an intermediate-risk group; and values greater than 3 mg/L, a high-risk group. Values over 10 mg/L should prompt a search for noncardiac sources of inflammation. At this point, there is insufficient evidence to recommend measurement of any other serum marker of inflammation (eg, fibrinogen, adhesion molecules, and cytokines) for widespread population screening.

SCREENING APPROACH BASED ON CURRENT DATA AND GUIDELINES

A practical approach to the use of screening tests is depicted in Figs 45-1 and 45-2. In both scenarios, there should be initial assessment of global risk based on clinical criteria and tools such as the Framingham risk score. For individuals who are about to start an exercise program

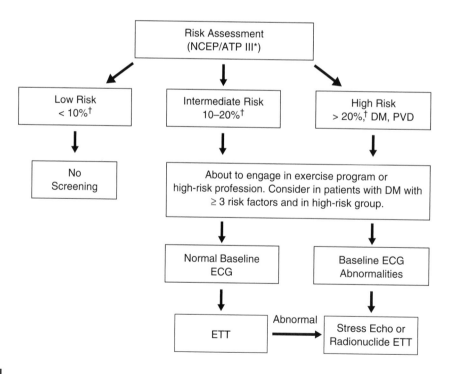

FIGURE 45-1

Screening for asymptomatic coronary artery disease (CAD): assessment for ischemia. DM indicates diabetes mellitus; PVD, peripheral vascular disease; ECG, electrocardiogram; ETT, exercise treadmill test; Echo, echocardiogram; *, National Cholesterol Education Program (NCEP) Expert Panel on Detection, Evaluation, and Treatment of High Blood Cholesterol in Adults (Adult Treatment Panel III)[16]; and †, 10-year absolute risk of coronary heart disease (risk of having a CHD event in 10 years).

or regularly engage in exercise programs or are in a profession in which their poor health would put the general public at risk, provocative exercise testing for occult obstructive CHD and ischemia has a role in individuals at intermediate risk (10% to 20% 10-year risk of MI or death); diabetic persons; or those with clinically significant noncardiac vascular disease, as assessed by symptoms, examination, or noninvasive testing such as ABI. General screening with stress testing should be considered in diabetic patients with multiple additional risk factors and in individuals in a high-risk subgroup (>20% 10-year risk) or with other comorbid illnesses associated with CHD. In the presence of a normal baseline ECG result, the exercise ECG is the most cost-effective approach. In individuals with baseline ECG abnormalities or to confirm ischemia in an asymptomatic individual with an abnormal result of stress ECG testing, stress echocardiography or radionuclide stress testing should be employed. Individuals with high-risk stress tests characterized by low workload, widespread ischemia, or reduced LV ejection fraction should be considered for aggressive pharmacologic therapy for ischemia or invasive evaluation, or both. In the low-risk population (less than 10% 10-year risk), no screening is recommended. Testing such as EBCT, hsCRP, and measures of systemic atherosclerosis may help identify individuals with increased atherosclerotic burden but not necessarily those with

ischemia producing coronary stenoses. The use of EBCT or inflammatory markers to influence decisions for stress testing is not recommended.

These newer imaging modalities and serum markers of CHD have a greater role in screening for presymptomatic CHD in order to make a judgment regarding the intensity of risk factor modification. Stress testing would often not identify these individuals. The initial approach is risk stratification. In the low-risk group, no additional screening but continued emphasis on lifestyle modification is recommended. If the risk score is in the intermediate range, additional standardized testing, such as hsCRP, EBCT, ABI, and IMT, may help identify a higher risk subgroup not identified by standard assessment. The most appropriate cutoffs in these various measurements for defining the at-risk group most likely to benefit from early intervention in not precisely known. However, based on the current information, in intermediate-risk individuals with an hsCRP above 3 mg/L or an age- and sex-corrected EBCT in the top quartile of risk or calcium scores greater than 400 H, goals for aggressive risk reduction that typically applied to the population with CHD or a CHD equivalent should be considered. A person in a high-risk group should be treated intensively regardless of the hsCRP or calcium score. Based on current data, additional testing would have little impact on treatment decisions in this group.

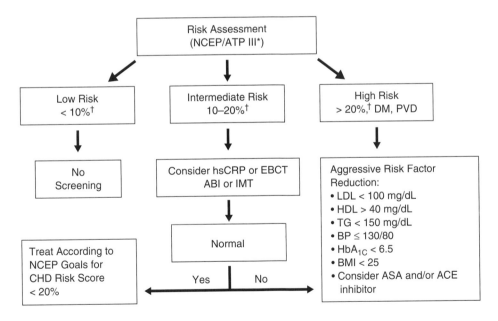

F I G U R E 45-2

Screening for asymptomatic coronary artery disease (CAD): assessment for cardiovascular risk for risk factor modification. DM indicates diabetes mellitus; PVD, peripheral vascular disease; hsCRP, high-sensitivity C-reactive protein; EBCT, electron beam computed tomography; ABI, ankle-brachial index; IMT, intimal medial thickness; CHD, coronary heart disease; LDL-C, low-density lipoprotein cholesterol; HDL-C, high-density lipoprotein cholesterol; TG, triglycerides; BP, blood pressure; HbA1c, glycosylated hemoglobin; BMI, body mass index; ASA, acetylsalicylic acid (aspirin); ACE, angiotensin-converting enzyme; *, National Cholesterol Education Program (NCEP) Expert Panel on Detection, Evaluation, and Treatment of High Blood Cholesterol in Adults (Adult Treatment Panel III)[16]; and †, 10-year absolute risk of coronary heart disease (risk of having a CHD event in 10 years).

SUMMARY

Coronary atherosclerosis remains a widespread problem that is responsible for substantial annual morbidity and mortality. Our changing understanding of the pathophysiology of atherosclerosis, combined with a not insignificant risk of adverse cardiac events in asymptomatic individuals with undiagnosed CAD, has motivated us to continue to develop screening tools that can be applied to the general population without accruing the adverse consequences of inaccurate testing.

Screening modalities to identify CHD fall into 2 main categories. The first includes provocative tests, such as stress testing, to identify substantial obstructive atherosclerotic lesions that cause silent myocardial ischemia (Fig 45-1). These tests are best suited to intermediate- to high-risk populations who are about to begin exercise programs or who have employment in which impairment may put the public at risk. The second is to identify subclinical nonobstructive CAD that is not severe enough to provoke measurable ischemia but is associated with an enhanced risk of MI or sudden cardiac death (Fig 45-2). Tests such as EBCT, hsCRP, and ABI appear to have value particularly in intermediate-risk populations as assessed by standard methods. Although these additional markers may help further refine risk stratification and help direct therapies, final recommendations regarding more widespread regular use await additional testing in the asymptomatic population. Ongoing studies examining the use of these newer testing modalities in assessing incremental prognostic value, the benefits of treatment-guided strategies, and the role of serial testing may lead to widening indications for their use in the future.

Many diagnostic tests, such as stress imaging studies, have proven value in the evaluation and treatment of patients with symptoms of CHD or known CHD. However, widespread application of these tests in the asymptomatic population is not appropriate. It is important to recognize that although many diagnostic tests for CHD are currently available or are being developed, the accuracy of each test may be affected by the low pretest probability of disease in the general asymptomatic population. Therefore, current screening recommendations should target patients deemed to be at intermediate to high risk of CHD, as a means of identifying patients likely to benefit from intensified primary prevention measures or from further invasive evaluations and treatments without accruing the risk and cost of false-positive test results.

REFERENCES

1. Cooper R, Cutler J, Desvigne-Nickens P, et al. Trends and disparities in coronary heart disease, stroke, and other cardiovascular diseases in the United States: findings of the national conference on cardiovascular disease prevention. *Circulation*. 2000;102:3137.

2. McGovern PG, Jacobs DR Jr, Shahar E, et al. Trends in acute coronary heart disease mortality, morbidity, and medical care from 1985 through 1997: the Minnesota Heart Survey. *Circulation*. 2001;104:19–24.

3. *Heart Disease and Stroke Statistics: 2003 Update.* Dallas, Tex: American Heart Association; 2002.

4. Murray C, Lopez AD, eds. *The Global Burden of Disease: A Comprehensive Assessment of Mortality and Disability from Diseases, Injuries, and Risk Factors in 1990 and Projected to 2020.* Cambridge, Mass: Harvard School of Public Health Press; 1996.

5. Rocco MB, Nabel EG, Campbell S, et al. Prognostic importance of myocardial ischemia detected by ambulatory monitoring in patients with stable coronary artery disease. *Circulation*. 1988;78:877–884.

6. Kannel W, Thomas HE Jr. Sudden coronary death: the Framingham Study. *Ann N Y Acad Sci*. 1982;382:3.

7. Deedwania P, Carbajal EV. Silent myocardial ischemia: a clinical perspective. *Arch Intern Med*. 1991;151:2373.

8. Falk E. Stable versus unstable atherosclerosis: clinical aspects. *Am Heart J*. 1999;138(5 pt 2):S421–425.

9. Berenson GS, Srinivasan SR, Bao W, Newman WP III, Tracy RE, Wattigney WA. Association between multiple cardiovascular risk factors and atherosclerosis in children and young adults: the Bogalusa Heart Study. *N Engl J Med*. 1998;338:1650–1656.

10. Tuzcu EM, Kapadia SR, Tutar E, et al. High prevalence of coronary atherosclerosis in asymptomatic teenagers and young adults: evidence from intravascular ultrasound. *Circulation*. 2001;103:2705–2710.

11. Scandinavian Simvastatin Survival Study Group. Randomised trial of cholesterol lowering in 4444 patients with coronary heart disease: the Scandinavian Simvastatin Survival Study (4S). *Lancet*. 1994;344:1383–1389.

12. Shepherd J, Cobbe SM, Ford I, et al, for the West of Scotland Coronary Prevention Study Group. Prevention of coronary heart disease with pravastatin in men with hypercholesterolemia. *N Engl J Med*. 1995;333:1301–1307.

13. Heart Outcomes Prevention Evaluation Study investigators. Effects of an angiotensin-converting-enzyme inhibitor, ramipril, on cardiovascular events in high-risk patients. *N Engl J Med*. 2000;342:145–153.

14. Sever PS, Dahlof B, Poulter NR, et al, for the ASCOT investigators. Prevention of coronary and stroke events with atorvastatin in hypertensive patients who have average or lower-than-average cholesterol concentrations, in the Anglo-Scandinavian Cardiac Outcomes trial-Lipid Lowering Arm (ASCOT-LLA): a multicentre randomized controlled trial. *Lancet*. 2003;361:1149–1158.

15. Fonarow GC, Gawlinski A. Rationale and design of the Cardiac Hospitalization Atherosclerosis Management Program at the University of California Los Angeles. *Am J Cardiol*. 2000;85:10A–17A.

16. Executive summary of the third report of the National Cholesterol Education Program (NCEP) Expert Panel on Detection, Evaluation, and Treatment of High Blood Cholesterol in Adults (Adult Treatment Panel III). *JAMA.* 2001;285:2486–2497.

17. Wilson PW, Castelli WP, Kannel WB. Coronary risk prediction in adults (the Framingham Heart Study). *Am J Cardiol.* 1987;59:91G–94G.

18. Haffner SM, Lehto S, Ronnemaa T, Pyorala K, Laakso M. Mortality from coronary heart disease in subjects with type 2 diabetes and in nondiabetic subjects with and without prior myocardial infarction. *N Engl J Med.* 1998;339:229–234.

19. Fontbonne AM, Eschwege EM. Insulin and cardiovascular disease: Paris Prospective Study. *Diabetes Care.* 1991;14:461–469.

20. Gibbons RJ, Balady GJ, Bricker JT, et al. ACC/AHA 2002 guideline update for exercise testing: summary article: a report of the American College of Cardiology/American Heart Association Task Force on Practice Guidelines (Committee to Update the 1997 Exercise Testing Guidelines). *Circulation.* 2002;106:1883–1892.

21. Kadish AH, Buxton AE, Kennedy HL, et al. ACC/AHA clinical competence statement on electrocardiography and ambulatory electrocardiography: a report of the ACC/AHA/ACP-ASIM Task Force on Clinical Competence (ACC/AHA Committee to develop a clinical competence statement on electrocardiography and ambulatory electrocardiography) endorsed by the International Society for Holter and Noninvasive Electrocardiology. *Circulation.* 2001;104:3169–3178.

22. Ritchie JL, Bateman TM, Bonow RO, et al. Guidelines for clinical use of cardiac radionuclide imaging: a report of the American College of Cardiology/American Heart Association Task Force on Assessment of Diagnostic and Therapeutic Cardiovascular Procedures (Committee on Radionuclide Imaging)—developed in collaboration with the American Society of Nuclear Cardiology. *J Nucl Cardiol.* 1995;2:172–192.

23. O'Rourke RA, Brundage BH, Froelicher VF, et al. American College of Cardiology/American Heart Association Expert Consensus document on electron-beam computed tomography for the diagnosis and prognosis of coronary artery disease. *Circulation.* 2000;102:126–140.

24. Pearson TA, Mensah GA, Alexander RW, et al. Markers of inflammation and cardiovascular disease: application to clinical and public health practice: a statement for healthcare professionals from the Centers for Disease Control and Prevention and the American Heart Association. *Circulation.* 2003;107:499–511.

25. Mark DB, Hlatky MA, Harrell FE Jr, Lee KL, Califf RM, Pryor DB. Exercise treadmill score for predicting prognosis in coronary artery disease. *Ann Intern Med.* 1987;106:793–800.

26. Lauer M, Francis GS, Okin PS, et al. Impaired chronotropic response to exercise stress testing as a predictor of mortality. *JAMA.* 1999;281:524–529.

27. Cole C, Foody JM, Blackstone EH, et al. Heart rate recovery after submaximal exercise testing as a predictor of mortality in a cardiovascularly healthy cohort. *Ann Intern Med.* 2000;132:552–555.

28. Knutsen R, Knutsen SF, Curb JD, et al. The predictive value of resting electrocardiograms for 12-year incidence of coronary heart disease in the Honolulu Heart Program. *J Clin Epidemiol.* 1988;41:293.

29. De Bacquer D, De Backer G, Kornitzer M, et al. Prognostic value of ischemic electrocardiographic findings for cardiovascular mortality in men and women. *J Am Coll Cardiol.* 1998;32:680.

30. *Unites States Preventive Services Task Force: Guide to Clinical Preventive Services.* 2nd ed. Baltimore, Md: Williams & Wilkins; 1996.

31. Coronary Artery Surgery Study (CASS): a randomized trial of coronary artery bypass surgery: survival data. *Circulation.* 1983;68:939–950.

32. Crawford MH, Bernstein SJ, Deedwania PC, et al. ACC/AHA guidelines for ambulatory electrocardiography: executive summary and recommendations: a report of the American College of Cardiology/American Heart Association Task Force on Practice Guidelines (Committee to Revise the Guidelines for Ambulatory Electrocardiography). *Circulation.* 1999;100:886–893.

33. De Lorenzo A, Lima RS, Siqueira-Filho AG, Pantoja MR. Prevalence and prognostic value of perfusion defects detected by stress technetium-99m sestamibi myocardial perfusion single-photon emission computed tomography in asymptomatic patients with diabetes mellitus and no known coronary artery disease. *Am J Cardiol.* 2002;90:827–832.

34. Penfornis A, Zimmerman C, Boumal D, et al. Use of dobutamine stress echocardiography in detecting silent myocardial ischaemia in asymptomatic diabetic populations: a comparison with thallium scintigraphy and exercise testing. *Diabetes Med.* 2001;18:900–905.

35. Tanenbaum S, Kondos GT, Veselik KE, et al. Detection of calcific deposits in coronary arteries by ultrafast computed tomography and correlation with angiography. *Am J Cardiol.* 1989;63:870–872.

36. Davies M. The composition of coronary artery plaque. *N Engl J Med.* 1993;69:377–381.

37. Janowitz WR, Agatston AS, Kaplan G, Viamonte M Jr. Differences in prevalence and extent of coronary artery calcium detected by ultrafast computed tomography in asymptomatic men and women. *Am J Cardiol.* 1993;72:247–254.

38. Wong ND, Kouwabunpat D, Vo AN, et al. Coronary calcium and atherosclerosis by ultrafast computed tomography in asymptomatic men and women: relation to age and risk factors. *Am Heart J.* 1994;127:422–430.

39. Shaw L, Callister T, Berman D, Raggi P. Is coronary taken as a measure of biologic age an improved predictor of risk? *Am J Cardiol*. 2002;90:64L.

40. Callister T, Cooil B, Raya SP, et al. Coronary artery disease: improved reproducibility of calcium scoring with an electron beam CT volumetric method. *Radiology*. 1998;208:807–814.

41. Callister T, Raggi P, Cooil B, et al. Effect of HMG-CoA reductase inhibitors on coronary artery disease as assessed by electron-beam computed tomography. *N Engl J Med*. 1998;339:1972–1978.

42. Yang P, McConnell MV, Nishimura DG, et al. Magnetic resonance coronary angiography. *Curr Cardiol Rep*. 2003;1:55–62.

43. Budoff MJ, Oudiz RJ, Zalace CP, et al. Intravenous three-dimensional coronary angiography using contrast enhanced electron beam computed tomography. *Am J Cardiol*. 1999;83:840–845.

44. Criqui M, Deneberg JO, Langer RD, et al. The epidemiology of peripheral artery disease: importance of identifying the population at risk. *Vasc Med*. 1997;2:221–226.

45. O'Leary D, Polak JF, Dronmal RA, et al. Carotid-artery intima and media thickness as a risk factor for myocardial infarction and stroke in older adults: Cardiovascular Health Study. *N Engl J Med*. 1999;340:14–22.

46. Danesh J, Whincup P, Walker M, et al. Low grade inflammation and coronary heart disease: prospective study and updated meta-analyses. *Br Med J*. 2000;321:199–204.

47. Ridker P, Haughie P. Prospective studies of C-reactive protein as a risk factor for cardiovascular disease. *J Invest Med*. 1998;46:391–395.

48. Ridker PM, Rifai N, Buring JE, Cook NR. Comparison of C-reactive protein and low density lipoprotein cholesterol levels in the prediction of first cardiovascular events. *N Engl J Med*. 2002;347:1557–1565.

49. Pearson TA. New tools for coronary risk assessment: what are their advantages and limitations? *Circulation*. 2002;105:886–892.

chapter 46

Screening for Asymptomatic Peripheral Arterial Disease

Felipe Navarro, MD, and J. Michael Bacharach, MPH, MD

INTRODUCTION

Peripheral arterial disease (PAD) is a broad term encompassing a variety of disorders. The most common cause of PAD is atherosclerosis, a systemic process that frequently causes narrowing of the arterial lumen secondary to accumulation of complex plaque material in the vessel wall leading to occlusion and/or aneurysm formation. Inflammatory disease, fibromuscular dysplasia, infection, or trauma also can cause occlusive and aneurysmal disease. For the purposes of this review, the etiologic focus will be atherosclerosis.

The extent of PAD varies and the location can involve many different arterial beds. Atherosclerotic involvement of the aorta may be associated with occlusive disease in the carotid, visceral, renal, subclavian, or iliac arteries. The location and extent of aneurysmal disease are also variable. The infrarenal aorta is the most common site. Aneurysms of the femoral, popliteal, and visceral segments can also occur but are less frequent.

SIGNIFICANCE OF ATHEROSCLEROTIC PAD

When caused by atherosclerosis, PAD has been shown to be an independent risk factor for premature death.[1] Atherosclerosis is a systemic process. Patients with PAD have a high prevalence of coronary artery disease as well as cerebrovascular disease and most often die of these conditions. A strong correlation exists between the severity of PAD and survival. Patients with mildly symptomatic PAD have a 5-year mortality of almost 30%, 50% at 10 years, and 70% at 15 years.[1,2] In patients with severe, symptomatic PAD of the lower extremities, the 10-year mortality rate reaches 75%.[3] Patients with carotid artery disease are at increased risk of cardiac death. The European Carotid Surgery Trial[4] study showed that symptomatic patients had high death rates due to nonstroke vascular disease,

regardless of the percent of carotid stenosis. Studies have shown that asymptomatic patients with at least 50% stenosis have a 10-year mortality rate of 10% to 51% due to cardiac death.[5-8]

Infrarenal abdominal aortic aneurysm and iliac artery aneurysm often are considered a single clinical entity given the frequent coexistence as well as anatomical continuum. An abdominal aorta measuring 3 cm or more is considered aneurysmal. Abdominal aortic aneurysm now ranks as the 13th most common cause of death in the Western world.[9] Abdominal aortic aneurysms most often are seen in white men over the age of 65 years, with a prevalence of 5%.[9] Peripheral aneurysms occur most frequently in the popliteal arteries. Patients with popliteal artery aneurysms have a 45% to 68% incidence of bilateral involvement.[10,11] Up to 70% of patients with popliteal or femoral artery aneurysms have an associated aortic aneurysm.[12] The presence of aortic aneurysmal disease is associated with a 50% increased risk in total mortality, cardiovascular disease mortality, and incident cardiovascular disease. This risk is independent of age, sex, other clinical cardiovascular disease, risk factors, and extent of atherosclerosis.[13]

Patients with PAD and resultant intermittent claudication (cramping and pain of muscles occurring with exertion, due to arterial blockage from atherosclerosis) have marked impairment in exercise performance and overall functional capacity. Their peak oxygen consumption is only 15 to 20 mL/kg/min, a value that approximates that of class III heart failure according to the New York Heart Association.[14] The inability to aerobically exercise because of PAD significantly contributes to morbidity and mortality (primarily cardiovascular).[15] Patients found to have vascular occlusive or aneurysmal disease need, in addition to treatment of their clinical manifestations, aggressive modification of cardiovascular risk factors. Screening for coronary and cerebrovascular disease is essential to improve survival benefit.

EPIDEMIOLOGY

Despite the recognized impact of PAD on survival and its importance as a marker of systemic disease, PAD is underdiagnosed. Peripheral arterial disease is prevalent but frequently goes unrecognized in primary care practices. Symptoms of claudication are often attributed to osteoarthritis or radiculopathy. Age has an important linear relationship to the prevalence of PAD. With increasing age, the prevalence of PAD increases rapidly; under age 60 years, the prevalence is less than 3%, and after age 60 years, prevalence steadily increases to more than 20%. Unlike coronary artery disease, there are no sex-related differences in the prevalence of PAD.[2,16]

Peripheral arterial disease represents a state of generalized atherosclerosis, which confers a high risk of fatal and nonfatal cardiovascular ischemic events. The increased risk of concomitant cardiovascular disease is not limited to the symptomatic patient. Asymptomatic patients with PAD are also at increased risk. Epidemiologic studies have demonstrated that up to 50% of the 8 to 12 million Americans with PAD are asymptomatic.[2,17] This results from lack of using objective methods for diagnosis and a generalized lack of awareness about PAD. Diagnosis of PAD by using a classic history of intermittent claudication alone, as defined by the Rose claudication questionnaire, will result in underrecognition. As many as 85% to 90% of cases of PAD are estimated to go undetected.[18] The PAD Awareness, Risk, and Treatment: New Resources for Survival (PARTNERS) study demonstrated an overall lack of awareness about PAD. Only 49% of physicians who voluntarily participated in the PARTNERS study were aware of the diagnosis of PAD in their symptomatic patients.[19]

RISK FACTORS

The risk factors leading to the development of vascular disease parallel those for coronary artery disease. These risk factors include increasing age, diabetes, tobacco use, hypertension, dyslipidemia (specifically elevated low-density lipoproteins and depressed high-density lipoproteins), obesity, sedentary lifestyle, family history of premature atherosclerosis, and genetic factors.

Cigarette Smoking

Tobacco use is thought to be the single most important independent risk factor for the development and progression of atherosclerosis. There is a strong association between the development of PAD and tobacco use. Data from the Framingham Study showed cigarette smoking, more than any other risk factor for atherosclerosis, to correlate with the incidence of intermittent claudication and even more closely with the development of intermittent claudication.[20] The risk of development of intermittent claudication doubled in both men and women who use tobacco products. In addition, smoking increases risk of

intermittent claudication 8-fold to 10-fold.[21] Similarly, Gardner[22] demonstrated that patients with intermittent claudication who smoked had onset of claudication symptoms earlier with exercise and that their symptoms required more time to resolve after resting compared with nonsmokers. Faulkner et al[23] followed the survival rates of 133 patients who underwent surgical revascularization of the lower extremities for treatment of symptomatic peripheral vascular disease. The survival rates for smokers were less than those for nonsmokers. The patients who stopped smoking had 5-year survival rates nearly double those who continued to smoke. Jonason and Bergstrom[24] looked at the effect of smoking cessation in 343 patients with intermittent claudication. In patients who quit smoking, 10-year survival was 82% compared with 46% in smokers. This parallels a higher rate of myocardial infarctions among smokers than in nonsmokers (53% vs 11%, respectively). In addition, progression to ischemic rest pain occurred in 18% of those with intermittent claudication who continued smoking, compared with none in those who quit smoking. The prevalence of PAD has been shown to drop with a decline in the prevalence of smoking.[25] The impact of tobacco use is not limited to occlusive arterial disease. Aneurysmal disease also is affected. In patients identified as having aneurysmal disease, those who smoked at the time of an initial screening for abdominal aortic aneurysm were 3 times more likely to have a new abdominal aortic aneurysm at a subsequent screening 4 years later.[26]

Diabetes Mellitus

Systemic atherosclerosis develops a decade earlier in diabetic patients than in nondiabetic individuals. Atherosclerosis is 11 times more prevalent in diabetic patients.[27] Due to this accelerated atherosclerotic process, diabetic patients have an aggressive pattern of disease that is often multisegmental. Compared with nondiabetic persons, diabetic patients have a lower incidence of aortoiliac disease and a higher incidence of disease in the profunda femoris and tibial vessels. Diabetics and individuals without diabetes share a similar incidence of occlusive disease of the superficial femoral artery. The foot vessels usually are spared.[28,29] Contrary to popular belief, diabetic patients do not have a higher tendency toward small-vessel disease than do nondiabetic persons. Moreover, diabetic patients have normal functional reactivity in the distal resistance vessels.[30] However, due to the aggressive nature of PAD in diabetic patients, both with respect to severity and rate of progression to critical limb ischemia, the relative risk of limb amputation is 40 times greater than for people without diabetes.[31] The presence of neuropathy in diabetic patients increases the risk of the development of ulcerations at pressure points in the foot. Neuropathy often allows the ulcer to progress undetected by the patient. The interplay among arterial insufficiency, neuropathy, and infection often culminates in loss of a limb.

Dyslipidemia

The development and progression of PAD are very dependent on abnormalities in lipid metabolism. In one study, almost 90% of patients with ASO have dyslipidemia.[32] Elevated levels of total cholesterol, low-density lipoprotein cholesterol (LDL-C), triglycerides, and lipoprotein(a) are independent risk factors for occlusive ASO and aneurysmal disease.[33-35] Depressed levels of high-density lipoprotein cholesterol (HDL-C) are prevalent in patients with intermittent claudication[36] and are an independent risk factor for cardiac morbidity and mortality.[37-39]

Hypertension

Hypertension increases the risk of intermittent claudication by 300%, as shown by the Framingham Study.[40] In addition, elevated systolic arterial blood pressure is independently associated with progression of PAD to rest pain or gangrene.[41]

CLINICAL PRESENTATION

The most common manifestation of lower-extremity occlusive PAD is intermittent claudication. Patients often report a gradual but progressive onset of their symptoms of intermittent claudication. The symptoms can seem insidious, since they may initially be attributed to a non-vascular cause such as arthritis, radiculopathy, or the aging process. Intermittent claudication typically is described as a consistent and reproducible ache, tightness, fatigue, or pain in a muscle group that occurs with exercise and is relieved with rest. A key feature of intermittent claudication is that symptoms occur predictably after walking a specific distance, provided there is no change in walking speed or surface grade. With rest, whether sitting or remaining standing, symptoms abate after 2 to 5 minutes. Resuming walking will again summon the symptoms. Patients who "walk through" the pain might require substantially more time for their symptoms to resolve after resting.

Occlusive disease in the aortoiliac segment occurs in all age groups but has typically been associated with younger patients, even before 40 years of age. Claudication symptoms occur in the buttock, thigh, or calf muscles. Sometimes, both the patient and health professional may mistake aortoiliac disease for hip arthritis. Lack of hip pain with prolonged standing and free range of passive motion of the hip found on examination can help shift the focus from the hip joint to the vascular system. Occlusion of the superficial femoral or popliteal arteries is more common in patients over age 40 years. Calf claudication is the most common site of claudication in such patients. Because of the crucial function of the profunda femoris in providing collateral flow around the occluded superficial femoral segment, these patients may initially have only minimal stable claudication symptoms

or no symptoms at all. Patients with multilevel disease will manifest symptoms initially in the distal muscle group. As the patient continues to walk, the more proximal muscle group will develop symptoms. As the severity of arterial occlusion progresses, patients may exhibit pallor of the feet with leg elevation and rubor with dependency. Ultimately, patients may exhibit ischemic rest pain, especially when in a supine position. They find that they must dangle their feet over the side of the bed to obtain relief. Some of these patients sleep in a chair to keep their legs in a dependent position.

An important differential diagnosis of vascular claudication is pseudoclaudication due to lumbar canal stenosis. These patients complain of buttock, hip, thigh, and calf pain. However, unlike patients with true vascular claudication, patients with pseudoclaudication experience leg pain with either walking or prolonged standing. The walking distance required to produce symptoms may vary from day to day. Relief usually is obtained by sitting or stooping forward, which decompresses the lumbar canal stenosis. Symptoms of pseudoclaudication can persist for at least 20 minutes. Additionally, because of nerve root involvement, these patients often experience associated numbness and tingling in the feet.

Clinical clues that suggest underlying renovascular disease include the onset of hypertension before the age of 30 years (due to fibromuscular dysplasia) or after age 55 years (due to atherosclerotic renal artery disease). Another clue is previously well-controlled essential hypertension that becomes difficult to control, accelerated, or even resistant to medical treatment. In elderly patients with atherosclerosis in other vascular beds, the development of azotemia may indicate the presence of renovascular disease.

The hallmark for chronic mesenteric ischemia is postprandial pain, which begins 30 to 90 minutes after meals and lasts for 2 to 3 hours. Such pain eventually causes patients to actively and consciously avoid food, which leads to weight loss, another hallmark of chronic mesenteric ischemia.

Symptoms of carotid artery disease relate to cerebral ischemia ipsilateral to the stenotic carotid artery. Such symptoms include transient ischemic attacks, strokes, or amaurosis fugax. These symptoms are due to hemodynamic factors related to the degree of (1) stenosis (usually at least 70%) in the internal carotid artery; (2) collateral flow, from both the circle of Willis and the external carotid artery; and (3) intracranial arterial disease. Alternatively, embolism from an ulcerated plaque in the internal carotid artery or from the stump of a completely occluded internal carotid artery may cause neurologic deficit.

About 75% of all abdominal aortic aneurysms are asymptomatic at initial diagnosis.[9] Abdominal aortic aneurysms may become symptomatic without rupturing. Symptomatic patients present with vague abdominal pain or low back pain which may herald the beginning of a rupture. Erosion of an abdominal aortic aneurysm into the duodenum causes gastrointestinal hemorrhage. Patients with embolization of mural thrombus from an abdominal aortic aneurysm may present with acute limb ischemia. Whereas aortic aneurysms culminate in rupture, arterial aneurysms in an extremity tend to thrombose. Acute limb ischemia ensues, and the patient requires urgent revascularization. As femoral and popliteal artery aneurysms enlarge, they compress the surrounding venous structures and cause unilateral leg edema, venous hypertension, venous thrombosis with occlusion, or pain due to local nerve compression.

SCREENING

Selection of Patients

Appropriate screening for PAD involves identification of high-risk patient groups and a targeted approach. In addition to consideration of risk factors, a thorough history and physical examination may help identify those with underlying PAD. Special attention to the presence and quality of pulses, auscultation for arterial bruits, palpation for abdominal and peripheral aneurysms, and inspection of skin in the toes and fingers for fissures or ulcerations all are essential. Based on PARTNERS study data, asymptomatic patients aged 50 to 69 years who have a history of smoking or diabetes and those aged 70 or older with any other cardiovascular risk factors should be considered for screening for PAD.[19] Patients who have leg pain on exertion, or have distal limb ulceration not attributed to obvious causes or an ulceration that is not healing properly merit screening for PAD. Asymptomatic patients with diminished or unequal pulses, arterial bruits, palpable arterial aneurysms, or ischemic fissures or ulcers should undergo screening for PAD.

The identification of patients at risk of carotid stenosis aims to prevent cerebrovascular events. In the Asymptomatic Carotid Atherosclerosis Study, the relative risk reduction for ipsilateral major stroke or perioperative death over 5 years was 53% in favor of carotid endarterectomy in patients with 80% to 99% stenosis found with duplex ultrasonography (DUS).[42] In the Framingham Study population, the incidence of carotid artery disease, as defined by stenosis of greater than 50%, was 8%. In another study of healthy volunteers 70 years of age or older, the incidence rate of carotid stenosis greater than 50% was 5.1% and 1.5% in younger individuals.[43,44] The low prevalence of carotid stenosis in the general population does not warrant screening of unselected patients. Patients with lower-extremity PAD are at risk of carotid disease. Patients with carotid bruits who are aged 65 years and older, hypertensive, smokers, and have advanced PAD have a higher prevalence rate of major carotid stenosis than the average population with asymptomatic carotid bruits. In patients 65 years of age and older with carotid bruits, their level of risk progressively increases when other cardiovascular risks are present.[45] Therefore, it is in this patient population that screening for asymptomatic disease should be considered.

Issues related to screening patients for abdominal aortic aneurysm include cost-effectiveness of screening and the lack of consensus on which patients should be screened. A recent study found "quick-screen" ultrasound to be accurate, compared with a full ultrasonographic examination, and cost-effective in men over age 70 years.[46] When other risk factors such as smoking, family history of abdominal aortic aneurysm, peripheral vascular disease, and cerebrovascular disease were present, cost effectiveness improved. A recent British trial followed up more than 61,000 men between the ages of 65 and 70 years, with half undergoing screening for abdominal aortic aneurysm.[47] After 4 years, the screened group had a 42% reduction in risk of death due to ruptured abdominal aortic aneurysms. However, by the end of the trial, all-cause mortality was similar, with 11% of the men in each group having died.[47]

Repeated screening of normal abdominal aortas is also controversial. Two recent studies suggest little practicality in rescreening men older than 65 years who had normal abdominal aortas on ultrasonograms. However, the development of new aneurysms in initially normal abdominal aortas is independently predicted by a history of smoking, coronary artery disease, or generalized atherosclerosis. In this patient population, rescreening every 4 years may be appropriate.[26,48]

In patients 65 years or older with a history of smoking, coronary artery disease, and PAD, screening for abdominal aortic aneurysm should be considered. Patients with multiple risk factors who are found on initial screening to have normal abdominal aortas should be rescreened no sooner than 4 years later. In addition, patients with a family history of abdominal aortic aneurysm, whether ruptured or not, should be included in the screening process. Patients with peripheral arterial or thoracic aortas should undergo screening for coexisting abdominal aortic aneurysm. Given enlargement rates of 0.3 to 0.57 cm/y for abdominal aortic aneurysms, patients who are found to have an abdominal aortic aneurysm should undergo yearly ultrasound monitoring.[49] Once the abdominal aortic aneurysm grows by 0.5 cm in 6 months (1 cm/y) or reaches a size of at least 5 cm, evaluation for surgical repair can be considered.[50,51]

Diagnostic and Screening Tools

Ankle-brachial index
One of the more effective screening tools for the diagnosis of PAD is the ankle-brachial index (ABI). The ABI has 90% sensitivity and 98% specificity for angiographically defined stenosis of 50% or greater.[18,52] The ABI can be obtained in the physician's office using a handheld 5-MHz Doppler device. Systolic blood pressure is

measured with the Doppler probe in each arm, and the higher of the 2 blood pressures is selected. A difference of approximately 10 mm Hg between the 2 arms may be seen. Next, the higher systolic pressure measured in the dorsalis pedis and posterior tibial arteries of each ankle is selected. The ABI is determined by dividing the higher ankle pressures in each leg by the higher arm pressure. Because arteries become stiffer in the distal vasculature, the ankle pressure may be slightly higher than the arm pressure. Therefore, an ABI of 0.91 to 1.2 is considered normal (Table 46-1). The ABI ratios for arterial disease also are shown in Table 46-1. An ABI greater than 1.2 suggests noncompressible, calcified vessels. In such circumstances, a toe-brachial index is more reliable, since digital vessels in the foot are less likely to be affected by medial calcinosis.

Pulse volume recordings

Instead of an ABI, pulse volume recordings (PVR) can be used to screen for PAD in asymptomatic patients with calcified tibial arteries. Pulse volume recordings are plethysmographic tracings that record pulsatile volume changes in the limb and are reliable in the context of medial calcinosis. Patients who have a normal ABI but have leg pain on exertion that is suggestive of claudication should undergo an exercise test. Exercise induces peripheral vasodilation, which results in a drop in the peripheral resistance. With hemodynamically significant stenosis, only a fixed amount of blood flow can be delivered and a compensatory increase in arterial flow cannot be achieved; therefore, distal systolic pressure falls. For the exercise test, a patient walks on a treadmill at 2 mph up a 10% to 12% grade for a maximum of 5 minutes. A postexercise ABI that decreases by 20% from baseline is diagnostic of PAD. Both the decline in ABI and the time for its return to baseline provide quantitative information about disease severity.

Duplex ultrasonography

Duplex ultrasonography can be used to assess the peripheral vasculature. Duplex ultrasound refers to B-mode technology, which provides real-time, gray-scale imaging, combined with velocity analysis using Doppler. Therefore, DUS renders both an anatomical and a functional assessment of the patient's anatomy. As blood flows through a stenotic lesion, its velocity increases. With DUS, peak systolic and end-diastolic velocities can be measured and used to estimate the severity of a focal arterial stenosis. Different velocity criteria apply to different vascular beds. This type of ultrasonography is an excellent screening tool for abdominal aortic aneurysms and carotid arteries. Limitations to adequate imaging include inability of ultrasound waves to pass through air. Doppler ultrasonography is limited due to difficulty in ascertaining

TABLE 46-1

Ankle-Brachial Index (ABI)*

ABI	Indicates
0.91–1.2	Normal arterial supply
0.76–0.90	Mild, possible asymptomatic PAD
0.51–0.75	Moderate PAD, usually symptomatic
0.26–0.50	Severe PAD, usually multisegmental
≤0.25	Critical PAD, often associated with rest pain and tissue loss

*PAD indicates peripheral arterial disease.

neighboring organs, and reliance on operator experience. Doppler ultrasonography of the renal arteries has been shown to have a sensitivity from 83% to 98% and a specificity of 95% to 100%.[53] Abdominal ultrasonography is an accurate screening tool to detect aneurysms, as it has a sensitivity close to 100%.[54]

Diagnostic modalities

Other modalities are used for diagnostic testing, rather than screening, in persons suspected of having or found to have PAD. Contrast-enhanced computed tomography (CT) is an accurate tool for obtaining precise information about the aorta and surrounding anatomical structures. It gives the most accurate measurement of an abdominal aortic aneurysm. Current technology is improving the ability to perform 3-dimensional reconstruction of arterial structures. Limitations of CT for screening include toxicity of contrast agents in patients with renal insufficiency as well as its high cost.

Magnetic resonance imaging (MRI) can delineate the aorta and its surrounding anatomical relationships, and provide good images of the carotid, renal, and lower-extremity arteries. Moreover, its 3-dimensional reconstruction is superior to that of CT. Magnetic resonance imaging is useful in patients with renal failure in whom intravenous contrast agents are not desirable. However, MRI cannot be used in patients who have implanted ferromagnetic equipment, such as pacemakers. Other limitations include cost and the potential for patient claustrophobia during scanning.

PREVENTIVE MEASURES

The preventive measures of persons found to have PAD or to be at risk of PAD include modification of atherosclerotic risk factors, as covered in Chapter 44, and improvement of functional status. The patient with intermittent claudication has marked impairment in exercise performance and overall functional capacity. Patients who participate in 3 to 6 months of supervised walking programs can increase their pain-free time by 165% and their peak walking time by 96%.[55] They also experience improvement in peak oxygen consumption. Well-supervised exercise programs do not increase the risk of morbidity or mortality. Functional capacity can be improved with percutaneous or surgical revascularization. Patients with isolated symptomatic aortoiliac disease can be treated with endovascular methods to achieve a lasting, normal functional capacity much quicker than with exercise walking programs. The return of a normal functional capacity can allow a patient to resume aerobic exercise, which can improve the patient's cardiovascular endurance and overall mortality. In cases of critical ischemia, the risk of tissue loss or amputation is high, and exercise-walking programs are inadequate to salvage the limb. Progression to critical ischemia is an indication to pursue surgical or endovascular revascularization.

Pharmacologic agents such as pentoxifylline (Trental, Pentoxil) and cilostazol (Pletal) are used in an attempt to increase walking distance. Pentoxifylline, a methylxanthine derivative, initially was approved in 1984 for the treatment of intermittent claudication. However, pentoxifylline has never been shown to provide a statistically significant advantage over placebo or a rigorous walking program. In 1999, the US Food and Drug Administration (FDA) approved the phosphodiesterase III inhibitor cilostazol for treatment of intermittent claudication. Cilostazol inhibits platelet aggregation, inhibits smooth-muscle proliferation, vasodilates, and increases HDL-C levels,[56-58] but its mechanism of action cannot be explained solely on any one of these properties. Cilostazol has been shown in several randomized trials to improve both pain-free and maximal walking distances compared with placebo.[56,59-61] In addition, cilostazol has been shown to be superior to both placebo and pentoxifylline.[60] Cilostazol has been issued a "black-box" warning from the FDA in patients with claudication who also have congestive heart failure, because this phosphodiesterase III inhibitor may be associated with increased mortality in patients with congestive heart failure.

Aspirin is recommended for secondary disease prevention in patients with cardiovascular disease. The Antiplatelet Trialists' Collaboration[62] studied 102,459 patients with evidence of established cardiovascular disease and concluded that aspirin therapy reduced risk of fatal or nonfatal cardiovascular events. A subgroup analysis of 3295 patients from the Antiplatelet Trialists' Collaboration did not show a statistically significant reduction in the risk of fatal or nonfatal cardiovascular events among those patients with claudication who took aspirin. However, 3226 patients with peripheral vascular disease treated with either saphenous-vein or prosthetic bypass grafting or peripheral angioplasty that took aspirin showed a 43% reduction in the rate of graft occlusion or angioplasty site occlusion.[63] Aspirin alone was as effective as the combination of aspirin and dipyridamole, sulfinpyrazone, or ticlopidine hydrochloride in preventing graft occlusion. Moreover, a daily regimen of low-dose aspirin (75 to 325 mg) appears to be as effective as high-dose aspirin (600 to 1500 mg). Ticlopidine (Ticlid) and clopidogrel bisulfate (Plavix) are both thienopyridine drugs that inhibit platelet adenosine diphosphate (ADP) receptors. Ticlopidine has been shown to be more effective than placebo in reducing risk of fatal or nonfatal myocardial infarction or stroke in patients with PAD.[64] In addition, ticlopidine has been shown to improve walking distance and function of the lower-extremity venous bypass graft.[65] Due to concerns of high rates of drug-induced thrombocytopenia, neutropenia, and thrombotic thrombocytopenia purpura, ticlopidine has fallen out of widespread use.[66] Clopidogrel does not have these associated hematologic side effects. The Clopidogrel versus Aspirin in Patients at Risk of Ischemic Events (CAPRIE) trial compared 75 mg/d of clopidogrel with 325 mg/d of aspirin in more than 19,000 patients with cardiovascular disease.[67] Patients receiving clopidogrel enjoyed an 8.7% reduction in the primary endpoint of fatal or nonfatal ischemic stroke, myocardial infarction, or vascular death. Patients with PAD, who had at least moderate arterial insufficiency, were found to have a relative risk reduction of approximately 24%, more so even in the subgroups of patients with myocardial infarction or ischemic stroke.

Several studies have shown that aggressive reduction of LDL-C reduces cardiovascular mortality by approximately 30% in patients with atherosclerosis.[68] Nonetheless, a recent study has shown that patients with PAD were less intensively managed for hyperlipidemia and lipid measurements were obtained less often than in patients with known coronary heart disease.[19] This finding emphasizes a prevailing sentiment by many health care providers that treating dyslipidemias does not affect the progression of PAD. Several studies have shown the favorable impact that treatment of dyslipidemias has on PAD. In the Cholesterol Lowering Atherosclerosis Study, the combination of colestipol hydrochloride and niacin halted progression or reversed femoral atherosclerotic plaque.[69] Both a recent trial and the Scandinavian Simvastatin Survival Study demonstrated that statin use is associated with improvement in claudication symptoms compared with no statin use.[70,71] This benefit was independent of cholesterol levels and attributed to the non–cholesterol-lowering properties of statins.

Smoking cessation similarly leads to improvement in symptoms of intermittent claudication. Quick and Cotton[72] evaluated patients with intermittent claudication over a 10-month period and found those who quit smoking had improved walking distances and ankle pressures compared with those who continued smoking. Inherent in both primary and secondary prevention of PAD are aggressive modification and treatment of these known atherosclerotic risk factors.

SUMMARY

Patients with peripheral arterial disease (PAD) may be asymptomatic or have various levels of impaired functional status. PAD may be manifested by arterial narrowing leading to end organ ischemia, or by aneurismal disease. The presence of PAD results not only in potential symptoms from arterial insufficiency, but also in increased cardiovascular morbidity and mortality. The risk of cardiovascular morbidity and mortality is directly proportional to the degree of peripheral ischemia. Therefore, it becomes important to be able to identify both symptomatic and asymptomatic patients with PAD. There are numerous screening modalities for PAD. Treatment is directed toward patient symptoms as well as toward reduction in risk factors for PAD. Medical treatment has been shown to improve survival in patients with PAD.

REFERENCES

1. Coffman JD. Intermittent claudication: not so benign. *Am Heart J.* 1986;112:1127–1128.

2. Criqui MH, Fronek A, Barrett-Connor E, Klauber MR, Gabriel S, Goodman D. The prevalence of peripheral arterial disease in a defined population. *Circulation.* 1985;71:510–515.

3. Criqui MH, Langer RD, Fronek A, et al. Mortality over a period of 10 years in patients with peripheral arterial disease. *N Engl J Med.* 1992;326:381–386.

4. Barnett HJ, Taylor DW, Eliasziw M, et al, for the North American Symptomatic Carotid Endarterectomy Trial Collaborators. Benefit of carotid endarterectomy in patients with symptomatic moderate or severe stenosis. *N Engl J Med.* 1998;339:1415–1425.

5. Group CS. Carotid surgery versus medical therapy in asymptomatic carotid stenosis. *Stroke.* 1991;22:1229–1235.

6. Group MACES. Results of a randomized controlled trial of carotid endarterectomy for asymptomatic carotid stenosis. *Mayo Clin Proc.* 1992;67:513–518.

7. Hobson RW II, Weiss DG, Fields WS, et al, for the Veterans Affairs Cooperative Study Group. Efficacy of carotid endarterectomy for asymptomatic carotid stenosis. *N Engl J Med.* 1993;328:221–227.

8. Executive Committee for the Endarterectomy for Asymptomatic Carotid Atherosclerosis Study. Endarterectomy for asymptomatic carotid artery stenosis. *JAMA.* 1995;273:1421–1428.

9. Thompson MM, Bell PR. ABC of arterial and venous disease: arterial aneurysms. *BMJ.* 2000;320:1193–1196.

10. Wychulis AR, Spittell JA Jr, Wallace RB. Popliteal aneurysms. *Surgery.* 1970;68:942–952.

11. Vermilion BD, Kimmins SA, Pace WG, Evans WE. A review of one hundred forty-seven popliteal aneurysms with long-term follow-up. *Surgery.* 1981;90:1009–1014.

12. Dent TL, Lindenauer SM, Ernst CB, Fry WJ. Multiple arteriosclerotic arterial aneurysms. *Arch Surg.* 1972;105:338–344.

13. Newman AB, Arnold AM, Burke GL, O'Leary DH, Manolio TA. Cardiovascular disease and mortality in older adults with small abdominal aortic aneurysms detected by ultrasonography: the cardiovascular health study. *Ann Intern Med.* 2001;134:182–190.

14. Hiatt WR, Nawaz D, Brass EP. Carnitine metabolism during exercise in patients with peripheral vascular disease. *J Appl Physiol.* 1987;62:2383–2387.

15. Blair SN, Kampert JB, Kohl HW III, et al. Influences of cardiorespiratory fitness and other precursors on cardiovascular disease and all-cause mortality in men and women. *JAMA.* 1996;276:205–210.

16. Newman AB, Sutton-Tyrrell K, Rutan GH, Locher J, Kuller LH. Lower extremity arterial disease in elderly subjects with systolic hypertension. *J Clin Epidemiol.* 1991;44:15–20.

17. Meijer WT, Hoes AW, Rutgers D, Bots ML, Hofman A, Grobbee DE. Peripheral arterial disease in the elderly: The Rotterdam Study. *Arteriosclerosis Thromb Vasc Biol.* 1998;18:185–192.

18. Criqui MH, Denenberg JO, Bird CE, Fronek A, Klauber MR, Langer RD. The correlation between symptoms and non-invasive test results in patients referred for peripheral arterial disease testing. *Vasc Med.* 1996;1:65–71.

19. Hirsch AT, Criqui MH, Treat-Jacobson D, et al. Peripheral arterial disease detection, awareness, and treatment in primary care. *JAMA.* 2001;286:1317–1324.

20. Freund KM, Belanger AJ, D'Agostino RB, Kannel WB. The health risks of smoking: The Framingham Study: 34 years of follow-up. *Ann Epidemiol.* 1993;3:417–424.

21. Kannel WB, McGee D, Gordon T. A general cardiovascular risk profile: the Framingham Study. *Am J Cardiol.* 1976;38:46–51.

22. Gardner AW. The effect of cigarette smoking on exercise capacity in patients with intermittent claudication. *Vasc Med.* 1996;1:181–186.

23. Faulkner KW, House AK, Castleden WM. The effect of cessation of smoking on the accumulative survival rates of patients with symptomatic peripheral vascular disease. *Med J Aust.* 1983;1:217–219.

24. Jonason T, Bergstrom R. Cessation of smoking in patients with intermittent claudication: effects on the risk of peripheral vascular complications, myocardial infarction and mortality. *Acta Med Scand.* 1987;221:253–260.

25. Ingolfsson IO, Sigurdsson G, Sigvaldason H, Thorgeirsson G, Sigfusson N. A marked decline in the prevalence and incidence of intermittent claudication in Icelandic men, 1968–1986: a strong relationship to smoking and serum cholesterol—the Reykjavik Study. *J Clin Epidemiol.* 1994;47:1237–1243.

26. Lederle FA, Johnson GR, Wilson SE, et al, for the Aneurysm Detection and Management Veterans Affairs Cooperative Study Investigators. Yield of repeated screening for abdominal aortic aneurysm after a 4-year interval. *Arch Intern Med.* 2000;160:1117–1121.

27. Beach KW, Brunzell JD, Strandness DE, Jr. Prevalence of severe arteriosclerosis obliterans in patients with diabetes mellitus: relation to smoking and form of therapy. *Arteriosclerosis.* 1982;2:275–280.

28. Strandness DE Jr, Priest RE, Gibbons GE. A combined clinical and pathologic study of diabetic and nondiabetic peripheral arterial disease. *Diabetes.* 1964;13:366.

29. Akbari CM, LoGerfo FW. Diabetes and peripheral vascular disease. *J Vasc Surg.* 1999;30:373–384.

30. Barner HB, Kaiser GC, Willman VL. Blood flow in the diabetic leg. *Circulation.* 1971;43:391–394.

31. Nathan DM. Long-term complications of diabetes mellitus. *N Engl J Med.* 1993;328:1676–1685.

32. Olin JW, Cressman MD, Young JR, Hoogwerf BJ, Weinstein CE. Lipid and lipoprotein abnormalities in lower-extremity arteriosclerosis obliterans. *Cleve Clin J Med.* 1992;59:491–497.

33. Johansson J, Egberg N, Johnsson H, Carlson LA. Serum lipoproteins and hemostatic function in intermittent claudication. *Arteriosclerosis Thromb.* 1993;13:1441–1448.

34. Murabito JM, D'Agostino RB, Silbershatz H, Wilson WF. Intermittent claudication: a risk profile from The Framingham Heart Study. *Circulation.* 1997;96:44–49.

35. Hiatt WR, Hoag S, Hamman RF. Effect of diagnostic criteria on the prevalence of peripheral arterial disease: The San Luis Valley Diabetes Study. *Circulation.* 1995;91:1472–1479.

36. Pomrehn P, Duncan B, Weissfeld L, et al. The association of dyslipoproteinemia with symptoms and signs of peripheral arterial disease: Lipid Research Clinics Program Prevalence Study. *Circulation.* 1986;73:100–107.

37. Assmann G, Schulte H, von Eckardstein A, Huang Y. High-density lipoprotein cholesterol as a predictor of coronary heart disease risk: the PROCAM experience and pathophysiological implications for reverse cholesterol transport. *Atherosclerosis.* 1996;124(suppl):S11–S20.

38. Gordon DJ, Probstfield JL, Garrison RJ, et al. High-density lipoprotein cholesterol and cardiovascular disease: four prospective American studies. *Circulation.* 1989;79:8–15.

39. Wilson PW, D'Agostino RB, Levy D, Belanger AM, Silbershatz H, Kannel WB. Prediction of coronary heart disease using risk factor categories. *Circulation.* 1998;97:1837–1847.

40. Kannel WB, McGee DL. Update on some epidemiologic features of intermittent claudication: the Framingham Study. *J Am Geriatr Soc.* 1985;33:13–18.

41. Jelnes R, Gaardsting O, Hougaard Jensen K, Baekgaard N, Tonnesen KH, Schroeder T. Fate in intermittent claudication: outcome and risk factors. *BMJ.* 1986;293:1137–1140.

42. Moore WS, Young B, Baker WH, et al, for the ACAS Investigators. Surgical results: a justification of the surgeon selection process for the ACAS trial. *J Vasc Surg.* 1996;23:323–328.

43. Wilson PW, Hoeg JM, D'Agostino RB, et al. Cumulative effects of high cholesterol levels, high blood pressure, and cigarette smoking on carotid stenosis. *N Engl J Med.* 1997;337:516–522.

44. Colgan MP, Strode GR, Sommer JD, Gibbs JL, Sumner DS. Prevalence of asymptomatic carotid disease: results of duplex scanning in 348 unselected volunteers. *J Vasc Surg.* 1988;8:674–678.

45. Marek J, Mills JL, Harvich J, Cui H, Fujitani RM. Utility of routine carotid duplex screening in patients who have claudication. *J Vasc Surg.* 1996;24:572–579.

46. Lee TY, Korn P, Heller JA, et al. The cost-effectiveness of a 'quick-screen' program for abdominal aortic aneurysms. *Surgery.* 2002;132:399–407.

47. Ashton HA, Buxton MJ, Day NE, et al. The Multicentre Aneurysm Screening Study (MASS) into the effect of abdominal aortic aneurysm screening on mortality in men: a randomised controlled trial. *Lancet.* 2002;360:1531–1539.

48. Crow P, Shaw E, Earnshaw JJ, Poskitt KR, Whyman MR, Heather BP. A single normal ultrasonographic scan at age 65 years rules out significant aneurysm disease for life in men. *Br J Surg.* 2001;88:941–944.

49. Delin A, Ohlsen H, Swedenborg J. Growth rate of abdominal aortic aneurysms as measured by computed tomography. *Br J Surg.* 1985;72:530–532.

50. Vardulaki KA, Prevost TC, Walker NM, et al. Growth rates and risk of rupture of abdominal aortic aneurysms. *Br J Surg.* 1998;85:1674–1680.

51. Hollier LH, Taylor LM, Ochsner J. Recommended indications for operative treatment of abdominal aortic aneurysms: report of a subcommittee of the Joint Council of the Society for Vascular Surgery and the North American Chapter of the International Society for Cardiovascular Surgery. *J Vasc Surg.* 1992;15:1046–1056.

52. Yao ST, Hobbs JT, Irvine WT. Ankle systolic pressure measurements in arterial disease affecting the lower extremities. *Br J Surg.* 1969;56:676–679.

53. Olin JW, Piedmonte MR, Young JR, DeAnna S, Grubb M, Childs MB. The utility of duplex ultrasound scanning of the renal arteries for diagnosing significant renal artery stenosis. *Ann Intern Med.* 1995;122:833–838.

54. LaRoy LL, Cormier PJ, Matalon TA, Patel SK, Turner DA, Silver B. Imaging of abdominal aortic aneurysms. *Am J Roentgenol.* 1989;152:785–792.

55. Hiatt WR, Regensteiner JG, Hargarten ME, Wolfel EE, Brass EP. Benefit of exercise conditioning for patients with peripheral arterial disease. *Circulation.* 1990;81:602–609.

56. Money SR, Herd JA, Isaacsohn JL, et al. Effect of cilostazol on walking distances in patients with intermittent claudication caused by peripheral vascular disease. *J Vasc Surg.* 1998;27:267–275.

57. Igawa T, Tani T, Chijiwa T, et al. Potentiation of anti-platelet aggregating activity of cilostazol with vascular endothelial cells. *Thromb Res.* 1990;57:617–623.

58. Tsuchikane E, Fukuhara A, Kobayashi T, et al. Impact of cilostazol on restenosis after percutaneous coronary balloon angioplasty. *Circulation.* 1999;100:21–26.

59. Dawson DL, Cutler BS, Meissner MH, Strandness DE Jr. Cilostazol has beneficial effects in treatment of intermittent claudication: results from a multicenter, randomized, prospective, double-blind trial. *Circulation.* 1998;98:678–686.

60. Dawson DL, Cutler BS, Hiatt WR, et al. A comparison of cilostazol and pentoxifylline for treating intermittent claudication. *Am J Med.* 2000;109:523–530.

61. Beebe HG, Dawson DL, Cutler BS, et al. A new pharmacological treatment for intermittent claudication: results of a randomized, multicenter trial. *Arch Intern Med.* 1999;159:2041–2050.

62. Antiplatelet Trialists' Collaboration. Collaborative overview of randomised trials of antiplatelet therapy: I. Prevention of death, myocardial infarction, and stroke by prolonged antiplatelet therapy in various categories of patients. *BMJ.* 1994;308:81–106.

63. Antiplatelet Trialists' Collaboration. Collaborative overview of randomised trials of antiplatelet therapy: II. Maintenance of vascular graft or arterial patency by antiplatelet therapy. *BMJ.* 1994;308:159–168.

64. Janzon L, Bergqvist D, Boberg J, et al. Prevention of myocardial infarction and stroke in patients with intermittent claudication; effects of ticlopidine: results from STIMS, the Swedish Ticlopidine Multicentre Study. *J Intern Med.* 1990;227:301–308.

65. Bergqvist D, Almgren B, Dickinson JP. Reduction of requirement for leg vascular surgery during long-term treatment of claudicant patients with ticlopidine: results from the Swedish Ticlopidine Multicentre Study (STIMS). *Eur J Vasc Endovasc Surg.* 1995;10:69–76.

66. Bennett CL, Davidson CJ, Raisch DW, Weinberg PD, Bennett RH, Feldman MD. Thrombotic thrombocytopenic purpura associated with ticlopidine in the setting of coronary artery stents and stroke prevention. *Arch Intern Med.* 1999;159:2524–2528.

67. CAPRIE Steering Committee. A randomised, blinded, trial of clopidogrel versus aspirin in patients at risk of ischaemic events (CAPRIE). *Lancet.* 1996;348:1329–1339.

68. LaRosa JC, He J, Vupputuri S. Effect of statins on risk of coronary disease: a meta-analysis of randomized controlled trials. *JAMA.* 1999;282:2340–2346.

69. Blankenhorn DH, Azen SP, Crawford DW, et al. Effects of colestipol-niacin therapy on human femoral atherosclerosis. *Circulation.* 1991;83:438–447.

70. McDermott MM, Guralnik JM, Greenland P, et al. Statin use and leg functioning in patients with and without lower-extremity peripheral arterial disease. *Circulation.* 2003;107:757–761.

71. Pedersen TR, Kjekshus J, Pyorala K, et al. Effect of simvastatin on ischemic signs and symptoms in the Scandinavian simvastatin survival study (4S). *Am J Cardiol.* 1998;81:333–335.

72. Quick CR, Cotton LT. The measured effect of stopping smoking on intermittent claudication. *Br J Surg.* 1982;69(suppl):S24–S26.

RESOURCES

American Heart Association
Web site: www.amhrt.org

Endovascular Forum
Web site: www.endovascular.org

Society of Vascular Medicine and Biology
Web site: www.sumb.org

Vascular Disease Foundation
Web site: www.vdf.org

PART 10

Cancer: Inheritance, Predisposition, Screening, and Prevention

chapter 47

Colorectal Cancer

Carol A. Burke, MD

INTRODUCTION

Colorectal cancer (CRC) is a major public health problem and remains the third leading cause of cancer and cancer-related deaths in American men and women. Approximately 147,500 new cases and 57,000 deaths occur each year.[1] Fewer than 40% of the cases are diagnosed before regional and distant spread occurs, when the disease is curable. The estimated costs associated with the care of patients with CRC are more than $5 billion annually.[2]

The incidence of CRC has been decreasing an average of 1.5% per annum since the mid-1980s and is paralleled by a diminution in CRC mortality[1]. The decline in mortality is likely due to the use of screening, which results in the detection of early-stage disease and better likelihood of survival (Table 47-1). The decrease in incidence is attributable to polypectomy of adenomatous polyps, thereby preventing their progression to cancer.

However, fewer than 40% of eligible Americans report having had recent CRC screening by fecal occult blood testing (FOBT), flexible sigmoidoscopy, or colonoscopy.[3] Inconvenience, risk perception for CRC, and failure of physicians to discuss screening were the most common patient-related reasons for noncompliance.[4] In a group of outpatients receiving primary care, less than one fourth reported that their physician had ever discussed CRC screening. Health care providers should understand the benefits, limitations, cost, and effectiveness of the available screening options and disseminate the information to patients, to make an impact on reducing the incidence and death rate due to CRC.

PATHOPHYSIOLOGY

Most, if not all, CRCs arise from an adenomatous polyp. *Polyp* is an inexact term that indicates a protuberance of tissue on the colonic mucosa. Polyps may be divided into 2 categories: neoplastic and nonneoplastic (Table 47-2). Neoplastic polyps may be benign or malignant. The most common polyp and the only known precursor to adenocarcinoma is the *adenomatous* polyp.[5] Most authorities agree that individuals with greatest risk of metachronous CRC are those with more than 2 adenomas or those with advanced neoplasia. *Advanced neoplasia* is usually defined as an adenoma with a diameter equal to or greater than 10 mm, or containing at least 25% villous component, or with high-grade dysplasia (also known as carcinoma in situ or intramucosal cancer), or an invasive adenocarcinoma. The nonneoplastic polyps include lymphoid, hamartomas, juvenile, inflammatory, and hyperplastic.

TABLE 47-1

Effect of Cancer Stage on Survival

Dukes Classification	Estimated 5-y Survival Rate (%)
A	95
B	80
C	35–60
D	<10

TABLE 47-2

Histologic Classification of Polyps

Neoplastic	Nonneoplastic
Benign	Hyperplastic
Tubular	Inflammatory
Tubulovillous	Lymphoid
Villous	Hamartoma
Severe dysplasia	Juvenile
Intramucosal cancer	
Carcinoma in situ	
Malignant	
Invasive adenocarcinoma	

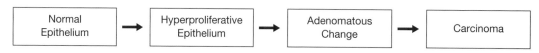

FIGURE 47-1

Histologic and genetic changes in sporadic adenoma-carcinoma sequence.

TABLE 47-3

Percentage of US Population With Diagnosed Invasive Colorectal Cancer*

Sex	Birth–39	Age, y 40–59	60–79	Lifetime Risk
Male	0.06 (1/1617)	0.88 (1/114)	4.00 (1/25)	5.88 (1/17)
Female	0.06 (1/1630)	0.69 (1/145)	3.03 (1/33)	5.56 (1/18)

*Adapted from Jemal et al.[1]

These polyps are not associated with increased risk of CRC and do not require special follow-up.

Hyperplastic polyps are the second most common type of polyp, accounting for up to 30% of colonic polyps. Hyperplastic polyps are most often found in the rectosigmoid. Unfortunately, hyperplastic polyps and adenomas are indistinguishable on endoscopy. Therefore, all polyps detected in the colon and rectum should be removed and sent for histologic analysis.

Whereas nearly 40% of Americans aged 50 years or older have adenomatous polyps, it is estimated that only 2% of adenomas will progress to cancer. Colorectal cancer results from complex interactions between genetic susceptibility and environmental factors. The environmental cofactors include advanced age, diet, smoking, physical inactivity, alcohol consumption, and obesity.[6-9] Sporadic CRC develops slowly and has a long precancerous and asymptomatic phase. Observational studies suggest that the adenoma-to-carcinoma sequence takes approximately 10 years. The progression from normal epithelium to adenoma to carcinoma occurs through a series of multiple somatic genetic and histologic changes.[10] When critical genes, such as oncogenes (k-ras) and tumor suppressor genes (APC, p53, 18q) are affected, normal controls on cellular proliferation and apoptosis are lost and cancer ensues (Fig 47-1). The genetic alterations are induced through at least 3 pathways. The first pathway, chromosomal instability, arises from an accumulation of allelic losses or mutations, resulting in gene inactivation.[11] A second pathway, microsatellite instability, involves inactivating mutations in the genes responsible for encoding a complex of proteins that repair mismatched DNA base pairs.[12] When the DNA mismatch repair system fails, widespread mutations at repetitive DNA sequences (microsatellites) in the genome occur. Microsatellite instability due to mismatch repair gene inactivation is present in approximately 15% of sporadic CRCs but is the major cause of hereditary nonpolyposis colorectal cancer

(HNPCC).[13] Some cancers have neither chromosomal nor microsatellite instability. Hypermethylation of promoter regions of genes can result in gene inactivation and is a third pathway of carcinogenesis.[14]

RISK FACTORS

The lifetime risk of an invasive CRC developing is 1 in 18 (Table 47-3). Colorectal cancer is uncommon under the age of 60 years, and the risk increases markedly thereafter.[1] Nearly 70% of cases are not associated with known risk factors. Known risk factors include the following:

- Prior personal history of CRC
- First-degree relative younger than 60 years with adenoma or CRC, or 2 first-degree relatives of any age with CRC
- Inherited CRC syndromes
- Hereditary nonpolyposis CRC
- Familial adenomatous polyposis (FAP)
- Ulcerative colitis and Crohn's colitis

Table 47-4 summarizes surveillance recommendations for CRC in high-risk groups.

A personal history of adenomatous polyps or CRC increases the risk of metachronous CRC twofold to threefold. First-degree relatives of patients with CRC have a twofold to threefold increased risk of colorectal neoplasia, including cancer and adenomatous polyps.[15,16] First-degree family members of patients with adenomatous polyps also have an increased risk of CRC, particularly when the relative's adenoma is diagnosed before age 60 years.[17]

People with the highest risk of CRC are those who have one of the dominantly inherited CRC syndromes: FAP or HNPCC. The diagnosis of these syndromes was purely clinical until their genetic bases were identified. Now, hereditary cancer risk assessment begins with an

TABLE 47-4

Colorectal Neoplasia Surveillance in Increased-Risk Groups*

Risk Factor	Recommendation	Interval
Moderate Risk		
<2, small (<1-cm) tubular adenoma and no family history of CRC	Colonoscopy	3–6 y after polyp removal; if normal, resume average-risk screening
>2, or >1-cm adenoma or adenomas with high-grade dysplasia or villous change	Colonoscopy	3 y after polyp removal; if normal, resume average-risk screening
Personal history of CRC	Colonoscopy	Within 1 year after surgery; if normal, repeat in 3 y. If normal, repeat every 5 y
CRC or adenomas in FDR aged <60 y, or ≥2 FDR of any age with CRC	Colonoscopy	Every 5–10 y beginning at age 40 y or 10 y younger than youngest FDR with CRC, whichever is earlier
High Risk		
Family history of familial adenomatous polyposis	Refer to specialty center for genetic counseling and consideration of genetic testing	At time of diagnosis
	Sigmoidoscopy or colonoscopy	Every 1–2 y beginning in puberty
Family history of hereditary nonpolyposis colorectal cancer	Refer to specialty center for genetic counseling and consideration of genetic testing	At time of diagnosis
	Colonoscopy	Every 1–2 y beginning at age 21 y until age 40 y, then annually
Inflammatory bowel disease	Colonoscopy with biopsy for dysplasia	Every 1–2 y beginning 8 y after start of pancolitis, 12–15 y after start of left-sided colitis

*Modified from Smith et al.[3] CRC indicates colorectal cancer; FDR, first-degree relative.

evaluation of the family pedigree, followed by genetic counseling and consideration of genetic testing for susceptibility genes for CRC.[18] Familial adenomatous polyposis is due to a germline mutation in the tumor suppressor gene *APC* on the long arm of chromosome 5. Genetic testing for mutations in *APC* is commercially available. The mutation causing FAP can be detected in approximately 90% of affected individuals. The *APC* mutation results in the development of hundreds to thousands of colonic adenomas, usually by the second decade of life. Colon cancer develops in all patients with FAP by age 40 years if prophylactic colectomy is not performed. Gastric fundic gland polyps and duodenal adenomas are common in all forms of FAP. Periampullary cancer is the second leading cause of cancer-related deaths in this population once colectomy has been performed.[19] Lifelong upper endoscopic surveillance is recommended, but the effectiveness of this approach has not been proved.[20] A form of polyposis with extraintestinal manifestations, called Gardner's syndrome, includes benign soft-tissue tumors, osteomas, supernumerary teeth, desmoid tumors, and congenital hypertrophy of the retinal pigment epithe-

lium. Phenotypic variation in the expression of FAP is noted and is related in part to the location of the mutation in the *APC* gene. A less severe form of colonic polyposis, named attenuated FAP, is characterized by fewer than 100 polyps at presentation and the age at onset of polyposis and cancer is shifted 1 to 2 decades later.

Hereditary nonpolyposis CRC is caused by microsatellite instability resulting from germline alterations in 1 of the 5 mismatch repair genes: MLH1, MSH2, MSH6, PMS1, and PMS2. Most families carry a mutation in MSH2 and MLH1 and testing for these genes is commercially available. Colorectal cancer occurs in up to 80% of those affected, usually by the age of 50 years, and is often right-sided. Extracolonic cancers such as endometrial, ovarian, small-bowel, transitional cell of the ureter or bladder, and gastric often occur in patients with HNPCC. The risk of endometrial carcinoma has been reported in up to 60% and ovarian carcinoma in up to 20% of patients with HNPCC. Therefore, aggressive gynecologic cancer screening is recommended in women in HNPCC kindreds.[21] The original clinical criteria set forth to unify the diagnosis of HNPCC families are referred to as the Amsterdam criteria.[22] They are as follows:

- Three or more relatives with CRC, with 1 a first-degree relative of the other 2
- At least 2 successive generations affected
- One cancer diagnosed before age 50 years

The Amsterdam criteria are specific for identifying HNPCC but insensitive because they do not consider the extracolonic cancer spectrum or account for small families.[23] The Amsterdam criteria were revised in an effort to recognize families that may benefit from genetic counseling and testing as well as intensive surveillance. The Amsterdam II criteria include extracolonic cancers (endometrial, small-bowel, ureter, and renal pelvis) in addition to CRC.[24] The Bethesda criteria for HNPCC established by the National Cancer Institute are primarily patient specific and include younger persons having adenomas, colorectal or endometrial cancers, and individuals with 2 HNPCC-related cancers (synchronous or metachronous) rather than focusing on an entire family group.[25]

The chronic inflammatory colitides, ulcerative colitis and Crohn disease, are associated with an increased risk of CRC.[26,27] Nearly all patients with inflammatory bowel disease (IBD) in whom CRC develops have dysplasia. The cancers are often multiple and arise from flat dysplastic mucosa. The proximal extent of colonic involvement and the duration of disease (not activity) stratify the level of risk. Risk is highest in patients with pancolitis and is negligible in patients with proctosigmoiditis. After a decade of disease, the cancer risk increases yearly by 1% to 2%. Colonoscopic surveillance every 1 to 2 years, with multiple biopsies at 10-cm intervals to assess for dysplasia, is recommended in these individuals.[3,27]

SCREENING

The American Cancer Society, the US Preventive Services Task Force, and a number of surgical and gastroenterologic associations have established guidelines for CRC screening and surveillance.[3,28-32] A variety of screening options are recommended for average-risk, asymptomatic individuals beginning at about age 50 years. These include FOBT, flexible sigmoidoscopy, double-contrast barium enema, or colonoscopy. A strategy for CRC screening guidelines is outlined in Table 47-5. The use of FOBT, sigmoidoscopy, and colonoscopy for screening is associated with a decrease in CRC mortality, and these procedures have been shown to be cost-effective.[33-39] The performance characteristics, compliance, complication rates, acceptability, effectiveness, and cost vary considerably between options.

Fecal Occult Blood Test

Fecal occult blood testing is recognized by its simplicity, low price, and cost-effectiveness. One study has found 31% of subjects preferring FOBT alone and declining all forms of invasive testing.[40] The major drawbacks of FOBT are low sensitivity and poor compliance. Poor compliance is likely due to a combination of physician and patient factors. Less than 35% of Americans eligible for screening were found to undergo FOBT in the previous 5 years.[41] Three randomized trials have demonstrated that use of FOBT decreases CRC mortality by up to 33%.[42-44] The reductions in mortality are associated with a shift to detection of cancer at earlier stages.

An indirect marker of CRC, FOBT is aimed at detecting hemoglobin from the bleeding neoplasm. Guaiac is the most common method used for FOBT in clinical practice today. The pseudoperoxidase activity of hemoglobin in the stool can be detected by a color change when it catalyzes the oxidation of guaiac by a peroxide reagent. To minimize false-positive test results, it is recommended that patients avoid ingesting red meat; peroxidase-containing vegetables, such as turnips and horseradish; melons; and high-dose nonsteroidal anti-inflammatory drugs (NSAIDs) 48 to 72 hours before stool collection.[45] A position paper reviewing clinical guidelines for hemoccult testing recommends preparation of 2 windows from different sites on a spontaneously passed stool on 3 separate occasions.[46] The rationale

TABLE 47-5

Colorectal Cancer Screening Guidelines for Average-Risk Individuals*

Screening Test†	Recommended Interval (beginning at age 50 y)
Fecal occult blood testing (FOBT) *or*	Annual
Flexible sigmoidoscopy (FS) *or*	Every 5 years
FOBT and FS *or*	FOBT annually and FS every 5 years
Double-contrast barium enema *or*	Every 5 years
Colonoscopy	Every 10 years

*Adapted from Jemal et al.[1]

†Both FOBT and FS are preferred to FOBT or FS alone.

behind 2 sites and multiple samples is based on concern that a colorectal neoplasm may bleed intermittently and blood is not admixed homogeneously throughout the bowel movement. There is controversy regarding whether FOBT performed on stools obtained by digital rectal examination is accurate. It has been postulated that digital trauma or dietary factors may decrease the specificity. Studies comparing the specificity of a single, in-office FOBT obtained on digital rectal examination vs spontaneously passed stools found no difference.[47,48] A "positive" (abnormal) FOBT result by either method generally warrants examination by colonoscopy.

A recent study of FOBT in patients undergoing screening colonoscopy found that only 24% of patients with advanced neoplasia were identified by a one-time rehydrated FOBT.[49] The reported sensitivity of a program of FOBT for cancer is 50% to 80%, and the specificity is reported to be up to 98%.[42,50] Rehydration increases the sensitivity but lowers the specificity of FOBT and is therefore not recommended.[42,51] Because the sensitivity of a single "negative" (normal) FOBT result by digital rectal examination is unclear, this generally should be followed by FOBT on 3 spontaneously passed stools. Any amount of blue coloration on an FOBT specimen is considered a positive test result and necessitates colonoscopy.

Sigmoidoscopy

No data exist from randomized, controlled trials as to the efficacy of sigmoidoscopy for CRC screening. However, several case-control studies have shown a reduction in deaths due to CRC in subjects who underwent sigmoidoscopic examinations.[52,53] At least 1, randomized controlled trial is examining the effect of a single, screening flexible sigmoidoscopy at age 60 years on the incidence and mortality of CRC.[54]

Sigmoidoscopy is safe and easy to perform, usually after 1 to 2 enemas and without sedation. A 60-cm flexible sigmoidoscope is advanced through the sigmoid, and occasionally into the descending colon. Diagnostic biopsy may be performed at the time of the examination. The sensitivity and the specificity for the detection of neoplasia in the segment of the bowel examined are high.

Although opinions do vary regarding the need for colonoscopy for patients in whom a single, small (<10-mm) tubular adenoma is found on flexible sigmoidoscopy, most experts advise a colonoscopy be performed in such situations because of the prevalence of proximal neoplasms. In one study, one third of patients with distal adenomas smaller than 5 mm were found to have more proximal adenomas and 6% had advanced lesions.[55] Another study found that 30% of subjects with advanced neoplasia would be missed if all patients with an adenoma in the distal colon did not undergo complete colonoscopy.[49] Additionally, the prevalence of proximal neoplasia can be based on the pathologic analysis of lesions in the distal colon. In one study, 7% of patients with distal tubular

adenomas and 11.5% with distal advanced adenomas had proximal advanced neoplasia detected on colonoscopy.[56] Studies using distal findings on colonoscopy as a surrogate for flexible sigmoidoscopy have found that approximately 50% of patients with advanced proximal neoplasia had no distal lesions that would have prompted colonoscopy,[49,56,57] thereby suggesting the advantage of colonoscopy as a better CRC screening modality.

Sigmoidoscopy Combined With FOBT

The rationale to use FOBT in combination with sigmoidoscopy is to benefit from the ability to assess for bleeding throughout the entire colorectum with FOBT and to visualize the distal colon and rectum with flexible sigmoidoscopy. In one controlled trial, 12,479 people underwent annual screening with either rigid sigmoidoscopy alone or rigid sigmoidoscopy combined with FOBT.[58] A reduction in the CRC mortality rate, detection of earlier-stage cancer, and longer survival were seen in patients undergoing both FOBT and rigid sigmoidoscopy. In contrast, the addition of a one-time rehydrated FOBT to sigmoidoscopy increased the detection of subjects with advanced neoplasms only an additional 5.5%.[49]

Barium Enema

Double-contrast barium enema has been included as an option for CRC screening. The double contrast is a better method than single contrast to assess fine colonic mucosal details and holds a theoretical advantage over FOBT or flexible sigmoidoscopy by the ability to image the entire colon.

Recent evidence suggests barium enema is inaccurate for detection of polyps and early cancers and is suboptimal for CRC screening or surveillance. In a prospective study comparing the accuracy of double-contrast barium enema and colonoscopy in a group of subjects undergoing postpolypectomy surveillance, the "miss" (false-negative) rate of barium enema for polyps larger than 1 cm was 52%.[59] If barium enema is to be used for screening or surveillance, it should be coupled with flexible sigmoidoscopy. The use of flexible sigmoidoscopy allows visualization of the rectosigmoid, which may not be seen well on barium enema because of the overlapping loops of bowel. Lesions detected on barium enema warrant colonoscopic evaluation.

Colonoscopy

Colonoscopy was adopted by expert panels as an alternative screening modality and first published as a screening option in clinical practice guidelines in 1997.[29,60] Various data have been used to support the recommendation for screening colonoscopy. Colonoscopic screening in average-risk individuals has been found to be cost-effective and similar to cervical or breast cancer screening techniques in cost-effectiveness per life-year saved.[33-37] The increasing recognition of the effectiveness of colonoscopy, limitations of FOBT and flexible sigmoidoscopy, and Medicare approval for screening colonoscopy have fostered a rapidly rising demand for the procedure. Unfortunately, the manpower and financial resources to perform screening colonoscopy in the eligible population are limited.

No randomized, controlled trials currently exist demonstrating the effectiveness of screening colonoscopy on CRC incidence or mortality. However, the incidence of CRC, which began to fall in 1986 and has continued to drop since, appears by analysis of population data on CRC risk factors and interventions to be likely due at least in part to the increased use of colonoscopic polypectomy.[61] The National Polyp Study compared the incidence of CRC in 1418 patients undergoing postpolypectomy surveillance with that in 3 reference groups, including 2 cohorts that were at increased risk of cancer (colonic polyps were not removed) and 1 general-population registry.[62] The group that had undergone polyp removal had a reduction in the incidence of CRC of 90%, 88%, and 76% vs the other cohorts, respectively. A case-control trial assessing the use of endoscopic procedures on the incidence of CRC found those who did not have CRC were about 50% more likely to have had endoscopic procedures than matched controls with CRC.[63]

Colonoscopy is the only technique with both diagnostic and therapeutic applications. The procedure can be completed in more than 95% of examinations with negligible risk. One study reported major morbidity related to therapeutic colonoscopy in 0.3% (9 of 3196 procedures), including bleeding of the lower gastrointestinal tract requiring intervention,[6] myocardial infarction and/or cerebrovascular accident,[2] and thrombophlebitis.[1,64] A study of 13,580 colonoscopies found a postprocedural complication rate of 0.2% bleeding (0.07%), perforation (0.07%), and death (0.007%).[65]

POSTPOLYPECTOMY SURVEILLANCE

Patients with adenomatous polyps are recommended to undergo postpolypectomy surveillance via colonoscopy because of the increased risk of metachronous neoplasia. When and how often to undergo such surveillance have been areas of debate, now being guided by information gained from studies of follow-up colonoscopies. A landmark study randomized 1418 patients who had undergone polypectomy to surveillance colonoscopy at 1 and 3 years or at 3 years alone. No difference was found in the proportion of advanced neoplasms (ie, >1 cm, high-grade dysplasia, invasive cancer) in the 2 groups.[66] To know

which patients merit more aggressive postpolypectomy surveillance and which may be more suitable to lengthened surveillance intervals requires understanding of risk stratification. Data suggest that the risk of advanced neoplasia (>1 cm, tubulovillous, villous, severe dysplasia, and CRC) after polypectomy can be predicted on the basis of the number, size, and pathologic findings of index adenomas. Atkin et al found a 3.6-fold risk of CRC in patients with baseline adenomas that were tubulovillous, villous, or 1 cm and a 6.6-fold risk if numerous (>2) adenomas were present.[67] The risk associated with small (<1-cm) tubular adenomas was 0.5, an incidence less than that in the age-matched general population. Another study confirmed that subjects with solitary, small adenomas are not at an increased risk of cancer compared with the age-matched population.[68] Patients with large (>1-cm) or numerous adenomas have a risk of metachronous cancer 2.7-fold and 5-fold greater than expected, respectively.[69]

It is possible to stratify the risk of metachronous, advanced neoplasia on a 3-year, postpolypectomy examination based on the characteristics of adenomas detected on the baseline colonoscopy. Subjects with fewer than 3 adenomas or small adenomas, or those younger than 60 years without a family history of neoplasia have a 3% risk of subsequent advanced neoplasia. Those with 3 or more adenomas or are older than 60 years and have a parent with CRC have a 10% risk.[70] Another study found that 70% of patients with fewer than 3 baseline adenomas had no recurrence and only 3.3% had advanced adenomas on a 3-year follow-up.[71] These authors concluded that patients with 1 or 2 tubular adenomas constitute a low-risk group for whom follow-up might be extended beyond 3 years. On the other hand, subjects with more than 2, or histologically advanced (tubulovillous, villous, severe dysplasia), or large (>1-cm) adenomas have an increased incidence of numerous or advanced adenomas on the first 3-year follow-up colonoscopy.

Based on data such as these, which allow for stratification of patients into low-risk and high-risk adenoma groups, postpolypectomy surveillance recommendations have changed. Low-risk patients are defined as those with 2 or fewer adenomas, an adenoma measuring less than 1 cm, and no family history of colorectal neoplasia. Low-risk patients should have their first postpolypectomy examination in 5 instead of 3 years.[51,72] Other expert guidelines have likewise extended the surveillance interval in the low-risk population from 3 years up to 6 years.[1,70] The high-risk group, consisting of subjects with greater than 2 polyps, or an adenoma measuring more than 1 cm, or adenomas of advanced disease, or a family history of colorectal neoplasia, is recommended to have the next colonoscopy examination in 3 years.[1,51,72] Table 47-4 summarizes surveillance recommendations in high-risk groups and after polypectomy.

EMERGING TECHNOLOGIES

Advances in molecular genetic techniques in concert with the understanding of the biologic progression of colorectal neoplasia has fostered the development of new, highly specific, stool-based DNA tests for CRC screening. Stool DNA testing is based on the ability to detect altered tumor DNA in stool samples of subjects with colorectal neoplasia. Testing fecal DNA provides a theoretical advantage over FOBT because it detects neoplasia directly. It is noninvasive, requires no bowel preparation or alteration in diet or medication, and is projected to be more sensitive than FOBT.

The basis of the test is due to the continual release of DNA into the fecal stream, more so from neoplasms than normal mucosa.[76] Since colorectal neoplasia is genetically heterogeneous it obviates the utility of a single marker as the sole target in fecal DNA assays. Combinations of multiple genetic markers have been studied in small numbers of subjects with known colorectal neoplasia.[75,77-79] Early clinical studies have found the specificity to be 90% to 100% with a sensitivity for adenomas and cancers of approximately 70% and 90%, respectively.[78,79] New molecular markers are being sought to maximize the sensitivity of fecal DNA testing. The utility of fecal DNA testing for CRC screening is being studied in 2 large, soon-to-be-completed trials.

Imaging techniques are increasingly being considered as alternative modalities for CRC screening. Virtual colonography makes use of helical computed tomographic (CT) scans to create 2- and 3-dimensional images of the colon that simulate conventional colonoscopy. Although the procedure is considered noninvasive and requires no sedation, the current strategy requires a bowel preparation and air insufflation of the colon, which may affect patient acceptability of the examination. Trials comparing the accuracy of colonoscopy vs CT colonography in average-risk populations are under way. Several of the largest studies from radiology centers with expertise in CT colonography have reported on the technique's sensitivity and specificity in the detection of colorectal polyps. These studies, performed in high-risk groups or subjects with symptoms, found that the sensitivity to detect polyps larger than 10 mm is between 85% and 100%, with a specificity approaching 90%.[80-82] The sensitivity worsens with decreasing polyp size to approximately 50% for polyps smaller than 5 mm. Before virtual colonography can be promoted for population-based screening for CRC, accuracy, availability, acceptability, and cost-effectiveness should be established.

Chemoprevention

An exciting area of research is the use of nutrients or medications for the primary and secondary prevention of colorectal cancer. In population-based observational studies, people taking non-steroidals (including aspirin), calcium, and folate had lower rates of colorectal cancer. Randomized, placebo-controlled trials have now demonstrated the efficacy of many of these agents.

Two recent, multi-center studies showed a modest effect of aspirin on recurrent adenoma development in patients who had previously had colorectal neoplasia. In the first study, of 1121 patients, patients with a previous adenoma were randomized to 80 or 325 mg of aspirin or placebo daily for 3 years. Those receiving 80 mg of aspirin had a 19% reduction in recurrent adenoma, as compared to the placebo group. No significant benefit was noted in the higher dose group.[81] Another study assessed the efficacy of 325 mg of aspirin in 635 patients with previous colorectal cancer. The adjusted relative risk of any recurrent adenoma in the aspirin group, as compared with the placebo group, was 0.65.[82] The use of aspirin solely to prevent colorectal neoplasia has not been studied and is currently not recommended. However, if patients require chronic aspirin therapy for other medical conditions, its chemopreventive benefit may be discussed with the patient.

Celecoxib, a selective COX-2 inhibitor, is the only FDA-approved agent for the regression of colorectal adenomas in patients with familial adenomatous polyposis (FAP) in conjunction with endoscopic surveillance and polypectomy. A 6-month, placebo-controlled trial in 77 FAP patients showed celecoxib 400 mg twice a day reduced the mean number of baseline polyps by 28% versus 5% with placebo.[83] Studies of the efficacy of COX-2 selective agents to prevent recurrent adenomas in the general population are currently underway.

Daily calcium supplements have been found to decrease recurrent adenomas in people who have had previous adenomas. One 4-year study in 930 participants found an adjusted risk ratio of recurrent adenomas of 0.85 in subjects taking 3 grams of calcium carbonate versus placebo.[84] The adjusted odds ratio for recurrent adenomas in a 3-year trial of 2 grams of elemental calcium was 0.66 vs placebo.[85]

Folate has not been proven in randomized, controlled trials to prevent colorectal neoplasia. However, the bulk of the observational and epidemiologic data suggests a beneficial effect.[86] Because it is nontoxic and low cost it is an attractive micronutrient to recommend at a dose of 400 µg/d.

REFERENCES

1. Jemal A, Murray T, Samuels A, et al. Cancer statistics 2003. *CA Cancer J Clin.* 2003;53:5–26.

2. *The Burden of Gastrointestinal Diseases.* Bethesda, Md: American Gastroenterological Association; 2001;51–59.

3. Smith D, Collinides V, Eyre H. American Cancer Society guidelines for the early detection of cancer, 2003. *CA Cancer J Clin.* 2003;53:27–43.

4. Lapin S, Abdullah M, Vlodov J, et al. Altering risk perception increases compliance with colorectal cancer screening guidelines. *Gastroenterology.* 2000;118:A262–1504.

5. Muto T, Bussey HJR, Morson BC. The evolution of cancer of the colon and rectum. *Cancer.* 1975;36:2252–2270.

6. Giovannucci E. An updated review of the epidemiological evidence that cigarette smoking increases risk of colorectal cancer. *Cancer Epidemiol Biol Prev.* 2001;10:725–731.

7. Michels KB, Giovannucci E, Joshipura KJ, et al. Prospective study of fruit and vegetable consumption and incidence of colon and rectal cancers. *J Natl Cancer Inst.* 2000;92:1740–1752.

8. Colbert LH, Hartman TJ, Malila N, et al. Physical activity in relation to cancer of the colon and rectum in a cohort of male smokers. *Cancer Epidemiol Biol Prev.* 2001;10:265–268.

9. Platz EA, Willett WC, Colditz GA, et al. Proportion of colon cancer risk that might be preventable in a cohort of middle-aged US men. *Cancer Causes Control.* 2000;11:579–588.

10. Vogelstein B, Fearon ER, Hamilton SR, et al. Genetic alterations during colorectal-tumor development. *N Engl J Med.* 1988;319:525–532.

11. Kern SE, Fearon ER, Tersmette KWF, et al. Allelic loss in colorectal carcinoma. *JAMA.* 1989;261:3099–3103.

12. Ionov Y, Peinado MA, Malkhosyan S, et al. Ubiquitous somatic mutations in simple repeated sequences reveal a new mechanism for colonic carcinogenesis. *Nature.* 1993;363:558–561.

13. Boland CR, Thibodeau SN, Hamilton SR, et al. A National Cancer Institute workshop on microsatellite instability for cancer detection and familial predisposition: development of international criteria for the determination of microsatellite instability in colorectal cancer. *Cancer Res.* 1998;58:5248–5257.

14. Toyota M, Ohe-Toyota M, Ahuja N, et al. Distinct genetic profiles in colorectal tumors with or without the CpG island methylator phenotype. *Proc Natl Acad Sci USA.* 200;97:71–75.

15. St John DJ, McDermott F, Hopper J, et al. Cancer risk in relatives of patients with common colorectal cancer. *Ann Intern Med.* 1993;118:785–790.

16. Bazzoli F, Fossi S, Sottili S, et al. The risk of adenomatous polyps in asymptomatic first-degree relatives of persons with colon cancer. *Gastroenterology.* 1995;109:783–788.

17. Winawer S, Zauber A, Gerdes H, et al. Risk of colorectal cancer in families of patients with adenomatous polyps. *N Engl J Med.* 1996;334:82–97.

18. Giardiello FM, Brensinger JD, Petersen GM. *American Gastroenterological Association Technical Review: Hereditary Colorectal Cancer and Genetic Testing.* Bethesda, Md: American Gastroenterological Association; April 2001.

19. Offerhaus GJ, Giardiello FM, Krush AJ, et al. The risk of upper gastrointestinal cancer in familial adenomatous polyposis. *Gastroenterology.* 1992; 102:1980–1982.

20. Burke CA. Risk stratification for periampullary carcinoma in patients with familial adenomatous polyposis: Does Theodore know what to do know? *Gastroenterology.* 2001;121:1246–1248.

21. Burke W, Petersen G, Lynch P, et al. Recommendations for follow-up of individuals with an inherited predisposition to cancer: I. Hereditary nonpolyposis colon cancer. *JAMA.* 1997;277:915–919.

22. Vasen HFA, Mecklin J-P, Khan MP, et al. The International Collaborative Group on Hereditary Non-Polyposis Colorectal Cancer (ICG-HNPCC). *Dis Colon Rectum.* 1991;34:424–425.

23. Syngal S, Fox EA, Eng C, et al. Sensitivity and specificity of clinical criteria for hereditary non-polyposis colorectal cancer associated mutations in MSH2 and MLH1. *J Med Genet.* 2000;37:641–645.

24. Vasen HF, Watson P, Mecklin JP, et al. New clinical criteria for hereditary nonpolyposis colorectal cancer (HNPCC, Lynch syndrome) proposed by the International Collaborative Group on HNPCC. *Gastroenterology.* 1999;116:1453–1456.

25. Rodriquez-Bigas MA, Boland CR, Hamilton SR, et al. A National Cancer Institute Workshop on hereditary nonpolyposis colorectal cancer syndrome: meeting highlights and Bethesda guidelines. *J Natl Cancer Inst.* 1997;89:1758–1762.

26. Judge TA, Lewis JD, Lichtenstein GR. Colonic dysplasia and cancer in inflammatory bowel disease. *Gastrointest Endosc Clin North Am.* 2002;12:495–523.

27. Friedman S, Rubin PH, Bodian C, et al. Screening and surveillance colonoscopy in chronic Crohn's colitis. *Gastroenterology.* 2001;120:820–826.

28. Colorectal cancer screening: recommendation statement from the Canadian Task Force on Preventive Health Care. *Can Med Assoc J.* 2001;165:206–207.

29. Winawer SJ, Fletcher R, Miller L, et al. Colorectal cancer screening: clinical guidelines and rationale. *Gastroenterology.* 1997;112:594–642.

30. Rex DK, Johnson DA, Lieberman DA, et al. Colorectal cancer prevention 2000: screening recommendations of the American College of Gastroenterology. *Am J Gastroenterol.* 2000;95:868–877.

31. American Society for Gastrointestinal Endoscopy. Guidelines for colorectal cancer screening and surveillance. *Gastrointest Endosc.* 2000;51:777–782.

32. Pignone M, Rich Melissa, Teutsch S, et al. Screening for colorectal cancer in adults at average risk: a summary of the evidence for the U.S. Preventive Services Task Force. *Ann Intern Med.* 2002;137:E132–E141.

33. Sonnenberg A, Delco F, Inadomi J. Cost-effectiveness of colonoscopy in screening for colorectal cancer. *Ann Intern Med.* 2000;133:573–584.

34. Frazier L, Colditz G, Fuchs C, Kuntz K. Cost-effectiveness of screening for colorectal cancer in the general population. *JAMA.* 2000;284:1954–1961.

35. Eddy DM. Screening for colorectal cancer. *Ann Intern Med.* 1990;113:373–384.

36. Wagner JL, Herdman RC, Wadhwa S. Cost effectiveness of colorectal cancer screening in the elderly. *Ann Intern Med.* 1991;115:807–817.

37. Lieberman DA. Cost-effectiveness model for colon cancer screening. *Gastroenterology.* 1995;109:1781–1790.

38. Eddy DM, Nugent FW, Eddy JF, et al. Screening for colorectal cancer in a high-risk population: results of a mathematical model. *Gastroenterology.* 1987;92:682–692.

39. Wagner JL, Tunis S, Brown M, Ching A, Almeida R. Cost-effectiveness of colorectal cancer screening in average-risk adults. In: Young GP, Rozen P, Levin B, eds. *Prevention and Early Detection of Colorectal Cancer.* Philadelphia, Pa: WB Saunders Co; 1996:321–356.

40. Leard LE, Savides TJ, Ganiats TG. Patient preferences for colorectal cancer screening. *J Fam Pract.* 1997;45:211–218.

41. *MMWR Morbid Mortal Wkly Rep.* February 9, 1996;45(5):107–110.

42. Mandel JS, Bond JH, Church TR, et al. Reducing mortality from colorectal cancer by screening for fecal occult blood: Minnesota Colon Cancer Control Study. *N Engl J Med.* 1993;328:1365–1371.

43. Kronborg O, Fenger C, Olsen J, Jorgensen OD, Sondergaard O. Randomised study of screening for colorectal cancer with faecal occult blood test. *Lancet.* 1996;348:1467–1471.

44. Hardcastle JD, Thomas WM, Chamberlain J, et al. Randomized, controlled trial of faecal occult blood screening for colorectal cancer: results for first 107,349 subjects. *Lancet.* 1989;1:1160–1164.

45. Ransohoff DF, Lang CA. Suggested technique for fecal occult blood testing and interpretation in colorectal cancer screening. *Ann Intern Med.* 1997;126:808–810.

46. Ransohoff D, Lang C. Clinical guideline: II. Screening for colorectal cancer with the fecal occult blood test: a background paper. *Ann Intern Med.* 1997;126:811–822.

47. Burke CA, Tadikonda L, Machicao V. Fecal occult blood testing for colorectal cancer screening: use the finger. *Am J Gastroenterol.* 2001;96:3175–3177.

48. Bini EJ, Rajapaksa RC, Weinshel EH. The findings and impact of nonrehydrated guaiac examination of the rectum (FINGER) study: a comparison of 2 methods of screening for colorectal cancer in asymptomatic average-risk patients. *Arch Intern Med.* 1999;159:2022–2026.

49. Lieberman D, Weiss D. One time screening for colorectal cancer with combined fecal occult blood testing and examination of the distal colon. *N Engl J Med.* 2001;345:555–560.

50. Kronborg O, Fenger C, Olsen J, et al. Repeated screening for colorectal cancer with fecal occult blood test. *Scand J Gastroenterol.* 1989;24:599–606.

51. Winawer S, Fletcher R, Rex D, et al. Colorectal cancer screening and surveillance: clinical guidelines and rationale—update based on new evidence. *Gastroenterology.* 2003;124:544–561.

52. Selby JV, Friedman GD, Quesenberry CP, et al. A case-control study of screening sigmoidoscopy and mortality from colorectal cancer. *N Engl J Med.* 1992;326:653–657.

53. Gilbertsen VA. Proctosigmoidoscopy and polypectomy in reducing the incidence of rectal cancer. *Cancer.* 1974;34:936–939.

54. UK Flexible Sigmoidoscopy Screening Trial Investigators. Single flexible sigmoidoscopy screening to prevent colorectal cancer: baseline findings of a UK multicentre randomised trial. *Lancet.* 2002;359:1291–1300.

55. Read TE, Read JD, Butterly LF. Importance of adenomas 5 mm or less in diameter that are detected by sigmoidoscopy. *N Engl J Med.* 1997;336:8–12.

56. Imperiale T, Wagner D, Lin C, et al. Risk of advanced proximal neoplasms in asymptomatic adults according to the distal colorectal findings. *N Engl J Med.* 2000;343:169–174.

57. Lieberman DA, Weiss D, Bond J, et al. Use of colonoscopy to screen asymptomatic adults for colorectal cancer. *N Engl J Med.* 2000;343:162–168.

58. Winawer SJ, Flehinger BJ, Schottenfeld D, et al. Screening for colorectal cancer with fecal occult blood testing and sigmoidoscopy. *J Natl Cancer Inst.* 1993;85:1311–1318.

59. Winawer SJ, Stewart ET, Zauber AG, et al. A comparison of colonoscopy and double-contrast barium enema for surveillance after polypectomy. *N Engl J Med.* 2000;342:1766–1772.

60. Byers T, Levin B, Rothenberger D, et al. American Cancer Society guidelines for screening and surveillance for early detection of colorectal polyps and cancer: update 1997. *CA Cancer J Clin.* 1997;47:154–160.

61. Nelson RL, Persky V, Turyk M. Determination of factors responsible for the declining incidence of colorectal cancer. *Dis Col Rectum.* 1999;42:741–752.

62. Winawer SJ, Zauber AG, Ho MN, et al, for National Polyp Study Work Group. Prevention of colorectal cancer by colonoscopic polypectomy. *N Engl J Med.* 1993;329:1977–1981.

63. Muller AD, Sonnenberg A. Protection by endoscopy against death from colorectal cancer: a case-control study among veterans. *Arch Intern Med.* 1995;155:1741–1748.

64. Nelson DB, McQuaid KR, Bond JH, et al. Procedural success and complications of large-scale screening colonoscopy. *Gastrointest Endosc.* 2002;55:307–314.

65. Wexner SD, Gargbus JE, Singh JJ, for SAGES Colonoscopy Study Outcomes Group. A prospective analysis of 13,580 colonoscopies: reevaluation of credentialing guidelines. *Surg Endosc.* 2001;15:251–261.

66. Winawer S, Zauber A, O'Brien M, et al. Randomized comparison of surveillance intervals after colonoscopic removal of newly diagnosed adenomatous polyps. *N Engl J Med.* 1993;328:901–906.

67. Atkin WS, Morson BC, Cuzick J. Long-term risk of colorectal cancer after excision of rectosigmoid adenomas. *N Engl J Med.* 1992;326:658–662.

68. Spencer RJ, Melton LJ, Ready RL, et al. Treatment of small colorectal polyps: a population-based study of risk of subsequent carcinoma. *Mayo Clin Proc.* 1984;59:305–310.

69. Lotfi AM, Spencer RJ, Illstrup DM, et al. Colorectal polyps and the risk of subsequent carcinoma. *Mayo Clin Proc.* 1986;61:337–343.

70. Winawer SJ. Appropriate intervals for surveillance. *Gastrointest Endosc.* 1999;49:S63–S66.

71. Van Stolk RU, Beck G, Baron J, Haile R, Summers R, for Polyp Prevention Study Group. Adenoma characteristics at first colonoscopy as predictors of adenoma recurrence and characteristics at follow-up. *Gastroenterology.* 1998:115;13–18.

72. Bond JH, for Practice Parameters Committee of the American College of Gastroenterology. *Am J Gastroenterol.* 2000;95:3053–3063.

73. Ahlquist DA, Harrington JJ, Burgart LJ, et al. Morphometric analysis of the mucocellular layer overlying colorectal cancer and normal mucosa: relevance to exfoliated stool screening markers. *Hum Pathol.* 2002;31:51–57.

74. Rengucci C, Maiolo P, Saragoni L, et al. Multiple detection of genetic alterations in tumors and stool. *Clin Cancer Res.* 2001;7:590–593.

75. Traverso G, Shuber A, Olsson L, et al. Detection of proximal colorectal cancers through analysis of faecal DNA. *Lancet.* 2002;359:403–404.

76. Dong S, Traverso G, Johnson C, et al. Detecting colorectal cancer in stool with the use of multiple genetic targets. *J Natl Cancer Inst.* 2001;93:858–865.

77. Ahlquist D, Skoletsky J, Boynton K, et al. Colorectal cancer screening by detection of altered human DNA in stool: feasibility of a multitarget assay panel. *Gastroenterology.* 2000;119:1219–1227.

78. Fenlon HM, Clarke PD, Ferrucci JT. Virtual colonoscopy: imaging features with colonoscopic correlations. *Am J Roentgenol.* 1998;170:1303–1309.

79. Fletcher JG, Johnson CD, Welch TJ, et al. Optimization of CT colonography technique: prospective trial in 180 patients. *Radiology.* 2000;216:704–711.

80. Yee J, Akerkar GA, Hung RK, et al. Colorectal neoplasia: performance characteristics of CT colonography for detection in 300 patients. *Radiology.* 2001;219:685–692.

81. Baron JA, Cole BF, Sandler RS, et al. A randomized trial of aspirin to prevent colorectal adenomas. *N Engl J Med.* 2003;348:891–899.

82. Sandler RS, Halabi S, Baron JA, et al. A randomized trial of aspirin to prevent colorectal adenomas in patients with previous colorectal cancer. *N Engl J Med.* 2003;348:883–890.

83. Steinbach G, Lynch P, Phillips R, et al. The effect of celecoxib, a cyclooxygenase-2 inhibitor, in familial adenomatous polyposis. *N Engl J Med.* 2000;342:1946–1952.

84. Baron JA, Beach M, Mandel J, et al. Calcium supplements for the prevention of colorectal adenomas. *N Engl J Med.* 2003;340:101–107.

85. Bonithon-Kopp C, Kronborg O, Giacosa A, et al. Calcium and fibre supplementation in prevention of colorectal adenoma recurrence: a randomized intervention trial. *Lancet.* 2000;356:1300–1306.

86. Giovannuci E, Stampfer MJ, Colditz GA, et al. Multivitamin use, folate and colon cancer in women in the Nurses' Health Study. *Ann Intern Med.* 1998;129:517–524.

RESOURCES

The American College of Gastroenterology
Web site: www.ACG.GI.org

The American Gastroenterological Association
Web site: www.gastro.org

The American Society of Gastrointestinal Endoscopy
Web site: www.ASGE.org

chapter 48

Lung Cancer

James L. Mulshine, MD, and Elizabeth E. Warner, MD

INTRODUCTION

In the United States, half of the adult population are current or former smokers, and both groups share a persistently elevated risk of lung cancer.[1-3] Recently it was appreciated that 50% of new lung cancer cases occur in former smokers.[4] Deaths due to lung cancer among former smokers exceed the combined cancer mortality of breast cancer and prostate cancer.[5-7] Therefore, public health measures beyond smoking cessation are urgently needed to reduce the mortality of lung cancer.

In considering the existing completed lung cancer screening trials, which generally evaluated the use of chest X-ray in conjunction with sputum cytomorphology, an international group of experts concluded that these trials formed an inadequate basis for current public policy. These trials neither support nor disprove the utility of chest X-ray–based early lung cancer detection.[8] The further recommendation of this assemblage was to expedite the evaluation of lung cancer screening with new imaging technology in clinical trials.

Based on promising pilot data, lung cancer screening with high-resolution spiral computed tomography (CT) has emerged as an option to apply to the problem of lung cancer mortality.[9,12] The National Cancer Institute recently announced its prospective randomized trial, the National Lung Screening Trial (NLST), to evaluate this new approach to lung cancer detection: www.newscenter. cancer.gov/BenchMarks/archives/2002_09/index.html or www.cancer.gov/NLST.[13] This randomized trial will enroll 50,000 high-risk individuals to compare lung cancer mortality outcomes using serial evaluation with either chest radiography or spiral CT as a tool for early detection of lung cancer.

Cancer screening is a demanding proposition. Even in a trial with a high-risk cohort, the challenge is typically to find cancers in a population with a single case of cancer per 100 or even 1000 high-risk individuals. From this perspective, a number of authors have suggested that the potential for harm with lung cancer screening is substantial.[14-16] From a research perspective, spiral CT-based lung cancer screening is the most promising development in the field for the last 30 years.[17] The theoretical possibility of routinely detecting primary lung cancer at a size of 3 mm, or even imaging the cellular infiltration of pre-invasive lung cancer, is a remarkable prospect. However, harnessing this technology in light of the major concerns about potential harm to misclassified screenees presents a profound challenge to the research community.

This is a public health problem in which each aspect of the care must be optimized to result in clinical benefit. However, there has been no systematic effort to define and implement optimized clinical management for individuals detected in spiral CT screening programs. The goal of this review is to discuss the components of lung cancer screening and how they interact. What research is required to elucidate a screening management algorithm that can be reliably delivered to achieve a significant reduction in lung cancer–related mortality? If such clinical benefit is possible, how can the management be refined to permit economical delivery to the vast at-risk population?

SCREENING CRITERIA

Because mass screening is a demanding public health process, formal criteria have been proposed to define the appropriate situation for such an approach. A classic description was proposed by Wilson and Jungner[18] in 1968 and includes the following criteria:

1. The condition sought should be an important health problem.
2. There should be an effective treatment for patients with recognized early disease.
3. Facilities for diagnosis and treatment should be available.
4. There should be a recognizable latent or early symptomatic stage.
5. There should be a suitable test or examination.
6. The test should be acceptable to the population.

7. The natural history of the condition, including development from latent to declared disease, should be adequately understood.

8. There should be an agreed policy on whom to treat as patients.

9. The costs of case finding (including diagnosis and treatment of patients) should be economically balanced in relation to possible expenditure on medical care as a whole, and case finding should be a continuing surveillance process, not a "once-and-for-all" effort.

These criteria provide a useful framework for discussing lung cancer screening.

Important Health Problem

Lung cancer is the world's leading cause of cancer-related death. This disease is typically diagnosed at a time when regional or distant metastatic disease is already established. Because metastatic disease is generally incurable, there is only a 15% 5-year survival. In the United States, more than 157,000 people died of lung cancer in 2002.[7] The outcomes with this disease have not improved over the last several decades despite intensive research efforts.[7,17,19] Recently, lung cancer has even outstripped heart disease as the leading cause of death due to tobacco use.[20]

The aggregate economic cost of tobacco use in our society has been reported in a recent analysis by the Centers for Disease Control and Prevention. The annual total of direct health care expenditures and economic losses from tobacco use amounts to more than $150 billion, with lung cancer accounting for a large amount of that cost.[20] On several scores then, lung cancer represents one of the foremost health care problems in our society.

Effective Treatment of Early Disease

The current standard of care for early-stage lung cancer is surgical resection. Anatomical lobectomy has been shown to be a highly curative option, especially for individuals with small primary lung cancers.[7,21,22] Nonetheless, this is a major operation in which operative mortality and morbidity present a major challenge for application in a screening context.[24] In many instances, the lung cancers detected by spiral CT are much smaller than conventionally diagnosed lung cancer, which raises the question of whether there are less morbid ways to manage CT-detected lung cancer. This issue was the focus of a recent National Cancer Institute workshop titled, "Diagnosis and Therapy of Screen-detected Lung Cancer." As outlined in the meeting report, experimental approaches ranging from video-assisted thoracic surgery and tailored radiation therapy to medical options are being explored in an effort to effectively and efficiently manage very small primary lung cancers (www.webtie.org/sots/meetings/lung/June%2019%202001/Default.htm). Assuming that the

NLST will take from 8 to 10 years to complete, sorting out the best management of screen-identified lung cancer is a formidable challenge.

Facilities for Diagnosis and Treatment

An apparent advantage of spiral CT screening for lung cancer is that CT imaging facilities are broadly available across the country. However, the presence of a CT scanner does not make a lung cancer screening center. As with mammographic screening, the process of screening, case identification, intervention, and follow-up requires a specialized set of interdisciplinary health care providers. To provide optimal care in this setting also requires a tight system integration to facilitate the process as well as thoughtful measures for informing the participants about the dynamics of the process, including potential costs and benefits.[24,25]

A critical factor in evaluating a screening program is cost-effectiveness. Once the health and economic outcomes of a target screening strategy (benefits, harms, and costs) are defined, the next question is whether the potential improvement of health outcomes justifies the additional costs.[15] Although the issues regarding cost-effectiveness influence the adoption of screening procedures, how a screening service is delivered also can have a profound influence on cost. The US population is aging, and the incidence of many cancers increases with age. Facilitating multiorgan cancer screening by bundling the delivery of validated cancer prevention services in an integrated imaging facility may reduce cost and enhance the ease of user access. In a cancer screening setting with fully ambulatory individuals, cost could be significantly reduced if the design of the spiral CT was optimized for the more mobile, otherwise healthy individual. Many aspects of the lung cancer screening process could be redesigned for maximal cost economy should the service emerge as efficacious in validation trials. Screening for lung cancer addresses such a large at-risk population that purpose-built tools designed to minimize the cost of the screening test are feasible and could decrease the cost impact of this potential cancer screening service. Considerable cost savings could be realized by the development of facilities capable of delivering integrated cancer prevention services along with other types of preventive services in a more rational and user-convenient fashion. There are many reasons to contemplate such a strategy, as it may facilitate both compliance with preventive services and provide an ongoing forum for tailored health communications. In addition, if an organized cancer screening infrastructure was available for the organ sites where benefit has already been established, the incremental work in testing and potentially adding screening for lung cancer or some other organ site would be considerably more straightforward than the current situation.

Latent or Early Symptomatic Stage

When lung cancer is symptomatic, the outcomes are not favorable. The goal with lung cancer is to find small primary lung cancers that are latent. Because this disease has a dominant etiologic agent, which is exposure to tobacco combustion products, use of these exposures can efficiently define very-high-risk cohorts to focus on for lung cancer screening.[26–28]

A recent report from a single institutional referral experience concluded that size of primary lung cancer does not affect outcome for primary cancers smaller than 3 cm.[29] This report implied that finding smaller primary lung cancer in a screening setting may not be useful. This view is consistent with the "systemic" hypothesis of carcinogenesis and arises from the field of breast cancer screening.[30] The "systemic" hypothesis is based on the notion that breast cancer is a metastatic process from its inception. This contrasts with the "progressive" hypothesis, which is based on the notion that cancer evolves through steps of progressively increasing aggressiveness and results in an invasive cancer capable of growing in remote sites as metastatic foci. For breast cancer, a disease that is routinely detected as a primary cancer smaller than 1 cm, the 85% 5-year survival found with the disease argues strongly against the systemic hypothesis.[7] Lung cancer has only a 15% 5-year survival but is typically found with much larger primary tumors, often with evidence of at least regionally metastatic disease.[7] In general, smaller primary lung cancers, even below 3 cm in diameter, have been consistently reported to be associated with a more favorable mortality outcome.[21,31-35]

In the reported pilot experiences with spiral CT screening in high-risk populations, the cases of lung cancer in the prevalence screens are typically less than 2 cm.[10,11,36] In cases found after repeated annual screening, the average size of detected primary cancer tends to be even smaller than the cases detected at baseline screening.[10,12] It is clear with even this preliminary experience that a small number of very small lesions will be metastatic at their initial detection. Historical experience suggests that only approximately 10% of the primary lung cancers measuring less than 1 cm in diameter would be expected to have metastatic involvement.[21,33,37] In light of the frequent curability of early-stage lung cancer, that spiral CT is able to detect stage I lung cancer with a frequency exceeding 70% is remarkable.[10-12,38] Because of the rapid evolution of spiral CT, coupled with refinement in image processing, the mean size of screen-detected primary lung cancer will continue to shrink. Ongoing research is essential to delineate the evolving natural history of spiral CT-detected lung cancer, especially regarding metastatic frequency at time of initial detection. For now, there is no substantial evidence to suggest that smaller primary lung cancers detected with spiral CT will not generally be associated with a more favorable outcome.

Acceptable Test

Spiral CT is likely to be considered a less intrusive test compared with stool sampling for presence of blood, sigmoidoscopy or colonoscopy, pelvic examination with cervical smear, mammography, or digital rectal examination. Diagnostic CT has been performed for a variety of indications for many years, and the general acceptance among the public is good. There is no major negative issue associated with this test, such as with screening tests for other major types of cancer. By virtue of the low density of lung parenchyma, the radiation required for a chest spiral CT is modest compared with more challenging locations, such as the colon. For radiation exposure, the lifetime risk of a CT scan has been compared with the lifetime risk of smoking a pack of cigarettes.[39] A recent American Cancer Society analysis found that smokers counseled by their doctors to undergo spiral CT did so with an unprecedented level of compliance. In advance of rigorous scientific evidence supporting the use of spiral CT in this regard, many people are already directly availing themselves of this technology at their own expense.[14]

Protection of public confidence in a cancer screening process is an enormous challenge, but in this embryonic situation there is even greater potential for hazard. The public is already hearing conflicting messages about the utility of breast cancer screening and despite renewed affirmation of benefit, the dissonance about the benefit of this approach undermines compliance with screening measures.[40,41] Although cancer screening strives for perfection, in a fast-moving, investigational area such as lung cancer screening, even if this screening approach proves to be beneficial, it is not going to be perfect. It may be particularly corrosive to public support for a screening procedure if the public perceives that a screening approach is being delivered in a suboptimal fashion. In this case, lives that could be saved will not be. The challenge to the health care community is to conduct the rigorous clinical research to define the "best practice" around all aspects of the care of patients with screen-detected lung cancer; in this way, maximal benefit of this approach can be routinely delivered even as the process is being refined. Clinical management factors for early-stage lung cancer are as follows:

- Relevant high-risk cohort
- Imaging protocol
- Diagnostic workup algorithm
- Surgical intervention
- Follow-up imaging algorithm
- Smoking cessation services
- Inclusion of other tobacco-related preventive services

Final acceptance of the screening test will reflect the confidence of the public in the totality of the clinical management process.

Natural History

Smaller lesions are expected to be associated with a more favorable outcome than larger nodules. The nuances of the natural history for very early lung cancer, however, are not well delineated. Although this information base is sufficient to allow for establishment of approaches to management of CT-detected lung cancer, further study will enable refinement of this screening management. Tailoring the early lung cancer management for distinct clinical entities to employ less intrusive interventions may improve the resultant screening benefit of cost, morbidity, or both.

Carcinogenesis is a complex, long-term, and generally progressive process. The rate of progression is defined by a poorly understood array of genetic and epigenetic factors. The ability to distinguish a progressive pulmonary nodule from latent pulmonary nodules is of considerable importance when using an operative intervention. A recent proposal from Cornell University researchers to identify clinically important pulmonary nodules based not only on their visual appearance but also on the biological feature of growth rate is important.[12,42] The progress in biomedical image processing applications for lung cancer screening has been recently reviewed.[43] The Cornell approach employs image processing software tools to reconstruct (or render) a nodule of interest in 3 dimensions. This can be done by stacking the relevant, sequential CT image sections acquired over the axial length of a pulmonary nodule. The volume of the nodule is generated by superimposing the elements of the imaged nodule from series of successive image sections. An example of a small peripheral tumor surrounded by interstitial changes (often ground-glass opacities) demonstrates the exquisite sensitivity of this technology in recapitulating the actual thoracic anatomy. The areas of interstitial change were shown on pathological review to be composed of cellular infiltrates of atypical alveolar hyperplasia. The accuracy of the image reconstruction to the actual topography of the nodule depends on the imaging technique. Specifically, the more sections through the volume, the greater the acquired imaging data and therefore the greater the congruence with the anatomical features of the original nodule.

The Cornell proposal is to use this volumetric reconstruction capability to look at dynamic changes in suspicious-appearing nodules.[12,42] By reconstructing the same nodule from CT scans taken at 2 different time points and comparing the change in volume from the first to the second time point, it is possible to calculate growth rate. Therefore, spiral CT becomes a discriminant of tumor growth and not just an anatomical imaging tool. Use of a dynamic criterion such as tumor growth rate parallels the efforts in prostate cancer using prostate-specific antigen (PSA) over 2 time points (PSA velocity) to allow this biomarker to become a much more reliably predictive test.[44] Determination of nodule growth based on image analysis, if independently validated to be a robust way to identify clinically important lung cancers, could be a major breakthrough in making case selection for lung cancer more clinically manageable.

The challenge with lung cancer screening is to identify a potential lung cancer at the smallest possible size to give the greatest probability for detecting premetastatic cancer. The mammography literature demonstrates that the measurement error with radiologists increases as the mean size of the breast nodule decreases.[45] The imaging capabilities of spiral CT are rapidly expanding, and so much information is generated from each study that it becomes a challenge for the radiologic world to keep up using conventional analyses. Image processing can provide a number of tools to assist the radiologist in this process. This includes both measurement tools and software to facilitate comparisons of regions of interest from sequential studies. Algorithms are also being developed to allow for progressively more competent and complete computer-assisted spiral CT images.[46,47] This is a profoundly important issue. The reading of radiologically based breast cancer screening studies has required substantial labor from the radiologic community, so it is essential to establish efficient methods to handle the workload of lung cancer screening.[48] The experience with image processing and computer-assisted diagnosis to assist in cervical cancer screening has been protracted, but cost-efficient and robust automated systems are just now emerging.[49]

Can image processing be used to achieve automated computer-assisted diagnosis for lung cancer screening? The answer to that question is currently no. With the remarkable strides that have occurred in this field over the last decade, this situation is highly likely to change. Computer-assisted tools have been reported to have greater success in breast cancer diagnosis, resulting in recent approvals by the US Food and Drug Administration of mammographic screening devices.[50,51] The data load with this planar imaging technique for breast cancer is much simpler than the data sets generated by spiral CT for the lung. However, the physics of spiral CT in being a 3-dimensional imaging tool evaluating a 3-dimensional disease provides a major advantage as the resolution of this tool evolves. At the current level of development, computer-assisted diagnostic approaches work best with simple cases, such as with a large nodules surrounded by normal lung. It is more difficult to resolve smaller nodules, especially if they are close to potentially confounding normal structures. This field is advancing rapidly, and a recent report suggests that the accuracy of a computer-assisted approach already matches experienced radiologists' accuracy in assessing changes in volume.[52]

A technical challenge is establishing the optimal strategies for classifying anatomical structures in the thorax. This segmentation function (distinguishing one structure from another) is a greater problem with older CT scanners since relatively few sections, or "slices" (1 scan per centimeter), were taken in the course of an imaging study. Only coarse features of anatomical detail could be resolved. Now with the typical spiral CT scanners, sections can obtain a scan for every millimeter, and, with the newer scanners, sections can be obtained as frequently as every 0.6 mm, permitting greater resolution of nodules measuring several millimeters. For screening to have the greatest benefit on mortality, the ideal sensitivity for a spiral CT scanner is not presently evident.[43] For now, if the state-of-the-art technology can resolve most nodules measuring several millimeters—roughly the size at which primary tumors develop vascular connection to the host— this seems a reasonable size window to explore. With these high-resolution studies comes an exponential increase in imaging data and file sizes. Fortunately, newer computers can readily handle this data load and permit rapid 3-dimensional reconstructions of suspicious-looking nodules. The additional imaging data provides computer-assisted diagnostic programs vastly more and better imaging data for evaluating an imaging study. In large measure, the rapid advances in lung imaging relate to breakthroughs in the availability of inexpensive micro-processing power.

Although the lung cancer specialists have experience in managing advanced cancer, many aspects of managing early-stage lung cancer are new. An effort to better elucidate the natural history of CT-detected early lung cancer is already under way with the lung cancer imaging program of the National Cancer Institute.[53] Leading imaging groups are following up cohorts of individuals with interesting CT findings through time in a systematic effort to define the natural history of various types of CT-detected nodules. This matrix of CT findings, coupled with clinical outcome data, is a responsible effort to inform clinicians about the malignant potential of very early lung cancer and to be a resource for assisting the development of better computer-assisted diagnostic approaches.

Policy for Treatment

Although improved sensitivity of CT means that the size of lung cancer at detection is shrinking, the standard pathological criteria for an invasive cancer remain the gold standard for identifying candidates for surgical resection. With the early pilot screening experience, there is a strong consensus that the diagnosis of lung cancer must be confirmed with either histology or cytology before operative intervention.[10–12,38]

However, as the number of cases of very small lung cancers increases, surgical management will require

more attention. Currently, lung cancer surgery is challenging not only because the cancer often aggressively invades local thoracic structures but also owing to the substantial comorbidity of underlying cardiovascular or pulmonary disease that is routinely present in smokers. As a result of these factors, the surgical management of early-stage lung cancer has a mortality rate ranging from 3% to 6%.[54,55]

The occurrence of lethal complications from a screening intervention constitutes an enormous impediment to the utility of the screening process. To allow the fullest potential benefit of lung cancer screening, rigorous quality control measures must be developed to ensure that the rate of operative mortality for patients with screen-identified lung cancer is as low as possible. Further research to elucidate effective and less morbid approaches to managing small screen-identified lung cancers is a major priority to enhance the prospect for ultimate success of lung cancer screening.

In the screening setting, especially with high-resolution spiral CT, a small fraction of primary lung cancers are detected while they are still confined to the luminal surface of the airway. Groups from Japan and Holland have shown that many of these small lung cancers, when confined to the airway, can be successfully managed with direct bronchoscopically delivered ablation using photo-dynamic therapy or electrocautery without thoracotomy resection.[56–60] In all of these pilot studies, an essential aspect of the research to develop less invasive techniques for lung cancer management is to routinely involve close patient follow-up with spiral CT. Thus, patients in whom less invasive treatment fails still can undergo potentially curative salvage thoracotomy.

The issue of how to determine which cases should be aggressively evaluated has been more problematic. A group from the Mayo Clinic has commented that the sensitivity of spiral CT in finding numerous pulmonary nodules has led to many complex diagnostic workups.[36,38] A group using screening data along the lines of the Mayo study for a cost-effectiveness modeling experience found the cost of screening to be remarkably high relative to improvement in lung cancer outcomes.[14]

In contrast, the imaging group from Cornell has reported the use of serial imaging to calculate tumor growth rates by volumetric analysis. With this approach, an invasive diagnostic workup is initiated only if the suspicious-looking tumor nodule is shown to be growing faster than a defined rate.[42] This approach to finding the cancer cases in their cohort has been more efficient than the experience reported by the Mayo group.[12,36] The screening cost analysis based on the Cornell approach appears to be more economical than that mentioned in the recent report of Mahadevia and colleagues.[61] In this new field, direct comparisons of cost analyses of pilot CT screening experiences should be done with great caution, since the clinical management approaches differ widely. The serial imaging approach proposed by the Cornell group has great theoretical and practical appeal because it involves far fewer invasive diagnostic workups. Independent validation of the Cornell volumetric imaging proposal is critical, as the efficiency of a diagnostic workup is a major determinant of the success of the screening approach. It is a pivotal issue if the proposed image processing strategies are to be capable of improving the problem with spiral CT screening, which was reported from the Mayo Clinic.[12,36,38,42]

Costs of Case Finding

Of the 2 published reports about the potential cost-effectiveness of lung cancer screening, one is promising and one is discouraging.[15,61] The benefit of spiral CT has not been definitively proved, and direct-to-consumer marketing of spiral CT is not appropriate at this time. There is considerable heterogeneity in operative mortality rates for lung cancer in different settings.[23] The success of lung cancer screening may require new measures to ensure that surgical care is delivered in settings that have the institutional expertise to perform routine lung cancer surgery with low complication rates. Cost-effectiveness analyses can be reliably performed only when the optimal process has been defined for case identification, workup, intervention, and follow-up. In a recent update of the cost effectiveness associated with the Cornell experience, the cost per person year-of-life-saved is even lower than the economic analysis.[61,62] The reported costs are reasonably stable, a variety of other scenarios were suggested in additional analyses from the recent report. It should be emphasized that this is the actual cost experience of the Cornell group and the reported number of diagnostic work-ups per numbers of screened individuals does differ sharply with the comparable reports from the Mayo group.

SUMMARY

The enthusiasm of some physicians about the future of lung cancer screening reflects favorable prospects for major improvement in almost every phase of the clinical management of early-stage lung cancer. Progress in lung cancer therapeutics over the last 20 years has been modest, and professionals in the field are demanding new approaches to the management of early-stage lung cancer.[18]

Cancer screening in general is an extraordinarily demanding process, and the challenges with lung cancer screening are even more daunting.[63] However, the fast-evolving features of spiral CT coupled with parallel refinement of medical image processing capabilities provide clinicians with a diagnostic tool that is clearly better suited for finding early-stage lung cancer than any previous tool. If this detection technology is developed rigorously as a public health strategy for the comprehensive and integrated management of early lung cancer, then there is a very hopeful prospect for success. In order to complete the clinical trials required to support such progress, robust participation in early lung cancer detection and management trials is essential. It is extremely unlikely that this type of progress can occur as a by-product of empiric management in a routine care setting.

Acknowledgments: The authors thank Robert A. Smith, MD, David F. Yankelevitz, MD, Claudia I. Henschke, MD, Daniel C. Sullivan, MD, and Robert J. Ginsberg, MD, for their helpful comments.

REFERENCES

1. Gaffney M, Altshuler B. Examination of the role of cigarette smoke in lung carcinogenesis. *J Natl Cancer Inst.* 1988;80:925.

2. Enstrom JE, Heath CW Jr. Smoking cessation and mortality trends among 118,000 Californians, 1960–1997. *Epidemiology.* 1999;10:500–512.

3. Enstrom JE. Smoking cessation and mortality trends among two United States populations. *J Clin Epidemiol.* 1999;52:813–825.

4. Tong L, Spitz MR, Freger JJ, Amos CA. Lung carcinoma in former smokers. *Cancer.* 1996;78:1004–1010.

5. RA Smith, TJ Glynn. Epidemiology of lung cancer. *Radiol Clin North Am.* 2000;38:453–470.

6. Burns DM. Primary prevention, smoking, and smoking cessation: implications for future trends in lung cancer prevention. *Cancer.* 2000;89:2506–2509.

7. Jemal A, Thomas A, Murray T, Thun M. Cancer statistics, 2002. *CA Cancer J Clin.* 2002;52:23–47.

8. Strauss G, Dominioni L. Varese meeting report. *Lung Cancer.* 1999;23:171–172.

9. Kaneko M, Kusumoto M, Kobayashi T, et al. CT screening for lung cancer in Japan. *Cancer.* 2000;89:2485.

10. Sobue T, Moriyama N, Kaneko M, et al. Screening for lung cancer with low-dose helical computed tomography: anti-lung cancer association project. *J Clin Oncol.* 2002;20:911–920.

11. Henschke CI, McCauley DI, Yankelevitz DF, et al. Early Lung Cancer Action Project: overall design and findings from baseline screening. *Lancet.* 1999;354:99–105.

12. Henschke CI, Naidich DP, Yankelevitz DF, et al. Early lung cancer action project: initial findings on repeat screenings. *Cancer.* 2001;92:153–159.

13. Marcus PM. Lung cancer screening: an update. *J Clin Oncol.* 2001;19:83S–86S.

14. Lee TH, Brennan TA. Direct-to-consumer marketing of high-technology screening tests. *N Engl J Med.* 2002;346:529–531.

15. Mahadevia PJ, Fleisher LA, Frick KD, Eng J, Goodman SN, Powe NR. Lung cancer screening with helical computed tomography in older adult smokers: a decision and cost-effectiveness analysis. *JAMA.* 2003;289:313–322.

16. Grann VR, Neugut AI. Lung cancer screening at any price? *JAMA.* 2003;289:357–358.

17. Carney DN. Lung cancer: time to move on from chemotherapy. *N Engl J Med.* 2002;346:126–128.

18. Wilson JM, Jungner YG. Principles and practice of mass screening for disease. *Bol Of Sanit Panam.* 1968;65:281–393.

19. Chute JP, Chen T, Feigal E, Simon R, Johnson BE. Twenty years of phase III trials for patients with extensive-stage small-cell lung cancer: perceptible progress. *J Clin Oncol.* 1999;17:1794.

20. Fellows JL, Trosclair A. Annual smoking-attributable mortality, years of potential life lost and economic cost: United States 1995–1999. *MMWR Morbid Mortal Wkly Rep.* 2002;51:300–303.

21. Martini N, Rusch VW, Bains MS, et al. Factors influencing ten-year survival in resected stages I to IIIa non-small cell lung cancer. *J Thorac Cardiovasc Surg.* 1999;117:32–38.

22. Miller DL, Rowland CM, Deschamps C, Allen MS, Trastek VF, Pairolero PC. Surgical treatment of non-small cell lung cancer 1cm or less in diameter. *Ann Thoracic Surg.* 2002;73:1545–1551.

23. Warner EE, Mulshine JL. Surgical considerations with lung cancer screening. *J Surg Oncol.* 2003. In press.

24. Cady B. Breast cancer in the third millennium. *J Surg Oncol.* 2001;77:225–232.

25. Aberle DR, Gamsu G, Henschke CI, Naidich DP, Swensen SJ. A consensus statement of the Society of Thoracic Radiology: screening for lung cancer with helical computed tomography. *J Thorac Imaging.* 2001;16:65–68.

26. Peto R, Lopez AD, Boreham J, et al. Mortality from tobacco in developed countries: Indirect estimation from national vital statistics. *Lancet.* 1992;339:1268.

27. Peto R, Chen ZM, Boreham J. Tobacco—the growing epidemic. *Nat Med.* 1999;5:15–17.

28. Van Klaveren RJ, de Koning HJ, Mulshine J, Hirsch FR. Lung cancer screening by spiral CT: what is the optimal target population for screening trials? *Lung Cancer.* 2002;38:243–252.

29. Heyneman LE, Herndon JR, Goodman PC, Patz EF Jr. Stage distribution in patients with a small (< or = 3 cm) primary nonsmall cell lung carcinoma: implication for lung carcinoma screening. *Cancer.* 2001;92:3051–3055.

30. Cady B, Michaelson JS. The life-sparing potential of mammographic screening. *Cancer.* 2001;91:1699–1703.

31. Asamura H, Nakayama H, Kondo H, Tsuchiya R, Shimosato Y, Naruke T. Lymph node involvement, recurrence, and prognosis in resected small, peripheral, non-small-cell lung carcinomas: are these carcinomas candidates for video-assisted lobectomy? *J Thorac Cardiovasc Surg.* 1996;111:1125–1134.

32. Inoue K, Sato M, Fujimura S, et al. Prognostic assessment of 1310 patients with non-small-cell lung cancer who underwent complete resection from 1980 to 1993. *J Thorac Cardiovasc Surg.* 1998;116:407–411.

33. Konaka C, Ikeda N, Hiyoshi T, et al. Peripheral non-small cell lung cancers 2.0 cm or less in diameter: proposed criteria for limited pulmonary resection based upon clinicopathological presentation. *Lung Cancer.* 1998;21:185–191.

34. Mountain CF. Revisions in the International System for Staging Lung Cancer. *Chest.* 1997;111:1710–1717.

35. Read RC, Schaefer R, North N, Walls R. Diameter, cell type, and survival in stage I primary non-small-cell lung cancer. *Arch Surg.* 1988;123:446–449.

36. Swensen SJ. CT screening for lung cancer. *Am J Roentgenol.* 2002;179:833–836.

37. Martini N, Bains MS, Burt ME, et al. Incidence of local recurrence and second primary tumors in resected stage I lung cancer. *J Thorac Cardiovasc Surg.* 1995;109:120–129.

38. Swensen SJ, Jett JR, Sloan JA, et al. Screening for lung cancer with low-dose spiral computed tomography. *Am J Respir Crit Care Med.* 2002;165:508–513.

39. Hirsch F, Bunn P, Dmitrovsky E, et al. IV international conference on prevention and early detection of lung cancer, Reykjavik, Iceland, August 9–12, 2001. *Lung Cancer.* 2002;37:325.

40. Duffy SW, Tabar L, Chen HH, et al. The impact of organized mammography service screening on breast carcinoma mortality in seven Swedish counties. *Cancer.* 2002;95:458–469.

41. Smith RA, Cokkinides V, von Eschenbach AC, et al. American Cancer Society guidelines for the early detection of cancer. *CA Cancer J Clin.* 2002;52:8–22.

42. Yankelevitz DF, Reeves AP, Kostis WJ, Zhao B, Henschke CI. Small pulmonary nodules: volumetrically determined growth rates based on CT evaluation. *Radiology.* 2000;217:251–256.

43. Mulshine J. Screening for lung cancer: in pursuit of pre-metastatic disease. *Nature Rev Cancer.* 2003;3:65–73.

44. Wieder JA, Belldegrun AS. The utility of PSA doubling time to monitor prostate cancer recurrence. *Mayo Clin Proc.* 2001;76:571–572.

45. Beam CA, Layde PM, Sullivan DC. Variability in the interpretation of screening mammograms by US radiologists: findings from a national sample. *Arch Intern Med.* 1996;156:209–213.

46. Kanazawa K, Kawata Y, Niki N, et al. Computer-aided diagnosis for pulmonary nodules based on helical CT images. *Comput Med Imaging Graph.* 1998;22:157–167.

47. Reeves AP, Kostis WJ. Computer-aided diagnosis of small pulmonary nodules. *Semin Ultrasound CT MR.* 2000;21:116–128.

48. Enzmann DR, Anglada PM, Haviley C, Venta LA. Providing professional mammography services: financial analysis. *Radiology.* 2001;219:467–473.

49. McQuarrie HG, Ogden J, Costa M. Understanding the financial impact of covering new screening technologies: the case of automated Pap smears. *J Reprod Med.* 2000;45:898–906.

50. Leung JW. New modalities in breast imaging: digital mammography, positron emission tomography, and sestamibi scintimammography. *Radiol Clin North Am.* 2002;40:467–482.

51. Castellino RA. Computer-aided detection in oncologic imaging: screening mammography as a case study. *Cancer J.* 2002;8:93–99.

52. Ko JP, Betke M. Chest CT: automated nodule detection and assessment of change over time: preliminary experience. *Radiology.* 2001;218:267–273.

53. Clarke LP, Croft BY, Staab E, Baker H, Sullivan DC. National Cancer Institute initiative: lung image database resource for imaging research. *Acad Radiol.* 2001;8:447–450.

54. Deslauriers J, Ginsberg RJ, Piantadosi S, Fournier B. Prospective assessment of 30-day operative morbidity for surgical resections in lung cancer. *Chest.* 1994;106:329S–330S.

55. Finlayson EV, Birkmeyer JD. Operative mortality with elective surgery in older adults. *Eff Clin Pract.* 2001;4:172–177.

56. Sutedja G, Postmus PE. Bronchoscopic treatment of lung tumors. *Lung Cancer.* 1994;11:1–17.

57. Van Boxem TJ, Westerga J, Venmans BJ, Postmus PE, Sutedja TG. Tissue effects of bronchoscopic electrocautery: bronchoscopic appearance and histologic changes of bronchial wall after electrocautery. *Chest.* 2000;117:887–891.

58. Kato H, Okunaka T, Shimatani H. Photodynamic therapy for early stage bronchogenic carcinoma. *J Clin Laser Med Surg.* 1996;14:235–238.

59. Konaka C, Okunaka T, Furukawa K, et al. Laser photodynamic therapy for central-type lung cancer. *Nihon Kyobu Shikkan Gakkai Zasshi.* 1996;34(suppl):107–110.

60. Nakamura H, Kawasaki N, Hagiwara M, et al. Early hilar lung cancer: risk for multiple lung cancers and clinical outcome. *Lung Cancer.* 2001;33:51–57.

61. Marshall D, Simpson KN, Earle CC, Chu C. Potential cost-effectiveness of one-time screening for lung cancer (LC) in a high risk cohort. *Lung Cancer.* 2001;32:227–236.

62. Wisnivesky JP, Mushlin AI, Sicherman N, Henschke CI. The cost-effectiveness of low-dose CT screening for lung cancer: preliminary results of the baseline screening.

63. Bailar JC. Screening for lung cancer: where are we now? *Am Rev Respir Dis.* 1984;130:541.

chapter 49

Skin Cancers

Jaeyoung Yoon, MD, PhD, and Randall K. Roenigk, MD

INTRODUCTION

The rationale for promoting preventive measures in skin cancer is based on its high incidence as well as the compelling evidence that it is directly related to sun exposure, a potentially avoidable behavior. The most common skin cancers are basal cell carcinoma (BCC), squamous cell carcinoma (SCC), and malignant melanoma. Together, these malignancies are the most prevalent worldwide in fair-complexioned populations and account for more than 1 million cases per year in the United States.[1] Of greater concern is that studies show a dramatic increase in each of these cancers over the last 50 years.[2,3] Although skin cancers, in general, result in relatively few deaths per year, mostly attributed to melanoma, advanced BCC and squamous cell carcinomas can cause substantial morbidity.

Basal cell carcinoma is the most frequent cancer of fair-skinned individuals, currently accounting for an estimated 900,000 million cases per year in the United States.[1] Squamous cell carcinoma is the second most common skin cancer with an incidence of approximately 100,000 to 200,000 cases per year in the United States.[1] It is the cancer most strongly associated with ultraviolet irradiation of all the common skin cancers. Malignant melanoma is a complicated and deadly tumor with increasing incidence worldwide. Although it is the third most common skin cancer in white populations, with an incidence of 47,700 cases annually, it is the deadliest and was responsible for 7700 deaths in the year 2000 in the United States.[4] The lifetime risk of melanoma in the United States has steadily increased over the last 70 years at a rate of 3% to 8% per year. In 1935 the risk of melanoma was 1 in 1500 but is currently 1 in 75.[2]

CLINICAL FEATURES

Basal cell carcinoma is believed to originate from hair follicles and presents predominantly on sun-exposed areas, although it can develop on any part of the skin. Classically, it presents as a pearly or translucent papule or nodule with overlying telangiectasias (Fig 49-1).

About 80% of BCCs occur on the head and neck. Superficial BCCs are thinner, more often found on the trunk and limbs, and have a "rolled" border or edge. The morpheaform subtype can simulate a scar and is more aggressive and infiltrative.

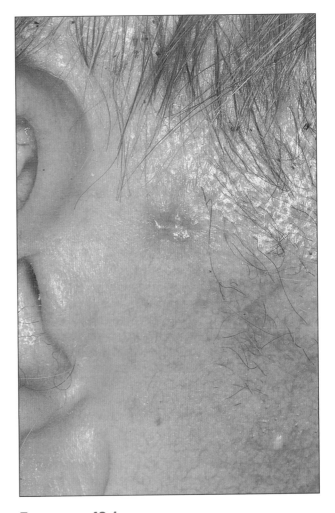

FIGURE 49-1

Nodular basal cell carcinoma. Translucent papule is surrounded by actinic damaged skin on right preauricular area of elderly patient.

Basal cell carcinomas are most often localized tumors, and they progressively destroy tissue until treated. Metastasis is rare, with a rate of less than 0.1%, and when it occurs, the tumor spreads to the lymph nodes, lung, and bone most frequently.[5] Metastatic tumors are usually those that have been neglected or are unusually large in size at presentation. Recurrent BCCs often behave more aggressively than the primary tumors, which emphasizes the importance of proper initial treatment. Patients who have had 1 BCC have a 45.2% chance of another BCC developing within 4 years, and they should be periodically screened for cancer recurrence and other primary tumors.[6]

Squamous cell carcinoma often presents on frequently sun-exposed surfaces of the skin as an erythematous scaly papule, plaque, or nodule (Fig 49-2). It also can present on mucosal surfaces. Subtypes include Bowen disease, an intraepidermal SCC; Marjolin tumor, which develops on a previous area of scarring; and erythroplasia of Queyrat, SCC of the glans penis. Other well-known asso-

ciated factors for the development of SCC are exposure to hydrocarbons, arsenic, X-ray radiation, and human papillomavirus types 16 and 18.

The metastasis rate of SCC varies widely in the literature from 0.5% to 31%.[7] Several factors are associated with increased propensity for metastasis. Tumors that are larger than 2 cm and those with poor histologic differentiation have metastasis rates near 30%. The location of the tumor is also important. Those located on the acral areas, penis, or lip are at higher risk, with metastasis from the lip occurring between 11% and 15% of the time.[7,8] In addition, SCCs developing in old scars, areas of chronic radiation dermatitis, sites of previously treated SCC, or immunosuppressed patients are also more aggressive.

Cutaneous melanoma is the result of malignant degeneration of melanocytes, the cells responsible for producing pigment in the skin (Fig 49-3). Malignant melanoma is classified into 4 main clinical subtypes: superficial spreading melanoma, nodular melanoma, acral-lentiginous melanoma, and lentigo maligna melanoma.

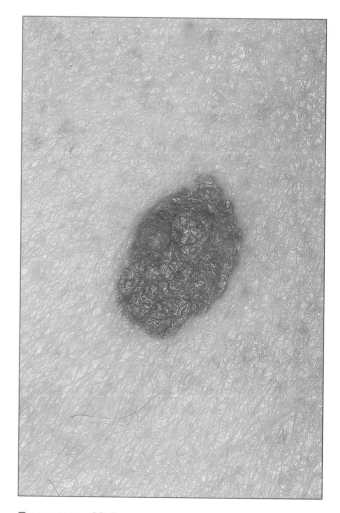

FIGURE 49-2

Squamous cell carcinoma. Erythematous and flesh-colored nodule has slight overlying hyperkeratosis.

FIGURE 49-3

Malignant melanoma. Large, thin plaque has brown and black variegation and slightly irregular border.

Superficial spreading is the most common and represents approximately 70% of melanomas. It is diagnosed most frequently on areas of intermittent sun exposure—the back and legs—and is a disease of middle age, with a mean age at diagnosis near 40 years.

Nodular melanoma is also a disease of middle age and represents about 15% of all melanomas. It is believed to enter a vertical growth phase more quickly than other subtypes and, therefore, has the worst prognosis.

In contrast, lentigo maligna is a disease of the elderly, affecting patients most commonly 70 to 80 years of age. It is a relatively slow-growing tumor and is usually found on frequently sun-exposed areas such as the face. Lentigo maligna represents approximately 5% of all melanomas.

Acral lentiginous melanoma is found on the extremities and is more common in Asian and African patients than in fair-skinned individuals. It has a poorer prognosis, and this is believed to result from a delay in diagnosis.

The single most important prognostic indicator for early melanoma is Breslow depth or tumor thickness. This is measured from the top of the granular cell layer of the epidermis to the deepest vertical extension of the tumor during histologic analysis of the biopsy specimen. This depth, measured in millimeters, correlates directly with 5- and 10-year survival rates (Table 49-1).[9] The 10-year survival for a patient with a Breslow depth under 1.0 mm is 94.5%. However, patients with a slightly deeper Breslow depth, between 2.0 and 4.0 mm, have a dramatically reduced 10-year survival of 59.9%. Other poor prognostic indicators include tumor ulceration[10] and elevated serum lactate dehydrogenase level.[11]

RISK FACTORS

The sun is a source of abundant energy in the form of electromagnetic radiation that supports life on earth through photosynthesis. Electromagnetic radiation is measured in nanometer wavelengths, which is inversely proportional to its energy (Table 49-2). This energy has deleterious effects on humans and is responsible, in large part, for promoting cutaneous neoplasms. The ultraviolet spectrum is most strongly associated with skin cancers and is divided into ultraviolet A, B, and C (UV-A, UV-B, and UV-C). The wavelength of UV-C ranges from 200 to 290 nm. It has the highest energy in the ultraviolet spectrum but minimally affects humans because the vast majority is absorbed by the ozone layer before reaching the earth's surface. The next highest energy level, UV-B, has a wavelength between 290 and 320 nm, and can penetrate into the upper layers of the dermis. The UV-A wavelength is subdivided into UV-A1, 320 to 340 nm, and UV-A2, 340 to 400 nm. Although it has the least energy potential, it is the most abundant ultraviolet radiation spectrum and penetrates most deeply, into the middermis.

The tumor-producing potential of ultraviolet radiation was demonstrated initially in laboratory animals in which skin cancers developed after exposure. Studies showed that the most effective carcinogenic portion of the spectrum is within the UV-B range between 295 nm and 305 nm, which is approximately 1000 times more potent than the ultraviolet radiation within the UV-A range.[12] Extrapolation of this data to humans contributed to the emphasis of UV-B protection to prevent skin cancers. However, although it is far less carcinogenic, several lines of evidence now support that protection from UV-A is also important in skin cancer prevention. When given in large enough doses, UV-A can produce tumors in mice.[13,14] This finding is particularly important because UV-A constitutes from 90% to 99% of the ultraviolet radiation at the earth's surface. Also, many sunscreens protect ultraviolet radiation within the UV-B range and inadvertently allow for prolonged exposure to UV-A. Tanning parlors, which are becoming increasingly popular, also use light within the UV-A spectrum. Further evidence of the carcinogenic potential of UV-A has been observed in dermatologic patients who undergo long-term photochemotherapy using UV-A and psoralen, a photosensitizer. Patients treated for many sessions for conditions such as psoriasis have a significantly increased incidence of skin cancers, SCC in particular.[15] Molecular studies show that UV-A may not act as a tumor initiator, as UV-B does, but rather as a tumor promoter that helps expand the initiated cells through modulation of protein kinase C, a signal transduction molecule.[16]

Clinical and epidemiologic evidence is compelling for the relationship between sun exposure and the formation of skin cancers. Almost all actinic keratoses, BCCs, and SCCs develop on frequently sun-exposed areas of the skin, including the head, neck, forearms, and dorsum of the hands. The most common sites of melanoma are the backs and legs, areas of intermittent sun exposure. The

T A B L E   49-1

Early-stage Melanoma Prognosis Based on Breslow Depth*

Breslow Depth, mm	5 y	10 y Survival, %
<1.00	98.0	94.5
1.00–2.00	90.0	83.3
2.00–4.00	70.0	59.9
>4.00	57.0	46.6

*Data from Buttner P, Garbe C, Bertz J, et al.[9]

T A B L E   49-2

Electromagnetic Radiation

Lower Energy (longer wavelength)			Higher Energy (shorter wavelength)		
Radio waves	Infrared	Visible	Ultraviolet (200–400 nm)	X-rays	Gamma rays

highest incidence of common skin cancers is in patients with fair skin complexion, who do not have the pigmentation that protects darker complexioned individuals from ultraviolet radiation. African albinos have a much higher incidence of skin cancers when compared with those in the same population who do not suffer from the pigmentary disorder.[17] Latitude studies also show that the incidence of the most common skin cancers within a country increases with proximity to the equator, where ultraviolet rays are most intense.[18] The highest incidence of BCC, SCC, and melanoma is in Australia, where the sun shines intensely for a substantial portion of the year and 92% of the population is Caucasian. The cumulative risk of melanoma in Queensland, Australia, is 1 in 14 for men and 1 in 17 for women.[19]

Factors that increase risk of melanoma include previous melanomas,[20] family history of melanoma, fair complexion (light-colored eyes and hair),[21] history of multiple blistering sunburns,[22] and proximity to the equator.[23] A small number of melanomas are hereditary and associated with a defect of the p16 gene, which produces a protein important for regulation of the cell cycle. A hereditary mutation of the nucleotide excision repair system (xeroderma pigmentosum) also increases the risk of melanoma. Another important risk factor is the presence of atypical melanocytic nevi. A multicenter study of 716 patients with newly diagnosed melanomas evaluated whether atypical nevi found on these patients increased their risk.[24] An atypical nevus was defined as being larger than 5 mm and having 2 of the following features: color variegation, irregular borders, or indistinct borders. The presence of 1 atypical nevus resulted in a twofold increased risk, and the presence of 10 or more atypical nevi increased the risk of melanoma by 12-fold. The presence of numerous (>50) small nevi resulted in a threefold increased risk. A final risk factor is immunosuppression such as that seen in organ transplant recipients.

PATIENT SCREENING

Screening for skin cancer is advocated because of the high prevalence and the improved prognosis with early detection, particularly in melanoma. The American Cancer Society recommends monthly skin self-examinations performed by the patient and a physician-performed skin examination every 3 years for those between the ages of 20 and 40 years, then annually after age 40.[25] The American College of Preventive Medicine recommends periodic screening and counseling for patients at high risk of skin cancer. These include patients with a personal or family history of skin cancer, fair-skinned individuals, and those with multiple melanocytic nevi.[26,27] The college further recommends education for pediatric patients regarding sun avoidance behaviors because protection is most critical in this age group. The greatest amount of sun exposure over one's lifetime is estimated to occur before age 18 years.

The pediatric population is at the highest risk of sunburns. A recent US telephone survey of 1192 youths between the ages of 11 and 18 years found that less than one third practiced effective sun protective measures.[28]

Although studies show that dermatologists are best at identifying skin cancers,[29,30] it is important that the practice of periodic screening is pursued by all physicians, particularly primary care physicians who see high volumes of patients. A full-body skin examination can take as little as 2 or 3 minutes of the office visit. Patients with suspicious lesions should undergo biopsy or be referred to a dermatologist. Men who are older than 50 years may be particularly important to target. In a recent study, 44% of newly diagnosed melanomas occurred in men 50 years of age or older, and these men had a disproportionately high mortality rate. This group, however, made up only 20% of all those who were screened.[31]

Self-examinations of skin may also be effective in identifying suspicious-looking cutaneous growths. One population-based case-control study investigated 1199 fair-skinned individuals in Connecticut, 650 with newly diagnosed melanoma and 549 matched control patients.[32] Although only 15% of patients practiced skin self-examinations, this practice was associated with a reduced risk of advanced disease. The study estimated that skin self-examinations may decrease melanoma mortality by as much as 63%, or approximately 4500 cases per year.

The dramatic difference in survival between early and late-stage melanoma underscores the importance of screening and early detection. Melanomas may be difficult to distinguish from benign melanocytic nevi, but certain criteria can aid in clinical diagnosis. This is known as the ABCDs of melanoma.[33] A represents *Asymmetry*. Melanomas usually do not grow uniformly, and when an imaginary line is drawn through the middle of the lesion, one side does not complement the other. B stands for *Border* irregularity. Benign lesions are usually well circumscribed, whereas melanomas can have ill-defined, notched, or even scalloped borders. C is *Color* variegation. Benign melanocytic nevi generally are uniform in color, whether tan, blue, brown, or black. Multiple colors within a lesion raises suspicion, as melanomas often have multiple colors, sometimes even with shades of red or blue. D is *Diameter*. Any melanocytic lesion larger than 6 mm, about the size of a pencil eraser head, should be examined and monitored for changes. Recent change in a previously healthy-appearing melanocytic nevus is especially concerning, and immediate excisional biopsy should be performed. In addition, signs or symptoms in the lesion such as pruritus, pain, bleeding, or fragility can be an indication of malignancy. Even given these standards, the clinical diagnosis of melanoma can still be extremely difficult in some cases. A high index of suspicion is required during skin screening to avoid missing a potentially lethal malignancy.

PREVENTION

Because of the strong relationship between sun exposure and cutaneous malignancies, guidelines on minimizing sun exposure have been established.[26,34,35] These include reducing daily outdoor activities during peak hours of ultraviolet radiation, between 10 AM and 4 PM, and wearing protective apparel—hats and clothes that cover the skin widely. The American Cancer Society and the American Academy of Dermatology further recommend regular use of sunscreen with a sun protection factor (SPF) of 15 or greater, especially for high-risk individuals.[35]

To date, only a few studies have shown that routine use of sunscreen reduces the incidence of actinic keratosis[36] and SCC.[37] Efficacy for reducing BCC[37] or melanoma[38] has not been shown with use of sunscreen. One possible explanation for the minimal benefit of sunscreens may be that its use actually increases exposure to the sun. Patients who use sunscreens may feel protected and more likely to spend time outdoors, including during peak hours, than they otherwise would. In addition, most sunscreen preparations in the past did not provide full-spectrum protection, with most absorbing only UV-B light. A final reason for greater overall accumulation of ultraviolet exposure in patients using sunscreen may be improper use of sunscreens. One study found that 73% of persons who applied sunscreen at a beach became sunburned due to incorrect use.[39]

Several practices can help maximize the benefit of sunscreen use. The American Academy of Dermatology recommends a broad-spectrum sunscreen, with an SPF of 15 or greater. It should be applied to the skin 15 to 30 minutes before going outdoors. This allows time for the active ingredients to diffuse evenly throughout the stratum corneum and for the sunscreen to dry, improving its adherence. People often use too little sunscreen, which results in reduction of the SPF. One ounce is necessary to cover the exposed area of the body, including the face, hands, arms, ears, and neck. Sunscreens should be re-applied on a regular basis every 2 hours, and immediately if the skin is exposed to water or after profuse sweating. Anyone who plans to participate in water activities should consider a water-resistant sunscreen.

Sunscreens are produced in a variety of vehicles, including lotion, gel, and applicator stick. They are divided into 2 general classes: chemical and physical. Chemical sunscreens contain molecules that are capable of absorbing ultraviolet radiation. The molecule is raised from a ground state to an excited state for a transient period before releasing the energy in another form, such as fluorescence or heat. These molecules absorb only portions and not the entire spectrum of ultraviolet radiation. Popular agents used today in chemical sunscreens include para-aminobenzoic acid (PABA) and cinnamates, which protect in the UV-B range, and avobenzone (Parsol 1789) and benzophenone, which protect in both the UV-A and UV-B ranges. Physical sunscreens produce a barrier to avoid penetration of ultraviolet radiation (UV-A and UV-B) and visible light, and result in light reflection or scattering. Popular agents used today in physical sunscreens include PABA, avobenzone, salicylates, benzophenone, and cinnamates. Previously, wide use of physical sunscreens was restricted by their opaque and cosmetically displeasing appearance on application. Newer compounding in micronized transparent formulations has popularized the use of physical sunscreens. The most common physical sunscreens available now include titanium dioxide and zinc oxide.

The SPF is defined by the ratio of a UV-B dose required for minimal erythema to develop with and without use of sunscreen. A UV-B dose 15 times greater, for example, is required to produce the same erythema on the skin when a sunscreen with an SPF of 15 is applied. This is based on a uniform application of 2 mg/cm^2 of sunscreen, according to the US Food and Drug Administration. Decreasing the thickness of this application also decreases the SPF value. Water resistance of a sunscreen is determined after 2 applications, each followed by 20 minutes of drying time, then a total of 40 minutes of water contact with 20 minutes of rest interval in between. If the SPF of the sunscreen after this test is the same before, it is considered water resistant. It is also important to note the expiration time of the sunscreen and to dispose any products past their expiration date. Chemical sunscreens become unstable and physical sunscreens can degrade when they are too old.

TREATMENT

Basal Cell Carcinoma

Several treatment options are available for low-risk BCCs. These include surgical excision using 4-mm margins, electrodesiccation and curettage, cryotherapy, and radiation therapy. Higher risk tumors are treated with Mohs micrographic surgery, a procedure where the tumor is harvested in a stepwise fashion with thin surrounding clinical margins until the entire perimeter of the tumor appears clear of malignant cells using analysis with light microscopy (Fig 49-4A–D).[40] This treatment method removes the tumor with minimal loss of healthy tissue and has the highest cure rate, with a 5-year recurrence of 1%.[41] Indications for Mohs surgery include tumors that are larger than 2 cm, have ill-defined borders, are recurrent, have an aggressive histologic subtype, or are located in cosmetically sensitive areas (Table 49-3).[42]

Squamous Cell Carcinoma

The approach to the treatment of primary cutaneous SCC is similar to that of BCC. The treatment of choice is

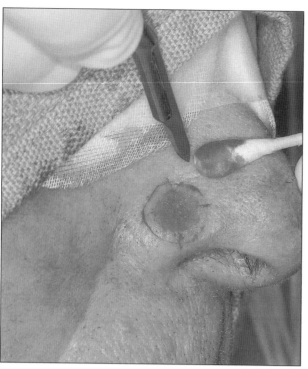

FIGURE 49-4A

During Mohs micrographic surgery, Mohs layer is taken from right nasal ala in patient with primary basal cell carcinoma. Hash marks are created at 12-, 3-, 6-, and 9-o'clock positions for orientation.

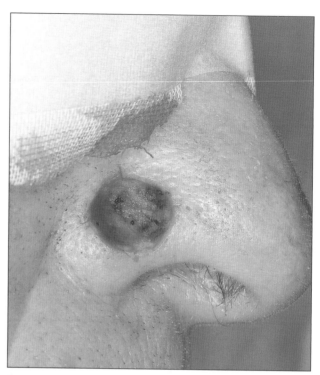

FIGURE 49-4B

Mohs defect after initial layer is taken during Mohs surgery.

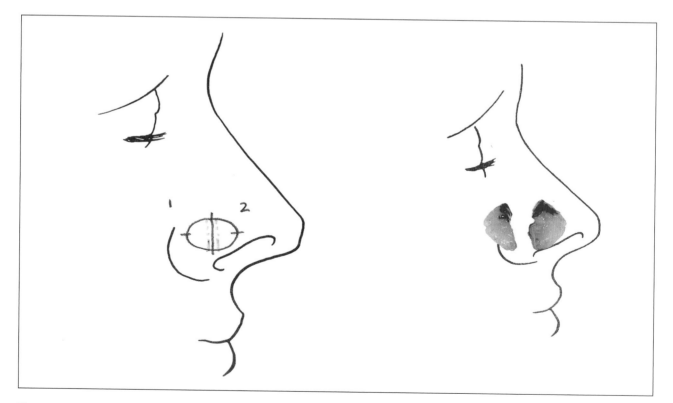

FIGURE 49-4C

Tissue harvested during Mohs surgery is divided vertically into 2 specimens and further orientated with different colored ink (right) according to Mohs map (left). Tissue is processed by histopathologic frozen section to examine entire peripheral margin for tumor. Process is repeated until clearance of tumor is verified.

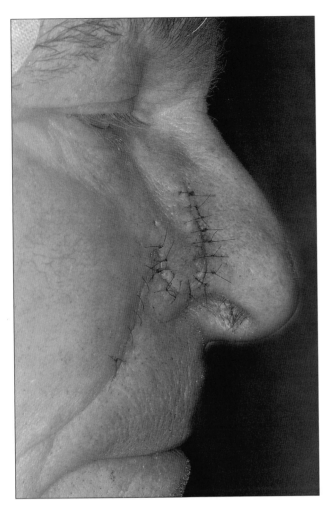

FIGURE 49-4D

Nasolabial transposition flap repair of Mohs defect after tumor clearance.

TABLE 49-3

Indications for Mohs Micrographic Surgery*

Location
  High recurrence rate if treated by traditional methods
  Embryonic fusion planes—sites of least resistance: nasolabial fold, philtrum, ala nasi, middle lower lip, chin, preauricular, retroauricular sulcus, temple, and periocular area
  Tissue conservation important on penis, digits, nose, and eyelids
Histology (subtype, aggressive)
  BCC—morpheaform, metatypical, micronodular
  SCC—grades II, III, and IV; Clark level IV and V
  Perineural
Tumor
  Marjolin
  Recurrent
  Large, invasive (>2 cm)
Immunosuppressed patient
Patient preference

*Data from Randle HW, Roenigk RK.[42]

surgery. Low-risk tumors may be treated using a variety of techniques, including electrodesiccation and curettage, wide excision with 4- to 6-mm margins, cryosurgery, and radiation therapy. High-risk tumors should be treated with Mohs micrographic surgery, similar to high-risk BCCs (Table 49-3). Mohs surgery has been shown to reduce the secondary recurrence rate of SCCs from 23% to 10% compared with other treatment methods[43] and to reduce the rate of metastasis from SCC of the lip from 15.8% to 7.4%.[8]

Melanoma

The treatment of choice for early-stage melanoma is wide local surgical excision, with the surgical margins determined by Breslow depth. In the early 1900s, melanomas were reexcised using margins of up to 5 cm. This method was based on data collected from autopsy results. Subsequent prospective randomized clinical trials have supported the safety of narrower margins[44,45] and have reduced the morbidity of intervention. Based on these studies, localized melanomas with a Breslow depth less than 1 mm are excised with 1-cm margins and those with a Breslow depth between 1 and 4 mm are excised with 2-cm margins. Sentinel lymph node biopsies are recommended for intermediate localized tumors with a thickness greater than 0.75 to 1.0 mm and without evidence of metastasis, to better stage the tumor. Subsequent lymph node dissection is performed if evidence of microscopic disease is identified.

The outlook for advanced or metastatic melanoma is grim. A number of biologic and conventional chemotherapeutic agents have been used but have done little to change long-term survival. Radiation usually is reserved for palliative therapy.

ORGAN TRANSPLANT RECIPIENTS

The prevention of skin cancer in recipients of solid organ transplants requires special consideration. Because these patients require long-term immunosuppression to avoid graft rejection, the incidence of internal and cutaneous cancers is significantly increased. One report from Norway studied 2561 kidney and heart transplant recipients. Compared with a healthy population, transplant recipients had a 65-fold increased risk of cutaneous SCC, an 84-fold increased risk of Kaposi sarcoma, a 20-fold increased risk of SCC of the lip, and a 3-fold increased risk of melanoma.[46] In addition, these cancers tend to be more aggressive, with increased metastasis and mortality.[47,48] A study of heart transplant recipients in Australia found that skin cancer was responsible for

TABLE 49-4

Dermatologic Follow-up Intervals for Transplant Recipients*

Patient Characteristic	Interval for Dermatologic Examination
No history of skin cancers or actinic keratosis	Initial dermatology consult, followed by annual examination by transplant physician until lesions arise. Patients at high risk of skin cancer may benefit from annual examination by dermatologist.
History of actinic keratosis	6 mo
History of 1 nonmelanoma skin cancer	6 mo
History of multiple nonmelanoma skin cancers	2–4 mo
History of high-risk squamous cell carcinoma or melanoma	3 mo
History of metastatic squamous cell carcinoma or melanoma	2 mo

*Data from Otley CC.[50]

27% of 41 deaths in 455 transplant recipients who were followed up.[49]

This increased morbidity makes education and screening particularly important. At the Mayo Clinic in Rochester, Minn, as a collaboration between the transplant service and the department of dermatology, a specialty clinic has been developed to optimize care of transplant recipients by emphasizing proactive education, prevention, and early detection of skin tumors.[50] Transplant physicians annually follow up patients with no history of actinic keratosis or skin cancers. Dermatologists more frequently follow up higher risk patients (Table 49-4). Prophylactic measures also are considered for higher risk patients. These include a daily topical retinoid using tretinoin, tazarotene, or adapalene (cream or gel) or a daily 2- to 8-week course of 5-fluorouracil cream. Patients at highest risk have multiple tumors (>5 per year), aggressive carcinomas, or melanoma. Systemic retinoid treatment using acitretin, 25 to 30 mg/d, may be considered to reduce the number of multiple SCCs.

REFERENCES

1. Miller DL, Weinstock MA. Nonmelanoma skin cancer in the United States: incidence. *J Am Acad Dermatol.* 1994;30:774–778.

2. Rigel DS, Friedman RJ, Kopf AW. The incidence of malignant melanoma in the United States: issues as we approach the 21st century. *J Am Acad Dermatol.* 1996;34:839–847.

3. Diepgen TL, Mahler V. The epidemiology of skin cancer. *Br J Dermatol.* 2002;146:1–6.

4. Greenlee RT, Murray T, Bolden S, Wingo PA. Cancer statistics, 2000. *CA Cancer J Clin.* 2000;50:7–33.

5. Domarus HV, Stevens PJ. Metastatic basal cell carcinomas: report of five cases and review 170 cases in the literature. *J Am Acad Dermatol.* 1984;10:1043–1060.

6. Marghoob A, Kopf AW, Bart RS, et al. Risk of another basal cell carcinoma developing after treatment of a basal cell carcinoma. *J Am Acad Dermatol.* 1993;28:22.

7. Melton JL, Hanke CW. Squamous cell carcinoma. In: Roenigk RK, Roenigk HH Jr, eds. *Roenigk and Roenigk's Dermatologic Surgery: Principles and Practice.* 2nd ed. New York, NY: Marcel Dekker Inc; 1996:503–521.

8. Dinehart SM, Pollack SV. Metastases from squamous cell carcinoma of the skin and lip: an analysis of 27 cases. *J Am Acad Dermatol.* 1989;21:241–248.

9. Buttner P, Garbe C, Bertz J, et al. Primary cutaneous melanoma: optimized cutoff points of tumor thickness and importance of Clark's level for prognostic classification. *Cancer.* 1995;75:2499–2506.

10. Balch CM. Cutaneous melanoma: prognosis and treatment results worldwide. *Semin Surg Oncol.* 1992;8:400–414.

11. Sirott MN, Bajorin DF, Wong GYC, et. al. Prognostic factors in patients with metastatic malignant melanoma: a multivariate analysis. *Cancer.* 1993;72:3091–3098.

12. Kripke ML. Carcinogenesis: ultraviolet radiation. In: Freedberg IM, Eisen AZ, Wolff K, et al, eds. *Fitzpatrick's Dermatology in General Medicine.* 5th ed. New York, NY: McGraw-Hill; 1999:467–468.

13. Strickland PF. Photocarcinogenesis by near-ultraviolet (UVA) radiation in sencar mice. *J Invest Dermatol.* 1986;87:272–275.

14. Sterenborg HJCM, van der Leun JC. Tumorigenesis by a long wavelength UV-A source. *Photochem Photobiol.* 1990;51:325–330.

15. Studniberg HM, Weller P. PUVA, UVB, psoriasis, and nonmelanoma skin cancer. *J Am Acad Dermatol.* 1993;29:1013–1022.

16. Matsui MS, DeLeo VA. Longwave ultraviolet radiation and promotion of skin cancer. *Cancer Cells.* 1991;3:8–12.

17. Kromberg JGR, Castle D, Zwane EM, Jenkins T. Albinism and skin cancer in southern Africa. *Clin Genet.* 1989;36:43–52.

18. Kricker A, Armstrong BK, English DR. Sun exposure and non-melanocytic skin cancer. *Cancer Causes Control.* 1994;5:367–392.

19. MacLennan R, Green AC, McLeod GRC, Martin NG. Increasing incidence of cutaneous melanoma in Queensland, Australia. *J Natl Cancer Inst.* 1992;84:1427–1432.

20. Ariyan S, Poo WJ, Bolognia J, et al. Multiple primary melanomas: data and significance. *Plast Reconstr Surg.* 1995;96:1384–1389.

21. Holly EA, Aston DA, Cress RD. Cutaneous melanoma in women: II. Phenotypic characteristics and other host-related factors. *Am J Epidemiol.* 1995;141:934–942.

22. Elwood JM. Melanoma and sun exposure: contrasts between intermittent and chronic sun exposure. *World J Surg.* 1992;16:157–165.

23. Armstrong BK. Epidemiology of malignant melanoma: intermittent or total accumulated exposure to the sun? *J Dermatol Surg Oncol.* 1988;14:835–849.

24. Tucker MA, Halpem A, Holly EA, Hartge P, Elder DE, Sagebiel RW. Clinically recognized dysplastic nevi: a central risk factor for cutaneous melanoma. *JAMA.* 1997;277:1439–1444.

25. Detecting skin cancer. [American Cancer Society website]. May 2002. Available at: www.cancer.org/docroot/PED/content/ped_7_1_Skin_Cancer_Detection_What_You_Can_Do.asp?sitearea=PED. Accessed January, 11, 2003.

26. Ferrini RL, Perlman M, Hill L. American College of Preventive Medicine policy statement: screening for skin cancer. *Am J Prev Med.* 1998;14:80–82.

27. Hill L, Ferrini RL. Skin cancer prevention and screening: summary of the American College of Preventive Medicine's practice policy statements. *CA Cancer J Clin.* 1998;48:232–235.

28. Cokkinides VE, Johnston-Davis K, Weinstock M, et al. Sun exposure and sun-protection behaviors and attitudes among U.S. youths, 11 to 18 years of age. *Prev Med.* 2001;33:141–151.

29. Wagner RF, Wagner D, Tomich JM, Wagner KD, Grande DJ. Diagnosis of skin disease: dermatologists vs. nondermatologists Residents' Corner. *J Dermatol Surg Oncol.* 1985;11:476–479.

30. Cassileth BR, Clark WH, Lusk EJ, Frederick BE, Thompson CJ, Walsh WP. How well do physicians recognize melanoma and other problem lesions? *J Am Acad Dermatol.* 1986;14:555–560.

31. Geller AC, Zhang Z, Sober AJ, et al. The first 15 years of the American Academy of Dermatology skin cancer screening programs: 1985–1999. *J Am Acad Dermatol.* 2003;48:34–41.

32. Berwick M, Begg CB, Fine JA, Roush GC, Barnhill RL. Screening for cutaneous melanoma by skin self-examination. *J Natl Cancer Inst.* 1996;88:17–23.

33. Friedman RJ, Rigel DS. The clinical features of malignant melanoma. *Dermatol Clin.* 1985;3:271–283.

34. Ferrini RL, Perlmann M, Hill L. American College of Preventive Medicine practice policy statement: skin protection from ultraviolet light exposure. *Am J Prev Med.* 1998;14:83–86.

35. McDonald CJ. American Cancer Society perspective on the American college of preventative medicine's policy statements on skin cancer prevention and screening. *CA Cancer J Clin.* 1998;48:229–231.

36. Thompson SC, Jolley D, Marks R. Reduction of solar keratoses by regular sunscreen use. *N Engl J Med.* 1993;329:1147–1151.

37. Green A, Williams G, Neale R, et al. Daily sunscreen application and betacarotene supplementation in prevention of basal-cell and squamous-cell carcinomas of the skin: a randomised controlled trial. *Lancet.* 1999;354:723–729.

38. Autier P, Dore JF, Schifflers E, et al. Melanoma and use of sunscreens: an EORTC case-control study in Germany, Belgium and France: the EORTC melanoma cooperative group. *Int J Cancer.* 1995;61:749–755.

39. Wright MW, Wright ST, Wagner RF. Mechanisms of sunscreen failure. *J Am Acad Dermatol.* 2001;44:781–784.

40. Mohs FE. *Chemosurgery: Microscopically Controlled Surgery for Skin Cancer.* Springfield, Ill: Charles C Thomas Publishers; 1978.

41. Rowe DE, Carroll RJ, Day CL. Long-term recurrence rates in previously untreated (primary) basal cell carcinomas: implications for patient follow-up. *J Dermatol Surg Oncol.* 1989;15:315–328.

42. Randle HW, Roenigk RK. Indications for Mohs micrographic surgery. In: Roenigk RK, Roenigk HH Jr, eds. *Roenigk and Roenigk's Dermatologic Surgery: Principles and Practice.* 2nd ed. New York, NY: Marcel Dekker, Inc; 1996:703–729.

43. Rowe DE, Carroll RJ, Day CL. Prognostic factors for local recurrence, metastasis, and survival rate in squamous cell carcinoma of the skin, ear, and lip. *J Am Acad Dermatol.* 1992;26:976–990.

44. Veronesi U, Cascinelli N, Adamus J, et al. Thin stage I primary cutaneous malignant melanoma: comparison of excision with margins of 1 or 3 cm. *N Engl J Med.* 1988;318:1159–1162.

45. Balch CM, Urist MM, Kara Kousis CP, et al. Efficacy of 2 cm surgical margins for intermediate-thickness melanomas (1 to 4 mm): results of a multi-institutional randomized surgical trial. *Ann Surg.* 1993;218:262–269.

46. Jensen P, Hansen S, Moller B, et al. Skin cancer in kidney and heart transplant recipients and different long-term immunosuppressive therapy regimens. *J Am Acad Dermatol.* 1999;40:177–186.

47. Veness MJ, Quinn DI, Ong CS. Aggressive cutaneous malignancies following cardiothoracic transplantation: the Australian experience. *Cancer.* 1999;85:1758–1764.

48. Euvrard S, Kanitakis J, Pouteil-Noble C, et al. Aggressive squamous cell carcinomas in organ transplant recipients. *Transplant Proc.* 1995;27:1767–1768.

49. Ong CS, Keogh AM, Kossard S, Macdonald PS, Spratt PM. Skin cancer in Australian heart transplant recipients. *J Am Acad Dermatol.* 1999;40:27–34.

50. Otley CC. Organization of a specialty clinic to optimize the care of organ transplant recipients at risk for skin cancer. *Dermatol Surg.* 2000;26:709–712.

RESOURCES

American Academy of Dermatology
930 E. Woodfield Rd., Schaumburg, IL 60173-4927
Correspondence address:
P.O. Box 4014, Schaumburg, IL 60168-4014
Phone: 847 330-0230
Fax: 847 330-0050
Web site: www.aad.org

American Society for Dermatologic Surgery
5550 Meadowbrook Dr.
Suite 120 Rolling Meadows, IL 60008
Phone: 847-956-0900
Fax: 847-956-0999
Email: info@aboutskinsurgery.com

Amercian College of Mohs Micrograghic Surgery and Cutaneous Oncology
611 East Wells Street
Milwaukee, WI 53202
Phone: 800 500-7224 or 414 347-1103
Web site: www.mohscollege.org

PART 11

Infectious Diseases

Adult Immunizations

Paul V. Targonski, MD, PhD, and Gregory A. Poland, MD

INTRODUCTION

Vaccination is one of the greatest public health interventions to positively affect the prevention of disease. Vaccination originated in the process of variolation, in which smallpox-naïve individuals were purposely exposed to small amounts of smallpox pustular material through either the nasal airway or incisions in the skin (scarification).[1] Although Edward Jenner is often considered synonymous with smallpox variolation, this practice was present in China, India, and the Ottoman Empire well before Jenner's fateful "n = 1" experiment in May 1796.[1] He injected exudative fluid from the vesicle of a milkmaid infected with what appeared to be cowpox into 2 incisions made into the arm of an 8-year-old smallpox-naïve boy. When the boy was subsequently exposed to variolation, he exhibited no clinical response and protection was inferred. In honor of Jenner, the term *vaccination* was coined 80 years later by Louis Pasteur to mean the artificial induction of immunity.[2] Sadly, one of the greatest public health and preventive medicine triumphs of humankind, the eradication of smallpox, is threatened in the 21st century by the specter of biological warfare using this very agent.

Prevention of disease through vaccination was a driving force for the remarkable advances in life expectancy observed during the 20th century. Life expectancy in the United States was 47 years in 1900 and 76.9 years by the year 2000.[3] Although vaccination alone was not solely responsible, decreases in infectious disease–related mortality accounted for most of the improvement in longevity in the first half of the 20th century.[4]

Most of these gains in life expectancy were the result of improving childhood survival, as the widespread use of vaccinations has remarkably diminished the occurrence of vaccine-preventable childhood diseases in the United States.[5] Preventing morbidity and mortality in adults through successful vaccination programs has been more difficult and limited.[6] For example, it was not until 2002 that the Advisory Committee on Immunization Practices (ACIP) approved a schedule for the routine vaccination of persons aged 19 years or older.[7]

Influenza, pneumococcal infections, and hepatitis B are the primary vaccine-preventable diseases affecting adults in the United States, resulting in 60,000 to 80,000 deaths per year. Treatment of these diseases and their complications costs in excess of $10 billion annually, excluding any consideration for years of potential life lost.[8] This disease and economic burden occurs despite the fact that vaccines are a safe, effective, and cost-saving way of preventing excess morbidity and mortality in adults, especially those who fall into "high-risk" categories due to lack of natural immunity or adequate previous vaccination, age (>65 years), lifestyle, immunosuppression, or chronic disease.

VACCINE COMPOSITION AND ADMINISTRATION

Viral vaccines are composed of live, attenuated viruses; inactivated viruses; or subunits of the virus or viruses against which the vaccine is directed. With attenuated vaccines, the virus is typically passaged repeatedly through an animal host or cell culture so that it retains a desirable level of immunogenicity yet is stripped of its virulence. An example is a live, attenuated intranasal influenza vaccine that has been cold-adapted through serial passage at successively lower temperatures, essentially restricting the virus to replication at 25°C to 33°C and limiting it to the upper respiratory tract,[9,10] where it is administered as an intranasal spray. Hepatitis A vaccine is an example of an inactivated virus vaccine, in which the virus is killed with chemical agents such as formaldehyde solution and used to induce an immune response. Hepatitis B vaccines use recombinant DNA techniques to produce hepatitis B surface antigen, a viral subunit that evokes an immune response in the vaccine recipient. Bacterial vaccines tend to be composed of toxoids—bacterial toxins neutralized via chemical processing but which retain immunogenicity—or capsular oligosaccharides or polysaccharides. These capsular carbohydrates are either used alone to induce a T-cell–independent humoral immune response or conjugated with proteins to invoke T-cell immunity and a resulting IgG response.

Most adult vaccinations are administered intramuscularly (IM), with the deltoid muscle routinely recommended for the injection site unless contraindicated.[11] Optimal antibody responses require administration of vaccines according to the manufacturer's instructions, or decreased efficacy and increased risk of adverse reactions could result.[11] When injecting vaccines into muscle, it should be remembered that different patients need different needle sizes.[12] In particular, IM administration requires that vaccines actually be deposited into muscle. Simultaneous administration of the most commonly used live, inactivated, subunit, toxoid, and polysaccharide vaccines is the favored approach when multiple vaccinations are required.[11] There does not appear to be an increased risk of adverse effects or seroconversion failure employing simultaneous vaccination, although most of these data are derived from studies in children. Live vaccines not administered on the same day should be administered at least 4 weeks apart, if possible, to minimize the risk of interference with production of immunity for either vaccine.[11]

VACCINE SAFETY AND ADVERSE EVENT REPORTING

For a vaccine to be approved for use in the United States, it must be considered safe, cause an appropriate and protective immune response, and retain potency during storage. However, safety is relative, as the severity of potential vaccine-related adverse effects may be weighed against the severity and complications of the illness the vaccine is engineered to prevent in the population.

Vaccine-related adverse events are categorized as either early or late reactions. Early reactions usually occur within the first 24 to 48 hours and may include mild events, such as fever, pain at the injection site, or swelling, or moderate to severe events, such as syncope, anaphylaxis, seizure, or cardiovascular collapse. Late reactions may occur after vaccination and may include such events as rashes, joint symptoms, encephalitis, or encephalopathy with subsequent brain damage. However, severe vaccination-related risks are quite small in individuals for whom vaccination is indicated. For example, rates of encephalitis secondary to infection with measles or mumps are 1 in 2000 and 1 in 300, respectively, yet the risk of vaccine-related encephalitis or a severe allergic reaction from the measles-mumps-rubella (MMR) vaccine is 1 in 1 million.[13] Unfortunately, potential adverse effects of new vaccines are not always observable until after licensing and administration of large numbers of doses.

The Vaccine Adverse Event Reporting System (VAERS) was activated on November 1, 1990, to replace separate systems previously run by the Centers for Disease Control and Prevention (CDC) and the US Food and Drug Administration (FDA) to survey vaccine-related adverse events in both the public and private sectors as mandated by the National Childhood Vaccine Injury Act of 1986.[14] Elements of the VAERS data are publicly available on the Internet (see "Resources" at the end of the chapter) and appear to validate the overall safety of vaccines, although the data suffer from incomplete ascertainment of all adverse events. During the period 1991 through 2001, more than 1.9 billion doses of human vaccines were distributed, and 128,717 adverse effect reports were filed with VAERS, or approximately 11.4 reports per 100,000 doses.[15] Events among adults (aged 18 years and older) comprised 37.5% of all reports filed, and reporting patterns varied temporally with the introduction of multiple new vaccines, such as those directed at pneumococcal diseases, varicella, and Lyme disease. Overall, the most commonly reported adverse events include fever (25.8%), hypersensitivity at the injection site (15.8%), and unspecified rash (11.0%), although life-threatening illness comprised 2.0% of all reports, and deaths were reported in 1.6% of all filings.[15] Of note, clinicians who are aware of VAERS can contribute to vaccine safety by reporting any adverse events related to vaccine administration in their patients.

Because life-threatening reactions such as anaphylaxis after vaccination occur rarely and may result in death,[15] vaccination providers should have appropriate training to recognize and provide initial care to persons with anaphylaxis or acute complications. Facilities should also have proper medications and equipment to allow appropriate treatment of early reactions. This includes both aqueous epinephrine and provision for instrumentation and management of the airway.[11] Furthermore, the risks and benefits as well as indications and contraindications for vaccines must be appropriately communicated to eligible adults before vaccination, and the opportunity for patient questions before vaccination must be provided to obtain informed consent. Vaccine Information Statements are available from the CDC's National Immunization Program Web site (see "Resources") to facilitate this process.

VACCINE COVERAGE AND BARRIERS TO ADULT IMMUNIZATION

The safest and most efficacious vaccines are clearly suboptimal unless they are adequately delivered to and used by the public. The influenza vaccination in adults is a prime example. In 2001, 64.9% of persons over the age of 64 years who responded to the US Behavioral Risk Factor Surveillance System (BRFSS) indicated that they had received an influenza vaccination in the previous year.[16] Although this meets goals for the US Department of Health and Human Services Healthy People 2000 influenza vaccination targets, the Healthy People 2010 coverage target is 90% of persons aged 65 years and older.[17] A recent examination of national Medicare data revealed that in a 3-month period in 1998, only 2.6% of fee-for-service Medicare patients aged 65 years and older (who were previously unvaccinated that year) received influenza vaccination during their hospitalization[18] in accordance with ACIP guidelines.[19] Low compliance with recommended annual inactivated vaccination against influenza in the elderly and inadequate programs to increase adult immunization rates are clear limitations of current vaccination strategies.[20]

Influenza vaccination rates among eligible adults under 65 years of age are also inadequate. The BRFSS observed that the median influenza coverage among persons aged 55 to 64 years was only 41% and in persons aged 54 years or younger was less than 30%.[21] Potter et al[22] demonstrated that vaccination of health care workers in geriatric long-term–care hospitals resulted in a significant reduction in both patient mortality and occurrence of influenza-like illness, even in settings where patients were not routinely vaccinated. This is another area of opportunity, as only about 38% of health care workers received influenza vaccinations in the year 2000, according to data from the National Health Interview Survey.[23] A recent cost-benefit analysis of influenza vaccination among healthy adults suggested that there may also be a population level benefit to vaccination of all adults aged 18 to 50 years.[24] Although this was an economic analysis focused primarily on symptom relief and lost work days due to influenza, substantial benefits were predicted for vaccination vs nonvaccination of this group in almost all cases examined.

There are also clear racial and socioeconomic disparities in the quality of health care and preventive services in the United States,[25,26] and vaccine delivery and receipt are not immune to these differences.[27] Among persons aged 65 years or older in the 1999 BRFSS, non-Hispanic black and Hispanic respondents were 30% to 60% less likely than non-Hispanic white respondents to report vaccination against influenza or pneumococcal disease[19] after adjustment for age, sex, education level, length of time since last check-up, self-reported health, and diabetes status. Subsequent studies have observed the persistence of racial disparities in influenza vaccination among adults in managed care and fee-for-service settings,[28] and there is no evidence to suggest that these disparities do not extend to other vaccine recommendations. Clearly, additional efforts are necessary to better understand and reduce these differences.

One effective strategy for improving vaccination coverage rates is simply recommending vaccination to patients when appropriate. A health care provider's recommendation is among the strongest determinants for inducing adult patients to receive vaccinations.[29] Additional strategies beyond the traditional outpatient medical clinic or inpatient settings to develop programs improving overall vaccination rates are currently being explored.

VACCINE-SPECIFIC INFORMATION

Immunization schedules are presented in Table 50-1 A and B, and indications and contraindications for adult vaccination are presented in Table 50-2. The following discussion provides additional details on vaccine-specific information.

Hepatitis A

Background
Hepatitis A is endemic in the United States, causing an estimated 143,000 new hepatitis infections in the year 2000,[30] with 13,397 clinical cases reported.[31] Although recent years have demonstrated a decline in reported prevalence overall,[31] hepatitis A results in approximately 100 deaths annually.[32] The National Health and Nutrition Examination Survey (NHANES) II sample of the US population (1976 to 1980) demonstrated that seroprevalence rates greatly increase with age, from 11% in children under 5 years to 74% in adults older than 50 years.[33]

Vaccine dose and administration
Currently licensed hepatitis A vaccines in the United States include Havrix, Vaqta, and Twinrix, all of which are killed, formaldehyde solution–inactivated vaccines prepared from whole virus. Guidelines for active or passive immunization to prevent hepatitis A were released in 1999,[34] and for the FDA-approved Twinrix, which is a combined hepatitis A and B vaccine, in 2001.[35]

The recommended adult dose of either vaccine is 1 mL IM, for adults, with booster doses 1 and 6 months later for Twinrix, 6 months later for Vaqta, and 6 to 12 months later for Havrix. Increasing the interval beyond the recommendation does not adversely affect the immunogenicity or efficacy of hepatitis A vaccines. However, persons traveling to highly endemic areas should receive the vaccine at least 2 weeks before departure. If this is not possible, administration of both vaccine and immune globulin at separate deltoid sites is reasonable, although high doses of immune globulin can depress the maximum antibody level obtained.[36]

Immunogenicity and efficacy
After 2 doses, essentially 100% of recipients seroconvert.[37,38] Sixty-nine percent to 98% of healthy, young adults seroconvert by 15 days after the first dose of

TABLE **50-1A**

Adult Immunization Schedule by Age Group

Recommended Adult Immunization Schedule, United States, 2003-2004
by Age Group

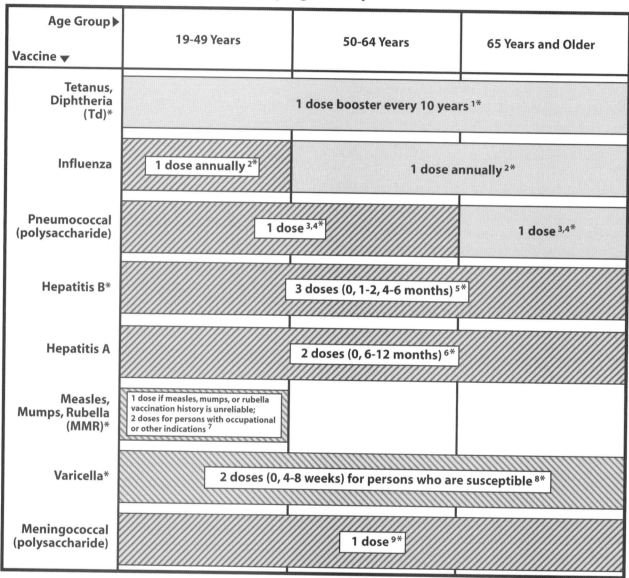

Age Group ▶ Vaccine ▼	19-49 Years	50-64 Years	65 Years and Older
Tetanus, Diphtheria (Td)*	1 dose booster every 10 years [1*]		
Influenza	1 dose annually [2*]	1 dose annually [2*]	
Pneumococcal (polysaccharide)	1 dose [3,4*]		1 dose [3,4*]
Hepatitis B*	3 doses (0, 1-2, 4-6 months) [5*]		
Hepatitis A	2 doses (0, 6-12 months) [6*]		
Measles, Mumps, Rubella (MMR)*	1 dose if measles, mumps, or rubella vaccination history is unreliable; 2 doses for persons with occupational or other indications [7]		
Varicella*	2 doses (0, 4-8 weeks) for persons who are susceptible [8*]		
Meningococcal (polysaccharide)	1 dose [9*]		

*See Footnotes for Recommended Adult Immunization Schedule, by Age Group and Medical Conditions, United States, 2003-2004 in full report

For all persons in this group   Catch-up on childhood vaccinations   For persons with medical / exposure indications

*Covered by the Vaccine Injury Compensation Program. For information on how to file a claim call 800-338-2382. Please also visit www.hrsa.gov/osp/vicp To file a claim for vaccine injury contact: U.S. Court of Federal Claims, 717 Madison Place, N.W., Washington D.C. 20005, 202-219-9657.

This schedule indicates the recommended age groups for routine administration of currently licensed vaccines for persons 19 years of age and older. Licensed combination vaccines may be used whenever any components of the combination are indicated and the vaccine's other components are not contraindicated. Providers should consult the manufacturers' package inserts for detailed recommendations.

Report all clinically significant post-vaccination reactions to the Vaccine Adverse Event Reporting System (VAERS). Reporting forms and instructions on filing a VAERS report are available by calling 800-822-7967 or from the VAERS website at www.vaers.org.

For additional information about the vaccines listed above and contraindications for immunization, visit the National Immunization Program Website at www.cdc.gov/nip/ or call the National Immunization Hotline at 800-232-2522 (English) or 800-232-0233 (Spanish).

Approved by the Advisory Committee on Immunization Practices (ACIP), and accepted by the American College of Obstetricians and Gynecologists (ACOG) and the American Academy of Family Physicians (AAFP)

TABLE 50-1B

Adult Immunization Schedule by Medical Conditions

Recommended Adult Immunization Schedule, United States, 2003-2004
by Medical Conditions

Medical Conditions ▼ Vaccine ▶	Tetanus-Diphtheria (Td)*,1	Influenza 2	Pneumo-coccal (polysacch-aride) 3,4	Hepatitis B*,5	Hepatitis A6	Measles, Mumps, Rubella (MMR)*,7	Varicella*,8
Pregnancy		A					
Diabetes, heart disease, chronic pulmonary disease, chronic liver disease, including chronic alcoholism		B	C		D		
Congenital Immunodeficiency, leukemia, lymphoma, generalized malignancy, therapy with alkylating agents, antimetabolites, radiation or large amounts of corticosteroids			E				F
Renal failure / end stage renal disease, recipients of hemodialysis or clotting factor concentrates			E	G			
Asplenia including elective splenectomy and terminal complement component deficiencies		H	E, I, J				
HIV infection			E, K			L	

See Special Notes for Medical Conditions below—also see Footnotes for Recommended Adult Immunization Schedule, by Age Group and Medical Conditions, United States, 2003-2004 in full report

▨ For all persons in this group	▨ For persons with medical / exposure indications
▨ Catch-up on childhood vaccinations	▨ Contraindicated

Special Notes for Medical Conditions

A. For women without chronic diseases/conditions, vaccinate if pregnancy will be at 2nd or 3rd trimester during influenza season. For women with chronic deseases/conditions, vaccinate at any time during the pregnancy.

B. Although chronic liver disease and alcoholism are not indicator conditions for influenza vaccination, give 1 dose annually if the patient is ≥ 50 years, has other indications for influenza vaccine, or if the patient requests vaccination.

C. Asthma is an indicator condition for influenza but not for pneumococcal vaccination.

D. For all persons with chronic liver disease.

E. For persons < 65 years, revaccinate once after 5 years or more have elapsed since initial vaccination.

F. Persons with impaired humoral immunity but intact cellular immunity may be vaccinated.

G. Hemodialysis patients: Use special formulation of vaccine (40 ug/mL) or two 1.0 mL 20 ug doses given at one site. Vaccinate early in the course of renal disease. Assess antibody titers to hep B surface antigen (anti-HBs) levels annually. Administer additional doses if anti-HBs levels decline to <10 milliinternational units (mIU)/ mL.

H. There are no data specifically on risk of severe or complicated influenza infections among persons with asplenia. However, influenza is a risk factor for secondary bacterial infections that may cause severe disease in asplenics.

I. Administer meningococcal vaccine and consider Hib vaccine.

J. Elective splenectomy: vaccinate at least 2 weeks before surgery.

K. Vaccinate as close to diagnosis as possible when CD4 cell counts are highest.

L. Withhold MMR or other measles containing vaccines from HIV-infected persons with evidence of severe immunosuppression. *MMWR* 1998; 47 (RR-8):21-22;

TABLE 50-2

Summary of Recommendations for Adult Immunization

Summary of Recommendations for Adult Immunization

Adapted from the recommendations of the Advisory Committee on Immunization Practices (ACIP)* by the Immunization Action Coalition, September 2003

Vaccine name and route	For whom it is recommended	Schedule for routine and "catch-up" administration	Contraindications (mild illness is not a contraindication)
Influenza Inactivated influenza vaccine (IIV) *Give IM* Live attenuated influenza vaccine (LAIV) *Give intranasally*	• All adults who are 50yrs of age or older. • People 6m–50yrs of age with medical problems (e.g., heart disease, lung disease, diabetes, renal dysfunction, hemoglobinopathies, immunosuppression) and/or people living in chronic-care facilities. • People (≥6m of age) working or living with at-risk people. • Pregnant women who have underlying medical conditions should be vaccinated before influenza season, regardless of the stage of pregnancy. • Healthy pregnant women who will be in their 2nd or 3rd trimesters during influenza season. • All health care workers and those who provide essential community services. • Travelers who go to areas where influenza activity exists or who may be among people from areas of the world where there is current influenza activity (e.g., on organized tours). • Anyone wishing to reduce the likelihood of becoming ill with influenza. **Special Note on Influenza Vaccines:** Inactivated influenza vaccine (IIV) may be given to any person ≥6 months of age for whom the vaccine is not contraindicated. Live attenuated influenza vaccine (LAIV) may be given to healthy, non-pregnant persons 5–49 years of age for whom the vaccine is not contraindicated.	• Given every year. • October through November is the *optimal* time to receive an annual influenza shot to maximize protection. • Influenza vaccine may be given at any time during the influenza season (typically December through March) or at other times when the risk of influenza exists. • May give with all other vaccines.	• Previous anaphylactic reaction to this vaccine, to any of its components, or to eggs. • Moderate or severe acute illness. • Do not give live attenuated influenza vaccine (LAIV) to persons ≥50 years of age, pregnant women, or to persons who have: asthma, reactive airway disease or other chronic disorder of the pulmonary or cardiovascular systems; an underlying medical condition, including metabolic diseases such as diabetes, renal dysfunction, and hemoglobinopathies; a known or suspected immune deficiency disease or who are receiving immunosuppressive therapy; a history of Guillain-Barré syndrome. **Note:** Use of inactivated influenza vaccine (IIV) is preferred for persons in close contact with immunosuppressed persons.
Pneumococcal polysaccharide (PPV23) *Give IM or SC*	• Adults who are 65yrs of age or older. • People 2–64yrs of age who have chronic illness or other risk factors, including chronic cardiac or pulmonary diseases, chronic liver disease, alcoholism, diabetes mellitus, CSF leaks, candidate for or recipient of cochlear implant, as well as people living in special environments or social settings (including Alaska Natives and certain American Indian populations). Those at highest risk of fatal pneumococcal infection are people with anatomic asplenia, functional asplenia, or sickle cell disease; immunocompromised persons including those with HIV infection, leukemia, lymphoma, Hodgkin's disease, multiple myeloma, generalized malignancy, chronic renal failure, or nephrotic syndrome; persons receiving immunosuppressive chemotherapy (including corticosteroids); and those who received an organ or bone marrow transplant. Pregnant women with high-risk conditions should be vaccinated if not done previously.	• Routinely given as a one-time dose; administer if previous vaccination history is unknown. • One-time revaccination is recommended 5yrs later for people at highest risk of fatal pneumococcal infection or rapid antibody loss (e.g., renal disease) and for people ≥65yrs of age if the 1st dose was given prior to age 65 and ≥5yrs have elapsed since previous dose. • May give with all other vaccines.	• Previous anaphylactic reaction to this vaccine or to any of its components. • Moderate or severe acute illness. **Note:** Pregnancy and breastfeeding are not contraindications to the use of this vaccine.
Hepatitis B (Hep B) *Give IM* Brands may be used interchangeably.	• All adolescents. • High-risk adults, including household contacts and sex partners of HBsAg-positive persons; users of illicit injectable drugs; heterosexuals with more than one sex partner in 6 months; men who have sex with men; people with recently diagnosed STDs; patients receiving hemodialysis and patients with renal disease that may result in dialysis; recipients of certain blood products; health care workers and public safety workers who are exposed to blood; clients and staff of institutions for the developmentally disabled; inmates of long-term correctional facilities; and certain international travelers. **Note:** Prior serologic testing may be recommended depending on the specific level of risk and/or likelihood of previous exposure. **Note:** In 1997, the NIH Consensus Development Conference, a panel of national experts, recommended that hepatitis B vaccination be given to all anti-HCV positive persons. **Ed. note:** Provide serologic screening for immigrants from endemic areas. When HBsAg-positive persons are identified, offer appropriate disease management. In addition, screen their sex partners and household members and, if found susceptible, vaccinate.	• Three doses are needed on a 0, 1, 6m schedule. • Alternative timing options for vaccination include 0, 2, 4m and 0, 1, 4m. • There must be 4wks between doses #1 and #2, and 8wks between doses #2 and #3. Overall there must be at least 16wks between doses #1 and #3. • **Schedule for those who have fallen behind:** If the series is delayed between doses, DO NOT start the series over. Continue from where you left off. • May give with all other vaccines.	• Previous anaphylactic reaction to this vaccine or to any of its components. • Moderate or severe acute illness. **Note:** Pregnancy and breastfeeding are not contraindications to the use of this vaccine.
Hepatitis A (Hep A) *Give IM* Brands may be used interchangeably.	• People who travel outside of the U.S. (except for Western Europe, New Zealand, Australia, Canada, and Japan). • People with chronic liver disease, including people with hepatitis C; people with hepatitis B who have chronic liver disease; illicit drug users; men who have sex with men; people with clotting-factor disorders; people who work with hepatitis A virus in experimental lab settings (not routine medical laboratories); and food handlers when health authorities or private employers determine vaccination to be cost effective. **Note:** Prevaccination testing is likely to be cost effective for persons >40yrs of age as well as for younger persons in certain groups with a high prevalence of hepatitis A virus infection.	For Twinrix™ (hepatitis A and B combination vaccine [GSK]), three doses are needed on a 0, 1, 6m schedule. • Two doses are needed. • The minimum interval between dose #1 and #2 is 6m. • If dose #2 is delayed, do not repeat dose #1. Just give dose #2. • May give with all other vaccines.	• Previous anaphylactic reaction to this vaccine or to any of its components. • Moderate or severe acute illness. • Safety during pregnancy has not been determined, so benefits must be weighed against potential risk. **Note:** Breastfeeding is not a contraindication to the use of this vaccine.

T A B L E 50-2—*Continued*

Vaccine name and route	For whom it is recommended	Schedule for routine and "catch-up" administration	Contraindications (mild illness is not a contraindication)
Td (Tetanus, diphtheria) *Give IM*	• All adolescents and adults. • After the primary series has been completed, a booster dose is recommended every 10yrs. Make sure your patients have received a primary series of 3 doses. • A booster dose as early as 5yrs later may be needed for the purpose of wound management, so consult ACIP recommendations.* • Use Td, not tetanus toxoid (TT), for all indications.	• Give booster dose every 10yrs after the primary series has been completed. • For those who are unvaccinated or behind, complete the primary series (spaced at 0, 1–2m, 6–12m intervals). Don't restart the series, no matter how long since the previous dose. • May give with all other vaccines.	• Previous anaphylactic or neurologic reaction to this vaccine or to any of its components. • Moderate or severe acute illness. • Note: Pregnancy and breastfeeding are not contraindications to the use of this vaccine.
MMR (Measles, mumps, rubella) *Give SC*	• Adults born in 1957 or later who are ≥18yrs of age (including those born outside the U.S.) should receive at least one dose of MMR if there is no serologic proof of immunity or documentation of a dose given on or after the first birthday. • Adults in high-risk groups, such as health care workers, students entering colleges and other post–high school educational institutions, and international travelers, should receive a total of two doses. • Adults born before 1957 are usually considered immune but proof of immunity may be desirable for health care workers. • All women of childbearing age (i.e., adolescent girls and premenopausal adult women) who do not have acceptable evidence of rubella immunity or vaccination. • Special attention should be given to immunizing women born outside the United States in 1957 or later.	• One or two doses are needed. • If dose #2 is recommended, give it no sooner than 4wks after dose #1. • May give with all other vaccines. • If varicella vaccine and MMR are both needed and are not administered on the same day, space them at least 4wks apart. • If a pregnant woman is found to be rubella-susceptible, administer MMR postpartum.	• Previous anaphylactic reaction to this vaccine or to any of its components. • Pregnancy or possibility of pregnancy within 4 weeks (use contraception). • Persons immunocompromised because of cancer, leukemia, lymphoma, immunosuppressive drug therapy, including high-dose steroids or radiation therapy. Note: HIV positivity is NOT a contraindication to MMR except for those who are severely immunocompromised. • If blood, plasma, and/or immune globulin were given in past 11m, see ACIP statement *General Recommendations on Immunization** regarding time to wait before vaccinating. • Moderate or severe acute illness. • Note: Breastfeeding is not a contraindication to the use of this vaccine. • Note: MMR is not contraindicated if a tuberculin skin test (i.e., PPD) was recently applied. If PPD and MMR not given on same day, delay PPD for 4–6wks after MMR.
Varicella (Var) (Chickenpox) *Give SC*	All susceptible adults and adolescents should be vaccinated. It is especially important to ensure vaccination of the following groups: susceptible persons who have close contact with persons at high risk for serious complications (e.g., health care workers and family contacts of immunocompromised persons) and susceptible persons who are at high risk of exposure (e.g., teachers of young children, day care employees, residents and staff in institutional settings such as colleges and correctional institutions, military personnel, adolescents and adults living with children, non-pregnant women of childbearing age, and international travelers who do not have evidence of immunity). Note: People with reliable histories of chickenpox (such as self or parental report of disease) can be assumed to be immune. For adults who have no reliable history, serologic testing may be cost effective since most adults with a negative or uncertain history of varicella are immune.	• Two doses are needed. • Dose #2 is given 4–8wks after dose #1. • May give with all other vaccines. • If varicella vaccine and MMR are both needed and are not administered on the same day, space them at least 4wks apart. • If the second dose is delayed, do not repeat dose #1. Just give dose #2.	• Previous anaphylactic reaction to this vaccine or to any of its components. • Pregnancy or possibility of pregnancy within 4 weeks (use contraception). • Persons immunocompromised because of malignancies and primary or acquired cellular immunodeficiency including HIV/AIDS. (See *MMWR* 1999, Vol. 48, No. RR-6.) Note: For those on high-dose immunosuppressive therapy, consult ACIP recommendations regarding delay time.* • If blood, plasma, and/or immune globulin (IG or VZIG) were given in past 11m, see ACIP statement *General Recommendations on Immunization** regarding time to wait before vaccinating. • Moderate or severe acute illness. • Note: Breastfeeding is not a contraindication to the use of this vaccine. • Note: Manufacturer recommends that salicylates be avoided for 6wks after receiving varicella vaccine because of a theoretical risk of Reye's syndrome.
Polio (IPV) *Give IM or SC*	• Not routinely recommended for persons 18yrs of age and older. • Note: Adults living in the U.S. who never received or completed a primary series of polio vaccine need not be vaccinated unless they intend to travel to areas where exposure to wild-type virus is likely. Previously vaccinated adults can receive one booster dose if traveling to polio endemic areas.	• Refer to ACIP recommendations* regarding unique situations, schedules, and dosing information. • May give with all other vaccines.	• Previous anaphylactic or neurologic reaction to this vaccine or to any of its components. • Moderate or severe acute illness. • Note: Pregnancy and breastfeeding are not contraindications to the use of this vaccine.
Meningococcal *Give SC*	Vaccinate people with risk factors. Discuss disease risk and vaccine availability with college students. Consult ACIP statement* on meningococcal disease (6/30/00) for details.		

* For specific ACIP immunization recommendations, refer to the statements, which are published in *MMWR*. To obtain a complete set of ACIP statements, call (800) 232-2522, or to access individual statements, visit CDC's website: www.cdc.gov/nip/publications/ACIP-list.htm or visit IAC's website: www.immunize.org

This table is revised yearly because of the changing nature of U.S. immunization recommendations. Visit the Immunization Action Coalition's website at www.immunize.org/adultrules to make sure you have the most current version. We extend our thanks to William Atkinson, MD, MPH, from CDC's National Immunization Program, and Linda Moyer, RN, from the Division of Viral Hepatitis, at CDC's National Center for Infectious Diseases for their assistance. This table is published by the Immunization Action Coalition, 1573 Selby Avenue, St. Paul, MN 55104, (651) 647-9009. Email: admin@immunize.org

www.immunize.org/catg.d/p2011b.pdf • Item #P2011 (09/03)

hepatitis A vaccines and greater than 95% convert after 30 days,[37,38] although not all trials have demonstrated this level of seroconversion.[39] Currently, there are no indications for additional booster doses. Long-term immune memory is thought to exist. Efficacy trials performed in pediatric age groups showed efficacy rates of 94% for the Havrix vaccine[40] and 100% for the Vaqta vaccine.[32]

Adverse effects and contraindications

Hepatitis A vaccines are considered exceptionally safe. In a review of 104 studies involving the Havrix vaccine, no serious adverse events were reported among the more than 50,000 people and over 120,000 doses of vaccine administered. Transient mild side effects (pain and tenderness at the injection site, headache, malaise) have been reported, and the frequency of side effects in vaccinees was similar to those who received placebo. Persons with known hypersensitivity to any component of the vaccine should not receive further injections.

Hepatitis B

Background

An estimated 1 to 1.25 million persons are chronically infected with hepatitis B in the United States, and approximately 4000 to 5000 deaths occur annually due to chronic hepatitis B-induced liver disease.[41] Since 1991, it has been mandatory for all health care facilities to offer hepatitis B vaccine to their employees,[42] and the estimated 79,000 new infections in 2001 represent 25% to 40% of the annual incidence in 1981, before hepatitis B vaccination programs were implemented in the United States.[43] Currently the greatest risk of hepatitis B infection among adults occurs for persons with multiple sex partners or diagnosis of a sexually transmitted disease, men who have sex with men, sex contacts of infected persons, injection drug users, household contacts of chronically infected persons, health care and public safety workers, and hemodialysis recipients.[44]

Vaccine dose and administration

Three recombinant DNA hepatitis B vaccines are licensed in the United States: Recombivax HB, Engerix-B, and Twinrix. Twinrix was licensed by the FDA in May 2001 and combines the antigenic components of Engerix-B with Havrix. Three IM doses of hepatitis B vaccine are routinely recommended to induce immunity (anti-hepatitis B virus levels >10 mIU/mL), with the second and third injections administered 1 and 6 months, respectively, after the first dose.[41] An increase in the interval between doses of hepatitis B vaccine does not adversely effect immunogenicity or efficacy. If the vaccination series is interrupted after the first dose, the second dose should be administered as soon as possible, with the second and third doses being separated by an interval

of at least 2 months. If the third dose is delayed, it should be administered when convenient. Both vaccines are interchangeable during the series,[41] and, as of the year 2000, neither contained thimerosal.[43]

Hepatitis B vaccine should be administered in the deltoid, rather than the gluteus, muscle, as injection in the gluteus is associated with a significantly increased risk of vaccine failure. This seems to be due to inadequate needle length, as studies have shown that if the hepatitis B vaccine is deposited into fat rather than the muscle, lower seroconversion rates result.[45] Deltoid fat pad thickness studies demonstrate that for men across all weight ranges, and women weighing between 60 and 90 kg, a 2.54-cm (1-in) needle is sufficient for muscle penetration. For women weighing over 90 kg, a 3.81-cm (1.5-in) needle was found to be adequate. For women weighing under 60 kg, a 1.59-cm (⅝-in) needle is capable of penetrating muscle.[46]

Immunogenicity and efficacy

The vaccine, when properly administered as a 3-dose schedule, induces immunity in 90% to 95% of healthy young adults.[41] Poorer immunogenicity may result in persons who received the vaccine in the gluteus, smokers, obese persons, males, immunocompromised persons, and people having certain HLA haplotypes.[45,47] In addition, seroconversion rates decrease with increasing age (>95% in 20-year-olds, 86% in 40-year-olds, and 47% in 60-year-olds).[42] Although antibody levels may wane with time, studies indicate that in healthy adults and children, immunologic memory persists and confers protection against chronic hepatitis B virus infection, even if anti-hepatitis B levels are not currently detectable.[41] Booster doses of vaccine are not recommended for adults with normal immune status at this time, nor is serologic testing after vaccination routinely recommended. However, in cases in which subsequent clinical management depends on knowledge of the immune status (eg, health care workers with a high risk of exposure to needle punctures, high risk of nonresponse, or a high risk of exposure to the hepatitis B virus), postvaccination serologic testing should be done 1 to 6 months after completion of the vaccine series.[41] An algorithm for managing vaccine nonresponse has been published.[42]

Adverse effects and contraindications

Although pain at the injection site and low-grade transient fever may occur, these side effects were reported no more frequently than in vaccinees who received placebo.[41] There is no known or verified association between recombinant hepatitis B vaccine and Guillain-Barré syndrome (GBS), multiple sclerosis, or other demyelinating disorders.[43,48,49] Persons who have had anaphylactic allergic reactions to yeast or those who have hypersensitivity to thimerosal should not receive a hepatitis B vaccine.

Influenza

Background

Influenza A and B viruses are responsible for epidemics of serious respiratory illness that occur every winter, causing approximately 40,000 deaths, up to 300,000 hospitalizations, and countless lost work and school days annually.[50] Morbidity and mortality are highest in the elderly; those with chronic medical conditions and persons aged 65 years or older account for more than 90% of the annual mortality associated with influenza in the United States each year.[51] In 2001, approximately 65% of persons aged 65 years or older received the vaccine in the United States,[16] but less than 30% of those aged 65 years or younger who are at risk of influenza complications receive the vaccine.[50]

Vaccine dose and administration

Influenza vaccine is generally trivalent, containing 2 type A strains and 1 type B strain of the viruses that are judged most likely to circulate in the upcoming season. Influenza vaccine should be administered annually as one 0.5-mL dose of the vaccine given IM in the deltoid region. Vaccination in the period before seasonal peaks occur is recommended.[50] Of note is that an influenza vaccine with different strains is often recommended in the Southern Hemisphere. The influenza vaccine can be given in conjunction with other vaccines such as the pneumococcal vaccine, provided that different anatomical sites and syringes are used.[11,50] A cold-adapted live intranasal influenza vaccine was available for the 2003–2004 season for people ages 5 to 49 years.

Immunogenicity and efficacy

When the viruses chosen for the vaccine resemble those of the circulating epidemic strains, vaccine efficacy for prevention of hospitalization and death approaches 70% to 90% among healthy young adults.[52] Significant reductions in morbidity also result after influenza immunization. A study of 849 healthy working adults, aged 18 to 64 years, who were randomly assigned to flu vaccine or placebo, demonstrated 25% fewer physician visits for upper respiratory tract infections (URIs), 43% fewer sick days off work due to URIs, 44% fewer doctor office visits for evaluation of URIs, and a cost savings of $46.85 per person immunized.[53]

Efficacy rates are often lower in the elderly than in younger adult populations due to chronic disease- and age-related decreases in immune function.[54-56] Studies among elderly persons living in nursing homes demonstrate a vaccine efficacy rate of 50% to 60% in protecting against hospitalization and up to 80% in preventing death.[50] The cost-benefits of vaccination among the elderly are well established as significantly favorable and improve with medical comorbidity and increasing age.[57,58]

Adverse effects and contraindications

Influenza vaccines are safe and are highly purified, containing only noninfectious viruses that cannot cause influenza.[50] Side effects in the elderly are nearly always mild, and immediate allergic reactions rarely occur. A randomized placebo-controlled study showed that the frequency of adverse reactions in elderly persons receiving the vaccine was no different from those who received placebo.[59] Other than the swine influenza vaccine of 1976, GBS has not been statistically associated with influenza vaccination, as vaccine-related increases in the incidence of GBS are over baseline rates on the order of only 1 case per 1 million persons vaccinated.[50] The vaccine is contraindicated in persons in whom GBS developed in association with influenza vaccination (defined as the development of GBS within 6 weeks of vaccine receipt).[50] Anaphylactic allergy to chicken eggs and sensitivity to thimerosal are also contraindications; however, persons at high risk of complications of influenza could benefit from vaccination after appropriate allergy evaluation and desensitization.[50]

The future

In mid-December 2002, the FDA Vaccines and Related Biological Products Advisory Committee recommended that the FDA approve FluMist, a live, attenuated intranasally administered influenza vaccine, for use in persons aged 5 to 49 years.[60] Because this vaccine provides a noninvasive alternative to IM vaccination, it may improve the coverage of children and young adults. This increased coverage may also result in better control of community-based influenza virus transmission, thereby diminishing morbidity and mortality of the elderly population as well.[61,62]

Measles, Mumps, and Rubella

Background

Since MMR vaccines were licensed in the United States in either monovalent or combination forms, the incidence of these diseases has decreased by 99%, with 86, 338, and 176 cases of measles, mumps, and rubella, respectively, reported in the year 2000 in the United States.[31,63]

Vaccine dose and administration

Monovalent measles (Attenuvax), mumps (Mumpsvax), and rubella (Meruvax II) vaccines are live virus vaccines, as are the combination vaccines (M-M-R II, M-R-Vax, and Biavax II). All vaccines are administered subcutaneously in a volume of 0.5 mL.[63]

Immunogenicity and efficacy

Efficacy in children ranges from 90% to 99% for each of the 3 vaccine components in this group, although lower (75%) efficacy rates have been noted in field trials.[63]

Adverse effects and contraindications

Local and systemic adverse reactions are well documented, although anaphylaxis after measles vaccination is reported to VAERS less than 1 time per million doses distributed.[63] The MMR vaccine may interfere with tuberculin skin testing, and it is recommended that any tuberculin testing be performed on the day of MMR vaccination or at least 4 weeks later.[63]

Meningococcal Disease

Background

Approximately 2000 to 3000 cases of meningococcal disease occur annually in the United States, with a 10% case fatality rate and substantial morbidity, including neurologic sequelae and hearing loss.[64] Almost all cases are sporadic, but the frequency of outbreaks has increased in the past decade.[64]

Vaccine dose and administration

A quadrivalent bacterial polysaccharide vaccine (Menomune) is available for use in adults and is administered subcutaneously as a 0.5-mL dose.[64]

Immunogenicity and efficacy

Efficacies of 85% or higher are reported, with antibody detectable in adults up to 10 years after vaccination.[64] Recommendations for use are presented in Table 50-2.

Adverse effects and contraindications

Fever, headache, dizziness, and injection site reactions are most commonly reported,[64] and pregnancy is not a contraindication for vaccine receipt.[64] Antimicrobial prophylaxis is a mainstay of prevention, with rifampin, ciprofloxacin, and ceftriaxone providing antibiotic options for chemoprophylaxis.[64]

Pneumococcus

Background

Streptococcus pneumoniae is the leading cause of bacterial pneumonia and meningitis in the United States and is responsible for 40,000 or more deaths per year in the United States.[65] An investigation of the CDC's Active Bacterial Core Surveillance data observed that 70.5% of invasive streptococcal illnesses from 1995 to 1998 in a multistate sample occurred among persons aged 18 years or older, and case fatality rates increased with age to 20.6% among persons aged 80 years or older.[66] These authors also noted that 76% of cases and 87% of all deaths occurred among pneumococcal vaccine-eligible individuals and that 85.9% of strains reported among persons aged 65 years or older were covered by the current 23-valent pneumococcal vaccine.[66]

In the United States, 60% of persons aged 65 or older reported receiving the pneumococcal vaccine in 2001.[16] This level is well below the Healthy People 2010 target of 90% and also below the 65% annual target vaccination rate for influenza in this age group. The statistics suggest continued missed opportunities for combined scheduling of vaccine administration (eg, with influenza vaccine) to optimize vaccination coverage rates. The reduction of morbidity and mortality through primary prevention via improved vaccination rates will become progressively more important as multidrug-resistant pneumococcal infections increase in the United States.[67]

Vaccine dose and administration

The current US-licensed pneumococcal vaccines include Pneumovax 23 and Pnu-Imune 23. Only the Pneumovax 23 vaccine is currently being manufactured. These vaccines are composed of purified capsular polysaccharide antigens of 23 different *S pneumoniae* serotypes, representing 85% to 90% of the serotypes that cause invasive bacterial disease in the United States.[68] Six serotypes (6B, 9V, 14, 19A, 19F, and 23F) included in the vaccine are the cause of most of the invasive drug-resistant infections in the United States.[69] The pneumococcal vaccine should be administered IM or subcutaneously as one 0.5-mL dose in the deltoid region. Intramuscular administration is recommended, as it decreases the rate of local side effects such as pain, swelling, induration, and erythema. Because 30% to 40% of adults have medical conditions that indicate the need for the pneumococcal vaccine, practitioners should use the patient's 50th birthday as a time to review all immunizations and to evaluate risk factors for pneumococcal vaccine.[69]

Revaccination is recommended only for persons who were aged less than 65 years when they first received the vaccine and who have not received the vaccine in the past 5 years. Immunosuppressed adults and adults with functional or anatomical asplenia should also be revaccinated once every 5 years after the first dose of vaccine. The need for more than 2 doses of vaccine is unclear and is currently not recommended.[69]

Immunogenicity and efficacy

The results of studies evaluating the efficacy of pneumococcal vaccine against pneumonia and pneumococcal bacteremia range widely from 57% to 100%, depending on the study design, vaccine, and groups evaluated.[69,70] The vaccine is not effective in protecting against nonvaccine serotype organisms. Efficacy against pneumococcal pneumonia is evident in young, high-risk persons but not conclusively present in elderly subjects.[70,71] Nonetheless, pneumococcal immunization does significantly decrease the risk of invasive disease (eg, bacteremia, meningitis), and this alone makes the vaccine a cost-saving measure in the elderly.[72]

Adverse effects and contraindications

The most common reactions include local side effects, such as tenderness and redness around the injection site (in up to 50% of recipients). These symptoms typically resolve within 48 hours. Severe systemic adverse events, such as anaphylactic reactions, are rare. In a meta-analysis of 9 randomized controlled trials of pneumococcal vaccine efficacy, approximately one third or fewer of the 7531 patients receiving the vaccine reported local reactions.[71] There were no reports of severe fever or anaphylactic reactions. Arthus-type symptoms may occur in persons who receive an additional dose of vaccine in a shorter interval than recommended. No serious neurologic disorders such as GBS have been causally linked with the pneumococcal vaccine.[69] Nonetheless, persons with a history of any type of neurologic symptom after vaccination should not receive further doses. In addition, the Pnu-Imune 23 vaccine contains thimerosal; persons who have allergic reactions to thimerosal should receive only Pneumovax 23, which contains phenol rather than thimerosal.

Smallpox

Background

Variola major has a mortality rate as high as 30%, and humans are the only natural host for the virus. Smallpox, or variola, was officially declared eradicated from the world in 1980.[73] Since then, recent world events have led to the conclusion that remaining stores of smallpox laboratory cultures may have been used in the development of biological weapons.[74] As a result, starting in December 2002, limited smallpox vaccination programs have been implemented among health care workers and first responders, and potentially perhaps for the public at large. For this reason, clinicians must be familiar with and knowledgeable about the vaccine, how to administer it, contraindications, and unique attributes of the vaccine in regard to potential and inadvertent transmission.

Vaccine dose and administration

Smallpox vaccine does not contain any smallpox virus. Rather, the vaccine contains vaccinia virus, a cowpoxlike strain, which cross-protects against smallpox.[75] Vaccinia is a live, attenuated vaccine virus, which typically undergoes limited replication in vivo and results in cross-protection against variola and other orthopox viruses. The vaccine strain used in the United States is known as the New York

City Board of Health (NYCBOH) strain. A bifurcated needle is dipped into reconstituted vaccine, causing approximately 0.0025 mL of vaccine to adhere between the 2 tines of the needle. The needle tines are then "jabbed" into the epidermis 3 times for primary vaccines and 15 times for repeated vaccinees.[75] Lower doses of vaccine (ie, diluted vaccine) have also been demonstrated to lead to acceptable success ("take") rates.[76]

Immunogenicity and efficacy

In approximately 95% of primary vaccinees, protective immunity develops, which is defined as detectable levels of neutralizing antibody. With the development of a "major reaction" (ie, the development of a jennerian pustule), protective immunity is assured. Any other reaction is labeled as a "no take" or "equivocal" reaction and cannot be assumed to indicate establishment of immunity.[75] Vaccination is recommended every 10 years if there is risk of ongoing exposure.[75] In Europe from 1950 to 1971, smallpox fatality rates varied from 1% among those vaccinated within 10 years to 10% among those immunized more than 20 years earlier, suggesting that waning immunity evidently occurs.[77]

Importantly, postexposure vaccination is effective if the vaccine can be administered within 3 to 4 days of variola exposure.[75] This relates to the shorter time from vaccination until development of neutralizing antibody (7 to 10 days) in vaccinees, compared with the incubation period of the virus (12 to 17 days).

Adverse effects and contraindications

Smallpox vaccination may lead to death in an estimated 1 primary vaccinee per million doses administered and in an estimated 0.1 repeated vaccinee per million doses administered.[78] Life-threatening complications may occur in 14 to 52 vaccinees per million doses administered. In addition, major complications such as eczema vaccinatum, progressive vaccinia, and postvaccinial encephalitis may occur.

The use of vaccinia vaccine may cause inadvertent or contact transmission of the virus to others,[79] and self-inoculation or autoinoculation to other areas of the body, including the eye.[79] Vaccine virus transmission has been documented from the time a papule forms after vaccination (typically days 2 to 4) until the scab falls off (typically days 21 to 28). Numerous case reports exist documenting substantial morbidity and mortality resulting from contact vaccinia.[79] This complication is completely preventable by hand hygiene measures, by contact infection control precautions, and by keeping the vaccination site covered with gauze and a semipermeable dressing.

After receipt of smallpox vaccine, the FDA currently recommends that blood donations from vaccinees without severe complications be deferred until after the vaccination scab falls off (or 21 days, whichever is longer) and at least 14 days after complete resolution of complications in vaccinees who experience severe complications.[80]

Preexposure vaccination is absolutely contraindicated in persons under age 1 year, pregnant or lactating women, persons who are immunocompromised for any reason, and persons with any history of eczema or atopic dermatitis. In addition, it is recommended that persons with any condition leading to substantial disruption of epidermal integrity (such as burns or severe acne) be deferred until resolution of the condition. No such contraindications exist if actual smallpox virus exposure has occurred (ie, postexposure vaccination), although some have demonstrated lower severe side effects if vaccine is coadministered with vaccinia immune globulin (VIG).[81] In addition, persons should not receive vaccine if any intimate partner or household members have any of the above contraindications. Finally, the ACIP does not currently recommend preexposure vaccination for persons under the age of 18 years.

Complications of vaccinia vaccination may be treated with VIG, which has been demonstrated to reduce morbidity and mortality,[82] and perhaps with cidofovir.[75] Exceptions to this statement include vaccinia keratitis and postvaccinia encephalitis.[75]

Tetanus-Diphtheria

Background

In developed countries, tetanus is almost exclusively a disease of elderly people who either did not complete a primary tetanus-diphtheria toxoid series or did not receive boosters. Although only 1 case of diphtheria was recognized in 2000 in the United States, 34 of 35 reported cases of tetanus in the United States occurred in persons aged 15 years or older and 34% of all cases occurred in persons aged 65 years or older.[31] This is disconcerting because approximately 27% of US adults older than 70 years of age are unprotected against diphtheria and tetanus.[83]

Vaccine dose and administration

The tetanus toxoid is a formaldehyde-inactivated toxoid vaccine. Single-antigen tetanus toxoid (fluid) and tetanus toxoid adsorbed are also available for persons 7 years or older, but tetanus and diphtheria toxoids, adult type (Td), are preferred for tetanus prophylaxis in adults, as most adults in need of tetanus toxoid are highly likely to be susceptible to diphtheria.[84] Only the adsorbed preparation should be used, unless there are documented reasons not to use it, as immunogenicity is better than the fluid preparation. The preparations are all given as 0.5-mL IM doses. The second dose should be administered 1 to 2 months after the first is given; the third dose should be given 6 to 12 months later. Doses should not be repeated if scheduled doses are delayed, as long intervals between doses do not adversely affect immunogenicity or efficacy. Tetanus toxoid vaccine can be administered with other vaccines,

provided that different syringes and different anatomical sites are used.[11,85]

Immunogenicity and efficacy

Essentially all adults who receive the tetanus-diphtheria vaccine in the proper series are protected against disease. A study performed in Sweden showed that when the vaccine was administered over a 3-dose schedule 4 to 6 weeks apart, it has a long-term efficacy rate of 94% after 10 years. Studies done in Denmark show efficacy rates of 96% after 13 to 14 years and 72% after 25 years. However, in one study, only 77% of elderly subjects had protective antitoxin levels 8 years after receiving a primary 3-dose series. Booster doses are therefore recommended every 10 years in the United States.[85]

Adverse effects and contraindications

Adverse effects such as local reactions are common and tend to increase with the number of doses given. For this reason, unnecessary doses of vaccine should not be given even for purposes of postexposure prophylaxis. Pain, tenderness, or localized erythema or edema at the injection site have been reported. Fever and other systemic symptoms such as headache are less common.[11]

Neurologic or anaphylactic sensitivity to a previous dose of vaccine is the only contraindication for this vaccine. Persons with a history of Arthus-type hypersensitivity reactions or a temperature higher than 39.4°C (103°F) after prior doses of tetanus toxoid should not receive booster doses of Td more frequently than every 10 years.[11,85] Persons with contraindications to tetanus-toxoid–containing preparations who require wound prophylaxis should be given only tetanus immune globulin.

Varicella

Background

Although infection with varicella-zoster virus (VZV) is typically viewed as a disease of children, varicella develops in approximately 45,000 US adults annually.[86] The severity of varicella is 25 times greater in adults than in children.[87] Adults account for only 5% of clinical cases, but they account for 10% of all encephalitis cases and 20% of all varicella-related deaths.[86] In the elderly population, postherpetic neuralgia after clinical zoster can result in substantial and extended disability.[88] Varicella disease also tends to be more severe in pregnancy, is associated with a risk of transmission to the fetus or newborn, and may result in congenital varicella syndrome or clinical varicella.[86]

Vaccine dose and administration

The varicella vaccine (Varivax) is a live, attenuated viral vaccine. Update recommendations for the use of varicella vaccine were published in 1999.[89] The schedule for an adult consists of 2 doses of 0.5 mL each, administered subcutaneously 4 to 8 weeks apart. To maintain vaccine potency, the vaccine must be stored frozen at $-15°$C or colder. Once reconstituted and ready for use, the vaccine may be stored at room temperature for no longer than 30 minutes. If not used within 30 minutes, the vaccine must be discarded. The vaccine does not contain preservatives.[90] Adults who have a reliable history of varicella are considered immune. Of adults in the United States who are uncertain of previous varicella infection, 71% to 93% are seropositive.[86] The value of laboratory testing to detect VZV depends on the rationale and method of testing (ie, assessment of susceptibility in high-risk exposed individuals vs response to previous vaccination); current cost-effectiveness analyses are mixed as to target populations of adults in whom testing before vaccination would be beneficial.[86,91]

New, expanded recommendations for use of this vaccine include the following[90]:

- postexposure protection against disease, if vaccine is administered within 3 to 5 days after exposure
- routine immunization of susceptible persons aged 13 years and older who live in households with children or who work in an environment where transmission is likely
- international travelers
- nonpregnant women of childbearing age
- persons with impaired humoral, but not cellular, immunity.

Immunogenicity and efficacy

Persistent VZV antibody levels are maintained from 6 to 20 years after vaccination in up to 90% of healthy children and adults,[92, 93] and VZV T-cell immunity may be boosted in adults as well.[94] Breakthrough infections (wild-type virus infection in vaccinated persons) can occur with a frequency in reported studies ranging from 2% to 20%, depending on patient characteristics, study design, and length of follow-up.[93,95,96] These infections typically result in asymptomatic or mild illness and generally occur only after intense household exposure to wild virus.[86] Although controlled efficacy trials have not been conducted for

adults, the vaccine has proved 95% effective in preventing severe disease in adults.[86]

Adverse effects and contraindications

Up to 10.2% of adults receiving the first dose and 9.5% of those receiving the second dose develop oral temperatures higher than 37.8°C (100°F). After the first and second doses, 24.4% and 32.5% of vaccinees, respectively, report injection-site symptoms such as soreness, erythema, rash, hematoma, induration, and numbness.[86]

Because varicella vaccine is a live viral vaccine, it is contraindicated in pregnant women or anyone having a malignancy affecting the bone marrow or lymphatic system.[86,89] Immunosuppressed persons or persons with active, untreated tuberculosis should not receive the vaccine.[32] Persons who have received blood products in the past 5 or 6 months also should not receive the vaccine due to the presence of passive immunity, which prevents the development of protective antibody.[86] Persons with anaphylactic allergic reactions to gelatin or neomycin should not receive the vaccine due to possible hypersensitivity reactions.[86]

SUMMARY

Vaccines are the most cost-effective and efficacious tool available in preventing infectious disease. It is estimated that more than 40,000 lives would be saved each year in the United States if routine adult vaccines against pneumococcus, influenza virus, and hepatitis B virus were fully utilized. Adults may require vaccines based on occupation, disease, lifestyle, or health condition. Multiple barriers to immunizing adults include inadequate access to health care, missed opportunities to vaccinate concomitant with any contact with a health care provider, fears concerning adverse events due to vaccination, lack of awareness of the seriousness of certain vaccine-preventable diseases, and inadequate reimbursement for immunization services. Advances in vaccine technology must be accompanied by decreased health disparities, improvements in access to health care, and effective programs for distribution and administration of vaccines to reach the Healthy People 2010 immunization goals.

REFERENCES

1. Barquet N, Domingo P. Smallpox: the triumph over the most terrible of the ministers of death. *Ann Intern Med.* 1997;127:635–642.

2. Plotkin SA. A hundred years of vaccination: the legacy of Louis Pasteur. *Pediatr Infect Dis J.* 1996;15:391–394.

3. Minino AM, Smith BL. Deaths: preliminary data for 2000. *Natl Vital Stat Rep.* 2001;49:1–40.

4. Lederberg J. Infectious history. *Science.* 2000;288:287–293.

5. Centers for Disease Control and Prevention. Achievements in public health, 1900–1999: impact of vaccines universally recommended for children: United States, 1990–1999. *Morb Mortal Wkly Rep.* 1999;48:243–248.

6. Centers for Disease Control and Prevention. Update on adult immunization: recommendations of the Immunization Practices Advisory Committee (ACIP). *MMWR Morb Mortal Wkly Rep.* 1991;40(RR-12):1–94.

7. Centers for Disease Control and Prevention. Notice to readers: recommended adult immunization schedule: United States, 2002–2003. *MMWR Morb Mortal Wkly Rep.* 2002;51:904–908.

8. Centers for Disease Control and Prevention. *Adult Immunization Action Plan: Report of the Workgroup on Adult Immunization.* Atlanta, Ga: Centers for Disease Control, US Dept of Health and Human Services; 1998.

9. Massab HF, Bryant ML. The development of live attenuated cold-adapted influenza virus vaccine for humans. *Rev Med Virol.* 1999;9:237–244.

10. Mills J, Chanock V, Chanock RM. Temperature-sensitive mutants of influenza virus. I. Behavior in tissue culture and in experimental animals. *J Infect Dis.* 1971;123:145–157.

11. Advisory Committee on Immunization Practices (ACIP), American Academy of Family Physicians (AAFP). General recommendations on immunization: recommendations of the Advisory Committee on Immunization Practices and the American Academy of Family Physicians. *MMWR Morb Mortal Wkly Rep.* 2002;51(RR-2):1–35.

12. Ipp MM, Gold R, Goldbach M, et al. Adverse reactions to diphtheria, tetanus, pertussis-polio vaccination at 18 months of age: effect of injection site and needle length. *Pediatrics.* 1989;83:679–682.

13. Centers for Disease Control and Prevention, National Immunization Program. Six common misconceptions about vaccination and how to respond to them. 2003. Available at: www.cdc gov/nip/publications/6mishome htm. Accessed January 28, 2003.

14. Public Health Service. National Childhood Vaccine Injury Act of the Public Health Service. 2125. 42 USC §300aa-26. (1986).

15. Zhou W, Pool V, Iskander JK, et al. Surveillance for safety after immunization: Vaccine Adverse Event Reporting System (VAERS): United States, 1991–2001. *MMWR Morb Mortal Wkly Rep.* 2003;52:1–24.

16. Centers for Disease Control and Prevention. Influenza and pneumococcal vaccination levels among person aged >65 years: United States, 2001. *MMWR Morb Mortal Wkly Rep.* 2003;51:1019–1024.

17. US Dept of Health and Human Services. *Healthy People 2010.* 2nd ed. Washington, DC: US Government Printing Office; 2000.

18. Bratzler DW, Houck PM, Jiang H, et al. Failure to vaccinate Medicare inpatients. *Arch Intern Med.* 2002; 162:2349–2356.

19. Centers for Disease Control and Prevention. Prevention and control of influenza: recommendations of the Advisory Committee on Immunization Practices (ACIP). *MMWR Morb Mortal Wkly Rep.* 2001;50:1–46.

20. van Essen GA, Kuyvenhoven MM, de Melker RA. Why do healthy elderly people fail to comply with influenza vaccination? *Age Ageing.* 1997;26:275–279.

21. National Center for Chronic Disease Prevention and Health Promotion, Centers for Disease Control and Prevention, US Dept of Health and Human Services. Behavioral Risk Factor Surveillance System. 1999. Available at: www.cdc.gov/ brfss/technical_infodata/surveydata.htm. Accessed October 2, 2003.

22. Potter J, Stott DJ, Roberts MA, et al. Influenza vaccination of health care workers in long-term-care hospitals reduces the mortality of elderly patients. *J Infect Dis.* 1997;175:1–6.

23. Walker FJ, Singleton JA, Strikas RA. Influenza vaccination of health care workers in the United States, 1989–1997 [abstract]. *Infect Control Hosp Epidemiol.* 2000;21:113.

24. Lee PY, Matchar DB, Clements DA, Huber J, Hamilton JD, Peterson ED. Economic analysis of influenza vaccination and antiviral treatment for healthy working adults. *Ann Intern Med.* 2002;137:225–231.

25. Fiscella K, Franks P, Gold MR, Clancy CM. Inequality in quality: addressing socioeconomic, racial, and ethnic disparities in health care. *JAMA.* 2000;283:2579–2584.

26. Gornick ME, Eggers PW, Reilly TW, et al. Effects of race and income on mortality and use of services among Medicare beneficiaries. *N Engl J Med.* 1996;335:791–799.

27. Centers for Disease Control and Prevention. Health objectives for the nation: race-specific differences in influenza vaccination levels among Medicare beneficiaries: United States. *MMWR Morb Mortal Wkly Rep.* 1995;44:24–27, 33.

28. Schneider EC, Cleary PD, Zaslavsky AM, Epstein AM. Racial disparity in influenza vaccination: does managed care narrow the gap between African Americans and whites? *JAMA.* 2001;286:1455–1460.

29. Centers for Disease Control and Prevention. Adult immunization: knowledge, attitudes, and practices: DeKalb

and Fulton Counties, Georgia, 1988. *MMWR Morb Mortal Wkly Rep.* 1988;37:657–661.

30. Armstrong GL, Bell BP. Hepatitis A virus infections in the United States: model-based estimates and implications for childhood immunization. *Pediatrics.* 2002;109:839–845.

31. Centers for Disease Control and Prevention. Summary of notifiable diseases, United States, 2000. *MMWR Morb Mortal Wkly Rep.* 2000;49:1–91.

32. Gardner P, Eickhoff T, Poland GA, et al. Adult immunizations. *Ann Intern Med.* 1996;124:35–40.

33. Koff RS. Seroepidemiology of hepatitis A in the United States. *J Infect Dis.* 1995;171:S19–S23.

34. Centers for Disease Control and Prevention. Prevention of hepatitis A through active or passive immunization: recommendations of the Advisory Committee on Immunization Practices (ACIP). *MMWR Morb Mortal Wkly Rep.* 1999;48:1–37.

35. Centers for Disease Control and Prevention. FDA approval for a combined hepatitis A and B vaccine. *MMWR Morb Mortal Wkly Rep.* 2001;50:806–807.

36. Koff RS. Hepatitis A. *Lancet.* 1998;351:1643–1647.

37. GlaxoSmithKline Biologicals. Havrix. US Prescribing Information; 2003.

38. Merck & Co Inc. Vaqta. US Prescribing Information; 2003.

39. Andre FE. Randomized, cross-over, controlled comparison of two inactivated hepatitis A vaccines. *Vaccine.* 2001;20:292–293.

40. Clemens R, Safary A, Hepburn A, Roche C, Stanbury WJ, Andre FE. Clinical experience with an inactivated hepatitis A vaccine. *J Infect Dis.* 1995;171(suppl 1):S44–S49.

41. Centers for Disease Control and Prevention, Advisory Committee on Immunization Practices. Protection against viral hepatitis. *MMWR Morb Mortal Wkly Rep.* 1990;39:1–26.

42. Poland GA. Hepatitis B immunization in health care workers: dealing with vaccine nonresponse. *Am J Prev Med.* 1998;15:73–77.

43. Centers for Disease Control and Prevention. Achievements in public health. *MMWR Morb Mortal Wkly Rep.* 2002;51:549–552.

44. National Center for Infectious Diseases, Centers for Disease Control and Prevention. Viral Hepatitis B Fact Sheet. 2003. Available at: www.cdc.gov/ncdod diseases/hepatitis/b/fact htm. Accessed January 23, 2003.

45. Shaw FE Jr, Guess HA, Roets JM, et al. Effect of anatomic injection site, age and smoking on the immune response to hepatitis B vaccination. *Vaccine.* 1989;7:425–430.

46. Poland GA, Borrud A, Jacobson RM, et al. Determination of deltoid fat pad thickness: implications for needle length in adult immunization. *JAMA.* 1997;277:1709–1711.

47. Hohler T, Reuss E, Evers N, et al. Differential genetic determination of immune responsiveness to hepatitis B surface antigen and to hepatitis A virus: a vaccination study in twins. *Lancet.* 2002;360:991–995.

48. Institute of Medicine Safety Review Committee. *Immunization Safety Review: Hepatitis B Vaccine and Neurological Demyelinating Disorders.* Washington, DC: National Academy Press; 2002.

49. Noseworthy JH, Poland GA. Multiple sclerosis. *N Engl J Med.* 2001;344:382.

50. Advisory Committee on Immunization Practices. Prevention and control of influenza: recommendations of the Advisory Committee on Immunization Practices. *MMWR Morb Mortal Wkly Rep.* 2002;51:1–31.

51. Williams GO. Vaccines in older patients: combating the risk of mortality. *Geriatrics.* 1980;35:55–64.

52. Couch RB. Summary of medical literature: review of effectiveness of inactivated influenza virus vaccine. In: *Cost-Effectiveness of Influenza Vaccination.* Washington, DC: US Congress, Office of Technology Assessment; 1981:43–45.

53. Nichol KL, Lind A, Margolis KL, et al. The effectiveness of vaccination against influenza in healthy, working adults. *N Engl J Med.* 1995;333:889–893.

54. Blumberg EA, Albano C, Pruett T, et al. The immunogenicity of influenza virus vaccine in solid organ transplant recipients. *Clin Infect Dis.* 1996;22:295–302.

55. Gross PA, Hermogenes AW, Sacks HS, Lau J, Levandowski RA. The efficacy of influenza vaccine in elderly persons: a meta-analysis and review of the literature. *Ann Intern Med.* 1995;123:518–527.

56. Beyer WEP, Palache AM, Baljet M, Masurel N. Antibody induction by influenza vaccines in the elderly: a review of the literature. *Vaccine.* 1989;7:385–394.

57. Nichol KL, Wuorenma J, von Sternberg T. Benefits of influenza vaccination for low-, intermediate-, and high-risk senior citizens. *Arch Intern Med.* 1998;158:1769–1776.

58. Office of Technology Assessment. *Cost-Effectiveness of Influenza Vaccination.* 1981. Washington, DC, US Congress, Office of Technology Assessment.

59. Margolis KL, Nichol KL, Poland GA, Pluhar RE. Frequency of adverse reactions to influenza vaccine in the elderly: a randomized, placebo-controlled trial. *JAMA.* 1990;264:1139–1141.

60. US Food and Drug Administration Vaccines and Related Biological Products Advisory Committee. *Summary Minutes of the U.S. Food and Drug Administration VRBPAC Meeting on December 17, 2002.* Rockville, Md: US Food and Drug Administration; 2002.

61. Glezen WP. Emerging infections: pandemic influenza. *Epidemiol Rev.* 1996;18:64–76.

62. Reichert TA, Sugaya N, Fedson DS, Glezen WP, Simonsen L, Tashiro M. The Japanese experience with vaccinating schoolchildren against influenza. *N Engl J Med.* 2001;344:889–896.

63. Watson JC, Hadler SC, Dykewicz CA, Reef S, Phillips L. Measles, mumps, and rubella:vaccine use and strategies for elimination of measles, rubella, and congenital rubella syndrome and control of mumps: recommendations of the Advisory Committee on Immunization Practices (ACIP). *MMWR Morb Mortal Wkly Rep.* 1998;47(RR-8):1–57.

64. Centers for Disease Control and Prevention. Prevention and control of meningococcal disease. *MMWR Morb Mortal Wkly Rep.* 2000;49:1–10.

65. National Immunization Program, Centers for Disease Control and Prevention. *Epidemiology and Prevention of Vaccine-Preventable Diseases.* 7th ed. Atlanta, Ga: Centers for Disease Control and Prevention; 2002.

66. Robinson KA, Baughman W, Rothrock G, et al. Epidemiology of invasive streptococcus pneumoniae infections in the United States, 1995–1998. *JAMA.* 2001;285:1729–1735.

67. Whitney CG, Farley MM, Hadler J, et al. Increasing prevalence of multidrug-resistant *Streptococcus pneumoniae* in the United States. *N Engl J Med.* 2000;343:1917–1924.

68. Division of Bacterial and Mycotic Diseases, Centers for Disease Control and Prevention. *Streptococcus pneumoniae* disease: technical information, 2002. 2003. Available at: www.cdc.gov/ncidod/dbmd/diseaseinfo/ streppneum_t.htm. Accessed January 28, 2003.

69. Centers for Disease Control and Prevention, Advisory Committee on Immunization Practices. Prevention of pneumococcal disease: recommendations of the Advisory Committee on Immunization Practices (ACIP). *MMWR Recomm Rep.* 1997;46(RR-8):1–24.

70. Koivula I, Sten M, Leinonen M, Makela PH. Clinical efficacy of pneumococcal vaccine in the elderly: a randomized, single-blind population-based trial. *Am J Med.* 1997;103:281–290.

71. Fine MJ, Smith MA, Carson CA, et al. Efficacy of pneumococcal vaccination in adults: a meta-analysis of randomized controlled trials. *Arch Intern Med.* 1994;154:2666–2677.

72. Vlasich C. Pneumococcal infection and vaccination in the elderly. *Vaccine.* 2001;19:2233–2237.

73. Breman JG, Arita I. The confirmation and maintenance of smallpox eradication. *N Engl J Med.* 1980;303:1263–1273.

74. Henderson DA, Inglesby TV, Bartlett JG, et al. Smallpox as a biological weapon: medical and public health management. *JAMA.* 1999;281:2127–2137.

75. Advisory Committee on Immunization Practices. Vaccinia (smallpox) vaccine recommendations of the Advisory Committee on Immunization Practices (ACIP), 2001. *MMWR Morb Mortal Wkly Rep.* 2001;50:1–22.

76. Frey SE, Couch RB, Tacket CO, et al. Clinical responses to undiluted and diluted smallpox vaccine. *N Engl J Med.* 2002;346:1265–1274.

77. Mack TM. Smallpox in Europe, 1950–1971. *J Infect Dis.* 1972;125:161–169.

78. Lane JM, Ruben FL, Abrutyn E, Millar JD. Deaths attributable to smallpox vaccination, 1959 to 1966, and 1968. *JAMA.* 1970;212:441–444.

79. Neff JM, Lane JM, Fulginiti VA, Henderson DA. Contact vaccinia: Transmission of vaccinia from smallpox vaccination. *JAMA.* 2002;288:1901–1905.

80. US Food and Drug Administration, US Dept of Health and Human Services. Guidance for Industry: recommendations for deferral of donors and quarantine and retrieval of blood and blood products in recent recipients of smallpox vaccine (vaccinia virus) and certain contacts of smallpox vaccine recipients. Rockville, Md: US Dept of Health and Human Services; December 2002:1–9. Available at: www.fda.gov/cber/gdlns/smpoxdefquar.pdf. Accessed October 2, 2003.

81. Goldstein JA, Neff JM, Lane JM, Koplan JP. Smallpox vaccination reactions, prophylaxis, and therapy of complications. *Pediatrics.* 1975;55:342–347.

82. Sussman S, Grossman M. Complications of smallpox vaccination. Effects of vaccinia immune globulin therapy. *J Pediatr.* 1965;67:1168–1173.

83. Gergen PJ, McQuillan GM, Kiely M, Ezzati-Rice TM, Sutter RW, Virella G. A population-based serologic survey of immunity to tetanus in the United States. *N Engl J Med.* 1995;332:761–766.

84. Centers for Disease Control and Prevention. Diphtheria, tetanus, and pertussis: recommendations for vaccine use and other preventive measures: recommendations of the Immunization Practices Advisory Committee (ACIP). *MMWR Morb Mortal Wkly Rep.* 1991;40:1–28.

85. Wassilak SGF, Orenstein WA, Sutter RW. Tetanus toxoid. In: Plotkin SA, Mortimer EA Jr, eds. *Vaccines.* Philadelphia, Pa: WB Saunders Co; 1994:57–90.

86. Centers for Disease Control and Prevention. Prevention of varicella: recommendations of the Advisory Committee on Immunization Practices (ACIP). *MMWR Morb Mortal Wkly Rep.* 1996;45:1–27.

87. Preblud SR. Varicella: complications and costs. *Pediatrics.* 1986;76:728–735.

88. Gilden DH. Herpes zoster with postherpetic neuralgia: persisting pain and frustration. *N Engl J Med.* 1994;330:932–934.

89. Centers for Disease Control and Prevention. Prevention of varicella: updated recommendations of the Advisory Committee on Immunization Practices (ACIP). *MMWR Morb Mortal Wkly Rep.* 1999;48:1–5.

90. Centers for Disease Control and Prevention. Vaccine management: recommendations for handling and storage of selected biologicals. Washington, DC, US Dept of Health and Human Services; 2001.

91. Smith KJ, Roberts MS. Cost effectiveness of vaccination strategies in adults without a history of chickenpox. *Am J Med.* 2000;108:723–729.

92. Arbeter AM, Starr SE, Plotkin SA. Varicella vaccine studies in healthy children and adults. *Pediatrics.* 1986;78(suppl):748–756.

93. Saiman L, LaRussa P, Steinberg SP, et al. Persistence of immunity to varicella-zoster virus after vaccination of healthcare workers. *Infect Control Hosp Epidemiol.* 2001;22:279–283.

94. Levin MJ, Barber D, Goldblatt E, et al. Use of a live attenuated varicella vaccine to boost varicella-specific immune responses in seropositive people 55 years of age and older: duration of booster effect. *J Infect Dis.* 1998;178(suppl 1):S109–S112.

95. Ampofo K, Saiman L, LaRussa P, Steinberg S, Annunziato P, Gershon A. Persistence of immunity to live attenuated varicella vaccine in healthy adults. *Clin Infect Dis.* 2002;34:774–779.

96. Johnson CE, Stancin T, Fattlar D, Rome LP, Kumar ML. A long-term prospective study of varicella vaccine in healthy children. *Pediatrics.* 1997;100:761–766.

RESOURCES

Centers for Disease Control and Prevention (CDC), Advisory Committee on Immunization Practices. Web site: www.cdc.gov/nip/ACIP.

CDC. Comprehensive and vaccine-specific Recommendations of the Advisory Committee on Immunization Practices. Web site: www.cdc.gov/nip/publications/ACIP-list.htm.

CDC, National Immunization Program. 800 232-2522. Web site: www.cdc.gov/nip.

CDC and Food and Drug Administration. Vaccine Adverse Event Reporting System. 800 822-7967. Web site: www.vaers.org.

Epidemiology and Prevention of Vaccine-Preventable Diseases. 7th ed. Atlanta, Ga: CDC National Immunization Program; 2003. Web site: www.cdc.gov/nip/publications/pink/default.htm#download.

US Dept of Health and Human Services. *Healthy People 2010.* 2nd ed. *With Understanding and Improving Health and Objectives for Improving Health.* 2 vols. Washington, DC: US Government Printing Office; November 2000. Web site: www.healthypeople.gov.

HIV and Sexually Transmissible Disease Prevention

Mary J. Kasten, MD

INTRODUCTION

Human immunodeficiency virus (HIV) is the most important sexually transmissible illness of our time. Globally, 5 million people were newly infected and 3.1 million people died of acquired immunodeficiency syndrome (AIDS) in 2002.[1] An estimated 900,000 adults and children were living with HIV infection in the United States at the end of 2001.[2] Wealthy nations, unlike the developing world, have seen a large decrease in AIDS-related deaths because of the widespread use of potent antiretroviral medications. Unfortunately, the success of antiretroviral treatment has shifted attention away from primary prevention. Many studies show that primary prevention can successfully decrease the spread of HIV. This chapter will emphasize the aspects of HIV prevention relevant to clinicians in the United States. The unique aspects of preventing other common sexually transmissible diseases also will be discussed in this chapter.

HUMAN IMMUNODEFICIENCY VIRUS

US Epidemiology and Transmission of HIV

In the United States, HIV was first recognized among white homosexual or bisexual men in the 1980s. Today, men who have sex with men remain at high risk of acquiring HIV, accounting for nearly 50% of new HIV infections in the United States in 2001. In contrast, heterosexual contact with an infected partner is the leading risk factor for acquiring HIV worldwide and is increasingly spreading HIV in the United States. Human immunodeficiency virus is transmitted through vaginal intercourse, and the risk is highest for the female partner. Oral-genital contact can transmit HIV but is much less risky than anal or vaginal intercourse. Nearly 30% of US adults and adolescents with newly acquired HIV in 2001

are thought to have acquired HIV through heterosexual contact. Approximately one third of new HIV infections in the United States occur in women, and heterosexual contact accounted for 68% of infections among women with identified risk factors as reported to the Centers for Disease Control and Prevention (CDC) in 2001. The other major risk factor for HIV infection in the United States is use of injectable drugs, which accounted for nearly 20% of new HIV infections in 2001.[3]

Not all exposures to HIV result in transmission of infection. The risk of infection depends on the amount of virus one is exposed to and the susceptibility of the exposed host. Sexual activity with a person with AIDS or primary HIV infection is associated with an increased risk of infection, presumably due to the large amount of virus in blood and body fluids in these conditions. People with certain rare genetic mutations appear to be resistant to infection.[4] The presence of a genital ulcer or another sexually transmitted illness increases one's susceptibility to HIV infection.

Screening, Counseling, and Testing for HIV

Counseling patients about how they can decrease their risk of becoming HIV infected and identifying and counseling those who are HIV infected about how they can prevent transmission to others are important pieces of the overall HIV prevention effort in the United States. Primary care providers need to be assertive in asking about HIV risk factors and in testing for HIV. They also need to be knowledgeable about counseling information and techniques that can help motivate patients to stop or change risky behavior. All patients should be questioned regarding high-risk behaviors. All patients with high-risk behaviors and the clinical signs listed in Table 51-1 should be encouraged to undergo HIV screening.[5] The CDC also recommends HIV screening for all pregnant women.[6] The visit in which screening for HIV is

T A B L E   51-1

Indications for HIV Screening*

High-risk Behaviors	Clinical Signs and Clues
Multiple sexual partners	Desires HIV screening
History of giving or obtaining sex for drugs or money	Active tuberculosis
History of anal intercourse	Herpes zoster in a healthy person <50 y old
History of sex with an intravenous drug user, person at risk of HIV, or person with known HIV infection	New severe psoriasis or other new unexplained severe skin disorder
History of a sexually transmitted disease	History of hepatitis B or C
History of intravenous drug use	Cervical cancer or HPV infection
History of having received blood or blood products before 1985	Thrush not related to recent antibiotic use
	Unexplained cachexia or weight loss
	Diffuse lymphadenopathy
	Unexplained thrombocytopenia, leukopenia, or anemia
	Unusual or prolonged unexplained viral-like illness (consider acute HIV)
	History of an opportunistic or unusual infection in an otherwise healthy individual
	Prolonged unexplained illness despite evaluation

*Reprinted with permission from Kasten MJ.[5] HIV indicates human immunodeficiency virus; HPV, human papillomavirus.

discussed also provides an opportunity to educate the patient about how HIV is, and is not, transmitted and about what the individual can do to lower his or her risk of infection.[5]

Recognition of and screening for primary acute HIV infection are challenging for primary care providers because the symptoms of primary HIV are similar to a number of other viral infections. Common symptoms include fever, sore throat, myalgias, and fatigue. Patients with primary HIV are usually very infectious and frequently engage in activity that promotes transmission of HIV infection. Therefore, appropriate screening and counseling of these individuals is an important part of HIV prevention in the United States.[7]

The serum enzyme-linked immunosorbent assay (ELISA) or enzyme immunoassay HIV antibody test is the most common HIV screening test used in the United States. When the result is positive, a highly specific confirmatory antibody test, most commonly the Western blot, is performed. This 2-step process takes from 2 days to 2 weeks to complete, depending on the institution. These antibody tests, when used together, are very accurate; however, false-negatives can occur during early infection. At least 95% of newly infected patients will have detectable HIV antibodies 3 months after infection.[8]

A single rapid antibody test was approved for use by the US Food and Drug Administration (FDA) in 2002.[9] Rapid antibody tests, when results are negative, can provide persons concerned about chronic infection reassurance on the day of testing. Positive results must be repeated, and a confirmatory test must be performed.

Diagnosis of primary HIV infection requires a negative result of an ELISA antibody test or an indeterminate Western blot test result, along with either a positive P24 antigen or a positive viral load assessment. The P24 is a more specific assay, but viral load assessment is more sensitive. False-positive viral loads are generally low, whereas true positive viral loads in a patient with acute HIV are generally more than 100,000 copies per milliliter.[10]

Prevention of Sexually Transmitted HIV

Primary care providers have an obligation to talk with their patients about their sexuality and assess their risk of sexually transmitted illness. Most patients want to talk with their health care givers about sexual concerns and AIDS.[11] Physician discomfort with these topics frequently leads to missed opportunities for providing appropriate counseling.[12] For most people who are sexually active, proper and consistent use of latex or polyurethane condoms is the best way of preventing HIV infection. The incidence and prevalence of HIV declines with increasing condom use.[13] However, condom use cannot provide complete protection. A meta-analysis among heterosexuals found condoms to be 87% effective in protecting against HIV transmission among consistent condom users.[14] Condom failure may be more common with anal intercourse. Receptive anal sex is more risky than receptive vaginal sex, insertive anal sex, or insertive vaginal sex.

Primary care providers should be able to counsel patients regarding the correct use of a condom. Patients need to know that adequate lubrication is important but only water-based lubricants should be used. Oil-based and petroleum-based lubricants, antifungal creams, and body lotion can all make the condom more prone to breakage. Old and damaged condoms should not be used. The condom should be unrolled onto an erect penis before genital contact. The penis should be withdrawn while still erect, and the condom should be held at the base to keep it from slipping off.[8] Condoms free of nonoxynol-9 are preferred for HIV prevention, since this chemical, which was hoped to be an effective vaginal microbicide, appears to have facilitated HIV transmission.[15] However, a condom containing nonoxynol-9 is certainly more effective than no condom.

Although primary care providers may lessen an individual's risk of acquiring HIV, such a strategy is not effective among populations that may have little interaction with physicians. Primary prevention efforts must be focused on communities at risk. Community-based prevention efforts have been successful, as evidenced by trends among homosexual and bisexual men in San Francisco. Early during the HIV epidemic, the gay community actively promoted condom use and a change in sexual behaviors. The incidence of HIV in this population sharply declined during the late 1980s, along with declines in the prevalence of sexual behaviors associated with HIV transmission.[16] A systematic review and meta-analysis of controlled HIV prevention trials aimed at reducing unprotected sex in men who have sex with men found the most favorable effects among trials that promoted interpersonal skills, were delivered in community-level formats, and focused on younger populations or those at higher behavioral risk.[17]

Drug use, particularly crack cocaine use, has been associated with high-risk sexual behaviors, including having sex with a partner at high risk of HIV, having multiple sexual partners, and not using condoms during sex.[18] Drug use often leads to behaviors that people would otherwise not engage in and is a major contributor to the spread of HIV in the United States. Effective substance abuse treatment is beneficial both for the drug user and as a primary and secondary HIV prevention measure.

Approximately half of all new HIV infections occur in the United States among people under age 25 years.[19] Interventions aimed at decreasing sexual activity are most successful in younger precoital teens.[20] Education programs for sexually active youth should not only promote abstinence but also focus on behaviors that lead to HIV infection and sexually transmitted diseases (STDs). School-based programs are among the most effective HIV prevention programs. These programs give students the

information to assess the benefits of delaying sexual intercourse and using a condom.[21] These programs have not led to increased sexual activity among youth;[21] rather, they have been credited with decreasing sexual risk-taking among teens.[22] Physicians can help educate parents regarding HIV risk and the realities of adolescent sexual behavior. Physicians also can encourage parents to openly discuss sexual activity with their children. Parents should know that clear communication with their children is important in helping adolescents adopt and maintain protective sexual behaviors.

Primary care providers with knowledge of safer sex practices can offer counseling tailored to the individual, which can affect an individual's risk of acquiring HIV and help prevent transmission. Physicians can also support community efforts that have been proved to successfully change behavior and decrease HIV transmission in at-risk populations.

Prevention of HIV Transmission Through Injection Drug Use

Injection drug use is a well-recognized risk factor for HIV but is often poorly understood by health professionals. Injection drug users put themselves at risk of HIV in many ways, including direct sharing of needles, syringes, and other drug injection equipment; indirect sharing of equipment; and risky sexual behavior. Appropriate counseling of injection drug users requires an understanding of the behaviors that place them at risk of HIV.

Drugs are frequently heated with water in a spoon or bottle cap, called a "cooker" and then drawn through a filter or cotton ball.[23] Drug users will determine that the needle is in a vein by pulling back on the plunger and seeing blood entering the syringe, that is, "registering." This contaminates the entire syringe with blood.[24] After injecting the drug, the user typically rinses the syringe with water. Contaminated rinse water is frequently shared or used to dissolve drugs in the cooker. Despite rinsing, the syringe frequently remains contaminated with HIV, and HIV can remain infectious at room temperature in used syringes for more than 4 weeks.[25] Many drug users are not aware that sharing equipment such as cotton balls, cookers, or rinse water in addition to syringes and needles puts them at risk of acquiring HIV and other bloodborne diseases.

Injection drug users are willing to change their drug injecting practices when educated and provided with sterile equipment.[26,27] Needle and syringe exchange programs have been very effective at reducing needle and syringe sharing. These programs also provide the opportunity to educate injection drug users regarding both safer drug use practices and safer sex. These programs have not resulted in increased drug use in the community.[28]

Patients who may share needles or other injection equipment should be educated on bleach disinfection. Household bleach is virucidal. The CDC, the National Institute on Drug Abuse, and the Center for Substance Abuse Treatment have published guidelines on bleach disinfection.[23] Unfortunately, a significant protective effect of bleach disinfection among intravenous (IV) drug users has not been demonstrated.[29] Physicians should ensure that patients understand that even with bleach disinfection any sharing of drug injection equipment is dangerous.

Effective substance abuse treatment eliminates the risk of HIV transmission from sharing contaminated equipment and frequently reduces risky sexual behaviors. Not all injection drug users are able or ready to quit. The need for substance abuse treatment is far greater than the availability of programs.[30,31] Efforts at preventing HIV among injection drug users must work to gain access to treatment for those ready to quit and also toward decreasing the risk of HIV acquisition and transmission for those who continue to use drugs.

Physicians, as leaders in communities, have an opportunity and responsibility to educate the general population and policy makers about the importance of substance abuse programs, the effectiveness of needle exchange programs, and the importance to the entire population of ensuring that injection drug users have access to sterile equipment. By providing knowledgeable and nonjudgmental HIV counseling and testing to injection drug users, the primary care provider plays another important role in the HIV prevention effort.

Prevention of HIV in Infants

The decrease in perinatal transmission of HIV in the United States over the last decade is an HIV prevention success story. However, the success is not complete since perinatal transmission still occurs. In 2001, there were 390 new HIV cases secondary to perinatal transmission.[3] Mother-to-child transmission of HIV can occur any time during pregnancy, at the time of delivery, and with breast-feeding.

Programs geared at preventing unwanted pregnancy and STDs will decrease the number of HIV-infected infants. Screening and identifying HIV before pregnancy or early in pregnancy when followed by appropriate HIV treatment is very effective in preventing HIV in infants. Treating HIV-infected pregnant mothers at any stage of HIV disease will decrease the chance of perinatal transmission. The longer the pregnant woman receives treatment, the more potent the treatment program, and the lower her viral load is at delivery, the less the risk of HIV transmission to the infant.[32] Risk of perinatal transmission is likely less than 1% in women receiving prolonged treatment and who have a plasma HIV viral load less than 400 HIV RNA copies per milliliter.[32] Having a cesarean section also reduces the risk of perinatal transmission.[33]

The Institute of Medicine concluded after a 1988 study that continued perinatal transmission was mainly caused by lack of awareness of HIV status among pregnant women. The Institute of Medicine concluded that the United States should adopt a national policy of voluntary universal testing as a routine component of prenatal care.[34] The CDC also encourages this approach.

Prevention of Nosocomial HIV

The current risk of HIV transmission from screened blood in the United States is very low, with an estimated range of 1 in 450,000 to 1 in 660,000.[35] Individuals who receive an HIV-contaminated unit of blood have a 90% likelihood of becoming infected.[36]

Transmission of HIV from infected health care workers to patients is possible but exceedingly rare.[37] An HIV-infected health care worker should not perform procedures if there is a substantial chance of injury that would result in exposure of the patient to the health care giver's blood. The CDC also recommends that HIV-infected health care workers with exudative skin lesions or dermatitis not have direct contact with patients. Nosocomial transmission of HIV is a much greater problem in developing countries, where equipment may not be able to be properly sterilized and where blood is more frequently HIV infected.

Prevention of HIV in Health Care Workers

The risk of transmission of HIV from patients to health care workers is small but real. As of June 2000, the CDC had received 194 reports of documented or possible cases of occupationally transmitted HIV. Transmission of HIV from patients to health care providers occurs most frequently via percutaneous injuries with sharp instruments. Mucosal splashes with HIV-infected blood or body fluids have also transmitted HIV.[38]

Gloves must be worn when there is any chance of exposure to blood or body fluids. Double gloving decreases the chance of blood exposure during surgery and is recommended when performing any invasive procedure.[39] Gowns, masks, and protective eyewear are recommended when there is the potential for a splash of blood or body fluids contacting the health care provider.[40] Used needles should not be recapped and should be disposed of immediately after use in puncture-proof containers. Safer needle devices and needle-free systems can help prevent needle injuries.[41]

Skin or wounds exposed to blood or other body fluids should be immediately washed with soap and water. Exposed mucous membranes should be rinsed with water and eyes flushed with sterile saline. Postexposure prophylaxis with antiretroviral agents should be considered if there is a potential HIV exposure.

Postexposure HIV Prophylaxis (PEP)

A retrospective case-control study of health care workers has shown that the use of zidovudine after exposure to HIV in the health care setting was associated with a reduction in the risk of HIV transmission by approximately 80%.[42] Both the exposed health care worker and the source patient should be tested for HIV. Ideally, PEP should be considered and treatment begun within hours of a potential exposure to HIV in the health care setting. Animal studies suggest that PEP is less effective when started more than 24 to 36 hours after exposure. Four weeks of PEP treatment is recommended by the CDC.[38]

Additionally, PEP is being used more frequently in nonoccupational settings, such as in the emergency room after rape, after condom failure with a partner known to have or be at risk of HIV, and occasionally after other potential HIV exposures. Because PEP is potentially toxic, it should not be used when the risk of transmission is minuscule. Therefore, PEP is not recommended for exposure of blood or other infected body fluid to intact skin.[38]

The most common PEP is a 2-drug program of zidovudine and lamivudine. Other combinations of nucleoside reverse transcriptase inhibitors can be used. The addition of a protease inhibitor or efavirenz is reasonable if the exposure was severe, such as a deep puncture with a large-bore hollow needle or exposure to a patient with known drug resistance or a very high viral load.[38]

Treatment of HIV

Treatment with multiple antiretroviral agents will decrease the amount of virus in blood and body fluids and decreases a person's infectiousness.[43] Increased sexual risk-taking activity due to the belief that sex is safe may offset prevention gains. Patients and physicians need to be aware that even when virus is undetectable in the blood, transmission of HIV may still occur.

HIV Vaccines

Although advances are occurring in our understanding of the immune responses that could prevent HIV infection, an effective and safe vaccine will not be available in the near future. Vaccines may be available that will augment the immune response to HIV in infected individuals in the next decade. However, a vaccine that can truly prevent infection in an uninfected person is likely decades away.

Summary of HIV Prevention

Successful prevention is key to gaining control over the HIV epidemic. A study published in 2002 estimated that HIV prevention efforts in the United States alone have prevented up to 1.5 million infections.[44] Much still remains to be accomplished, however, as 40,000 new infections occur annually in the United States. The primary health care provider in the United States has an important role to play in educating, screening, and counseling patients about HIV. Physicians need to be comfortable talking with patients about sensitive issues, including sex and drug use. They need to be knowledgeable regarding HIV transmission so they can provide patients with appropriate counsel and provide leadership that advances HIV prevention in their communities.

OTHER STDS

Many STDs, including syphilis, chlamydia, herpes simplex virus type 2 (HSV-2), gonorrhea, and chancroid, appear to facilitate HIV transmission. Infection with HIV may prolong symptomatic STDs and increase the likelihood of STD transmission. These interrelationships are currently believed to be responsible for the explosive spread of HIV among some populations.[45] Sexually transmitted diseases other than HIV can have serious long-term consequences, including infertility, a stillborn or ill infant, cancer, and premature death. A 1996 study estimated that 15.3 million new cases of non-HIV STDs occurred in the United States in 1996, and an estimated 1 in 4 Americans will contract an STD during their lifetime.[46] The remainder of this chapter will briefly review common STDs and prevention information unique to each organism and disease.

Genital Herpes

Genital herpes is very common, with at least 500,000 new cases estimated to occur annually in the United States.[47] The major cause of genital herpes is HSV-2. A recent survey indicated that more than 20% of US adults have antibodies to HSV-2.[48] This virus causes painful ulcers, sometimes associated with systemic symptoms, and may lead to severe illness and death when transmitted perinatally to an infant. Transmission occurs through close contact with a person who is shedding virus from an ulcer or genital or oral secretions.[47] Infected persons are frequently asymptomatic and unaware of being infectious, and most transmission occurs when there is no evidence of infection. Treatment of the primary infection cannot eradicate latent virus and does not prevent future recurrences or decrease overall infectiousness.[47] Daily antiviral therapy can prevent clinical recurrences and reduce viral shedding. Despite effective suppression of clinical disease, viral shedding is not eliminated. A study in progress is assessing the effect of suppressive valacyclovir treatment on sexual transmission of genital HSV infection; however, currently suppression is not yet a proven preventive therapy. Afflicted individuals should be counseled to abstain from sexual activity with uninfected partners when lesions or prodromal symptoms are present, since this is when they are most likely to be infectious. Patients and their partners, however, need to understand that sexual transmission can occur even when they are asymptomatic.[8]

Latex condoms are effective physical barriers against HSV-2.[49] Heterosexual men are less protected against transmission of HSV-2 by condoms than are women. An explanation for this sex difference is that men shed HSV-2 primarily from penile epithelial cells, and with appropriate use of condoms, these cells should be nearly completely covered. Women, however, shed HSV from a greater area, and despite correct use of condoms, a man may be exposed to the virus.[50]

Currently, preventing genital HSV-2 infections is challenging, since anyone who is sexually active with a partner who has had a previous partner is potentially at risk. Several investigators are working on developing an effective vaccine against genital HSV-2 infection. This approach has the potential of greatly decreasing the spread and possibly eliminating HSV-2 in the future.

Syphilis

The United States has made substantial progress toward the goal of eliminating syphilis from the country. Unfortunately, despite an overall decline in syphilis in the United States, an increasing incidence rate of syphilis has been reported recently in several urban areas, primarily among men who have sex with men.[51] High proportions of these men were also infected with HIV and were engaging in high-risk sexual behavior. Syphilis increases the risk of HIV transmission by threefold to fivefold.[52]

Syphilis remains a major cause of spontaneous abortion and morbidity globally. Syphilis can cause a multitude of clinical symptoms and needs to be considered in the differential diagnosis of many illnesses, despite its decreasing prevalence in the United States. Any woman who delivers a stillborn infant should be tested for syphilis.[8] Primary care providers should screen patients for syphilis who have a history of sexually transmitted illness, those who are HIV infected, and those at high risk of sexually transmitted illness.

Several studies suggest that condoms decrease the risk of acquiring or transmitting syphilis, although no rigorous assessment has been conducted. The organism responsible for syphilis, *Treponema pallidum*, is much larger than HIV and should not pass through an intact condom. Unfortunately, the bacteria are transmitted through contact with moist, infectious lesions, and condoms will not always prevent contact with infectious lesions. Syphilis is very infectious, and only a few organisms are required to transmit infection. Transmission risk is greatest during the first few months of infection.

Prevention efforts have, in the past, concentrated on identifying people with syphilis, treating them, and notifying, testing, and treating their sexual partners. The current outbreaks of syphilis in communities that share common behaviors suggest that behavioral interventions that have worked to decrease HIV transmission are likely to be effective at decreasing transmission of syphilis. Increased primary prevention efforts directed at high-risk communities are necessary to achieve the goal of eradication of syphilis from the United States.

Chlamydia

Chlamydia trachomatis is the most common sexually transmitted bacterial pathogen in the United States, with an estimated 3 million new sexually transmitted chlamydia infections annually.[53] Chlamydial infections increase the risk of a woman acquiring HIV.[53] Chlamydial infections may cause urethritis, cervicitis, pelvic inflammatory disease, ectopic pregnancy, and infertility in adults. The sequelae of chlamydial infection in women are estimated to cost $4 billion annually in the United States.[54] Most chlamydial infections in both men and women are asymptomatic.[54,55]

Risk factors for chlamydial infections include multiple sexual partners, a new sexual partner, unprotected sexual intercourse, and young age for women.[55] Latex condoms are effective physical barriers against *C trachomatis*.[49] Screening women at high risk and treating those infected have been shown to decrease pelvic inflammatory disease, ectopic pregnancy, and overall prevalence of chlamydia in targeted populations. Screening for chlamydia is much simpler since sensitive and specific polymerase chain reaction (PCR) urine-based tests have become available. The following are indications for chlamydia screening:[8,53]

- Women who present for an induced abortion
- Women admitted to a juvenile detention facility
- All sexually active women under 20 years of age
- Sexually active women aged 20 to 24 years who have more than one or a new partner in the last 3 months
- Sexually active women aged 20 to 24 who have not consistently used barrier contraceptives
- Sexually active women older than 24 who have not consistently used barrier contraceptives and have more than one or a new sexual partner in the last 3 months
- Prenatal screening at the first prenatal visit
- Testing during the third trimester for women younger than 25 and those at increased risk of infection
- Men or women with symptoms suggestive of infection
- Signs consistent with chlamydial infection during pelvic examination, including discharge, cervical erythema, and cervical friability

Screening of women who have had a recent chlamydia infection on an every-6-month basis is reasonable, because reinfection is common.[53] Screening and treating infected, asymptomatic young men is potentially a powerful preventive strategy that should be explored.[55]

Notification and treatment of infected partners is an important element of chlamydia prevention in the United States. Prevention efforts targeting high-risk populations, when sustained and aggressive, have been effective at decreasing the prevalence of chlamydia infections and clinical illness.[56]

Gonorrhea

Gonorrhea is a major cause of pelvic inflammatory disease. It can cause disseminated infection and can be transmitted to infants with resulting blindness if not treated. Most cases of gonorrhea cause symptomatic urethritis or cervicitis. Symptoms generally lead to medical evaluation and appropriate treatment shortly after acquisition of infection. However, women may have minimal symptoms or be asymptomatic.

Gonorrhea rates in the United States steadily declined from 1980 to 1997 by 74%. In 1998, the incidence of gonorrhea in the United States increased by 7.8% and has remained essentially unchanged through 2001 at 128.5 cases per 100,000 population.[57] Gonorrhea is thought to be spread in a population by a core group of effective transmitters.[58] High rates of partner change are therefore required to maintain infection in a population.

Condoms are effective physical barriers against *Neisseria gonorrhoeae*. Several studies have demonstrated a protective effect of condoms for men, but the degree of protection for women has not been well demonstrated. Behavioral interventions that were primarily used to decrease the transmission of HIV have been successful at decreasing the incidence of gonorrhea.[59] This has been well documented among men who have sex with men. Behavioral relapse in this group has been associated with an increased incidence of STDs, including gonorrhea, in the 1990s. Behavioral interventions need to be reinvigorated for continued success in this population.[59,60]

Because high rates of partner change are required to perpetuate a gonorrhea epidemic, partner notification and treatment are important and effective preventive measures. Reporting of cases also allows public health officials to concentrate preventive efforts where needed. Screening sexually active women at risk at the time of routine pelvic examinations and routine screening of pregnant women living in areas where the prevalence of *N gonorrhoeae* is high is recommended.[8] Screening outside the medical setting is now possible with PCR urine-based tests. Community-based screening of high-risk populations is feasible and may be an effective preventive measure.

Because outbreaks of gonorrhea require a rapid turnover of sexual partners to gain a foothold in a community, the incidence of gonorrhea within population subgroups can serve as a proxy for high-risk sexual behaviors. This has obvious implications for the transmission of other STDs, including HIV. Communities in which this happens are in need of culturally appropriate behavioral intervention strategies to decrease the rate of high-risk behaviors that are likely to lead to additional illness.[61]

Hepatitis B

Hepatitis B virus (HBV) infects an estimated 150,000 to 400,000 persons annually in the United States.[62] Hepatitis B is a major cause of chronic liver disease, hepatocellular carcinoma, and necrotizing vasculitis. Hepatitis B may be transmitted through intimate contact, sexual contact, exposure to blood, and from mother to child. Hepatitis B is much more efficiently transmitted through sexual contact than is HIV. Unlike HIV, in which receptive anal intercourse is the major risk factor, insertive anal intercourse is the major risk factor for HBV infection among homosexual men.[63] Only 50% of acute HBV infections are symptomatic, and many people are unaware of being infected.[8]

Sexual transmission accounts for approximately 55% of HBV infections in the United States.[8] The likelihood of sexual transmission of HBV is probably reduced with the correct use of condoms. Behavioral interventions that result in a decrease in high-risk sexual practices should be effective preventive measures for hepatitis B as well as for other STDs. A decline in hepatitis B cases among men who have sex with men was temporally associated with a decline in high-risk sexual practices in the mid-1980s.[62]

Hepatitis B is the only major sexually transmitted illness for which a safe and effective vaccine exists. Universal vaccination has already decreased the rate of infection in Taiwan and other countries.[64] Hepatitis B vaccination is now recommended for all children in the United States. Since hepatitis B is transmitted not only through sexual contact but also by other types of close contact and exposure to blood, the indications for vaccination are many. They include all newborn infants, all children and adolescents who have not been vaccinated, and adults at increased risk of infection, such as:

- Men who have sex with men
- Adults with multiple sexual partners
- Adults with a sexually transmitted illness
- Household contacts and sexual contacts of infected persons
- Injection drug users
- Health care workers
- Police officers, laboratory workers, and others with exposure to human blood

- Hemodialysis recipients
- Patients who will need multiple infusions of blood or blood products
- Prison inmates and staff
- Patients and staff of institutions for mentally disabled individuals
- Members of highly HBV-endemic populations (eg, Alaskan natives)
- Travelers to highly endemic areas with anticipated exposure to blood or sexual contact with local residents.
- Prolonged travel to highly endemic areas (>1 month)

Details regarding hepatitis B vaccination are reviewed in Chapter 50. Primary care providers should take an aggressive stance in screening and counseling patients. All patients at risk of hepatitis B need to be vaccinated.

Sexual contacts of a person with acute hepatitis B should receive postexposure immunization with hepatitis B immune globulin and the hepatitis B vaccine within 14 days of sexual contact. Simultaneous administration does not reduce effectiveness.[8]

Human Papillomavirus (HPV)

Genital HPV is the most common viral sexually transmitted illness in the United States, with an estimated 20 million people infected.[65] Strong evidence links certain types of HPV to cervical carcinoma and also suggests that HPV has a role in vaginal, vulvar, anal, and penile squamous cell cancers.[66,67]

Genital HPV is transmitted through contact with infected lesions, mucosal surfaces, or fluids of subclinical lesions. Human papillomavirus that causes genital infection can occur not only in the genital area but also on the inner thighs and around the anus. Condom use may decrease the risk of HPV infection, but this has not been proved by studies. This is not surprising, since HPV can be transmitted thorough contact with areas not covered by a condom.

Currently, prevention efforts for avoiding genital warts are limited to avoiding contact with infectious lesions. Vaccines are in development and have shown excellent protection against animal papillomavirus diseases.[68] Hopefully, human vaccines against HPV will eventually make cervical cancer an illness of the past.

SUMMARY

Primary behavioral interventions directed at high-risk groups have been successful at decreasing the rates of unprotected sex. This has resulted in a decrease in STDs and in HIV transmission in many studies. In the past, STD prevention has concentrated on diagnosis, appropriate treatment, and partner notification. These secondary prevention efforts are critical, but preventing the illness from occurring in the first place is preferable. The replication of successful primary behavioral interventions in communities at high risk of STDs, and integrating these messages into the private sector, where most individual with STDs receive treatment, will be key to decreasing the overall incidence and prevalence of STDs in the United States.

Prevention of HIV infection requires many approaches. Primary prevention, aimed at decreasing risky sexual behavior and reducing the incidence and prevalence of sexually transmitted infections, is likely to be among the most potent and cost-effective approaches for the United States and the world. Assessment of HIV risk, followed by testing when appropriate, needs to become part of routine preventive care. Clinicians who want to have an impact on the HIV epidemic can play a role with their individual patients, in the community, and even nationally by educating policy makers regarding the effectiveness and safety of HIV prevention programs.

REFERENCES

1. AIDS epidemic update—December 2002: Joint United Nations Program on HIV/AIDS (UNAIDS) and World Health Organization (WHO). Available at: www.unaids.org/worldaidsday/2002/press/ Epiupdate.html. Accessed July 9, 2003.

2. Epidemiological Fact Sheets on HIV/AIDS and Sexually Transmitted Infections— United States of America 2002 Update: UNAIDS/WHO. Available at: www.unaids.org/hivaidsinfo/statistics/ fact_sheets/pdfs/USA_en.pdf. Accessed July 9, 2003.

3. Centers for Disease Control and Prevention. HIV/AIDS Surveillance Report 2001;13 (No. 2):1–44.

4. Paxton WA, Kang S, Koup RA. The HIV type 1 coreceptor CCR5 and its role in viral transmission and disease progression. *AIDS Res Hum Retroviruses.* 1998;14 (suppl 1):S89–S92.

5. Kasten MJ. Human immunodeficiency virus: the initial physician-patient encounter. *Mayo Clin Proc.* 2002;77:957–963.

6. Centers for Disease Control and Prevention. Revised guidelines for HIV counseling, testing, and referral. *MMWR Morb Mortal Wkly Rep.* 2001;50(RR-19):1–54.

7. Koopman JS, Jacquez JA, Welch GW, et al. The role of early HIV infection in the spread of HIV through populations. *J Acquir Immune Defic Syndr.* 1997;14:249–258.

8. Centers for Disease Control and Prevention. Sexually transmitted diseases treatment guidelines: 2002. *MMWR Morb Mortal Wkly Rep.* 2002;51(RR06):1–80.

9. Centers for Disease Control and Prevention—Approval of a new rapid test for HIV antibody. *JAMA.* 2002;288:2960.

10. Daar ES, Little S, Pitt J, et al. Diagnosis of primary HIV-1 infection. *Ann Intern Med.* 2001;134:25–29.

11. Gerbert B, Maguire BT, Coates TJ. Are patients talking to their physicians about AIDS? *Am J Public Health.* 1990;80:467–468.

12. Epstein RM, Morse DS, Frankel RM, Frarey L, Anderson K, Beckman HB. Awkward moments in patient-physician communication about HIV risk. *Ann Intern Med.* 1998;128:435–442.

13. Nelson KE, Celentano DD, Eiumtrakol S, et al. Changes in sexual behavior and a decline in HIV infection among young men in Thailand. *N Engl J Med.* 1996;335:297–303.

14. Davis KR, Weller SC. The effectiveness of condoms in reducing heterosexual transmission of HIV. *Fam Plann Perspect.* 1999;31:272–279.

15. Kreiss J, Ngugi E, Holmes K, et al. Efficacy of nonoxynol 9 contraceptive sponge use in preventing heterosexual acquisition of HIV in Nairobi prostitutes. *JAMA.* 1992;268:477–482.

16. Winkelstein W, Wiley JA, Padian NS, et al. The San Francisco Men's Health Study: continued decline in HIV seroconversion rates among homosexual/bisexual men. *Am J Public Health.* 1988;78:1472–1474.

17. Johnson WD, Hedges LV, Ramirez G, et al. HIV prevention research for men who have sex with men: a systematic review and meta-analysis. *J Acquir Immune Defic Syndr.* 2002;30(Supplement 1):118–129.

18. Wang MQ, Collins CB, Kohler CL, DiClemente RJ, Wingood G. Drug use and HIV risk-related sex behaviors: a street outreach study of black adults. *South Med J.* 2000;93:186–190.

19. Youth and HIV/AIDS 2000: a new American agenda: White House Office of National AIDS Policy, October 2000. Available at: www.thebody.com/whitehouse/ youthreport/contents.html. Accessed July 9, 2003.

20. Aten MJ, Siegel DM, Enaharo M, Auinger P. Keeping middle school students abstinent: outcomes of a primary prevention intervention. *J Adolesc Health.* 2002;31:70–78.

21. Kirby D, Short L, Collins J, et al. School-based programs to reduce sexual risk behaviors: a review of effectiveness. *Public Health Rep.* 1994;109:339–360.

22. Centers for Disease Control and Prevention, National Center for HIV, STD, and TB Prevention. Young people at risk: HIV/AIDS among America's youth, 2002. Available at: www.cdc.gov/hiv/pubs/facts/youth.htm. Accessed July 9, 2003.

23. *Preventing HIV transmission: the role of sterile needles and bleach.* Washington, DC: National Academy Press; 1995.

24. Koester S. Following the blood: syringe reuse leads to blood-borne virus transmission among injection drug users. *J Acquir Immune Defic Syndr.* 1998;18(suppl 1):S139.

25. Abdala N, Stephens PC, Griffith BP, Heimer R. Survival of HIV-1 in syringes. *J Acquir Immune Defic Syndr.* 1999;20:73–80.

26. Sears C, Guydish JR, Weltzien EK, Lum PJ. Investigation of a secondary syringe exchange program for homeless young adult injection drug users in San Francisco, California, U.S.A. *J Acquir Immune Defic Syndr.* 2001;27:193–201.

27. Coyle SL, Needle RH, Normand J. Outreach-based HIV prevention for injecting drug users: a review of published outcome data. *Public Health Rep.* 1998;113(suppl 1):19–30.

28. Shalala D. Evidence-based findings on the efficacy of syringe exchange programs: an analysis from the Assistant Secretary for Health and Surgeon General of the scientific research completed since April 1998, Department of Health and Human Services. Available at: www.harmreduction.org/ issues/surgeongenrev/surgreview.html. Accessed July 9, 2003.

29. Titus S, Marmor M, Des Jarlais D, Kim M, Wolfe H, Beatrice S. Bleach use and HIV seroconversion among New

York City injection drug users. *J Acquir Immune Defic Syndr.* 1994;7:700–704.

30. *Preventing Blood-borne Infections Among Injection Drug Users: A Comprehensive Approach.* Atlanta, Ga: Academy for Educational Development, Centers for Disease Control and Prevention; 2000.

31. Epstein J, Gfroerer J. *Changes Affecting NHSDA Etimates of Treatment Need for 1994–1996.* Rockville, Md: Office of Applied Studies, Substance Abuse, and Mental Health Services Administration, US Dept of Health and Human Services; 1998.

32. Cooper ER, Charurat M, Mofenson L, Hanson C. Combination antiretroviral strategies for the treatment of pregnant HIV-1-infected women and prevention of perinatal HIV-a transmission. *J Acquir Immune Defic Syndr.* 2002;29:484–494.

33. American College of Obstetricians and Gynecologists (ACOG). ACOG committee opinion: scheduled cesarean delivery and the prevention of vertical transmission of HIV infection. *Int J Gynaecol Obstet.* 1999;66:305–306.

34. Rogers MF, Fowler MG, Lindegren ML. Centers for Disease Control and Prevention—Revised recommendations for HIV screening of pregnant women. *MMWR Morb Mortal Wkly Rep.* 2001;50(RR-19):63–85.

35. Lackritz EM, Satten GA, Aberle-Grasse J, et al. Estimated risk of transmission of the human immunodeficiency virus by screened blood in the United States. *N Engl J Med.* 1995;333:1721–1725.

36. Donegan E, Stuart M, Niland JC, et al. Infection with human immunodeficiency virus type 1 (HIV-1) among recipients of antibody-positive blood donations. *Ann Intern Med.* 1990;113:733–739.

37. Robert LM, Chamberland ME, Cleveland JL, et al. Investigations of patients of health care workers infected with HIV: the Centers for Disease Control and Prevention database. *Ann Intern Med.* 1995;122:653–657.

38. Centers for Disease Control and Prevention. Updated US Public Health Service guidelines for the management of occupational exposures of HBV, HCV, and HIV and recommendations for postexposure prophylaxis. *MMWR Morb Mortal Wkly Rep.* 2001;50(RR-11).

39. Gerberding JL, Littell C, Tarkington A, Brown A, Schecter WP. Risk of exposure of surgical personnel to patients' blood during surgery at San Francisco General Hospital. *N Engl J Med.* 1990;322:1788–1793.

40. Centers for Disease Control and Prevention. Recommendations for prevention of HIV transmission in health-care settings. *MMWR Morb Mortal Wkly Rep.* 1987;36(suppl 2).

41. Centers for Disease Control and Prevention. Evaluation of safety devices for preventing percutaneous injuries among health-care workers during phlebotomy procedures: Minneapolis-St. Paul, New York City, and San Francisco,

1993–1995. *MMWR Morb Mortal Wkly Rep.* 1997;46:21–25.

42. Cardo DM, Culver DH, Ciesielski CA, et al. A case-control study of HIV seroconversion in health care workers after percutaneous exposure. *N Engl J Med.* 1997;337:1485–1490.

43. Quinn TC, Wawer MJ, Sewankambo N, et al. Viral load and heterosexual transmission of human immunodeficiency virus type 1. *N Engl J Med.* 2000;342:921–929.

44. Holtgrave DR. Estimating the effectiveness and efficiency of US HIV prevention efforts using scenario and cost-effectiveness analysis. *AIDS.* 2002;16:2347–2348.

45. Centers for Disease Control and Prevention. HIV prevention through early detection and treatment of other sexually transmitted diseases—United States: recommendations of the Advisory Committee for HIV and STD prevention. *MMWR Morb Mortal Wkly Rep.* 1998;47(RR-12):1–24.

46. American Social Health Association for Kaiser Family Foundation. Sexually transmitted disease in America: How many cases and at what cost? 1998. Available at: www.kff.org/content/archive/1445/std_rep.html. Accessed July 9, 2003.

47. Whitley RJ, Kimberlin DW, Roizman B. Herpes simplex virus. *Clin Infect Dis.* 1998;26:541–555.

48. Fleming DT, McQuillan GM, Johnson RE, et al. Herpes simplex virus type 2 in the United States, 1976 to 1994. *N Engl J Med.* 1997;337:1105–1111.

49. Judson FN, Ehret JM, Bodin GF, Levin MJ, Riet-Meijer CA. In vitro evaluations of condoms with and without nonoxynol 9 as physical and chemical barriers against *Chlamydia trachomatis,* herpes simplex virus type 2 and human immunodeficiency virus. *Sex Transm Dis.* 1989;16:51–56.

50. Casper C, Wald A. Condom use and prevention of genital herpes acquisition. *Herpes.* 2002;9:10–14.

51. Centers for Disease Control and Prevention. Primary and secondary syphilis: United States, 2000–2001. *MMWR Morb Mortal Wkly Rep.* 2002;51:971–973.

52. Fleming DT, Wasserheit JN. From epidemiological synergy to public health policy and practice: the contribution of other sexually transmitted diseases to sexual transmission of HIV infection. *Sex Transm Dis.* 1999;75:3–17.

53. US Preventive Services Task Force—Screening for chlamydial infection: recommendations and rationale. *Am J Nursing.* 2002;102:87–92.

54. Stamm WE. *Chlamydia trachomatis* infections: progress and problems. *J Infect Dis.* 1999;179(suppl 2):S380–S383.

55. Ku L, St. Louis M, Farshy C, et al. Risk behaviors, medical care, and chlamydial infection among young men in the United States. *Am J Public Health.* 2002;92:1140–1143.

56. Addiss DG, Vaughn ML, Ludka D, Pfister J, Davis JP. Decreased prevalence of *Chlamydia trachomatis* infection associated with a selective screening program in family

planning clinics in Wisconsin. *Sex Transm Dis.* 1993;20:28–35.

57. Centers for Disease Control and Prevention. STD surveillance 2001. Available at: www.cdc.gov/std/stats/toc2001.htm. Accessed July 9, 2003.

58. Rothenberg RB. The geography of gonorrhea: empirical demonstration of core group transmission. *Am J Epidemiol.* 1983;117:688–694.

59. Centers for Disease Control and Prevention—Gonorrhea among men who have sex with men: selected sexually transmitted diseases clinics, 1993–1996. *JAMA.* 1997;278:1228–1229.

60. Centers for Disease Control and Prevention. Increases in unsafe sex and rectal gonorrhea among men who have sex with men: San Francisco, California, 1994–1997. *MMWR Morb Mortal Wkly Rep.* 1999;48:45–48.

61. Rice RJ, Roberts PL, Handsfield HH, Holmes KK. Sociodemographic distribution of gonorrhea incidence: implications for prevention and behavioral research. *Am J Public Health.* 1991;81:1252–1258.

62. Goldstein ST, Alter MJ, Williams IT, et al. Incidence and risk factors for acute hepatitis B in the United States, 1982–1998: implications for vaccination programs. *J Infect Dis.* 2002;185:713–719.

63. Kingsley LA, Rinaldo CR, Lyter DW, Valdiserri RO, Belle SH, Ho M. Sexual transmission efficiency of hepatitis B virus and human immunodeficiency virus among homosexual men. *JAMA.* 1990;264:230–234.

64. Ni Y-H, Change M-H, Huang L-M, et al. Hepatitis B virus infection in children and adolescents in a hyperendemic area: 15 years after mass hepatitis B vaccination. *Ann Intern Med.* 2001;135:796–800.

65. Cates W Jr, for American Social Health Association Panel. Estimates of the incidence and prevalence of sexually transmitted diseases in the United States. *Sex Transm Dis.* 1999;26(suppl 4):S2–S7.

66. Frisch M, Glimelius B, Van de Brule A, et al. Sexually transmitted infection as a cause of anal cancer. *N Engl J Med.* 1997;337:1350–1358.

67. Franco EL. Epidemiology of anogenital warts and cancer. *Obstet Gynecol Clin North Am.* 1996;23:597–623.

68. Hines JF, Ghim S-J, Schlegel R, Jenson AB. Prospects for a vaccine against human papillomavirus. *Obstet Gynecol.* 1995;86:860–866.

RESOURCES

UCSF Web site, which has much general information regarding HIV and is linked to other AIDS sites, is http://hivinsite.ucsf.edu.

The Web site of the Center for Disease Control and Prevention's National Center for HIV, STD and TB Prevention is www.cdc.gov/nchstp/od/nchstp.html.

chapter 52

The Immunocompromised Host

Priya Sampathkumar, MD

INTRODUCTION

Immunocompromised hosts are individuals who have 1 or more defects in the body's normal defense mechanisms that put them at increased risk of infection. Categories of immunocompromise include (1) severely immunocompromised, but no human immunodeficiency virus (HIV) infection, such as congenital immunodeficiency, hematopoietic stem cell transplantation, corticosteroid therapy, hematologic malignancy, chemotherapy, radiation, and neutropenia; (2) HIV infection; and (3) conditions with limited immune defect, such as asplenia or hyposplenia, diabetes, renal failure, and alcoholism. The number of immunocompromised individuals has increased in recent years for various reasons. The HIV epidemic has resulted in unprecedented numbers of people who have severely impaired immune function. More aggressive therapy is being administered to patients with cancer, and greater numbers of organ transplants are being performed, resulting in the emergence of specific patient populations with chronically depressed immune function. Relatively common diseases such as asthma, inflammatory bowel disease, and rheumatoid arthritis are being treated with cytotoxic medications, such as methotrexate and cyclosporine, or with anti-inflammatory monoclonal agents that are profoundly immunosuppressive.[1]

Infections contribute greatly to morbidity and mortality in immunocompromised hosts. Not only is the risk of infection greater in these individuals, but also once infection develops, it is often severe, rapidly progressive, and potentially life-threatening. In addition, microorganisms that are not usually pathogenic in the normal host may cause serious disease in the compromised patient. Depending on the specific immune defect, the infectious complications in these patients are often predictable (Table 52-1) and may be preventable.

The following interventions can prevent infections in the immunocompromised host:

- Identification and correction of risk factors in advance
- Augmentation of host defenses (eg, vaccine administration, use of immune globulin, and use of colony-stimulating factors to reduce duration of neutropenia)
- Reduction of exposure to exogenous pathogens
- Prophylaxis against specific pathogens with antimicrobials

This chapter will provide an overview of each of these interventions.

IDENTIFICATION AND CORRECTION OF RISK FACTORS IN ADVANCE

A thorough medical history and physical examination are essential to identify potential problems and apply remedial measures that may prevent serious infections. The place of birth and areas that the patient has resided in or traveled to can suggest potential latent infections such as tuberculosis and strongyloidosis. Hobbies and recreational activities such as spelunking, camping outdoors, and fishing as well as animal ownership may expose the patient to specific infections, as described later in this chapter. The patient's sexual history should be obtained, including history of prior sexually transmitted disease and alcohol or substance abuse. A meticulous systems review and physical examination should be performed. Specific attention should be given to skin integrity, oral hygiene, and presence of onychomycosis.

Any needed dental work should be carried out before administering immunosuppressive treatment. Smokers should be encouraged to quit smoking. Chronic skin conditions or infections of the nail bed should be treated as well as possible. A tuberculin skin test or tests for other

T A B L E 52-1

Defects of Natural Host Defense System and Associated Pathogens*

Component	Host Defense Defects or Conditions Predisposing to Infection	Pathogen
Anatomical barriers		

Skin	Skin diseases
	Iatrogenic factors
	   Intravascular catheters
	   Surgical wounds
	   Burns
		Staphylococci, streptococci, corynebacteria, *Pseudomonas* species, *Candida* species

Mucous membranes	Tumors
	Iatrogenic factors
	   Mucositis
	   Surgery
	   Catheters (urinary tract)
		Viridans streocci, coagulase-negative staphylococci, *Enterococcus* species, anaerobes, *Pseudomonas* species, herpes simplex virus, *Candida* species

T cells	Primary immunodeficiencies
	   Severe combined immunodeficiency
	   Adenosine deaminase deficiency
	Secondary deficiencies
	   Malnutrition
	   Chemotherapy
	   Radiation therapy
	   Immunosuppressive therapy
	      (corticosteroids, azathioprine,
	      methotrexate, cyclosporine, etc)
	   HIV infection
		Viruses: herpes simplex, varicella, cytomegalovirus
		Bacteria: *Legionella* species, *Listeria monocytogenes*, *Salmonella typhi*, *Mycobacterium tuberculosis*
		Fungi: *Candida* species, *Histoplasma, Cryptococcus, Pneumocystis carinii*
		Parasites: *Toxoplasma gondii, Cryptosporidium* species, *Leishmania*

Humoral immunity	Primary
	   X-linked agammaglobulinemia
	   Severe combined immunodeficiency
	   Selective IgA and IgG deficiency
	Secondary
	   Malignancies (CLL, multiple myeloma)
	   Nephrotic syndrome
	   Severe burns
	   Protein-losing enteropathy
	   Splenectomy
	   HSCT
		Streptococcus pneumoniae, other streptococci, *Haemophilus influenzae, Neisseria meningitidis, Capnocytophaga canimorsus*

Granulocytes	Quantitative defects: granulocytes <1000/mL
	   Chemotherapy
	   Radiation therapy
	   Myelodysplastic syndromes
	   Bone marrow infiltration
	Qualitative defects
	   Leukocyte adhesion deficiency
	   Chronic granulomatous disease
	   Chédiak-Higashi syndrome
		Viridans streptococci, *Staphylococcus aureus*, coagulase-negative staphylococci, gram-negative bacilli, *Candida* species, *Aspergillus*

Complement	Complement deficiencies
	   Classic pathway
	   Alternate pathway
	   C3
	   Terminal pathway
	Deficiencies in plasma or membrane proteins regulating complement activation
		S pneumoniae, H influenzae, N meningitidis, S aureus (C3), *Pseudomonas* species (C3)

*HIV indicates human immunodeficiency virus; IgA and IgG, immunoglobulins A and G; CLL, chronic lymphocytic leukemia; and HSCT, hematopoietic stem cell transplantation.

latent infections should be administered, if indicated by history or physical examination, and appropriate prophylaxis or treatment should be given.

AUGMENTATION OF HOST RESISTANCE

Vaccinations

The Advisory Committee on Immunization Practices divides immunocompromised patients into 3 categories:

1. Patients with HIV infection
2. Patients with severe immunosuppression not due to HIV
3. Patients with other conditions that cause limited immune deficits, such as asplenia, renal failure, diabetes, and alcoholism

In general, killed vaccines can be given to all patients. Live vaccines such as yellow fever, oral poliovirus, and measles-mumps-rubella (MMR) vaccines are contraindicated in patients in category 2 and some patients in category 1.[2] Some vaccines may not be efficacious (able to prevent infection or its complications) in patients with impaired immunity. Safety and efficacy of vaccines in immunocompromised patients are summarized in Table 52-2. Vaccine recommendations for specific immunosuppressive conditions are discussed below.

HIV infection

The risk of invasive pneumococcal disease is 50-fold to 100-fold greater in the HIV-infected population than in the general population. Therefore, all HIV-infected patients should receive the 23-valent polysaccharide pneumococcal vaccine. If the initial vaccination is given when the CD4 cell count is less than 200/mL, it should be repeated when the CD4 cell count is above 200/mL. Some experts recommend revaccination at 3- to 5-year intervals.[3] The 7-valent, protein-conjugated pneumococcal vaccine approved by the US Food and Drug Administration (FDA) in 2000 currently is recommended only in children. However, studies are ongoing in HIV-infected adults,

TABLE 52-2

Vaccine Safety and Efficacy in Immunocompromised Hosts

Vaccine	Safety	Efficacy

Toxoid vaccines
  Tetanus toxoid
  Diphtheria toxoid
Polysaccharide vaccines
  Haemophilus influenzae b
  Pneumococcus
  Meningococcus
Inactivated bacterial vaccines
  Pertussis
  Inactivated typhoid vaccine
Inactivated and subunit vaccines
  Inactivated poliovirus vaccine
  Influenza vaccine
  Hepatitis A
  Rabies
  Hepatitis B
	Safe for use in all patients	Not efficacious in patients with severely impaired humoral immunity
		
		Polysaccharide vaccines not as efficacious in asplenic patients, after HSCT, or in HIV-infected patients but should still be administered because of their potential benefit
		
		Additional or larger doses of hepatitis B vaccine may be needed to produce adequate antibody response to Hepatitis B. Periodic boosters may be necessary.

Live virus vaccines
  Oral poliovirus vaccine
  Measles
  Mumps
  Rubella
  Varicella
  Yellow fever
	Not safe for persons with severely impaired humoral or cellular immunity	Contraindicated in general.
		Varicella and yellow fever vaccines may be administered to selected patients if benefits outweigh risks.

Live bacterial vaccines
  BCG
  Typhoid (oral)
	Not safe for persons with severely impaired cellular immunity	Inactivated typhoid vaccine available for travelers. Less efficacious than live oral vaccine but safer.

since this vaccine may be more immunogenic in immuno-suppressed patients.

All susceptible patients (ie, anti–hepatitis B negative) should receive the hepatitis B series vaccine. Persons with HIV infection may have an impaired response to hepatitis B vaccine. The anti–hepatitis B surface antigen response of these patients should be tested after they are vaccinated, and those who have not responded should be revaccinated with 1 to 3 additional doses.[4] All susceptible patients at increased risk of hepatitis A infection (eg, illegal drug users, men who have sex with men, and hemophiliacs) or patients with chronic liver disease, including chronic hepatitis B or C, should receive the hepatitis A series.[5] All HIV-infected patients should receive the influenza vaccine annually, before the influenza season begins.

Severe immunosuppression not due to HIV

The classic patient with this type of immunosuppression is the recipient of a hematopoietic stem cell transplant. Hematopoietic stem cell transplantation (HSCT) is the infusion of hematopoietic stem cells from a donor into a patient who has received chemotherapy and often radiation in bone marrow ablative doses. Physicians prescribe HSCT to treat a variety of neoplastic diseases, hematologic disorders, immunodeficiency syndromes, and autoimmune disorders. Antibody titers to vaccine-preventable diseases decline during the 1 to 4 years after HSCT if the recipient is not revaccinated. Vaccine recommendations and the schedule for administration are outlined in Table 52-3.

Other conditions that cause limited immune deficits

Asplenia. Absence of the spleen or splenic function predisposes individuals to risk of overwhelming infection. These infections most often are due to encapsulated organisms, especially *Streptococcus pneumoniae*, *Haemophilus influenzae* type b, and *Neisseria meningitidis*, but any bacterial agent may cause the rapid onset of septicemia, meningitis, pneumonia, or shock characteristic of the asplenic-hyposplenic condition. The risk is greatest in infants and young children, but asplenic-hyposplenic adults also have an increased risk of infection. Splenectomy incidental to other operations, such as gastrectomy, results in the lowest risk of overwhelming infection, but it is still 35-fold greater than that in the general population. In increasing order of risk of infections, the other main indications for surgical removal of the spleen are idiopathic thrombocytopenia purpura, trauma, transplantation procedures, hereditary spherocytosis, staging Hodgkin disease, portal hypertension with hypersplenism, and thalassemia.[6]

If splenectomy is planned, pneumococcal vaccine should be administered at least 2 weeks before the surgical procedure (Table 52-4). If this is not feasible, patients should be vaccinated as soon as possible after recovery from surgery. Vaccination after splenectomy is less immunogenic, and patients should be aware that they may not be completely protected. Reimmunization of asplenic patients with the pneumococcal vaccine is recommended every 5 years. *Haemophilus influenzae* type b

TABLE 52-3

Vaccine Recommendations for HSCT Recipients*

Disease	Type of Vaccine	Schedule (months after HSCT)
Diphtheria, tetanus, pertussis		
Children <7 y	Diphtheria toxoid-tetanus toxoid-acellular pertussis vaccine (DTaP)	12, 14, 24
Age ≥7 y	Tetanus-diphtheria toxoid (Td)	12,14, 24
Haemophilus influenzae b	Polysaccharide conjugate vaccine	12, 14, 24
Streptococcus pneumoniae	23-valent polysaccharide vaccine	12, 24
Hepatitis B	Inactivated recombinant vaccine	12,14, 24
Poliomyelitis	Enhanced inactivated poliovirus vaccine	12, 14, 24
Mumps, measles, rubella	Live attenuated vaccine	≥24 mo if patient is deemed immunocompetent
Influenza	Inactivated trivalent influenza virus vaccine	Lifelong seasonal administration beginning before HSCT and resuming ≥6 mo after HSCT

*HSCT indicates hematopoietic stem cell transplantation.

and meningococcal vaccines also are recommended for asplenic adults who have not been previously vaccinated.[7-9] Patients should be educated about the potential risks of splenectomy and should be given written information to carry to alert health professionals of the risk of overwhelming infection. They should be cautioned about the potential risks of overseas travel, particularly regarding malaria and unusual infections such as those resulting from animal bites.

Diabetes.   An estimated 7% of the US adult population, or 8 million adults, have diabetes mellitus. Infections pose a serious threat to individuals with diabetes and account for up to 22% of deaths. Phagocytosis, intracellular killing of bacteria, is depressed in the neutrophils of patients with diabetes. However, these patients have normal adaptive immunity and normal responses to vaccines. Besides getting routine vaccines, diabetic persons should receive the pneumococcal vaccine and yearly influenza vaccine.

Renal failure.   Uremia has a profound immunosuppressive effect. Phagocytic activities of neutrophils and macrophages are depressed in patients with advanced renal failure.[10-12] Certain modalities of dialysis may make patients more susceptible to infections.[13,14] In addition to getting routine vaccines, patients with renal failure should receive pneumococcal and influenza vaccines. Hepatitis B vaccine also is recommended for patients whose renal disease is likely to lead to long-term hemodialysis or to renal transplantation. Such patients are at increased risk of hepatitis B because of their need for blood products and hemodialysis access. In these and other immunosuppressed patients, higher vaccine doses or increased numbers of doses are required. A special formulation of the hepatitis B vaccine is now available (Recombivax HB, 40 µg/mL). In addition, periodic boosters usually are needed after successful immunization with the timing being determined by serologic testing at 12-month intervals.[4]

Alcoholic cirrhosis   Patients with alcoholism and alcoholic liver disease have an increased incidence of infections, especially pneumonia. These patients have many defects in host defenses, including leukopenia, decreased complement activity, chemotactic defects, and impaired cell-mediated immunity. In cirrhotic patients, portosystemic shunting can diminish the clearance of bacteria and increase the severity of infection. These patients should receive a one-time pneumococcal vaccine and yearly influenza vaccine.[4]

Vaccination of household contacts.   Immunocompromised persons are at risk of acquiring infection through person-to-person transmission from household contacts and nosocomial acquisition from health care workers. Therefore, it is reasonable to consider vaccination of household contacts and health care workers against contagious and pathogenic organisms to provide an additional means of protecting immunocompromised persons from infection.

Varicella vaccine is specifically recommended for susceptible health care workers and household contacts of immunocompromised persons. Because varicella is a live-virus vaccine, transmission of vaccine virus can occur. However, the risk of transmission of vaccine virus is very low and disease caused by the vaccine virus in

TABLE 52-4

Vaccine Recommendations for Splenectomized Patients

Pathogen	Vaccine	Vaccination Strategy	Revaccination
Streptococcus pneumoniae	23-valent polysaccharide vaccine	Single dose, ideally 14 d before splenectomy. If not, give 14 d after surgery for best functional antibody response	Every 5 years
Haemophilus influenzae b	Polysaccharide-protein conjugate	2–6 mo old: 3 doses 4 weeks apart plus booster at 12 mo 7–11 mo old: 2 doses plus booster >15 mo: single dose	None recommended
Neisseria meningitidis	Quadrivalent vaccine	Single dose	May be considered 3–5 years after initial dose, especially in high-risk groups such as college students and those who plan to travel to or reside in endemic regions

immunocompromised persons is mild. Recipients of varicella vaccine on whom a rash develops should avoid direct contact with immunocompromised persons for the duration of the rash.[15]

Immunization against influenza and MMR is recommended. Although MMR is a live attenuated vaccine, persons who receive MMR vaccine or its component vaccines do not transmit measles, rubella, or mumps viruses. Thus, MMR vaccine can be administered safely to susceptible children or other persons with household contact with immunocompromised hosts to help protect these persons from exposure to wild virus.

Household contacts of persons with severely impaired humoral or cellular immunity should not receive live oral poliovirus vaccine (OPV) because of the risk of transmitting virulent poliovirus and development of vaccine-associated paralytic poliomyelitis. Instead, inactivated poliovirus vaccine should be used. If live OPV is inadvertently given to a household member, close contact should be limited for 4 to 6 weeks after vaccination, the duration of poliovirus shedding. Increased attention to good hygiene, particularly hand washing, also will reduce the risk of poliovirus transmission.

Passive Immunization

Passive immunization refers to the administration of preformed donor antibody by either the intramuscular route or intravenous route. This is indicated as postexposure prophylaxis in susceptible patients exposed to hepatitis A or B or to varicella or measles virus. Intravenous immune globulin also is indicated at regular intervals for patients with humoral deficiency syndromes and chronic lymphocytic leukemia. It also is used as prophylaxis in certain high-risk recipients of a solid organ transplant to prevent or ameliorate cytomegalovirus (CMV) and Epstein-Barr virus infections.[16,17]

Use of Colony-Stimulating Factors

Cancer chemotherapeutic regimens routinely lead to granulocytopenia and coincident risk of serious infection. Colony-stimulating factors such as granulocyte colony-stimulating factor (filgrastim, pegfilgrastim) and granulocyte-macrophage colony-stimulating factor (sargramostim) have been shown to reduce the duration and severity of neutropenia. American Society of Clinical Oncology guidelines suggest that these agents be used only in high-risk patients.[18] However, in many centers physicians routinely use these agents in patients who are expected to become neutropenic because of the benefits of reduced hospital stay and fewer days of antimicrobial therapy.[19] Treatment with filgrastim has lessened neutropenia, reduced bacterial infections, and shortened hospital stay in patients with HIV infection.

REDUCTION OF EXPOSURE TO EXOGENOUS PATHOGENS

Food and Water

Food and water are potential modes of acquisition of enteric and other infections. The immunosuppressed patient should avoid tap water and ice made from tap water, or should boil water for longer than 1 minute before consumption to reduce the risk of cryptosporidiosis. Well water should be avoided unless it is tested frequently for microbial contamination.

Fresh fruit and vegetables can be colonized with gram-negative bacteria, including *Pseudomonas aeruginosa, Escherichia coli,* and *Klebsiella* species. These organisms can cause invasive disease after ingestion. The low-bacteria diet or the cooked food diet, when combined with other modalities, may reduce the risk of these infections in neutropenic patients.[20]

The use of cold cuts has been implicated in outbreaks of listeriosis in susceptible populations. In general, immunocompromised patients should not eat raw or undercooked meat, including beef, poultry, lamb, or venison. In addition, foods that contain raw or undercooked eggs (eg, hollandaise sauce, Caesar and other salad dressings, mayonnaise, and eggnog) should be avoided because of the risk of infection with *Salmonella enteritidis.* To prevent viral gastroenteritis and exposure to *Vibrio* species and *Cryptosporidium parvum,* these patients should be advised to not consume raw or undercooked seafood, such as oysters or clams.[21,22]

Plants and Fresh Flowers

Plants and fresh cut flowers have multiple resistant bacteria as part of their normal flora and shed these into vase water. It has been shown that colony counts of these organisms in vase water rise with time.[23] Fresh flowers should be completely avoided by severely immunocompromised patients, such as stem cell transplant recipients. For less severely immunosuppressed individuals, the handling of flowers and vase water should be done with great care.

Potted plants can harbor pathogenic fungi, including *Aspergillus, Fusarium,* and *Scedosporium* species.[24] *Aspergillus terreus* has been implicated in at least one outbreak of hospital-acquired fungal infection in patients undergoing myeloablative therapy.[25] Hence, it is recommended that plants not be allowed in the hospital rooms of severely immunosuppressed patients and also be avoided at home.

Hand Washing and Related Issues

Hand hygiene

Hand hygiene is the single most effective procedure for preventing nosocomial infection. All persons, especially health care workers, should wash their hands before and after any interaction with a patient. Immunocompromised patients must be encouraged to practice good hand hygiene—washing hands before eating, after using the toilet, and before and after touching a wound. Hands should be washed with antimicrobial soap and water or an alcohol-based hand rub.[26]

Artificial nails

The use of artificial nails has become a popular fashion trend, and many health care workers are following this trend. There is debate whether artificial nails are putting patients at risk of nosocomial infections. Research has shown that the colony counts on artificial nails are greater than the colony counts on natural nails. Artificial nails also have been linked to poor hand washing practices and more tears in disposable gloves.[27,28] These factors lead to an increased risk of transmitting bacteria to patients. The use of artificial nails by health care workers caring for immunocompromised patients should be discouraged.[26,29]

Animal Exposure

Pet therapy is increasingly being recognized as being of psychologic benefit to hospitalized patients, and many institutions now have well-established pet therapy programs.[30] However, pets pose potential infection control hazards because of the number of microorganisms that they can transmit to humans (Table 52-5).[31]

Patients who have undergone a splenectomy are at high risk of overwhelming, fatal infection with *Capnocytophaga canimorsus*, a gram-negative bacterium present in dog and cat saliva. Turtles, lizards, and snakes harbor *Salmonella* organisms. Dogs can be asymptomatic excreters of *Leptospira* in urine; mice and hamsters can excrete lymphocytic choriomeningitis virus. Careful hand washing after contact with body fluids of these animals is important. Immunocompromised hosts should be advised to not clean animal litter boxes or dispose of animal waste. Gloves should be worn when handling items contaminated with bird droppings, as these can be a source of *Cryptococcus neoformans, Mycobacterium avium,* or *Histoplasma capsulatum.* To minimize potential exposure to *Mycobacterium marinum,* immunocompromised individuals should not clean fish tanks and, if they must handle a fish tank, should wear gloves and wash hands thoroughly afterward.

Physicians should advise patients of the potential infection risks posed by pet ownership. Immunocompromised patients who choose to own pets should be more vigilant regarding maintenance of their pets' health than are immunocompetent pet owners. All pets should be housebroken, up to date on their immunizations, and pronounced disease-free by a veterinarian.

Visitation

Visitors to hospitalized, immunocompromised individuals should be screened for active infections and instructed in the importance of proper infection control. Children under the age of 12 years can transmit infection unknowingly; hence, they should have only controlled, limited access. Children should be screened for exposure in the previous 4 weeks to chickenpox, rubella, mumps, hepatitis A, streptococcal throat infection, whooping cough, viral upper respiratory tract infection, diarrhea, and live-virus immunization with oral poliovirus vaccine. Patients should wash hands carefully after contact with pediatric visitors. Visitors with respiratory or diarrheal illnesses should be discouraged from visiting the patient.

Construction and Renovation

Ongoing hospital construction and renovation have been associated with an increased risk of nosocomial fungal infections, especially aspergillosis, among severely immunocompromised patients. Patients with prolonged

T A B L E 52-5

Animals and Associated Pathogens That Can Be Transmitted to Humans

Animal	Pathogen
Dogs	Rabies, *Pasteurella multocida, Brucella canis, Capnocytophaga canimorsus, Campylobacter jejuni, Toxocara canis, Giardia lamblia, Cryptosporidium parvum*
Cats	Rabies, *P multocida, Toxocara cati, G lamblia, C parvum, Toxoplasma gondii*
Rabbits	*P multocida, Francisella tularensis, Yersinia pestis,* dermatophytes
Rats and mice	*Hantavirus,* lymphocytic choriomeningitis virus, *Streptobacillus moniliformis, Leptospira species*
Turtles	*Salmonella species, Aeromonas species*
Fish	*Mycobacterium marinum, Streptococcus iniae, Erysipelothrix rhusiopathiae,* fish tapeworm
Birds	*Chlamydiae psittaci, Cryptococcus neoformans, Histoplasma capsulatum*
Reptiles	*Salmonella species*

neutropenia are those at highest risk of invasive aspergillosis.[32] Whenever possible, immunocompromised patients should avoid construction and renovation areas. Hospital planners should ensure that rooms for neutropenic patients have the ability to minimize fungal spore counts using:

1. High-efficiency particulate air (HEPA) filtration
2. Directed airflow rooms (positive air pressure in patient rooms so that air from patient rooms flows into corridor)
3. High rates of air exchange (ie, >12 exchanges per hour)
4. Barriers (eg, sealed plastic) between patient care areas and renovation or construction sites that prevent dust from entering patient care areas and reduce exposure to aspergillus spores[33-35]

With the trend toward early dismissal from the hospital, patients often leave the hospital while still neutropenic. They must be reminded about avoiding activities at home that may result in exposure to dust and molds and advised to use a mask if such activity is inevitable.

SPECIFIC ANTIMICROBIAL PROPHYLAXIS

In addition to the general precautions described above, specific antimicrobial prophylaxis targeted against pathogens most likely to cause disease in certain types of immunocompromised patients may be indicated. One such group where clear guidelines exist is the HIV-infected population. Individuals infected with HIV have varying levels of immunity that depend on CD4 counts. The current recommendations regarding primary prophylaxis with antimicrobials against opportunistic pathogens in HIV-infected patients are summarized in Table 52-6. The use of antimicrobial prophylaxis in other settings is discussed below.

TABLE 52-6

Antimicrobial Prophylaxis to Prevent First Episode of Opportunistic Infection Among HIV-Infected Adults*

Pathogen	Indication	First-choice Preventive Regimen	Alternative Choice
Pneumocystis carinii	CD4 <200/μL or oropharyngeal candidiasis	TMP-SMZ, 1 DS or SS po daily	Dapsone, 50 mg po twice daily or 100 mg once daily; aerosolized pentamidine, 300 mg/mo or atovaquone, 1500 mg/d po
Toxoplasma gondii	Immunoglobulin G antibody to Toxoplasma and CD4 <100/μL	TMP-SMZ, 1 DS po daily	TMP-SMZ, 1 SS po daily; dapsone, 50 mg/d po or 200 mg/wk po, plus pyrimethamine, 50 mg/wk po, plus leucovorin calcium, 25 mg/wk po; atovaquone, 1500 mg/d po with or without pyrimethamine, 25 mg/d po, plus leucovorin, 10 mg/d po
Mycobacterium avium-intracellulare	CD4 <50/μL	Azithromycin dihydrate, 1200 mg/wk po, or clarithromycin, 500 mg po twice daily	Rifabutin, 300 mg/d po; azithromycin, 1200 mg/d po, plus rifabutin, 300 mg/d po
Mycobacterium tuberculosis Isoniazid-sensitive	Tuberculin skin test reaction ≥5 mm or prior positive test without treatment or contact with person with active tuberculosis, regardless of skin test result	Isoniazid, 300 mg po, plus pyridoxine hydrochloride, 50 mg/d po for 9 mo; or isoniazid, 900 mg, plus pyridoxine, 100 mg po twice weekly for 9 mo	Rifampin, 600 mg, or rifabutin, 300 mg/d po for 4 mo; or pyrazinamide, 15–20 mg/kg of body weight po daily for 2 mo with either rifampin, 600 mg/d, or rifabutin, 300 mg/d for 2 mo
Mycobacterium tuberculosis Isoniazid-resistant	Same as above; increased probability of exposure to isoniazid-resistant tuberculosis	Rifampin, 600 mg/d, or rifabutin, 300 mg/d for 4 mo	Pyrazinamide, 15–20 mg/kg body weight po daily for 2 mo with either rifampin, 600 mg, or rifabutin, 300 mg daily for 2 mo

*HIV indicates human immunodeficiency virus; TMP-SMZ, trimethoprim-sulfamethoxazole; SS, single strength; DS, double strength; and po, orally. Data from 2001 guidelines of US Public Health Service and Infectious Diseases Society of America.

Antibacterials

Penicillin

Patients who are hyposplenic or asplenic may benefit from prophylaxis with oral antibiotics. The usual regimen is penicillin V potassium, 500 mg, or amoxicillin, 500 mg once daily. This may not be appropriate in areas of the world where there are high rates of penicillin resistance in pneumococci, which are the main organisms being targeted. Most authorities recommend antibiotic prophylaxis for asplenic or hyposplenic children for the first 2 years after splenectomy. Some investigators advocate continuing chemoprophylaxis in children for at least 5 years or until the age of 21 years.[36] The value of such an approach in older children or adults has not been adequately evaluated in a clinical trial; compliance is frequently a problem. Another shortcoming of antibiotic prophylaxis is the inevitable selection for colonization with nonsusceptible pathogens.

Because cases of overwhelming postsplenectomy sepsis involving pneumococcal infection have been reported in patients who have received both penicillin prophylaxis and vaccination, the use of prophylactic measures should never be allowed to engender a false sense of security.

Trimethoprim-sulfamethoxazole

Persons receiving long-term treatment with corticosteroids in doses of more than 15 mg/d of prednisone are at risk of *Pneumocystis* infection and should receive prophylaxis with trimethoprim-sulfamethoxazole or an alternative agent. (See Table 52-6 for alternatives.[37]) Studies of prophylaxis with trimethoprim-sulfamethoxazole in neutropenic patients have shown decreased rates of infection but no impact on infection-related mortality. In some studies, the duration of neutropenia was prolonged and there was an increased rate of fungal colonization in patients receiving prophylactic trimethoprim-sulfamethoxazole.[38] For these reasons, along with the availability of alternative drugs, this agent is no longer routinely used as a prophylactic agent in neutropenic patients.

Oral fluoroquinolones

Fluoroquinolones have several features that make them attractive as prophylactic agents in patients with neutropenia. They are well absorbed orally and are ineffective against anaerobes, thus helping to preserve normal gut flora and reducing the risk of colonization with nosocomial pathogens. A meta-analysis of studies that used fluoroquinolones in cancer-affected patients with neutropenia concluded that fluoroquinolones alone were effective in preventing gram-negative bacteremia but not gram-positive bacteremia, fever-related morbidity, and infection-related mortality.[39] Since then, several newer

quinolones with enhanced activity against gram-positive organisms have been introduced and are being studied in neutropenic patients.[40,41] Emergence of antibiotic-resistant organisms, including methicillin-resistant *Staphylococcus aureus* and more virulent viridans streptococci, is a concern in patients receiving prolonged quinolone prophylaxis. Therefore, current guidelines from the Infectious Diseases Society of America (IDSA) recommend that quinolone use be reserved for patients with profound and prolonged neutropenia that outweighs the risk of resistant organisms.[42]

Antifungal Prophylaxis

During the last decade, with better control of opportunistic infections such as CMV infection, invasive fungal disease has emerged as an important cause of death in HSCT recipients. Fluconazole prophylaxis has been shown to reduce the incidence of both mucosal and systemic yeast infections when administered to HSCT recipients from the time of transplant to engraftment.[43,44] However, opportunistic infections due to fungi other than *Candida* are being increasingly reported in patients receiving systemic antifungal prophylaxis with fluconazole.[45] Despite this, current guidelines from the IDSA, Centers for Disease Control and Prevention (CDC), and American Society of Blood and Marrow Transplantation recommend the use of fluconazole prophylaxis from the day of HSCT until engraftment.[46] Studies are under way to assess whether newer antifungal drugs such as itraconazole and voriconazole can be used for prophylaxis, particularly because they have additional activity against aspergilli and other molds. Prophylactic antifungal therapy is not recommended routinely in other immunosuppressed patients.

Antivirals

Influenza

The CDC recommends antiviral chemoprophylaxis against influenza in persons at risk of complications under certain circumstances. They are as follows: (1) persons who were vaccinated after influenza activity began, because the development of antibodies can take as long as 2 weeks; (2) outbreaks caused by variant strains of influenza that are not covered by the vaccine; (3) patients whose immunodeficiency causes them to have an inadequate response to influenza vaccine; and (4) patients in whom influenza vaccine is contraindicated, including persons with anaphylactic hypersensitivity to egg proteins or other vaccine components.

Options available for chemoprophylaxis are M2 protein channel inhibitors—amantadine hydrochloride and rimantadine hydrochloride—or a neuraminidase inhibitor such as oseltamivir phosphate (Tamiflu) or zanamivir

(Relenza). Neuraminidase inhibitors have the advantage of efficacy against both influenza A and B. Only oseltamivir is currently FDA approved for prophylaxis. Prophylaxis should be continued for 10 days after exposure. When an antiviral agent is used in conjunction with the vaccine, prophylaxis should be continued for 2 weeks after administration of the vaccine.

Herpes simplex virus (HSV)

Acyclovir prophylaxis should be routinely offered to all HSV-seropositive allogeneic HSCT recipients in the early post-transplant period. The standard approach is to begin acyclovir prophylaxis at the start of the conditioning therapy and to continue it until engraftment occurs or until mucositis resolves, whichever is longer. Continued acyclovir prophylaxis can be considered for patients with frequent, recurrent HSV infections.[46] In other immunosuppressed patients, antiviral medications are indicated only if there is evidence of HSV disease.

CMV

Various regimens of antivirals are used for prophylaxis against CMV infections in recipients of a solid organ transplant, HSCT recipients, and HIV-infected patients. New oral drugs, including ganciclovir and valganciclovir hydrochloride, that are well absorbed after oral administration have made prophylactic regimens easier. However, emergence of ganciclovir-resistant strains of CMV have been reported in both HIV-infected patients and transplant recipients receiving long-term prophylaxis with these drugs.[47]

SUMMARY

Immunocompromised hosts vary greatly in the type and degree of immunocompromise. Mechanisms of immunocompromise include alterations in skin and mucosal barriers, normal oral and intestinal flora, splenic function, and number or function of T cells, B cells, granulocytes, and monocytes. To prevent adverse outcomes in the immunocompromised host, the practitioner must find ways of maintaining those defenses, minimizing the environmental risks to the patient, anticipating potential infections in order to institute appropriate prophylactic measures, and diagnosing and aggressively treating infections as they occur.

REFERENCES

1. Lee JH, Slifman NR, Gershon SK, et al. Life-threatening histoplasmosis complicating immunotherapy with tumor necrosis factor alpha antagonists infliximab and etanercept. *Arthritis Rheum.* 2002;46:2565–2570.

2. Atkinson WL, Pickering LK, Schwart B, Weniger BA, Islander SK, Watson JC. General recommendations on immunization: recommendations of the Advisory Committee on Immunization Practices (ACIP) and the American Academy of Family Physicians (AAFP). *MMWR Morb Mortal Wkly Rep.* 2002;51(RR-2):1–35.

3. Kovacs JA, Masur H. Prophylaxis against opportunistic infections in patients with human immunodeficiency virus infection. *N Engl J Med.* 2000;342:1416–1429.

4. Advisory Committee on Immunization Practices (ACIP). ACIP issues recommendations for vaccines and immune globulins in immunocompromised persons. *Am Fam Physician.* 1993;48:337–340.

5. Prevention of hepatitis A through active or passive immunization: recommendations of the Advisory Committee on Immunization Practices (ACIP). *MMWR Morb Mortal Wkly Rep.* 1996;45(RR-15):1–30. Erratum appears in *MMWR Morb Mortal Wkly Rep.* 1997;46(25):588.

6. Hansen K, Singer DB. Asplenic-hyposplenic overwhelming sepsis: postsplenectomy sepsis revisited. *Pediatr Dev Pathol.* 2001;4:105–121.

7. Davies JM, Barnes R, Milligan D. Update of guidelines for the prevention and treatment of infection in patients with an absent or dysfunctional spleen. *Clin Med.* 2002;2:440–443.

8. Prevention of pneumococcal disease: recommendations of the Advisory Committee on Immunization Practices (ACIP). *MMWR Morb Mortal Wkly Rep.* 1997;46 (RR-8):1–24.

9. Control and prevention of meningococcal disease: recommendations of the Advisory Committee on Immunization Practices (ACIP). *MMWR Morb Mortal Wkly Rep.* 1997;46(RR-5):1–10.

10. Cohen G, Haag-Weber M, Horl WH. Immune dysfunction in uremia. *Kidney Int.* 1997;62(suppl):S79–S82.

11. Saeki A, Kaito K, Kobayashi M. Impaired neutrophil function in chronic renal failure: dysregulation of surface adhesion molecule expression and phagocytosis. *Nippon Jinzo Gakkai Shi.* 1996;38:585–594.

12. Haag-Weber M, Horl WH. Dysfunction of polymorphonuclear leukocytes in uremia. *Semin Nephrol.* 1996;16:192–201.

13. Schiffl H, Lang SM, Haider M. Bioincompatibility of dialyzer membranes may have a negative impact on outcome of acute renal failure, independent of the dose of dialysis delivered: a retrospective multicenter analysis. *ASAIO J.* 1998;44:M418–M422.

14. Schiffl H, et al. Bioincompatible membranes place patients with acute renal failure at increased risk of infection [comment]. *ASAIO J.* 1995;41:M709–M712.

15. Prevention of varicella: update recommendations of the Advisory Committee on Immunization Practices (ACIP). *MMWR Morb Mortal Wkly Rep.* 1999;48(RR-6):1–5.

16. Lories RJ, et al. The use of polyclonal intravenous immunoglobulins in the prevention and treatment of infectious diseases. *Acta Clin Belg.* 2000;55:163–169.

17. Fischer GW. Uses of intravenous globulin to prevent or treat infections. *Adv Pediatr Infect Dis.* 1992;7:85–108.

18. American Society of Clinical Oncology. Update of recommendations for the use of hematopoietic colony-stimulating factors: evidence-based clinical practice guidelines [comment]. *J Clin Oncol.* 1996;14:1957–1960.

19. Bennett CL, et al, for the Health Services Research Committee of the American Society of Clinical Oncology. Use of hematopoietic colony-stimulating factors: the American Society of Clinical Oncology survey. *J Clin Oncol.* 1996;14:2511–2520.

20. Todd J, et al. The low-bacteria diet for immunocompromised patients: reasonable prudence or clinical superstition? *Cancer Pract.* 1999;7:205–207.

21. Martin G, Wright AM, Banakarim K. A case of fatal food-borne septicemia: can family physicians provide prevention? *J Am Board Fam Pract.* 2000;13:197–200.

22. Gholami P, Lew SQ, Klontz KC. Raw shellfish consumption among renal disease patients: a risk factor for severe *Vibrio vulnificus* infection. *Am J Prev Med.* 1998;15:243–245.

23. Kates SG, et al. Indigenous multiresistant bacteria from flowers in hospital and nonhospital environments. *Am J Infect Control.* 1991;19:156–161.

24. Summerbell RC, Krajden S, Kane J. Potted plants in hospitals as reservoirs of pathogenic fungi. *Mycopathologia.* 1989;106:3–22.

25. Lass-Florl C, et al. *Aspergillus terreus* infections in haematological malignancies: molecular epidemiology suggests association with in-hospital plants. *J Hosp Infect.* 2000;46:31–35.

26. Boyce JM, et al. Guidelines for hand hygiene in health-care settings: recommendations of the Healthcare Infection Control Practices Advisory Committee and the HICPAC/SHEA/APIC/IDSA Hand Hygiene Task Force [Society for Healthcare Epidemiology of America/Association for Professionals in Infection Control/Infectious Diseases Society of America]. *MMWR Morb Mortal Wkly Rep.* 2002;51(RR-16):1–45.

27. McNeil SA, et al. Effect of hand cleansing with antimicrobial soap or alcohol-based gel on microbial colonization of artificial fingernails worn by health care workers. *Clin Infect Dis.* 2001;32:367–372.

28. Hedderwick SA, et al. Pathogenic organisms associated with artificial fingernails worn by healthcare workers. *Infect Control Hosp Epidemiol.* 2000;21:505–509.

29. Toles A. Artificial nails: are they putting patients at risk? A review of the research. *J Pediatr Oncol Nurs.* 2002;19:164–171.

30. Brodie SJ, Biley FC, Shewring M. An exploration of the potential risks associated with using pet therapy in healthcare settings. *J Clin Nurs.* 2002;11:444–456.

31. Plaut M, Zimmerman EM, Goldstein RA. Health hazards to humans associated with domestic pets. *Annu Rev Pub Health.* 1996;17:221–245.

32. Oren I, et al. Invasive pulmonary aspergillosis in neutropenic patients during hospital construction: before and after chemoprophylaxis and institution of HEPA filters. *Am J Hematol.* 2001;66:257–262.

33. O'Dea TJ. Protecting the immunocompromised patient: the role of the hospital clinical engineer. *J Clin Eng.* 1996;21:466–482.

34. Perry P. Dust busters protect patients during construction. *Materials Manage Health Care.* 1997;6:20.

35. Loo VG, et al. Control of construction-associated nosocomial aspergillosis in an antiquated hematology unit. *Infect Control Hosp Epidemiol.* 1996;17:360–364.

36. Waghorn DJ. Overwhelming infection in asplenic patients: current best practice preventive measures are not being followed. *J Clin Pathol.* 2001;54:214–218.

37. Russian DA, Levine SJ. *Pneumocystis carinii* pneumonia in patients without HIV infection. *Am J Med Sci.* 2001;321:56–65.

38. Hughes WT, et al. Successful intermittent chemoprophylaxis for *Pneumocystis carinii* pneumonitis. *N Engl J Med.* 1987;316:1627–1632.

39. Cruciani M, et al. Prophylaxis with fluoroquinolones for bacterial infections in neutropenic patients: a meta-analysis [comment]. *Clin Infect Dis.* 1996;23:795–805.

40. Maertens J, Boogaerts MA. Anti-infective strategies in neutropenic patients. *Acta Clin Belg.* 1998;53:168–177.

41. Kerr KG, Armitage HT, McWhinney PH. Activity of quinolones against viridans group streptococci isolated from blood cultures of patients with haematological malignancy. *Supportive Care Cancer.* 1999;7:28–30.

42. Hughes WT, et al. 2002 guidelines for the use of antimicrobial agents in neutropenic patients with cancer [comment]. *Clin Infect Dis.* 2002;34:730–751.

43. Wakerly L, et al. Fluconazole versus oral polyenes in the prophylaxis of immunocompromised patients: a cost-minimization analysis. *J Hosp Infect.* 1996;33:35–48.

44. Klastersky J. Prevention and therapy of fungal infections in cancer patients: a review of recently published information [comment]. *Supportive Care Cancer.* 1995;3:393–401.

45. Oliveira JS, et al. Fungal infections in marrow transplant recipients under antifungal prophylaxis with fluconazole. *Braz J Med Biol Res.* 2002;35:789–798.

46. Centers for Disease Control and Prevention. Guidelines for preventing opportunistic infections among hematopoietic stem cell transplant recipients. *MMWR Morb Mortal Wkly Rep.* 2000;49(RR-10):1–125.

47. Ljungman P. Prophylaxis against herpesvirus infections in transplant recipients. *Drugs.* 2001;61:187–196.

chapter 53

Preventing Common Infections

Robert Orenstein, DO

INTRODUCTION

One of the great breakthroughs of the 20th century has been the ability to prevent and control many infectious diseases via improved public health and sanitation, personal preventive measures, widespread use of vaccines, and antimicrobial agents. Near the end of the 20th century, it appeared that humans had nearly conquered all the common infectious diseases. However, the convergence of the worldwide pandemic of human immunodeficiency virus (HIV) infection, the reemergence of tuberculosis, the spread of multiresistant bacteria, and the potential use of biological weapons such as anthrax and smallpox have tempered that hubris. In some respects, we have relied on technologic breakthroughs, vaccines, and antimicrobial agents to outwit infectious agents, with little regard for the role of personal health behaviors. The epidemics of HIV, sexually transmitted diseases (STDs), hepatitis C, and antimicrobial resistance illustrate the need for greater individual responsibility to prevent common infections.

What, then, might be the role of the primary care physician in establishing these behaviors? First, we need to ask patients the appropriate questions; second, we should use the office visit to counsel patients on ways to reduce risk behaviors. This may be accomplished by making the patient-physician relationship a partnership in which the patient assumes greater responsibility. This personal empowerment and its impact are reflected by the increasing use of alternative therapies to treat common health problems. Physicians need to use primary care visits as an opportunity to deliver preventive services. Examples of such interactions include offering influenza prophylaxis to family members to halt a household and community outbreak or discussing safe sex with adolescents. The purpose of this chapter is to focus on infections commonly seen in a primary care practice and to illustrate measures shown to be effective for primary or secondary prevention. Each section will address the burden of disease and then discuss preventive measures. Previous chapters have addressed the prevention of HIV and STDs as well as general aspects of immunization and infections in travelers. Therefore, this chapter will focus on the common community-acquired infections seen in the office and hospital, which may be preventable.

Common preventable infections include the following:

- Upper respiratory tract infections (URIs), such as common colds, streptococcal pharyngitis, acute sinusitis, otitis media (OM), and influenza
- Lower respiratory tract infections (LRIs), such as pneumonia and tuberculosis
- Urinary tract infections (UTIs)
- Herpetic eye infections
- Enteric and diarrheal diseases
- Skin and soft-tissue infections (SSTIs)
- Zoonoses
- Ulcer disease and *Helicobacter pylori*
- Coronary disease and Chlamydia
- Endocarditis and prosthetic infections
- Health care–associated infections

Infectious diseases account for 19% of all physician encounters and 129 million annual ambulatory care visits in the United States.[1] The top 4 categories of infectious diseases in the National Ambulatory Medical Care Survey—URI, OM and otitis externa (OE), LRI, and SSTI—accounted for 77% of all visits for care of infectious disease. Of these, URIs account for 38%, followed by OM and LRIs.[1] Most of these visits are for children below 4 years of age and for patients aged 65 to 84 years. In adults, URIs, UTIs, SSTIs, and enteric infections are frequent reasons for office visits.

RESPIRATORY TRACT INFECTIONS

Upper respiratory tract infections are an important target for preventive measures in the primary care setting (Table 53-1) since they account for 37 million physician office and emergency care visits.[2] They are the second leading condition for which antibiotics are prescribed, often inappropriately, and account for 10% of all outpatient antibiotic prescriptions.[3] Most URIs resolve spontaneously after 1 or 2 weeks. Of those affected, around 2% develop bacterial rhinosinusitis, and preventive antibiotic therapy does not alter this.[4] Thus, the patient who requests antibiotics to prevent his cold from becoming a sinus infection should be counseled as such. A systematic review of studies that looked at the use of antibiotics to treat adults, children, and college students with URI or the common cold showed there to be no benefit for this practice.[5] Unfortunately, physicians and patients both rely on the purulence of nasal or sputum secretions to determine whether antibiotics are appropriate. However, this indicator fails to predict a bacterial cause or, when it's treated with antibiotics, it does not alter outcomes.[6,7]

The Common Cold

The most common respiratory tract infection seen by physicians is the common cold. This syndrome, caused by a variety of viruses, including rhinoviruses, coronavirus, parainfluenza, influenza, respiratory syncytial virus, and adenoviruses, accounts for substantial morbidity and lost workdays and is a leading cause of widespread antibiotic misuse.[8] Numerous studies have looked at anti-infectives, immune stimulation, and other measures to treat or prevent the common cold; however, few have proved effective.[8-10] Antibiotics are often prescribed for the common cold under the pretenses that it will prevent progression into a more serious illness, that it will shorten the disease duration, and that it is difficult to discern mycoplasma or chlamydial infections, which may be antibiotic responsive. A Cochrane review of 9 trials of antibiotics for URI lasting less than 7 days, which involved more than 2000 patients, found that persons who received antibiotics did no better than those who received placebo but did experience an increased number of adverse events.[5]

Because no approved medications exist for treatment of the common cold, sufferers have sought a variety of alternative and nonconventional therapies. Most data supporting these treatments are anecdotal and shrouded in superstition. A few of the therapies reported to be effective are chicken soup, zinc lozenges, vitamin C, vitamin E, echinacea, and exercise. Recently, several of these have been more rigorously evaluated. Trials of prevention found that echinacea had minimal impact on the incidence of colds.[8] A recent randomized placebo-controlled trial of echinacea for the treatment of common cold in a group of college students found no demonstrable benefit in duration or symptom severity.[8]

Another agent believed to prevent or decrease the severity and duration of colds is zinc.[10] This is based on the premise that zinc inhibits rhinovirus replication in vitro. However, in vivo studies have not demonstrated this effect, and clinical trials of oral and intranasal zinc gluconate have failed to prevent or decrease the severity of experimental rhinovirus colds.[11] Despite encouraging results from some clinical trials of zinc lozenges, overall, the data do not support the use of zinc to treat or prevent colds. Others have suggested that antioxidant vitamins might be beneficial. Studies have shown that almost 50% of elderly persons use dietary supplements, such as a multivitamin or vitamin E, to ward off a variety of ailments.[12] A recent placebo-controlled study of multivitamins and vitamin E in noninstitutionalized adults over age 60 years to prevent respiratory tract infections found no decrease in the incidence of URI.[12] In fact, those who took vitamin E and acquired a URI experienced an increased severity and duration of symptoms.

Sinusitis

Acute sinusitis is one of the 10 most common diagnoses in ambulatory care, accounting for 25 million visits.[1] It is the fifth most common reason for antibiotic prescription, and 97% of those who see a physician because of this diagnosis receive antibiotics despite the fact that sinusitis develops in less than 5% of people with rhinovirus colds.[13,14] Because of the difficulty distinguishing viral and bacterial rhinosinusitis, antibiotics should be reserved for those persons with greater than 1 week of symptoms, maxillary pain or facial tenderness, and purulent nasal secretions.[14] (Mucus produced in the sinuses normally wicks away germs and debris. With inflammation, the drainage slows.) The common predisposing factors for rhinosinusitis are as follows:

- Viral respiratory tract infection
- Allergic rhinitis
- Anatomical obstruction of the ostia
- Environmental pollutants
- Pregnancy
- Immune compromise
- Ciliary function defects

TABLE **53-1**

Preventive Practices

Preventive Practice	Examples
Personal protective measures	Hand washing; gloves, masks, eyewear; condoms; repellants
Public health measures	Safer needles, sanitation, vector control, education
Immunization	Vaccines, immunoglobulin
Antimicrobials	Antibiotic prophylaxis, preemptive therapy

The 3 major precipitating causes are allergies, structural abnormalities, and environmental irritants, especially tobacco. Management of each of these may help prevent acute bacterial sinusitis. Simple preventive measures include avoiding cigarette smoke, dust, and pollutant exposure; maintaining household humidity between 45% and 65% in the winter; and avoiding alcohol, which can cause rebound nasal vasodilation. Other helpful measures include avoidance of antihistamines, which dry and thicken mucus; use of decongestants to help improve nasal congestive symptoms; and use of a plain saline nasal spray several times daily to loosen mucus and remove bacteria. Another preventive measure is to avoid the predisposing viral illness such as influenza through appropriate vaccination and chemoprophylaxis.

Sore Throat

Sore throat is another common complaint in primary care practice, accounting for 1% to 2% of all outpatient visits.[1,2] The diagnosis of acute pharyngitis precipitates an antibiotic prescription in up to 75% of adults even though less than 5% to 15% of cases in adults are due to β-hemolytic group A streptococci (GAS).[15] So, how does one differentiate these illnesses to provide the best prevention and treatment? The most reliable clinical criteria are the presence of tonsillar exudates, tender anterior cervical adenopathy, the absence of cough, and a history of fever.[15] The sensitivity and specificity of the presence of either 3 or 4 of these criteria are 75%.[15] The use of rapid antigen screening for GAS improves the specificity.

Bronchitis

Acute bronchitis also ranks among the top 10 reasons for office visits. This illness, most often due to a viral infection, in which cough and phlegm are predominant, accounted for almost 10 million visits in 1997.[16] The most important viral pathogen is influenza, which causes 50 million infections annually in the United States resulting in 24 million patient visits, 300,000 hospitalizations, and between 20,000 and 50,000 deaths.[17] Important host factors for the control of influenza are hydration to maintain loose secretions; fever, which may inhibit viral replication; and rest, which decreases the risk of aspirating virus from the upper respiratory tract. For centuries, mothers have advocated the use of chicken soup to improve symptoms of respiratory illness. Recent studies show there to be some truth to this, in that chicken soup may inhibit neutrophil chemotaxis.[18] Treatment of influenza within 48 hours of onset may shorten the duration of symptoms by 1 to 2 days. A strategy for early detection and treatment of influenza may help prevent epidemic spread and limit antimicrobial use.[19] In a study of winter Olympic athletes with flulike symptoms, 2 rapid diagnostic tests were done. If the result of either test was positive, therapy with oseltamivir phosphate was initiated. This both reduced inappropriate antibiotic use and prevented secondary influenza cases.[19]

INFLUENZA

Influenza affects 10% to 20% of the US population annually and accounts for up to 20,000 deaths per year in those at highest risk. Vaccination, which is underused, is highly effective at reducing the risk of acquiring influenza and decreasing its morbidity, loss of productivity, and mortality.[20-22] Although rates of influenza illness are greatest in children, the morbidity of influenza is greatest in those above 65 years of age.[23] Of even greater concern are institutionalized elderly individuals, for whom influenza attack rates may range from 5% to 20% and more than 70% during an epidemic.[23] Compared with the 70% to 90% of young, healthy adults who develop protective antibody titers, only about half of institutionalized elderly persons develop influenza titers, which are protective. Thus, the goal in high-risk institutionalized elderly patients is to develop herd immunity via broad vaccination and to promptly initiate chemoprophylaxis in case of an outbreak.

For unvaccinated or vaccine nonresponders, other strategies are needed. Two classes of agents are effective for the prophylaxis of influenza: neuraminidase inhibitors and M2 channel inhibitors. The M2 channel inhibitors are effective only against strains of influenza A, whereas the newer, neuraminidase inhibitors protect against both A and B strains. Amantadine hydrochloride, rimantadine hydrochloride, oseltamivir, and zanamivir are equally effective as prophylaxis in healthy adults, with a relative risk reduction of almost two thirds compared with placebo.[24,25] However, there are few data on the use of these agents in the well elderly population.

With regard to household outbreaks of influenza, children commonly introduce influenza into the home and cause family outbreaks. Preventing household spread may be an effective way to control community outbreaks. The M2 inhibitors amantadine and rimantadine have been effective at limiting household spread but are associated with the development of M2 inhibitor-resistant isolates, poor tolerance, and lack of activity against B strains. In a randomized, placebo-controlled, double-blinded, multicenter study, inhaled zanamivir, 10 mg/d for 10 days, given to other family members after identification of a suspected household case provided a protective efficacy of 81%.[26] This agent was not used in children under age 5 years, which may have lessened the impact. The frequency of adverse effects with zanamivir was lower than that reported in trials of oseltamivir and M2 inhibitors.[27,28] In household outbreaks, oseltamivir phosphate given at 75 mg/d orally for 7 days provided a protective efficacy between 84% and 89% if given within 48 hours of onset of symptoms.[29] This strategy of early institution of influenza prophylaxis to limit spread might also be applied in the workplace when a suspected case is identified.

Upper and lower respiratory tract infections are common complications of influenza illness.[30] The alterations in nasal patency and eustachian tube function caused by influenza may predispose to bacterial sinusitis and OM.[31] Thus, early detection and treatment of influenza might reduce the incidence of these complications and the need for antibiotics. A study of inhaled zanamivir for acute influenza illness in healthy adults demonstrated a 31% reduction in the need for antibiotics for lower respiratory tract complications.[31] The choice of specific agent, zanamivir or oseltamivir, depends on its respective tolerance and ease of administration. Oseltamivir may be associated with gastrointestinal intolerance unless the patient takes it on a full stomach. Zanamivir may be difficult for patients with bronchospasm. In older adults with respiratory disease and visual or cognitive difficulties, the oral agent oseltamivir may be more easily administered.

OTITIS MEDIA

Otitis media is diagnosed more than 5 million times annually and is the most common reason for antibiotic use in children.[1,2] Concurrent with the widespread use of antibiotics for treatment of OM, a large increase in the antimicrobial-resistant flora of young children has emerged. There is controversy over the optimal approach to management of OM in children and the use of antibiotics. Otitis media predictably follows a viral infection of the upper respiratory tract, which causes eustachian tube dysfunction. Thus, the opportunity to prevent OM lies in the prevention of either the preceding URI or eustachian tube dysfunction. Acute OM imposes a substantial burden on preschool children, their parents, and the health care system. The widespread use of antibiotics for the treatment of acute OM has been the driving force for the emergence of antibiotic-resistant *Streptococcus pneumoniae*. There may be several opportunities to reduce this burden via pneumococcal vaccine and seasonal immunization against influenza. Children in day care who received influenza vaccine had a 33% to 36% reduction in cases of OM during the influenza season.[32] Similarly, early treatment with oseltamivir of children with influenza reduced the incidence of OM by 40% during the influenza season.[33]

The ability of the pneumococcal vaccine to prevent the complication of acute OM has also been evaluated. In trials of children below age 2 years, the 7-valent pneumococcal conjugate vaccine (PNCRM7) had a 56% efficacy

rate against vaccine serotypes but only 6% overall due to increases in infection from nonvaccine strains.[34-36] Immunization with PNCRM7 could decrease the overall risk of acute OM episodes by up to 6%, office visits by up to 9%, and the risk of recurrent acute OM and tympanostomy tube placement by up to 22%.[36] Furthermore, vaccination decreased the risk of pneumococcal acute OM caused by vaccine serotype-specific and serogroup-specific isolates by more than 50%, which are also the serotypes most frequently associated with antibiotic resistance. The clustering of resistance among vaccine-specific serogroups, in combination with the association between pneumococcal antibiotic resistance and persistent and/or recurrent acute OM, explains the greater efficacy of vaccination in preventing frequently recurrent acute OM compared with acute OM overall. This vaccine-related reduction in recurrent acute OM may also be responsible for the 20% reduction in tympanostomy tube insertion among vaccine recipients.

The pneumococcal conjugate vaccine may have the additional benefit of herd immunity. A study found a 58% reduction in invasive pneumococcal disease among all ages, including a 58% decline in people 20 to 39 years old, suggesting that immunization of children might also be protective for parents.[36] The 7 serotypes in the vaccine cover 80% to 90% of invasive strains in children, and many others are cross-reactive.

Recurrent OM is another common infection that may be preventable. Proposed measures include chemoprophylaxis vs influenza, use of inactivated parenteral influenza vaccine, environmental controls, and placement of tympanostomy tubes. Another approach to prevention of recurrent OM is to attempt to eradicate the nasopharyngeal carriage of organisms that cause acute OM, as failure to eradicate these organisms may lead to recurrent infections and development of resistance.

New approaches to the prevention of acute OM include nasal vaccines and immunotherapy. An intranasal virosomal influenza vaccine reduced the number of episodes of acute OM by 44% and reduced antibiotic use by 39% during a 6-month follow-up.[37] This intranasal vaccine reduced the persistence of middle ear effusion and was most effective in children 2 to 5 years old. Another investigational approach to acute OM prevention is the use of immunotherapy with bacterial ribosomes such as the biologic response modifier Immucytal, which is a ribosomal extract of 4 common bacteria. Bacterial ribosomes may enhance immune responses against the common pathogens that cause acute OM.[38]

STREPTOCOCCAL PHARYNGITIS

Acute pharyngitis is one of the most common illnesses seen by practicing physicians. Although GAS represent the most important bacterial cause of acute pharyngitis, these bacteria account for only a small percentage of cases of pharyngitis; GAS are the only indication for prescribing antibiotics for treatment of pharyngitis.[39] Group A streptococci are uncommon in adults, causing pharyngitis in only 5% to 10% of adults compared with 15% to 30% of pharyngitis in children.[39] Thus, it is important to exclude acute GAS pharyngitis with rapid antigen testing. Group A streptococci may be important to consider in parents or teachers of school-aged children. Other less common but important causes of pharyngitis are diphtheria and STDs. Because the clinical manifestations of GAS pharyngitis overlap with nonbacterial causes, empirical therapy is a leading cause of excessive antimicrobial use for viral respiratory tract infections.

Treatment

The primary reasons to treat GAS pharyngitis are to prevent the suppurative complications of GAS, prevent rheumatic fever, reduce clinical symptoms, and decrease potential infectivity to others. Rheumatic fever may be prevented even if therapy is delayed up to 9 days after onset of symptoms.[40]

The standard regimens for GAS pharyngitis are 10 days of oral penicillin, erythromycin, or cephalosporin or a single dose of intramuscular (IM) benzathine penicillin G. Treatment is highly effective at preventing the suppurative and nonsuppurative complications. Except under the special circumstances noted in the next paragraph, patients who have been successfully treated for GAS pharyngitis should not undergo repeated cultures or antigen testing at the completion of therapy. In the small percentage of patients with a clinical relapse, if poor adherence is suspected, another course of therapy may be indicated with the initial agent or with benzathine penicillin. In those with recurrent episodes, it may be difficult to establish whether these are viral and the person is a GAS carrier or has symptomatic GAS pharyngitis. In these cases, an attempt at eradication with amoxicillin-clavulanate potassium or clindamycin may be reasonable. Intramuscular benzathine penicillin has been shown to reduce cases of rheumatic fever in epidemics among military recruits.[41] Usually 48 hours of therapy greatly diminishes the risk of infectivity. Approximately 25% of asymptomatic persons in the household of each index patient harbor GAS in their respiratory tract.

The indications for follow-up throat cultures after treatment of GAS pharyngitis are:

- Patients with a personal history of rheumatic fever
- Patients with acute pharyngitis during an outbreak of rheumatic fever or poststreptococcal glomerulonephritis
- Outbreaks of pharyngitis in closed communities
- Recurrent familial spread of GAS pharyngitis

In these circumstances, cultures should be obtained from household contacts, and those who test positive for GAS should be treated.

Streptococcal carriers generally do not require treatment. In those requiring therapy, either amoxicillin (40 mg/kg/d) for 10 days with 4 days of rifampin (15 mg/kg/d) or cefpodoxime proxetil (10 mg/kg/d) for 10 days was equally efficacious: 83% at eradicating carriage.[42] Up to 20% of asymptomatic school-aged children may harbor GAS during the winter and early spring. During this time, they may have multiple bouts of pharyngitis and may be colonized for months. These carriers are unlikely to spread the disease to close contacts, and eradication is more difficult.[39]

For those with multiple documented episodes of symptomatic disease, tonsillectomy may be considered.[39] Children who undergo tonsillectomy have lower rates of recurrent pharyngitis. However, there is no significant change in the number of moderate or severe episodes of pharyngitis, and there is an 8% risk of intraoperative or postoperative complications.[43] Performance of adenoidectomy along with tonsillectomy appears to offer no additional benefit over tonsillectomy alone.[43] Guidelines from the American Academy of Otolaryngology—Head and Neck Surgery for the year 2000 suggest surgery for children with 3 or more episodes of tonsillitis per year despite adequate medical therapy, but this recommendation may need revision.

Invasive GAS Disease

News reports of invasive GAS disease and "flesh-eating bacteria" have struck fear into many communities despite the low incidence of these strains. In the United States, 8800 cases and 1000 deaths due to invasive GAS occurred in 2000.[44] The case fatality rate was 12% to 13% overall and 30% to 80% among persons with toxic shock syndrome. Those experiencing the greatest morbidity are elderly individuals.

Risk factors for sporadic invasive GAS are as follows:

- Age greater than 65 years
- HIV infection
- Diabetes
- Chickenpox
- Cancer
- Heart disease
- Use of injection drugs
- Corticosteroid use
- Native American

Two prospective studies evaluated the risk of subsequent GAS cases of household contacts of persons with invasive GAS and found only 5 confirmed cases.[44] On the basis of these data, it has been estimated that if chemoprophylaxis were offered to 12,000 to 22,000 household contacts annually and it was 100% effective, only 8 to 64 cases of invasive disease would be prevented.[44] Because of this low risk and the untoward effects of providing antibiotics to large numbers of contacts, antibiotic prophylaxis is recommended only to those at the highest risk of invasive disease. No controlled studies of prophylaxis in preventing invasive GAS disease among household contacts exist. However, data extrapolated from studies of pharyngeal eradication of GAS carriers suggest that therapy with benzathine penicillin G, penicillin G plus rifampin, oral clindamycin, or azithromycin might be effective (Table 53-2).[44]

The Centers for Disease Control and Prevention (CDC) recommendation is to inform all household contacts about the manifestations of invasive GAS (fever, sore throat, and myalgia) and to seek immediate medical attention. Household contacts should be monitored for 30 days after diagnosis of the index case. Because of the increased morbidity in those older than 65 years, prophylaxis could be offered to the entire household in which they reside. Routine cultures for GAS are not indicated because asymptomatic carriage may occur and may be unrelated to the source of the outbreak.

COMMUNITY-ACQUIRED PNEUMONIA

Approximately 4 million cases of community-acquired pneumonia occur annually in the United States, resulting in 1 million hospitalizations.[45,46] It is the fifth leading cause of death in persons over 65 years of age. Pneumococcal pneumonia accounts for 150,000 to 570,000 cases

T A B L E 53-2

Chemoprophylaxis of Invasive Group A Streptococcal Infection in Household Contacts

Drug	Dosage
Benzathine penicillin G	600,000 U intramusculariy if <27 kg; 1.2 million units if ≥27 kg
plus rifampin	20 mg/kg/d in 2 divided doses for 4 days (maximum, 600 mg/d)
or clindamycin	20 mg/kg/d orally (maximum daily dosage, 900 mg) in 3 divided doses for 10 d
or azithromycin	12 mg/kg/d orally (maximum daily dosage, 500 mg/d) single dose for 5 d

per year, with an estimated mortality rate of 12% to 39%.[45,46] Over the past decade, a number of studies and guidelines have been developed to enhance the quality and costs of care associated with this common complication.[45,46] Annual influenza vaccination and pneumococcal vaccination are effective at reducing this burden of disease. These vaccines are covered in Chapters 50 and 59.

PREVENTION OF LATENT TUBERCULOSIS

Although not considered a common infection in the United States, tuberculosis remains one of the leading causes of infectious morbidity worldwide. Because some clinicians may practice in regions with large immigrant populations and other high-risk groups, it is important to understand how the spread of tuberculosis is prevented in the United States. The frequently used terms *preventive therapy* and *chemoprophylaxis* for tuberculosis mean the treatment of latent tuberculosis infection (LTBI). Recent CDC guidelines for LTBI have focused on targeted tuberculin skin testing of those at highest risk and, hence, those who should be treated if they test positive for tuberculosis.[47] High-risk adults who have received BCG vaccination and have a positive result of a purified protein derivative (PPD) skin test should receive therapy for LTBI. The recommended skin test cutoffs and treatment regimens for LTBI are found in Tables 53-3 and 53-4.[47]

URINARY TRACT INFECTIONS

Urinary tract infections account for more than 7 million annual office visits, over 1 million emergency room visits, and 100,000 hospitalizations at a cost of more than $1 billion per year.[48] Catheter-associated UTIs account for 40% of all nosocomial infections. Thus, UTIs are an increasing source of morbidity for older men and women. Several strategies have been developed to prevent recurrent infections in younger women as well as postmenopausal women. In sexually active women, postcoital antimicrobial prophylaxis 3 times weekly or daily is both safe and effective.[49] Recent studies have also shown that motivated women with recurrent UTIs may effectively initiate their own antimicrobial therapy after self-diagnosis of an uncomplicated UTI.[50] In postmenopausal women, topical estrogen therapy may reduce the frequency of recurrent UTIs.[51] A vaginal ring that releases estradiol locally (Estring) led to a 25% reduction in UTIs in a group of postmenopausal women.[52]

Prevention in the geriatric population poses a particular challenge since UTIs are second only to respiratory infections in the healthy elderly population, accounting for 24% of all infections.[53] This high frequency of UTIs in elderly individuals may be related to bladder dysfunction

T A B L E 53-3

Criteria for Positive PPD Skin Test Result by Risk Group and Millimeters of Induration*

	Induration	
>5 mm	**>10 mm**	**>15 mm**
HIV positive	Immigrant 5 y from high-prevalence area	Persons with *no* risk factors for TB
Recent contact of TB case	Injectable drug users	
Fibrotic changes on CXR consistent with prior TB	Residents and employees of high-risk institutions (eg, prisons, health care, homeless)	
Organ transplant recipients	Patients with silicosis; diabetes; renal failure; leukemia; lymphoma; cancers of head, neck, and lung; weight loss of >10%; after gastrectomy or jejunoileal bypass; children <4 y; children exposed to high-risk adults	
Patients receiving >15 mg/d prednisone >1 mo		

*PPD indicates purified protein derivative; HIV, human immunodeficiency virus; TB, tuberculosis; and CXR, chest X-ray. Adapted from American Thoracic Society.[47]

and incontinence. Asymptomatic bacteriuria is common, affecting 50% and 35% of elderly women and men, respectively.[53] Urinary tract infections arise from perineal colonization with fecal bacteria, followed by adherence and induction of an inflammatory reaction.

Preventive strategies that interfere with this pathway include the use of probiotics, lactobacillus vaginal suppositories, and oral cranberry juice.[54,55] In a study of Finnish university students, [a lactobacillus GG drink 5 days per week was compared with] 300 mL/d (50 mL of concentrate) of cranberry-lingonberry juice for 6 months. The cranberry drink reduced recurrent *Escherichia coli* UTIs by a relative risk reduction of 56%.[56] This particular product is no longer available, although other evidence supports the use of cranberry juice for prevention. Cranberry juice works by preventing adherence of P-fimbriated *E coli* bacteria to the urothelial cells.[57,58] This may then cause selection of less adherent strains. Fifty-eight berries of the *Vaccinium* species produce proanthocyanidins, which are believed to be the agents that inhibit adherence. Cranberry juice tablets, 300 to 400 mg twice daily, or 224 to 448 g (8 to 16 oz) of at least 30% juice is needed to achieve these results.

Up to 60% of women experience a UTI. Recurrent UTIs occur in one third of women affected, especially those aged 25 to 29 years and those over 55 years.[59] Women with 3 or more symptomatic UTIs may be candidates for antibiotic prophylaxis using low doses for long-term secondary prevention following treatment. Both continuous use of daily antibiotics for 6 months and postcoital antibiotic therapy have been effective. Effective

T A B L E 53-4

Treatment of Latent Tuberculosis Infection in Adults*

Drug	Interval and Duration	Comment
Isoniazid	300 mg/d for 9 mo or	Preferred regimen
	900 mg twice weekly for 9 mo via directly observed therapy	Alternate regimen
Rifampin	600 mg/d for 4 mo	Alternate regimen
Rifampin plus pyrazinamide	Daily for 2 mo	Limited by hepatotoxicity

*Adapted from American Thoracic Society.[47]

antibiotics include nitrofurantoin (50 mg/d), daily or thrice weekly trimethoprim-sulfamethoxazole, 100 mg daily of trimethoprim, and oral fluoroquinolones. Other potential candidates for antibiotic prophylaxis include pregnant women with bacteriuria, men with chronic prostatitis, and men before and after prostatectomy.

Asymptomatic bacteriuria (ASB) is a common target for prophylactic antibiotics. The overall prevalence of ASB is estimated at 3.5%, but some groups have an increased frequency: elderly persons, those with a history of UTI, and pregnant or diabetic women.[60] Until recently, it had been suggested that diabetic women with asymptomatic bacteriuria were at high risk of UTI complications and should be treated. However, a prospective, randomized trial in 2002 showed a reduction in ASB among those treated but no difference in symptomatic UTI or time to first symptomatic UTI.[61] Thus, there appears to be no benefit in screening asymptomatic diabetic women for ASB. New preventive strategies in development include vaccines to immunize those at highest risk. One such vaccine is directed at the E coli type 1 fimbriated adhesin and its chaperone protein.[62]

Even some of the common strategies for UTI prevention have come under scrutiny. Aggressive oral hydration is often recommended to "flush out" the bladder. A 1999 study actually found that increased water intake may dilute Tamm-Horsfall glycoprotein (which acts as an antibacterial) and thus may increase the risk of infection.[63] Other commonly used therapies for UTI prevention include the use of methenamine hippurate. However, a recent study found limited support for its use.[64] Other suggested measures that lack strong evidence include washing the perineal area before sex, urinating before intercourse, avoiding the use of a diaphragm with spermicides, and wiping from front to back after urinating or defecating.[65]

HERPES INFECTIONS

Infections due to herpes viruses affect 60% to 90% of the world's population.[66] Thirty million people are infected with herpes simplex 2 (HSV-2), most of whom are asymptomatic. Symptomatic herpes infections are most often characterized by recurrent oral-labial or genital ulcers or, in the case of varicella-zoster, shingles in adults and chickenpox in children. Antiviral prophylaxis with acyclovir is effective at reducing recurrence rates of genital and orofacial lesions in healthy and immunosuppressed persons. Varicella vaccine may be another effective measure to prevent primary infection.

In the United States, herpes simplex infection of the eye is the most common cause of corneal blindness.[67] The use of antivirals such as acyclovir, famciclovir, and valacyclovir have been shown to prevent recurrent disease and blindness.[67] In Rochester, Minn, the incidence of herpetic eye disease was 8.4 per 100,000 person-years.[68] Fifty percent of these individuals had recurrences over 5 years. Oral acyclovir at a dose of 400 mg twice daily reduced the recurrence rate by 45% over 12 months.[67] The results of this study suggest that patients with recurrent disease and stromal keratitis are good candidates for oral acyclovir therapy, whereas those with epithelial keratitis may be managed with topical agents. The risk of stromal keratitis in this study was strongly related to the number of previous episodes of stromal involvement. This may be important in that recent animal studies show that photoradial keratotomy (PRK) treatment may reactivate herpetic disease, and this can be prevented with valacyclovir.[69]

INFECTIOUS DIARRHEA

Infectious diarrhea is a common problem, causing 1 or 2 episodes per person annually on average. Children younger than 3 years old and those in day care are at greatest risk, with a seasonal peak in winter. Infectious diarrheal diseases are the second leading cause of global morbidity and in the United States result in 28 million office visits, 45 million telephone consultations, 1.8 million hospitalizations, 19 million prescriptions for antimicrobial agents, and 3100 deaths each year.[70] The globalization of our food supply and ease of world travel have led to an increasing spectrum of diarrheal disease. Some of these diarrheal pathogens may cause substantial long-term morbidity such as hemolytic uremic syndrome (HUS) after enterohemorrhagic E coli 0157-H7 (EHEC) infection, Guillain-Barré syndrome after Campylobacter jejuni infection, aortitis after Salmonella infection, and listeriosis in pregnant women and immunosuppressed hosts.

Preventive measures for these pathogens focus on avoidance of undercooked food (burgers, fish, and poultry: Salmonella, Campylobacter, and EHEC), avoidance of unpasteurized dairy products (milk and cheese: listeriosis), and thorough hand washing. Other preventive strategies include safe swimming (pool sanitation and infants wearing clean diapers: EHEC) and appropriate counseling of travelers (Norwalk outbreak, vaccines against typhoid). The enteric pathogens—EHEC, Salmonella, Shigella, C jejuni, Clostridium difficile, Giardia, Cyclospora, caliciviruses, and others—account for more than 200 million cases of diarrhea per year in the United States. Many of these are foodborne or waterborne or are spread from person to person. In the health care environment, C difficile reigns as the most common cause of infectious diarrhea. This is preventable by prudent use of antimicrobial agents, routine hand washing, disinfection of potentially contaminated objects, isolation of infected patients, and use of contact precautions.

Antibiotics may be indicated in specific circumstances to prevent the spread of infectious diarrheal agents. Examples include the early treatment of persons with Campylobacter infection with erythromycin to reduce shedding.[71] In children less than 6 months of age or when there is a major risk of spread of Salmonella infection, treatment should be offered. The EHEC infections should not be treated with antibiotics or motility agents as these may increase the risk of complications such as HUS.

Most of the common diarrheal diseases are best prevented by good personal hygiene and safe food preparation. The kitchen and home bathroom are reservoirs for potential diarrheal pathogens. Studies show that Enterobacteriaceae counts are highest in mops, used sponges, cleaning cloths, cutting boards, and sinks. The dishcloth used to wipe up is a frequent source for disseminating these bacteria. Hand washing with soap and water is the most important measure for preventing diarrhea in the normal host. However, plain soap and water may not be particularly effective for cleaning inanimate surfaces. In immunosuppressed persons, a variety of other measures may be important. These include water filtration to prevent cryptosporidiosis in HIV-affected patients as well as avoidance of shellfish in patients with chronic liver disease to prevent *Vibrio* infections, unpasteurized milk and soft cheeses to prevent brucellosis and listeriosis, and uncooked meats to prevent toxoplasmosis and EHEC.

Prevention of foodborne and waterborne disease includes the following strategies:

- Avoid undercooked meats, poultry, or seafood
- Avoid soft cheeses and unpasteurized dairy products
- Avoid raw eggs
- Wash or peel fruits
- Boil water longer than 1 minute when there is a community outbreak
- Wash hands after handling animals and waste products
- Avoid drinking from streams or lakes

Travelers should:

- Drink only bottled water or carbonated or hot beverages
- Avoid ice cubes
- Eat only fruit that they peel themselves
- Avoid eating fresh, raw vegetables and salads
- Eat no food obtained from street vendors

PROPHYLAXIS FOR SPLENECTOMY

Approximately 25,000 splenectomies are performed annually.[72] Physicians who see patients after splenectomy or other patients with functional asplenia need to be aware of applicable preventive measures. The risk of sepsis after splenectomy is estimated to be more than 50 times that of the general population. The spleen primarily functions to prevent infection with encapsulated bacteria. Infections with *Streptococcus pneumoniae, Haemophilus influenzae,* and *Neisseria meningitidis* account for 25% of infections in asplenic patients. The overall incidence of postsplenectomy sepsis is approximately 2% in adults and 5% to 9% in children, with mortality rates approaching 50% to 80%.[72] The younger the patient at the time of splenectomy, the greater the risk. Vaccination against these organisms is recommended and preferably is given more than 2 weeks before elective splenectomy. There are limited data on the conjugate *H influenzae* or the new conjugate 7-valent pneumococcal vaccine, although they are recommended before splenectomy. Older children and adults should receive the 23-valent pneumococcal vaccine at 5-year intervals.

Asplenic persons should carry identification that they are asplenic and should have antibiotics available in the event they cannot reach medical attention promptly. Individuals with temperatures above 38.9°C should seek immediate medical attention. These patients should have blood cultures drawn and begin immediate therapy. Two measures shown to reduce mortality in these patients are the pneumococcal vaccine and immediate antibiotic prophylaxis with penicillins. Amoxicillin, 250 to 500 mg daily, is recommended for children under age 5 years for up to 3 years.[72] In adults, antibiotic prophylaxis is not indicated unless patients have experienced recurrent episodes despite vaccination.

RECURRENT CELLULITIS

Recurrent cellulitis most often occurs in association with chronic venous or lymphatic obstruction. Risk factors include use of injection drugs, venous ulcerations, chronic venous stasis after vein graft harvest, lymphedema, and chronic skin conditions. Preventive measures involve treating the underlying or predisposing factors. Persons with multiple episodes of cellulitis after lymphedema may benefit from the use of prophylactic antibiotics. Recurrent erysipelas may be associated with chronic venous or lymphatic diseases of an extremity. Persons with a first episode have a 10% annual recurrence rate and episodes tend to be stereotypical. In cases of multiple relapses, oral penicillin prophylaxis, 250 mg/d for 1 week per month, or benzathine penicillin G, 1.2 million U IM monthly for 3 to 6 months, may be effective.[73] If recurrences happen after this regimen is discontinued, long-term prophylaxis may be considered.

ANTIBIOTIC PROPHYLAXIS AND PROSTHETIC DEVICES

As our population ages and technology improves, the number of persons with prostheses continues to escalate. Infections of these devices are associated with substantial morbidity, and hence preventive approaches have been proposed. The predisposing factors for these infections include dental, urinary tract, and skin infections. In certain circumstances, perioperative or periprocedural antibiotics may reduce this risk. Approximately 500,000 prosthetic joint arthroplasties are performed annually in the United States.[74] The periods of greatest risk of infection are the perioperative period and for the first 2 years after implantation. There is no evidence that antibiotic prophylaxis before dental procedures prevents hematogenous seeding of the prosthesis, yet this is a common practice. The American Academy of Orthopaedic Surgery and the American Dental Association recently drafted a consensus statement regarding the appropriate use of antibiotics in patients at risk.[74]

Patients at risk of hematogenous prosthetic joint infection include the following:

- Those with inflammatory arthropathies, such as rheumatoid arthritis and lupus erythematosus
- Patients with disease-, drug-, or radiation-induced immunosuppression
- Individuals with type 1 diabetes
- Anyone who has had joint replacement in the previous 2 years
- Patients with prior prosthetic joint infection
- Malnourished persons
- Hemophiliac patients

BITES

From arthropods to snakes, bites occupy a major portion of primary care practice. Mammalian bites account for 1% of ER visits, with bites from cats and dogs being the most frequent.[75] There are 57 million pet cats who inhabit one third of US households and cause 400,000 bites per year.[75] Cat bites commonly lead to infection, especially when there is skin penetration. Prophylaxis of dog and cat bites is controversial since only 5% to 20% of dog bites and 50% of cat bites become infected.[76] Although there is no definitive evidence to support postbite prophylaxis, most authorities recommend antibiotics. The antibiotic of choice for these bite wound infections is amoxicillin-clavulanate potassium, 500 mg 3 times a day or 875 mg twice daily for 3 to 5 days. Prophylactic antibiotics have been shown to reduce infections in human bites.[76]

Prevention of rabies, tetanus, and bacterial infection is an important consideration. Bites from wild animals such as raccoons, skunks, bats, coyotes, and other carnivores should be considered for rabies prophylaxis, whereas those due to squirrels, chipmunks, and rodents are rarely rabid. Rabies prophylaxis after exposure consists of passive receipt of rabies immune globulin—half at the site of the bite and half IM in the buttock (20 IU/kg total) and administration of the human diploid rabies vaccine.

Candidates for antibiotic prophylaxis of bite wounds include the following settings:

- Moderate to severe injury less than 8 hours old
- Bone or joint penetration
- Wounds of the face, hands, genitals, or periprosthesis
- Immunosuppressed hosts
- Cat bites
- Human bites

Bites of venomous and nonvenomous snakes do not require prophylaxis.[77,78] Arthropods are common vectors of human diseases from malaria to Lyme disease. Common infections include tickborne diseases such as Lyme disease, ehrlichiosis, Rocky Mountain spotted fever, and babesiosis and the mosquitoborne diseases such as dengue, malaria, and arboviral encephalitides. Mosquitoes alone transmit diseases to more than 700 million people annually. In the United States, periodic epidemics of mosquitoborne arbovirus infections, such as West Nile, Eastern equine, St Louis, and La Crosse encephalitides, create major health concerns. Public health measures to reduce mosquitoborne and tickborne exposures include the use of insecticides or reducing the deer population to control tick density. The optimal ways to prevent these diseases are by avoidance of infested habitats, wearing light-colored clothing that allows easier indication of the arthropod, daily inspection of skin after outdoor exposure and prompt removal of ticks, and use of insect repellants containing diethyltoluamide (deet) and permethrin.[79] In some circumstances, prophylactic antimicrobials are beneficial, such as for malaria, and in others, such as Lyme disease, far more controversial. Lyme disease is the most common arthropodborne zoonosis in the United States. A vaccine was available from 1998 to 2001 for preventing Lyme disease but was removed by the manufacturer due to lack of demand. This has led to consideration of alternate prophylactic strategies in those at highest risk. Even in Lyme-endemic areas, the incidence of infection after a deer tick bite is 1% to 4%. Thus, the efficacy of antibiotic prophylaxis has been difficult to prove. It has been estimated that 83 patients would need to be treated with antibiotics to prevent 1 case of Lyme disease.[80] However, a recent CDC study found that a single 200-mg dose of doxycycline given to persons who had removed a partially engorged *Ixodes* tick within the past 72 hours had an efficacy of 87% in preventing Lyme disease.[81]

SUMMARY

Despite the resurgence of infectious diseases during the past decade, many of these may be prevented by simple infection control measures and appropriate and selective use of antimicrobial prophylaxis. This chapter has reviewed some of the common infections seen in a primary care setting and some key strategies that may be effective for prevention.

REFERENCES

1. Armstrong GL, Pinner RW. Outpatient visits for infectious disease in the United States, 1980 through 1996. *Arch Intern Med.* 1999;459:2531–2536.

2. Schappert SM. Ambulatory care visits to physicians offices, hospital outpatient departments: United States, 1997. *Vital and Health Statistics.* Series 13, No. 143. Hyattsville, Md: National Center for Health Statistics, US Dept of Health and Human Services; 1999. DHS publication 2000–1714.

3. McCaig LF, Hughes JM. Trends in antimicrobial drug prescribing among office-based physicians in the United States. *JAMA.* 1995;273:214–219.

4. Hickner JM, Bartlett JG, Besser RE, Gonzales R, Hoffman JR, Sande MA. Principles of appropriate antibiotic use for acute rhinosinusitis in adults: background. *Ann Emerg Med.* 2001;37:703–710.

5. Arroll B, Kenealy T. Antibiotics for the common cold. *Cochrane Database Syst Rev.* 2000;CD000247.

6. Stott B, West RR. Randomized controlled trial of antibiotics in patients with cough and purulent sputum. *Br Med J.* 1976;2:556–559.

7. Verheij TJ, Hermans J, Mulder JD. Effects of doxycycline in patients with acute cough and purulent sputum: a double-blind placebo controlled trial. *Br J Gen Pract.* 1994;44:400–404.

8. Barrett BP, Brown RL, Locken K, Maberry R, Bobula JA, D'Alessio D. Treatment of the common cold with unrefined echinacea: a randomized double-blind placebo-controlled trial. *Ann Intern Med.* 2002;137:939–946.

9. Melchart D, Linde K, Fischer P, Kaesmayr J. Echinacea for preventing and treating the common cold. *Cochrane Database Syst Rev.* 2000;CD000530.

10. Marshall I. Zinc for the common cold. *Cochrane Database Syst Rev.* 2000;CD001364.

11. Turner RB. Ineffectiveness of intranasal zinc gluconate for prevention of experimental rhinovirus colds. *Clin Infect Dis.* 2001;33:1865–1873.

12. Graat JM, Schouten EG, Kok FJ. Effect of vitamin E and multivitamin supplementation on acute respiratory tract infections in elderly persons. *JAMA.* 2002;288:715–721.

13. Ambulatory care visits to physicians offices, hospital outpatient departments and emergency departments: United States, 1996. *Vital and Health Statistics.* Series 13, No. 134, Hyattsville, Md: National Center for Health Statistics, US Dept of Health and Human Services; 1998.

14. Antimicrobial treatment guidelines for acute bacterial rhinosinusitis: sinus and allergy health partnership. *Otolaryngol Head Neck Surg.* 2000;123:5–31.

15. Cooper RJ, Hoffman JT, Bartlett JG, et al. Principles of appropriate antibiotic use for acute pharyngitis in adults: background. *Ann Emerg Med.* 2001;37:711–719.

16. Gonzales R, Bartlett JG, Besser RE, et al. Principles of appropriate antibiotic use for the treatment of uncomplicated acute bronchitis: background. *Ann Emerg Med.* 2001;37:720–727.

17. Centers for Disease Control and Prevention. Prevention and control of influenza: recommendations of the Advisory Committee on Immunization Practices (ACIP). *MMWR Morb Mortal Wkly Rep.* 2002;51(RR-3):1–31.

18. Rennard BO, Ertl RF, Gossman GL, et al. Chicken soup inhibits neutrophil chemotaxis in vitro. *Chest.* 2000;118:1150–1157.

19. Gundlapalli AV, Rubin M, Lopanski B, et al. Prospective surveillance for upper respiratory viruses promotes reduced antibiotic use at the 2002 winter Olympics and Paralympics. Presented at 40th IDSA meeting; October 24–27, 2002; Chicago, Ill. Abstract 591.

20. Lee PY, Matchar DB, Clements DA, et al. Economic analysis of influenza vaccination and antiviral treatment for healthy working adults. *Ann Intern Med.* 2002;137:225–231.

21. Couch RB. Prevention and treatment of influenza. *N Engl J Med.* 2000;343:1778–1787.

22. Bratzler DW, Houck PM, Jiang H, et al. Failure to vaccinate Medicare inpatients. *Arch Intern Med.* 2002;162:2349–2356.

23. Gravenstein S, Davidson HE. Current strategies for management of influenza in the elderly population. *Clin Infect Dis.* 2002;35:729–737.

24. Jefferson TO, Demicheli V, Deeks JJ, Rivetti D. Amantidine and rimantidine for preventing and treating influenza A in healthy adults. *Cochrane Database Syst Rev.* 2000;CD001169.

25. Jefferson TO, Demicheli V, Deeks JJ, et al. Neuraminidase inhibitors for preventing and treating influenza in healthy adults. *Cochrane Database Syst Rev.* 2000;CD0001265.

26. Monto AS, Pichicero ME, Blanckenberg SJ, et al. Zanamivir prophylaxis: an effective strategy for prevention of influenza types A and B within households. *J Infect Dis.* 2002;186:1582–1588.

27. Treanor JJ, Hayden FG, Vrooman PS. Efficacy and safety of the oral neuraminidase inhibitor oseltamivir in treating acute influenza: a randomized controlled trial. *JAMA.* 2000;283:1016–1024.

28. Hayden FG, Gwaltney JM Jr, van de Castle RL, Adams KF, Gioglani B. Comparative toxicity of amantadine hydrochloride and rimantadine hydrochloride in healthy adults. *Antimicrob Agents Chemother.* 1981;19:226–237.

29. Welliver R, Monto AS, Carewicz O, et al. Effectiveness of oseltamivir in preventing influenza in household contacts: a randomized controlled trial. *JAMA.* 2001;285:748–754.

30. Henderson FW, Collier AM, Sanyal MA, et al. A longitudinal study of respiratory viruses and bacteria in the

etiology of acute otitis media with effusion. *N Engl J Med.* 1982;306:1377–1383.

31. Kaiser L, Keene ON, Hammond JMJ, et al. Impact of zanamivir on antibiotic use for respiratory events following acute influenza in adolescents and adults. *Arch Intern Med.* 2000;160:3234–3240.

32. Heikkinen T, Ruuskanen O, Waris M, et al. Influenza vaccination in the prevention of acute otitis media in children. *Am J Dis Child.* 1991;145:445–448.

33. Hendley JO. Otitis media. *N Engl J Med.* 2002;347:1169–1174.

34. Eskola J, Kilpi T, Palmu L, et al. Efficacy of a pneumococcal conjugate vaccine against acute otitis media. *N Engl J Med.* 2001;344:403–409.

35. Straetmans M, Sanders EA, Veenhoven RH, et al. Pneumococcal vaccines for preventing otitis media. *Cochrane Database Syst Rev.* 2002;CD001480.

36. Jacobs MR. Prevention of otitis media: role of pneumococcal conjugate vaccines in reducing incidence and antibiotic resistance. *J Pediatr.* 2002;141:287–293.

37. Marchisio P, Cavagna R, Maspes B, et al. Efficacy of intranasal virosomal influenza vaccine in the prevention of recurrent acute otitis media in children. *Clin Infect Dis.* 2002;35:168–174.

38. Mora R, Barbieri M, Passali GC, et al. A preventive measure for otitis media in children with upper respiratory tract infections. *Int J Pediatr Otorhinolaryngol.* 2002;63:111–118.

39. Bisno AL, Gerber MA, Gwaltney JM Jr, et al. Practice guidelines for the diagnosis and management of group A streptococcal pharyngitis. *Clin Infect Dis.* 2002;35:113–125.

40. Denny FW, Wannamaker LW, Brink WR, et al. Prevention of rheumatic fever: treatment of the preceding streptococcal infection. *JAMA.* 1950;143:151–153.

41. Frank PF, Stollerman GH, Miller LF. Protection of a military population from rheumatic fever. *JAMA.* 1965;193:755–783.

42. Perry RF, Maher MT, Cockerill FR, et al. Management of pharyngeal carriers of group A streptococcal organisms. *JAMA.* 1997;277:1203.

43. Paradise JL, Bluestone CD, Colborn DK, et al. Tonsillectomy and adenotonsillectomy for recurrent throat infection in moderately affected children. *Pediatrics.* 2002;110:7–14.

44. Prevention of invasive group A streptococcal infections in workshop participants. Prevention of invasive group A streptococcal disease among household contacts of case patients and among postpartum and postsurgical patients: recommendations from the Centers for Disease Control and Prevention. *Clin Infect Dis.* 2002;35:950–959.

45. Bartlett JG, Dowell SF, Mandell LA, et al. Practice guidelines for the management of community-acquired pneumonia in adults. *Clin Infect Dis.* 2000;31:347–382.

46. American Thoracic Society. Guidelines for the initial management of adults with community-acquired pneumonia: diagnosis, assessment of severity, and initial antimicrobial therapy. *Am Rev Respir Dis.* 1993;148:1418–1426.

47. American Thoracic Society. Targeted tuberculin testing and treatment of latent tuberculosis infection. *Am J Respir Crit Care Med.* 2000;161:S221–S247.

48. Stamm WE. Scientific and clinical challenges in the management of urinary tract infections. *Am J Med.* 2002;113:1S–4S.

49. Stapleton A, Latham RH, Johnson C, Stamm WE. Postcoital antimicrobial prophylaxis for recurrent urinary tract infection: a randomized, double-blind, placebo-controlled trial. *JAMA.* 1990;264:703–706.

50. Gupta K, Hooton TM, Roberts P, Stamm WE. Patient-initiated treatment of uncomplicated recurrent urinary tract infections in young women. *Ann Intern Med.* 2001;135:9–16.

51. Raz R, Stamm WE. A controlled trial of intravaginal estradiol in postmenopausal women with recurrent urinary tract infections. *N Engl J Med.* 1993;329:753–756.

52. Eriksen B. A randomized, open, parallel-group study on the preventative effect of an estradiol releasing vaginal ring (Estring) on recurrent urinary tract infections in postmenopausal women. *Am J Obstet Gynecol.* 1999;180:1072–1079.

53. Shortliffe LMD, McCue JD. Urinary tract infection at the age extremes: pediatrics and geriatrics. *Am J Med.* 2002;113:55S–66S.

54. Reid G, Bruce AW, Taylor M. Influence of three day antimicrobial treatment and lactobacillus vaginal suppositories on recurrence of urinary tract infections. *Clin Ther.* 1992;14:11–16.

55. Avorn J, Moinane M, Gurwitz JH, et al. Reduction of bacteriuria and pyuria after ingestion of cranberry juice. *JAMA.* 1994;271:751–754.

56. Kontiokari T, Sundqvist K, Nuutinen M, Pokka T, Koskela M, Uhari M. Randomized trial of cranberry-lingonberry juice and Lactobacillus GG drink for the prevention of urinary tract infections in women. *BMJ.* 2001;322:1571–1573.

57. Ahuja S, Kaak B, Roberts J. Loss of fimbrial adhesion with the berries of *Vaccinium macrocarpo* to the growth medium of P-fimbriated *Escherichia coli. J Urol.* 1998;159:559–562.

58. Howell AB, Vorsa N, Der Marderosian A, Foo LY. Inhibition of adherence of P-fimbriated *Escherichia coli* to uroepithelial-cell surfaces by proanthocyanidin extracts from cranberries. *N Engl J Med.* 1998;339:1085–1086.

59. Foxman B, Gillespie B, Koopman J, et al. Risk factors for second urinary tract infection among college women. *Am J Epidemiol.* 2000;151:1194–1205.

60. Foxman B. Epidemiology of urinary tract infections: incidence, morbidity, and economic costs. *Am J Med.* 2002;113:5S–13S.

61. Harding GKM, Zhanel GG, Nicolle LE, Cheang M. Antimicrobial treatment in diabetic women with asymptomatic bacteriuria. *N Engl J Med.* 2002:347:1576–1583.

62. Hopkins WJ, Uehling DT. Vaccine development for the prevention of urinary tract infections. *Curr Infect Dis Rep.* 2002;4:509–513.

63. Habash MB, Mei HC, van der Reid G, Busscher R. The effect of water, ascorbic acid and cranberry derived supplementation on human urine and uropathogen adhesion to silicone rubber. *Can J Microbiol.* 1999;45:691–694.

64. Lee B, Bhuta T, Craig J, Simpson J. Methenamine hippurate for preventing urinary tract infections. *Cochrane Database Syst Rev.* 2002;CD003265.

65. Orenstein R, Wong ES. Urinary tract infections in adults. *Am Fam Physician.* 1999;59:1225–1234.

66. Smith JS, Robinson NJ. Age-specific prevalence of infection with herpes simplex virus types 2 and 1: a global review. *J Infect Dis.* 2002;186:S3–S28.

67. Herpetic Eye Disease Study Group. Acyclovir for the prevention of recurrent herpes simplex virus eye disease. *N Engl J Med.* 1998;339:300–306.

68. Liesegang TJ, Melton LJ 3rd, Daly PJ, Ilstrup DM. Epidemiology of ocular herpes simplex. Incidence in Rochester, Minnesota, 1950–1982. *Arch Ophthalmol.* 1989;107:1155–1159.

69. Asbell PA. Valacyclovir for the prevention of recurrent herpes simplex virus eye disease after excimer laser photokeratectomy. *Trans Am Ophthalmol Soc.* 2000;98:285–303.

70. Guerrant RL, VanGilder T, Steiner TS, et al. Practice guidelines for the management of diarrhea. *Clin Infect Dis.* 2001;32:331–350.

71. Williams MD, Schorling JB, Barrett LJ, et al. Early treatment of *Campylobacter jejuni* enteritis. *Antimicrob Agents Chemother.* 1989;33:248–250.

72. Brigden ML, Patullo AL. Prevention and management of overwhelming postsplenectomy infection: an update. *Crit Care Med.* 1999;27:836–842.

73. Wang JH, Liu YC, Cheng DL, et al. Role of benzathine penicillin G in prophylaxis for recurrent streptococcal cellulitis of the lower legs. *Clin Infect Dis.* 1997;25:685–689.

74. Advisory Statement of American Academy of Orthopaedic Surgeons and American Dental Association. Antibiotic prophylaxis for dental patients with total joint replacements. January 2003. Available at: www.aaos.org/wordhtml/papers/advistmt/denta.htm. Accessed 2/03/03.

75. Kravetz JD, Federman DG. Cat-associated zoonoses. *Arch Intern Med.* 2002;162:1945–1952.

76. Medeiros I, Saconato H. Antibiotic prophylaxis for mammalian bites. *Cochrane Database Syst Rev.* 2001;CD001738.

77. Terry P, Mackway-Jones K. Towards evidence-based emergency medicine: best BETs from the Manchester Royal Infirmary: antibiotics in non-venomous snakebite. *Emerg Med J.* 2002;19:142.

78. Blalock RS. Antibiotic use and infection in snakebite victims. *South Med J.* 1999;89:874–876.

79. Fradin MS, Day JF. Comparative efficacy of insect repellants against mosquito bites. *N Engl J Med.* 2002;347:13–18.

80. Warshafsky S, Nowakowski J, Nadelman RB et al. Efficacy of antibiotic prophylaxis for prevention of Lyme disease. *J Gen Intern Med.* 1996;11:329–333.

81. Nadelman RB, Novakowski J, Fish D, et al. Prophylaxis with single dose doxycycline for the prevention of Lyme disease after an *Ixodes scapularis* tick bite. *N Engl J Med.* 2001;345:79–84.

PART 12

Prevention in Common Clinical Problems

chapter 54

Gastrointestinal Diseases

John A. Schaffner, MD

INTRODUCTION

Prevention of gastrointestinal (GI) and liver disorders can be approached from both the patient and physician standpoint. Behavioral patterns and diet can be employed to avoid symptoms and diseases. Screening for some diseases has been useful for early detection, treatment, and the prevention of complications. This chapter will cover a wide range of GI symptoms and diseases and the approach to their prevention.

GAS

Belching is rarely a sign of severe disease. It results from excessive air swallowing, either voluntarily or involuntarily. Circumstances that lead to aerophagia include anxiety, eating too fast, carbonated beverages, drinking with straws, and poorly fitting dentures. Patients with oral movement disorders such as tardive dyskinesia may also swallow excessive air. On occasion, belching can be a symptom associated with gastroesophageal reflux, motility disorders, and bowel obstructions. Treatment of belching is targeted at the underlying disorder. Symptoms can sometimes be reduced by simethicone, which causes gas to coalesce and can be taken liberally.

Flatus is almost always related to diet and may or may not reflect severe disease. Undigested carbohydrate is the source of fuel for intestinal bacteria. Individuals vary in the amount of gas-producing organisms they possess, which is one explanation for the difference in tolerance to specific foods. High-fiber foods tend to promote gas production and the amount of gas correlates with the amount of fiber. Thus, bran, while it has many benefits, produces large quantities of gas in some individuals.

Apart from high-fiber foods, other sugars may produce gas and increased frequency of bowel movements. Lactose intolerance is a very common cause of flatus, with onset occurring at almost any age. The ability to tolerate lactose is quite variable among individuals. Patients often overlook the possibility that milk is the culprit because

before that time they had always been able to tolerate milk without problems. Age, infection, or illness affecting the small bowel can cause adults to lose enough lactase to become intolerant. Symptoms can be greatly reduced in many people by using lactase-treated milk, by taking lactase supplements, or by consuming lactose-containing foods near the end of the meal.

Other carbohydrates that may produce gas are lactulose, sorbitol, mannitol, and fructose. Symptoms can be reduced by consuming more complex carbohydrates or by taking exogenous α-galactosidase in over-the-counter preparations. Flatus is usually present in diseases characterized by malabsorption. However, other symptoms such as diarrhea or steatorrhea are usually much more prominent. On occasion, gas can be a presenting symptom of celiac disease.

ESOPHAGEAL DISEASES

Gastroesophageal reflux disease (GERD) is a common disorder, affecting as many as 30% of individuals on a monthly basis and 7% of individuals on a daily basis. There are 5 major factors that contribute to the damage of the refluxate.[1] These factors include decreased lower esophageal sphincter (LES) pressure, altered esophageal motility, delay in gastric emptying or altered gastric accommodation, increased frequency of transient LES relaxation, and alteration of the crural diaphragm. The exact reason why some individuals develop symptomatic reflux and esophagitis is unclear. There is generally a poor correlation between the appearance of the esophagus and symptoms.

Little can be done to change the pathophysiologic defects that lead to reflux. However, preventive lifestyle measures can be helpful in many people (Table 54-1). Most measures are aimed at affecting the LES and the pressures across the sphincter. Avoiding the supine position after eating until the stomach has emptied or sleeping with one's head elevated can be most useful. Avoiding increased abdominal pressure by tight-fitting clothing or weight loss can be helpful for occasional symptoms, but

TABLE 54-1

Lifestyle Changes That Will Help Prevent
Gastroesophageal Reflux

Weight loss
Reduce or discontinue dietary intake of:
Caffeine-containing drinks (eg, coffee, tea, soda)
Carbonated drinks
Chocolate
Citrus fruits
Fatty or spicy foods
Alcohol
Mint
Onions, tomatoes
Do not eat within 3 hours of lying down, including before bedtime
Eat smaller meals at night
Stop smoking
Raise head of bed 10.2–15.2 cm (4–6 in), or sleep on a firm wedge (pillows tend to sag)

often does not benefit patients with frequent problems. The LES can be affected by certain foods and medications, as well as pregnancy. Stress also may play a role in reflux disease.

Barrett esophagus is one of the major consequences of long-standing GERD and is associated with an increased risk of esophageal adenocarcinoma.[2] Currently, the factors that promote Barrett esophagus are unclear. There are presently 2 types of Barrett epithelial patterns that are recognized, short-segment Barrett (<3 cm from the gastroesophageal junction) or traditional or long-segment Barrett (>3 cm above the gastroesophageal junction) esophagus. The pathogenesis of these 2 types may be different. The risk of adenocarcinoma in Barrett epithelium is estimated at 0.5% per year. Whether the risk of cancer in short-segment and long-segment Barrett epithelium is the same has not been convincingly answered. At present, both lesions are managed in the same way.

Patients with Barrett esophagus cannot be distinguished from patients with GERD alone based on symptoms. As many as 3% to 5% of individuals with reflux may have long-segment Barrett esophagus, and 10% to 15% may have short-segment Barrett esophagus. Individuals at greater risk of Barrett esophagus are white men over the age of 50 years with a history of more than 5 years of symptoms. Unfortunately, up to 40% of patients with adenocarcinoma of the esophagus will have no reflux history. There is no convincing evidence that medical or surgical therapy for GERD reduces the risk of development of esophageal adenocarcinoma due to Barrett esophagus. Endoscopy is required to determine the presence of Barrett esophagus. However, if endoscopy does not reveal Barrett esophagus, it is highly unlikely

that an individual will ever develop it, so repeated endoscopic examinations for reflux are rarely indicated if symptoms remain unchanged.

There is, as yet, little evidence that screening patients with Barrett epithelium has reduced deaths due to esophageal adenocarcinoma. Furthermore, only 5% of patients with adenocarcinoma of the esophagus were known to have Barrett esophagus. However, because it is a known premalignant condition, screening surveillance is performed. Currently, for patients with Barrett esophagus, screening for dysplasia and malignancy is recommended at 2- to 3-year intervals in the absence of dysplasia and every 6 to 12 months if low-grade dysplasia is found, although the optimal interval has not been determined. Biopsy specimens should be obtained from 4 quadrants every 2 cm within the involved area. Finding high-grade dysplasia requires choosing between esophagectomy, endoscopic ablative therapy, or intensive surveillance.[3] Endoscopic therapy using photodynamic therapy or thermal ablation is still considered experimental.

One particular form of esophagitis is related to pills lodging in the esophagus, usually at the level of the aortic arch. Ulcerations that occur because of direct contact are usually associated with the abrupt onset of odynophagia and chest pain. The most common medication associated with pill esophagitis is tetracycline. This is preventable by ensuring that the pill passes into the stomach through adequate ingestion of liquid. Once an ulcer is present, antacid therapy is not effective. Topical analgesia provides the most symptomatic benefit for the patient.

ULCER DISEASE

Nearly all ulcers in the stomach and duodenum are associated with either *Helicobacter pylori* or nonsteroidal anti-inflammatory drug (NSAID) use. The incidence of *H pylori* varies with age, socioeconomic status, and country of origin. Unfortunately, the source of the infection among most individuals is unknown. There is an increased incidence among health care workers and family members of infected individuals. Only a small percentage of individuals with infection come to medical attention, which is one of the main reasons why controversy exists as to how aggressively to screen for the organism. Three primary indications for screening for *H pylori* are ulcer disease, mucosa-associated lymphoid tissue (MALT) lymphoma, and gastric cancer. In these situations, symptoms are often present and esophagogastroduodenoscopy (EGD) is performed. A biopsy for *H pylori* can be performed during the EGD. There is still controversy over the role of the organism in nonulcer dyspepsia. However, once proved, the organism should be treated with triple therapy (2 antibiotics and high-dose acid suppression). Eradication does not have to be proved, except in the circumstances of complicated ulcer disease, MALT lymphoma, and gastric cancer. Breath tests are the most sensitive way to prove eradication, although stool antigen is much cheaper.

Ingestion of NSAIDs is a common cause of GI symptoms. As many as 25% of individuals may have dyspeptic symptoms when receiving NSAID therapy, although symptoms do not necessarily correlate with anatomical findings. The US Food and Drug Administration estimates that 1% to 4% of people taking NSAIDs will experience complications. All NSAIDs have been associated with GI mucosal damage, most of which occurs in the stomach and to a lesser degree in the duodenum. However, more extensive injury of the small bowel as well as colonic damage occur both as silent and symptomatic disease. Mucosal injury is directly related to higher doses and drugs with longer half-lives. Cyclooxygenase-2 inhibitors are associated with significantly less GI damage than are other NSAIDs but are still capable of producing mucosal injury.[4] Aspirin is one of the most common causes of mucosal damage and can induce major changes even at low doses prescribed for cardiovascular indications.[5] It is unknown if enteric coating reduces risk. It does appear that H pylori may increase the risk of gastric injury due to aspirin and NSAID intake.[6]

Prevention of NSAID-induced injury could result in substantial reduction in health care costs, morbidity, and lives lost due to bleeding and perforation. Factors that increase the risk of NSAID gastric injury include age over 60 years, female sex, history of dyspepsia or ulcer disease, multiple NSAID use or use of NSAID and aspirin, concomitant use of steroids, and smoking. There is no convincing evidence that taking medication with food will alter the mucosal damage. Although dyspeptic symptoms may be reduced, actual ulcerations may not be altered.

Misoprostol has been shown to reduce NSAID-induced gastric and duodenal injury and complications. Diarrhea is a frequent side effect of this medication. It must be used cautiously or avoided in women of childbearing age. Proton pump blockers have also been shown to be effective in reducing gastric and duodenal injury. Judicious use of NSAIDs and using as low a dose as possible should also be beneficial.

Stress-related mucosal disease (SRMD) is usually not related to gastric hypersecretion. It is associated with multisystem failure, sepsis, extensive burns, head injury, and trauma. The lesion of SRMD usually affects the proximal stomach and is never associated with pain. Except in head injury (Cushing ulcer) or patients with burns (Curling ulcer), there is rarely a single ulcer causing bleeding.

Usually SRMD is present on admission to the intensive care unit. Overall, the incidence of this lesion seems to be decreasing, most likely related to improved medical care in the severely ill patient. There is no treatment of this disorder other than to improve the overall status of the patient. The mortality is related to the underlying illness, not the presence of gastric bleeding.

Prevention of SRMD has been most successful using acid suppression with H_2 receptor antagonists. The target of therapy has been maintaining gastric pH above 4.0, which can be accomplished with continuous infusion of ranitidine or cimetidine, or bolus therapy with famotidine. Intravenous pantoprazole will also elevate the pH to the desired level. Concerns about gastric colonization and nosocomial pneumonia in ventilator-dependent patients due to lack of acid had been raised in the past, but acid suppression is still the main form of SRMD prophylaxis. In addition to acid suppression, there may be benefit in feeding patients early in their hospital course.

DIVERTICULAR DISEASE

Diverticular disease has been associated with the diet of Western civilization. Affecting nearly 40% of individuals in the United States over the age of 50 years, this disorder is almost nonexistent in cultures where consumption of a high-fiber diet is the norm. Approximately 10% to 25% of people with this disorder will experience a complication of the disease, either diverticulitis or bleeding of the lower GI tract.

Once a patient has had an attack of diverticulitis, there is approximately a 25% to 30% chance of recurrence, although a range of 7% to 62% has been reported.[7] Usually, 2 documented attacks of diverticulitis warrant consideration of surgery, since subsequent attacks are less likely to respond to therapy and are associated with a higher mortality rate. Surgery is clearly best performed when the patient is symptom free. Care must be taken not to perform surgery for symptoms of lower left quadrant pain alone, since this frequently represents irritable bowel syndrome (IBS) and is unlikely to improve with surgery. Diverticulitis, when it occurs at an early age, is often more aggressive and requires surgical intervention. Recommended treatments of attacks of diverticulitis include amoxicillin plus clavulanic acid, trimethoprim-sulfamethoxazole with metronidazole, or a quinolone with metronidazole. Patients who have had an attack of diverticulitis should have their colon examined after recovery to exclude other disease.

Prevention of diverticulitis likely requires intervention early in life. Whether institution of a high-fiber diet is effective in prevention of complications once the individual is aware of the condition or once symptoms occur is not clear. One of the unsubstantiated dietary theories in GI diseases is that a diet excluding seeds or nuts will prevent episodes of diverticulitis or bleeding. Unfortunately, there is no proof that there is any benefit to such an exclusion diet, and many patients will avoid anything that has even a miniscule seed such as tomatoes or poppy seeds. Whether any substance, including popcorn, can precipitate an attack is far from certain. Generally, a high-fiber diet is recommended that contains 20 to 30 g/d of fiber. Fiber reduces intraluminal pressure and theoretically may reduce impaction of material in a diverticulum.

ANAL DISEASES

Hemorrhoids and fissures are a common cause of discomfort and concern for many people. While typically associated with perirectal burning, itching, or pain, they can result in substantial morbidity due to bleeding or infection. Hemorrhoids are a dilation of the normal vascular bed in the anal canal at the point where the arterial and venous systems intersect. Both hemorrhoids and fissures can cause problems secondary to constipation, diarrhea, straining, and even normal defecation. Increased fiber intake, either by diet or with over-the-counter supplements, improves rectal function and should be a mainstay of therapy for individuals prone to problems. Prolonged defecation should be avoided to reduce increased pressure predisposing to prolapse. If hemorrhoids should protrude after bowel movements, manual attempts to reduce them may help reduce the chance of thrombosis. Submersing the perianal area in hot water (sitz bath) may promote healing of fissures by increasing local blood flow in addition to improving perirectal symptoms. Surgical treatment can be offered to individuals whose disease cannot be managed with medical treatment alone.

IRRITABLE BOWEL SYNDROME

Irritable bowel syndrome is a name given to a host of symptoms that are part of a group of functional disorders of the GI tract. Several criteria have been useful for characterizing this group of patients[8-10] (Table 54-2). Recognition of this disorder is important to administer appropriate treatment, avoid unnecessary testing and doctor visits, and prevent unwarranted and unsuccessful surgery. Care should be taken to avoid labeling patients as having IBS when they may have other disorders, such as microscopic colitis, pelvic floor dysfunction, or chronic abdominal pain.

The prevalence of IBS has been evaluated in several studies to be between 6% and 20% of the US population and accounts for a large percentage of visits to primary care providers and gastroenterologists. The origins of this disorder are as yet unknown. Several potential explanations include a learned response of the GI tract to stresses, GI tract infections, previous surgical procedures, and exposure to "irritants" such as lactose.

Evaluation of patients suspected of having irritable bowel may vary but should start with an extensive history.[11] Presently, universal recommendations include a complete blood cell count and basic biochemical studies. On the other hand, additional studies such as thyroid evaluation, stool studies for ova and parasites, and sedimentation rate have repeatedly demonstrated a very low yield and are not routinely recommended. The usefulness of endoscopic evaluation and imaging studies remains controversial. Several investigators believe that the routine use of colon histology in patients who meet clinical criteria for IBS is not helpful. Symptoms that should provoke a more intensive investigation include weight loss, nocturnal symptoms, anemia, or blood in the stool. Patients with a family history of colon cancer or inflammatory bowel disease, or recent onset of symptoms in patients over age 50 years should also prompt an investigation.

T A B L E 54-2

Criteria for Irritable Bowel Syndrome

ROME Criteria[8]	ROME II Criteria[9]	Manning Criteria[10]
At least 12 wk of continuous or recurrent symptoms of the following: Abdominal pain or discomfort: 1. relieved with defecation, or 2. associated with a change in frequency of stool, or 3. associated with a change in consistency of stool Two or more of the following, at least on one fourth of occasions or days: 1. altered stool frequency 2. altered stool form 3. altered stool passage 4. passage of mucus 5. bloating or feeling of abdominal distension	At least 12 wk, which need not be consecutive, in preceding 12 mo of abdominal discomfort or pain that has 2 or more of these 3 features: 1. relieved with defecation 2. onset associated with a change in frequency of stool 3. onset associated with a change in form of stool	Abdominal pain relieved by defecation Looser stools with onset of pain More frequent stools with onset of pain Abdominal distension Passage of mucus in stools Sensation of incomplete evacuation

Treatment of IBS requires a good patient-physician relationship, which can then focus therapy toward the patient's complaints. It is important to establish with the patient that this is not a curable disorder, that symptoms will continue to persist, and that medical therapy is aimed at controlling the symptoms.[12] Although widely used, there is no proven benefit of fiber for symptoms of IBS except for relieving constipation. Care must be taken when prescribing fiber to warn of potential bloating and excessive gas. Antidiarrheal agents should be used when patients experience diarrhea, but it is important to avoid excessive use that could enhance the swings between constipation and diarrhea. Antispasmodics appear to have a role in patients with abdominal cramping but lose their effectiveness when used over long periods instead of on an as-needed basis. Tricyclic antidepressants or serotonin reuptake inhibitors may also have a role in the treatment of IBS. The 5-hydroxytryptamine-3 antagonist alosetron was shown to be effective in women with diarrhea-predominant IBS but must be used cautiously given the severe side effects of bowel ischemia. The partial 5-HT4 agonist tegaserod may have a role in patients with constipation.

LIVER DISEASE

Hepatitis

Hepatitis related to viral infections poses major health problems throughout the world. Hepatitis A, B, C, D, and E have been identified as causes of infection, with varying frequency in different populations. Hepatitis A has been associated with poor sanitation and foodborne spread. Hepatitis E is not present in the United States or Western Europe. Its greatest threat of severe disease is among pregnant women. Hepatitis B and D, while diminishing in frequency because of blood screening and vaccination, is still prevalent among intravenous drug users. Hepatitis C is the cause of most transfusion-related hepatitis and is associated with needle stick exposure. Many cases of hepatitis C have no known exposure. It is apparent that alcohol ingestion markedly enhances the liver damage wrought by hepatitis C.

Prevention of viral hepatitis can be approached from 2 fronts: avoidance of at-risk behavior and vaccination. Hepatitis A vaccine is recommended for patients entering endemic areas, patients with chronic liver disease, recipients of clotting factor concentrates, homosexual men, and illicit drug users. Some also advocate its use in schoolchildren and food handlers. Hepatitis B vaccine is effective and is now recommended for all newborns and children as well as adults at high risk. It is also recommended that all pregnant women be screened for hepatitis B surface antigen (HBsAg) to identify women at risk so that treatment can be administered to prevent transmission to the newborn.

Nonalcoholic Fatty Liver Disease

Nonalcoholic fatty liver disease (NAFLD) encompasses a group of disorders that includes steatosis and nonalcoholic steatohepatitis (NASH).[13] These disorders account for a large percentage of the patients with mildly abnormal liver tests and may be a major contributor to more advanced liver disease. Reports from Japanese and European studies estimate the prevalence of NAFLD to be 14% to 21%. Severe fibrosis has been noted in 15% to 50% of patients with NASH undergoing liver biopsy, and 7% to 26% of patients are found to have cirrhosis at diagnosis. Risk factors for NAFLD include obesity, insulin resistance and type 2 diabetes mellitus, and dyslipidemias. The presence of NAFLD may interact with other liver diseases. Patients with hepatitis C and NAFLD are more likely to have progression to cirrhosis than are those with hepatitis C alone. Similarly, patients with NAFLD who carry the hemochromatosis genotype are also more likely for their disease to progress to cirrhosis.

Aggressive treatment of NAFLD may reduce the progression to more advanced liver disease.[14] Weight loss improves liver enzyme abnormalities in patients with obesity and NAFLD as well as reduces the risk of type 2 diabetes. Treatment with metformin has been shown to decrease hepatic steatosis and improve liver enzymes in some patients. Other possible therapies such as antioxidants, ursodeoxycholic acid, and lipid-lowering drugs need further study to demonstrate beneficial effect on liver histology.

Alcoholic Liver Disease

Alcoholic liver disease is a major health problem in many countries, although only a small percentage of the greater public health problem of alcohol abuse and alcoholism. Cirrhosis remains a major cause of death in the United States, particularly among men in the 25- to 64-year age group. Alcoholic liver disease can range from fatty liver to alcoholic hepatitis to end-stage cirrhosis. Only about 10% of alcoholics will go on to have alcoholic hepatitis or cirrhosis, although reported percentages vary considerably. The important factors leading to liver disease are the amount and duration of alcohol use, with the pattern of consumption not clearly important. In one study, as little as 40 g of alcohol daily in men and 20 g in women for more than 10 years was associated with a significant increase in cirrhosis. This translates into 4 bottles of beer or 112 g (4 oz) of whiskey daily for men. In the presence of hepatitis C, progression to cirrhosis is more rapid and may occur with lower intake of alcohol.

Additional factors may increase susceptibility to alcoholic liver injury. Nutritional deficiencies may play a role, although the exact nature of these relationships is unclear. Genetic factors may also be important. Interest is currently focused on polymorphisms of genes encoding cytokines and ethanol metabolism, which may be important factors in determining development of alcoholic liver disease. Overall, prevention of alcoholic liver disease at this time can be accomplished only by reducing consumption.

Hemochromatosis

Hemochromatosis is an autosomal recessive disorder associated with iron overload causing liver, heart, joint, and endocrine disease. The incidence of the disease is approximately 1 in 200 to 300 people of Northern European descent. The liver is the most frequently affected organ, with cirrhosis being the most common manifestation. In as many as 30% of untreated patients with hemochromatosis, hepatocellular carcinoma will develop. The gene for hereditary hemochromatosis *(HFE)* was identified in 1996. Two mutations have been recognized: *C282Y,* present in more than 90% of individuals with the disease, and *H63D,* present in a small number of patients. Only 1.5% of patients with the disease have neither mutation. The presence of these gene mutations results in an abnormal iron transport protein that leads to intracellular iron accumulation.

One current recommendation for screening is measurement of transferrin saturation in patients of Northern European ancestry.[15] Serum iron and ferritin may be helpful in certain instances. If the saturation is greater than 45%, an assay for the *HFE* genotype can be performed. Genetic counseling should be considered before genetic testing. If genotyping is consistent with *HFE,* a liver biopsy is recommended for individuals older than 40 years of age and in patients with markedly elevated transaminase levels. A liver biopsy can also be performed if the diagnosis is uncertain based on transferrin saturation, ferritin levels, liver function test results, and *HFE* genotyping. When the diagnosis is established, further genetic counseling should be considered and family members of affected individuals should be screened. Institution of therapy before the onset of end-organ damage may avoid later complications, including hepatocellular carcinoma.

Gallstones

Gallstone prevalence varies considerably by the population surveyed and by the method of detection. The Framingham study found a prevalence of 3.9% among adults aged 30 to 62 years.[16] In Denmark, the prevalence varied from 4.8% to 22.4% among women of similar age intervals.[17] The prevalence in men increased from 1.8% at age 30 years to 12.9% at age 60. Among the Pima Indians in the southwestern United States, the prevalence was 12.7% in females aged 15 to 24 years and 89.5% in women older than 65.[18] While Pima men had a lower prevalence than women, they still had a prevalence of 67.8% over age 65.

The risk factors associated with gallstones include age, obesity, female sex, ethnicity, heredity, and parity. Specific factors that can lead to gallstone formation include rapid weight loss and certain medications, including estrogens, clofibrate, and octreotide. Diseases associated with stone formation include cirrhosis, hemolytic diseases, ileal disease or resection, cystic fibrosis, and parenteral alimentation.

Most patients with gallstones are asymptomatic. As shown in several long-term studies, the rate at which patients with gallstones experience symptoms is approximately 1% to 2% per year. The risk of presenting with a complication such as gallstone pancreatitis is very low. These findings have led to the recommendation that asymptomatic gallstones should be left alone. In addition, there is currently no evidence to support prophylactic cholecystectomy for the prevention of gallbladder cancer, except in patients with a porcelain gallbladder (calcifications in the wall of the gallbladder).

SUMMARY

The prevention of GI disorders requires proper nutrition, avoidance of harmful substances, and early detection of illness. Identification of patients at risk of diseases such as Barrett esophagus, NSAID-induced gastric injury, NAFLD, hemochromatosis, diverticular disease, and IBS could greatly lower health care costs, reduce morbidity and mortality, and prevent development of future disease.

REFERENCES

1. Sarosiek J, McCallum RW. Mechanisms of oesophageal mucosal defence. *Baillieres Clin Gastroenterol.* 2000;14:701–717.

2. Falk GW. Barrett's esophagus. *Gastroenterology.* 2002;122:1569–1591.

3. Spechler SJ. Clinical practice: Barrett's esophagus. *N Engl J Med.* 2002;346:836–842.

4. Bombardier C, Laine L, Reicin A, et al, for VIGOR Study Group. Comparison of upper gastrointestinal toxicity of rofecoxib and naproxen in patients with rheumatoid arthritis. *N Engl J Med.* 2000;343:1520–1528.

5. Chan FKL, Chung S, Suen BY, et al. Preventing recurrent upper gastrointestinal bleeding in patients with *Helicobacter pylori* infection who are taking low-dose aspirin or naproxen. *N Engl J Med.* 2001;344:967–973.

6. Hawkey CJ, Wilson I, Naesdal J, et al. Influence of sex and *Helicobacter pylori* on development and healing of gastroduodenal lesions in non-steroidal anti-inflammatory drug users. *Gut.* 2002;51:344–350.

7. Stollman NH, Raskin JB. Diagnosis and management of diverticular disease of the colon in adults: Ad Hoc Practice Parameters Committee of the American College of Gastroenterology. *Am J Gastroenterol.* 1999;94:3110–3121.

8. Thompson WG, Dotewall G, Drossman DA, et al. Irritable bowel syndrome: guidelines for the diagnosis. *Gastroenterol Int.* 1989;2:92–95.

9. Thompson WG, Longstreth GF, Drossman DA, et al. Functional bowel disorders and functional abdominal pain. *Gut.* 1999;45(suppl 2):1143–1147.

10. Manning AP, Thompson WG, Heaton KW, et al. Towards a positive diagnosis of the irritable bowel syndrome. *BMJ.* 1978;2:653–654.

11. Olden KW. Diagnosis of irritable bowel syndrome. *Gastroenterology.* 2002;122:1701–1714.

12. Camilleri M, Heading RC, Thompson WG. Consensus report: clinical perspectives, mechanisms, diagnosis and management of irritable bowel syndrome. *Aliment Pharmacol Ther.* 2002;16:1407–1430.

13. Angulo P. Nonalcoholic fatty liver disease. *N Engl J Med.* 2002;346:1221–1231.

14. Clark JM, Brancati FL, Diehl AM. Nonalcoholic fatty liver disease. *Gastroenterology.* 2002;122:1649–1657.

15. Maddrey WC. Update in hepatology. *Ann Intern Med.* 2001;134:216–223.

16. Sampliner RE, Bennett PH, Comess LJ, Rose FA, Burch TA. Gallbladder disease in Pima Indians: demonstration of high prevalence and early onset by cholecystography. *N Engl J Med.* 1970;283(25):1358–1364.

17. Jensen KH, Jorgensen T. Incidence of gallstones in a Danish population. *Gastroenterology.* 1991;100:790.

18. Friedman GD, Kannel WB, Dawber TR. The epidemiology of gallbladder disease: observations in the Framingham Study. *J Chronic Dis.* 1966;19(3):273–292.

chapter 55

Kidney Disorders

Stephen B. Erickson, MD

INTRODUCTION

It is probably human nature to look for a panacea for our problems. This is no less true for medicine in general and kidney disorders in particular. It is the author's impression that there are 2 prevalent misconceptions regarding kidney cure-alls. One has to do with cranberries and the other with water.

MISCONCEPTIONS

Cranberry

Popular opinion has it that cranberries are effective in preventing or treating urinary tract infections. Proanthocyanidins in cranberries inhibit the attachment of *Escherichia coli* to the uroepithelial cells of the urinary tract by blocking the adherence of their p-fimbria. Lack of adherence allows the bacterial colonization to be voided with each emptying of the bladder. There is also evidence that cranberry juice may weaken the attachment of *E coli* to urinary catheters. However, a Cochrane review found no evidence to support the use of cranberry products for either the prevention or treatment of urinary tract infections.[1] Since then, 2 additional studies have been published suggesting effectiveness for prevention, although they suffer from small size, inadequate blinding, and, in one of them, industry sponsorship.[2] No study has compared cranberry products to antibiotics in a head-to-head trial. The use of cranberry products appears clinically safe. If effective, the dose of cranberry product required is unknown. A typical dose is 3 glasses (8 oz or 224 g) of cranberry juice per day, which contains a substantial number of calories because sugar is virtually always added. The cranberry product used should contain proanthocyanidins. To the extent that cranberries contain oxalate, the same therapy might be deleterious in the prevention of nephrolithiasis. Although there is suggestive evidence that cranberry products may help prevent (not treat) urinary tract infections, there is no scientific evidence that cranberries are helpful in the treatment of any other kidney disorder.

Water

It is generally regarded that a large intake of water, roughly eight 8-oz (224-g) glasses daily, will ward off all potential disorders of the kidney. This belief is clearly unfounded. For example, patients with end-stage renal disease and oliguria can easily become water overloaded, with subsequent congestive heart failure and pulmonary edema requiring more intensive dialysis. Patients prone to euvolemic hyponatremia, such as in the syndrome of inappropriate antidiuretic hormone, are often treated with water restriction to avoid aggravating their hyponatremia. It is true that a large fluid intake is beneficial for prevention of nephrolithiasis. It is also probably true that large water intake increases urinary frequency, which will decrease the risk of urinary tract infection. However, water is no panacea for renal disorders.

Although a panacea does not exist for the prevention of renal diseases, there are preventive measures that may be quite helpful for a variety of individual kidney disorders. The rest of this chapter will first focus on various interventions that may be helpful in the primary prevention of specific kidney disorders. Then, selected kidney diseases will be discussed with regard to secondary prevention.

PRIMARY PREVENTION

Angiotensin-Converting Enzyme Inhibitors

Angiotensin-converting enzyme (ACE) inhibitors were initially introduced for the treatment of resistant hypertension. It was discovered soon thereafter that ACE inhibitors could cause acute renal failure in patients with high-grade bilateral renal artery stenoses. Later it was discovered that ACE inhibitors have a hypoproteinuric effect. This occurs by the same mechanism as does acute renal failure: a dilation of the efferent arteriole with a decrease in intraglomerular pressure and filtration. Much research has shown that hypertension is a leading cause of renal failure and that the degree of proteinuria predicts an adverse outcome for glomerular diseases. Thus, ACE inhibitors and the similar angiotensin receptor blockers (ARBs) are the antihypertensive agents of choice for many nephrologists.

It is key to either look for bilateral high-grade renal artery stenosis before initiating treatment with an ACE inhibitor or ARB or, more commonly, to check a measure of glomerular filtration rate, such as serum creatinine, before and a few weeks after initiation of treatment with the ACE inhibitor or ARB. A mild increase in the serum creatinine level of 38.1 mol/L (0.5 mg/dL) or less is commonly observed. This relates to the reversible, hemodynamic effect of the vasodilation of the efferent artery and "depressurization" of the glomerulus. It is a short-term loss for long-term gain.[3]

Antioxidants

Among certain segments of the American population, antioxidant therapy is held in high regard. The rationale for the use of antioxidants in the prevention of renal disease is that oxidative stress appears to mediate inflammation. Unfortunately, well-done human studies are virtually nonexistent. There are limited animal data for vitamins C and E. In rats with diabetic nephropathy, vitamin C appears to be helpful, and a dose extrapolated to 200 mg/d has been recommended for humans.[4] Vitamin E also has been found helpful in amelioration of proteinuria in diabetic rats.[5] In clinical practice, it is probably premature to recommend antioxidants for the prevention of human renal disease.

Aspirin

There is weak evidence that prolonged high-dose aspirin may contribute to analgesic-associated nephropathy, but low-dose aspirin may be another matter. Low-dose aspirin has been shown to be beneficial in the primary and secondary prevention of cardiovascular disease. It is reasonable to wonder if low-dose aspirin might also have preventive properties for a highly vascular organ such as the kidney. However, human data on the beneficial effects of low-dose aspirin on the kidney are lacking. In theory, the anticoagulant effect of aspirin could blunt the procoagulant effects of various types of nephritis and might also retard the progression of atherosclerotic disease. On the other hand, low-dose aspirin should probably be avoided by people with polycystic kidney disease for fear of exacerbating cyst hemorrhage. It should also be avoided by patients with uncontrolled hypertension because of the potential for cerebral hemorrhage. Thus, whereas low-dose aspirin has theoretical attractiveness as

a preventive medication for certain kidney disorders, there is little evidence to make a firm recommendation to use it on a renal basis only.

Blood Pressure

The kidney is a target organ for hypertensive damage. In no group does this appear truer than African American males. Hypertension is disproportionately represented as a cause for end-stage renal disease in this group. Prevention or adequate treatment of hypertension will prevent hypertensive nephrosclerosis and is one of the most effective ways to prevent renal failure in the United States. Although nephrologists are increasingly treating patients with ACE inhibitors or ARBs as a first step in patients without preexisting renal injury, it is not as important which class of antihypertensive medication is chosen as it is to reach the treatment goal. As noted in the Seventh Report of the Joint National Committee on Prevention, Detection, Evaluation, and Treatment of High Blood Pressure, lifestyle modifications should precede drug treatment in patients with high normal or stage 1 (mild) hypertension who do not have target organ damage, clinical cardiovascular disease, or diabetes.[6] In patients with preexisting renal disease as defined by an elevated serum creatinine level, the blood pressure goal should be 130/85 mm Hg or less; those with more than 1 g/d of proteinuria should aim for a blood pressure of 125/75 mm Hg or less.[6] Otherwise, a targeted blood pressure below 140/90 mm Hg is acceptable.

Diabetes Mellitus

The primary cause of end-stage renal disease in the United States is diabetes mellitus. Although patients with either type 1 or type 2 diabetes can ultimately reach end-stage renal failure because of their illness, those with type 2 diabetes predominate simply because they comprise 90% of diabetic patients. With the worsening of the obesity epidemic in the United States and the increased incidence of type 2 diabetes at earlier ages, nephrologists await the consequences with growing concern. Fortunately, end-stage renal failure due to diabetic nephropathy is rarely inevitable. It is well known that tight glycemic control coupled with tight hypertensive control will prevent the development of diabetic nephropathy in most diabetic patients.

As mentioned earlier, the blood pressure goal in a patient with normal renal function and diabetes should be 130/80 mm Hg or less according to the Seventh Report of the Joint National Committee.[6] Data, primarily from subset analysis of the Hypertension Optimal Treatment (HOT) trial,[7] have also led to suggestions by the National Kidney Foundation for blood pressure below 130/80 mm Hg.[8] Euglycemia would be ideal from the preventive aspect of diabetic nephropathy. However, this may cause an unacceptable risk of hypoglycemic reactions, particularly in brittle type 1 diabetes; thus, more moderate goals are usually adopted by the clinical nephrologist. Most nephrologists recommend glycosylated hemoglobin of 7% or less. If the diabetic patient has hypoglycemic unawareness, even this goal may be too rigorous. The detection of microalbuminuria is a strong predictor of incipient clinical diabetic nephropathy. The urinary microalbumin determination should be a standard part of monitoring for all diabetic patients.

Diet

Diet is an important lifestyle risk factor for many illnesses and organ systems, including the renal system. This section will consider selected dietary components as they relate to kidney disorders.

Calcium

Traditionally, dietary calcium has been presumed to aggravate the risk of calcium-containing kidney stones. This view was upended a decade ago by the publication of a prospective, cohort study of 45,000 males[9] and later by a similar study of 90,000 females.[10] These studies showed that the risk of kidney stones was actually increased by a low-calcium diet. Paradoxically, calcium supplementation increased the risk of kidney stones by approximately 20%. There was no dose-response trend with the calcium supplement data, however, casting some doubt on their validity. The findings have not been confirmed in a large randomized and blinded study. Nonetheless, it is current nephrologic practice to recommend moderation in the consumption of dairy products to patients who are prone to the development of calcium stones ("calcium stone formers"). "Moderation" means the consumption of approximately 1200 mg of dietary calcium daily. Calcium supplements are not recommended if patients can consume the necessary calcium through food. If not, calcium supplements should be taken with meals on the theory that calcium will bind dietary oxalate and diminish stone risk. On theoretical grounds only, calcium citrate might be the preferred supplement because various citrate preparations have been efficacious in the prevention of nephrolithiasis.

Magnesium

Some studies have shown that magnesium supplementation is effective in preventing the formation of calcium-containing kidney stones. No adequate studies exist using dietary sources of magnesium.

Oxalate

Calcium oxalate stones are the most common type of stone in westernized society. Oxalate enters the urine both from dietary sources and endogenous metabolism.

Patients with surgical modification of their small bowel, as in various bypasses for obesity or inflammatory illnesses of the small bowel such as Crohn disease, may hyperabsorb dietary oxalate. This condition is known as enteric hyperoxaluria. For patients with enteric hyperoxaluria in particular, and for calcium oxalate stone formers in general, diets restricted in oxalate are generally recommended. Double-blind randomized studies have not been done to confirm these recommendations. Foods traditionally restricted include chocolate products, nuts of all types, rhubarb, and dark-green leafy vegetables such as spinach. The bioavailability of oxalate varies from food to food and depends on what other foods are ingested (eg, calcium-containing ones), leaving specific recommendations for dietary oxalate reduction more art than science. Oxalate has no known benefit for humans, although in theory a diet entirely free of oxalate might promote hypercalciuria, another risk factor for stones.

Sugar

There are animal data strongly suggesting that the ingestion of sugar (but not artificial sweeteners) increases hypercalciuria. Human data are sparse. Diets low in sugar are often recommended for the prevention of calcium-containing stones.

Lipids

Lipid disorders are relatively common in kidney diseases. By definition, patients with nephrotic syndrome are hyperlipidemic. Typically, the hyperlipidemia is that of elevated total cholesterol and low-density lipoprotein cholesterol (LDL-C). Frequently, elevated triglycerides and low high-density lipoprotein cholesterol (HDL-C) levels also occur. In chronic renal failure, lipid elevation is also relatively common. Compared with other nutrients, the effect of lipids on progression of renal disease has been reported in a small amount of the literature, which was summarized in a recent meta-analysis.[11] There was a reported lower rate of decline in the glomerular filtration rate in the low cholesterol group treated with 3-hydroxy-3-methylglutaryl coenzyme A (HMG CoA) reduction inhibitors compared with the controls. Although it seems reasonable that cholesterol lowering by dietary methods would give the same results, this has not been shown in a scientific study. Nonetheless, a low-cholesterol diet generally is recommended for patients with nephrotic syndrome and those with progressive renal failure.

Protein

Ingestion of dietary protein promotes hypercalciuria. A diet containing approximately 52 g/d of protein proved superior to a random diet for prevention of nephrolithiasis.[12] Dietary protein consumption has also been studied with respect to progression of renal insufficiency. The largest and best performed study was the Modification of

Diet in Renal Disease (MDRD). Initial analysis of these data failed to find benefit of a low-protein diet over a 2- to 3-year period in slowing the progression of renal disease.[13] However, numerous secondary analyses have been performed. In the aggregate, they tend to show a small beneficial effect of dietary protein restriction in slowing the rate of renal failure.[14,15]

In theory, dietary protein would be expected to worsen renal failure. An increase in dietary protein causes an increase in the glomerular filtration rate because of an increase in glomerular pressure and flow rate. Hyperfiltration causes glomerular damage. As more glomeruli are damaged, the remaining glomeruli need to function at even higher glomerular filtration rates to maintain the status quo. Thus, dietary protein starts a progressive downward spiral of renal failure. Studies to prove the hyperfiltration theory have largely been done in animals. There is no evidence that humans with 2 or even 1 normal kidney are susceptible to hyperfiltration damage. Studies that have found an adverse effect of dietary protein were in patients with moderate to severe renal failure. In standard nephrology practice, low-protein diets are recommended for prevention of calcium-containing nephrolithiasis and in secondary prevention of chronic renal failure.

Salt

Sodium chloride is clearly hypercalciuric in laboratory animals. A recent study confirmed that diets high in sodium and protein were associated with higher rates of stone formation compared with diets restricted in the substances.[12] An increase in dietary salt also increases the urinary excretion of cystine in patients with cystinuria, an unusual genetic error of dibasic amino acid metabolism. Dietary sodium tends to increase blood pressure in approximately one half of our population who are "salt sensitive." The hypertensive effect of sodium is mediated, at least in part, by its osmotic increase in the volume of the extracellular space. Thus, dietary sodium promotes the formation of edema, particularly in patients with a low glomerular filtration rate or with nephrotic syndrome. Clinically, for these reasons, low-sodium diets are commonly recommended as preventive measures in standard nephrology practice.

Diuretics

Many patients and a few physicians believe that diuretics damage renal function. Although this is largely untrue, there are 2 situations in which damage can occur. The first situation occurs when the patient is allergic to the diuretic. An allergic interstitial nephritis has been reported in association with almost all of the thiazide and loop diuretics. Presumably, there is an allergy to the sulfa moiety present in all these drugs. Thus, one would prescribe such diuretics only with great caution in patients who have a known sulfa allergy. Discontinuation of therapy with the offending

drug should allow complete resolution of the acute renal failure. There are anecdotal reports that moderate doses of a glucocorticoid, such as prednisone, 20 mg daily, may hasten the resolution, but there is no good scientific evidence to support this practice.

A second situation wherein diuretics may cause acute or acute on chronic renal failure is when these drugs are overdosed. If the patient loses enough extracellular volume, a situation known as "prerenal" azotemia may develop. As renal perfusion falls, the glomerular filtration rate follows. Since this is a hemodynamic situation, it is potentially entirely reversible if detected before acute tubular necrosis (ATN) supervenes. Treatment involves simply a reduction in dose or temporary cessation of the diuretic with careful rehydration. When used judiciously, diuretics are a trusted tool in nephrology practice and do not worsen renal failure. Carefully prescribed diuretics will relieve the morbidity of mild to moderate edema and the mortality of congestive heart failure and pulmonary edema.

Herbs

Approximately 10% of the American public is reported to use herbal therapy, and this number is growing. Simply because herbs are natural does not mean that they are safe. Just as there are nephrotoxic drugs, there are nephrotoxic herbs. An excellent example is *Aristolochia fangii*.[16] Its use in a Belgian weight loss compound led to multiple cases of renal failure secondary to a tubulo-interstitial fibrosis. Many of these patients progressed to end-stage renal disease. Later, an unusual number of uroepithelial carcinomas were noted in this patient population.[16] Other herbs known to have renal toxicity are noted in Table 55-1.

In the United States, herbs are not subject to US Food and Drug Administration regulations concerning medication. Thus, the quality and quantity of any given herbal preparation may vary not only from one manufacturer to another but also from one lot to another. Additionally, the pharmacokinetics of herbs has been poorly studied. Their renal handling is largely unknown. Because of the potential for decreased excretion in renal failure, the clinician would be wise to discourage the use of herbal products in this population.

Nephrotoxic Drugs

Many medicines have the idiosyncratic potential to cause renal damage. Most of these are dealt with in the Interstitial Nephritis section later in this chapter. Many other drugs need dose modification in renal failure because they are renally metabolized or excreted. Some drugs, however, are inherently nephrotoxic. Examples are the calcineurin inhibitors cyclosporine and tacrolimus.

TABLE 55-1

Herbal Remedies and Their Major Constituents That Potentially Cause Renal Toxicity*

β-Aescin (saponin mixture from horse-chestnut seed)
Cape aloes
Cat's claw
Certain essential oils
Chaparral leaf or stem
Chinese yew
Herbs rich in aristolochic acids
Impila root
Jering fruit
Pennyroyal oil
Squirting cucumber
Star fruit

*Modified from De Smet PAGM. Herbal remedies. *N Engl J Med.* 2002;347:2046-2056. Copyright 2002 Massachusetts Medical Society. All rights reserved. The full version of this table is available from the National Auxiliary Publications Service (NAPS). See NAPS document 05609 for 33 pages of supplementary material. Order from NAPS, c/o Microfiche Publications, 248 Hempstead Turnpike, West Hempstead, NY 11552. Adverse effects of multiple-herb therapies are not included. Case reports do not always provide adequate evidence that the remedy in question was labeled correctly. As a result, it is possible that some of the adverse events reported for a specific herb were actually due to a different, unidentified botanical or another adulterant or contaminant. A single case was reported without reference to previous cases.

Another example is the aminoglycoside class of antibiotics, of which gentamicin is the most commonly used. Other nephrotoxic drugs are amphotericin B and cisplatin. To the extent that use of these drugs can be avoided, kidney damage will be prevented. When the use of such drugs is necessary, careful attention to dosing, determination of serum drug levels when appropriate, and close monitoring of renal function will minimize the chances of renal toxicity.

Nonsteroidal Anti-inflammatory Drugs

Nonsteroidal anti-inflammatory drugs (NSAIDs) have become very popular with the American public. All the NSAIDs are cyclooxygenase inhibitors and decrease the production of renal prostaglandins. On the whole, renal prostaglandins are vasodilatory and therefore affect renal blood flow and glomerular filtration rate.[17] By inhibiting renal prostaglandins, NSAIDs have a renal hemodynamic effect of decreasing renal blood flow and glomerular filtration rate, which is reversible after stopping treatment with the drug. The mechanism that mediates the hemodynamic effect is constriction of the afferent arteriole.

Another universal effect of NSAIDs is renal sodium retention.[17] Again, this is caused by decreased production of renal prostaglandins that tend to be natriuretic. With retention of sodium by the kidney comes retention of water to maintain plasma osmolality. This is also reversible upon stopping the medication regimen. Obviously, the retention of salt and water will antagonize the action of diuretics, including their antihypertensive effect.

Through the above-mentioned effects on renal prostaglandins as well as a tendency to decrease the production of renin and aldosterone, NSAIDs tend to produce a mild renal retention of potassium.[17] This can be important in the presence of preexisting renal insufficiency. There is also an idiosyncratic effect of NSAIDs. Proteinuria will develop in a very small percentage of the population as a result of taking NSAIDs, which can reach nephrotic range. On a renal biopsy specimen, minimal change disease (nil lesion) is usually present. Unlike patients with nil lesion not due to NSAIDs, some of these patients will go on to have chronic renal failure, even to the point of requiring renal replacement therapy. Even this is potentially reversible, although recovery from severe renal failure may take several months.

In clinical nephrology practice, NSAIDs are generally avoided. Obviously, the tendency to decrease renal blood flow and glomerular filtration rate will worsen preexisting renal failure. The tendency to retain salt and water will exacerbate hypertension, which is rampant with renal parenchymal disease, and will worsen the fluid overload that typically occurs with both nephrotic and nephritic syndromes. The fear that NSAIDs will increase proteinuria and worsen renal failure through their idiosyncratic effect is real, although its frequency is probably overestimated. Actually, through decreasing renal blood flow and glomerular filtration rate by constriction of the afferent renal arteriole, proteinuria generally diminishes. At one time, NSAIDs actually were used therapeutically in this regard. However, ACE inhibitors and ARBs are at least as hypoproteinuric as NSAIDs and are preferred because of favorable effects on blood pressure and a better safety profile. For the reasons mentioned earlier, it is easy to see why clinical nephrologists discourage the use of NSAIDs.

Potassium

Hypokalemia is commonly seen in patients receiving diuretics, particularly when they do not follow a dietary sodium restriction. It is generally thought that hypokalemic nephropathy can develop after long periods of sustained hypokalemia. This condition can ultimately progress to renal failure. The patients most at risk are those who abuse diuretics. Typically, these patients are women with idiopathic edema or characteristics of anorexia nervosa who have resorted to diuretics as an aid to weight control. Prevention of hypokalemic nephropathy should be uniformly possible through careful prescribing of diuretics, proper follow-up, instruction in sodium-restricted diets for those receiving diuretics, and, if necessary, the addition of potassium supplements or potassium-sparing agents such as amiloride hydrochloride or triamterene.

Hyperkalemia typically supervenes in severe renal failure. Drugs that cause hyperkalemia include the following:

- ACE inhibitors
- ARBs
- β-blockers
- NSAIDs
- potassium supplements

Although β-blockers, ACE inhibitors, and ARBs tend to worsen hyperkalemia, they play important roles in the treatment of chronic renal failure. Nonsteroidal anti-inflammatory drugs, which also worsen hyperkalemia, have little, if any, role in the treatment of renal diseases and are therefore generally avoided. Hyperkalemia can be ameliorated with a low-potassium diet or diuretics.

Proteinuria

Proteinuria is deleterious to glomerular filtration rate. A small amount of proteinuria in humans is normal. Typically, humans excrete less than 150 mg/d of protein in their urine. The precise threshold above which damage begins to occur is unknown but is generally regarded as approximately 1000 mg/d. It has further been noted that reduction of proteinuria decreases the rate at which glomerular filtration is lost. Thus, the reduction of proteinuria is becoming increasingly important in current practice.[18,19] The drugs of choice to reduce proteinuria are the ACE inhibitors and ARBs (see Fig 55-1). Both of them selectively increase dilation of the efferent renal arteriole. This hemodynamically decreases the intra-glomerular pressure and the glomerular filtration rate. It should be noted that the observed benefits on protection of glomerular filtration rate from ACE inhibitors and ARBs exceed those predicted to occur by reduction of proteinuria alone. Other mechanisms are present, and there are some emerging data that this may be via an antifibrotic action. Although the doses of ACE inhibitors and ARBs necessary to interrupt the positive feedback cycle are unknown and although the level of proteinuria below which no further renal damage is speculative, it is becoming common nephrologic practice to use ACE inhibitors and ARBs to minimize proteinuria.

Smoking Cessation

There are many excellent reasons to discourage the use of tobacco products. It has long been recognized that smoking is a major risk factor for uroepithelial carcinomas. More recently, it has also been recognized that smoking predisposes to the development of hypernephromas. Data are also emerging that smoking accelerates the progression of certain types of chronic renal failure, such as diabetic nephropathy.[20,21] Smoking also appears to be a risk factor in the development of Goodpasture syndrome.

The following section will look at specific renal diseases with an emphasis on secondary prevention.

SECONDARY PREVENTION OF RENAL DISEASES

Analgesic-Associated Nephropathy

The association between heavy analgesic consumption and renal disease has long been recognized. The primary culprit was identified as phenacetin.[22] As the evidence mounted, phenacetin was withdrawn from the market and ultimately banned in westernized countries. Subsequent studies generally showed a decrease, but not elimination, of analgesic-associated nephropathy. The failure of the phenacetin ban to completely resolve the problem raised suspicion that other analgesics, either

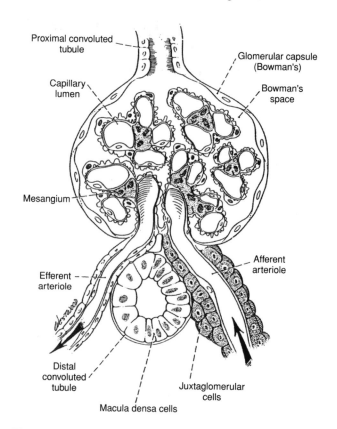

FIGURE 55-1

Anatomy of glomerulus.

Original source: Knox FG. Textbook of renal pathophysiology, 1978. Reprinted by permission from Lippencott, Williams and Wilkins.

alone or in combination, were the cause. The major suspect was acetaminophen, the major metabolite of phenacetin. Studies in this area are difficult to perform because they depend on the patient's history of exposure over many years before the illness becomes clinically apparent. Patients commonly minimize or deny analgesic abuse. Several well-designed studies have found an association between acetaminophen and chronic renal failure.[23,24]

An association between aspirin use and chronic renal failure has also been reported, although the correlation is more tenuous.[25,26] Concerns have also been raised regarding the role of combination analgesics because of the concern that multiple drugs may potentiate each other's toxicities. Again, studies are conflicting. It seems reasonably clear that habitual, heavy use of various analgesics is potentially harmful to kidney function and should be discouraged. Patients with chronic pain problems need to be evaluated by a physician familiar with treatment of chronic pain and managed accordingly. Drugs not related to analgesic nephropathy include propoxyphene, tramadol hydrochloride, and codeine (schedule II drugs). Use of NSAIDs is discouraged for this reason as well as other reasons noted earlier in this chapter.

Renal Cancer

Fortunately, cancer of the kidney accounts for only 2% to 3% of new malignancies in the United States. Approximately 80% of renal cancers are parenchymal (renal cell, also known as hypernephromas). Most of the remainder are in the renal pelvis (transitional cell, also known as uroepithelial). Transitional cell carcinomas predominate in the bladder. The same risk factors and preventive techniques are thought to apply to all uroepithelial malignancies regardless of location.

Renal cell carcinoma

Common risk factors include male sex, black race, obesity, smoking, and hypertension.[27] Renal cell carcinomas are prone to develop in patients with the acquired cystic disease of renal failure and von Hippel-Lindau disease. Although it seems plausible that prevention of hypertension, smoking, and obesity would decrease the incidence of renal cell carcinoma, this has never been tested scientifically. Surgery is the only chance of cure. Surveillance for recurrence typically consists of periodic contrast radiographs.

Transitional cell carcinoma

The major risk factor for transitional cell carcinoma of the renal pelvis is smoking, which is responsible for 40% to 70% of all such cancers. Smoking increases the risk of transitional cell carcinoma approximately threefold over nonsmokers.[28] Other recognized, but less common, risk factors are noted in Table 55-2.[28] Certain analgesics, the

herb *Aristolochia,* and cyclophosphamide are medications that increase transitional cell carcinoma risk. Chronic mechanical irritation of the upper urinary tract is also said to be associated with transitional cell carcinoma, although given the prevalence of stones in the United States, the association must be very weak.

Transitional cell carcinomas of the upper urinary tract are typically discovered through investigation of hematuria. Fortunately, contralateral tumors are rare, occurring in 2% to 4% of cases. Surveillance for recurrence is mandatory, as this tends to be a multicentric carcinoma. Cystoscopy, urine cytology, and contrast radiography of the upper urinary tract are required for surveillance. Avoidance of smoking, occupational exposures, and causative medications should reduce the incidence of transitional cell carcinoma, although this preventive plan has not been tested scientifically.

Interstitial Nephritis

Interstitial nephritis may be a primary or secondary renal disease and can be of an allergic or nonallergic variety. The underlying process can proceed to fibrosis and end-stage renal disease. Broad categories of instigating factors are kidney stones, obstructive uropathies, renal infections, drugs, and electrolyte disturbance, primarily hypercalcemia and hypokalemia. Kidney stones and urinary tract infections will be discussed below. A list of drugs that have been implicated as a cause for interstitial nephritis is provided in Table 55-3. Obviously, when a drug therapy is suspected of causing interstitial nephritis, it should be withdrawn.

Renal Failure

Acute renal failure

Acute renal failure does not have a standard definition. It is characterized by a sudden rise in the serum creatinine or fall in the glomerular filtration rate. Acute renal failure may be the final common pathway for multiple pathophysiologic processes. Acute tubular necrosis occurs when renal arterial blood flow or oxygen tension drops below the levels necessary to sustain renal tubular epithelial cells. Many cases of acute tubular necrosis occur postoperatively. Careful attention to perioperative hydration, blood pressure, and oxygenation have the potential to prevent a substantial amount of ATN. Recovery typically occurs within 6 weeks.

Contrast nephrotoxicity is another form of acute renal failure. It is different from acute tubular necrosis in that typically there is no cell death. Instead, there is an intense vasoconstriction, which usually is reversible within a few days to a week. Only occasional cases progress to end-stage renal failure. As the name implies, contrast nephrotoxicity is caused by the use of high-osmolality

TABLE 55-2

Relative Risks for Development of Transitional Cell Carcinoma of Upper Urinary Tract*

Factor	Relative Risk (odds ratio)
Analgesic abuse	2.4–4.2
Coffee consumption	1.0–1.3
Industrial exposure	
Health care	0.4
Office work	1.0
Metal industries	1.4
Rubber industry	1.6
Paint manufacture	1.8
Leather and tanning	2.2
Chemical, coke (coal residue), and coal industries	4.0
Tobacco	
Never smoked	1.0
Cigars only	1.3
Pipe only	2.2
Cigarettes only	2.6–3.1
Mixed, including cigarettes	3.8
Mixed, excluding cigarettes	6.5

*From Klein EA.[28]

TABLE 55-3

Acute Interstitial Nephritis: Causative Factors*

Antibiotics
  Penicillins
  Rifampin
  Sulfa
  Vancomycin hydrochloride
  Ciprofloxacin
  Cephalosporins E
  Erythromycin
  Minocycline hydrochloride
  Trimethoprim-sulfamethoxazole
  Acyclovir
  Ethambutol hydrochloride
Nonsteroidal anti-inflammatory drugs
Diuretics
  Thiazides
  Furosemide
  Triamterene
Miscellaneous agents
  Captopril
  Cimetidine
  Ranitidine hydrochloride
  Phenobarbital
  Nitrofurantoin
  Phenindione
  Phenytoin
  Allopurinol
  Interferon
  Interleukin-2
  Anti-CD4 antibody
  Hairy vetch poisoning

*Modified with permission from Kelly CJ, Neilson EG. In: Brenner BM, ed. *The Kidney*. 6th ed. Philadelphia, Pa: WB Saunders Co; 2000:1519.

iodinated radiographic contrast agents. Although many risk factors have been described, including age, left ventricular failure, and diabetes, the 2 major ones are preexisting impairment of glomerular filtration rate and decreased intravascular volume. When the serum creatinine level indicates moderate to severe renal failure (roughly greater than 1.5 mg/dL), the clinician and radiologist should carefully assess the risk-to-benefit ratio of the intended procedure. The use of nonionic iodinated contrast material may reduce the risk of contrast nephrotoxicity. Careful precontrast hydration is essential. Diuretics should be used with care or not at all to avoid dehydration. Multiple drugs have been tried to prevent contrast nephrotoxicity and, essentially, all have failed.

Nonsteroidal anti-inflammatory drugs also predispose an individual to acute renal failure. The typical clinical scenarios where this may occur are in patients with severe congestive heart failure or intravascular volume depletion. Nonsteroidal anti-inflammatory drugs inhibit the production of vasodilatory renal prostaglandins at a time when they are most necessary. Clearly, NSAIDs should be withheld in the event of renal hypoperfusion.

Chronic renal failure

Chronic renal failure is the final common pathway for a wide variety of primary and systemic diseases affecting the kidney. After the initial injury, renal disease may progress in the absence of ongoing injury. The processes at work seem to be increased glomerular pressures and heavy proteinuria. These pathophysiologic processes create a positive feedback loop, wherein injury begets increased glomerular pressures and proteinuria, which in turn produce more injury. For the purposes of discussion, chronic renal failure will be considered as due to either diabetic or nondiabetic causes.

Diabetic nephropathy. With the advent of insulin, type 1 diabetes was no longer a rapidly fatal illness. However, it soon became apparent that insulin was not a cure for diabetes. Microvascular and macrovascular complications occurred. Microvascular complications include neuropathy, retinopathy, and nephropathy. Macrovascular complications are those of atherosclerosis. The Diabetes Control and Complications Trial showed a reduction in the microvascular but not macrovascular complications of diabetes with tight glycemic control.[29] At this point it appeared possible to prevent the development of diabetic nephropathy in many patients. However, once established, diabetic nephropathy still invariably progressed to end-stage renal disease (see Fig. 55-2).

The next major improvement in the prevention of diabetic nephropathy was the use of ACE inhibitors. Not only did the agents reduce blood pressure but they markedly decreased proteinuria, a hallmark of diabetic nephropathy, and slowed progression to end-stage renal disease. In recent years, several papers have appeared showing that in a subgroup of patients with type 1 diabetic nephropathy, tight blood pressure control over a period of several years will cause a remission and even a regression in diabetic nephropathy.[30-32]

Type 2 diabetes typically develops at later ages than does type 1 diabetes. Patients with type 2 diabetes are characteristically more obese and sedentary. However, they have in common the same microvascular and macrovascular complications. In type 2 diabetes as well, tight glucose control will minimize the risk of microvascular complications. Tight glucose control can often be

achieved with oral hypoglycemic agents, although some patients with type 2 diabetes will require insulin, especially as they approach end-stage renal disease. Both ACE inhibitors and ARBs are effective in reducing hypertension and proteinuria.[33,34] The data for the use of ARBs in type 2 diabetes are stronger than for type 1 diabetes.[35-37] However, because of the beneficial effect of ACE inhibitors on cardiovascular mortality in type 2 diabetes, a nephrologist typically will start patients with type 2 diabetes on treatment with an ACE inhibitor.[38] Angiotensin receptor blockers tend to be reserved in current practice for those who do not tolerate ACE inhibitors.

Compared with only 10 years ago, there is a great deal nephrologists have to offer both for primary and secondary prevention of type 1 and type 2 diabetic nephropathy. There are data to support starting patients with type 1 diabetes on treatment with ACE inhibitors at first presentation of the illness, even if they are not hypertensive. It is also common practice to start a patient with type 2 diabetes on treatment with an ACE inhibitor when diabetes is first detected. Most of the time these patients will already be hypertensive. If not already on an ACE inhibitor, a diabetic patient should have his or her microalbumin level monitored closely and start ACE inhibitor therapy in the event of microalbuminuria. Tight

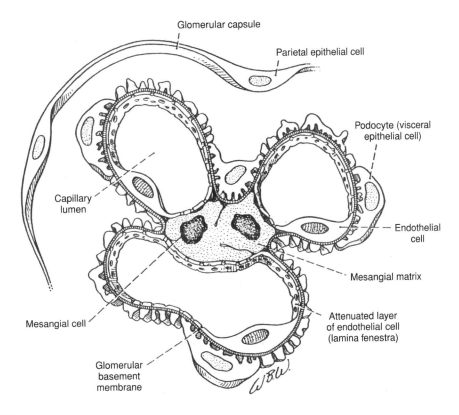

FIGURE 55-2

A portion of a glomerular lobule.

Original source: Knox FG. Textbook of renal pathophysiology, 1978. Reprinted by permission from Lippencott, Williams and Wilkins.

blood pressure control and maximal lowering of protein-uria with ACE inhibitors or ARBs may induce remission or even regression of established diabetic nephropathy. The question as to whether there is an advantage of combining an ACE inhibitor with an ARB is not yet satis-factorily answered, but evidence to date suggests a mild additive effect. As noted earlier, the clinician needs to be alert for the development of hyperkalemia with the use of ACE inhibitors or ARBs. As previously mentioned, there is limited evidence that control of hyperlipidemia, antico-agulation with aspirin, and possibly use of antioxidants might confer additional benefit. Clearly, smoking should be strongly discouraged in this patient population.

Nondiabetic nephropathy.   There are scant data to sepa-rate the preventive treatment of the different types of nondiabetic nephropathy. This section will combine hypertensive, nephrotic, and nephritic causes. Features of nephrotic syndrome are as follows:

- proteinuria more than 3.0 g/24 h
- hypoalbuminemia
- hyperlipidemia

Features of nephritic syndrome are glomerular hema-turia (dysmorphic red cells, red cell/hemoglobin casts) and hypertension.

Polycystic kidney disease will be covered separately, and other hereditary nephritides will be omitted for lack of effective prevention. Presently, there are 2 basic approaches a clinician can take. Most of the nephrotic and nephritic renal diseases have potentially curative therapy. Although description of these treatment regimens is beyond the scope of this chapter, generally these pro-grams include a combination of a corticosteroid, such as prednisone, with a cytotoxic agent, such as cyclophos-phamide. In more recent years, immune-modulating agents, such as cyclosporine, and mycophenolate mofetil have established themselves in some curative treatment regimens. The programs, however, are still very blunt instruments and predictably cause substantial toxicity without guarantee of improvement. Therefore, this author strongly recommends that such treatment programs be undertaken only under the supervision of an experienced clinical nephrologist.

The second treatment approach is within the realm of nearly all practicing physicians. It involves breaking the cycle of hypertension and proteinuria that so often propels the patient to end-stage renal disease even if the primary injury has resolved. As with the treatment of diabetic nephropathy, ACE inhibitors and ARBs are a cornerstone of therapy. These agents are preferentially started as first-line drugs for the treatment of hypertension, and the dose is titrated upward to minimize proteinuria if present. As is also true with the treatment of diabetic nephropathy, prolonged tight control of blood pressure and reduction of proteinuria may actually induce disease remission in a

subset of these patients.[39-41] As with diabetes, a multifac-eted treatment approach may offer further benefit.[42-44] Smoking cessation, reduction of dietary salt and protein, effective treatment of hyperlipidemia with a statin and possibly low-dose aspirin therapy, and the use of antioxi-dants all have some evidence to support their use.

Polycystic Kidney Disease

The discovery of the genes for type 1 and type 2 auto-somal dominant polycystic kidney disease and their gene products, known as polycystin 1 and 2, has greatly enhanced the probability of primary or secondary preven-tion for this relatively common genetic disease.[45] At this point, the single best preventive measure there is to offer for progression of renal failure due to polycystic kidney disease is control of nearly universally present hyperten-sion. If renal insufficiency is present, the targeted blood pressure should be 130/85 mm Hg or below. Unlike with diabetic or nondiabetic nephropathies, ACE inhibitors and ARBs do not appear to be any more effective than other agents, probably because proteinuria is typically minimal. Avoidance of instrumentation to prevent renal parenchymal or cyst infections is advisable. Smoking should be strongly discouraged. Low-dose aspirin may be avoided for fear of inciting cyst hemorrhage. Cere-bral aneurysms occur in 5% of patients but tend to cluster in families. A family history of aneurysm or hemor-rhagic stroke should prompt a cerebral magnetic resonance angiogram.[46]

Stones

Nephrolithiasis is the final common pathway for super-saturated crystal systems. Usually this occurs when the mineral component is excreted into the urine in excessive amounts, when there is a low urine volume in which to dissolve it, or a combination of these 2 factors. However, in the calcium crystal systems, there may also be the lack of naturally occurring inhibitors of crystallization. The most therapeutically relevant of these is citrate. In west-ernized society, kidney stones are very common and are caused by lifestyle, metabolic, and genetic factors. The most common type of kidney stone composition is cal-cium oxalate, generally with variable amounts of calcium phosphate. These stones account for roughly 70% of the total. Relatively pure calcium phosphate stones comprise roughly 10%, uric acid stones another 10%, and struvite stones the remaining 10%. Cystine and a multitude of even rarer stones comprise 1% or less of the total stone production.

Prevention of stones is best guided by their composi-tion. Stone composition is most easily ascertained by analysis of a captured stone or stone fragment. When these data are not available, one can make an educated guess as to the stone composition by looking at which crystal systems are supersaturated in a 24-hour urine collection. Other clues as to stone composition come from the individual urinary analytes and radiographic appearance. Major stone types will be discussed here in terms of prevention.

Calcium oxalate

It is a rare stone former who cannot lessen his or her chance of stone recurrence by increasing urine volume. Multiple studies provide a scientific basis for this seemingly obvious recommendation.[47,48] The concern that a large urine volume would dilute naturally occurring inhibitors of crystallization has proved untrue. In this author's opinion, probably the single largest risk factor for the production of calcium oxalate stones is a diet high in animal protein. Stone formers seem excessively sensitive to such a diet in terms of developing hypercalciuria. This diet also promotes hyperuricosuria, which is a risk factor for both calcium oxalate and uric acid nephrolithiasis. It also indirectly increases hyperoxaluria. A high-protein diet tends to lower urinary pH, which will increase the supersaturation of organic acids, which at least hypothetically can cause a nidus around which a calcium oxalate stone may form.

Diets low in animal protein have been shown to reduce the risk of calcium-containing nephrolithiasis.[49,50] Diets high in sodium have also been shown to promote hypercalciuria, and reduction of dietary sodium has been shown to prevent calcium stones. Hypercalciuria, a risk factor for the development of calcium stones, can be counteracted directly with thiazide diuretics. Hyperuricosuria, another risk factor for calcium oxalate stones, can be reduced with allopurinol. Hypocitraturia, yet another risk factor for calcium stone production, can be improved with the addition of potassium citrate supplementation. Hyperoxaluria may be reduced by the judicious use of dietary calcium supplementation (to promote gastrointestinal oxalate binding) and a low-oxalate diet. Finally, evidence has shown that the time-honored advice for calcium stone formers to follow a low-calcium diet is bad advice. A progressive decrease in the risk of stone formation occurs with calcium consumption up to about 1200 mg/d. It is still theoretically possible that extremely high-calcium diets may be lithogenic. The author does not use sodium cellulose phosphate to lower hypercalciuria because it causes hyperoxaluria and hypomagnesuria, both risk factors for stone formation. Neither does the author use magnesium salts for calcium stone prevention because of their laxative effect predisposing to chronic diarrhea, which increases the risk of stone formation.

Calcium phosphate

Calcium phosphate is soluble in urine of normal pH. The formation of calcium phosphate stones implies a relatively alkaline urine. This situation can occur with the ingestion of absorbable alkali, such as Tums, Rolaids, Alka Seltzer, and sodium bicarbonate. Metabolic causes of calcium phosphate stones include distal renal tubular acidosis, which can be treated with supplemental alkali, and primary hyperparathyroidism, which can be treated by removal of the overactive tissue. In idiopathic cases, anecdotal evidence suggests the efficacy of urinary acidification with ammonium chloride.

Uric acid

Contrary to calcium phosphate stones, the discovery of uric acid nephrolithiasis indicates an unusually acid urine pH. In fact, three fourths of uric acid stone formers have normal uricosuria. Only one fourth of the uric acid stone formers consume excess purines. For the prevention of uric acid stones in these patients, a diet low in purine is strongly indicated. Allopurinol may be a useful adjunct. For patients with unusually acidic urine, urinary alkalinization with potassium citrate is the most rational treatment.

Struvite

Struvite nephrolithiasis is proof of a urease-producing urinary tract infection. Urease splits urea, normally present in urine, into ammonium. This raises the urinary pH with the precipitation of calcium magnesium ammonium phosphate (triple phosphate). The appropriate treatment for struvite stones is that of an infected foreign body: removal. If this is not possible or fragments are left postoperatively, the infection can be suppressed with long-term, low-dose antibiotic therapy based on antimicrobial sensitivity of the organism. Acetohydroxamic acid is another treatment that inhibits bacterial urease. Unfortunately, this medication increases the risk of deep venous thrombosis. Thus, its use in patients with paraplegia, a common population for struvite stones, is relatively contraindicated.

Cystine

Typically, heterozygotes for cystinuria do not excrete enough cystine into the urine to be stone formers, with occasional exceptions. The amount of cystine excreted is somewhat dependent on the dietary content of methionine, its precursor, as well as sodium. Thus, a diet to minimize the urinary excretion of cystine in affected patients will be low in sodium and protein. The excretion of cystine also can be decreased by the use of D-penicillamine or tiopronin. Because the solubility of cystine in urine increases rapidly above a pH of 7.0, aggressive urinary alkalinization is a mainstay in the prevention of cystine stones.

Urinary Tract Infections

Except at the very beginning and terminal years of life, women are much more prone to the development of urinary tract infections. This is because of the anatomical proximity of the female anus and urethral meatus. Symptomatically, most urinary tract infections seem to be confined to the bladder. However, there is a subset of patients who seem particularly prone to upper urinary tract infections. There are host factors that allow bacterial fimbria to adhere to the uroepithelium. Otherwise, urinary colonization is cleared within a day or two by voiding. Urinary colonization appears to occur relatively frequently. Trauma to the female urethra, such as during vaginal intercourse, regularly causes bladder colonization. In addition to the host factors that govern bacterial adhesion, other risk factors for the development of symptomatic urinary tract infection include vesicoureteral reflux, obstructive uropathy, neurogenic bladder, and pregnancy. One study showed that a decreased frequency of bladder emptying, whether because of low fluid intake or deferred micturition, resulted in an increased frequency of urinary tract infection.[51]

Prevention of urinary tract infection may include various hygienic measures to avoid spreading colonic flora toward the female vulva. However, the effectiveness of these measures has not undergone rigorous scientific testing. Urging patients to void at least every 3 hours has been shown to decrease the incidence of urinary tract infection.[51] The daily use of estrogen cream in the vagina of postmenopausal women may be helpful.[52] The most effective prevention of urinary tract infection, however, is antibiotic prophylaxis. Effective prophylaxis can be given to a woman as a single dose immediately after vaginal intercourse or as nightly, long-term, low-dose therapy.[53]

Sulfamethoxazole-trimethoprim, plain trimethoprim, cephalosporins, nitrofurantoin, and nalidixic acid have been shown to be efficacious in the prevention of recurrent urinary tract infections.[54,55] Typically, treatment is given for 6 months and then discontinued. Reinfection should prompt reinstitution of treatment, preferably for 2 more years.

The fact that urinary tract infections can be prevented does not answer the question whether urinary tract infections *should* be prevented. A cost-benefit analysis has suggested that women who have 3 or more symptomatic urinary tract infections a year benefit from antibiotic prophylaxis. Scientific studies have also shown that the treatment of asymptomatic urinary tract infections in debilitated nursing home residents and diabetic outpatients does not influence morbidity or mortality.[56,57] The exception is in the pregnant diabetic female, in whom acute pyelonephritis is more likely to develop.

Acknowledgment: The author thanks Donna Bamlet for her expert secretarial assistance in the preparation of the chapter manuscript.

REFERENCES

1. Jepson RG, Mihaljevic L, Craig J. Cranberries for preventing urinary-tract infections. *Cochrane Database System Rev.* 2001;(3):CD001321.

2. Alschuler M, Ring M. Cranberry (*Vaccinium macrocarpon*) and urinary tract infection. *Alternative Med Alert.* 2002;5(11):125–136.

3. Palmer BF. Renal dysfunction complicating the treatment of hypertension. *N Engl J Med.* 2002;347:1256–1262.

4. Craven PA, Derubertis FR, Kagan VE, Melhem M, Studer RK. Effects of supplementation with vitamin C or E on albuminuria, glomerular TGF-, and glomerular size in diabetes. *J Am Soc Nephrol.* 1997;8:1405–1414.

5. Koya D, Lee In-Kyu, Ishii H, Kanoh H, King GL. Prevention of glomerular dysfunction in diabetic rats by treatment with a D-tocopherol. *JASN.* 1997;8:426–435.

6. The Seventh Report of the Joint National Committee on Prevention, Detection, Evaluation, and Treatment of High Blood Pressure. *JAMA.* 2003;289:2560–2572.

7. Hansson L, Zanchetti A, Carruthers SG, et al. Effects of intensive blood-pressure lowering and low-dose aspirin in patients with hypertension: principal results in the Hypertension Optimal Treatment (HOT) randomised trial. *Lancet.* 1998;351:1755–1762.

8. Bakris GL, Williams M, Dworkin L, et al, for National Kidney Foundation Hypertension and Diabetes Executive Committees Working Group. Preserving renal function in adults with hypertension and diabetes: a consensus approach. *Am J Kidney Dis.* 2000;36:646–661.

9. Curhan GC, Willett WC, Rimm EB, Stampfer MJ. A prospective study of dietary calcium and other nutrients and the risk of symptomatic kidney stones. *N Engl J Med.* 1993;328:833–838.

10. Curhan GC, Willett WC, et al. Comparison of dietary calcium with supplemental calcium and other nutrients as factors affecting the risk for kidney stones in women. *Ann Intern Med.* 1997;126:497–504.

11. Fried LF, Orchard TJ, Kasiske BL, for Lipids and Renal Disease Progression Meta-Analysis Study Group. Effect of lipid reduction on the progression of renal disease: a meta-analysis. *Kidney Int.* 2001;59:260–269.

12. Borghi L, Schianchi T, Meschi T, Guerra A. Comparison of two diets for the prevention of recurrent stones in idiopathic hypercalciuria. *N Engl J Med.* 2002;346:77–84.

13. Klahr S, Levey AS, Beck GJ, et al. The effects of dietary protein restriction and blood-pressure control on the progression of chronic renal disease. *N Engl J Med.* 1994;330:877–884.

14. Levey AS, Adler S, Caggiula AW. Effects of dietary protein restriction on the progression of moderate renal disease in the modification of diet in renal disease study. *JASN.* 1996;7:2616–2626.

15. Levey AS, Greene T, Beck GJ, et al. Dietary protein restriction and the progression of chronic renal disease: what have all the results of the MDRD study shown? *JASN.* 1999;10:2426–2439.

16. Yang CS, Lin CH, Chang SH, Hsu HC. Rapidly progressive fibrosing interstitial nephritis associated with Chinese herbal drugs. *Am J Kidney Dis.* 2000;35:313–318.

17. Schlondorff D. Renal complications of nonsteroidal anti-inflammatory drugs. *Kidney Int.* 1993;44:643–653.

18. Remuzzi G, et al. Understanding the nature of renal disease progression: in proteinuric nephropathies enhanced glomerular protein traffic contributes to interstitial inflammation and renal scarring. *Kidney Int.* 1997;51:2–15.

19. Keane WF, Eknoyan G. Proteinuria, albuminuria, risk, assessment, detection, elimination (PARADE): a position paper of the National Kidney Foundation. *Am J Kidney Dis.* 1999;33:1004–1010.

20. Orth SR, Stockmann A, et al. Smoking as a risk factor for end-stage renal failure in men with primary renal disease. *Kidney Int.* 1998;54:926–931.

21. Orth SR, Ritz E, Schrier RW. The renal risks of smoking. *Kidney Int.* 1997;51:1669–1677.

22. Dubach UC, Rosner B, Pfister E. Epidemiologic study of abuse of analgesics containing phenacetin. *N Engl J Med.* 1983;308:357–362.

23. Dubach UC, Rosner B, Sturmer T. An epidemiologic study of abuse of analgesic drugs. *N Engl J Med.* 1991;324:155–160.

24. Sandler DP, Smith JC, Weinberg CR, et al. Analgesic use and chronic renal disease. *N Engl J Med.* 1989;320:1238–1243.

25. Perneger TV, Whelton PK, Klag MJ. Risk of kidney failure associated with the use of acetaminophen, aspirin, and nonsteroidal anti-inflammatory drugs. *N Engl J Med.* 1994;331:1675–1679.

26. Fored CM, Ejerblad E, Lindblad P, et al. Acetaminophen, aspirin, and chronic renal failure. *N Engl J Med.* 2001;345:1801–1808.

27. Chow WH, Gridley G, Fraumeni JF, Jarvholm B. Obesity, hypertension, and the risk of kidney cancer in men. *N Engl J Med.* 2000;343:1305–1312.

28. Klein EA. Cancers of the kidney and bladder. In: Matzen RN, Lang R, Mayshark C, eds. *Clinical Preventive Medicine.* St Louis, Mo: Mosby; 1993:965–972.

29. The Diabetes Control and Complications Trial Research Group. The effect of intensive treatment of diabetes on the development and progression of long-term complications in insulin dependent diabetes mellitus. *N Engl J Med.* 1993;329:977–986.

30. Wilmer WA, Hebert LA, et al. Remission of nephrotic syndrome in type 1 diabetes: long-term follow-up of patients in the captopril study. *Am J Kidney Dis.* 1999;34:308–314.

31. Lewis JB, Berl T, et al. Effect of intensive blood pressure control on the course of type 1 diabetic nephropathy. *Am J Kidney Dis.* 1999;34:809–817.

32. Hovind P, Rossing P, Tamow L, Smidt UM, Parving HH. Remission and regression in the nephropathy of type 1 diabetes when blood pressure is controlled aggressively. *Kidney Int.* 2001;60:277–283.

33. Lacourciere Y, Belanger A, et al. Long-term comparison of losartan and enalapril on kidney function in hypertensive type 2 diabetics with early nephropathy. *Kidney Int.* 2000;58:762–769.

34. Kasiske BL, Kalil RS, Ma JZ, Liao M, Keane WF. Effect of antihypertensive therapy on the kidney in patients with diabetes: a meta-regression analysis. *Ann Intern Med.* 1993;118:129–138.

35. Brenner BM, Cooper ME, et al. Effects of losartan on renal and cardiovascular outcomes in patients with type 2 diabetes and nephropathy. *N Engl J Med.* 2001;345:861–868.

36. Parving HH, Lehnert H, et al. The effect of irbesartan on the development of diabetic nephropathy in patients with type 2 diabetes. *N Engl J Med.* 2001;345:870–878.

37. Lewis EJ, Hunsicker LG, et al. Renoprotective effect of the angiotensin-receptor antagonist irbesartan in patients with nephropathy due to type 2 diabetes. *N Engl J Med.* 2001;345:851–860.

38. The Heart Outcomes Prevention Evaluation Study Investigators. Effects of an angiotensin-converting-enzyme inhibitor, ramipril, on cardiovascular events in high-risk patients. *N Engl J Med.* 2000;342:145–153.

39. Remuzzi G, Ruggenenti P, Perico N. Chronic renal diseases: renoprotective benefits of renin-angiotensin system inhibition. *Ann Intern Med.* 2002;136:604–615.

40. Jafar TH, Schmid CH, et al. Angiotensin-converting enzyme inhibitors and progression of nondiabetic renal disease. *Ann Intern Med.* 2001;135:73–87.

41. Ruggenenti P, Perna A, et al. In chronic nephropathies prolonged ACE inhibition can induce remission: dynamics of time-dependent changes in GFR. *JASN.* 1999;10:997–1006.

42. Levey AS. Nondiabetic kidney disease. *N Engl J Med.* 2002;347:1505–1511.

43. Zoja C, Coma D, et al. How to fully protect the kidney in a severe model of progressive nephropathy: a multidrug approach. *JASN.* 2002;13:2898–2908.

44. Hebert LA, Wilmer WA, et al. Renoprotection: one or many therapies? *Kidney International,* 2001;59:1211–1226.

45. Igarashi P, Somlo S. Genetics and pathogenesis of polycystic kidney disease. *JASN.* 2002;13:2384-2398.

46. Huston J, Torres VE, Sulivan PP, Offord KP, Wiebers DO. Value of magnetic resonance angiography for the detection of intracranial aneurysms in autosomal dominant polycystic kidney disease. *JASN.* 1993;3:1871–1877.

47. Curhan GC, Willett WC, Rimm EB, Spiegelman D, Stampfer MJ. Prospective study of beverage use and the risk of kidney stones. *Am J Epidemiol.* 1996;143:240–247.

48. Curhan GC, Willett WC, Speizer FE, Stampfer MJ. Beverage use and risk for kidney stones in women. *Ann Intern Med.* 1998;128:534–540.

49. Rotily M, Leonetti F, et al. Effects of low animal protein or high-fiber diets on urine composition in calcium nephrolithiasis. *Kidney Int.* 2000;57:1115–1123.

50. Hiatt RA, Ettinger B, Caan B, Quesenberry CP, Duncan D, Citron JT. Randomized controlled trial of a low animal protein, high fiber diet in the prevention of recurrent calcium oxalate kidney stones. *Am J Epidemiol.* 1996;144:25–33.

51. Adatto K, Doebele KG, Galland L, Granowetter L. Behavorial factors and urinary tract infection. *JAMA.* 1979;241:2525–2526.

52. Raz R, Stamm WE. A controlled trial of intravaginal estriol in postmenopausal women with recurrent urinary tract infections. *N Engl J Med.* 1993;329:753–756.

53. Vosti KL. Recurrent urinary tract infections. *JAMA.* 1975;231:934–940.

54. Stamm WE, Counts GW, et al. Antimicrobial prophylaxis of recurrent urinary tract infections. *Ann Intern Med.* 1980;92:770–775.

55. Stamm WE. Prevention of urinary tract infections. *Am J Med.* 1984;148–154.

56. Nordenstam GR, Brandberg CA, et al. Bacteriuria and mortality in an elderly population. *N Engl J Med.* 1986;314:1152–1156.

57. Harding GKM, Zhanel GG, Nicolle LE, Cheang M. Antimicrobial treatment in diabetic women with asymptomatic bacteriuria. *N Engl J Med.* 2002;347:1576–1583.

RESOURCES

American Society of Nephrology.
Web site: www.asn-online.org/

International Society of Nephrology.
Web site: www.isn-online.org/

Report of the Seventh Joint National Committee on Treatment of Hypertension.
Web site: www.nhlbi.nih.gov/guidelines/hypertension/

chapter 56

Musculoskeletal Disorders

Daniel J. Mazanec, MD, and Peter Sinks, MD

INTRODUCTION

Musculoskeletal disorders are the most common cause of functional impairment and disability in the United States. More than 7 million Americans report impairment in performance of daily activities because of arthritis.[1] With an aging population, this number is expected to approach 12 million persons by 2020. Presently, approximately 21 million Americans have osteoarthritis.[2] A review of chronic conditions causing disability ranked arthritis as number 1 and back pain as number 2, accounting for almost one third of all disability.[3] The annual incidence of low back pain in the US population is 5%.[4] Nonarticular rheumatic complaints ranging from shoulder pain to plantar fasciitis account for substantial morbidity in the working and nonworking populations as well.

OSTEOARTHRITIS

Epidemiology

Osteoarthritis (degenerative joint disease) is the most common form of arthritis. The disease is recognized by the presence of typical symptoms—joint pain, stiffness, and swelling—and confirmed radiographically by the presence of joint space narrowing, osteophyte formation, and subchondral sclerosis. Many people with radiographic changes of degenerative joint disease are asymptomatic. The prevalence of degenerative joint disease increases with age—twofold to tenfold between the ages of 30 and 65 years.[5] By age 65 years, 11% of persons have symptoms of knee osteoarthritis.[6] Almost 3 times as many individuals older than age 65 years have radiographic evidence of the disease.[7] Before age 50 years, the prevalence of osteoarthritis in most joints is more common in men, whereas after 50, women are more commonly affected with hand, foot, and knee disease.[8]

Although osteoarthritis can affect virtually any joint, involvement of the knees or hips probably accounts for most of the functional disability related to the condition. Osteoarthritis of the hips or knees is the most common reason persons over 65 years old have difficulty with walking or stairs[9] and is the most common indication for total knee or hip replacement surgery.[8]

Pathogenesis and Risk Factors

The pathogenesis of osteoarthritis involves systemic and local (mechanical) factors. Mechanisms of degenerative disease in the small joints of the hands and wrists are different from larger weight-bearing joints. Systemic factors in pathogenesis include ethnicity and genetics, age and sex, nutrition, hormones, and bone density.[6] Local contributors to pathogenesis of degenerative joint disease include joint injury or congenital abnormality, periarticular ligamentous or muscular weakness, repetitive overuse of the joint, and obesity.

Genetic factors play a significant role in osteoarthritis, particularly in the hands and hips.[10] Features suggestive of a strong genetic basis for osteoarthritis include early or premature onset of the disease in some families; polyarticular involvement, especially including the hands; and ethnic or racial differences in severity and prevalence of disease. For example, Asian Americans have a much lower rate of total hip replacement than do other groups.[11] Genetic factors may be more important in women than men.[12]

Free oxygen radicals and other oxidants may play a role in the pathogenesis of osteoarthritis. In the Framingham study, persons in the lowest tertile of vitamin C consumption were noted to have a 3 times greater risk of osteoarthritic progression in the knee than persons in the highest tertile.[13] In this study, however, vitamin E, another potent dietary antioxidant, was not associated with lower osteoarthritis risk. Even stronger evidence suggests that vitamin D is important in protecting against incident and progressive osteoarthritis, particularly in the hip.[14] Vitamin D is required for normal bone metabolism, including remodeling. In addition, vitamin D may have direct effects on chondrocytes in osteoarthritic cartilage.[12] Subjects in the Framingham study who were in the lower tertile for vitamin D intake were at significantly greater risk of progression of osteoarthritis.[15]

Numerous studies have reported an inverse relationship between estrogen use in women and osteoarthritis.[6] Somewhat paradoxically, however, osteoarthritis is also inversely associated with osteoporosis.[8] Interestingly, data from the Framingham study suggest that although higher bone density is associated with increased risk of osteoarthritis, it may also protect against radiographically proven progression of degenerative disease.[16] It has been proposed that osteoporotic bone is more deformable and, therefore, more resistant to mechanical stresses associated with osteoarthritis. Alternatively, bone growth factors might be a common factor responsible for superior bone density as well as tendency to osteophyte formation.

Antecedent hip or knee injury is strongly associated with development of osteoarthritis. Previous hip injury increases the risk of subsequent hip osteoarthritis fourfold.[17] Men with a history of previous knee injury—anterior cruciate or meniscal tears—have a 5 to 6 times increased risk of osteoarthritis.[18] A history of a severe knee or hip injury as a young adult increases the risk of subsequent osteoarthritis at that site by threefold to fivefold.[19] Developmental or congenital joint dysplasias are strongly associated with osteoarthritis development in the affected joints. Risk of posttraumatic osteoarthritis is increased by obesity, high levels of physical activity, joint surface incongruity, and joint instability.[8] Although quadriceps muscle weakness may occur in association with existing knee osteoarthritis as a result of disuse atrophy, it is also a risk factor for degenerative joint disease itself.[20] Adequate muscular strength and balance support joint stability and attenuate joint impact loading.[21]

Regular sports participation, particularly at the top level in soccer or running, is associated with increased risk of osteoarthritis in the weight-bearing joints.[22-24] Risk factors for sport-related osteoarthritis include higher levels of participation, sports that involve rapid acceleration and deceleration such as track and field or tennis, a prior sport-related injury, and an occupation with high physical demands.[25] The presence of biomechanical abnormality or anatomical variance may increase further the risk of osteoarthritis. These anatomical risk factors include knee valgus or varus deformity, leg length discrepancy, or mild hip dysplasia.[26] Moderate, regular, high-impact recreational activities such as jogging or running do not appear to increase the risk of knee or hip osteoarthritis.[27,28]

Occupational risk factors are particularly important in the genesis of hip and knee osteoarthritis in men, in whom work-related joint stress may be responsible for almost one third of knee osteoarthritis.[29] Risk factors include repetitive bending, lifting, squatting, and heavy lifting. Farming, for example, is associated with a significant increase in hip osteoarthritis.[30] Osteoarthritis of smaller hand joints may be accelerated in occupations requiring repetitive grasping or pinching.

Obesity is clearly associated with osteoarthritis of the hips and knees.[17,31,32] The association is stronger with knee arthritis than hip osteoarthritis and greater in women than men. In persons with existing osteoarthritis, obesity increases the risk of disease progression shown radiographically.[33] The effect of obesity on joint integrity is probably related to the fact that with weight-bearing activity, 3 times a person's body weight is transmitted directly to the knees and hips.[12] An alternative explanation for the effect of obesity on arthritis risk beyond purely increased mechanical stress is suggested by the association of obesity with hand osteoarthritis.[6] Production of a "metabolic" factor by adipose tissue deleterious to cartilage has been proposed. Weight change significantly affects the risk of osteoarthritis developing in the knee. Data from the Framingham study suggest that weight loss of 5.1 kg over 10 years decreased the risk of symptomatic osteoarthritis by over 50%.[34]

Prevention

Primary prevention of osteoarthritis focuses on addressing the major modifiable risk factors, including obesity, joint injury, and occupational overuse. Even modest weight reduction significantly reduces the risk of osteoarthritis of the knee. Avoiding joint injury, particularly in the middle-aged athlete, clearly reduces arthritis risk in weight-bearing joints. This may be achieved by maintaining muscular strength and tone, reducing abnormal, fatigue-related joint stress. Appropriate training, warm-up, and equipment may reduce the risk of injury. Alternating activities with different joint loading patterns may further decrease the stress on joints at risk.[25] Finally, careful rehabilitation of articular injuries, including modification of subsequent sports activities, is crucial to reducing the possibility of posttraumatic degenerative joint disease. Early recognition of joint instability and prompt repair should reduce the chances of secondary osteoarthritis. For example, unrecognized rotator cuff tear with abnormal glenohumeral motion may result in cuff tear arthropathy, a condition of severe, almost Charcot-like degenerative joint disease.[35] A similar situation may occur in a knee rendered unstable by severe meniscal or cruciate injury. In the occupational realm, modification and rotation of job tasks to minimize repetitive stress and heavy lifting are reasonable but untested strategies to lessen the likelihood of osteoarthritis in weight-bearing joints.

Based on the Framingham data reviewed earlier, the potential benefit of vitamin D and vitamin C supplementation for osteoarthritis prophylaxis deserves consideration. Clearly further study is required to define more precisely the clinical parameters of this approach. Similarly, the role of estrogen in osteoarthritis prevention in women needs further study before a definitive recommendation can be made.

Glucosamine, a constituent of proteoglycan found in articular cartilage, has been proposed as an agent to retard development or progression of osteoarthritis. Loss of cartilage matrix, including proteoglycan, is characteristic of degenerative joint disease. Exogenous glucosamine may be incorporated into joint cartilage as well as stimulate additional proteoglycan synthesis.[36] Recent reviews have suggested that glucosamine is as effective as ibuprofen in symptomatic treatment of osteoarthritis.[36] More importantly, from a preventive standpoint, a recent 3-year, placebo-controlled clinical trial in patients with severe knee osteoarthritis found less progression of disease in patients receiving 1500 mg of glucosamine daily.[37] Further confirmatory studies are necessary to validate this finding.

THE PAINFUL SHOULDER

Although shoulder pain can originate from the glenohumeral joint itself or from extra-articular sites such as with cervical radiculopathy or diaphragmatic irritation, 90% of nontraumatic shoulder pain is a result of inflammation of the rotator cuff and associated subacromial bursa.[38] The supraspinous tendon and the tendon of the biceps muscle are most vulnerable to trauma or impingement between the head of the humerus and the coracoacromial arch. When the arm is raised to the position in which most upper extremity functions are performed, with the hand in front of the shoulder, the supraspinatus passes under the anterior edge of the acromion and the acromioclavicular joint.[39] Repetitive motions or overuse of the upper extremity may result in injury with edema and swelling in the cuff tendons. The pain of impingement syndrome is usually anterolateral and may extend down the lateral arm. Diagnosis is confirmed by the presence of a positive impingement sign. This is demonstrated with the examiner behind the patient, using one hand to prevent scapular rotation while the other hand raises the arm in forced forward elevation.[39] Three stages of impingement syndrome progressing from pain and inflammation (stage 1) through fibrosis and tendonitis (stage 2) to rotator cuff tear (stage 3) have been described.[39] Although in younger persons rotator cuff tear is usually traumatic, in older persons it may occur near the end of this degenerative cascade. Individuals at risk of impingement syndrome include workers engaging in repetitive activities with the arm above shoulder level, such as overhead assemblers, carpenters, painters, or welders. Athletic pursuits, including swimming, baseball, tennis, and golf, may also be associated with development of impingement symptoms.

Prevention of rotator cuff inflammation, including impingement syndrome, bicipital tendonitis, bursitis, and

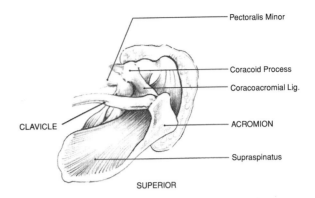

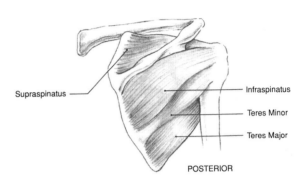

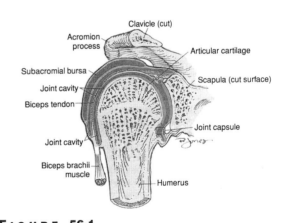

F I G U R E 56-1

The Painful Shoulder

even rotator cuff tear, involves identification of activities, occupational or athletic, that expose the vulnerable components of the rotator cuff to injury, inflammation, and subsequent degenerative changes. Suspension of recreational activities that may be producing symptoms to permit resolution of inflammation, may limit risk of progression to a more advanced stage of cuff injury. Training programs, which emphasize proper technique and isokinetic strengthening, may benefit athletes. Assessment of work tasks with job modification to reduce the work required with overhead arm use should be considered. Alternatively, rotation of job tasks may limit risk of repetitive trauma injury.

CARPAL TUNNEL SYNDROME

Carpal tunnel syndrome (CTS) is a common nerve entrapment, which occurs in about 3% of adult women and 2% of men.[40] The syndrome results from increased pressure in the carpal tunnel, resulting in ischemia of the median nerve. Symptoms may be sensory or motor. Typically, patients report nocturnal pain or paresthesias in the distribution of the median nerve—the palmar aspect of the thumb, index finger, middle finger, and radial half of the ring finger. Similar symptoms may occur while driving or reading a newspaper. Late signs of CTS include thenar atrophy and loss of 2-point discrimination in the distribution of the nerve. Diagnosis of CTS is suggested by the presence of Tinel and Phalen signs. Tinel sign is "positive" when light tapping over the volar flexor crease of the wrist reproduces symptoms—pain or paresthesias—in the median nerve distribution. The Phalen sign is present when full flexion of the wrists for 60 seconds produces similar symptoms. The Phalen sign is the more sensitive of the 2 tests, but Tinel sign is more specific.[41,42] If the diagnosis is uncertain, electrodiagnostic studies are the gold standard, although false-positive and false-negative results do occur.

Pathogenesis and Risk Factors

Considerable controversy exists regarding the role of occupational factors in the genesis of CTS. Since 1986 when the National Institute for Occupational Health and Safety (NIOSH) recognized repetitive microtrauma in the workplace as a cause of CTS, the reported cases have risen dramatically. Fifty percent to 90% of all cases of CTS have been attributed to work-related factors by some authors.[43-45] Repetitive activities of the hand and wrist, particularly in awkward postures and involving forceful use or vibrating tools, have been suggested as predisposing to CTS. Higher risk occupations may include food processing, manufacturing, logging, and construction.[40]

The methodology of studies purporting to demonstrate an association between occupational factors and CTS has been critically reviewed by Hadler,[46] who concluded: "To declare carpal tunnel syndrome an injury or occupational disease is not science. It is policy and we need to query who is served by such policy." Furthermore, medical illnesses associated with CTS or substantial obesity have been identified in almost two thirds of persons whose CTS had been previously attributed to occupational injury.[47,48] Others have pointed out that despite considerable efforts at improving workplace ergonomics, the incidence of CTS has continued to increase, raising questions about the role of occupational factors in causation.[49] These authors surveyed 64 articles on CTS, including those cited as demonstrating an association between CTS and work. The primary risk factors for CTS identified were menopausal status in women, obesity or lack of fit-

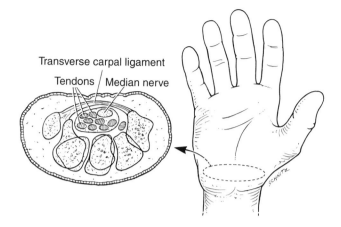

F I G U R E   56-2
Carpal Tunnel Syndrome

ness, diabetes or family history of diabetes, osteoarthritis of the carpometacarpal joint of the thumb, smoking, and lifetime alcohol intake.

Conditions associated with CTS include pregnancy, hypothyroidism, obesity, inflammatory arthritis, diabetes mellitus, acromegaly, history of Colles fracture, and amyloidosis.[50] In some patients, CTS is the presenting manifestation of hypothyroidism.[46] Other conditions that may mimic CTS include diabetic neuropathy, motor neuron disease, multiple sclerosis, cervical radiculopathy, and thoracic outlet syndrome.[51]

Prevention

Modification of mechanical and lifestyle factors may have a role in prevention of CTS. Minimizing excessive repetitive forceful flexion and extension in the workplace is advisable. Further studies are required, however, to demonstrate the effectiveness of risk factor modification in the workplace as primary prevention of CTS. Obesity is clearly a risk factor for CTS, and weight control should be encouraged. Identification and treatment of hypothyroidism will prevent or reverse associated CTS. In patients with inflammatory arthritis, aggressive treatment with disease-modifying agents may prevent CTS by minimizing wrist synovitis. Risk of wrist fracture and associated CTS should be reduced by optimizing bone density and encouraging fall prevention strategies, particularly in older patients.

PAINFUL HEEL SYNDROME AND PLANTAR FASCIITIS

The clinical syndrome of plantar fasciitis is a common cause of foot pain. The classical symptoms include focal pain and tenderness over the plantar aspect of the foot, particularly the medial calcaneus. Pain is typically worse on arising in the morning or after prolonged sitting. In persons with this history, the condition is clinically confirmed by demonstration of point tenderness at the insertion of the plantar fascia on the medial tuberosity of the calcaneus.

Pathophysiology and Risk Factors

Plantar fasciitis is believed to result from repetitive microtrauma at the insertion point of the plantar fascia on the medial calcaneal tuberosity. Pathologic changes described include collagen necrosis, angiofibroblastic hyperplasia, chondroid metaplasia, and matrix calcification.[52] A calcaneal spur is observed in up to 50% of patients with the syndrome but is probably uninvolved in pathogenesis.[53] The condition, which is most common in people between 40 and 60 years of age and occurs with equal frequency in both sexes, is associated with obesity in more than one third of patients and pes planus in almost 25%.[54] Approximately 10% of runners report symptoms of plantar fasciitis.[55] Occupations requiring prolonged standing (or jumping) on hard floors increase the risk of developing the syndrome, probably explaining the increased incidence of the condition in dancers. The presence of bilateral fasciitis in association with articular involvement elsewhere should suggest the possibility of an underlying systemic inflammatory condition, such as rheumatoid arthritis or seronegative spondyloarthropathy.

Prevention

Prevention of plantar fasciitis requires avoidance of obesity and treatment of pes planus if present. Exercises to strengthen the intrinsic muscles of the foot may be of benefit in some persons. Fabrication of orthotics designed to correct foot deformity, including excessive pronation and pes planus, should be helpful, particularly in runners, dancers, or individuals working in occupations requiring prolonged standing or walking on hard floors. The natural history of plantar fasciitis is favorable, with resolution of symptoms in more than 80% of patients within 12 months.[56]

LOW BACK PAIN

Epidemiology and Pathogenesis

Low back pain is a very common complaint, affecting up to 80% of adults during their lifetime.[57] More than 10 million people annually seek treatment of low back pain from physicians, chiropractors, and physical therapists, at a cost exceeding $50 billion per year.[58] Fortunately, although low back pain affects nearly all adults and affects all aspects of daily living, including work, family, and recreational activities, it is usually benign and self-limited. In fact, nonspecific low back pain can be considered a normal life event. The prognosis is excellent almost irregardless of the specific treatment.[59,60] About 80% of sufferers will be better in 2-4 weeks and 90% will be better by 3 months.[59–61]

Despite advances in diagnostic imaging such as computed tomography (CT) and magnetic resonance imaging (MRI), the specific anatomical cause of any single episode of low back pain remains unclear in as many as 80% to 90% of case.[62] Sciatica, with true nerve root compression, occurs in less than 1% of episodes of acute low back pain.[63] Further confounding the diagnostician is the fact that many abnormal physical and X-ray findings are as common in asymptomatic individuals as those with back pain. These findings may include spondylolisthesis, increased lumbosacral angle, leg length discrepancy, transitional lumbosacral vertebrae, single disk space narrowing, Schmorl nodes, mild to moderate scoliosis, spina bifida occulta, and disk space calcification. Furthermore, MRI studies in asymptomatic individuals reveal abnormalities in about 50%, including herniated disk, spinal stenosis, and facet degenerative changes. Careful clinical correlation is required before attribution of clinical significance to a specific imaging finding.[64] Errors of symptom attribution may lead to unnecessary treatment.

The most common findings in acute low back pain are nonspecific and often attributed to a mechanical injury to myofascial tissues (ie, lumbosacral strain or sprain). As such, mechanical pain syndromes can be thought to arise out of abnormal forces applied to abnormal structures. That end result is an anatomical structure that is overstretched or overcompressed, resulting in regional pain.[65] Examples include exerting normal force on a degenerative disk, joint, or ligament or excessive stretch or compression of an otherwise normal structure. These forces may arise during performance of ordinary activities with poor posture or poor body mechanics on a repeated basis, increasing the mechanical load to the low back.

Prevention

Despite the fact that the specific anatomical abnormality or, in some cases, the specific event responsible for an episode of low back pain cannot be determined, modifiable risk factors may be identified. People who are more physically fit have fewer episodes of low back pain.[66] More recent studies have concluded that increased general fitness or spinal flexibility may have a slight protective benefit against the future development of back pain.[67]

Furthermore, workplace studies support the notion that regular physical activity can reduce the impact of back pain disability.[68] The maintenance of lumbar lordosis while lifting, sitting, or standing has been advocated by McKenzie[69] to help prevent back pain.

Another modifiable risk factor for increased low back pain is cigarette smoking.[63] Possible mechanisms include increased coughing causing increased intradiskal pressure as well as nicotine-induced vertebral vasoconstriction with reduced blood flow and reduced oxygen tissue delivery. Smoking-related lifestyle factors, such as deconditioning, also may play a role.

There is no convincing evidence that lumbar support braces or belts help prevent low back pain. Finally, according to Waddell,[70] reduction of anxiety and stress can help prevent back pain disability.

NECK PAIN

Many of the same principles described in low back pain prevention apply to neck pain as well. Neck pain is less common than back pain. Neck pain occurs most often from a mechanical disorder of the cervical spine. The disorders range from muscle and ligament strain, disk abnormalities, and osteoarthritis.[71,72] Often no specific trauma is identified. Sometimes, an awkward sleeping position, poor posture, or rapid head movements may trigger pain.[73] The most commonly affected muscles are the trapezius and the sternocleidomastoid.[74]

Strategies for preventing neck pain are similar to those for preventing back pain. They include performing regular stretching and strengthening exercises, maintaining good posture, avoidance of awkward positions or postures, and stress and anxiety reduction.[75] In addition, the use of a supportive cervical pillow while sleeping has been shown to prevent neck pain.[72]

SUMMARY

Musculoskeletal disorders are common and typically a consequence of repetitive overuse behavior as well as age-related degenerative change. In some cases, modification of risk factors, eg smoking cessation, may slow progression. In general, active, customized exercise programs are often effective in both prevention and treatment of these diverse conditions.

REFERENCES

1. Centers for Disease Control and Prevention. Arthritis prevalence and activity limitations—United States, 1990. *MMWR Morb Mortal Wkly Rep.* 1994;43:433–438.

2. Lawrence RC, Helmick CG, Arnett FC, et al. Estimates of the prevalence of arthritis and selected musculoskeletal disorders in the United States. *Arthritis Rheum.* 1998;41:778–799.

3. Centers for Disease Control and Prevention. Prevalence of disabilities and associated health conditions—United States 1991–1992. *MMWR Morb Mortal Wkly Rep.* 1994;43:730–739.

4. Malanga GA, Nadler SF, Agesen T. Epidemiology. In: Cole AJ, Hering SA, eds. *Low Back Pain Handbook.* 2nd ed. Philadelphia, Pa: Hanley and Belfus; 2003:1–7.

5. Oliveria SA, Felson DT, Reed JI, Cirillo PA, Walker AM. Incidence of symptomatic hand, hip, and knee osteoarthritis among patients in a health maintenance organization. *Arthritis Rheum.* 1995;38:1134–1141.

6. Felson DT, Zhang Y. An update on the epidemiology of knee and hip osteoarthritis with a view to prevention. *Arthritis Rheum.* 1998;41:1343–1355.

7. Felson DT. The epidemiology of knee osteoarthritis: results from the Framingham Study. *Semin Arthritis Rheum.* 1990;20:42–50.

8. Felson DT, Lawrence RC, Dieppe PA, et al. Osteoarthritis: new insights: I. The disease and its risk factors. *Ann Intern Med.* 2000;133:635–646.

9. Guccione AA, Felson DT, Anderson JJ, et al. The effects of specific medical conditions on functional limitations of elders in the Framingham Study. *Am J Public Health.* 1994;84:351–358.

10. Spector TD, Cicuttini F, Baker J, Loughlin J, Hart D. Genetic influences on osteoarthritis in women: a twin study. *BMJ.* 1996;312:940–943.

11. Hoagland FT, Oishi CS, Gialamas GG. Extreme variations in racial rates of total hip arthroplasty for primary coxarthrosis: a population-based study in San Francisco. *Ann Rheum Dis.* 1995;54:107–110.

12. Felson DT. Preventing knee and hip osteoarthritis. *Bull Rheum Dis.* 1998;47:1–4.

13. McAlindon TE, Jacques P, Zhang Y, et al. Do antioxidant micronutrients protect against the development and progression of knee osteoarthritis? *Arthritis Rheum.* 1996;39:648–656.

14. Lane NE, Gore LR, Cummings SR, et al, for Osteoporotic Fractures Research Group. Serum vitamin D levels and incident changes of radiographic hip osteoarthritis: a longitudinal study. *Arthritis Rheum.* 1999;42:854–860.

15. McAlindon TE, Felson DT, Zhang Y, et al. Relation of dietary intake and serum levels of vitamin D to progression of osteoarthritis of the knee among participants in the Framingham study. *Ann Intern Med.* 1996;125:353–359.

16. Zhang Y, Hannan MT, Chaisson CE, et al. Bone mineral density and risk of incident and progressive radiographic knee osteoarthritis in women: the Framingham study. *J Rheumatol.* 2000;27:1032–1037.

17. Cooper C, Inskip H, Croft P, et al. Individual risk factors for hip osteoarthritis: obesity, hip injury, and physical activity. *Am J Epidemiol.* 1998;147:516–522.

18. Zhang Y, Glynn RJ, Felson DT. Musculoskeletal disease research: should we analyze the joint or the person? *J Rheumatol.* 1996;23:1130–1134.

19. Gelber AC, Hochberg MC, Mead LA, et al. Joint injury in young adults and risk for subsequent knee and hip osteoarthritis. *Ann Intern Med.* 2000;133:321–328.

20. Slemenda C, Heilman DK, Brandt KD, et al. Reduced quadriceps strength relative to body weight: a risk factor for knee osteoarthritis in women? *Arthritis Rheum.* 1998;41:1951–1959.

21. Felson DT, Lawrence RC, Hochberg MC, et al. Osteoarthritis: new insights: II. Treatment options. *Ann Intern Med.* 2000;133:726–737.

22. Roos H, Lindberg H, Gardsell P, Lohmander LS, Wingstrand H. The prevalence of gonarthrosis in former soccer players and its relation to meniscectomy. *Am J Sports Med.* 1994;22:219–222.

23. Spector TD, Harris PA, Hart DJ, et al. Risk of osteoarthritis associated with long-term weight bearing sports: a radiologic survey of the hips and knees in female ex-athletes and population controls. *Arthritis Rheum.* 1996;39:988–995.

24. Marti B, Knowbloch M, Eschopp A, Jucker A, Howald H. Is excessive running predictive of degenerative hip disease? Controlled study of former elite athletes. *BMJ.* 1989;299:91–93.

25. Saxon L, Finch C, Bass S. Sports participation, sports injuries, and osteoarthritis. Implications for prevention. *Sports Med.* 1999;2:123–135.

26. Lane N. Exercise in osteoarthritis. *Bull Rheum Dis.* 1991;41:5–7.

27. Lane NE, Michel B, Bjorkengren A, et al. The risk of osteoarthritis with running and aging: a 5-year longitudinal study. *J Rheumatol.* 1993;20:461–468.

28. Lane NE, Block DA, Wood PD, Fries JF. Aging, long-distance running, and the development of musculoskeletal disability: a controlled study. *Am J Med.* 1987;82:772–780.

29. Felson DT, Hannan MT, Naimark A, et al. Occupational physical demands, knee bending, and knee osteoarthritis: results from the Framingham Study. *J Rheumatol.* 1991;18:1587–1592.

30. Coggon D, Kellingray S, Inskip H, Croft P, Campbell L, Cooper C. Osteoarthritis of the hip and occupational lifting. *Am J Epidemiol.* 1998;147:523–528.

31. Hartz AJ, Fisher ME, Bril G, et al. The association of obesity with joint pain and osteoarthritis in the HANES data. *J Chron Dis.* 1986;39:311–319.

32. Cooper C, Snow S, McAlindon TE, et al. Risk factors for the incidence and progression of radiographic knee osteoarthritis. *Arthritis Rheum.* 2000;43:995–1000.

33. Dougados, M, Gueguen A, Nguyen M, et al. Longitudinal radiographic evaluation of osteoarthritis of the knee. *J Rheumatol.* 1992;19:378–383.

34. Felson DT, Zhang Y, Anthony JM, Naimark K, Anderson JJ. Weight loss reduces the risk for symptomatic knee osteoarthritis in women. *Ann Intern Med.* 1992;116:535–539.

35. Neer CS, Craig EV, Fukuda H. Cuff-tear arthropathy. *J Bone Joint Surg.* 1983;65A:1232–1244.

36. Delafuente JC. Glucosamine in the treatment of osteoarthritis. *Rheum Dis Clin N Am.* 2000;26:1–11.

37. Pavelka K, Gatterova J, Olejarova M, Machacek S, Giacovelli G, Rovati LC. Glucosamine sulfate use and delay of progression of knee osteoarthritis. *Arch Intern Med.* 2002;162:2113–2123.

38. Steinfeld R, Valente RM, Stuart MJ. A commonsense approach to shoulder problems. *Mayo Clin Proc.* 1999;74:785–794.

39. Neer CS. Impingement lesions. *Clin Orthop.* 1983;173:70–77.

40. Katz JN, Simmons BP. Carpal tunnel syndrome. *N Engl J Med.* 2002;346:1807–1812.

41. Golding DN, Rose DM, Selvarajah K. Clinical tests for carpal tunnel syndrome: an evaluation. *Br J Rheumatol.* 1986;25:388–390.

42. Buch-Jaeger N, Foucher G. Correlation of clinical signs with nerve conduction tests in the diagnosis of carpal tunnel syndrome. *J Hand Surg Br.* 1994;19:720–724.

43. Rossignol M, Stock S, Patry L, Armstrong B. Carpal tunnel syndrome: what is attributable to work? The Montreal Study. *Occup Environ Med.* 1997;54:519–523.

44. Hagberg M, Morgenstern H, Kelsh M. Impact of occupations and job tasks on the prevalence of carpal tunnel syndrome. *Scand J Work Environ Health.* 1992;18:337–345.

45. Miller RS, Iverson DC, Fried RA, Green LA, Nutting PA. Carpal tunnel syndrome in primary care: a report from ASPN. *J Fam Pract.* 1994;38:337–344.

46. Hadler NM. *Occupational Musculoskeletal Disorders.* New York, NY: Raven Press; 1993.

47. Yocum DE. The many faces of carpal tunnel syndrome [editorial]. *Arch Intern Med.* 1998;158:1496.

48. Atcheson SG, Ward JR, Lowe W. Concurrent medical disease in work-related carpal tunnel syndrome. *Arch Intern Med.* 1998;158:1506–1512.

49. Falkiner S, Myers S. When exactly can carpal tunnel syndrome be considered work-related? *ANZ J Surg* 2002;72:204–209.

50. Solomon DH, Katz JN, Bahn R, Mogun H, Avorn J. Nonoccupational risk factors for carpal tunnel syndrome. *J Gen Intern Med.* 1999;14:310–314.

51. Witt JC, Stevens JC. Neurologic disorders masquerading as carpal tunnel syndrome: 12 cases of failed carpal tunnel release. *Mayo Clin Proc.* 2000;75:409–413.

52. Voloshin I, DiGiovanni BF, Baumhauer JF. Plantar heel pain: making a difficult diagnosis. *J Musculoskeletal Med.* 2002;19:373–380.

53. Lapidus P, Guidotti F. Painful heel: report of 323 patients with 364 painful heels. *Clin Orthop.* 1965;39:178–186.

54. Furey JG. Plantar fasciitis, the painful heel syndrome. *J Bone Joint Surg Am.* 1975;57:672–673.

55. Kibler W, Goldberg C, Chandler T. Functional biomechanical deficits in running athletes with plantar fasciitis. *Am J Sports Med.* 1991;19:66–71.

56. Buchbinder R, Ptasznik R, Gordon J, Buchanan J, Prabaharan V, Forbes A. Ultrasound-guided extracorporeal shock wave therapy for plantar fasciitis: a randomized controlled trial. *JAMA.* 2002;288:1364–1372.

57. Waddell G. A new clinical model for the treatment of low back pain. *Spine.* 1987;12:623–644.

58. Hall H, Iceton J. Back School: An overview with specific reference to the Canadian back education units. *Clin Orthop.* 1983;179:10–17.

59. Nachemson AL. The lumbar spine: an orthopedic challenge. *Spine.* 1976;1:59–71.

60. Quinet RJ, Hadler NM. Diagnosis and treatment of backache. *Semin Arthritis Rheum.* 1979;8:261–287.

61. Anderson GJB, Svensson HO, Oden A. The intensity of work recovery in low back pain. *Spine.* 1983;8:880–884.

62. Nachemson AL. Advances in low back pain. *Clin Orthop.* 1985;200:266–278.

63. Frymoyer JW, Clements JH, Wilder DG, MacPherson B, Ashikaga T. Risk factors in low back pain. *J Bone Joint Surg.* 1983;65A:213–218.

64. Modic M, Ross JM. Dental magnetic resonance imaging of the lumbar spine in people without back pain. *N Engl J Med.* 1994;331:69–73.

65. McKenzie R. *Treat Your Own Back.* 7th ed. New Zealand: Spinal Publications Ltd; 1997:7–12.

66. Cady LD, Bischoff DP, O'Connell ER, Thomas PC, Allan JH. Strength and fitness and subsequent back injuries in fire fighters. *J Occup Med.* 1979;21:269–272.

67. Harreby M, Hesselsoe G, Kjer J, Neergaard K. Low back pain and physical exercise in leisure time in 38-year-old men and women: a 25-year prospective cohort study of 640 school children. *Eur Spine J.* 1997;6:181–186.

68. Underwood MR. Exercise and the prevention of back pain disability. *Br J Sports Med.* 2000;34:5.

69. McKenzie R. *The Lumbar Spine: Mechanical Diagnosis and Therapy.* Upper Hutt, New Zealand: Wright and Carmen Ltd; 1981:6–8.

70. Waddell G. *The Back Pain Revolution.* Edinburgh, Scotland: Churchill Livingston; 1998.

71. Helliwell PS, Evans PF, Wright V. The straight cervical spine: does it indicate muscle spasm? *J Bone Joint Surg.* 1994;76B:103–106.

72. Bernhardt M, Hynes RA, Blume HW, White AA III. Cervical spondylotic myelopathy. *J Bone Joint Surg.* 1993;75A:119–128.

73. McKenzie R. *The Cervical and Thoracic Spine, Mechanical Diagnosis and Therapy.* Upper Hutt, New Zealand: Wright and Carmen Ltd; 1981.

74. Borenstein DG. Disorders of the low back and neck. In: *Primer on the Rheumatic Diseases.* 11th ed. Atlanta, Ga: Arthritis Foundation; 1997:134–135.

75. McKinney LA. Early mobilization and outcome in acute sprains of the neck. *BMJ.* 1989;299:1006–1008.

RESOURCES

The Arthritis Foundation
This foundation provides information and materials related to osteoarthritis and many other rheumatic disorders.
Web site: www.arthritis.org/

American Physical Therapy Association
This association provides information for patients related to the role of physical therapy and the management of musculoskeletal disorders.
Web site: www.apta.org/

North American Spine Society
This society provides some educational material for spinal disorders.
Web site: www.spine.org/

The American College of Rheumatology
This organization offers information to physicians who evaluate and treat musculoskeletal disorders.
Web site: www. Rheumatology.org/

chapter 57

Headache

Glen D. Solomon, MD

INTRODUCTION

Headache is the seventh most common presenting complaint for ambulatory care encounters in the United States. The problem of headache generates 18.3 million outpatient physician visits in the United States annually.[1]

Headaches are generally differentiated into primary (idiopathic) headache syndromes, which include migraine, tension-type, and cluster headache, and secondary headaches caused by underlying disease. Migraine is a syndrome of intermittent, moderate- to severe-intensity headaches, lasting from 4 to 72 hours.[2] The headaches are typically unilateral, throbbing, and associated with nausea or vomiting and sensitivity to light and/or noise. Aura, usually scintillating scotomata or fortification spectra, precede the headache in approximately 15% of patients.

Tension-type headache is typically described as a bandlike pressure headache without associated symptoms. The International Headache Society (IHS)[2] defines tension-type headache as a bilateral headache having a pressing or tightening quality of mild to moderate severity. Unlike migraine, it is not aggravated by physical activity, nor is it associated with vomiting. Phonophobia or photophobia may be present, but not both. In chronic tension-type headache, but not episodic tension-type headache, patients may experience nausea. By definition, chronic tension-type headache occurs at least 15 days per month for at least 6 months,[2] although in clinical practice it is usually a daily or almost daily headache.

The clinical presentation of cluster headache is a unilateral headache of excruciating severity accompanied by certain autonomic phenomena, is more common in men, and is strikingly periodic in occurrence.[2] Cluster headache is marked by cycles of headache lasting 1 to 4 months, separated by remissions of 6 to 24 months. The cluster headache attacks are always unilateral, located around the eye, temple, or upper part of the jaw. Associated symptoms include reddening and tearing of the eye, drooping of the eyelid, nasal stuffiness, and rhinorrhea. The attacks generally last from 15 minutes to 2 hours, occur 1 to 8 times daily, and often awaken the patient after 90 to 120 minutes of sleep.

EPIDEMIOLOGY

The advent of sophisticated epidemiologic methodology and the widespread acceptance of the International Headache Society (IHS) criteria[2] (Table 57-1) for the diagnosis of headache disorders stimulated a new understanding of the epidemiology of headache. Four key studies,[1,3-5] each using a different methodology, definition of migraine, and population group, were performed in the late 1980s and early 1990s to detail the prevalence of headache disorders.

To determine the overall prevalence of headache in the general population, Rasmussen and colleagues[4] performed a study of a representative sample of the population of Copenhagen, Denmark, and found a lifetime prevalence of headache of 96%, significantly higher among women (99%) than among men (93%), with men aged 55 to 64 years having the lowest lifetime prevalence and last-year prevalence of headache. The overall lifetime prevalence of migraine was 16%: 25% among women and 8% among men. The male-to-female ratio was approximately 1:3. There were no significant differences in migraine prevalence rates according to age.

Of migraineurs, 15% had migraine 8 to 14 days per year and 9% had it more than 14 days per year. Eighty-five percent of migraineurs reported severe pain intensity. The lifetime prevalence of tension-type headache was 78%: 88% among women and 69% among men. The male-to-female ratio was about 4:5. Men aged 55 to 64 years had the lowest lifetime prevalence of tension-type headache. Among women, there was a significant decrease in prevalence of tension-type headache with increasing age. Of people with tension-type headache

T A B L E   57-1

IHS Criteria for Diagnosis of Primary Headache Disorders*

Migraine Without Aura	Migraine With Aura
A. At least 5 attacks fulfilling B–D.	A. At least 2 attacks fulfilling B.
B. Attacks lasting 4–72 hours (untreated or unsuccessfully treated).	B. At least 3 of the following characteristics:
C. At least 2 of the following characteristics:	1. One or more fully reversible aura symptom indicating focal cerebral cortical and/or brain-stem dysfunction.
1. Unilateral location	2. At least one aura symptom develops gradually over more than 4 minutes or 2 or more symptoms occur in succession.
2. Pulsating quality	
3. Moderate or severe intensity (inhibits or prohibits daily activities)	3. No aura symptom lasts more than 60 minutes. If more than 1 aura symptom present, accepted duration is proportionally increased.
4. Aggravation by walking stairs or similar routine activity	4. Attack follows aura with a free interval of <60 minutes. (It may also begin before or simultaneously with aura.)
D. At least one of the following:	
1. Nausea and/or vomiting	C. At least one of the following:
2. Photophobia and phonophobia	1. History and physical and neurologic findings do not suggest disorders in groups 5–11 of IHS classification.
E. At least one of the following:	
1. History and physical and neurologic findings do not suggest disorders in groups 5–11 of IHS classification.	2. History and/or physical and/or neurologic findings do suggest such disorder but are ruled out by appropriate investigations.
2. History and/or physical and/or neurologic findings do suggest such disorder but are ruled out by appropriate investigations.	3. Such disorder is present, but attacks do not occur for the first time in close temporal relation to the disorder.
3. Such disorder is present, but attacks do not occur for the first time in close temporal relation to the disorder.	

Chronic Tension-type Headache	Cluster Headache
A. Average frequency of attacks >15 days/month (180/year) for >6 months fulfilling criteria B–D below.	A. At least 5 attacks fulfilling B–D below.
B. At least 2 of the following pain characteristics:	B. Severe unilateral orbital, supraorbital, and/or temporal pain lasting 15–180 minutes when untreated.
1. Pressing or tightening quality	C. Attack is associated with at least one of the following signs on the side of pain:
2. Mild or moderate severity (may inhibit but does not prohibit activities)	1. Conjunctival injection
3. Bilateral location	2. Lacrimation
4. No aggravation by walking stairs or similar routine physical activity	3. Nasal congestion
C. Both of the following:	4. Rhinorrhea
1. No vomiting	5. Forehead and facial sweating
2. No more than 1 of the following: nausea, photophobia, or phonophobia	6. Miosis
D. At least one of the following:	7. Ptosis
1. History and physical and neurologic findings do not suggest disorders in groups 5–11 of IHS classification.	8. Eyelid edema
	D. Frequency: 1 every other day to 8 per day.
2. History and/or physical and/or neurologic findings do suggest other disorder but are ruled out by appropriate investigations.	E. At least one of the following:
	1. History and physical and neurologic findings do not suggest disorders in groups 5–11 of IHS classification.
3. Such disorder is present, but tension-type headache does not occur for the first time in close temporal relation to the disorder.	2. History and/or physical and/or neurologic findings do suggest other disorder but are ruled out by appropriate investigations.
	3. Such disorder is present, but tension-type headache does not occur for the first time in close temporal relation to the disorder.

*IHS indicates International Headache Society. From the Headache Classification Committee of the International Headache Society.[2]

23% had headache 8 to 14 days per year and 36% had it several times per month. Chronic tension-type headache (tension-type headache occurring 180 or more days per year) was noted by 3% of the population. Only 1% of patients with tension-type headache reported severe pain intensity, while moderate pain was noted by 58% and mild pain was reported by 41%.

To assess the prevalence of headache in young adults and their utilization of medical care, Linet and associates[1] performed a population-based telephone interview study of 10,169 young adults in Washington County, Maryland. Greater than 90% of males and 95% of females had a history of headache during their lifetime. Of the subjects, 57.1% of males and 76.5% of females reported that their most recent headache occurred within the previous 4 weeks. Only 9% of males and 5% of females had no headache during the previous year. Just over 6% of males and 14% of females noted 4 or more headaches in the preceding month. Migraine headache within the previous month was reported by 3% of males and 7.4% of females. Headaches caused substantial disability. Almost 8% of males and 14% of females reported missing work or school. Disability was greatest for women aged 24 to 29 years. Women described headaches that were more severe and longer in duration than men. Despite the disabling nature of their headaches, 85% of male and 72% of female headache sufferers never consulted a physician for a headache-related problem.

Headache prevalence in the elderly population (age, ≥ 65 years) is less than in younger age groups. Cook et al[6] found that 53% of women and 36% of men reported headache in the past year. Headaches occurring several times a month or more were reported by 17% of their elderly population. The overall prevalence of migraine was 12% among women and 7% among men. The prevalence of migraine fell with advancing age from 14% in women aged 65 to 69 years to 6% in women over 90 years old. In men, the prevalence fell from 10% in those aged 65 to 69 to 0% in men over 90 years old. Solomon et al[7] found that older individuals with headache attending a referral medical center had more tension-type headache and less migraine headache compared with younger headache-affected patients.

To understand the magnitude and distribution of the public health problem posed by migraine, Stewart et al[5] sent a self-administered questionnaire to 15,000 households representative of the US population. The large sample allowed the authors to evaluate migraine prevalence, frequency, and disability by sex, age, race, household income, and geographic factors. Migraine prevalence was 5.7% of males and 17.6% of females. Female blacks and whites had the same prevalence of migraine, but migraine was less common in either black or white males. Migraine prevalence was highest in both men and women between ages 35 and 45 years. Migraine prevalence was strongly associated with household income; prevalence in the lowest income group was more than 60% higher than in the 2 highest income groups. Females aged 30 to 49 years from lower-income households were at especially high risk of having migraines and were more likely to use emergency care services for their treatment.

Stewart et al[5] proposed several theories to explain the higher prevalence of migraine in lower-income groups. Diet, stress, and other factors associated with poverty may have precipitated migraine attacks. Alternatively, access to good health care by higher-income groups may have decreased the duration and, therefore, the prevalence of migraine. In some sufferers, the frequency of debilitating headaches may have led to loss of job or income, resulting in a downward drift of socioeconomic status.

To determine trends in the prevalence of chronic migraine and the impact on disability and utilization of medical care, the National Health Interview Survey (NHIS) collected data through personal interviews conducted with a representative sample of the US population.[3] This study compared migraine prevalence for 1980 and 1989. In contrast to Linet et al,[1] who showed that about three fourths of individuals with headache did not seek medical care for their headaches, the NHIS study showed that more than 80% of female and 70% of male migraineurs had at least one physician contact per year because of migraine headaches. In addition, 8% of female and 7% of male patients with migraine were hospitalized at least once per year for migraine. Long-term limitations in functional capacity due to migraines were reported by 3% of females and 4% of males.

The NHIS reported the prevalence rate of migraine in the United States in 1989 to be 41 per 1000 persons. This represented a 60% increase from 10 years earlier. These figures are considerably lower than the 10% previous-year prevalence reported by the Danish group.[4] The difference in prevalence rate likely represents the method used to diagnose migraine, rather than a difference in the populations studied. The NHIS study used self-diagnosis, while the Danish study used physician evaluation, to diagnose migraine. Patients often mistakenly self-diagnose their headache as "sinus headache" or "stress headache" when migraine is the appropriate medical diagnosis. The NHIS report found that 71% of the increase in migraine occurred among persons younger than 45 years of age.[3] In each year of the study, the prevalence of migraine was greater in women than in men, and the rate of increase in migraine was greater in women than in men.

Although recent studies have clarified the epidemiology of migraine headache, there are fewer data on other types of headache. Chronic daily headache encompasses a group of headache disorders lasting longer than 6 months, marked by a frequency of 4 hours or more, for at least half of the days of the month.[8] It is not a diagnostic entity included in the International Headache Society's (IHS) classification of headache.[2] The most common daily headache syndromes include chronic tension-type headache with or without medication overuse, chronic (or transformed) migraine (migraine with concomitant chronic tension-type headache), or medication overuse headache in patients with frequent migraine attacks. Five percent of the population has severe headache on a daily basis.[9]

In the Danish population study, the 1-year prevalence of chronic tension-type headache was 3%, with approximately 4% saying they had headaches occurring at least half the days of the year.[10] The prevalence of tension-type headache decreased with increasing age. The severity of tension-type headache increased significantly with its frequency. Fifty-nine percent of people with tension-type headache said it interfered with their daily activities. People with tension-type headache rarely sought medical attention. Consultation rates were higher in women than in men; in addition, people were more likely to see a doctor if their headaches were more frequent.[10]

Population-based studies report that the most common cause of chronic daily headache is chronic tension-type headache, followed by chronic migraine.[11] In tertiary headache centers, the most common cause of chronic daily headache is chronic (transformed) migraine. Studies report that chronic daily headache is roughly twice as prevalent in women as in men.[12] The average age at onset of chronic daily headache is in the 30s. The prevalence of chronic daily headache appears consistent across all age groups from childhood to the elderly.[12] This is in contrast to migraine, which decreases in prevalence after the sixth decade.

Patients with chronic tension-type headache, like patients with other chronic pain disorders, have about a 25% likelihood of developing secondary depression. Half of these patients develop depression simultaneously with the pain, whereas in the other half, the development of depression is more insidious.[13] Tension-type headache may be present in almost all psychiatric disturbances.[14] This should not suggest, however, that most tension-type headaches are associated with psychiatric or psychological disorders.

Psychiatric comorbidity is more frequent in patients with migraine. Anxiety, depression, panic disorder, and bipolar disease have all been found to be more common in migraineurs.[15,16] Depression has been reported in 25% to 80% of patients with "chronic migraine."[17,18] Generalized anxiety was reported in 70% of those with "chronic migraine," and somatoform disorders (including somatization, conversion disorder, and hypochondriasis), in 5.7%.[18] The somatoform disorders were always concomitant with anxiety and mood disorders.

In evaluating patients with comorbid migraine and major depression, Breslau[11] has reported that major depression does not influence the persistence of migraine, increase the frequency of migraine episodes, or exacerbate migraine disability over time. In addition, migraine does not influence the recurrence of major depression. This suggests that chronic headache is not the result of major depression in migraineurs.

In contrast to migraine and tension-type headache, cluster headache is uncommon. At specialized headache centers, the incidence of cluster headache has ranged from 2% to 16% of headache-affected patients.[19] Cluster headache is the only major primary headache disorder that is more common in males. Studies suggest a male-to-female ratio of between 5 and 9 males to every 1 female cluster headache sufferer.[19] The average age at onset of cluster headache is 26 years. Although migraine is a hereditary disorder, familial cluster headache is unusual, reportedly occurring in only 3% of patients with cluster headache. A family history of migraine is reported in 15% to 17% of those with cluster headache, a figure compatible with the frequency of migraine in the general population.[19]

There is a significant association between cluster headache and cigarette smoking. Diamond et al[19] found that 71% of patients with episodic cluster and 93% of patients with chronic cluster smoked cigarettes at the time of initial presentation. Sadjapour[20] found that, with few exceptions, patients with cluster headache were long-term, heavy cigarette smokers who began smoking during adolescence. He suggested that cigarette smoking may be etiologically related to cluster headache. Only a small percentage of patients with cluster headache, however, have been nearly lifelong nonsmokers.

SCREENING

Headache is a symptom rather than a disease. Headache usually is categorized as primary (idiopathic) or secondary (organic), meaning that the headache is a symptom of an underlying disease (ie, giant cell arteritis, meningitis). Primary (benign) headaches are classified based on patterns and accompanying symptoms. Because headache is always symptomatic, screening for asymptomatic disease does not occur. Screening in headache disorders is performed for 2 key purposes: (1) to separate primary headaches from those caused by another disease and (2) to ensure that patients with headache-related disability are receiving appropriate treatment.

Patient History

Headache history

The first step in evaluating any patient with headache is to obtain a thorough headache history.[21] The history is the key to making the correct diagnosis. Because the physical and neurologic examination, laboratory tests, and radiographic studies are usually normal, the headache history determines whether a headache is migraine, cluster, or tension-type or whether it represents a symptom of underlying disease (secondary headache). Most often, a careful and complete history will provide a presumptive diagnosis, which can then be confirmed by physical examination and laboratory or radiographic studies.

Evaluating factors such as age at onset, temporal pattern, quality and location of pain, and settings that trigger headaches usually allow the physician to diagnose the headache problem and initiate therapy. Duration of the headache problem, or age at onset, is often a key indicator as to probable underlying cause. Severe headache of sudden onset, especially if associated with focal neurologic signs or changes in level of consciousness, suggests serious illness, such as hemorrhage or meningitis. Recurrent episodic headache dating back many years, on the other hand, more likely reflects a type of vascular headache—migraine or cluster. A long history of daily headaches without associated symptoms suggests chronic tension-type headache. Among the most difficult headaches to interpret are those developing over weeks or months. These may be benign or arise from conditions as diverse as sinusitis, ocular disease, subdural hematoma, mass lesion, hydrocephalus, or—in the patient over age 60 years—giant cell arteritis.

After establishing the frequency and duration of the headache, the timing with respect to other physiological events can be crucial to correct diagnosis of the recurrent headache. One should inquire as to the time of day the headache occurs and its relationship to puberty, menses, pregnancy, menopause, or use of hormones. Migraine often initially occurs during puberty and may resolve after menopause. It may occur irregularly for months to years or it may follow a regular pattern of occurring with menses. An acute migraine can last from 4 to 72 hours, with headache-free intervals between attacks.

Episodic cluster headache follows a pattern of cyclic bouts or clusters, lasting from 2 weeks to several months. These bouts are separated by quiescent periods lasting from months to years. During these bouts, severe headaches lasting from 15 minutes to 3 hours may occur from 1 to 8 times a day, often awakening the patient from sleep. The duration of the cluster headache distinguishes it from trigeminal neuralgia, which presents with recurrent jabs of pain lasting less than a minute. Cluster variant headaches, such as chronic paroxysmal hemicrania, show a pain pattern similar to that of cluster headache, but attacks are more frequent and occur predominantly during the day.

Chronic tension-type headaches show no periodicity and have rare headache-free intervals. The patient typically describes a daily, unrelenting headache. The chronic daily headache syndrome is characterized by intermittent paroxysms of severe, throbbing, "sick" (migraine) headache superimposed on a constant daily headache.

Location of the head pain can sometimes aid in diagnosis, such as in cluster headache or trigeminal neuralgia. Migraine is unilateral two thirds of the time. Chronic tension-type headache is usually bilateral but may be uni-

lateral. Cluster headaches, trigeminal neuralgia, and headaches linked to local disease of the eye, nose, sinuses, or scalp are always unilateral. Headaches arising from hemorrhage or space-occupying lesions may begin unilaterally but usually become bilateral. Migraine usually alternates sides with different attacks but may be predominantly unilateral throughout life. Cluster headache is invariably unilateral and affects only one side during a series of attacks.

The patient's description of the quality of the pain can be valuable. Migraine is usually throbbing or pulsatile, whereas a constant ache suggests tension-type headache, and deep, boring intense pain points to cluster headache. Trigeminal neuralgia is marked by short, intense, shock-like jabs.

The intensity of pain in cluster headache and trigeminal neuralgia is invariably described as so severe that the person experiencing the cluster headache usually cannot remain still. The migraineur, by contrast, often seeks to rest in a quiet, darkened room.

If the patient tells of an aura or warning signs, this generally means migraine with aura (classic migraine), the only type of headache with a recognizable prodrome. Visual or neurologic symptoms commonly precede the headache by 10 to 60 minutes (usually 20 minutes). Premonitory symptoms, which can include euphoria, fatigue, yawning, and craving for sweets, may occur 12 to 24 hours before an attack. Associated symptoms that may accompany migraine include photophobia, phonophobia, anorexia, nausea, vomiting, and focal neurologic signs. Seen with cluster headache are partial Horner syndrome, constricted pupils, injected conjunctiva, and unilateral lacrimation and rhinorrhea. Rhinorrhea and nasal congestion are also common in sinusitis. Neck stiffness or other signs of meningeal irritation can signal meningitis, encephalitis, or hemorrhage. A mass lesion, hydrocephalus, or encephalitis may be suggested by decreased level of consciousness or obtundation. Seizures can reflect cortical irritation, resulting from a mass or arteriovenous malformation. Fever and sweating suggest an infectious process.

Precipitating factors

One also should consider precipitating factors. Fatigue, particularly loss of sleep, may trigger either migraine or tension-type headache. Stress may exacerbate tension-type headache, whereas migraine may occur after a period of stress, often occurring on weekends or vacations. Migraineurs may associate their headaches with menses, missing meals, or imbibing foods rich in tyramine, such as red wine or aged cheese. Alcohol may trigger a cluster headache during a series but will have no effect during a quiescent period. Weather changes can be associated with migraine or exacerbation of sinusitis. Commonly associated with chronic tension-type headache are symptoms of depression, such as sleep and appetite disturbances. One also should assess possible exposure to occupational toxins, chemicals, or infectious agents. Carbon monoxide poisoning, for example, often manifests as headache. Certain chemicals such as nitrates induce withdrawal and reintroduction headache. It should be emphasized that exposure to infectious agents in immunosuppressed patients or those with acquired immunodeficiency syndrome (AIDS) may induce encephalitis or meningitis unaccompanied by classic fever and stiff neck.

Family history

A review of the patient's family history may prove rewarding. Migraine is a familial disorder, with a "positive" family history in two thirds of cases. Three fourths of patients will have a family history of migraine on the maternal side only, 20% on the paternal side only, and 6% on both the maternal and paternal sides. Based on a number of studies, there is approximately a 70% risk of migraine in offspring when both parents suffer from migraine, 45% risk when only one parent is affected, and less than 30% risk when both parents are unaffected. The risk for sibs of an affected child but with unaffected parents is estimated at 20%. The genetic basis for migraine is probably multifactorial where the genetic component is polygenic; there is an additive effect of a number of genes that render the individual more or less susceptible to the disorder in response to a number of environmental trigger factors. In tension-type headache, a family history of depression or alcohol abuse is common. This may reflect a hereditary abnormality of serotonin neurotransmission, which has been associated with those having tension-type headaches, depressed patients, and alcohol and physical abuse.

Medical-surgical history

The patient's medical-surgical history and history of current and previous medications can aid in diagnosis. Head trauma, for instance, may suggest subdural hematoma or skull fracture. Certain medications can trigger the onset of headache or exacerbate headache in patients with an underlying headache disorder. Askmark and colleagues[22] evaluated data from the World Health Organization Collaborating Centre for International Drug Monitoring. Medication-induced headache was most frequently reported with the following medications: indomethacin, nifedipine, cimetidine, atenolol, trimethoprim-sulfamethoxazole, zimeldine, nitroglycerin, isosorbide dinitrate, ranitidine hydrochloride, isotretinoin, captopril, piroxicam, metoprolol, and diclofenac sodium. When the frequency of headache was compiled with respect to the amount of drug sold, the drugs most likely to cause headache were zimeldine, nalidixic acid, trimethoprim, griseofulvin, ranitidine, and nifedipine. Certain medications were found to initiate migraine headaches. These included cimetidine, oral contraceptives, atenolol,

indomethacin, danazol, nifedipine, diclofenac, and ranitidine. Medications that may aggravate existing migraine include vitamin A; its retinoic acid derivatives; and hormonal therapy, such as oral contraceptives, clomiphene citrate, and postmenopausal estrogens. Both migraine and cluster headaches may be exacerbated by vasodilators such as sildenafil citrate, nitrates, hydralazine hydrochloride, minoxidil, nifedipine, and prazosin hydrochloride.

Indomethacin, while useful in treating cluster variant headaches, can cause a generalized headache. Long-term use of some drugs, including narcotics, barbiturates, caffeine, and ergots, can lead to analgesic overuse (rebound) headaches.[23]

Psychological function

Comprehensive history taking includes assessment of psychological functioning. It is necessary to identify or rule out psychiatric disease or personality disorders. If these are present, concomitant psychological or psychiatric management must be considered. Second, the psychological reaction to pain should be recounted. The reaction to pain reflects the underlying personality or coping style. Third, general health behaviors are reviewed (ie, exercise, alcohol use, recreational drug use, sleep and eating habits, and smoking). These may reflect patients' perceived locus of control for their health. Previous health behaviors, as well as patients' reactions to the suggestion that they modify current health behaviors, can be important data in predicting success with nonpharmacologic therapy for headache.

The final step in evaluating the patient's history is a measurement of headache-related disability. It is valuable to assess whether the patient has absenteeism or decreased productivity at work, family, or social events due to headache. This assessment can be performed by simple questioning or with the use of disability questionnaires. Patients with severe headache-related disability are candidates for aggressive therapeutic interventions.

Differential Considerations

In primary care, most headaches are not caused by underlying disease. It is important to recognize, however, that headache can be the presenting symptom of several diseases. Fever, regardless of cause, is probably the most common medical problem that causes headache. Less common causes include pheochromocytoma, chronic renal failure, hyperthyroidism, and malignant hypertension.[23] Rheumatologic diseases may have headache as an early manifestation. Headache is common in systemic lupus erythematosus, polyarteritis nodosa, and giant cell arteritis. About two thirds of patients with fibrositis or fibromyalgia report headache, usually tension-type headache. Many types of vasculitis can also present with headache.[23] Headache upon awakening may be the initial symptom of sleep apnea syndrome. The headache often will improve as the day progresses. Associated symptoms include snoring, daytime somnolence, hypertension, and arrhythmias.[23]

Physical Examination

After evaluating the headache history, the physician should perform a targeted physical examination. This should include mental status examination, blood pressure and pulse measurement, examination of the cranial nerves, funduscopy, palpation of the head and neck, auscultation of the carotid arteries and heart, evaluation of motor and balance, and palpation of peripheral pulses (Tables 57-2 and 57-3).

Diagnostic Testing

Diagnostic testing of the patient with headache should be determined based on the results of the history and physical examination. In a patient with a typical headache history of several years' duration and normal findings of

the neurologic examination, no further evaluation may be needed. All patients older than 60 years with new-onset headache or change in their headache pattern should have a sedimentation rate or C-reactive protein measurement to evaluate for giant cell arteritis.

Screening laboratory studies may occasionally be obtained to rule out the more likely diseases that present with headache. Testing may include thyrotropin (thyroid-stimulating hormone) and sedimentation rate in patients with symptoms of rheumatologic disease and those over 60 years old. Patients suspected of sleep apnea should be evaluated by sleep study (polysomnography).

Several commonly ordered tests have little or no value in the headache evaluation.[24] "Routine" laboratory screening with complete blood cell count, urinalysis, and chemistry profile adds little diagnostic information. Electroencephalography (EEG) may be abnormal in some

---

TABLE 57-2

Key Aspects of Physical Examination*

1. Observation and palpation of head for signs of trauma, tenderness, and adequacy of temporal artery pulses
2. Assessment of cranial nerves, including funduscopic evaluation
3. Examination of oral cavity for dental disease; tongue for midline positioning; palette for symmetrical movement
4. Assessment of temporomandibular joints for alignment, ease of mobility, and "clicking"
5. Palpation of neck for lymphadenopathy and thyromegaly; auscultation over carotids
6. Assessment of cervical motion for meningeal irritation or spinal abnormalities
7. Palpation of areas, including suboccipital and sternocleidomastoid for "trigger points"
8. Assessment of muscle strength in upper extremities (biceps, triceps, hand grip) and in lower extremities (leg extension and flexion; ankle and toe dorsiflexion)
9. Assessment of tactile sense with pinprick to face, hand, and foot
10. Testing of deep-tendon reflexes of arm, knees, and ankle; Babinski response
11. Examination of ears, throat, lungs, heart, and abdomen for systemic disease
12. Screening for postural abnormalities, skeletal asymmetry, scoliosis, spasm, and additional trigger points in shoulders and back

*From Solomon et al.[60]

TABLE 57-3

Red Flags in Diagnosis of Headache*

1. Onset of headache after age 50 years
2. Onset of new or different headache
3. "Worst" headache ever experienced
4. Onset of subacute headache that progressively worsens over time
5. Onset of headache with exertion, sexual activity, coughing, or sneezing
6. Headache associated with any of the following changes in neurologic evaluation:
   a. Drowsiness, confusion, memory impairment
   b. Weakness, ataxia, loss of coordination
   c. Numbness and/or tingling in extremities
   d. Paralysis
   e. Sensory loss associated with headache
   f. Asymmetry of pupillary response, deep tendon reflexes, or Babinski response
   g. Signs of meningeal irritation
   h. Progressive visual or neurologic changes
   i. Other evidence to suggest an underlying neurologic disorder, such as persistent tinnitus, loss of sense of smell, loss of sensation over the face, and dysphagia
7. Abnormal medical evaluation:
   a. Fever
   b. Stiff neck
   c. Hypertension
   d. Weight loss
   e. Tender, poorly pulsatile temporal arteries
   f. Papilledema
   g. Chronic cough, lymphadenopathy, recurrent nasal drainage or discharge, or other evidence to suggest a systemic illness

*From Solomon et al.[60]

migraineurs, but EEG changes are neither specific for nor diagnostic of migraine. As a screening test to localize organic lesions, EEG has been supplanted by more specific computed tomographic (CT) and magnetic resonance imaging (MRI). Evoked potentials (visual, auditory, and somatosensory) fail to show specific findings in migraine. Like EEG, evoked potentials have no utility as a screening test for headache. Thermography has been touted by some practitioners as diagnostic for vascular headache and other pain states, but review of the medical literature fails to support the use of thermography in generating a diagnosis, in guiding therapy, or in determining prognosis for headache disorders.[25] Therefore, the use of thermography in headache should be discouraged.

Neuroradiology has little role in the diagnosis of headache beyond ruling out occult lesions such as neoplasm, hemorrhage, vascular malformations, brain abscesses, hydrocephalus, or congenital malformations. Neither MRI nor CT will pick up other organic causes of headache, such as idiopathic intracranial hypertension (pseudotumor cerebri), meningitis or other infections, glaucoma or other eye disease, and metabolic or toxic causes of headache.[24] Guidelines for use of CT and MRI in the setting of headache are outlined in Table 57-4.

Parenchymal brain lesions, described as well-defined, high-intensity T2 foci in the periventricular white matter, have been reported on MRI in 12% to 46% of migraineurs.[26,27] These "unidentified bright objects," or UBOs, also have been reported in patients with demyelinating disease (multiple sclerosis) and small vessel atherosclerotic disease (lacunar infarcts). These white-matter abnormalities increase in frequency with patient age and may reflect low-grade vascular insufficiency with resulting perivascular gliosis.[28] Neither multiple sclerosis nor atherosclerotic cerebrovascular disease typically presents with headache as a dominant clinical feature. Further workup for these conditions is not necessary if UBOs are noted on an MRI in a patient with symptoms of migraine.[26] The advent of CT and MRI has replaced plain film radiography of the skull in evaluating

headache-affected patients. The use of cervical spine radiography is rarely useful in the diagnosis and management of headache.[24]

Expected Outcome of Screening

The stated goal of screening patients with headache is to separate the rare patients with secondary causes from the patients with a primary headache disorder. Once a primary (benign) headache diagnosis is made, the major role of the physician is to initiate a therapeutic plan. Important goals of the therapeutic plan are to limit disability caused by headache and to prevent the development of analgesic overuse headache. Because headache is often a disorder of otherwise healthy young adults, the physician often is able to use the headache evaluation to encourage a healthy lifestyle. Patients are usually relieved when their headache evaluation shows no abnormalities, and this can open the door to a dialogue on maintaining health.

EFFECTIVENESS OF EARLY DETECTION

The purpose of early detection of headache is to diagnose the organic (secondary) causes of headache, initiate therapy, and reduce the morbidity and disability caused by chronic headache disorders. The disability resulting from chronic headache leads to absenteeism and decreased productivity ("presenteeism") at work. Osterhaus and coworkers[29] reported that 55% of migraineurs missed 2 workdays per month, and 88% worked 5.6 days per month with migraine symptoms that reduced their productivity. Stewart et al[5] found that migraine was more prevalent in the lowest income group. This was postulated to be due to downward socioeconomic drift caused by disruption of function at school or work related to recurrent migraines. Early intervention may stop the downward economic spiral caused by recurrent migraine headaches. The value of early intervention is largely determined by

TABLE 57-4

Guidelines for Use of CT and MRI*

Neuroimaging Procedures May Be Indicated When *Any* of the Following Is Present:	Neuroimaging Procedures May *Not Be* Indicated When *All* of the Following Are Present:
1. Decreased alertness or cognition	1. History of similar headaches
2. Normal vital signs	2. Onset of pain with exertion, coitus, coughing, or sneezing
3. Worsening under observation	3. Alertness and cognition intact
4. Nuchal rigidity	4. Supple neck
5. Focal neurologic signs	5. No neurologic signs
6. First headache in patient >50 years	6. Improvement in headache without analgesics or abortive medications
7. Worst headache ever experienced	
8. Headache not fitting a defined pattern	

*From Solomon et al.[60]

the effectiveness of therapy. Some therapies appear to be more effective if used early in treatment. Biofeedback therapy for headaches is more effective in younger subjects who are not chronically habituated to pain medications.[30] Patients older than 60 years had a poor response to biofeedback and relaxation therapy, with only 18% noting clinical improvement.[31] Therefore, if persons with headache are identified at a young age and before they become habituated to pain medications, biofeedback therapy has a 60% to 65% likelihood of inducing improvement.[30] The percentage of patients reporting continued major improvement at 3 to 5 years after treatment with biofeedback ranges from 30% to 80%.

Prophylactic drug therapy for migraine effectively reduces headache frequency for about two thirds of patients. Because the efficacy of drug therapy, like biofeedback, is reduced in patients taking large amounts of habituating pain medication, early intervention with appropriate prophylactic therapy is quite valuable.

HEADACHE DUE TO ANALGESIC MEDICATION OVERUSE

An extremely important condition contributing to the development of headaches in a chronic daily pattern is overuse of analgesic medication. This is most likely to occur in patients with frequent headaches. Analgesic overuse was reported in 25% to 38% of the population with chronic daily headache.[12] In headache referral centers, rates of analgesic overuse range from 46% to 87% of patients who have chronic daily headache.[12] Headache induced by long-term substance use is defined as headache occurring during the daily use of symptomatic headache medication or long-term intake of other substances, as well as headache occurring in the withdrawal phase after such substance use.[2] The headache is daily or almost daily and disappears within a few weeks of medication withdrawal. Headache induced by long-term substance use occurs after daily doses of a substance for at least 3 months. According to the IHS, the doses of medication required to induce analgesic abuse headache are greater than 50 g of aspirin or equivalent mild analgesic per month (approximately 150 tablets per month), more than 100 tablets per month of combination analgesics (barbiturate or other nonopioid), or 1 or more opioid analgesics daily. Daily uses of ergotamine (>2 mg orally or 1 mg rectally) can cause ergotamine-induced headache. The IHS criteria[2] for analgesic overuse are arbitrary and unsupported by medical evidence. There is no compelling scientific research that simple analgesics such as aspirin, acetaminophen, or nonsteroidal anti-inflammatory drugs (NSAIDs) induce headaches with daily use, and there is some evidence that daily NSAID or aspirin use may reduce headache frequency.[32]

Medication overuse headache in migraineurs presents as a constant, diffuse, dull headache without associated symptoms.[33] Clinically, this syndrome cannot be differentiated from migraine with chronic tension-type headache or from chronic migraine. Withdrawal headache in migraineurs resembles a severe and prolonged migraine attack. In patients with chronic tension-type headache or post-traumatic headache, medication overuse headache cannot be discriminated from the characteristics of the primary headache.[33]

Daily use of ergots may lead to a throbbing, pulsating headache in the early morning, sometimes with nausea. The headache disappears between 30 and 60 minutes after intake of ergotamine. It may be distinguished from migraine by the absence of an attack pattern or associated migraine symptoms.[33]

In their meta-analysis of studies on chronic medication overuse headache, Diener and Dahlof[33] found 65% of patients had migraine as their underlying headache disorder, 27% had tension-type headache, and 8% had mixed headache. Women were 3.5 times more likely than men to have headache due to long-term medication overuse. Patients with this type of medication overuse headache had an average duration of primary headache exceeding 20 years and frequent drug intake for greater than 10 years. The mean duration of daily headache was almost 6 years. Patients used either combination drugs or multiple products, averaging 2.5 to 5.8 different pharmacologic components taken simultaneously.

Because the efficacy of prophylactic therapy is reduced by excessive use of habituating medications, early intervention permits the selection of nonhabituating medications to treat acute headache attacks. Furthermore, early intervention may reduce the morbidity caused by frequent use of over-the-counter analgesics, such as peptic ulcer diseases and analgesic nephropathy.

FOLLOW-UP SCREENING

Benign headache disorders tend to be chronic illnesses, offering the physician many opportunities for follow-up care. The major questions in the continuing care of the headache-affected patient are as follows:

1. Has the prescribed intervention been effective?
2. Has the therapy caused adverse effects?
3. Is the patient with headache experiencing new medical problems that require treatment?
4. Has an organic cause of headache developed that was missed on initial screening?

Certain medical illnesses are more common in patients who experience headaches. Featherstone[34] evaluated the prevalence of concomitant medical diseases in people with chronic headache by reviewing 1414 life insurance applications, obtaining 200 headache cases with matched controls without chronic headaches. Six conditions were found to occur more often in the chronic headache group: hypertension, dizziness or vertigo, gastroesophageal reflux, depression or anxiety, peptic ulcer disease, and irritable bowel syndrome. Three conditions were significantly more common in the population without headache: nephrolithiasis, alcohol abuse in men, and abdominal pain in women. Several conditions or health risk factors had the same prevalence in both headache and nonheadache groups: ischemic heart disease, mitral valve prolapse, cardiovascular disease, central nervous system ischemia, cigarette smoking, emphysema, and previous surgery.

Other investigators have found associations between specific headache diagnoses and medical diseases. To examine the association between migraine and other conditions, Merikangas[35] found the following conditions to be strongly associated with migraine: stroke, heart attack, bronchitis, colitis, nervous breakdown, urinary tract disorders, and ulcers. Migraine also has been associated with an increased prevalence of coronary vasospasm, Raynaud phenomenon, aspirin-sensitive asthma, mitral valve prolapse, and hypertension.[23] Cluster headache is associated with a threefold increase in the prevalence of peptic ulcer disease.[19] Chronic tension-type headache sufferers have an increased prevalence of depression.[13]

A controversy in headache management is the issue of repeated evaluations to look for organic causes of headache. Most physicians agree that repeating the pertinent headache history and the targeted physical examination is important to pick up clues for new diagnoses and diagnoses missed at initial evaluation. The issue of obtaining additional CT scans or MRIs is unsettled. Neuroradiographic imaging would be prudent to consider in a patient whose condition is deteriorating or when history or physical examination has revealed new neurologic abnormalities, but it offers little yield in patients whose headache course is stable, even if the patient is not responding well to treatment.

THERAPEUTIC INTERVENTIONS

Drug Habituation and Detoxification

Drug habituation may accompany many chronic headache syndromes. Analgesic overuse must be considered early in patient management. Medications that are known to cause analgesic overuse (rebound) headaches include narcotics, barbiturates, ergotamine tartrate compounds, benzodiazepines, and caffeine preparations.[36] There is no evidence that simple analgesics such as aspirin, acetaminophen, or NSAIDs cause rebound headaches with daily use. Discontinuation of habituating drugs should be the initial step in the treatment of patients who are taking excessive pain medications (ie, using daily or almost daily habituating pain medication, or taking ergotamine or triptans more than twice weekly). Prophylactic medication is

ineffective in patients experiencing analgesic overuse headaches. Frequently, patients will say that they "would stop taking pain medication if only the preventive medication prevented the headaches." Patients must be instructed that the "pain medication" is part of the cause of the headaches and that headache therapy is futile until the rebound/habituation cycle is resolved. Typical analgesic withdrawal symptoms last 2 to 10 days (average, 3.5 days) and include headache, nausea, vomiting, hypotension, tachycardia, sleep disturbances, restlessness, and anxiety. Seizures and hallucinations are rare, even for patients using barbiturate-combination drugs.

Management of the habituated patient can be difficult, and the medical literature offers limited insight into proper techniques of detoxification. Hering and Steiner[37] reported successful outpatient management of patients with analgesic overuse headache using the technique of (1) abrupt drug withdrawal, (2) explanation of the disorder, (3) regular follow-up, (4) 10 mg of amitriptyline hydrochloride at bedtime for prophylaxis, and (5) 500 mg of naproxen for acute relief. Smith[38] reported an effective outpatient treatment plan for analgesic rebound headache, which included (1) abrupt drug withdrawal; (2) 2 mg of tizanidine hydrochloride at bedtime, titrated every 3 to 5 days to 2 to 16 mg at bedtime; and (3) a long-acting NSAID or coxib in the morning.

Patients who are habituated to opioids may benefit from clonidine hydrochloride to prevent physical signs and symptoms of withdrawal. In the absence of good scientific evidence, glucocorticoids and phenothiazines are sometimes prescribed for outpatient detoxification from butalbital, ergotamine, or low doses of opioids. Generally, a 6- to 14-day tapering course of glucocorticoid is given, and phenothiazine suppositories are prescribed for severe withdrawal headaches associated with vomiting. For patients with concomitant medical problems, a history of seizures, or prior unsuccessful outpatient detoxification, inpatient detoxification may be required. Prevention of relapse after detoxification is critical to prevent recurrence. About one third of patients will relapse into drug overuse within the first 5 years after detoxification. Almost 90% of patients who relapse use the same drug that they initially overused.[33]

An approach to reduce relapse should include the following:

- Use specific antimigraine drugs only for migraine attacks
- Restrict the dose of ergots and triptans weekly and for each attack
- Avoid mixed analgesics, butalbital, opioids, and tranquilizers
- Start prophylactic drugs early ($\geq$ 2–3 attacks per month)

Treatment of Chronic Headache

The first step in the treatment of the "chronic daily headache" syndrome is to split the problem into manageable headache components. While there is no specific treatment of "chronic daily headache," there are potentially effective approaches for medication-overuse headache, chronic tension-type headache, and migraine. The management approach may include treatment of the analgesic overuse by abrupt analgesic withdrawal, prophylactic therapy for the chronic tension-type headaches, and abortive and prophylactic therapy for the migraine attacks.

In clinical practice, it is not uncommon to see improvements in some components of the headache syndrome and intractability in other components. After drug withdrawal and initiation of abortive and prophylactic therapies, patients may improve in their ability to manage their acute migraine attacks but continue to be burdened by the frequency of their migraine or tension-type headaches. Their quality of life and functional ability are often greatly improved, yet they may still report having frequent headaches. Practitioners should rely on quality of life or functional (disability) measures, rather than number of headache days, to judge the outcome of therapy. Only by splitting the "chronic migraine" into its component parts can the practitioner modify therapy to improve the poorly controlled component or components without giving up the gains achieved in other aspects of the headache syndrome.

There are no drugs currently approved by the US Food and Drug Administration (FDA) specifically for the treatment of chronic tension-type or chronic daily headache. However, given the chronic nature of the disorder and the risk of medication overuse headache in patients with frequent headaches, prophylactic therapy seems warranted for most patients. Since chronic headache is a disorder of central pain processing, medications with central pain modulating effects tend to be the most effective.[36]

Preventive medications

Tricyclic antidepressants are the drugs of choice for chronic tension-type headache, and several of these agents are also effective in migraine prophylaxis. The antidepressants that have been tested in double-blind, placebo-controlled studies of patients with chronic tension-type headache include amitriptyline, doxepin hydrochloride, and maprotiline hydrochloride.[39] Other tricyclic antidepressants may also be effective, although they have not been studied in this population. In children and elderly patients, the usual starting dose of amitriptyline hydrochloride (or a similar drug) is 10 mg at bedtime. In adults, the usual starting dose is 25 mg at bedtime. The dosage can be increased every few days until a thera-

peutic result is obtained or side effects become intolerable. Antidepressants usually take from 4 to 6 weeks to show beneficial effects.

The selective serotonin reuptake inhibitors (SSRIs) fluoxetine hydrochloride, paroxetine hydrochloride, and citalopram hydrochloride[40-42] have not shown efficacy in controlled studies. Since they lack efficacy in headache prophylaxis, they should be considered only for patients with headache who cannot tolerate or who fail to respond to tricyclic therapy.

Cyclobenzaprine hydrochloride is a muscle relaxant that is related structurally to amitriptyline. In a 1972 double-blind study,[43] 10 of 20 patients receiving cyclobenzaprine showed a 50% or greater improvement in chronic tension-type headache, whereas only 5 of 20 patients receiving placebo were improved. The usual dosage of cyclobenzaprine hydrochloride is 10 mg at bedtime. Tizanidine hydrochloride, an α-adrenergic blocker, was reported to be effective for chronic tension-type headache in a single placebo-controlled study.[44] The dosage was titrated from 2 mg at bedtime to 20 mg each day, divided into 3 doses. Sedation is the most common adverse effect of this agent.

Nonsteroidal anti-inflammatory drugs are widely prescribed both as adjunctive therapy for tension-type headache and for the prophylaxis of migraine headache.[45] There are no randomized controlled trials of their efficacy in the prophylaxis of chronic tension-type headache, but several NSAIDs have shown efficacy for migraine prophylaxis.[46]

Valproate sodium, a GABA agonist anticonvulsant, has been evaluated for efficacy in migraine[47,48] and "chronic daily headache"[49] and found to lead to significant improvement in many patients. Commonly reported side effects include weight gain, tremor, hair loss, and nausea. Results have not been replicated in a randomized controlled trial.

Botulinum toxin A injections into the muscles of the head and neck have been studied for the relief of chronic tension-type headache and migraine. A review of the studies using evidence-based medicine criteria[50] concluded that the results did not support the prophylactic treatment of primary headaches with botulinum toxin A.

Abortive therapy

Treatment of the daily, tension-type headache with abortive medications is difficult. Muscle relaxants such as chlorzoxazone, orphenadrine citrate, carisoprodol, and metaxalone, either alone or in combinations with aspirin, acetaminophen, and/or caffeine, are commonly prescribed to patients with chronic tension-type headache; however, they have not been shown to be effective for acute headache relief.[36] Nonsteroidal anti-inflammatory drugs may be useful as analgesics for daily headache, and they lack the potential for causing medication-induced headache.[32] Sumatriptan succinate has been evaluated in several studies in tension-type headache.[51,52] The drug was no more effective than placebo in acute attacks for patients with chronic tension-type headache; however, severe episodic tension-type headaches in patients with coexisting migraine appear to respond to this agent.[53]

Benzodiazepines, butalbital combinations, and opioids should be avoided, or their use should be carefully controlled, because of the risk of habituation and analgesic overuse headache with frequent use.

Nonpharmacologic Therapy

Many clinical studies have supported the utility of relaxation therapy and electromyographic (EMG) biofeedback in the management of chronic tension-type headache.[46] Averaging the results of 37 trials that used daily headache recordings to evaluate relaxation or EMG biofeedback therapy, each therapy or the combination yielded a 50% reduction in tension-type headache activity. Studies have not found differences between the efficacy of relaxation, biofeedback, or the combination. Stress management therapy utilizing cognitive-behavior therapy is as effective as relaxation or biofeedback therapy in reducing tension-type headache. Cognitive therapy may be most likely to enhance the effectiveness of relaxation or biofeedback therapies when chronic stress, depression, or adjustment problems aggravate the patient's headaches.[46]

The combination of nonpharmacologic therapy and pharmacotherapy provides greater benefit than either therapy used alone. The addition of guided imagery to pharmacologic therapy resulted in significant improvements in both health-related quality of life and headache-related disability.[54] In a placebo-controlled study comparing tricyclic antidepressant medication with stress management therapy, both modalities were modestly effective by themselves in treating chronic tension-type headache, but combined therapy was better than monotherapy.[55]

Nonpharmacologic therapy is particularly useful for patients who are reluctant to take medications due to desire for pregnancy, previous adverse reactions to medications, or concomitant medical problems. Although biofeedback and stress management usually require referral to psychologists, guided imagery and relaxation therapy can be learned from audiotapes available at most book stores.[36]

Treatment of Migraine

Trigger factors

It is important to understand how trigger factors work in precipitating migraine. Most migraines are precipitated only when several triggers occur in close temporal proximity, usually in the 12 hours preceding the migraine onset. The simultaneous elimination of multiple headache triggers has an additive effect in decreasing the probability that the migraine threshold will be crossed. Migraines are rarely induced 100% of the time after exposure to individual triggers. For example, alcohol exposure will precipitate migraine 60% to 80% of the time in headache-prone individuals. The triggers may vary from one migraine attack to another in the same patient, although patients may have their own typical triggers. The combination of trigger elimination with medication management will improve headache control in more patients than either approach alone.[56]

Identification and elimination of triggers of headache has been found to be a highly effective and long-lasting migraine treatment. The most common migraine trigger factors are alcohol, tyramine (found in aged cheese, fermented foods), aspartame (found in many diet soft drinks), monosodium glutamate (MSG, found in Chinese restaurant food and flavor enhancers), and phenylethylamine (found in chocolate).[56] Additional common trigger factors are hormonal changes (eg, menses, climacteric), alterations in sleep patterns (eg, shift changes, jet lag, sleeping late on weekends), fasting, weather changes, and "let down" after stress (occurring on weekends and vacations).

Medications

A wide variety of medications have been used in the prophylaxis of migraine, including methysergide, β-blockers, calcium channel blockers, NSAIDs, tricyclic antidepressants, and cyproheptadine. Methysergide is rarely used today for migraine prophylaxis due to the risk of serious complications, such as retroperitoneal fibrosis. Cyproheptadine is generally used for migraine prophylaxis in children. Adults often find the side effects of fatigue and weight gain from this antihistamine-antiserotonin drug to be intolerable.

β-blockers, tricyclic antidepressants, calcium channel blockers, and NSAIDs are valued as first-line drugs for the prophylaxis of migraine.

Several β-blockers have been shown to be effective in migraine prophylaxis. Among these are propranolol hydrochloride and timolol maleate (the only beta blockers approved by the FDA for migraine prophylaxis), nadolol, metoprolol, and atenolol. β-blockers with intrinsic sympathomimetic activity, such as pindolol and acebutolol hydrochloride, have not been found useful in migraine prophylaxis. Side effects of β-blockers include depression, fatigue, and sleep disorders. Depression is more commonly reported with propranolol than with other β-blockers. These side effects may worsen the tension-type headache component of the chronic daily headache syndrome. Patients should not abruptly discontinue β-blocker therapy, since abrupt discontinuation may lead to myocardial infarction, even in patients with no prior history of heart disease.[23]

Calcium entry blockers are useful in the prophylaxis of migraine and cluster headache. Several calcium entry blockers have been shown to be effective in migraine prophylaxis, including verapamil hydrochloride, diltiazem hydrochloride, flunarizine, nimodipine, and nicardipine hydrochloride. Nifedipine is either weakly effective or ineffective for migraine prophylaxis and can exacerbate migraine in some patients because of profound vasodilation. In the United States, verapamil is considered the calcium channel blocker of choice for migraine and cluster prophylaxis.[57] Adverse effects with calcium entry blockers include constipation with verapamil; sedation, weight gain, and parkinsonism with flunarizine; flushing and edema with nifedipine; and gastrointestinal upset and parkinsonism with diltiazem.

Nonsteroidal anti-inflammatory drugs are valuable in both the prophylaxis of migraine headache and as adjunctive therapy for tension-type headache.[45] This dual effect on migraine and tension-type headache allows for NSAIDs to be used as single drug therapy in some patients with the chronic daily headache syndrome. Several NSAIDs have been reported to have prophylactic activity in migraine. Among these are aspirin, naproxen, flurbiprofen, ketoprofen, flufenamic acid, tolfenamic acid, and fenoprofen calcium. Adverse effects from NSAIDs are relatively common. They may include gastrointestinal symptoms, such as dyspepsia, heartburn, nausea, vomiting, diarrhea, constipation, generalized abdominal pain, bleeding of the upper gastrointestinal tract, altered kidney function, and fluid retention. Renal problems are most likely to occur in patients who are elderly, who are hypertensive, who have renovascular or advanced atherosclerotic disease, or who take diuretics. Indomethacin and fenoprofen appear to be more nephrotoxic than other NSAIDs. Analgesic nephropathy, the most common cause of drug-induced renal failure, has been associated with excessive use of NSAIDs along with phenacetin or acetaminophen.

For the abortive (acute) treatment of migraine headaches, guidelines suggest starting with a NSAID. The most effective NSAIDs to abort migraine attacks are naproxen sodium, flurbiprofen, and meclofenamate sodium. Generally, a dose is given at the onset of the headache (naproxen sodium, 550 mg; flurbiprofen, 100 mg; or meclofenamate sodium, 200 mg) and is repeated in 1 hour if the headache is still present. Many patients will have self-treated with over-the-counter NSAIDs before seeking medical consultation.

Patients whose migraines are associated with moderate to severe disability or whose attacks fail to respond to simple analgesics or NSAIDs may be candidates for a triptan (sumatriptan, zolmitriptan, naratriptan hydrochloride, rizatriptan benzoate, almotriptan maleate, frovatriptan, eletriptan). These "migraine-specific" therapies are structurally related to the neurotransmitter, serotonin (5-hydroxytryptamine, 5-HT). They are potent and selective agonists for the 5-HT$_{1B/1D}$ receptors, which are largely restricted to blood vessels, particularly in the internal carotid and middle cerebral arteries, and the trigeminal nerve. The triptans have no known analgesic effect per se. These agents relieve not only head pain but also associated symptoms of nausea, vomiting, photophobia, and phonophobia.

The triptans are often effective even if given far after the onset of migraine, during the peak intensity of headache. This feature makes these drugs useful for patients who frequently awaken with a fully evolved migraine. Triptans are prescribed to abort a migraine attack. If a triptan fails to do that with one dose, or in some cases with one more dose given 2 to 4 hours later, it is unlikely that this medication will help this attack. Rescue medications to reduce pain and the migraine's accompanying symptoms should then be used. Additional doses, beyond 1 to 2, should be kept in reserve only for headache recurrence (when a headache occurs within 24 hours of relief of the initial attack). In other words, triptans are never used "as needed for pain." Use of these medications more than 2 times during a treatment day (24 hours) or more than 6 to 8 treatment days per month signals a need for patient reevaluation. A triptan should not be given concurrently or within 24 hours of other triptans, related ergot-containing preparations, or ergotlike medications (dihydroergotamine mesylate, methysergide) due to the potential for additive vasoconstrictor effects.

Triptans may cause mild, transient elevation of blood pressure and may cause coronary vasospasm. They are contraindicated in patients with documented or suspected ischemic heart disease, history of myocardial infarction, documented silent ischemia, Prinzmetal angina, suspected coronary heart disease, and uncontrolled hypertension. These drugs have not been studied for management of basilar or hemiplegic migraine, nor have they been studied in pregnant women.

Ergotamine tartrate is usually effective for migraine but, because of the problem of adverse effects and ergotamine rebound with frequent use, is used only if the other medications are ineffective. When ergotamine is prescribed, it should be given no more often than every 4 days to prevent rebound headaches.

For patients suffering a migraine attack, their primary goal is rapid resolution of symptoms to permit a return to normal function. The pharmacologic features that they most desire are rapid onset of action, effectiveness to stop the head pain and associated symptoms, and few debilitating adverse effects. Despite the nausea that accompanies migraine, patients generally prefer an oral formulation for its convenience and ease of use.

Medical Treatment of Cluster Headache

Medications used in the prophylaxis of cluster headache include ergotamine, corticosteroids, methysergide, verapamil, and lithium carbonate. Verapamil hydrochloride, 240 to 480 mg daily, is useful in both episodic and chronic cluster headache, and it is generally considered the drug of choice for cluster prophylaxis. Corticosteroids and methysergide are used only in episodic cluster headache because of the potential adverse effects with long-term use. Lithium carbonate, 300 mg 3 times daily, is reserved for patients with chronic cluster headache. The drug of choice for the acute treatment of cluster headache is oxygen, given at 8 to 10 L/min by mask for 10 minutes. Other useful abortive medications include ergotamine and dihydroergotamine, sumatriptan subcutaneous injections, and lidocaine nosedrops.[58]

Counseling and Compliance

In an effort to evaluate the nature of consumer expectations, barriers to care, and levels of satisfaction with headache treatment, Klassen and Berman[59] surveyed subjects attending an educational seminar on headache. Three out of 4 subjects indicated the presence of factors that made it difficult to see physicians for headache, including attitudes and behaviors of physicians ("doctors won't listen") and high cost or inconvenience. A lack of satisfaction with treatments received from physicians for their headaches was indicated by 34% of subjects. The most frequently cited reasons for dissatisfaction were ineffectiveness of medications and physician behaviors. The most frequent suggestion made by subjects to improve medical care for headache was to change physician behavior or performance ("know more," "listen more," or "try harder").

It is estimated that nearly half of all migraineurs have given up seeking help for their headaches from their physicians. Although patients sometimes find their headache medications to be ineffective, it is physician behavior toward the headache-affected patient that discourages continuity of care. Counseling the patient on the mechanisms of headache, trigger factors, expected outcome of therapy ("control" of headaches and improvement in lifestyle without "cure" of disease), and reassurance of the absence of serious disease should help to cement the therapeutic relationship. Further discussion on the wide variety of medications available to aid headaches should encourage the patient to continue care if the initial therapy is ineffective or poorly tolerated.

Compliance rarely is a problem when the patient and physician have formed a good relationship based on an understanding of the disease as well as the patient's response to her or his illness, and knowledge of the risks, benefits, and goals of therapy. Limiting the dietary and lifestyle restrictions (reduction of trigger factors) to those that apply to a given patient will improve compliance. For example, a woman who gets migraines only with menses should not be asked to eliminate chocolate and cheese from her diet. Patients with cluster headache must eliminate alcohol during the cluster cycle, but abstinence between cycles will not influence the headache pattern. Smoking cessation, however, may benefit the headache problem. The physician treating patients with headache must be available to handle the episodic exacerbations of headache and the occasional headache that does not respond to usual medications. Additionally, the patient and physician must forge a long-term relationship to deal with the chronic nature of headaches.

SUMMARY

Headache, one of the most frequent complaints in the outpatient setting, tends to be a recurrent, chronic medical problem. As physicians become more involved in the management of headache, they will find that headache medicine fits well within the long-term care ideals of preventive medicine. Physicians, hospitals, and, most important, patients can only benefit from physicians assuming a preventive approach to the care of chronic headaches.

REFERENCES

1. Linet MS, Stewart WF, Celentano DD, Ziegler D, Sprecher M. An epidemiologic study of headache among adolescents and young adults. *JAMA.* 1989; 261:2211–2216.

2. Headache Classification Committee of the International Headache Society. Classification and diagnostic criteria for headache disorders, cranial neuralgias, and facial pain. *Cephalalgia.* 1988;8(suppl 7):1–96.

3. *MMWR Morb Mortal Wkly Rep.* 1991;40:331–338.

4. Rasmussen BK, et al. Epidemiology of headache in a general population: a prevalence study. *J Clin Epidemiol.* 1991;44:1147–1157.

5. Stewart WF, et al. Prevalence of migraine headache in the United States. *JAMA.* 1992;267:64–69.

6. Cook NR, et al. Correlates of headache in a population-based cohort of elderly. *Arch Neurol.* 1989;46:1338–1344.

7. Solomon GD, Kunkel RS, Frame J. Demographics of headache in elderly patients. *Headache.* 1990;30:273–276.

8. Silberstein SD, Lipton RB, Sliwinski M. Classification of daily and near-daily headaches: field trial of revised HIS criteria. *Neurology.* 1996;47:871–875.

9. Newman LC, Lipton SB, Solomon S, et al. Daily headache in a population sample: results from American Migraine Study. *Headache.* 1994;34:295.

10. Rasmussen BK, Jensen R, Olesen J. Epidemiology of tension-type headache in a general population. In: Olesen J, Schoenen J, eds. *Tension-type Headache: Classification, Mechanisms, and Treatment.* New York, NY: Raven Press; 1993:9–13.

11. Scher AI. Natural history of and risk factors for headache transformation. Paper presented at: American Headache Society annual meeting; June 21, 2002; Seattle, Wash.

12. Bech P, Langemark M, Loidrup D, et al. Tension-type headache: psychiatric aspects. In: Olesen J, Schoenen J, eds. *Tension-type Headache: Classification, Mechanisms, and Treatment.* New York, NY: Raven Press; 1993:143–146.

13. Goncalves JA, Monteiro P. Psychiatric analysis of patients with tension-type headache. In: Olesen J, Schoenen J, eds. *Tension-type Headache: Classification, Mechanisms, and Treatment.* New York, NY: Raven Press; 1993:167–172.

14. Merikangas KR, Angst J, Isler H. Migraine and psychopathology: results of the Zurich cohort study of young adults. *Arch Gen Psychiatry.* 1990;47:849–853.

15. Breslau N, Davis GC. Migraine, physical health and psychiatric disorders: a prospective epidemiologic study of young adults. *J Psychiatr Res.* 1993;27:211–221.

16. Silberstein DS, Lipton RB. Chronic daily headache, including transformed migraine, chronic tension-type headache, and medication overuse. In: Silberstein SD, Lipton RB, Dalessio DJ, eds. *Wolff's Headache.* 7th ed. Oxford, England: Oxford University Press; 2001:247–282.

17. Verri AP, Cecchini P, Galli C, et al. Psychiatric comorbidity in chronic daily headache. *Cephalalgia.* 1998;18:45–49.

18. Breslau N. New insights into the comorbidity of migraine. Paper presented at: American Headache Society annual meeting; June 21, 2002; Seattle, Wash.

19. Diamond S, Solomon GD, Freitag FG. Cluster headache. *Clin J Pain.* 1987;3:171–176.

20. Sadjapour K. Cluster headache. Paper presented at: Bergen Migraine Symposium; 1975; Bergen, Norway.

21. Diamond S, Solomon GD, Freitag FG. Differential diagnosis of headache pain. In: Tollison CD, ed. *Handbook of Chronic Pain Management.* Baltimore, Md: Williams & Wilkins; 1988.

22. Askmark H, Lundberg PO, Olsson S. Drug-related headache. *Headache.* 1989;29:441–444.

23. Solomon GD. Concomitant medical disease and headache. *Med Clin North Am.* 1991;75:631–639.

24. Donohoe CD, Waldman SD. The targeted physical examination. *Intern Med Special.* 1991;12:30–39.

25. Cotton P. AMA's Council on Scientific Affairs takes a fresh look at thermography. *JAMA.* 1992;267:1885–1887.

26. Soges LJ, et al. Migraine: evaluation by MR. *Am J Neuroradiol.* 1988;9:425–429.

27. Osborn RE, Alder DC, Mitchell CS. MR imaging of the brain in patients with migraine headaches. *Am J Neuroradiol.* 1991;12:521–524.

28. Prager JM, et al. Evaluation of headache patients by MRI. *Headache Q.* 1991;2:192–195.

29. Osterhaus JT, Gutterman DL, Plachetka JR. Labor costs associated with migraine headaches. *Headache.* 1990;30:302–303.

30. Chapman SL. A review and clinical perspective on the use of EMG and thermal biofeedback for chronic headaches. *Pain.* 1986;27:1–43.

31. Blanchard EB, et al. Biofeedback and relaxation treatments for headache in the elderly: a caution and a challenge. *Biofeedback Self Regul.* 1985;10:69–73.

32. Lipton RB. Frequent headaches: a far too frequent problem. Paper presented at: Headache World 2000; September 2000; London, England.

33. Diener HC, Dahlof CG. Headache associated with chronic use of substances. In: Olesen J, Tfelt-Hansen P, Welch KMA, eds. *The Headaches.* 2nd ed. Philadelphia, Pa: Lippincott Williams & Wilkins; 2000:871–878.

34. Featherstone HJ. Medical diagnoses and problems in individuals with recurrent idiopathic headaches. *Headache.* 1985;25:136–140.

35. Merikangas KR. Comorbidity of migraine and other conditions in the general population of adults in the United States. *Cephalalgia.* 1991;11(suppl 11):108–109.

36. Solomon GD. Tension-type headache: advice for the vice-like headache. *Cleve Clin J Med.* 2002;69:167–172.

37. Hering R, Steiner T. Abrupt outpatient withdrawal from medication in analgesic-abusing migraineurs. *Lancet.* 1991;337:1442–1443.

38. Smith TR. Low-dose tizanidine with non-steroidal anti-inflammatory drugs for detoxification from analgesic rebound headache. *Headache.* 2002;42:175–177.

39. Mathew N, Bendtsen L. Prophylactic pharmacotherpy of tension-type headache. In: Olesen J, Tfelt-Hansen P, Welch KMA, eds. *The Headaches.* Philadelphia, Pa: Lippincott Williams & Wilkins; 2000:667–673.

40. Saper J, Silberstein S, Lake A, Winters M. Double blind trial of fluoxetine: chronic daily headache and migraine. *Headache.* 1994;34:497–502.

41. Foster CA, Bafaloukos J. Paroxetine on the treatment of chronic daily headache. *Headache.* 1994;34:587–589.

42. Bendtsen L, Jensen R, Olesen J. A nonselective (amitriptyline), but not a selective (citalopram), serotonin reuptake inhibitor is effective in the prophylactic treatment of chronic tension-type headache. *J Neurol Neurolsurg Psychiatry.* 1996;61:285–290.

43. Lance JW, Anthony M. Cyclobenzaprine in the treatment of chronic tension headache. *Med J Aust.* 1972;2:1409–1411.

44. Fogelholm R, Murros K. Tizanidine in chronic tension-type headache: a placebo-controlled double-blind cross-over study. *Headache.* 1992;32:509–513.

45. Solomon GD. Pharmacology and use of headache medications. *Cleve Clin J Med.* 1990;57:627–635.

46. Sorensen K. Valproate: a new drug in migraine prophylaxis. *Acta Neurol Scand.* 1988;78:346–348.

47. Herring R, Kuritzky A. Sodium valproate in the prophylactic treatment of migraine: a double-blind study versus placebo. *Cephalalgia.* 1992;12:81–84.

48. Mathew NT, Ali S. Valproate in the treatment of persistent chronic daily headache: an open label study. *Headache.* 1991;31:71–74.

49. Evers S, Rahman A, Vollmer-Hasse J, Husstedt I-W. Treatment of headache with botulinum toxin A: a review according to evidence-based medicine criteria. *Cephalalgia.* 2002; 22:699–710.

50. Brennum J, Kjeldsen M, Olesen J. The 5-HT 1-like agonist sumatriptan has a significant effect in chronic tension-type headache. *Cephalalgia.* 1992;12:375–379.

51. Brennum J, Brinck T, Schriver L, et al. Sumatriptan has no clinically relevant effect in the treatment of episodic tension-type headache. *Eur J Neurol.* 1996;3:23–28.

52. Cady R, Gutterman D, Saiers JA, Beach ME. Responsiveness of non-IHS migraine and tension-type headache to sumatriptan. *Cephalalgia.* 1997;17:588–590.

53. Holyroid KA. Behavioral treatment strategies. In: Olesen J, Schoenen J, eds. *Tension-type Headache: Classification, Mechanisms, and Treatment.* New York, NY: Raven Press; 1993:245–254.

54. Mannix LK, Chandurkar RS, Rybicki LA, Tusek DL, Solomon GD. Effect of guided imagery on quality of life for patients with chronic tension-type headache. *Headache.* 1999;39:326–334.

55. Holroyd K, O'Donnell F, Stensland M, Lipchik G, Cordingley G, Carlson B. Management of chronic tension-type headache with tricyclic antidepressant medication, stress management therapy, and their combination. *JAMA.* 2001;285:2208–2215.

56. Scopp AL. Headache triggers: theory, research, and clinical application. *Headache Q.* 1992;3:32–37.

57. Elkind AH. Interval therapy of migraine: the art and science. *Headache Q.* 1990;1:280–289.

58. Solomon GD. Pharmacology and use of headache medications. *Cleve Clin J Med.* 1990;57:627–635.

59. Klassen AC, Berman ME. Medical care for headache: a consumer survey. *Cephalalgia.* 1991;11(suppl 11):85–86.

60. Solomon GD, Cady R, Klapper J, Ryan R. National Headache Foundation: standards of care for treating headache in primary care practice. *Cleve Clin J Med.* 1997;64:373–383.

RESOURCES

American Council for Headache Education (ACHE), 19 Mantua Road, Mount Royal, NJ 08061; 800 255-ACHE (outside New Jersey) or 609 845-0322.
Web site: www.achenet.org. (A nonprofit organization whose goal is to educate the public that headache is a valid and treatable disease.)

American Headache Society, 19 Mantua Road, Mount Royal, NJ 08061; 856 423-0043.
Web site: www.ashnet.org. (Professional and scientific organization dedicated to headache.)

National Headache Foundation, 428 W St James Pl, 2nd Floor, Chicago, IL 60614-2750; 888 NHF-5552 (643-5552).
Web site: www.headaches.org. (A national nonprofit group dedicated to educating the public, promoting research, and serving as an information resource. It has a referral list of member physicians.)

chapter 58

Asthma and Allergic Disorders

Benjamin J. Ansell, MD, and Kenneth J. Serio, MD

INTRODUCTION

Allergic diseases are a major contributor to medical expenses in the United States, with asthma alone accounting for approximately $6 billion in annual health care costs.[1] Over the last half century, there has been a marked increase in the prevalence of allergic diseases, such as asthma,[2,3] allergic rhinitis,[3,4] and atopic dermatitis.[3,5] The exact reasons for this trend are unclear. However, multiple factors appear to be involved, including the decreased exposure to bacteria early in life, broader use of antibiotics, increased indoor and outdoor air pollution, and dietary changes. Among these, the "hygiene hypothesis," related to the diminished early life exposure to bacterial infections in developed countries, has recently been proposed to attempt to explain the rising prevalence of asthma.[6] Studies in support of this theory indicate that serologic evidence of certain foodborne and orofecal infections is associated with a decreased likelihood of developing atopic sensitization to airborne allergens, hay fever, and asthma.[7,8]

Although exposure to bacterial products early in life has been a focus of many epidemiologic investigations of allergic disease, other factors are also believed to play a major role. There are geographic differences in the prevalence of allergic disease, with the southern regions of Europe having a higher rate of disease than the northern regions.[9] The observed geographic variations may be due to differences in genetics, dietary factors, or climate. Despite concerns over urban air pollutants contributing to an increase in respiratory allergic disease, the rural lifestyle has not been shown, by itself, to afford any protection against the development of allergy.[10] In addition, despite considerable evidence suggesting that air pollution is a factor in the trend in prevalence of allergic disease,[11] some studies suggest that increased levels of air pollution may not specifically be responsible for the increased prevalence of allergic disease when factors such as atopy and exposure to indoor allergens are considered.[12,13] The prevalence of asthma is strongly correlated with national

socioeconomic status, as reflected by the gross national product of a country.[12] Dietary influences, particularly the early exposure to farm milk products, are also associated with a decreased likelihood of subsequent allergy.[9] Smaller family size, with a resultant decreased exposure to siblings, has been linked to an increase in atopy.[14] Finally, some have suggested that the perceived increasing incidence of allergic disease may reflect increased patient awareness[15] or improved medical recognition of these conditions in affluent societies.

PREVENTION OF ALLERGIC DISEASE

Prevention of allergic disease has traditionally focused on altering either the exposure or immunologic response to environmental allergens. Although the acute allergic (immediate hypersensitivity-type) reaction results from an interaction of an allergen with IgE, bound to the surface of mast cells and basophils,[16] it is clear that antigen-specific IgE alone is not sufficient to cause allergy. Not all persons who demonstrate IgE response to an antigen later become clinically allergic to that antigen. Likewise, a minority of asthmatic adults possess antigen-specific IgE against airborne allergens.[17] After IgE binding, mast cell degranulation occurs with the secretion of prostaglandins, leukotrienes, and platelet-activating factor. These contribute to the late-phase reaction involving recruitment of neutrophils, T cells, eosinophils, and basophils.[18]

The interaction between an extrinsic allergic antigen and the immune system requires the presence of the antigen both during the initial sensitization and again during a subsequent challenge. As a result, prevention of allergic symptoms typically involves the avoidance of environmental contact with the antigen. Given the facts that skin tests positive for allergens occur in up to 30% of children of atopic parents within the first 3 months of life[19] and that children born during an allergen season have higher allergen-specific IgE levels,[17] early life sensitization to antigens likely occurs. With presumed sensitization early in life, the prevention of clinical allergic reactions in adults primarily focuses on awareness and avoidance of the suspected allergen. Where avoidance is not possible, antigen-specific immunotherapy and pharmacologic therapy may provide a means to diminish the allergic response to the antigen.

ALLERGIC RHINITIS

Epidemiology

Allergic rhinitis is defined as an IgE-mediated disorder of the nose that results in mucosal inflammation. Allergic rhinitis is believed to affect 10% to 25% of the population,[20] and its prevalence has notably been increasing.[21] The onset of disease is typically before 20 years of age.[22] Allergic rhinitis has a substantial impact on quality of life, work productivity,[23] and health care costs.[24]

Similar to asthma, the pathogenesis of allergic rhinitis involves the IgE-mediated production of cysteinyl leukotrienes and other inflammatory mediators.[25] Also similar to asthma, allergic rhinitis has a known genetic component.[26] Interestingly, approximately 60% to 78% of asthmatic patients have coexisting allergic rhinitis.[27] This significant disease association has been recognized since the 19th century and has led some to recently propose the "one airway, one disease" model.[27] Such a concept suggests that both the upper and lower airways may exhibit parallel immunologic responses to the inciting aeroallergen. Commonly implicated indoor aeroallergens include dust mites, domestic animals (eg, cats), insects, and plants (eg, *Ficus*). Outdoor aeroallergens consist primarily of pollens and molds, thus contributing to seasonal variations in the prevalence of allergic rhinitis.[28] Occupational rhinitis has also been recognized as a disease entity, and its symptoms may precede the onset of associated occupational asthma.[29] Outdoor and indoor air pollution (including tobacco smoke) have been linked to the exacerbation of allergic rhinitis.[30,31]

Diagnosis

Current guidelines recommend confirmatory testing consisting of allergen-specific skin testing or radioallergosorbent testing (RAST) when empiric symptomatic therapy is unsuccessful or the diagnosis of allergic rhinitis is suspect.[22] Skin testing consists of the epidermal injection of allergen extracts, with a wheal and flare reaction within 15 minutes indicating a positive response. In contrast, RAST employs an in vitro assay that uses the patient's serum. While both of these tests are based on the detection of allergen-specific IgE, skin testing is the less expensive method and is believed to have a higher sensitivity than does RAST.

The most commonly tested substances are ragweed, grass pollen, molds, animal danders, and dust mites.

Testing is generally targeted to assess reactivity to a battery of allergens to which a patient may reasonably be exposed. However, the presence of skin test positivity by itself does not confirm the diagnosis; nor does a clinical history of sensitivity always correlate with a positive skin test reaction. As in other allergic diseases, skin testing and RAST should be related to the clinical symptoms and can be expected to provide data that may allow targeted avoidance of the allergen and/or subsequent immunotherapy.

Symptomatic Therapy

Although confirmatory testing may be useful, many clinicians opt for an empiric trial of medications. Nasal corticosteroids are generally believed to be the most effective medications in the management of allergic rhinitis, owing to their effects on decreasing nasal inflammation. The nonsedating antihistamines (loratadine, fexofenadine hydrochloride, and others) represent an alternate primary or secondary therapy for allergic rhinitis. These agents are well tolerated and exhibit few of the side effects that had been reported with the first generation of nonsedating antihistamines. Cromolyn sodium, when used regularly, has been proved in randomized trials to prevent the onset of symptoms in allergic rhinitis.[32] The leukotriene modifier montelukast has been shown to be as effective as the antihistamine loratadine in providing relief of disease symptoms.[33]

Decongestants may be helpful in providing relief from the common symptom of nasal congestion but do little to treat the underlying inflammatory process. Subcutaneous immunotherapy, targeted against specific allergens to which the patient manifests a reaction, has demonstrated proven and sustained clinical efficacy in the treatment of allergic rhinitis in multiple controlled trials, even years after therapy is discontinued.[34] Avoidance of potential aeroallergens is an especially important component of therapy. This may include the washing of pets and use of high-efficiency particulate air (HEPA) filtration devices. However, these latter measures have not been proved to improve patient outcomes in allergic rhinitis.[35]

ASTHMA

Epidemiology

Asthma is a common disease, with 10.5 million Americans reporting a diagnosis of asthma in 1999.[36] Both the prevalence and severity of asthma in the United States has been increasing in recent decades.[37,38] Between 1980 and 1999, physician office visits due to asthma increased from 5.9 million to 10.8 million visits annually.[36] The cause or causes of these trends remain to be clarified but may involve multiple environmental factors, including the role of decreased early-life bacterial exposure, according to the hygiene hypothesis.[6]

Viral and bacterial airway infections have long been cited as factors that acutely exacerbate preexisting asthma.[39,40] Reports also indicate that chronic airway infection with organisms such as *Chlamydia pneumoniae* may be responsible for persistent asthmatic symptoms.[41] However, many current investigations have focused on the role of the environmental bacterial exposure that occurs early in life, supporting the hygiene hypothesis.

Consistent with a protective role of bacterial exposure against the later development of asthma, exposure to day care and siblings[42] and living on a farm as a child are associated with decreased risk of developing asthma.[10] This observed protective effect may relate to the presence of increased bacterial endotoxin levels in bedding materials.[43] Similarly, in cross-sectional studies of children from anthroposophic families in Sweden, the restricted use of routine vaccinations and antibiotics early in life has been associated with decreased risk of later developing asthma.[44] However, the increased prevalence of asthma in children living in poor urban areas appears to conflict with the hygiene hypothesis.[45] Recent studies have attempted to reconcile these observations by demonstrating that these children exhibit increased sensitization to house dust mites and cockroach antigens.[46,47] The role of airway infection and bacterial exposure in contributing to the pathogenesis of asthma remains an area of substantial research interest.

Factors other than diminished early-life bacterial exposure have been linked with the rising prevalence of asthma. Many studies report an increased prevalence of asthmatic symptoms in urban areas associated with increased levels of air pollution.[48-50] Although a direct causal effect has been difficult to prove,[51,52] some have suggested that air pollutants enhance the airway response to respiratory allergens.[53] Consistent with this theory, multiple studies cite an epidemiologic association between locally increased air pollution levels and acute asthma exacerbations.[54,55] Secondhand tobacco smoke exposure has been associated with the exacerbation of asthma in adults[56] and increased asthma severity in children,[57,58] providing a large opportunity for prevention. Childhood obesity is also associated with asthma prevalence,[59,60] especially in females, and is increasing in prevalence in developed countries.[61,62]

Gastroesophageal reflux disease (GERD) has been found to be associated with asthma.[63] However, this association is variable, with anywhere between 34% and 89% of asthmatic patients having GERD, depending on the diagnostic criteria and subject population.[64] Although investigations of the link between GERD and asthma remain brisk, the etiologic relationship between these diseases still remains unclear. Certain dietary factors, such as the increased intake of saturated fats[65] and the decreased ingestion of flavonoid antioxidants,[66] have been suggested to play a role in an increased risk of asthma. Interestingly, increased low-density lipoprotein cholesterol levels have

been associated with airway obstruction, as measured by spirometry,[67] although it is not clear whether any causal relationship exists between these variables.

Clinical Variants of Asthma

Asthma is a multifactorial disease, clinically characterized by reversible airway obstruction that results from multiple pathogenetic pathways. Asthma is believed to have a genetic basis in many individuals.[68] Although distinct clinical variants of asthma have been described, there is substantial overlap between these entities. Recognized variants include atopic asthma, aspirin-intolerant asthma (AIA), cold-induced asthma, exercise-induced asthma, cough-variant asthma, and occupational asthma.

Atopic asthma is the best described of these entities and is characterized by a family history of asthma, onset of disease early in life, and suspected exacerbation in response to environmental aeroallergens. Although the incidence of atopy as assessed by skin testing is high in asthma, only 40% to 50% of asthmatic adults demonstrate antigen-specific IgE against an identified airborne antigen.[17] The entity of AIA, which affects up to 10% of asthmatic individudals[69] and may be associated with concomitant rhinitis symptoms, has been extensively investigated.[70] Although the mechanism for the development of asthma symptoms in response to nonsteroidal anti-inflammatory drug (NSAID) administration is poorly understood, the phenomenon has long been believed to involve an abnormality in cyclooxygenase pathway regulation.[71] However, recent studies note that a polymorphism in the leukotriene C_4 synthase gene promoter has been found to occur at higher frequency in some populations of patients with AIA, providing a genetic predisposition to an enhanced biologic response in these individuals.[72]

Multiple environmental exposures have been reported to be associated with occupational asthma (Table 58-1), with the prevalence of work-related asthma being 3.7%, according to the National Health and Nutrition Examination Survey III.[73] However, many investigators believe that this is an underestimate, given the lack of a standardized definition across studies and the work-related exacerbation of asthma that has been attributed to other causes.

Diagnosis

The range of reported symptoms in asthma varies from acute, infrequent exacerbations of dyspnea and wheezing to chronic, unrelenting breathlessness with severely limited exercise tolerance. In cases in which asthmatic symptoms occur in association with occupational exposures, the clinical pattern of symptoms may give important clues as to the cause of the airway obstruction. The diagnosis of asthma in difficult cases has classically been confirmed by the presence of bronchoconstriction, as

T A B L E 58-1

Common Etiologies of Occupational Asthma With Typical Sources of Exposure

Agent	Occupation
Animal	Veterinary medicine
	Laboratory animal handling
	Farming
Metals	Metal refining
	Plating
	Chemical manufacturing
Isocyanates	Auto body repair (polyurethanes)
	Roofing (roofing foams)
Acid Anhydrides	Paint industry
	Polyester/Polymer industry
	Circuit boards
Wood	Furniture manufacturing
Dusts	Cabinet manufacturing
Grain	Bakery
Dusts	Milling
Acrylates	Paint industry
	Adhesive industry
Cobalt	Carbide-tipped tool Manufacturing
Latex	Health care
Formaldehyde and Glutaraldehyde	Medical instrument sterilization

quantified by a decrease in the forced expiratory volume in 1 second (FEV_1) of at least 20%, in response to inhaled agents such as methacholine or histamine. Clinical monitoring of disease activity is typically accomplished using the ongoing assessment of clinical symptoms and physical examination, pulmonary function tests, regular peak flow measurements, and the frequency of short-acting rescue medication use. Although early studies suggested that regular and repeated use of short-acting β-2-agonist inhalers was associated with increased mortality in asthma,[74] most clinicians now believe that repeated use of these medications is a marker for poorly controlled disease.

The revised 1997 National Asthma Education and Prevention Program (NAEPP) guidelines for the treatment of asthma recommend that all patients with persistent asthma be tested with skin tests or in vitro assays for perennial allergens, such as house dust mite, cat, dog, cockroach, and *Alternaria*.[75] The results of such testing allow targeted avoidance of exposure to specific allergens and the subsequent modification of the allergic response to that allergen through immunotherapy. Immunotherapy has been reported to influence the development of the Th1 cytokine response to antigens, perhaps modifying the ongoing pathogenesis of allergy in asthma.[40] This technique has been proved particularly beneficial in treating seasonal asthma and decreasing the need for controller medications, while allowing the simultaneous treatment of both upper and lower airway disease.[76]

Symptomatic Therapy

An algorithmic, stepwise approach to asthma management, dependent on defined stratifications of disease severity, has evolved as the standard clinical approach recommended by the NAEPP[77] (Table 58-2). Asthma medications are generally classified as either maintenance or rescue therapies. For patients with mild, intermittent asthma (defined by asthma symptoms ≤2 days per week or ≤2 nights per month), initial treatment with as-needed inhaled bronchodilators, such as short-acting β-2-agonists with an accompanying spacer device, is typically recommended. In patients with mild persistent asthma (defined by asthma symptoms >2 times per week, but <1 time per day, or >2 nights per month), the addition of a maintenance medication is recommended, with inhaled steroids having emerged as the preferred first-line agent. For patients with moderate, persistent (asthma symptoms >1 night per week) or severe, persistent (continuous or frequent asthma symptoms) disease, the addition of other maintenance medications, such as the leukotriene modifiers, long-acting β 2-agonists, and/or theophylline, is beneficial.

Over the last decade, inhaled corticosteroids (fluticasone, beclomethasone, flunisolide, etc) have become the cornerstone of maintenance therapy for asthma, given their specific roles in modulating airway inflammation[78] and their potential role in affecting airway remodeling.[79] These agents have been shown to be effective in all clinical variants of asthma to decrease the risk of hospitalization for treatment of exacerbation.[80] However, there is no evidence suggesting that early intervention with inhaled corticosteroids in mild to moderate asthma prevents long-term disease progression.[81]

The long-acting β-2-agonists (salmeterol xinafoate and formoterol fumarate) and the leukotriene modifier agents (zafirlukast, montelukast, etc) have emerged as particularly effective maintenance therapies for the prevention of episodic asthmatic symptoms, as occur in exercise-induced asthma,[82] nocturnal asthma,[83] and AIA.[84] In addition, a recent update to the NAEPP guidelines indicates that in poorly controlled patients on inhaled steroids, the addition of a long-acting β-2-agonist is preferred over increasing the inhaled steroid dose.[81] The leukotriene modifier agents, which include inhibitors of the 5-lipoxygenase enzyme or cysteinyl leukotriene receptor antagonists, have been reported to improve lung function[85] and decrease the need for β-2 agonist rescue.[84] Although these agents

TABLE 58-2

Stepwise Approach to Asthma Maintenance Therapy*

Asthma Severity	Recommended Maintenance Medications	
Severe Persistent	**High-Dose Inhaled Corticosteroids and Long-Acting β-Agonists** Optional additional agent: Oral corticosteroids	
Moderate Persistent	**Medium-Dose Inhaled Corticosteroids and Long-Acting β-Agonists** Alternative agent: Medium-dose inhaled corticosteroids and either Leukotriene Receptor Antagonist or Theophylline	
	Low-Dose Inhaled Corticosteroids and Long-Acting β-Agonists Alternative agent: Medium-dose inhaled corticosteroids and either Leukotriene Receptor Antagonist or Theophylline	
Mild Persistent	**Low-Dose Inhaled Corticosteroids** Alternative agent: Cromolyn or Leukotriene Receptor Antagonist	
Mild Intermittent	None	

*Adapted from NAEPP Expert Panel Report: Guidelines for the Diagnosis and Management of Asthma—Update on Selected Topics. Bethesda, Md: National Institutes of Health; 2002. NIH Publication 02-5075.

have an excellent safety profile, the selection of optimal patient candidates for these agents must be determined with an empiric trial.[84,86] The ability to predict clinical responsiveness to these agents may be related to the presence of polymorphisms within the 5-lipoxygenase promoter region.[87] Other maintenance medications, such as cromolyn sodium, continue to have a role in the management of mild, persistent disease.[81]

The first-line acute, rescue medications for asthma remain the short-acting β-2-agonists (albuterol, pirbuterol, bitolterol, and terbutaline) and anticholinergic agents (eg, ipratropium bromide). Given findings suggesting that the use of regularly scheduled inhaled β-2-agonists is equivalent to as-needed use, administration of these medications on an as-needed basis remains the preferred therapeutic approach.[88] Although the use of bronchodilators in nebulized form remains common, the use of metered-dose inhalers (MDIs) in conjunction with a spacer device has been proved to be as effective as nebulization in most patients and is less expensive.[89] Recent advances in the inhaled delivery of medications include breath-actuated MDIs (which may be useful for patients who have difficulty timing inhalations with MDIs), as well as multidose dry powder and chlorofluorocarbon-free aerosol MDIs (which may offer the benefit of avoiding the use of chlorofluorocarbon propellants). Systemic steroids are reserved for the management of the acute, severe asthma exacerbation or chronic, persistent asthma that is unresponsive to other maintenance medications.

Treatment Efficacy

Nonpharmacologic preventive measures for asthma include annual influenza vaccination (in patients with persistent asthma), avoidance of tobacco smoke and inciting aeroallergens, and avoidance of NSAID use (in patients with AIA). In addition, frequent reevaluation of the asthma treatment regimen and the clinical response is vital to maintaining good control of the disease. Although studies have not been able to define a clear benefit for written medical action plans (which include patient education and the interpretation of home peak flow values) in the care of asthma, these assisted-management strategies are nonetheless recommended for the optimal treatment of asthma.[81]

Patients should routinely assess peak flow measurements to determine baseline "personal best" values and should seek medical attention when these values fall below predefined thresholds, particularly when the flows are unresponsive to rescue medication administration. Treatment of coexistent GERD is suggested, although controlled trials are conflicting as to whether this has a long-term beneficial impact on the control of asthma.[90] Studies suggest that patients with allergies and asthma experience more significant improvements in health-related quality of life when treated by allergy specialists, as compared with treatment by primary care physicians.[91] Both quality of life and functional employment status in patients with asthma have been found to be associated with the likelihood of the treating physician to engage the patient in the formulation of the treatment plan.[92]

FOOD ALLERGY

Introduction

Food allergy represents a constellation of adverse immunologic reactions to food, ranging from atopic dermatitis and airway reactivity to overt anaphylaxis. The prevalence of food allergy has been reported to be increasing in conjunction with that of other allergic diseases, with a range of 3.5%[93] to 12%[94] of the population reporting having a food allergy. The variable nature of food allergies suggests that these disorders result from a variety of immune responses to food antigens. The IgE-dependent food allergies, such as angioedema and anaphylaxis, typically result in the acute onset of symptoms after exposure. These disorders can affect a wide variety of target organs, including the skin (with urticarial reactions), gastrointestinal tract (with diarrhea), airway (with asthma or rhinitis symptoms), and cardiovascular system (with shock). Other food allergies are variably associated with IgE elevations and include subacute disease entities such as atopic dermatitis. T-cell–mediated food allergies, such as celiac disease, typically demonstrate a delayed onset after exposure and exhibit chronic symptoms related primarily to the gastrointestinal tract. Immune response–related food allergies should be differentiated from a wide variety of food intolerances, which are not directly mediated by the immune system.

The link between food allergy in childhood and the occurrence of atopic dermatitis has long been known.[95] Atopic dermatitis is characterized by the presence of a pruritic, papular, or urticarial rash, which may develop confluent regions. Approximately 35% of children with at least moderately severe atopic dermatitis have also been diagnosed with a food allergy.[96] Reports also indicate that 80% to 90% of infants with atopic dermatitis will develop positive skin test reactions to aeroallergens and food allergens.[17] These findings suggest that the early exposure to food antigens may increase the probability of an allergy developing later. In this respect, food allergy is often seen as the precursor to the later development of other allergic diseases. In young children with food allergy, symptoms typically diminish with age, giving rise to asthma and allergic rhinitis.[97]

Prevention Strategies

Efforts aimed at the prevention of the development of food allergy and atopic dermatitis have produced limited success. Strategies aimed at reducing maternal-fetal and neonatal exposure to particular food antigens in those at high risk of atopy appeared to decrease the prevalence of atopic dermatitis and food allergy in the first year of life.[98] However, longitudinal follow-up demonstrated no difference in the prevalence of food allergy, atopic dermatitis, asthma, or allergic rhinitis later in childhood.[99] Infants who are exclusively breast-fed have a decreased risk of later food allergy.[17] This protective effect has been theorized to originate from either maternal-infant transfer of IgA or decreased early exposure to food antigens.[17] The delayed introduction of solid food has also been reported to protect against the development of atopy.[100] The most widely accepted recommendations include the employment of breast-feeding for 6 to 12 months, the delayed introduction of solid foods (until after 4 months of age), and the use of hypoallergenic formula in children at high risk of atopy.[101]

Preventive strategies aimed at decreasing the adverse consequences of food allergy are guided by the use of clinical history, skin testing, and oral food challenge. The most common food allergens, including eggs, soy, milk, wheat, and nuts, should be suspected first. In addition, because many foods may contain these allergens in a form that the patient may not readily recognize (Table 58-3), the patient should examine food labels.

The medical history is rarely diagnostic by itself; therefore, skin testing (with the appropriate negative controls) is commonly employed to assay for food-specific IgE. Alternatively, RAST is commonly used to detect the presence of food-specific IgE. The presence of positive responses by skin testing and/or RAST should be correlated with the clinical reaction to a suspected food allergen. The absence of a positive skin test reaction can be helpful in excluding a food as being the cause of a reaction. The results from this testing and those obtained from medically supervised oral food challenges allow for the creation of a more limited list of foods that a patient should avoid. An alternative diagnostic strategy is to employ an elimination diet, in which a simple diet is initially instituted, with vigilance for reactions during the gradual reintroduction of potentially offensive foods.

Treatment

Although most children typically lose their allergy to the most common food allergens within the first 5 years of life, the persistence of childhood food allergy has been increasing in frequency.[102] In contrast, adults with food allergy generally demonstrate a persistent sensitivity to the allergen, mandating lifelong preventive measures and vigilance. However, dietary adjustment is often difficult, due to food labeling errors by manufacturers,[3] cross-contamination of foods during the commercial preparation process, and social obstacles to food avoidance. Antihistamines are generally indicated for the symptomatic treatment of mild to moderate reactions. In cases that result in more severe reactions or in anaphylaxis, corticosteroids, epinephrine, and other supportive medical care may be required. Many clinicians will advise patients to carry a prophylactic epinephrine pen device in cases in which a history of severe and potentially life-threatening food allergy exists.

TABLE 58-3

Label Ingredients Indicating Presence of Common Food Allergens*

Food Allergen	Label Ingredient	
Milk	Milk Solids	Lactalbumin
	Casein	Sour cream
	Caseinates	Whey
	Butter	Curds
	Butter fat	Cheese
	Yogurt	
	Artificial butter flavor	
Egg	Egg yolk	Mayonnaise
	Egg white	Ovalbumin
	Albumin	Ovomucoid
	Eggnog	
Soy	Soy flour	Soy sauce
	Soy protein	Tofu
	Soy nuts	
	Textured vegetable protein	
Wheat	Wheat flour	Couscous
	Graham flour	Farina
	Bread flour	Gluten
	Enriched flour	Bran
	High-Protein flour	Bulgar
	Cracker meal	Spelt
	Semolina	Kamut
	Bread crumbs	Soy sauce
	Cereal extract	Starch
	Vegetable gum	Wheat gluten
	Wheat bran	
	Wheat germ	
	Wheat starch	
	Wheat malt	

*Adapted from Koerner CB, Sampson HA. Diets and nutrition. In: Metcalfe KK, Sampson, HA, Simon RA, eds. *Food Allergy: Adverse Reactions to Foods and Food Additives*. Boston, Mass: Blackwell Scientific Publications; 1991.

DRUG ALLERGY

Introduction

Allergic reactions to drugs are relatively common, with 3.1% to 6.2% of hospital admissions being due to an adverse drug reaction[103] and women being more commonly affected than men (65% to 70% vs 30% to 35%).[104] Although atopic patients do not appear to be affected with an increased frequency, they have been reported to have more severe reactions.[105] An increased frequency of drug reactions has been reported in patients with systemic lupus erythematosus[106] and acquired immunodeficiency syndrome (AIDS).[107] Drug allergies can present with a wide variety of clinical manifestations, ranging from maculopapular rash to anaphylaxis. These reactions occur as the result of IgE, IgG, IgM, and T-cell–mediated immunologic mechanisms. The clinical history should address the nature of the symptoms, medication use history, chronology of the reaction, and medical history of previous drug reactions. However, the clinical history is often not diagnostic, as many patients will have ingested multiple medications before the onset of symptoms.

Preventive Strategies

The prevention of drug-related allergy involves identification of the offending agent. Skin testing, while valuable in other allergic disease, can be problematic in the assessment of drug allergy owing to the lack of standardization of protocols and test concentrations across centers. However, the latency of the response to the medication can give valuable insight into the immunologic mechanism, with IgE-mediated reactions giving positive results within 20 minutes and T-cell–mediated reactions producing a positive reaction hours to days later.[108]

Provocation testing demonstrates the highest sensitivity but is restricted to centers that can administer the appropriate supportive care in the event of a positive reaction. This type of testing is most valuable with agents such as NSAIDs, local anesthetics, and nonpenicillin antibiotics when skin testing may be negative.[108] Provocation testing should be avoided in cases with dermal blistering-type skin reactions or when the offending agent can be easily avoided. The demonstration of drug-specific IgE (available only against a limited number of agents, such as penicillins or tetanus toxoid) may be useful in conjunction with positive skin testing reactions and the clinical history. After identification of the responsible drug, avoidance is generally possible. Where avoidance cannot be maintained, desensitization therapy is an alternative to allow the use of the medication.

VENOM ALLERGY

Venom allergy can represent an uncommon but potentially life-threatening reaction to a sting from the insect order *Hymenoptera*. Although this class of insects includes wasps and hornets, the most commonly encountered stings are those from the honeybee and bumblebee. *Hymenoptera* venom is known to contain various allergenic components, including enzymes, biogenic amines, and basic peptides. The diagnosis of bee venom allergy is typically made by clinical history in conjunction with the presence of positive skin testing reaction to venom or the presence of venom-specific IgE in the patient's serum. The severity of the reaction to the sting is not correlated with the results of skin testing or serum venom-specific

IgE levels.[109] Although the presence of prior atopy increases the risk of anaphylaxis,[110] most patients who die of insect sting anaphylaxis have not manifested prior systemic allergic reactions to stings.[111] The avoidance of exposure to *Hymenoptera* stings remains the cornerstone of management. Venom immunotherapy is frequently used to decrease the risk of anaphylaxis due to a sting[109] and is recommended in patients with a history of severe reactions. However, many patients lose their sensitivity to stings over time, without having received immunotherapy.[112] An epinephrine injection pen device can be lifesaving in patients with a history of severe reactions.

SUMMARY

Although the modern practice of medicine in developed countries has resulted in major advances in the treatment of infectious diseases over the last half-century, this has occurred in conjunction with a marked increase in the prevalence of allergic disease. The reasons for this increase are unclear but are likely related to a number of environmental factors, including the decreased environmental exposure to bacteria and the increased exposure to airborne and food allergens. Management of allergic disease includes the identification of the inciting allergen, followed by avoidance and medication therapy aimed at treating the underlying inflammatory process. Immunotherapy remains a therapeutic tool to allow targeted avoidance and to modify the immune response to the allergen. The aggressive treatment of allergic disease can have a substantial positive impact on quality of life for many patients.

REFERENCES

1. Smith DH, Malone DC, Lawson KA, Okamoto LJ, Battista C, Saunders WB. A national estimate of the economic costs of asthma. *Am J Respir Crit Care Med.* 1997;156:787–793.

2. Woolcock AJ, Peat JK. Evidence for the increase in asthma worldwide. *Ciba Found Symp.* 1997;206:122–134; discussion 134–139, 157–159.

3. Aberg N, Hesselmar B, Aberg B, Eriksson B. Increase of asthma, allergic rhinitis and eczema in Swedish schoolchildren between 1979 and 1991. *Clin Exp Allergy.* 1995;25:815–819.

4. Upton MN, McConnachie A, McSharry C, et al. Intergenerational 20-year trends in the prevalence of asthma and hay fever in adults: the Midspan family study surveys of parents and offspring. *BMJ.* 2000;321:88–92.

5. Williams HC. Is the prevalence of atopic dermatitis increasing? *Clin Exp Dermatol.* 1992;17:385–391.

6. Matricardi PM, Bonini S. High microbial turnover rate preventing atopy: a solution to inconsistencies impinging on the hygiene hypothesis? *Clin Exp Allergy.* 2000;30:1506–1510.

7. Matricardi PM, Rosmini F, Ferrigno L, et al. Cross sectional retrospective study of prevalence of atopy among Italian military students with antibodies against hepatitis A virus. *BMJ.* 1997;314:999–1003.

8. Matricardi PM, Rosmini F, Panetta V, Ferrigno L, Bonini S. Hay fever and asthma in relation to markers of infection in the United States. *J Allergy Clin Immunol.* 2002;110:381–387.

9. Weiland SK, von Mutius E, Husing A, Asher MI, for ISAAC Steering Committee. Intake of trans fatty acids and prevalence of childhood asthma and allergies in Europe. *Lancet.* 1999;353:2040–2041.

10. Riedler J, Braun-Fahrlander C, Eder W, et al. Exposure to farming in early life and development of asthma and allergy: a cross-sectional survey. *Lancet.* 2001;358:1129–1133.

11. Salvi S. Pollution and allergic airways disease. *Curr Opin Allergy Clin Immunol.* 2001;1:35–41.

12. von Mutius E, Martinez FD, Fritzsch C, Nicolai T, Roell G, Thiemann HH. Prevalence of asthma and atopy in two areas of West and East Germany. *Am J Respir Crit Care Med.* 1994;149:358–364.

13. Nowak D, Heinrich J, Jorres R, et al. Prevalence of respiratory symptoms, bronchial hyperresponsiveness and atopy among adults: west and east Germany. *Eur Respir J.* 1996;9:2541–2552.

14. von Mutius E, Martinez FD, Fritzsch C, Nicolai T, Reitmeir P, Thiemann HH. Skin test reactivity and number of siblings. *BMJ.* 1994;308:692–695.

15. Barraclough R, Devereux G, Hendrick DJ, Stenton SC. Apparent but not real increase in asthma prevalence during the 1990s. *Eur Respir J.* 2002;20:826–833.

16. Kinet JP. The high-affinity IgE receptor (Fc epsilon RI): from physiology to pathology. *Annu Rev Immunol.* 1999;17:931–972.

17. Peden DB. Influences on the development of allergy and asthma. *Toxicology.* 2002;181–182:323–328.

18. Ying S, Robinson DS, Meng Q, et al. C-C chemokines in allergen-induced late-phase cutaneous responses in atopic subjects: association of eotaxin with early 6-hour eosinophils, and of eotaxin-2 and monocyte chemoattractant protein-4 with the later 24-hour tissue eosinophilia, and relationship to basophils and other C-C chemokines (monocyte chemoattractant protein-3 and RANTES). *J Immunol.* 1999;163:3976–3984.

19. Peden DB. Development of atopy and asthma: candidate environmental influences and important periods of exposure. *Environ Health Perspect.* 2000;108(suppl 3):475–482.

20. Strachan D, Sibbald B, Weiland S, et al. Worldwide variations in prevalence of symptoms of allergic rhinoconjunctivitis in children: the International Study of Asthma and Allergies in Childhood (ISAAC). *Pediatr Allergy Immunol.* 1997;8:161–176.

21. Lundback B. Epidemiology of rhinitis and asthma. *Clin Exp Allergy.* 1998;28(suppl 2):3–10.

22. Dykewicz MS, Fineman S, Skoner DP, et al. Diagnosis and management of rhinitis: complete guidelines of the Joint Task Force on Practice Parameters in Allergy, Asthma and Immunology, American Academy of Allergy, Asthma, and Immunology. *Ann Allergy Asthma Immunol.* 1998;81:478–518.

23. Cockbum IM, Bailit HL, Bemdt ER, Finkelstein SN. Loss of work productivity due to illness and medical treatment. *J Occup Environ Med.* 1999;41:948–953.

24. Malone DC, Lawson KA, Smith DH, Arrighi HM, Battista C. A cost of illness study of allergic rhinitis in the United States. *J Allergy Clin Immunol.* 1997;99:22–27.

25. Taylor GW, Taylor I, Black P, et al. Urinary leukotriene E4 after antigen challenge and in acute asthma and allergic rhinitis. *Lancet.* 1989;1:584–588.

26. Barnes KC, Marsh DG. The genetics and complexity of allergy and asthma. *Immunol Today.* 1998;19:325–332.

27. Grossman J. One airway, one disease. *Chest.* 1997;111(suppl):11S–16S.

28. Pedersen PA, Rung Weeke E. Seasonal variation of asthma and allergic rhinitis. Consultation pattern in general practice related to pollen and spore counts and to five indicators of air pollution. *Allergy.* 1984;39:165–170.

29. Malo JL, Lemiere C, Desjardins A, Cartier A. Prevalence and intensity of rhinoconjunctivitis in subjects with occupational asthma. *Eur Respir J.* 1997;10:1513–1515.

30. Health effects of outdoor air pollution. Committee of the Environmental and Occupational Health Assembly of the American Thoracic Society. *Am J Respir Crit Care Med.* 1996;153:3–50.

31. Burr ML, Anderson HR, Austin JB, et al. Respiratory symptoms and home environment in children: a national survey. *Thorax*. 1999;54:27–32.

32. LaForce C. Use of nasal steroids in managing allergic rhinitis. *J Allergy Clin Immunol*. 1999;103:S388–S394.

33. Meltzer EO, Malmstrom K, Lu S, et al. Concomitant montelukast and loratadine as treatment for seasonal allergic rhinitis: a randomized, placebo-controlled clinical trial. *J Allergy Clin Immunol*. 2000;105:917–922.

34. Durham SR, Walker SM, Varga EM, et al. Long-term clinical efficacy of grass-pollen immunotherapy. *N Engl J Med*. 1999;341:468–475.

35. Eggleston PA, Bush RK. Environmental allergen avoidance: an overview. *J Allergy Clin Immunol*. 2001;107(suppl):S403–S405.

36. Mannino DM, Homa DM, Akinbami LJ, Moorman JE, Gwynn C, Redd SC. Surveillance for asthma—United States, 1980–1999. *MMWR Surveill Summ*. 2002;51:1–13.

37. Asthma—United States, 1982–1992. *MMWR Morb Mortal Wkly Rep*. 1995;43:952–955.

38. Mannino DM, Homa DM, Pertowski CA, et al. Surveillance for asthma—United States, 1960–1995. *MMWR Surveill Summ*. 1998;47:1–27.

39. Stenius-Aarniala B. The role of infection in asthma. *Chest*. 1987;91(suppl):157S–160S.

40. Fernandez-Benitez M, Ano M, Maselli JP, Sanz ML. Respiratory infection in asthma. *J Investig Allergol Clin Immunol*. 2002;12:48–51.

41. von HL. Role of persistent infection in the control and severity of asthma: focus on *Chlamydia pneumoniae*. *Eur Respir J*. 2002;19:546–556.

42. Ball TM, Castro-Rodriguez JA, Griffith KA, Holberg CJ, Martinez FD, Wright AL. Siblings, day-care attendance, and the risk of asthma and wheezing during childhood. *N Engl J Med*. 2000;343:538–543.

43. Braun-Fahrlander C, Riedler J, Herz U, et al. Environmental exposure to endotoxin and its relation to asthma in school-age children. *N Engl J Med*. 2002;347:869–877.

44. Alm JS, Swartz J, Lilja G, Scheynius A, Pershagen G. Atopy in children of families with an anthroposophic lifestyle. *Lancet*. 1999;353:1485–1488.

45. Call RS, Smith TF, Morris E, Chapman MD, Platts-Mills TA. Risk factors for asthma in inner city children. *J Pediatr*. 1992;121:862–866.

46. Korsgaard J, Iversen M. Epidemiology of house dust mite allergy. *Allergy*. 1991;46(suppl 11):14–18.

47. Rosenstreich DL, Eggleston P, Kattan M, et al. The role of cockroach allergy and exposure to cockroach allergen in causing morbidity among inner-city children with asthma. *N Engl J Med*. 1997;336:1356–1363.

48. Delfino RJ. Epidemiologic evidence for asthma and exposure to air toxics: linkages between occupational, indoor, and community air pollution research. *Environ Health Perspect*. 2002;110(suppl 4):573–589.

49. Desqueyroux H, Pujet JC, Prosper M, Squinazi F, Momas I. Short-term effects of low-level air pollution on respiratory health of adults suffering from moderate to severe asthma. *Environ Res*. 2002;89:29–37.

50. D'Amato G, Liccardi G, D'Amato M, Cazzola M. Outdoor air pollution, climatic changes and allergic bronchial asthma. *Eur Respir J*. 2002;20:763–776.

51. Anderson HR. Air pollution and trends in asthma. *Ciba Found Symp*. 1997;206:190–202; discussion 203–197.

52. Koenig JQ. Air pollution and asthma. *J Allergy Clin Immunol*. 1999;104:717–722.

53. D'Amato G. Environmental urban factors (air pollution and allergens) and the rising trends in allergic respiratory diseases. *Allergy*. 2002;57(suppl 72):30–33.

54. Koenig JQ, Covert DS, Marshall SG, Van Belle G, Pierson WE. The effects of ozone and nitrogen dioxide on pulmonary function in healthy and in asthmatic adolescents. *Am Rev Respir Dis*. 1987;136:1152–1157.

55. Abbey DE, Petersen F, Mills PK, Beeson WL. Long-term ambient concentrations of total suspended particulates, ozone, and sulfur dioxide and respiratory symptoms in a non-smoking population. *Arch Environ Health*. 1993;48:33–46.

56. Eisner MD. Environmental tobacco smoke and adult asthma. *Clin Chest Med*. 2002;23:749–761.

57. Martinez FD, Antognoni G, Macri F, et al. Parental smoking enhances bronchial responsiveness in nine-year-old children. *Am Rev Respir Dis*. 1988;138:518–523.

58. Mannino DM, Homa DM, Redd SC. Involuntary smoking and asthma severity in children: data from the Third National Health and Nutrition Examination. Survey. *Chest*. 2002;122:409–415.

59. von Mutius E, Schwartz J, Neas LM, Dockery D, Weiss ST. Relation of body mass index to asthma and atopy in children: the National Health and Nutrition Examination Study III. *Thorax*. 2001;56:835–838.

60. Epstein LH, Wu YW, Paluch RA, Cemy FJ, Dorn JP. Asthma and maternal body mass index are related to pediatric body mass index and obesity: results from the Third National Health and Nutrition Examination Survey. *Obes Res*. 2000;8:575–581.

61. Chen Y, Dales R, Tang M, Krewski D. Obesity may increase the incidence of asthma in women but not in men: longitudinal observations from the Canadian National Population Health Surveys. *Am J Epidemiol*. 2002;155:191–197.

62. Alexander JA, Hunt LW, Patel AM. Prevalence, pathophysiology, and treatment of patients with asthma and gastroesophageal reflux disease. *Mayo Clin Proc*. 2000;75:1055–1063.

63. Harding SM. Acid reflux and asthma. *Curr Opin Pulm Med.* 2003;9:42–45.

64. Harding SM, Richter JE. The role of gastroesophageal reflux in chronic cough and asthma. *Chest.* 1997;111:1389–1402.

65. Huang SL, Pan WH. Dietary fats and asthma in teenagers: analyses of the first Nutrition and Health Survey in Taiwan (NAHSIT). *Clin Exp Allergy.* 2001;31:1875–1880.

66. Shaheen SO, Steme JA, Thompson RL, Songhurst CE, Margetts BM, Bumey PG. Dietary antioxidants and asthma in adults: population-based case-control study. *Am J Respir Crit Care Med.* 2001;164:1823–1828.

67. Cirillo DJ, Agrawal Y, Cassano PA. Lipids and pulmonary function in the Third National Health and Nutrition Examination Survey. *Am J Epidemiol.* 2002;155:842–848.

68. Skadhauge LR, Christensen K, Kyvik KO, Sigsgaard T. Genetic and environmental influence on asthma: a population-based study of 11,688 Danish twin pairs. *Eur Respir J.* 1999;13:8–14.

69. Szczeklik A. Mechanism of aspirin-induced asthma. *Allergy.* 1997;52:613–619.

70. Szczeklik A. The cyclooxygenase theory of aspirin-induced asthma. *Eur Respir J.* 1990;3:588–593.

71. Picado C. Aspirin-intolerant asthma: role of cyclo-oxygenase enzymes. *Allergy.* 2002;57(suppl 72):58–60.

72. Sanak M, Simon HU, Szczeklik A. Leukotriene C4 synthase promoter polymorphism and risk of aspirin-induced asthma. *Lancet.* 1997;350:1599–1600.

73. Arif AA, Whitehead LW, Delclos GL, Tortolero SR, Lee ES. Prevalence and risk factors of work related asthma by industry among United States workers: data from the third National Health and Nutrition Examination Survey (1988–94). *Occup Environ Med.* 2002;59:505–511.

74. Spitzer WO, Suissa S, Ernst P, et al. The use of beta-agonists and the risk of death and near death from asthma. *N Engl J Med.* 1992;326:501–506.

75. *Guidelines for the Management of Asthma: Expert Panel Report II.* Bethesda, Md: National Institutes of Health; 1997. NIH Publication No. 97-4051.

76. Ramirez NC, Ledford DK. Immunotherapy for allergic asthma. *Med Clin North Am.* 2002;86:1091–1112.

77. *Practical Guide for the Diagnosis and Management of Asthma.* Bethesda, Md: National Institutes of Health; 1997. NIH Publication 97-4053.

78. Barnes PJ. Mechanisms of action of glucocorticoids in asthma. *Am J Respir Crit Care Med.* 1996;154:S21–S26; discussion S26–S27.

79. Lieberman P, Yates SW, Welk K. Pulmonary remodeling in asthma. *J Investig Allergol Clin Immunol.* 2001;11:220–234.

80. Donahue JG, Weiss ST, Livingston JM, Goetsch MA, Greineder DK, Platt R. Inhaled steroids and the risk of hospitalization for asthma. *JAMA.* 1997;277:887–891.

81. National Asthma Education and Prevention Program expert panel report: guidelines for the diagnosis and management of asthma, update in selected topics 2002. *J Allergy Clin Immunol.* 2002;110:S141–S219.

82. Nelson JA, Strauss L, Skowronski M, Ciufo R, Novak R, McFadden ER Jr. Effect of long-term salmeterol treatment on exercise-induced asthma. *N Engl J Med.* 1998;339:141–146.

83. Fitzpatrick MF, Mackay T, Driver H, Douglas NJ. Salmeterol in nocturnal asthma: a double blind, placebo controlled trial of a long acting inhaled beta 2 agonist. *BMJ.* 1990;301:1365–1368.

84. Drazen JM, Israel E, O'Byrne PM. Treatment of asthma with drugs modifying the leukotriene pathway. *N Engl J Med.* 1999;340:197–206.

85. Barnes NC, Pujet JC. Pranlukast, a novel leukotriene receptor antagonist: results of the first European, placebo controlled, multicentre clinical study in asthma. *Thorax.* 1997;52:523–527.

86. Reiss TF, Chervinsky P, Dockhorn RJ, Shingo S, Seidenberg B, Edwards TB, for Montelukast Clinical Research Study Group. Montelukast, a once-daily leukotriene receptor antagonist, in the treatment of chronic asthma: a multicenter, randomized, double-blind trial. *Arch Intern Med.* 1998;158:1213–1220.

87. Drazen JM, Yandava CN, Dube L, et al. Pharmacogenetic association between ALOX5 promoter genotype and the response to anti-asthma treatment. *Nat Genet.* 1999;22:168–170.

88. Drazen JM, Israel E, Boushey HA, et al, for Asthma Clinical Research Network. Comparison of regularly scheduled with as-needed use of albuterol in mild asthma. *N Engl J Med.* 1996;335:841–847.

89. Blake KV, Hoppe M, Harman E, Hendeles L. Relative amount of albuterol delivered to lung receptors from a metered-dose inhaler and nebulizer solution: bioassay by histamine bronchoprovocation. *Chest.* 1992;101:309–315.

90. Field SK, Sutherland LR. Does medical antireflux therapy improve asthma in asthmatics with gastroesophageal reflux?: a critical review of the literature. *Chest.* 1998;114:275–283.

91. Kanter LJ, Siegel CJ, Snyder CF, Pelletier EM, Buchner DA, Goss TF. Impact of respiratory symptoms on health-related quality of life and medical resource utilization of patients treated by allergy specialists and primary care providers. *Ann Allergy Asthma Immunol.* 2002;89:139–147.

92. Adams RJ, Smith BJ, Ruffin RE. Impact of the physician's participatory style in asthma outcomes and patient satisfaction. *Ann Allergy Asthma Immunol.* 2001;86:263–271.

93. Kanny G, Moneret-Vautrin DA, Flabbee J, Beaudouin E, Morisset M, Thevenin F. Population study of food allergy in France. *J Allergy Clin Immunol.* 2001;108:133–140.

94. Woods RK, Abramson M, Bailey M, Walters EH. International prevalences of reported food allergies and intolerances: comparisons arising from the European Community Respiratory Health Survey (ECRHS) 1991–1994. *Eur J Clin Nutr.* 2001;55:298–304.

95. Sampson HA. Role of immediate food hypersensitivity in the pathogenesis of atopic dermatitis. *J Allergy Clin Immunol.* 1983;71:473–480.

96. Sicherer SH. Food allergy. *Lancet.* 2002;360:701–710.

97. Wahn U, von Mutius E. Childhood risk factors for atopy and the importance of early intervention. *J Allergy Clin Immunol.* 2001;107:567–574.

98. Zeiger RS, Heller S, Mellon MH, et al. Effect of combined maternal and infant food-allergen avoidance on development of atopy in early infancy: a randomized study. *J Allergy Clin Immunol.* 1989;84:72–89.

99. Zeiger RS, Heller S. The development and prediction of atopy in high-risk children: follow-up at age seven years in a prospective randomized study of combined maternal and infant food allergen avoidance. *J Allergy Clin Immunol.* 1995;95:1179–1190.

100. Fergusson DM, Horwood LJ, Shannon FT. Early solid feeding and recurrent childhood eczema: a 10-year longitudinal study. *Pediatrics.* 1990;86:541–546.

101. American Academy of Pediatrics Committee on Nutrition. Hypoallergenic infant formulas. *Pediatrics.* 2000;106:346–349.

102. Kokkonen J, Haapalahti M, Laurila K, Karttunen TJ, Maki M. Cow's milk protein-sensitive enteropathy at school age. *J Pediatr.* 2001;139:797–803.

103. Lazarou J, Pomeranz BH, Corey PN. Incidence of adverse drug reactions in hospitalized patients: a meta-analysis of prospective studies. *JAMA.* 1998;279:1200–1205.

104. Barranco P, Lopez-Serrano MC. General and epidemiological aspects of allergic drug reactions. *Clin Exp Allergy.* 1998;28(suppl 4):61–62.

105. Haddi E, Charpin D, Tafforeau M, et al. Atopy and systemic reactions to drugs. *Allergy.* 1990;45:236–239.

106. Petri M, Allbritton J. Antibiotic allergy in systemic lupus erythematosus: a case-control study. *J Rheumatol.* 1992;19:265–269.

107. Coopman SA, Johnson RA, Platt R, Stem RS. Cutaneous disease and drug reactions in HIV infection. *N Engl J Med.* 1993;328:1670–1674.

108. Demoly P, Bousquet J. Drug allergy diagnosis work up. *Allergy.* 2002;57(suppl 72):37–40.

109. Annila I. Bee venom allergy. *Clin Exp Allergy.* 2000;30:1682–1687.

110. Lockey RF, Turkeltaub PC, Baird-Warren IA, et al. The *Hymenoptera* venom study: I. 1979–1982: demographics and history—sting data. *J Allergy Clin Immunol.* 1988;82:370–381.

111. Bamard JH. Studies of 400 *Hymenoptera* sting deaths in the United States. *J Allergy Clin Immunol.* 1973;52:259–264.

112. Reisman RE, Dvorin DJ, Randolph CC, Georgitis JW. Stinging insect allergy: natural history and modification with venom immunotherapy. *J Allergy Clin Immunol.* 1985;75:735–740.

RESOURCES

American Academy of Allergy, Asthma, and Immunology (AAAAI).
Web site: www.aaai.org

American College of Allergy, Asthma, and Immunology (ACAAI).
Web site: www.acaai.org/index.shtml

Global Initiative for Asthma.
Web site: www.ginasthma.com

Joint Council of Allergy, Asthma, and Immunology (JCAAI).
Web site: www.jcaai.org

National Asthma Education and Prevention program (NIH/NHLBI).
Web site: www.nhlbi.nih.gov/about/naepp/index.htm

Chronic Obstructive Pulmonary Disease

Clayton T. Cowl, MD, MS

INTRODUCTION

Chronic obstructive pulmonary disease (COPD) has been used by clinicians to describe a constellation of overlapping terms, including emphysema, chronic bronchitis, and asthma with variable degrees of airflow obstruction (see Chapter 58). Although patients with COPD all have some component of airway obstruction, the characteristics and severity in an individual patient may be quite variable. A clinician should consider each patient with COPD to fall within a spectrum of disease pattern and severity (Fig 59-1) and understand that this spectrum is dynamic throughout the patient's life.

Emphysema causes irreversible loss of elasticity of the alveoli and, ultimately, alveolar destruction and larger airway collapse with progressive obstruction. *Chronic bronchitis* refers to an inflammatory process that begins typically in the smaller airways and may progress to larger airway involvement. It is associated with increased mucous production, respiratory tract infections, and chronic cough. *Asthmatic bronchitis* indicates chronic persistent asthma with inflammatory airway changes, which is clinically relevant because of the potential to achieve some airway reversibility with bronchodilators and inhaled corticosteroids. Although chronic bronchitis is the most prevalent component of the disease, most patients experience a combination of these factors.

EPIDEMIOLOGY

The Centers for Disease Control and Prevention estimate that in 2000 there were 44.9 COPD-related deaths per 100,000 individuals in the United States,[1] making it the fourth largest cause of mortality. More than 16 million patients have been diagnosed with the condition, and perhaps an additional 16 million more are symptomatic but undiagnosed.[2] The significance from a public health perspective hinges on the fact that the natural history of COPD is chronic and progressive, resulting in severe and prolonged disability. Chronic obstructive pulmonary disease led to $23.9 billion in US health care spending in

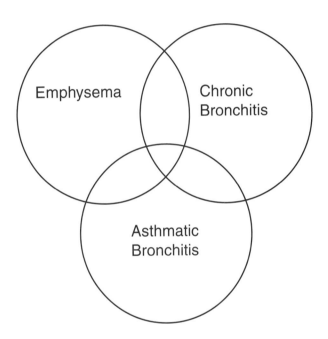

F I G U R E   59-1

Disease patterns of patients with chronic obstructive pulmonary disease (COPD).

1993, with $14.7 billion in direct expenses and an additional $9.2 billion in indirect expenses through lost wages or time away from work.[3] As health care spending escalates, management of this disease will likely play a larger role in public health initiatives.

RISK FACTORS

A combination of individual risk factors and environmental exposures determines the probability of developing COPD as well as its severity and prognosis. Cigarette smoking is the most common cause of COPD, accounting for more than 80% of all cases. However, the disease is associated with certain host characteristics that may predispose some individuals to development of the disease. Familial clusters of patients with certain demographic and socioeconomic

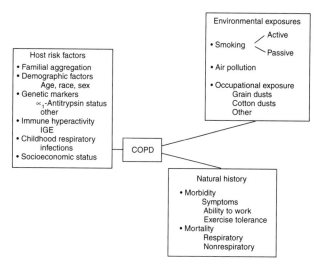

FIGURE 59-2

Conceptual schematic demonstrating major hereditary and environmental factors affecting pathogenesis, course, and prognosis of chronic obstructive pulmonary disease (COPD).

variables have been identified with a higher prevalence of COPD; genetic factors such as α_1-antitrypsin deficiency also can increase disease risk (Fig 59-2). The presence of early childhood respiratory tract infections may also predispose some individuals to COPD development. Environmental factors such as occupational exposures (eg, organic dusts, or intense exposure to upper respiratory tract irritants), air pollution, and passive smoking combine to affect the pathogenesis and natural history of the illness.

DIAGNOSTIC ASSESSMENT

History and Physical Examination

The history and physical examination findings of the patient with COPD often reveal exertional dyspnea, which may later occur at rest as the disease advances, along with wheezing, sputum production, and chronic cough. These symptoms are nonspecific but, when combined with appropriate laboratory and radiographic testing, a diagnosis can be confirmed. Auscultation typically reveals expiratory prolongation, and diminished thoracic excursion is often noted in more advanced disease. Weight loss, tachypnea, pursed-lip breathing, and use of accessory muscles of respiration may be seen in patients with severe emphysema. Signs of cor pulmonale may be present in cases of end-stage disease. In patients with severe hypercapnia, asterixis is occasionally identified.

Radiographs and Imaging

Chest radiographs in patients with COPD often reveal flattened diaphragms due to hyperinflation and air trapping.

In severe emphysema, areas of hyperlucency may be identified along with bullae and absence of vascular markings in these regions. *Centrilobular emphysema*, which is most frequently associated with cigarette smoking, involves the lung apices and parenchymal periphery. Marked hyperinflation and obstructive airway changes are often noted. *Panacinar emphysema* is associated with α_1-antitrypsin deficiency and involves the lower lung zones. *Paraseptal emphysema* is commonly seen with spontaneous pneumothoraces of young adults. In this type of emphysema, the distal acinus is involved and, as a result, airway obstruction is evident only occasionally. Computed tomography (CT) of the chest also helps to delineate emphysematous changes of the pulmonary parenchyma as well as pleural and mediastinal abnormalities, if present. Recently, 3-dimensional CT imagery has been used to calculate the extent of emphysematous changes in patients considering lung volume reduction surgery.

Pulmonary Function Testing

Spirometry is used to measure the rate at which lung volumes change during a forced breathing maneuver. These tests are underused but provide an abundance of important clinical information, often years before clinical presentation of symptoms (Fig 59-3). The most commonly performed spirometric testing procedure requires the patient to inhale maximally and then exhale as rapidly and completely as possible, referred to as the *forced expiratory vital capacity* (FVC). These volume measurements are frequently plotted against time. An expiratory effort of 6 seconds is considered a minimum for ensuring adequate measurements.[4] The FVC test may also be plotted as a flow-volume curve. This expiratory flow-volume curve measurement is important in that for any given person there is an individual limit to the maximal flow that may be attained for any specific lung volume. This limit is reached with only moderate expiratory efforts, and increasing individual expiratory force does not increase the flow. What results is a "signature" maximal expiratory flow curve that is highly reproducible for each individual because the curve defines a limit to flow. The maximal flow is also quite sensitive to changes encountered with the earliest forms of respiratory disease.[5]

The most common measurement taken from the FVC is the forced expiratory volume in 1 second (FEV_1), or the volume of air exhaled in the first second of the FVC test. This is the most reproducible and possibly the most useful measurement obtained during spirometry. Similar to the FVC, the normal values for the FEV_1 depend on the patient's size, age, sex, and race. Equations have been formulated to establish predicted norms for each spirometric value.[6] These equations account for the demographic variables noted above. A reduced ratio of FEV_1 to

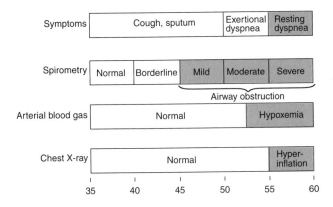

Symptoms	Cough, sputum			Exertional dyspnea	Resting dyspnea
Spirometry	Normal	Borderline	Mild	Moderate	Severe
			Airway obstruction		
Arterial blood gas	Normal				Hypoxemia
Chest X-ray	Normal				Hyper-inflation

35   40   45   50   55   60

FIGURE 59-3

Progression of symptoms in chronic obstructive pulmonary disease (COPD) shown schematically by spirometry, arterial blood-gas analysis, and chest radiographs. Spirometry may detect COPD years before severe dyspnea occurs. From PL Enright, RE Hyatt, eds. *Office Spirometry: A Practical Guide to the Selection and Use of Spirometers.* Philadelphia, Pa: Lea & Febiger; 1987. By permission of Mayo Foundation.

FVC (FEV$_1$/FVC, expressed in a percentage) aids in identifying patients with airway obstruction in whom the FVC is also reduced. It may also help to separate an obstructive airway disease from a restrictive process in which FEV$_1$/FVC would be normal. Peak expiratory flow (PEF), also known as maximal expiratory flow, occurs shortly after the onset of expiration. This measurement is obtained frequently in the outpatient setting using inexpensive handheld devices but is plagued by reproducibility problems due to its dependence on patient effort. However, this method of measuring maximal expiratory flow has proved useful for compliant patients in the management of obstructive airway diseases. Measurements of PEF are most useful when analyzing measurement trends rather than specific flow rates, due to the imprecise nature of the test.

In patients with COPD, the FEV$_1$ will typically be proportionally lower than the FVC (a reduced FEV$_1$/FVC) and the terminal portion of the flow-volume curve is "scooped out" or concave. Patients with substantial emphysema may have a reduction in diffusing capacity, suggesting progressive alveolar destruction. Even if the clinical diagnosis of COPD is established, spirometric measurements help to define the degree of impairment of pulmonary function. For example, an FEV$_1$ of 50% of predicted or less suggests future disabling disease. An FEV$_1$ of less than 800 mL predicts respiratory insufficiency manifested by carbon dioxide retention. Periodic spirometry every 1 to 2 years in frequency helps to establish excessive rates of FEV$_1$ decline beyond the 25 to 30 mL per year expected in normal subjects. Those with FEV$_1$ declines of 60 mL or greater may have a substantial reversible component of bronchospastic airway disease and may benefit from

chronic therapy with inhaled corticosteroids and/or longer-acting bronchodilators.[5]

SCREENING

Unfortunately, at this time there are no tests with adequate specificity and positive predictive value to screen for COPD or other chest conditions, including lung carcinoma, in the general population. The diagnosis of COPD in asymptomatic individuals is frequently overlooked and underestimated.

PREVENTION OF COPD

Primary Prevention: Smoking Cessation

The effects of tobacco abuse and strategies for smoking cessation are outlined in detail in Chapter 11. Smoking cessation is undoubtedly the single greatest action to reduce the risk of COPD and manifestations of chronic lung disease. The ability to establish rapport with the patient, ask questions about the individual's insight or desire to quit smoking, and make appropriate recommendations for ending tobacco abuse are the key factors in directing individual and population-based health improvements from the preventive perspective.

Secondary Prevention

The earliest stages of COPD are not associated with symptoms. Thus, the role of preventive medicine practitioners in recognizing impending disease and direct lifestyle and therapeutic modifications is even more important. Cough and expectoration are typically described as the first noticeable symptoms in COPD. However, by the time a patient presents with dyspnea with minimal exertion or at rest, their disease stage is already advanced and severe. Although the result of the physical examination is frequently normal during the early stages of COPD with the exception of prolonged expiratory airflows, spirometry remains the most sensitive and specific diagnostic tool to identify patients with obstructive airflow abnormalities. Obviously, smoking cessation is again the most important modifiable factor to delay progression of COPD.

Vaccines

With reduction in baseline spirometric airflow resulting from chronic effects on the body's immune system and mucociliary escalator of the upper respiratory tract, patients with COPD are especially susceptible to influenza epidemics and to infections caused by streptococcal pneumonitis. For this reason and because of antigenic shift, COPD-affected patients should receive a pneumococcal vaccination as well as an annual influenza vaccination administered in October or November or within 1 to 3 months of the anticipated epidemic. This is thought to provide 80% protection from the virus. A pneumococcal vaccination may be administered once, and a booster may be given 7 years after the initial vaccine, although advocates for this vaccine suggest a 5-year booster interval may be appropriate.[7]

Exercise

Individuals with chronic lung disease should be encouraged to participate in regular aerobic exercise programs with an emphasis on high-intensity training as tolerated. Regular physical conditioning has been shown to improve maximum exercise tolerance. Programs that emphasize upper body conditioning as well as lower extremity workouts have demonstrated consistent improvement in maximum exercise tolerance.[8]

Nutritional counseling

Nearly one fourth of patients with COPD have been reported to have a body weight of less than 90% of ideal body weight (BMI <20 kg/m^2).[9] Many patients remain undernourished, even when taking enteral supplements. Although once thought to exacerbate the hypercapnia noted in severe disease, intake of carbohydrates does not generate excessive carbon dioxide unless caloric (energy) intake greatly exceeds individual energy requirements. These requirements are frequently greater than one would expect, resulting from the increased work of breathing. Patients with COPD should eat a well-balanced diet that includes carbohydrates and focuses on appropriate weight targets (see Chapters 16–18)

Patient and family education

Education is vital in the care of the patient with COPD. Not only do educated patients recognize exacerbations more quickly and understand when to seek professional medical evaluation, they tend to be more compliant with daily medication regimens that prevent or attenuate COPD triggers.[8]

TERTIARY PREVENTION AND TREATMENT

A variety of potential environmental and systemic triggers lead to exacerbations of bronchospasm and increased mucous production with airway plugging, which increases the work of breathing. This results in worsening dyspnea, fatigue, and, in some cases, respiratory failure. Although infections are the most prevalent cause of COPD exacerbations, other causes such as pulmonary emboli, sedative

drug narcosis, pneumothorax, or pulmonary edema may increase breathlessness and cause worsened gas exchange. Treatment of the underlying exacerbating factor is key toward reducing morbidity and mortality in patients who experience exacerbations of COPD. In addition, there are a number of therapeutic modalities available to treat COPD symptoms that are outlined in this section.

Bronchodilators

β-Andrenergic agonists increase cyclic adenosine monophosphate (cAMP) formation, causing a shift in calcium ion concentration intracellularly and a reduction in airway tone. They are rapidly acting and used frequently in treatment of COPD, although they have a relatively short half-life. Because of the risk of tachyphylaxis due to downregulation of β2 receptors, these drugs are often used only intermittently with symptoms of wheezing or shortness of breath, and as the primary therapy for certain patients with infrequent symptoms. There are several formulations of the drug available, including metered-dose inhalers, and nebulized forms. Oral dosing is used rarely because of an increased side-effect profile that includes tachycardia, dysrhythmias, tremor, agitation, and insomnia. Longer acting β-andrenergic agents have been developed but have been associated recently with increased mortality in asthmatic patients.

Anticholinergic agents inhibit the effects of acetylcholine at parasympathetic cholinergic synapses by competing for acetylcholine receptors. This causes a reduction in the intracellular guanosine 3',5'-cyclic monophosphate (cGMP) levels, which in turn causes a decrease in bronchial smooth-muscle tone. Although atropine was used originally for bronchodilation, its side-effect profile was vast and included dry mouth, blurred vision, tachycardia, urinary retention, and in some cases mental status changes. Ipratropium bromide, a quaternary ammonium atropine derivative, has less mucosal absorption and fewer side effects and is the only anticholinergic agent available in the United States.

Theophylline, the prototype methylxanthine, has been used in obstructive airway disease for years, but its mechanism is unknown. It is thought to relax airway smooth muscle, stimulate diaphragmatic contractility, and reduce pulmonary vascular resistance.[8] However, use of the medication has fallen out of favor because of its potentially lethal toxic side effects and its low therapeutic index. These potential side effects have been exacerbated by the fact that many commonly prescribed medications such as macrolide and quinolone antibiotics as well as histamine blockers have been associated with increase in theophylline half-life. Serum theophylline levels must be monitored during administration of the drug (therapeutic levels are 10 to 20 μg/mL). Despite this, certain patients with severe disease have tolerated slow-release theophylline in long-term maintenance medication regimens.[10]

Corticosteroids

The role of systemic corticosteroids (methylprednisolone) for patients with COPD remains controversial. For acute exacerbations, airflow improvement has been demonstrated in some patients. However, it is difficult to predict prospectively who will benefit from the use of oral glucocorticoids and for this reason, they are not prescribed routinely for prolonged administration. Hyperglycemia, skin bruising, bone demineralization, oral candidiasis, insomnia, and fluid retention are just a few of the untoward side effects that may develop due to long-term systemic therapy. Inhaled corticosteroids have been used in certain patients with a major component of airway reversibility. Although inhaled corticosteroids involve fewer systemic side effects, their long-term efficacy in patients with COPD is unclear.

Leukotriene Inhibitors

Drugs such as montelukast cause inhibition of airway cysteinyl leukotriene receptors, inhibiting the physiologic action of the cysteinyl leukotriene LTD_4. This receptor inhibition reduces early- and late-phase bronchoconstriction resulting from antigen challenge and has been used successfully in asthmatic patients. Initial studies in patients with COPD have shown modest reductions in some measures of neutrophilic bronchial inflammation using leukotriene inhibitors.[11] However, there are few published studies that demonstrate clear objective improvement using leukotriene inhibitors in this population, and additional research is ongoing.

Treatment of Infections

Because bronchial infection is the most common precipitating factor for acute exacerbation of COPD, treatment with oral antibiotics has been studied extensively. Antibiotics appear to have beneficial effects for patients with COPD who are experiencing acute exacerbation: shortened length of time to recovery and improved expiratory airflows.[12,13]

Pulmonary Rehabilitation

Pulmonary rehabilitation is designed to assist patients with COPD who experience frequent respiratory exacerbations despite optimal medical management. Most programs combine patient education of appropriate nutrition recommendations, exercise programs, and psychosocial support with retraining programs focused on

techniques of chest physiotherapy, pursed-lip breathing, and diaphragmatic breathing.

Oxygen Therapy

Supplemental oxygen therapy has been shown to be effective in decreasing mortality in patients with severe COPD.[14] The current indications for long-term supplemental oxygen include a resting PaO_2 of 55 mm Hg or less, or evidence of tissue hypoxia or end-organ damage manifested as secondary polycythemia, cor pulmonale, signs of right ventricular failure, or impaired mental status. The need for nocturnal supplemental oxygen should also be evaluated because some patients with COPD experience nocturnal desaturation without evidence of sleep-related disordered breathing. Supplemental oxygen therapy, typically administered through a nasal cannula, may be supplied via compressed oxygen cylinders, a ready source of liquid oxygen, or an oxygen concentrator. The concentrator is the least expensive and most reliable delivery system, requiring little maintenance. However, backup oxygen sources are recommended in the event of power failure and to allow patients added mobility.

Antiprotease Replacement

Antiprotease therapy for patients with α_1-antitrypsin deficiency has been studied extensively in the past decade and hinges on the theory that replacement of appropriate levels of antiproteases in the body may help to minimize symptoms or reduce mortality rates. Weekly or monthly infusions have been used with little or no side effects.[15,16] Although a number of trials have shown stabilization of subjective symptoms, there have been no clear long-term benefits identified, and treatments have been cost-prohibitive in many cases.

Surgical Treatment of Emphysema

Lung volume reduction surgery

In the 1950s, wedge resections of parenchymal lung tissue were performed on patients with diffuse emphysema with hopes to relieve small airways radial traction.[17] However, at that time surgical risks tended to outweigh the benefits of wedge resection. In the past decade, there has been a variety of studies assessing the efficacy and safety of lung volume reduction surgery in select patients with emphysema. In the more recent procedures, a midline sternotomy is performed and about one third of each lung is removed. Alternatively, video-assisted thoracoscopy (VATS) is used. Strips of bovine pericardium are stapled to the pulmonary suture line to reduce the risk of postoperative air leaks.[18] Although initial studies showed improvements in subjective dyspnea, pulmonary function tests,[14] and overall quality of life, the mortality rates for individuals with low FEV_1 and homogenous emphysematous disease were shown to be remarkably high by the National Emphysema Treatment Trial (NETT) Research Group.[19] The procedure is reserved for patients with severe emphysema and has been used recently as a bridging procedure or in place of lung transplantation.

Lung transplantation

Since methods of immunosuppression have been improved substantially in the past decade, lung transplantation has become a reasonable alternative for some patients with severe end-stage emphysema. Chronic obstructive pulmonary disease with severe emphysema has become the most prevalent indication for lung transplantation today and can restore pulmonary function and reverse dyspnea in may cases. Although selection criteria for transplant candidates were initially quite stringent,

these restrictions have gradually lessened over time. Cost and availability of transplant organs have been the greatest barriers to this avenue of treatment.

SUMMARY

In the future, COPD will continue to be a substantial health and economic burden as long as tobacco abuse remains prevalent throughout the world. Although efforts to decrease environmental contaminants in the atmosphere and smoking prevalence in the United States in the past 2 decades have been considered successful, increased rates of teenage and young adult smokers in the past 5 years will likely result in a corresponding increased incidence of this disease in the future. For this and other reasons, continuing educational efforts to eliminate smoking are paramount, especially with younger smokers and youth before they begin smoking.

REFERENCES

1. *Deaths: Preliminary Data for 2000.* Atlanta, Ga: Centers for Disease Control and Prevention. 2001;49:1–40. Publication HS 2001–1120.

2. Petty TL. A new strategy for COPD. *J Res Dis.* 1997;18:365–369.

3. Hurd S. The impact of COPD on lung health worldwide: epidemiology and incidence. *Chest.* 2000;117(suppl):1S–4S.

4. American Thoracic Society. Standardization of spirometry: 1987 update. *Am Rev Respir Dis.* 1987;136:1285–1298.

5. Hyatt RE, Scanlon PD, Nakamura M. *Interpretation of Pulmonary Function Tests: A Practical Guide.* Philadelphia, Pa: Lippincott-Raven Publishers; 1997.

6. American Thoracic Society. Lung function testing: selection of reference values and interpretative strategies. *Am Rev Respir Dis.* 1991;144:1202–1218.

7. Shapiro ED, et al. The protective efficacy of polyvalent pneumococcal polysaccharide vaccine. *N Engl J Med.* 1991;325:1453–1460.

8. Celli BR, Snider GL, Heffner J, et al. Standards for the diagnosis and care of patients with chronic obstructive pulmonary disease. *Am J Respir Crit Care Med.* 1995;152(suppl):S77–S120.

9. Ferguson GT, Cherniak RM. Management of chronic obstructive pulmonary disease. *New Engl J Med.* 1993;328:1017–1022.

10. Ramsdell J. Use of theophylline in the treatment of COPD. *Chest.* 1995;107(suppl):206S–209S.

11. Gompertz S, Stockle RA. A randomized, placebo-controlled trial of a leukotriene synthesis inhibitor in patients with COPD. *Chest.* 2002;122:289–294.

12. Anthonisen NR, Connett JE, Kiley JP, et al. Antibiotic therapy in exacerbations of chronic obstructive pulmonary disease. *Ann Intern Med.* 1987;106:196–204.

13. Saint S, Bent S, Vittinghoff E, Grady D. Antibiotics in chronic obstructive pulmonary disease exacerbations: a meta-analysis. *JAMA.* 1995;273:957–960.

14. Nocturnal Oxygen Therapy Trial Group. Continuous or nocturnal oxygen therapy in hypoxemic chronic obstructive lung disease: a clinical trial. *Ann Intern Med.* 1980;93:391–398.

15. Wewers MA, et al. Replacement therapy for alpha-1-antitrypsin deficiency associated with emphysema. *N Engl J Med.* 1987;316:1055–1062.

16. Hubbard RC, et al. Biochemical efficacy and safety of monthly augmentation therapy for alpha-1-antitrypsin deficiency. *JAMA.* 1988;260:1259–1264.

17. Brantigan OC, Mueller E, Kress MB. A surgical approach to pulmonary emphysema. *Am Rev Respir Dis.* 1959;80:194–202.

18. Cooper JD, Trulock EP, Triantafillou AN, et al. Bilateral pneumonectomy (volume reduction) for chronic obstructive pulmonary disease. *J Thorac Cardiovasc Surg.* 1995;109:106–199.

19. Koebe HG, Kugler C, Dienemann H. Evidence-based medicine: lung volume reduction surgery (LVRS). *J Thorac Cardiovasc Surg.* 2002;50:315–322.

RESOURCES

Rakel RE, Bope ET, eds. *Conn's Current Therapy,* 2003, 55th edition. Philadelphia, Pa: WB Saunders; 2002.

Mandell GL, Douglas RG, Bennett JE, Dolin R. *Principles and Practice of Infectious Diseases,* 5th edition. London, England: Churchill Livingstone; 1995.

Sin DD, McAlister FA, Man SF, Anthonisen NR. Contemporary management of chronic obstructive pulmonary disease. *JAMA.* 2003;290(17):2301–2312.

Calverley PM, Walker P. Chronic destructive pulmonary disease. *Lancet.* 2003;362(9389):1053–1061.

chapter 60

Disorders of the Ear, Nose, and Throat

Catherine A. Henry, MD, FACP

THE EAR

The ear is divided anatomically into external, middle, and inner components (Fig 60-1). The external ear directs sound to the tympanic membrane, which vibrates in response to sound waves, transmitting them to the cochlea via the ossicles. The middle ear functions as both a transmitter of sound and an amplifier, recovering most of the 30 dB of sound energy lost when sound waves are passed from air to liquid in the inner ear. Vibration of the perilymph is transmitted to the basilar membrane, which stimulates the hair cells in the organ of Corti. These cells convert the sound waves to neural impulses that are transmitted via the eighth cranial nerve to the brain, where sound is perceived and interpreted. Each component is important to normal hearing, and disorders of each part can contribute to hearing loss.

The brain perceives balance and motion by a complex system. Baseline signals emitted by the right and left vestibular system stimulate the brain equally. When motion occurs, the hair cells in each vestibule are stimulated differently, sending impulses to each vestibular nucleus. This results in the vestibulo-ocular reflex, which allows the eyes to remain focused on an object while the head is in motion. When one side of the vestibular system does not function properly, the brain perceives this as persistent stimulation, resulting in a subjective sensation of movement (vertigo) and its objective manifestation of slow alternating with fast eye movement (nystagmus). In addition, the vestibulospinal reflex results in muscle contraction on the ipsilateral side and relaxation on the contralateral side, causing leaning or falling to the side of the vestibular deficit. Additional connections throughout the brain stem and cerebellum contribute to the nausea, vomiting, and salivation frequently seen in vestibular disorders.[1]

Hearing Testing and Screening

Whereas most individuals have had their eyes examined at one time or another, many people have never had a hearing test. There are no universally accepted guidelines for routine hearing testing in the general adult population. Screening questionnaires, such as the Hearing Handicap Inventory for the Elderly—Screening Version (HHIE-S),

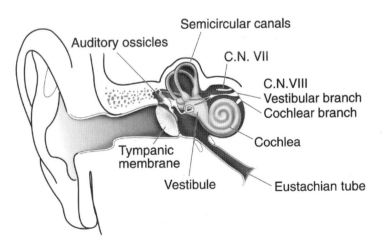

FIGURE 60-1

Anatomy of the ear.

TABLE 60-1

Screening Version of the Hearing Handicap Inventory for the Elderly (HHIE-S)*

Item No.	Item	Yes (4 points)	Sometimes (2 points)	No (0 points)
E-1	Does a hearing problem cause you to feel embarrassed when you meet new people?			
E-2	Does a hearing problem cause you to feel frustrated when talking to members of your family?			
S-3	Do you have difficulty hearing when someone speaks in a whisper?			
E-4	Do you feel handicapped by a hearing problem?			
S-5	Does a hearing problem cause you difficulty when visiting friends, relatives, or neighbors?			
S-6	Does a hearing problem cause you to attend religious services less often than you would like?			
E-7	Does a hearing problem cause you to have arguments with family members?			
S-8	Does a hearing problem cause you difficulty when listening to TV or radio?			
E-9	Do you feel that any difficulty with your hearing limits or hampers your personal or social life?			
S-10	Does a hearing problem cause you difficulty when in a restaurant with relatives or friends?			

Raw score _____

Interpreting the Raw Score

0–8 = 13% probability of hearing impairment (no handicap/no referral)

10–24 = 50% probability of hearing impairment (mild to moderate handicap)

26–40 = 84% probability of hearing impairment (severe handicap)

*E indicates emotional items; S, social or situational items; and raw score, sum of points assigned to each item. Adapted with permission from Ventry IM, Weinstein BE. The Hearing Handicap Inventory for the Elderly: a new tool. *Ear Hear.* 1982;3:128-134.

are available to estimate the degree of hearing loss in the elderly and select patients for audiometric testing (Table 60-1). However, one study demonstrated that patient self-report (answering yes to the question "Do you feel you have a hearing loss?") is a more sensitive indicator of hearing loss than the HHIE-S.[2]

Audiometric testing is appropriate for any patients who express concern regarding their hearing and who do not have an obvious cause of hearing loss, such as cerumen impaction. Pure tone audiometry assesses the sound pressure level (SPL) in decibels that a patient can perceive at a variety of frequencies, generally between 250 and 8000 Hz (Fig 60-2A). Speech discrimination testing measures a patient's ability to recognize 1- and 2-syllable words at an SPL high enough for the patient to hear (based on pure tone testing). Additional tests can be performed to measure middle ear function, acoustic reflexes, and other aspects of hearing. Periodic screening of hearing is appropriate for patients exposed to loud noise on a regular basis.

Presbycusis

Approximately 40% of the US population over the age of 75 years experiences measurable hearing loss, making presbycusis or hearing loss due to the aging process the most common cause of sensorineural hearing loss in the United States. Hearing declines beginning in middle age, progressing twice as fast in men as in women. Several pathophysiologic mechanisms contribute to hearing loss in the aging ear, but the most common pattern is that of sensory hearing loss, a sharply downsloping high tone loss with well-preserved speech discrimination (Fig 60-2B). Presbycusis is frequently combined with noise-induced hearing loss, resulting in a superimposed "notch" at 4000 Hz on pure tone audiometry. The 2 sources of hearing loss are, in practical terms, impossible to separate.[3]

There are currently no effective medical or surgical treatments of presbycusis. However, early detection in high-risk individuals (those with noise exposure, prior ear disease, exposure to ototoxic medications, or family

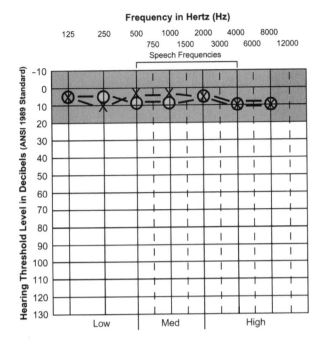

FIGURE 60-2A

Normal hearing thresholds.

Key: Right ear = O═O═O
      Left ear = X═X═X

history of adult-onset hearing loss) can be helpful in reducing additional risks to hearing (principally noise). Early detection also affords the opportunity for timely use of assistive devices and hearing aids, where appropriate. Ototoxic drugs should be avoided where possible. Risk factors for cardiovascular disease (hypertension, hyperlipidemia, and diabetes mellitus) are also associated with hearing loss; maintenance of good general health is associated with better hearing with age.

Noise-Induced Hearing Loss

The world is a noisy place. Many sounds, even those not perceived by the listener as loud, are sufficient to result in measurable, permanent hearing loss. Patients should be questioned about exposure to noise in the workplace, the home, and with recreational activities, especially if they have symptoms of hearing loss or tinnitus. In general, any environment noisy enough to result in difficulty communicating by speech is sufficient to cause hearing loss, and measures to conserve hearing should be initiated. Reduction of environmental noise and use of hearing protection adequate for the anticipated noise level are vital in preventing noise-induced hearing loss.

Factors that may predispose individuals to noise-induced hearing loss include genetic factors, fair complexion with blue eyes, diabetes, nutritional deficien-

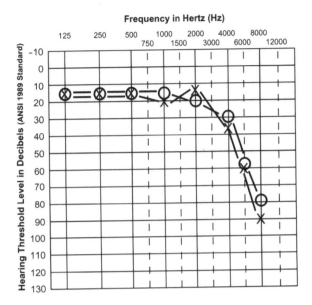

FIGURE 60-2B

Presbycusis.

Key: Right ear = O═O═O
      Left ear = X═X═X

cies (iron, vitamin A), age, prematurity, atherosclerosis and its risk factors (atherogenic diet, smoking), cochlear hydrops, and ototoxic drug therapy (aminoglycosides, cisplatinum).[1] Excessive noise can produce both biochemical alterations in the inner ear and anatomical disruption of inner ear structures to result in temporary or permanent hearing impairment.

With short-term exposure to loud noise, such as a rock concert, affected individuals may experience temporary hearing loss, aural fullness, and/or tinnitus, with resolution over a period of days. With repeated exposure over time, however, hearing thresholds do not return to normal and permanent hearing loss results. Noise-induced hearing loss typically occurs at sound frequency of 4000 Hz but extends to higher and lower frequencies as it progresses (Fig 60-2C).

The Occupational Safety and Health Administration has published standards for noise exposure in the workplace.[4] These should also serve as a guide for patients with recreational or home noise exposure (Table 60-2). In general, employees with noise exposure of 85 dB or higher for an 8-hour period on a regular basis require annual screening for hearing loss. For every 5-dB increase in sound level, the allowed exposure time is cut in half. Employees with a 10-dB decrement in hearing thresholds compared with baseline, or those with greater than 8-hour daily exposure to 85 dB or higher, must be fitted with hearing protectors. Maximum sound level without protection should not exceed 115 dB.

Various devices are available to reduce noise exposure for occupational or recreational activities, including earmuffs, earplugs, or molds (Fig 60-3). Earplugs made of

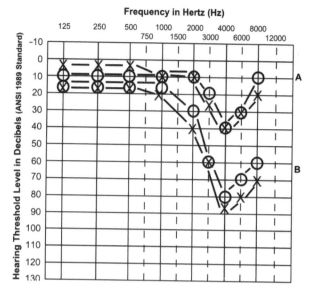

FIGURE 60-2C

Noise-induced hearing loss early (left) and late (right).

Key: Right ear = O═O═O
       Left ear = X═X═X

silicone putty or moldable foam are popular and easy to use, and can be worn with earmuffs for additional protection. Custom-fitted earplugs can be made for those who require consistent, comfortable protection. Whatever device the person chooses, good fit and consistent use are key to obtaining maximum benefit. Even 1 hour a day (in 8 hours of exposure) without protection can reduce effectiveness by 50%. Users also should note that the manufacturer's rating of noise reduction is usually 10 dB greater than the actual benefit with typical use.

The key to hearing protection is wearing proper protection during noise exposure. Therefore, patients should be counseled about recreational and home situations where noise is likely to be encountered in addition to occupational protection. Such situations include concerts; sporting events; hunting; and use of power tools, motors, and lawnmowers.

Hearing Aids

The most common types of hearing loss involve loss in the midrange to high frequencies (1 to 8 kHz) that are critical for speech discrimination, particularly consonant sounds. Since background noise is primarily of low frequency (250 to 1000 Hz), it often drowns out what the patient is trying to hear. Therefore, most individuals with a moderate or greater hearing impairment can benefit from amplification and, if they are willing, should be referred for audiologic assessment and trial of a hearing aid. Many elderly persons with hearing loss exhibit social

TABLE 60-2

Noise Levels and Sources

Noise Level, dB	Source
150	Jet takeoff
140	Shotgun, jet engine
130	Jackhammer
120	Thunder clap
115	Sandblasting, auto horn
110	Chain saw, rock concert
100	Snowmobile, pneumatic drill
90	Power lawn mower, shop tools*
80	Heavy traffic, noisy restaurant
60	Normal conversation
30	Whisper
0	Faintest audible sound

*Hearing protection required at this level and above (see text).

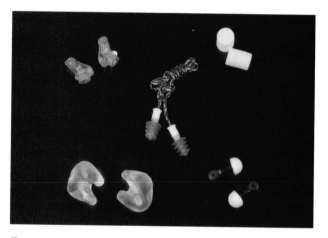

FIGURE 60-3

Various earplugs available to reduce exposure to noise.

withdrawal, depression, and pseudodementia related to their hearing loss, which can often be greatly improved with hearing aids.[5] Predictors of success include the type and severity of hearing loss, perceived difficulty hearing by the patient, lifestyle factors, motivation, and patient expectations. Patients and family members should understand that hearing aids will improve hearing by about half on average but will not restore normal hearing.

Many different types and sizes of hearing aids are available. Figure 60-4 illustrates the difference in size between hearing aids that go behind the ear, in the ear, in the canal, and completely in the canal. Choosing between them depends on the cosmetic desires of the patient, electronic features available for each model, and the patient's

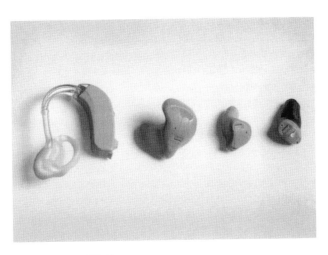

FIGURE 60-4

Hearing aids (L-R): behind ear, in ear, in ear canal, and completely in canal.

budget. In general, smaller aids are less powerful, have shorter battery life, and are more expensive.

Hearing aids fall into 3 categories based on their electronic circuitry: nonprogrammable, programmable analog, and digital.[6] Nonprogrammable aids are the oldest generation and are ordered based on the closest match to the patient's hearing loss. Small adjustments can be made by the hearing-aid fitter. Programmable analog aids use additional circuitry that can be fine-tuned via computer to adjust for the patient's individual needs. Digital aids convert the analog signal into computer code, where advanced programming allows sound processing not possible with analog devices.

Two hearing aids are generally recommended for symmetric hearing loss, as this improves speech discrimination in noise and sound localization. There is some evidence that speech discrimination deteriorates in the unaided ear, making an even stronger argument for binaural amplification.

Cerumen Impaction

Contrary to popular belief by many laypersons, the presence of earwax does not indicate that the ears are not clean; rather, cerumen is critical for cleansing the canal and promoting resistance to infection. Wax is formed by the ceruminous glands of the skin in the cartilaginous portion of the external canal and normally migrates outward, providing normal skin pH and lubrication. Individuals vary greatly in the amount and consistency of wax produced; hence, some ears do not self-cleanse as well as others.

Wax impaction is commonly precipitated by use of cotton swabs inserted into the external canal in attempts

to clean it. Wax impaction is also more common in the elderly and those with prior mastoid surgery. It is usually not perceptible to the patient until the canal is completely obstructed or nearly so, as even a small opening to transmit sound waves will allow normal hearing. Nearly complete impaction, however, often causes intermittent or abrupt hearing loss when a small drop of water occludes the opening. Other symptoms of wax impaction include ear fullness, tinnitus, or sometimes pain (when wax is extremely hard) causing inflammation.

Ceruminolytic agents, such as Debrox, Ceruminex, Murine eardrops, and even the liquid stool softener docusate,[7] will soften and loosen small amounts of cerumen, which can then be irrigated with a bulb syringe using lukewarm water, generally by the patient or a family member. If the cerumen is completely impacted, deep within the canal, or very hard, removal by a medical professional is recommended. Suction is most effective for very soft wax. Curettage under direct visualization is preferred for firm wax.

In primary care settings, irrigation of the canal is most often performed. This should be done with a large-volume, handheld syringe, using lukewarm water and can be preceded by peroxide drops to loosen the wax. Powered devices for irrigation are available, but only those specifically designed for irrigating the ear should be used. Irrigation of the canal should not be performed in the presence of known or suspected tympanic membrane perforation, if there is substantial otalgia, or if there are signs of infection.[8]

The most important preventive measure for cerumen impaction is to instruct patients to avoid the use of cotton swabs, which tend to impact the wax deeper into the canal and aggravate the problem. For patients with a history of repeated impaction, regular use of ceruminolytic drops may decrease the frequency of impaction. Patients with substantial wax accumulation on physical examination should have it removed at that visit to prevent complete impaction. The use of the home remedy ear candles is not recommended because of lack of evidence of effectiveness and potential for injury (burns, candle wax deposition in the ear, and tympanic membrane perforation).[9]

Tinnitus

Tinnitus is any sound perceptible to the patient when no external stimulus exists.[10] Tinnitus affects an estimated 35 million people in the United States, of which approximately 10 million have severe or troubling symptoms. It is most common between the ages of 40 and 70 years, with no sex predominance.

Objective tinnitus is tinnitus caused by a variety of physiological and pathological processes that are audible to the patient and sometimes the physician. These include vascular abnormalities, neuromuscular disorders, and eustachian tube dysfunction. Objective tinnitus is often described as a pulsatile or clicking sound. Although many of the disorders that cause objective tinnitus are benign, many can be successfully treated, and some are associated with underlying medical conditions (hypertension, carotid stenosis, and benign intracranial hypertension). Patients with objective tinnitus should therefore be referred to an otolaryngologist for evaluation and discussion of treatment options.

Subjective tinnitus is tinnitus not associated with any disorder external to the auditory system; it is far more common than objective tinnitus. Although tinnitus is often equated with "ringing in the ears," it may take the form of humming, buzzing, roaring, hissing, clicking, or other sounds. Subjective tinnitus can be associated with nearly any disorder that causes hearing loss, metabolic abnormalities, use of certain drugs (eg, nonsteroidal anti-inflammatory drugs [NSAIDs], salicylates, aminoglycosides, benzodiazepines, anticonvulsants, local anesthetics, alcohol, antidepressants), heavy metals, musculoskeletal disease (temporomandibular joint dysfunction, cervicalgia), neurologic disease (head injury, multiple sclerosis, meningitis), and psychiatric disorders, or it may be idiopathic. Patients with subjective tinnitus should have a thorough history as well as head and neck and otologic examinations, hearing testing, and identification and treatment of underlying medical conditions before tinnitus is classified as idiopathic.

For patients with idiopathic tinnitus or tinnitus that persists after the underlying disorder has been treated, many drugs have been tried,[11] with evidence of effectiveness remaining anecdotal or disappointing. Multiple nonmedical therapies, however, have shown variable levels of effectiveness. These include masking (ear level and environmental), biofeedback, cognitive therapy, and tinnitus retraining therapy. Masking applies white noise at either the ear level (with an instrument similar to a hearing aid) or environmentally (with a sound generator). Tinnitus retraining therapy uses education, counseling, and low-level noise generators to facilitate auditory habituation,[12] with a success rate approaching 80%. For patients with hearing loss sufficient to consider amplification, hearing aids alone may be sufficient to reduce tinnitus to a tolerable level.

Eustachian Tube Dysfunction

The eustachian tube connects the middle ear space to the nasopharynx. It is normally closed, preventing flow of secretions and bacteria into the middle ear, and protecting the ear from fluctuations in nasopharyngeal pressure associated with swallowing, sneezing, coughing, and other respiratory events. The middle ear maintains a slight negative pressure, and the eustachian tube opens with each swallow to equalize pressure. Eustachian tubes can be abnormally patent (patulous), but eustachian tube dysfunction most commonly signifies obstruction or reduced opening function of the tube, leading to increased negative pressure in the middle ear and its complications.

Although more common in children, eustachian tube dysfunction and serous otitis media in adults occurs most commonly associated with nasal obstruction due to upper respiratory tract infection, allergic rhinitis, sinusitis, or adenoiditis. It is also more common in those with cleft palate. Patients with a history of serous otitis media who present with upper respiratory tract infection should be encouraged to use decongestants (unless contraindicated) to prevent recurrent middle ear effusion. Allergy therapy should be optimized, including the use of immunotherapy if necessary, for allergic patients with a history of middle ear disease. Recurrent or persistent (>1 month) middle ear effusion requires direct visualization of the nasopharynx to rule out eustachian tube obstruction due to tumor.[13]

Barotrauma occurs when the eustachian tube cannot compensate for rapid pressure changes, such as those that occur during airplane descent or underwater diving. This common occurrence usually presents with ear fullness, pain, and a popping sensation. Mild cases require no treatment and should resolve in several days. More persistent cases or those associated with middle ear effusion should be treated with oral or topical nasal decongestants. For patients with a history of barotrauma or recurrent serous otitis media, preventive measures can be employed to prevent recurrence with future flights. Oral decongestants, such as pseudoephedrine 60 mg, can be administered before takeoff (repeated 30 to 60 minutes before landing for longer flights), with or without topical decongestant sprays (oxymetazoline or phenylephrine). Patients should be instructed to actively open the jaw (yawning, chewing gum) and autoinflate the ears (holding the nose, closing the glottis and mouth, and "popping" the ears) frequently during descent, and to continue oral decongestant therapy after landing if symptoms persist. Patients with severe symptoms who must fly frequently for business can be helped by placement of ventilating tubes, but this is rarely necessary and requires the patient to keep the ears dry to prevent middle ear infection and drainage.

Motion Sickness

Motion sickness is so well known throughout history that even the word nausea is derived from the Greek word for ship (naus).[14] Motion sickness is generally thought to be caused by a mismatch between visual, vestibular, and proprioceptive stimuli. Hence, symptoms can be produced by situations where there is no actual movement, including flight simulators, video games, and movies. Symptoms most often include epigastric distress, warmth, and increased salivation, followed by delayed gastric emptying, nausea, pallor, sweating, and eventually emesis. A second type of motion sickness is characterized by drowsiness, headache, apathy, depression, and general malaise. Prevalence of motion sickness peaks between the ages of 4 and 10 years, gradually declining thereafter, and is more common in women at all ages. Recent food ingestion, high level of aerobic conditioning, oral contraceptives, menses, pregnancy, and anxiety are all predisposing factors. Prevalence varies depending on conditions but occurs in up to 100% of ship passengers in rough seas, 50% of shuttle astronauts, and 29% of airline pilots.[15]

Patients who have experienced motion sickness in the past should be instructed to eat a light meal at least 3 hours before travel, avoiding dairy products and foods high in calories, sodium, and protein. Focusing on a stable horizon or external object, limiting head movements, lying supine, and staying in a central location (if on a boat or plane) or in the front seat (if in a car) will also help reduce symptoms. Alcohol and tobacco should be avoided.

Medications to prevent and treat motion sickness target the high levels of dopamine in the chemoreceptor trigger zone and acetylcholine in the vomiting center of the medulla oblongata, although the precise action of these drugs remains unclear. Treatments generally fall into antidopaminergic, anticholinergic, and antihistamine classes, sometimes combined with sympathomimetics to counteract drowsiness (Table 60-3). The most popular agent in use is the scopolamine hydrobromide patch (Transderm-Scop), which delivers a continuous dose of scopolamine over 3 days. Scopolamine is a centrally acting antimuscarinic that inhibits vestibular input to the central nervous system and may have a direct effect on the vomiting center. Typical anticholinergic side effects are common, including mucosal dryness, blurred vision, and sedation. Scopolamine is contraindicated in patients at risk for narrow-angle glaucoma and should be used with caution in individuals with impaired renal or hepatic function and in those with gastrointestinal or urinary obstruction. Prolonged use is associated with a withdrawal syndrome characterized by nausea, disequilibrium, and headache.

Alternative therapies have become popular for motion sickness, and a variety of herbal and homeopathic remedies are purported to prevent or relieve motion sickness.[14] Ginger is the most popular, but a controlled trial showed no effect.[16] Acupressure at a point 3 cm proximal to the palmar crease of the head using a wristband is popular but in a study performed no better than placebo.[17]

For patients willing to take medication, one of the antihistamines taken 1 hour before exposure should be sufficient to prevent symptoms for activities of short duration. Meclizine has a longer duration of action and is suitable for longer (transoceanic) flights. For longer exposures, such as cruises, transdermal scopolamine is appropriate. The patch should be applied at least 4 hours before exposure. Patients should be specifically instructed to wash their hands after applying it to avoid ocular symptoms if drug from the patch is transferred directly to the eye. Promethazine or trimethobenzamide can be added for severe nausea. Promethazine or scopolamine can be combined with ephedrine (50 mg) when mental alertness is required.

THE NOSE AND SINUSES

The nose performs 4 important functions: olfaction, filtration, temperature control, and humidity control. The filtration and "climate control" functions of the nose are served primarily by the turbinates, which are covered with

TABLE 60-3

Common Drugs for Motion Sickness*

Drug (Trade Name)	Class	Adult Dosage
Promethazine (Phenergan)	Antidopaminergic	12.5–25 mg q12h (PO, PR, IM, IV)
Metoclopramide (Reglan)	Antidopaminergic	10 mg qid (PO, IM, IV)
Scopolamine (Transderm-Scop)	Anticholinergic	1 patch q72h
Meclizine (Antivert)	Antihistamine	25–50 mg q24h (PO)
Diphenhydramine hydrochloride (Benadryl)	Antihistamine	50–100 mg q4–6h (PO, IM, IV), maximum 400 mg/d
Dimenhydrinate (Dramamine)	Antihistamine	50–100 mg q4–6h (PO, IM, IV), maximum 400 mg/d
Trimethobenzamide (Tigan)	Other	250 mg tid/qid (PO) 200 mg tid/qid (PR, IM)

*PO indicates by mouth; PR, per rectum (suppository); IM, intramuscular; IV, intravenous; q, every; qid, 4 times a day; and tid, 3 times a day.

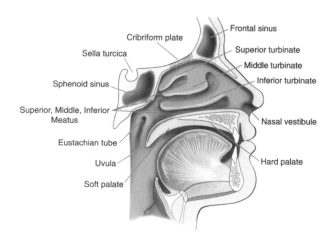

FIGURE 60-5

Anatomy of lateral nasal wall.

ciliated respiratory mucosa rich in submucosal glands and goblet cells. Mucociliary clearance replaces nasal mucus approximately every 20 minutes, moving the mucous blanket and trapped particles into the nasopharynx, where it is swallowed. A normal nose produces up to 1 L of mucus daily. Normal nasal function is required for warm, humidified air that is free of most particulate matter to be delivered to the lungs. The paranasal sinuses supplement these functions but also serve to provide resonance for the voice, lighten the skull, provide a level of protection from facial trauma, and act as a temperature buffer for the brain. Figure 60-5 illustrates nasal and sinus structures.

Epistaxis

Epistaxis is the most common complaint in otolaryngology practice, with estimates of between 10% and 60% of persons having had at least one serious nosebleed.[18] Although most nosebleeds are self-limited, older patients may require hospital admission to control bleeding and prevent complications. Almost all nosebleeds are anterior, with the most common site being the anteroinferior septum (Little's area). This area is easily accessible to environmental irritants (principally dry air) and mechanical trauma (nose picking), and is supplied by both the external and internal carotid systems via the Kiesselbach plexus. Nosebleeds posterior to this area are more difficult to control with pressure and are more likely to require specialty care.

Nosebleeds occur year round but are more common in winter, when the air is dry.[19] Local factors that contribute to the development of epistaxis include trauma, septal deviation or perforation, medical procedures, inflammation (allergy and infection), irritants (chemicals, cocaine, and cigarette smoke), and tumor.[20] Anticoagulants and antiplatelet agents also may contribute to propensity for

nosebleeds. One case-control study, however, found no association between NSAID use and epistaxis.[21] Systemic disorders associated with epistaxis include coagulation disorders, renal disease, heavy alcohol consumption, and hereditary hemorrhagic telangiectasia (Osler-Weber-Rendu disease).[22]

Hypertension is often cited as a cause of epistaxis, but most patients with epistaxis are normotensive. Two studies, however, have shown an increased prevalence of sustained hypertension in patients presenting with active epistaxis and elevated blood pressure in the emergency department.[23,24] It is therefore reasonable to monitor blood pressures in patients with epistaxis that is severe enough to require medical attention, especially if they are hypertensive at presentation. Conversely, however, a history of epistaxis does not correlate with severity of hypertension or other evidence of end-organ damage in known hypertensive patients.[25]

Although initial management of simple anterior epistaxis is fairly straightforward, the general public is largely ignorant of the correct steps to take to stop a nosebleed.[18] Patients should be instructed to keep the head elevated above the heart (leaning forward to minimize drainage of blood into the pharynx is permissible). The patient should apply firm pressure, pinching the nose shut for at least 5 uninterrupted minutes or 10 to 15 if the patient is receiving antiplatelet agents or anticoagulants. If bleeding persists, cotton soaked in oxymetazoline or phenylephrine can be placed in the nostril and pressure applied again. Ice packs over the dorsum of the nose will facilitate vasoconstriction. In general, if bleeding persists beyond 20 minutes, the patient should seek medical attention. Once bleeding stops, patients should be instructed not to blow the nose for at least 48 hours to prevent dislodging the clot.

Most anterior nosebleeds can be prevented with careful attention to keeping the nose moist and avoiding trauma. Nasal saline spray (eg, Ocean, NaSal, or Simply Saline) should be applied several times daily. Nasal emollient gels or ointments can be applied once or twice daily. These should not be applied directly to the septum but rather to the lateral wall of the nasal vestibule and then the nostrils should be rubbed together. Environmental humidification, especially in the bedroom, can be helpful.

Rhinitis, Sinusitis, and Nasal Obstruction

Many otherwise healthy patients have acute, recurrent, or persistent complaints of nasal stuffiness (congestion or obstruction) and/or rhinorrhea. Causes range from trivial, such as the common cold, to life-threatening. Most patients with continuous, fixed nasal congestion suffer from an anatomical obstruction, principally septal deviation and turbinate enlargement. Nasal polyposis and adenoid hypertrophy are also common, with neoplasm, vasculitis, and granulomatous diseases being less common.[26] Patients with fixed obstruction should be referred to an otolaryngologist for evaluation and management.

Many patients with nasal congestion refer to this symptom as sinus, especially if combined with facial discomfort or headache. Most patients with this complaint, however, do not have acute or chronic sinusitis, which is more appropriately termed rhinosinusitis.[27] Acute rhinosinusitis develops when the natural sinus ostia are obstructed by mucosal swelling and/or thick secretions. It can progress to subacute or chronic rhinosinusitis when diseased mucosa with impaired mucociliary clearance fails to clear infected secretions from the sinus cavity. Patients with anatomical obstruction of the sinus ostia or ostiomeatal complex due to polyps or anatomical variations often require surgery for complete resolution. Patients can take the following steps to prevent acute rhinosinusitis triggered by uncomplicated upper respiratory tract infections:

- Moisturization: adequate hydration, humidification, nasal saline spray
- Decongestion: topical (3 days maximum) or oral
- Improved clearance of mucus: mucolytics (guaifenesin, SSKI [potassium iodide]), nasal saline washes

In addition, optimal allergy management can reduce the frequency of infections in those with allergic rhinitis. Patients with recurrent episodes of congestion should be questioned about symptoms suggestive of allergy or infection. Those without allergic triggers or evidence of infection often have vasomotor rhinitis, an imbalance of autonomic innervation to the nose. These patients experience variable nasal congestion and clear rhinorrhea, often in response to minor triggers such as eating (gustatory rhinorrhea), temperature or humidity changes, and even change in body position (nocturnal nasal obstruction). This common condition is often refractory to treatment, requiring lysis of autonomics for relief. Some patients with rhinorrhea will improve with ipratropium bromide nasal spray. Patients with new-onset vasomotor rhinitis should be checked for hypothyroidism, which can cause excess parasympathetic tone.[28] Nasal congestion due to estrogen (oral contraceptives, hormone therapy) or α-blockers can also be confused with vasomotor rhinitis.

Rhinitis medicamentosa is a condition of persistent nasal obstruction characterized by striking mucosal hyperemia and nasal congestion, which responds poorly to topical nasal decongestants. This is caused by continuous use of topical nasal decongestants, such as oxymetazoline or phenylephrine, which are available without prescription, and can begin within a few days of use. To prevent this, patients should be instructed not to use topical decon-

gestants for more than a few days (usually 3) without taking a break. Cessation of decongestant use will resolve the problem over a period of days to weeks depending on length of abuse; this may be made somewhat easier by use of oral decongestants and possibly nasal steroids.

THE THROAT, VOICE, AND SWALLOWING

The oral cavity, oropharynx, and hypopharynx perform the critical functions of maintaining unimpeded air entry into the respiratory tract (cough and gag), facilitating nutrition (swallowing), and communication (speech). The pharynx is responsible for both deglutition and respiration, but these functions, under normal circumstances, occur at different times, avoiding aspiration.

Voice is produced when the vocal processes of the arytenoid cartilages adduct during expiration, causing vibration of the vocal folds. Voice production and quality depend on adequacy of breath support, position and mobility of laryngeal structures, and properties of the laryngeal mucosa itself.

Normal swallowing begins with mastication, followed by propulsion of the bolus of food into the oropharynx by the tongue. The palate elevates, preventing regurgitation of food into the nasopharynx. The superior pharyngeal constrictor muscle then contracts as the larynx elevates and epiglottis retroflexes (diverting the bolus around the larynx and into the esophagus). As the food is propelled farther into the hypopharynx, the cricopharyngeal muscle relaxes, allowing passage of food into the thoracic esophagus, where peristaltic contractions propel it into the stomach.

Voice Disorders

Transient hoarseness is common, and most people have experienced it at one time or another. Hoarseness lasting longer than 2 weeks, while most often due to benign disease, always raises the possibility of neoplasm, even in nonsmokers. As there is no reliable way to distinguish hoarseness due to neoplasm from that due to benign causes based on history or voice quality, these patients require a thorough head and neck examination and direct visualization of the larynx for accurate diagnosis. Patients with frequently recurring episodes of hoarseness also require evaluation by an otolaryngologist, as many causes of recurrent and chronic hoarseness are preventable or at least modifiable.

Chronic laryngitis is common in smokers, producing a polypoid degeneration of laryngeal mucosa called Reinke edema. The voice changes in Reinke edema are impossible to distinguish from those of early laryngeal cancers. As long as the patient continues to smoke or the voice does not improve, periodic visualization of the larynx should be performed to assess for possible precancerous changes. Smoking cessation is critical, along with reduction of other factors contributing to dysphonia such as voice abuse or acid reflux.

Gastroesophageal reflux is a common cause of hoarseness, often referred to as laryngopharyngeal reflux (LPR) when the predominant symptoms are intermittent or continuous hoarseness, cough, throat irritation, frequent throat clearing, and globus sensation. Acid clearance and mucosal resistance protect the esophagus from acid exposure, so many patients with severe LPR do not have prominent esophageal symptoms.[29] Prevention and initial treatment of LPR begin with lifestyle changes, including weight loss; avoiding late-night meals (last full meal at least 2 to 3 hours before bed and no food at least 1 hour before bed); avoidance of caffeine, alcohol, tobacco, and peppermint; and elevation of the head of the bed. These measures are appropriate for those with classic symptoms and are sufficient for approximately 50% of patients.[29] Those who do not respond or who present with severe symptoms should be offered acid suppressive therapy with H2 blockers or proton pump inhibitors. Failure to respond to drug therapy in 2 months should prompt additional evaluation.

Given the number of hours daily that we use our voices, it is no surprise that voice abuse and vocal hyperfunction are also common causes of hoarseness. Voice abuse consists of vocal behaviors, such as screaming, hard glottal attacks, or singing, in the face of existing laryngeal injury or inflammation. Nonspeech behaviors such as chronic cough, throat clearing, grunting, or even laughing[30] also contribute to voice abuse. These behaviors can lead to vocal fold edema, nodule, polyps, or ulcers. Vocal hyperfunction occurs when supraglottic structures contract inappropriately during speech, making the voice sound strained and effortful. This is often referred to as muscle tension dysphonia, and may occur in the absence of an organic process or begin with another source of laryngeal irritation but persist after the original problem resolves. Vocal hyperfunction and voice abuse generally respond to speech therapy, although surgery may be required if polyps or ulcers are present.

Many occupations are associated with vocal disorders, among them teachers, politicians, ministers, translators, telephone operators, salespersons, tour guides, and others.[31] Most occupational voice disorders are related to vocal hyperfunction, voice abuse, or an underlying medical disorder. However, several workplace inhalants have been reported to cause dysphonia,[32] including Freon gas, formaldehyde, organic mercury, diquat, sulfuric acid, and solvents, and exposure should be minimized.

A variety of medications can cause or contribute to voice disorders, primarily by drying the upper airway mucosa.[33] These are outlined in Table 60-4. Of note, although dysphonia in asthmatic patients is frequently attributed to use of inhaled corticosteroids, the mechanism remains unknown, and use of spacer devices with metered-dose inhalers is not protective.[34]

For patients who use their voices professionally or who have experienced hoarseness in the past, vocal hygiene is critical to preventing voice problems.[35] Good vocal hygiene includes general measures such as avoidance of tobacco and other inhaled irritants, adequate hydration, humidification, avoidance or reduction of alcohol intake, avoidance of offending drugs, antireflux measures, stress reduction, adequate sleep, aerobic exercise, and avoidance of speaking in noisy environments. Singers and other professional voice users can benefit from vocal exercises focusing on breath support, pitch flexibility, and resonance. Singing while sick should be avoided, as already irritated vocal folds are more prone to hemorrhage and the development of polyps or cysts.

Choking

Although choking and aspiration are more often concerns in pediatric, elderly, and neurologically impaired populations, everyone is at risk for acute airway obstruction, primarily during meals. This "café coronary" is an uncommon but clearly preventable cause of sudden death. The Heimlich maneuver, introduced in 1974, is an effective, easy-to-learn technique to dislodge foreign material from the upper airway,[36] which is now taught in American Heart Association Heartsaver and American Red Cross first aid and cardiopulmonary resuscitation (CPR) courses. It has been successfully administered by untrained persons with coaching over the telephone by emergency personnel[37] and can be self-administered if necessary. The Heimlich maneuver is credited with saving thousands of lives but may have adverse effects due to the chest trauma.

Salivary Gland Disorders

There are 3 pairs of major salivary glands, the parotid, submaxillary (also called submandibular), and sublingual glands. The parotid gland produces primarily serous secretions, which drain into the mouth via the Stensen's duct. The sublingual gland produces primarily mucous secretions, which drain via several small ducts into the floor of the mouth. The submaxillary gland produces a mixture of serous and mucous secretions, and it drains via the Wharton duct on either side of the lingual frenulum. The oral cavity, pharynx, and larynx are also lined with hundreds of minor salivary glands. Saliva provides lubrication to facilitate speech and swallowing, prevents tooth decay and oral soft-tissue infection, and begins the process of digestion.

TABLE 60-4

Selected Medications Causing Iatrogenic Dysphonia

Medication	Effect
Anticholinergics (antihistamines, scopolamine, Parkinson's agents	Drying
Antidepressants (tricyclics, SSRIs, others)	Drying
Lithium	Hypothyroidism, tremor
Diuretics	Drying
Antihypertensives	
ACE inhibitors	Chronic cough
Most others	Drying
Antacids	Drying
H2 blockers	Drying
High-dose vitamin C	Drying
Antiplatelet agents	Vocal fold hemorrhage
Analgesics	Increased vocal fold damage (voice abusers)
Androgens	Coarsening of voice, lowered frequencies
Inhaled corticosteroids	Candidiasis, vocal fold bowing

Xerostomia, or dry mouth, is a common symptom due to a wide variety of primary and secondary causes. Causes of secondary xerostomia include head and neck irradiation, dehydration, depression, medications (more than 400 have been identified,[38] mostly with anticholinergic properties), and central nervous system disorders. A variety of systemic disorders can cause swelling and inflammation of the salivary glands, which is generally painless, symmetrical, and often associated with dry mouth. These include diabetes mellitus, gout, alcoholism, sarcoidosis, and malnutrition. Benign lymphoepithelial sialadenopathies produce unilateral or bilateral salivary gland enlargement with lymphocytic infiltration of the gland. The most well known, Sjögren's syndrome, causes xerostomia and keratoconjunctivitis sicca, and is the second most common autoimmune disorder.[39] Management of patients with xerostomia should include good oral hygiene, treatment of the underlying cause, and use of a saliva substitute. The use of fluoride is particularly important because of the propensity for progressive dental caries in patients with xerostomia.

Head and Neck Cancer Screening and Prevention

Head and neck cancers (HNC) are about one fourth as common as the common cancers for which regular screening is generally advised and provided. Although important advances have been made in recent years in the treatment of carcinomas of the upper aerodigestive tract, the 5-year survival rate remains disappointing at 53%.[40]

Sixty percent of tumors are diagnosed at stages III and IV, with a 30% 5-year survival, compared with more than 90% for stages I and II cancers. Early detection therefore appears to be a key to improved survival and reduced morbidity. Unfortunately, symptoms are a poor indicator in early cancers,[41] with the exception of hoarseness in the case of glottic cancers. Ninety percent of HNC occur in locations accessible to examination by a primary care physician or dentist. Universal screening with physical examination, however, is of low yield. High-risk populations may be identified by the following factors:

- Age greater than 40 years
- Substance abuse: tobacco (including smokeless), alcohol, betel nut chewing
- Environmental exposures: wood and metal dusts, asbestos, radon, arsenic, herbicides
- Infections: human papillomavirus, human immunodeficiency virus (HIV), tuberculosis, syphilis
- Poor oral hygiene or poorly fitting dental prostheses
- Previous radiation therapy
- Organ transplantation
- Family history of lung cancer or HNC
- Prior HNC

Even in high-risk groups, however, screening has had limited impact. Compliance with screening programs has been poor in these groups.

One promising screening technology under investigation is polymerase chain reaction (PCR) to identify abnormal DNA sequences associated with HNC, such as p53 tumor suppressor gene mutations. If genes that mutate early in the progression to cancer can be identified, screening for these mutations might identify high-risk patients for further evaluation. Currently, the sensitivity and specificity of PCR screening make this too cost ineffective for routine use.

SUMMARY

Until reliable, cost-effective screening methods are available, clinicians must remain vigilant, especially in high-risk patients, for abnormalities that may indicate an early cancer: hoarseness, neck pain, otalgia, oral ulcers, and persistent white or red lesions (leukoplakia, erythroplakia). Attention to risk factor reduction (particularly tobacco and alcohol use) is particularly key to reducing the incidence of these devastating cancers.

REFERENCES

1. Shulman JB, Lambert PR, Goodhill V. Acoustic trauma and noise-induced hearing loss. In: Canalis RF, Lambert PR, eds. *The Ear: Comprehensive Otology.* Philadelphia, Pa: Lippincott, Williams & Wilkins; 2000:773–783.

2. Nondahl DM, Cruickshanks KJ, Wiley TL, Tweed TS, Klein R, Klein BE. Accuracy of self-reported hearing loss. *Audiology.* 1998;37:295–301.

3. Gates GA, Rees TS. Hear ye? Hear ye! Successful auditory aging. *West J Med.* 1997;167:247–252.

4. Hearing conservation. Occupational Safety and Health Administration, US Department of Labor [Web site]; 1995. Available at: www.osha.gov/Publications/osha3074.html. Accessed January 18, 2003.

5. Weinstein BE. Age-related hearing loss: how to screen for it, and when to intervene. *Geriatrics.* 1994;49:40–47.

6. Klein AJ, Weber PC. Hearing aids. *Med Clin North Am.* 1999;83:139–151.

7. Singer AJ, Sauris E, Viccellio AW. Ceruminolytic effects of docusate sodium: a randomized, controlled trial. *Ann Emerg Med.* 2000;36:228–232.

8. Grossan M. Safe, effective techniques for cerumen removal. *Geriatrics.* 2000;55:80, 83–86.

9. Seely DR, Quigley SM, Langman AW. Ear candles—efficacy and safety. *Laryngoscope.* 1996;106:1226–1229.

10. Fortune DS, Haynes DS, Hall JW. Tinnitus: current evaluation and management. *Med Clin North Am.* 1999;83:153–162.

11. Seidman MD, Jacobson GP. Update on tinnitus. *Otolaryngol Clin North Am.* 1996;29:455–465.

12. Jastreboff PJ, Gray WC, Gold SL. Neurophysiological approach to tinnitus patients. *Am J Otol.* 1996;17:236–240.

13. Sperling NM, Kumra V, Madell JR. Hearing loss and its rehabilitation. In: Lucente FE, Har-El G, eds. *Essentials of Otolaryngology.* Philadelphia, Pa: Lippincott, Williams & Wilkins; 1999:63–76.

14. Gahlinger PM. Motion sickness: how to help your patients avoid travel travail. *Postgrad Med.* 1999;106:177–184.

15. James M, Green R. Airline pilot incapacitation survey. *Aviat Space Environ Med.* 1991;62:1068–1072.

16. Stewart JJ, Wood MJ, Wood CD, Mims ME. Effects of ginger on motion sickness susceptibility and gastric function. *Pharmacology.* 1991;42:111–120.

17. Bruce DG, Golding JF, Hockenhull N, Pethybridge RJ. Acupressure and motion sickness. *Aviat Space Environ Med.* 1990;61:361–365.

18. Strachan D, England J. First-aid treatment of epistaxis—confirmation of widespread ignorance. *Postgrad Med J.* 1998;74:113–114.

19. Manfredini R, Gallerani M, Portaluppi F. Seasonal variation in the occurrence of epistaxis. *Am J Med.* 2000;108:759–760.

20. Tan LK, Calhoun KH. Epistaxis. *Med Clin North Am.* 1999;83:43–56.

21. Tay HL, Evans JM, McMahon AD, MacDonald TM. Aspirin, nonsteroidal anti-inflammatory drugs, and epistaxis: a regional record linkage case control study. *Ann Otol Rhinol Laryngol.* 1998;107:671–674.

22. Shah RK, Dhingra JK, Shapshay SM. Hereditary hemorrhagic telangiectasia: a review of 76 cases. *Laryngoscope.* 2002;112:767–773.

23. Herkner H, Havel C, Mullner M, et al. Active epistaxis at ED presentation is associated with arterial hypertension. *Am J Emerg Med.* 2002;20:92–95.

24. Herkner H, Laggner AN, Mullner M, et al. Hypertension in patients presenting with epistaxis. *Ann Emerg Med.* 2000;35:126–130.

25. Lubianca Neto JF, Fuchs FD, Facco SR, et al. Is epistaxis evidence of end-organ damage in patients with hypertension? *Laryngoscope.* 1999;109:1111–1115.

26. Fornadley JA. The stuffy nose and rhinitis. *Med Clin North Am.* 1999;83:1–12.

27. Lanza DC, Kennedy DW. Adult rhinosinusitis defined. *Otolaryngol Head Neck Surg.* 1997;117:S1–S7.

28. Pinczower EF. Nasal obstruction. In: Calhoun KH, Eibling DE, Wax MK, eds. *Expert Guide to Otolaryngology.* Philadelphia, Pa: American College of Physicians; 2001:145–160.

29. Ulualp SO, Toohill RJ. Laryngopharyngeal reflux: state of the art diagnosis and treatment. *Otolaryngol Clin North Am.* 2000;33:785–801.

30. Garrett CG, Ossoff RH. Hoarseness. *Med Clin North Am.* 1999;83:115–123.

31. Mattiske JA, Oates JM, Greenwood KM. Vocal problems among teachers: a review of prevalence, causes, prevention, and treatment. *J Voice.* 1998;12:489–499.

32. Williams NR. Occupational voice disorders due to workplace exposure to irritants—a review of the literature. *Occup Med.* 2002;52:99–101.

33. Spiegel JR, Hawkshaw M, Sataloff RT. Dysphonia related to medical therapy. *Otolaryngol Clin North Am.* 2000;33:771–784.

34. Williamson IJ, Matusiewicz SP, Brown PH, Greening AP, Crompton GK. Frequency of voice problems and cough in patients using pressurized aerosol inhaled steroid preparations. *Eur Respir J.* 1995;8:590–592.

35. Murry T, Rosen CA. Vocal education for the professional voice user and singer. *Otolaryngol Clin North Am.* 2000;33:967–982.

36. Heimlich HJ, Patrick EA. The Heimlich maneuver: best technique for saving any choking victim's life. *Postgrad Med.* 1990;87:38–48, 53.

37. Lapostolle F, Desmaizieres M, Adnet F, Minadeo J. Telephone-assisted Heimlich maneuver. *Ann Emerg Med.* 2000;36:171.

38. Ettinger RL. Review: xerostomia: a symptom which acts like a disease [comment]. *Age Ageing.* 1996;25:409–412.

39. Eibling DE. Salivary gland disorders. In: Calhoun KH, Eibling DE, Wax MK, eds. *Expert Guide to Otolaryngology*. Philadelphia, Pa: American College of Physicians; 2001:429–449.

40. Ellison MD, Campbell BH. Screening for cancers of the head and neck: addressing the problem. *Surg Oncol Clin North Am.* 1999;8:725–734.

41. Dolan RW, Vaughan CW, Fuleihan N. Symptoms in early head and neck cancer: an inadequate indicator. *Otolaryngol Head Neck Surg.* 1998;119:463–467.

RESOURCES

American Academy of Otolaryngology–Head & Neck Surgery, 1 Prince St, Alexandria, VA 22314.
Web site: www.entnet.org. (Information for patients and professionals on a variety of ear, nose, and throat disorders, including online educational programs and multiple links to other sites.)

American Rhinologic Society.
Web site: www.american-rhinologic.org. (Information for patients and professionals on nasal and sinus disease.)

American Speech-Language-Hearing Association, 10801 Rockville Pike, Rockville, MD 20852; 800 498-2071 (professionals); 800 638-8255 (public).
Web site: www.asha.org. (Patient information about hearing loss and voice disorders.)

American Tinnitus Association, PO Box 5, Portland, OR 97207; 800 634-8978.
Web site: www.ata.org. (Self-help, support, and advocacy for those with tinnitus.)

Hearing Education and Awareness for Rockers.
Web site: www.hearnet.com. (Interactive site oriented toward rock musicians, providing information and resources on tinnitus, hearing loss, hearing evaluation referrals, and hearing aids and assistive listening devices, as well as a referral service of audiology affiliates, physicians, and entertainment links.)

Heimlich HJ. How to do the Heimlich maneuver [The Heimlich Institute Web site].
Available at: www.heimlichinstitute.org/howtodo.html.

chapter 61

Ophthalmologic Disorders

Leonid E. Lerner, MD, PhD, and Hilel Lewis, MD

INTRODUCTION

Physiologic visual acuity is remarkably consistent among healthy humans and is limited by retinal anatomy. Normal acuity reflects accurate resolution of an object that subtends an angle of 1 degree on the human retina. The 20/20 line on the Snellen visual acuity chart comprises letters that subtend an angle of 5 degrees when held 20 ft from the subject. However, individual segments of each letters subtend an angle of 1 degree and must be resolved to identify the letter. When patients are unable to resolve letters that subtend 1 degree of arc, their vision is considered impaired. For example, when a patient views the Snellen chart from the standard test distance of 20 ft and is able to distinguish the line of letters that is supposed to be seen from 40 ft, he or she is noted to have 20/40 vision.

Visual impairment describes useful residual vision that is less than 20/20 (Table 61-1). An impairment may result from a number of ophthalmologic or neurologic disorders and may include a variety of different disorders of the visual function. The cause may lie anywhere along the visual pathway from the tear film to the visual cortex

TABLE 61-1

Visual Acuity Required for Common Daily Activities

Activity or Status	Visual Acuity
Physiologic vision	20/20
Obtain driver's license (varies by state)	20/30–20/100
Read newspaper print	20/50
Read large print (eg, *Reader's Digest*)	20/70
Write a check	20/100
Legal blindness	20/200
Distinguish denomination of paper currency	20/400

of the occipital lobe (Fig 61-1). Most commonly, visual impairment is described in terms of remaining visual acuity or visual field. Other aspects of impaired visual function may be equally important in activities of daily living such as reading, ambulation, and driving. A central scotoma or diplopia (double vision) also would profoundly affect vision. Glare and reduced contrast sensitivity are recognized as important factors that influence

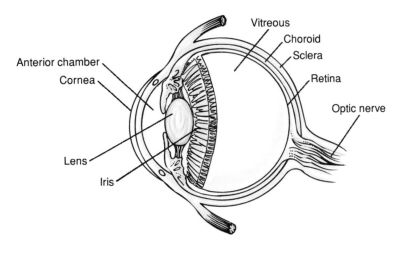

FIGURE 61-1

Anatomy of the human eye.

performance and should be considered in the evaluation of ophthalmic diseases and treatments.

EPIDEMIOLOGY OF VISUAL IMPAIRMENT

Although visual impairment may occur at any age, its incidence and prevalence generally increases with age. In general, eye disorders are very common among the adult population. Eighty million Americans, or approximately one third of the US population, have some ocular abnormality that affects visual function.[1] In addition, at least one fourth of all Americans have refractive errors that require correction to achieve best vision. In the Baltimore Eye Survey, an urban community study, half of adults 40 years of age and older reported improved vision with new prescription glasses, with 7.5% improving 3 or more lines.[2]

Impaired visual function is most prevalent among the elderly. It is estimated that 13.5 million Americans over the age of 45 years have visual impairments, and more than two thirds of them are more than 65 years old.[3] The highest prevalence of visual impairment is found in individuals 85 years and older; about 13% of them are reported to be legally blind (defined in the United States as best corrected visual acuity of 20/200 or worse in the better eye, or a visual field equal to or less than 20 degrees). As the proportion of elderly in the population rises, the number of individuals with low vision is likely to increase as well.

Race plays a role as well. Visual impairment and legal blindness are twice as common among African Americans compared with white Americans.[2]

The impact of eye disease on public health is great because vision affects daily functioning. Preserving eyesight through effective eye care and treatment of ocular disease enhances quality of life and improves physical function. Several studies have shown that improvement in visual function that results from treatment of ocular disorders is accompanied by improvement in life satisfaction, mental health, home activities, and community activities.[4,5] After arthritis and heart disease, vision loss has been ranked the third most common chronic condition requiring assistance in activities of daily living among individuals over age 70 years.[6] In addition, acquired brain injury, including trauma, stroke, and tumors, may be associated with major functional limitations resulting from visual impairment.

DIAGNOSIS OF OCULAR DISEASES AND PREVENTION OF VISUAL LOSS

Routine Ocular Evaluation

A comprehensive ocular examination by an ophthalmologist is recommended for asymptomatic adult patients who have never been examined. Based on the results of the evaluation, patients could be placed into 1 of 3 categories:

TABLE 61-2

Comprehensive Ocular Evaluation for Patients Without Ocular Risk Factors[*]

Age, y	Frequency of Evaluation
20–29	At least once during this period
30–39	At least twice during this period
40–64	Every 1 to 2 y
≥65	Every 1 to 2 y

[*]From American Academy of Ophthalmology.[94]

patients with no risk factors for eye disease, patients with risk factors for eye disease, and patients with established conditions requiring therapeutic intervention.

Even in the absence of ocular risk factors, patients should be reexamined periodically (Table 61-2) to prevent visual loss by detecting and treating disease in its early stages before symptoms develop. A thorough eye evaluation may uncover important abnormalities of the visual system or detect evidence of certain systemic diseases with ophthalmic manifestations. With early diagnosis and appropriate intervention, potentially blinding illnesses such as glaucoma, cataract, and diabetic retinopathy, all of which increase in prevalence with age, may have a much more favorable outcome. Studies have indicated that up to 40% of legal blindness found among nursing home residents[7] in both urban[8] and rural[9] communities could have been prevented or ameliorated by appropriate ophthalmologic care.

A number of common ocular diseases may develop without the patient being aware of any problem. These include the most common causes of low vision in the United States: primary open-angle glaucoma, diabetic retinopathy, age-related macular degeneration (AMD), and peripheral retinal breaks and degenerations.[2] In addition, a thorough ophthalmic evaluation may aid the ophthalmologist in making the initial diagnosis of a number of systemic diseases.

A patient is considered to be at risk when the evaluation reveals signs that suggest a potentially abnormal condition or when risk factors for ocular disease are identified, but no intervention is yet required. In these situations, patients require close follow-up to monitor their ocular health and to detect early signs of disease. In general, appropriate follow-up intervals should be determined for each patient based on clinical signs, risk factors, incidence of disease, and potential rate of disease progression. Some common conditions and risk factors are summarized in Table 61-3 with the recommended follow-up schedules.

Refractive Errors

Ametropia, or refractive error, occurs when parallel rays of light entering the nonaccommodating eye fail to focus

TABLE 61-3

Comprehensive Ocular Evaluation for Patients With Ocular Risk Factors[*]

Condition/ Risk Factor	Frequency of Evaluation[†]
Diabetes without retinopathy	
Onset after age 30 y[‡]	Once a year
Onset before age 30 y[‡]	5 y after onset and yearly thereafter
Pregnancy	Before conception or early in first trimester and every 3 mo thereafter
Risk factors for glaucoma[§]	
Age 20–29 y	Every 3–5 y
Age 30–64 y	Every 2–4 y
Age ≥65 y	Every 1–2 y

[*]From American Academy of Ophthalmology.[94]

[†]Abnormal findings may dictate more frequent follow-up examinations.

[‡]As indicated in Wisconsin Epidemiologic Study of Diabetic Retinopathy, these are operational definitions of type 1 and 2 diabetes based on age (age <30 years at diagnosis indicates type 1; age ≥30 years, type 2) and not pathogenetic classification.

[§]Examples include African descent and family history of glaucoma. See text for full list of glaucoma risk factors.

on the retina. High refractive errors are defined as myopia (nearsightedness) of 6 diopters or greater, hyperopia (farsightedness) of 4 diopters or greater, and astigmatism of 3 diopters or greater. Presbyopia is characterized as insufficient accommodation for near vision in a patient whose distance refractive error is zero or fully corrected. It develops as part of the normal ocular aging process usually beginning at about age 40 years. Although not truly a refractive error, its correction is similar to the correction of refractive errors.

Almost three fourths of adults over age 42 years have a refractive error.[10] More than 100 million Americans would benefit from correction of refractive errors. Associations of both hereditary and environmental factors have been reported in studies of patients with refractive errors. Asians seem to have higher rates of myopia in general and high, degenerative myopia in particular than do whites or African Americans.[11] The prevalence of myopia in African Americans is 25% less than in whites.[12] However, genetics alone cannot account for the prevalence patterns and phenotypic variations of refractive errors. Several environmental factors have been implicated in the development or progression of myopia, including the amount of near work and[13,14] visual deprivation[15] as well as socioeconomic factors such as a higher educational level and greater household income.[10,12,16] However, despite a number of associations reported in

epidemiologic studies, the underlying etiology and pathogenic mechanisms of myopia are still unclear.

Individuals with severe refractive errors are more likely to experience pathologic ocular changes over time. Patients with high myopia have an increased incidence of retinal thinning, peripheral retinal degeneration, retinal detachment, and early cataract.[17] Hyperopic patients have an increased incidence of angle-closure glaucoma.[18]

Although treatments that claim to prevent progression of refractive errors, particularly myopia, have been reported, none have been conclusively proved. Optical correction has been evaluated in a prospective randomized clinical trial, but no benefit was demonstrated.[19] Atropine has been proposed to inhibit accommodation and thus theoretically prevent axial elongation of the eye, and it may also inhibit certain growth factors that act to elongate the eye independent of accommodation.[20] Although atropine has been used in trials in the United States and Canada and appeared to provide some benefit,[21,22] no definitive conclusion could be drawn about its efficacy due to the methodological difficulties such as poor patient compliance, lack of appropriate controls, and unclear techniques of analysis. Visual training by convergence exercises and near-far focusing exercises[23] has never been tested in a scientifically acceptable study and, therefore, cannot be recommended. At present, no scientifically valid studies are available regarding the effects of nutrition or nutritional supplements on progression of myopia. Nutrition modification to influence myopia is not recommended.

Amblyopia

Amblyopia is defined as reduced visual acuity due to abnormal central visual processing. It represents a functional disorder of visual development that is caused by an optical, physical, or ocular alignment defect that occurs during early childhood. The visual pathways continue to develop from birth to approximately age 9 years, at which time the plasticity of the visual pathways ceases. The most rapid progression occurs in infancy.

Amblyopia is a common public health problem. Although the prevalence of amblyopia depends on the population studied and the definition used, the incidence in the US population is generally estimated at 2%. Approximately 50% of cases of unilateral amblyopia are associated with strabismus, and there is a significant but somewhat smaller association of amblyopia with anisometropia (cortical suppression of vision due to a marked difference in refractive error of the 2 eyes).[24] Early diagnosis and treatment of amblyopia minimizes loss of vision. Unfortunately, infants and preverbal children are at greatest risk of amblyopia, but they are unable to complain of unilateral poor vision and are often difficult to examine. Because treatment is more effective at younger ages, early screening is recommended for all children beginning in the newborn period and continuing through the early school-age years.

Cataract

A cataract is a degradation of the optical quality of the crystalline lens through the loss of clarity or change in color. Cataract is the leading cause of blindness worldwide.[25,26] The Salisbury Eye Evaluation Study found that, after refractive error, cataract was the leading cause of visual impairment in both whites and African Americans.[26] In a study of nursing home residents in the Baltimore area, cataract was found to be the leading cause of blindness, contributing to blindness in 30% of eyes.[7]

There are several different types of age-related cataract: nuclear, cortical, posterior subcapsular (PSC), and combination. Each type has its own anatomical location within the crystalline lens, pathology, and risk factors for development. Nuclear cataract represents a central opacification of the lens and tends to progress slowly. In general, it affects distance vision more than near vision. In advanced cases, the lens becomes brown and opaque. Cortical cataracts are caused by opacification of the lens cortex and can be central or peripheral. Patients often complain of glare. A mature cortical cataract appears white and opaque. Posterior subcapsular cataracts are found more often in young patients, and the near vision tends to be more affected than distance vision. Of the 3 cataract types, PSC cataract is associated with the greatest visual impairment and the highest rate of cataract surgery.[27] Age-related cataract is a multifactorial disease, and the cataract development has been linked to many potential risk factors.[28] However, most studies on age-related cataracts are observational, which means that they can suggest an association but cannot prove a causative effect.

For all cataract types, lower education status and higher alcohol use appear to be associated with higher rates of cataract. There are several risk factors for both PSC and cortical cataracts, including a history of diabetes[29] and the use of systemic or inhaled corticosteroids.[30,31] Patients receiving long-term corticosteroid therapy and those with diabetes should be informed about the risks of cataract formation.

Patients who are exposed to high levels of solar radiation are 2.5 times more likely to later have cortical cataracts, 4 times more likely to get mixed cataracts, and almost 3 times more likely to need cataract surgery.[32] To reduce the cumulative lifetime exposure to ultraviolet radiation, patients should be advised to wear sunglasses and hats when outside during daylight. For nuclear cataracts, smoking appears to be a significant risk factor that can be reversed with smoking cessation.[33,34] Other factors that increase the risk of lens opacification include blunt trauma to the eye, exposure to ionizing radiation, chemical or electrical injuries to the ocular surface,

and conditions such as chronic uveitis and prior intraocular surgery, particularly vitrectomy or glaucoma filtration procedures.

High doses of vitamin and mineral supplementation did not slow the development or progression of cataract in the prospective, randomized, placebo-controlled Age-Related Eye Disease Study (AREDS).[35] Therefore, the use of vitamin or nutritional supplementation to delay the onset or progression of cataracts cannot be recommended at this time due to the lack of supporting evidence.[36]

Glaucoma

Primary open-angle glaucoma and glaucoma suspect

Glaucoma is a disease in which elevated intraocular pressure damages the optic nerve. Glaucoma is a major health problem worldwide; in the United States, glaucoma is the second most common cause of legal blindness overall and the leading cause of legal blindness among African Americans.[8] The Baltimore Eye Survey showed that approximately 2.5 million Americans have primary open-angle glaucoma, and about half of them are unaware that they have the disease.[37,38] More than 1 in 10 African Americans and 1 in 50 white Americans who are 80 years of age or older has glaucoma.[38]

Primary open-angle glaucoma, the most common form of glaucoma, is a multifactorial optic neuropathy in which there is a characteristic acquired primary loss of retinal ganglion cells and atrophy of the optic nerve. It is a chronic, generally bilateral, but often asymmetrical disease. Primary open-angle glaucoma is characterized by progressive optic nerve damage as evident on funduscopic examination and/or by the presence of a typical visual field abnormality, an adult onset, open and normal-appearing anterior chamber angle, and the absence of other known explanations for progressive optic nerve changes. While most patients with glaucoma have elevated intraocular pressure, approximately 15% to 40% of patients will have characteristic glaucomatous damage with intraocular pressure below 21 mm Hg.[39] These patients are commonly referred to as having normal-tension or low-tension glaucoma. Strong risk factors for the development of primary open-angle glaucoma are:

1. Elevated intraocular pressure.[40,41]
2. Advancing age.[37,42,43]
3. African descent.[37]
4. Family history of glaucoma.[44-46]

The following conditions have been implicated as possible risk factors for the development of glaucoma, although their respective associations with the disease have not been consistently demonstrated:[42,46-51]

1. Diabetes mellitus.
2. Systemic hypertension.
3. Cardiovascular disease.
4. Myopia.
5. Migraine headache and peripheral vasospasm.

Neither intraocular pressure measurement nor any other single test is an effective method for primary screening of the general population for glaucoma. Therefore, screening generally involves evaluating a patient's race, age, family history, and general health status. In addition, an ophthalmologist should perform an eye examination that includes evaluation of the optic nerve and visual field testing.

Screening may be more efficient and cost-effective when targeted toward specific groups that have a high risk of the disease. In defining such groups for screening, race and age have been found to be particularly important factors.[8,38-40,43,49,52] The frequency of age- and race-specific screening examinations recommended by the American Academy of Ophthalmology is listed in Table 61-4. Early detection of glaucoma is important because progressive visual loss may be prevented or retarded by therapy aimed at lowering the intraocular pressure from the level associated with optic nerve damage; this level should be determined for each patient.[47,53,54] The less optic nerve damage that is present at the time of diagnosis, the better the chances are for long-term preservation of visual function.

Primary angle-closure glaucoma

Primary angle-closure glaucoma (PACG) results from pupillary block, whereby complete iris-lens apposition occurs, which impedes the flow of aqueous humor from the posterior chamber to the anterior chamber and the outflow pathway. The accumulation of the aqueous humor in the posterior chamber causes a forward bowing of the peripheral iris so that the iris occludes the anterior chamber angle and the filtering portion of the trabecular meshwork, leading to elevation of intraocular pressure.

TABLE 61-4

Recommended Frequency of Age- and Race-specific Glaucoma Screening Examinations[*]

Age, y	Asymptomatic African Americans	Asymptomatic Other Patients
20–29	Every 3–5 y	At least once
30–39	Every 2–4 y	At least twice
40–64	Every 2–4 y	Every 2–4 y
≥65	Every 1–2 y	Every 1–2 y

[*]From American Academy of Ophthalmology.[39]

Primary angle-closure glaucoma generally is a bilateral condition, although patients often present with the condition in only one eye.

There are large variations in the prevalence of PACG among racial and ethnic groups. The highest prevalence has been reported in Alaskan Inuits (2.65% of people aged 40 years and older)[55] and the lowest rates have been found in whites (0.17% in England among patients aged 40 years and older).[56] It is estimated that PACG accounts for approximately 10% of glaucoma cases in the United States.[39] However, PACG may account for the majority of glaucoma in some Asian populations.[57] Presenting symptoms may vary from pressure-induced corneal edema (experienced as blurred vision and occasionally as multicolored halos around lights), conjunctival vascular congestion, pain, and nausea and vomiting in cases of acute angle closure, to the absence of symptoms in cases of chronic angle-closure glaucoma. In the latter form of PACG, the slow progressive closure of the angle may gradually elevate intraocular pressure and lead to glaucomatous optic nerve damage.

The following have been implicated as risk factors for the development of PACG:

1. Hyperopia.[58,59]
2. Family history of PACG.[60,61]
3. Advancing age.[62,63]
4. Female sex.[64,65]
5. Eskimo or Far Eastern Asian extraction.[57,63]

Patients who present with PACG are at high risk of visual loss if they do not receive treatment by a trained ophthalmologist. Approximately half of untreated fellow eyes develop angle closure within 5 years.[66,67] During the natural history of this disease, painful bilateral blindness will develop in untreated patients.

Diabetic Retinopathy

Diabetic retinopathy is a disorder of the retinal vasculature due to the damage from diabetes mellitus. The risk of diabetic retinopathy increases with the duration of diabetes. Most patients who have had diabetes for 20 or more years will have some degree of retinopathy. During its early stages, diabetic retinopathy manifests as retinal microaneurysms and intraretinal hemorrhages. Vascular changes may progress to increasing numbers of hemorrhages, the focal areas of axoplasmic stasis in the nerve fiber layer described clinically as cotton-wool spots, and intraretinal microvascular abnormalities. Pathologic vasopermeability of the retinal vessels results in focal areas of retinal edema (thickening), which when present in the center of the macula, results in significant visual impairment. Increasing retinal capillary nonperfusion leads to progressive retinal ischemia, which results in pathologic proliferation of new blood vessels. Visual loss in diabetic retinopathy results primarily from the following:

1. Macular edema.
2. Macular ischemia due to capillary nonperfusion.
3. Vitreous hemorrhage.
4. Traction retinal detachment.

Diabetic retinopathy is broadly categorized as nonproliferative or proliferative. The severity of non-proliferative retinopathy is largely determined by the extent of intraretinal hemorrhages, microaneurysms and microvascular abnormalities and by the presence of venous beading. Proliferative diabetic retinopathy is characterized by the onset of retinal neovascularization induced by the retinal ischemia. Proliferative diabetic retinopathy is further divided into low-risk and high-risk based on the extent and location of neovascularization as well as the presence of vitreous hemorrhage.[68] This division is important in predicting severe visual loss and providing the appropriate guidelines and timing for pho-tocoagulation treatment of diabetic retinopathy by an ophthalmologist.[69,70]

The most important modifiable risk factor for the development and progression of diabetic retinopathy is the degree of hyperglycemia. Strong evidence for this association has been provided by epidemiologic studies as well as by clinical trials that have evaluated the long-term effects on diabetic retinopathy of intensive treatment of diabetes.[71-73] Thus, it is important to educate and re-emphasize to patients the value of safely maintaining normal or near-normal levels of blood glucose. Although both severity of hyperglycemia and duration of diabetes are major risk factors for development of retinopathy, the duration of diabetes becomes a less important predic-tive factor than the level of hyperglycemia for the progression of diabetic retinopathy once the diagnosis has been made.[73]

Current treatment approaches for diabetic retinopathy may be 90% effective in preventing severe vision loss.[74] Therefore, it is important that patients with diabetes be referred for ophthalmic care according to the guidelines of the American Diabetes Association and the American Academy of Ophthalmology.[75] Both physicians and patients need to be educated about indications for referral. A comprehensive eye examination by an ophthalmologist who is experienced in managing diabetic retinopathy is the standard of care.

Age-related Macular Degeneration

Age-related macular degeneration is the leading cause of irreversible severe visual loss in whites 50 years of age or older in the United States and in most of the developed world. Both the incidence and progression of AMD increase significantly with age. Approximately 10% of people who are 65 to 74 years have manifestations of AMD compared with 30% in people who are 75 to 85 years of age.[76-78] Overall, 2% of people 65 years or older have visual acuity of 20/200 or less in one eye due to AMD.[78] Although most patients with AMD have the nonneovascular (atrophic, or "dry") form, most patients (up to 90%) with severe visual loss due to AMD have the neovascular (exudative, or "wet") form associated with choroidal neovascularization (CNV). The incidence of AMD, particularly its neovascular form, is higher among whites than African Americans.[79]

Some of the risk factors reported in association with AMD include genetic factors[80,81] and smoking.[82,83] Other potential risk factors possibly associated with increased risk include diet, cardiovascular disease, hypertension, and hyperopia.[84-93] The AREDS recently reported benefits for some patients with AMD from high-dose antioxidants and zinc supplementation (Table 61-5).[92] This multicenter randomized clinical trial evaluated the value of high-dose antioxidant vitamins and minerals in 4757 participants with various stages of AMD. Based on the results of this study, the AREDS group recommended that these supple-ments be taken by patients with soft drusen, geographic atrophy, or neovascular AMD with a visual acuity of 20/32 or better in at least one eye.

The AREDS also showed that for patients who pre-sented with advanced AMD (defined as geographic atrophy involving the center of the fovea or the presence of CNV) in one eye, the rate of development of either geographic atrophy in the fovea or neovascular AMD in the other eye without treatment was 43%. However, only 1.3% of the patients in the low-risk AREDS category progressed to advanced AMD in 5 years, and there was no benefit of treatment with antioxidant vitamins and minerals in delaying progression of AMD in those patients who entered the AREDS at this low-risk stage of the disease. Thus, if the patient has only small drusen (>63 μm), there is no benefit from taking these vitamins and minerals. Likewise, no treatment benefit was demon-strated for patients who present with severe bilateral

TABLE 61-5

High-dose Antioxidant Vitamins and Minerals Recommended for Age-related Macular Degeneration*

Supplement	Daily Dose
Vitamin C	500 mg
Vitamin E	400 IU
Beta carotene†	15 mg (25,000 IU)
Zinc oxide	80 mg
Cupric oxide	2 mg

*From Age-Related Eye Disease Study.[35,92]

†Beta carotene should not be given to smokers.

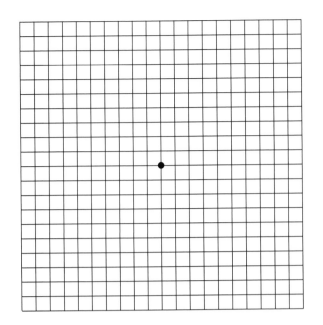

FIGURE 61-2

Macular degeneration vision test: Amsler grid. Patients are instructed to fixate on central dot while wearing their reading glasses and to observe for any distortion or absence of vertical or horizontal lines. Patients should test each eye separately on daily basis.

visual loss resulting from either nonneovascular or neovascular AMD.

Primary public screening for AMD is not indicated. For patients with early stages of AMD as documented by an ophthalmologist, regular dilated funduscopic eye examinations are recommended. Patients with AMD who have an increased risk of visual loss or progression to advanced AMD should be educated by an ophthalmologist regarding the methods of self-testing and detection of new symptoms of CNV. One useful way to test vision, which can detect even the smallest changes when they first appear, is to use the Amsler grid on a daily basis (Fig 61-2). A person with new symptoms of progression of AMD may notice new distortion of the grid pattern such as bent lines and irregular box shapes or a gray shaded area. Such symptoms warrant an immediate appointment with an ophthalmologist. Current therapies for treatable neovascular lesions can improve the visual outcome provided that the lesions are detected early. Patients with risk factors for visual loss can be detected if those between the ages of 40 and 64 years undergo a comprehensive eye examination every 2 to 4 years and those who are older than 65 years undergo such an examination every 1 to 2 years.[94,95]

Hypertensive Retinopathy

Systemic arterial hypertension is one of the most prevalent diseases in industrialized countries. The retinal vascular changes caused by systemic hypertension may overlap with those seen with other retinal vascular disease, such as diabetes. The overall incidence of hypertensive retinopathy in a population of hypertensive patients who do not have coexisting, confounding vascular diseases is approximately 15%.[96] Elevated blood pressure that persists despite the use of antihypertensive medications results in a higher risk of retinal vascular changes.

Chronic hypertensive retinopathy is a clinical diagnosis made when the characteristic fundus findings are seen in a patient who has a history of systemic arterial hypertension. The most common clinical manifestations include focal constriction and dilation of the retinal arterioles, an increase in the arteriolar light reflex, and loss of transparency of the intra-arterial blood column. Prominent arteriovenous crossings (nicking) are the hallmark of hypertensive retinopathy and represent a pathognomonic finding. The course of the vein may change to a more perpendicular direction. When venous flow is impeded, certain signs may develop, including dilation and tortuosity of the vein distal to the arteriovenous crossing, intraretinal hemorrhages, cotton-wool spots, and macular edema. Secondary ocular complications of chronic systemic hypertension include retinal vascular occlusive disease and nonarteritic anterior ischemic optic neuropathy (NAION).

Chronic hypertensive retinopathy alone rarely results in substantial loss of vision. Treatment of the underlying systemic hypertension can halt the progression of the retinal changes. Arteriolar narrowing and prominent arteriovenous crossings are usually permanent. Both treatment and prevention of various ocular manifestations of chronic and accelerated systemic hypertension consist of lowering blood pressure. No specific ocular therapy exists to reverse the changes associated with systemic hypertension. Blood pressure should be lowered to a level that minimizes the chance of acute end-organ damage in accelerated hypertension and the long-term vascular changes in the chronic disease. In the setting of accelerated hypertension, the actual level of blood pressure is less important in gauging the urgency of the situation than is the impending end-organ damage.

Retinal Vascular Obstructive Disorders

Systemic hypertension has also been implicated as a major underlying condition in retinal venous occlusions. Venous obstructive disease of the retina is relatively common and its incidence is second only to diabetic retinopathy. It typically affects individuals who are 50 years of age or older. In contrast to venous occlusive disease, retinal artery occlusions are not generally associated with systemic hypertension. Most retinal arterial obstructions are either thrombotic or embolic. Thrombus formation in a retinal artery is usually a result of atherosclerosis. Medical examinations such as carotid angiography and angioplasty as well as manipulations such as chiropractic neck manipulation may rarely lead to embolic central retinal artery occlusion. It is of paramount importance to rule out giant cell (temporal) arteritis as a cause of central retinal artery occlusion in all patients over 50 years of age, although it is present in less than 5% of cases. Risk factors for embolic retinal arterial disease include predisposing family history, hypertension, elevated lipid levels, cigarette smoking, and diabetes mellitus.

Three main types of retinal arterial emboli are cholesterol (Hollenhorst plaque), platelet-fibrin, and calcific. Cholesterol emboli typically originate from atheromatous plaques in the ipsilateral carotid artery, although the aorta or heart valves may also be a source. Platelet-fibrin emboli typically are associated with carotid or cardiac thromboses. Calcific emboli are solid, white, nonrefractile plugs associated with calcification of heart valves or the aorta. Prevention of retinal arterial emboli and their consequences rests in prevention of atherosclerosis and surveillance and management of carotid artery disease and valvular heart disease.

Ischemic Optic Neuropathy

Optic nerve ischemia occurring at the optic nerve head is termed anterior ischemic optic neuropathy (AION). This neuropathy is further categorized as (1) arteritic or in association with giant cell (temporal) arteritis (AAION) and (2) nonarteritic (NAION). In patients 60 years of age and older, NAION is the most prevalent acute optic neuropathy, with an estimated 6000 to 8000 new cases each year (3.25 per 100,000 population) in the United States.[97]

Anterior ischemic optic neuropathy manifests with the rapid onset of painless, monocular visual loss. In the initial management of AION, the most important step is the differentiation of the arteritic from the nonarteritic type of the disease. Active giant cell arteritis is typically but not always associated with an elevation of the erythrocyte sedimentation rate (ESR) up to 70 to 120 mm/h and is associated with other characteristic clinical symptoms. Although the specificity and sensitivity of ESR is far from perfect and may be affected by many unrelated factors, such elevation should prompt immediate corticosteroid therapy and confirmatory temporal artery biopsy. Levels of plasma fibrinogen and C-reactive protein may aid in the diagnosis, as they tend to parallel ESR only in vasculitis. The diagnosis of giant cell arteritis should be confirmed by superficial temporal artery biopsy and is recommended in any case of AION in which a clinical suspicion of arteritis exists. A normal biopsy result does not rule out arteritis, and consideration should be given to a contralateral biopsy. Patients with AAION typically note

other general symptoms, such as headache (most common), jaw claudication, scalp tenderness, malaise, anorexia, weight loss, fever, proximal joint arthralgia, and myalgia. Occasionally, the disease manifests with visual loss in the absence of overt systemic symptoms. The contralateral eye is eventually involved in up to 95% of cases without treatment.

Approximately 95% of cases of AION are unrelated to giant cell arteritis and are classified as NAION. Whereas AAION represents a manifestation of giant cell arteritis, NAION has been reported in association with a number of diseases that could predispose an individual to reduced perfusion pressure or increased resistance to flow within the optic nerve head. Systemic hypertension has been documented in up to 47% and diabetes in up to 24% of patients with NAION.[98]

Trauma

Ocular injuries caused by accidental events include corneal abrasions, hyphema, vitreous hemorrhage, retinal detachment, orbital fractures, and ruptured globe. Many cases of ocular trauma are preventable. Ocular trauma typically occurs in individuals below the age of 30 years. Thus, the socioeconomic impact of ocular injuries is substantial.[99]

Many causes of ocular injuries such as work-related accidents, sports-related injuries, and domestic accidents are preventable by using simple safety measures. Occupations that have a high incidence of severe ocular injuries include automobile-repair and construction-related work.[99]

Sports-related eye injuries occur most commonly in baseball, softball, basketball, and racquetball. Overall, sports-related injuries are thought to be responsible for about 33,000 eye injuries each year.[100] Well-designed sports goggles can prevent many of these injuries. Standard dress spectacles not only fail to provide ocular protection but their components may break and cause more damage than the projectile itself. Safety frames must be constructed as a 1-piece unit without hinges and made of polycarbonate or stronger material. Lenses made of polycarbonate provide effective eye protection and are available with prescription.[101] Lens-free eye guards should not be used for protection from a small ball in any competitive sport because the ball can deform through the guard and strike the eye.

A large number of severe ocular injuries result from gunshot wounds. Air-powered guns are associated with substantial ocular morbidity.[102] In addition, many accidental facial gunshot wounds occur during each hunting season. It has been demonstrated, however, that polycarbonate protective eyewear with integral side shields and a secure headband can virtually eliminate injuries from shotguns fired at more than 22.5 m (25 yd).[103]

TABLE 61-6

Ocular Manifestations of Vitamin Deficiencies

Vitamin	Ocular Manifestations
A	Bitot spots, conjunctival and corneal xerosis, keratomalacia, night blindness, xerophthalmic fundus
B_1	Corneal epithelial changes, ophthalmoplegia, nystagmus, optic atrophy
B_2	Peripheral corneal vascularization, angular blepharoconjunctivitis
B_3	Optic neuropathy
B_6	Optic neuritis, angular blepharoconjunctivitis, gyrate atrophy (rare)
B_{12}	Optic neuropathy, central scotoma, flame-shaped and dot-blot retinal hemorrhages
C	Hemorrhages in eyelids, conjunctiva, anterior chamber, and retina; proptosis in infantile scurvy
D	Exophthalmos

Visual Loss Associated With Nutritional Disorders

Ocular manifestations of nutritional disorders, predominantly vitamin deficiencies, are generally seen in developing countries and are a major worldwide cause of visual loss and blindness. Ocular manifestations of different hypovitaminoses are summarized in Table 61-6.

Among different nutritional deficiencies, hypovitaminosis A is the greatest cause of ocular disease. Approximately 20,000 to 100,000 new cases of blindness each year in the world are due to complications associated with vitamin A deficiency leading to xerophthalmia. A vitamin A deficiency is defined as a plasma level of 0.35 μmol/L or less.[104] Triangular, perilimbal, gray plaques of keratinized conjunctiva called Bitot spots are often used as a clinical sign of vitamin A deficiency. However, this sign also may be present due to generalized malnutrition and may persist despite normal vitamin A

levels.[105] Thus, it may not be an adequate indicator of vitamin A deficiency.

Another useful laboratory technique that correlates closely with serum vitamin A levels and with clinical improvement is conjunctival impression cytology. It may be particularly useful in developing countries where direct laboratory measurement of serum vitamin A levels is not readily available. Because vitamin A deficiency is typically accompanied by concurrent malnutrition, both protein and vitamin A should be administered.[106] Hypovitaminosis A can also occur in developed countries, most often as a result of decreased absorption of vitamin A. In patients with malabsorption secondary to gastrointestinal diseases and primary liver diseases (eg, alcoholic cirrhosis, hepatitis, bowel resections, abetalipoproteinemia, or cystic fibrosis) or self-imposed dietary restrictions, vitamin A–related ocular disease may develop. In particular, corneal ulcers that are persistent and unresponsive to treatment in elderly, debilitated patients may be due to vitamin A deficiency and malnutrition. To prevent hypovitaminosis A, vitamin A should be supplemented orally or by intramuscular injections.[104]

Hypervitaminoses with ocular manifestation have been described for vitamins A and D. Excessive vitamin A ingestion can lead to strabismus and diplopia, and is associated with pseudotumor cerebri. Excessive ingestion of vitamin D can result in scleral, conjunctival, or corneal calcifications (band keratopathy).

SUMMARY

A thorough eye evaluation, even in the absence of ocular complaints, may detect important abnormalities of the visual system, or uncover certain systemic diseases with ophthalmic manifestations. In fact, a number of common ocular diseases may develop without the patient being aware of any problem. With early diagnosis and appropriate intervention, potentially blinding illnesses such as glaucoma, cataract, and diabetic retinopathy, all of which increase in prevalence with age, may have a much more favorable outcome. Therefore, a comprehensive ocular examination by an ophthalmologist is recommended for any symptomatic patient as well as for asymptomatic patients who have not had a recent ocular examination.

REFERENCES

1. American Academy of Ophthalmology. Eye care for the American people. *Ophthalmology.* 1987(suppl).

2. Tielsch JM, Sommer A, Witt K, Katz J, Royall RM. Blindness and visual impairment in an American urban population: the Baltimore Eye Survey. *Arch Ophthalmol.* 1990;108:286–290.

3. US Dept of Commerce, Economics, and Statistics Administration, Bureau of the Census. *Sixty-five plus in the United States: Statistical Brief.* Washington, DC: US Bureau of the Census; May 1995.

4. Applegate WB, Miller ST, Elam JT, et al. Impact of cataract surgery with lens implantation on vision and physical function in elderly patients. *JAMA.* 1987;257:1064–1066.

5. Brenner MH, Curbow B, Javitt JC, Legro NW, Sommer A. Vision change and quality of life in the elderly: response to cataract surgery and treatment of other chronic ocular conditions. *Arch Ophthalmol.* 1993;111:680–685.

6. Silverstone B, et al. *The Lighthouse Handbook on Vision Impairment and Vision Rehabilitation.* New York, NY: Oxford University Press Inc; 2000:517–539.

7. Tielsch JM, Javitt JC, Coleman A, Katz J, Sommer A. The prevalence of blindness and visual impairment among nursing home residents in Baltimore. *N Engl J Med.* 1995;332:1205–1209.

8. Sommer A, Tielsch JM, Katz J, et al. Racial differences in the cause-specific prevalence of blindness in east Baltimore. *N Engl J Med.* 1991;325:1412–1417.

9. Dana MR, Tielsch JM, Enger C, et al. Visual impairment in a rural Appalachian community: prevalence and causes. *JAMA.* 1990;264:2400–2405.

10. Wang Q, Klein BE, Klein R, Moss SE. Refractive status in the Beaver Dam Eye Study. *Invest Ophthalmol Vis Sci.* 1994;35:4344–4347.

11. Lin LL, Chen CJ, Hung PT, Ko LS. Nation-wide survey of myopia among schoolchildren in Taiwan, 1986. *Acta Ophthalmol.* 1988;185(suppl):29–33.

12. Katz J, Tielsch JM, Sommer A. Prevalence and risk factors for refractive errors in an adult inner city population. *Invest Ophthalmol Vis Sci.* 1997;38:334–340.

13. Zylbermann R, Landau D, Berson D. The influence of study habits on myopia in Jewish teenagers. *J Pediatr Ophthalmol Strabismus.* 1993;30:319–322.

14. Richler A, Bear JC. Refraction, nearwork and education: a population study in Newfoundland. *Acta Ophthalmol [Copenh].* 1980;58:468–478.

15. Robb RM. Refractive errors associated with hemangiomas of the eyelids and orbit in infancy. *Am J Ophthalmol.* 1977;83:52–58.

16. Sperduto RD, Seigel D, Roberts J, Rowland M. Prevalence of myopia in the United States. *Arch Ophthalmol.* 1983;101:405–407.

17. Curtin BJ. *The Myopias: Basic Science and Clinical Management.* New York, NY: Harper & Row Publishers; 1985:284–292, 299–300, 333–348.

18. Lowe RF. Causes of shallow anterior chamber in primary angle-closure glaucoma: ultrasonic biometry of normal and angle-closure glaucoma eyes. *Am J Ophthalmol.* 1969;67:87–93.

19. Parssinen O, Hemminki E, Klemetti A. Effect of spectacle use and accommodation on myopic progression: final results of a three-year randomized clinical trial among schoolchildren. *Br J Ophthalmol.* 1989;73:547–551.

20. Oishi T, Lauber JK. Chicks blinded with formoguanamine do not develop lid suture myopia. *Curr Eye Res.* 1988;7:69–73.

21. Brodstein RS, Brodstein DE, Olson RJ, Hunt SC, Williams RR. The treatment of myopia with atropine and bifocals: a long-term prospective study. *Ophthalmology.* 1984;91:1373–1379.

22. Dyer JA. Role of cycloplegics in progressive myopia. *Ophthalmology.* 1979;86:692–694.

23. Bates WH. *The Cure of Imperfect Sight by Treatment Without Glasses.* New York, NY: Central Fixation Publishing Co; 1920.

24. National Society to Prevent Blindness. *Vision Problems in the U.S.: Data Analysis: Definitions, Data Sources, Detailed Data Tables, Analysis, Interpretation.* New York, NY: National Society to Prevent Blindness; 1980. Publication P-10.

25. Foster A, Johnson GJ. Magnitude and causes of blindness in the developing world. *Int Ophthalmol.* 1990;14:135–140.

26. Munoz B, West SK, Rubin GS, et al. Causes of blindness and visual impairment in a population of older Americans: the Salisbury Eye Evaluation Study. *Arch Ophthalmol.* 2000;118:819–825.

27. Klein BE, Klein R, Moss SE. Incident cataract surgery: the Beaver Dam Eye Study. *Ophthalmology.* 1997;104:573–580.

28. Taylor HR. Epidemiology of age-related cataract. *Eye.* 1999;13:445–448.

29. Leske MC, Wu SY, Hennis A, et al. Diabetes, hypertension, and central obesity as cataract risk factors in a black population: the Barbados Eye Study. *Ophthalmology.* 1999;106:35–41.

30. Urban RC Jr, Cotlier E. Corticosteroid-induced cataracts. *Surv Ophthalmol.* 1986;31:102–110.

31. Cumming RG, Mitchell P, Leeder SR. Use of inhaled corticosteroids and the risk of cataracts. *N Engl J Med.* 1997;337:8–14.

32. Delcourt C, Carriere I, Ponton-Sanchez A, et al. Light exposure and the risk of cortical, nuclear, and posterior subcapsular cataracts: the Pathologies Oculaires Liees a l'Age (POLA) study. *Arch Ophthalmol.* 2000;118:385–392.

33. Christen WG, Glynn RJ, Ajani UA, et al. Smoking cessation and risk of age-related cataract in men. *JAMA.* 2000;284:713–716.

34. Christen WG, Manson JE, Seddon JM, et al. A prospective study of cigarette smoking and risk of cataract in men. *JAMA.* 1992;268:989–993.

35. AREDS Report No. 9: a randomized, placebo-controlled, clinical trial of high-dose supplementation with vitamins C and E and beta carotene for age-related cataract and vision loss. *Arch Ophthalmol.* 2001;119:1439–1452.

36. Congdon NG, West KP Jr. Nutrition and the eye. *Curr Opin Ophthalmol.* 1999;10:464–473.

37. Tielsch JM, Sommer A, Katz J, et al. Racial variations in the prevalence of primary open-angle glaucoma: the Baltimore Eye Survey. *JAMA.* 1991;266:369–374.

38. Quigley HA, Vitale S. Models of open-angle glaucoma prevalence and incidence in the United States. *Invest Ophthalmol Vis Sci.* 1997;38:83–91.

39. American Academy of Ophthalmology. *Primary Open-Angle Glaucoma: Preferred Practice Pattern.* San Francisco, Calif: American Academy of Ophthalmology; 2000.

40. Sommer A, Tielsch JM, Katz J, et al. Relationship between intraocular pressure and primary open angle glaucoma among white and black Americans: the Baltimore Eye Survey. *Arch Ophthalmol.* 1991;109:1090–1095.

41. Mitchell P, Smith W, Attebo K, Healey PR. Prevalence of open-angle glaucoma in Australia: the Blue Mountains Eye Study. *Ophthalmology.* 1996;103:1661–1669.

42. Armaly MF, Krueger DE, Maunder L, et al. Biostatistical analysis of the collaborative glaucoma study: I. Summary report of the risk factors for glaucomatous visual-field defects. *Arch Ophthalmol.* 1980;98:2163–2171.

43. Mason RP, Kosoko O, Wilson MR, et al. National survey of the prevalence and risk factors of glaucoma in St. Lucia, West Indies: I. Prevalence findings. *Ophthalmology.* 1989;96:1363–1368.

44. Wolfs RC, Klaver CC, Ramrattan RS, et al. Genetic risk of primary open-angle glaucoma: population-based familial aggregation study. *Arch Ophthalmol.* 1998;116:1640–1645.

45. Tielsch JM, Katz J, Sommer A, Quigley HA, Javitt JC. Family history and risk of primary open angle glaucoma: the Baltimore Eye Survey. *Arch Ophthalmol.* 1994;112:69–73.

46. Mitchell P, Smith W, Chey T, Healey PR. Open-angle glaucoma and diabetes: the Blue Mountains Eye Study, Australia. *Ophthalmology.* 1997;104:712–718.

47. The Advanced Glaucoma Intervention Study (AGIS): III. Baseline characteristics of black and white patients. *Ophthalmology.* 1998;105:1137–1145.

48. Tielsch JM, Katz J, Quigley HA, Javitt JC, Sommer A. Diabetes, intraocular pressure, and primary open-angle glaucoma in the Baltimore Eye Survey. *Ophthalmology.* 1995;102:48–53.

49. Wu SY, Leske MC. Associations with intraocular pressure in the Barbados Eye Study. *Arch Ophthalmol.* 1997;115:1572–1576.

50. Mitchell P, Hourihan F, Sandbach J, Wang JJ. The relationship between glaucoma and myopia: the Blue Mountains Eye Study. *Ophthalmology.* 1999;106:2010–2015.

51. Leske MC, Connell AM, Wu SY, Hyman LG, Schachat AP. Risk factors for open-angle glaucoma: the Barbados Eye Study. *Arch Ophthalmol.* 1995;113:918–924.

52. Klaver CC, Wolfs RC, Vingerling JR, Hofman A, de Jong PT. Age-specific prevalence and causes of blindness and visual impairment in an older population: the Rotterdam Study. *Arch Ophthalmol.* 1998;116:653–658.

53. Jay JL, Allan D. The benefit of early trabeculectomy versus conventional management in primary open angle glaucoma relative to severity of disease. *Eye.* 1989;3:528–535.

54. Collaborative Normal-Tension Glaucoma Study Group. The effectiveness of intraocular pressure reduction in the treatment of normal-tension glaucoma. *Am J Ophthalmol.* 1998;126:498–505.

55. Arkell SM, Lightman DA, Sommer A, et al. The prevalence of glaucoma among Eskimos of northwest Alaska. *Arch Ophthalmol.* 1987;105:482–485.

56. Bankes JLK, Perkins ES, Tsolakis S, Wright JE. Bedford glaucoma survey. *BMJ.* 1968;1:791–796.

57. Congdon N, Wang F, Tielsch JM. Issues in the epidemiology and population-based screening of primary angle-closure glaucoma. *Surv Ophthalmol.* 1992;36:411–423.

58. Van Herick W, Shaffer RN, Schwartz A. Estimation of width of angle of anterior chamber: incidence and significance of the narrow angle. *Am J Ophthalmol.* 1969;68:626–629.

59. Lowe RF. Etiology of the anatomical basis for primary angle-closure glaucoma. *Br J Ophthalmol.* 1970;54:161–169.

60. Leighton DA. Survey of the first-degree relatives of glaucoma patients. *Trans Ophthalmol Soc UK.* 1976;96:28–32.

61. Perkins ES. Family studies in glaucoma. *Br J Ophthalmol.* 1974;58:529–535.

62. Bengtsson B. The prevalence of glaucoma. *Br J Ophthalmol.* 1981;65:46–49.

63. Foster PJ, Baasanhu J, Alsbirk PH, et al. Glaucoma in Mongolia: a population-based survey in Hovsgol province, northern Mongolia. *Arch Ophthalmol.* 1996;114:1235–1241.

64. Seah SK, Foster PJ, Chew PT, et al. Incidence of acute primary angle-closure glaucoma in Singapore: an island-wide survey. *Arch Ophthalmol.* 1997;115:1436–1440.

65. Wolfs RC, Grobbee DE, Hofman A, de Jong PT. Risk of acute angle-closure glaucoma after diagnostic mydriasis in nonselected subjects: the Rotterdam Study. *Invest Ophthalmol Vis Sci.* 1997;38:2683–2687.

66. Bain WES. The fellow eye in acute closed-angle glaucoma. *Br J Ophthalmol.* 1957;41:193–199.

67. Lowe RF. Acute angle-closure glaucoma: the second eye: an analysis of 200 cases. *Br J Ophthalmol.* 1962;46:641–650.

68. Diabetic Retinopathy Study Research Group. Four risk factors for severe visual loss in diabetic retinopathy: the third report from the Diabetic Retinopathy Study. *Arch Ophthalmol.* 1979;97:654–655.

69. Diabetic Retinopathy Study Research Group. Indications for photocoagulation treatment of diabetic retinopathy: Diabetic Retinopathy Study Report no. 14. *Int Ophthalmol Clin.* 1987;27:239–253.

70. Early Treatment Diabetic Retinopathy Study Research Group. Early photocoagulation for diabetic retinopathy: ETDRS report number 9. *Ophthalmology.* 1991;98(suppl):766–785.

71. Klein R, Klein BE, Moss SE, Davis MD, DeMets DL. Glycosylated hemoglobin predicts the incidence and progression of diabetic retinopathy. *JAMA.* 1988;260:2864–2871.

72. Diabetes Control and Complications Trial Research Group. The effect of intensive treatment of diabetes on the development and progression of long-term complications in insulin-dependent diabetes mellitus. *N Engl J Med.* 1993;329:977–986.

73. Davis MD, Fisher MR, Gangnon RE, et al. Risk factors for high-risk proliferative diabetic retinopathy and severe visual loss: Early Treatment Diabetic Retinopathy Study Report #18. *Invest Ophthalmol Vis Sci.* 1998;39:233–252.

74. Ferris FL III. How effective are treatments for diabetic retinopathy? *JAMA.* 1993;269:1290–1291.

75. Kraft SK, Marrero DG, Lazaridis EN, et al. Primary care physicians' practice patterns and diabetic retinopathy: current levels of care. *Arch Fam Med.* 1997;6:29–37.

76. Klein R, Klein BE, Jensen SC, Meuer SM. The five-year incidence and progression of age-related maculopathy: the Beaver Dam Eye Study. *Ophthalmology.* 1997;104:7–21.

77. Klein R, Klein BE, Linton KL. Prevalence of age-related maculopathy: the Beaver Dam Eye Study. *Ophthalmology.* 1992;99:933–943.

78. Leibowitz HM, Krueger DE, Maunder LR, et al. The Framingham Eye Study monograph: An ophthalmological and epidemiological study of cataract, glaucoma, diabetic retinopathy, macular degeneration, and visual acuity in a general population of 2631 adults, 1973–1975. *Surv Ophthalmol.* 1980;24(suppl):335–610.

79. Schachat AP, Hyman L, Leske MC, Connell AM, Wu SY. Features of age-related macular degeneration in a black population: the Barbados Eye Study Group. *Arch Ophthalmol.* 1995;113:728–735.

80. Meyers SM, Greene T, Gutman FA. A twin study of age-related macular degeneration. *Am J Ophthalmol.* 1995;120:757–766.

81. Seddon JM, Ajani UA, Mitchell BD. Familial aggregation of age-related maculopathy. *Am J Ophthalmol.* 1997;123:199–206.

82. Christen WG, Glynn RJ, Manson JE, Ajani UA, Buring JE. A prospective study of cigarette smoking and risk of age-related macular degeneration in men. *JAMA.* 1996;276:1147–1151.

83. Vingerling JR, Hofman A, Grobbee DE, de Jong PT. Age-related macular degeneration and smoking: the Rotterdam Study. *Arch Ophthalmol.* 1996;114:1193–1196.

84. Sandberg MA, Tolentino MJ, Miller S, Berson EL, Gaudio AR. Hyperopia and neovascularization in age-related macular degeneration. *Ophthalmology.* 1993;100:1009–1013.

85. Mares-Perlman JA, Klein R, Klein BE, et al. Association of zinc and antioxidant nutrients with age-related maculopathy. *Arch Ophthalmol.* 1996;114:991–997.

86. Eye Disease Case-Control Study Group. Risk factors for neovascular age-related macular degeneration. *Arch Ophthalmol.* 1992;110:1701–1708.

87. Seddon JM, Ajani UA, Sperduto RD, et al for Eye Disease Case-Control Study Group. Dietary carotenoids, vitamins A, C, and E, and advanced age-related macular degeneration. *JAMA.* 1994;272:1413–1420.

88. Stur M, Tittl M, Reitner A, Meisinger V. Oral zinc and the second eye in age-related macular degeneration. *Invest Ophthalmol Vis Sci.* 1996;37:1225–1235.

89. Teikari JM, Laatikainen L, Virtamo J, et al. Six-year supplementation with alpha-tocopherol and beta-carotene and age-related maculopathy. *Acta Ophthalmol Scand.* 1998;76:224–229.

90. Smith W, Mitchell P, Webb K, Leeder SR. Dietary antioxidants and age-related maculopathy: the Blue Mountains Eye Study. *Ophthalmology.* 1999;106:761–767.

91. Snow KK, Seddon JM. Do age-related macular degeneration and cardiovascular disease share common antecedents? *Ophthalmic Epidemiol.* 1999;6:125–143.

92. AREDS Report No. 8: a randomized, placebo-controlled, clinical trial of high-dose supplementation with vitamins C and E, beta carotene, and zinc for age-related macular

degeneration and vision loss. *Arch Ophthalmol.* 2001;119:1417–1436.

93. Delcourt C, Cristol JP, Terrier F, et al, for POLA Study Group. Age-related macular degeneration and antioxidant status in the POLA study: Pathologies Oculaires Liees a l'Age. *Arch Ophthalmol.* 1999;117:1384–1390.

94. American Academy of Ophthalmology. *Comprehensive Adult Medical Eye Evaluation: Preferred Practice Pattern.* San Francisco, Calif: American Academy of Ophthalmology; 2000.

95. Grey RH, Bird AC, Chisholm IH. Senile disciform macular degeneration: features indicating suitability for photocoagulation. *Br J Ophthalmol.* 1979;63:85–89.

96. Klein R, Klein BE, Moss SE, Wang Q. Hypertension and retinopathy, arteriolar narrowing, and arteriovenous nicking in a population. *Arch Ophthalmol.* 1994;112:92–98.

97. Johnson LN, Arnold AC. Incidence of nonarteritic and arteritic anterior ischemic optic neuropathy: population-based study in the State of Missouri and Los Angeles County, California. *J Neuro Ophthalmol.* 1994;14:38–44.

98. Ischemic Optic Neuropathy Decompression Trial Research Group. Characteristics of patients with nonarteritic anterior ischemic optic neuropathy eligible for the Ischemic Optic Neuropathy Decompression Trial. *Arch Ophthalmol.* 1996;114:1366–1374.

99. Schein OD, Hibberd PL, Shingleton BJ, et al. The spectrum and burden of ocular injury. *Ophthalmology.* 1988;95:300–305.

100. Larrison WI, Hersh PS, Kunzweiler T, Shingleton BJ. Sports-related ocular trauma. *Ophthalmology.* 1990;97:1265–1269.

101. Feigelman MJ, Sugar J, Jednock N, Read JS, Johnson PL. Assessment of ocular protection for racquetball. *Arch Ophthalmol.* 1992;110:1701–1708.

102. Sternberg P Jr, de Juan E Jr, Green WR, Hirst LW, Sommer A. Ocular BB injuries. *Ophthalmology.* 1984;91:1269–1277.

103. Varr WF III, Cook RA. Shotgun eye injuries: ocular risk and eye protection efficacy. *Ophthalmology.* 1992;99:867–872.

104. World Health Organization (WHO). *Report of a Joint WHO/UNICEF/USAAID/HKI/IVACG Meeting: Control of Vitamin A Deficiency.* Geneva, Switzerland: WHO; 1982.

105. Semba RD, Wirasasmita S, Natadisastra G, Muhilal, Sommer A. Response of Bitot's spots in preschool children to vitamin A treatment. *Am J Ophthalmol.* 1990;110:416–420.

106. Baisya DC, Dutta LC, Goswami P, Saha SK. Role of serum protein in the ocular manifestations of vitamin A deficiency. *Br J Ophthalmol.* 1971;55:700–703.

RESOURCES

American Academy of Ophthalmology
Web site: www.aao.org

Medical Library online (Medem)
Web site: www.medem.com/MedLB/sub

Eyecare programs and international public service
Web site: www.eyecareamerica.org

Diabetes Mellitus

John P. Campbell, MD, and Douglas G. Rogers, MD

INTRODUCTION

Diabetes mellitus (DM) can be a devastating disease. Once DM occurs, it may be controlled but never cured. Similarly, once diabetic complications develop, they may be controlled but cannot be reversed. Although DM can occur at any age, the different types of the disease can be classified by etiology and often are found more commonly in certain age groups, ethnic backgrounds, and body types. Diabetes mellitus can be classified into 2 major types. *Type 1* DM is characterized by inadequate insulin production secondary to autoimmune destruction of pancreatic β-cells more commonly developing in thin individuals under age 25 years of age. *Type 2* DM is characterized by insulin resistance and abnormal insulin secretion more commonly developing in overweight individuals over 45 years of age. Gestational DM, often considered a subgroup of type 2 DM, develops at the onset of pregnancy or during a pregnancy. Secondary types of diabetes are associated with genetic defects in B-cell function or insulin action, genetic syndromes such as Down syndrome, infections, drugs such as diuretics, nonautoimmune damage to the pancreas associated with pancreatitis or surgery, and endocrinopathies such as Cushing disease. Diabetic complications occur much more often in the more prevalent type 2 DM and less prevalent type 1 DM than in the other types of diabetes.

Type 2 DM fulfills the criteria required for useful strategies of preventive intervention. It represents a major public health and economic burden. Secondly, type 2 DM has an identifiable predisease state. Studies also have demonstrated that interruption of the natural course of type 2 DM by decreasing disease duration and level of hyperglycemia results in a decrease in microvascular complications. Finally, studies have shown evidence that nonpharmacologic and/or pharmacologic protocols can delay or prevent type 2 DM. Unfortunately, type 1 DM does not fulfill these same criteria for aggressive preventive strategies at this time because no protocols have been found to delay or prevent the disease onset.

PREVALENCE AND EPIDEMIOLOGY

Diabetes mellitus is one of the most burdensome and costly chronic diseases and is increasing in epidemic proportions throughout the world. The global prevalence of DM was 150 million in the year 2000 and is estimated to be 300 million by 2025. The rate of increase is projected to be greater in developing countries than in developed countries because of the greater change in lifestyle and increase in obesity.[1] In the United States, 17 million individuals, or 6.2% of the total population, were estimated to have DM in 2000. Unfortunately, only 11.1 million individuals were aware of having DM, and 5.9 million had not yet received a diagnosis. Approximately 151,000 individuals under 20 years of age, or 0.19% of all individuals in this age group, have DM. Approximately 16.9 million individuals in the United States over age 20 years, or 8.6% of this age group, have DM. In the United States, 7.8 million men (8.3%) have DM and 9.1 million women (8.9%) have DM.[2]

The prevalence of DM varies by race and ethnicity. In individuals older than 20 years who reside in the United States, DM can be found in 15.1% (105,000) of all American Indians and Alaskan natives receiving care from the Indian Health Service, 13% (2.8 million) of all non-Hispanic blacks, 10.2% (2 million) of all Hispanics and Latin Americans, and 7.8% (11.4) million) of all non-Hispanic whites.[2] Although prevalence data are limited for Asian Americans and native Hawaiians or Pacific Islanders, native Hawaiians appear to be 2.5 times more likely to have a diagnosis of DM than do whites in Hawaii in the same age group. Similarly, non-Hispanic blacks, Hispanics and Latin Americans, and Alaskan natives have a 1.9- to 2.6-fold increased risk of having DM than do non-Hispanic whites in the same age group. Furthermore, 1 million new cases of DM are diagnosed each year in individuals older than 20 years.[2]

MORBIDITY AND MORTALITY

Diabetes mellitus is a major cause of morbidity and mortality. In 1999, approximately 19% (450,000) of all deaths in the United States occurred in diabetic individuals over age 25 years. In general, the risk of death is twofold greater in diabetic than nondiabetic individuals. However, the risk is not uniform for both sexes and all age groups. For example, the risk of death in the age group 25 to 44 years old is increased 3.6 in diabetic persons compared with nondiabetic individuals, but in the age group 65 to 74 years the risk falls to 1.5-fold. Diabetic women aged 45 to 64 years old have a 2.7-fold increased risk of death compared with a twofold increased risk in diabetic men over the same nondiabetic age group and sex.[2]

Diabetes mellitus can cause damage to every tissue and organ in the body. The disease is the leading cause of new cases of blindness in adults aged 20 to 74 years old. In addition, DM is the leading cause of end-stage renal disease. Greater than 60% of diabetic individuals have mild to severe neuropathy, which can be associated with paresthesias; balance disturbance; and bowel, bladder, and/or sexual dysfunction. Severe neuropathy is a major contributor to lower-extremity amputations. Periodontal, or gum, disease is twofold more common among diabetic than nondiabetic individuals. Approximately 33% of diabetic individuals have or will have severe periodontal disease. Hyperglycemia before or during the first trimester of pregnancy can lead to major birth defects in 5% to 10% of these babies and spontaneous abortion in 15% to 20% of these pregnancies. In addition, poorly controlled blood glucose levels during the second and third trimesters can result in large babies weighing more than 4 kg at term and thus raising the risk of delivery problems.[2]

Often, DM is associated with hypertension, low high-density lipoprotein cholesterol (HDL-C), hypertriglyceridemia, and central abdominal obesity. This cluster of findings is known as metabolic syndrome X, which is associated with a threefold increase in cardiovascular disease over the general population. Like other chronic disease, DM with complications often is associated with depression.[2]

The total (direct and indirect) costs of DM in the United States approach $98 billion. Approximately $44 billion account for direct medical costs, and $54 billion make up indirect costs, including disability, work loss, and premature death.[2]

STUDIES OF PREVENTION AND COMPLICATIONS OF DM

Several large studies in individuals with known diabetes (The Diabetes Control and Complications Trial, studying type 1 DM,[3] and the United Kingdom Prospective Diabetes Study, or UKPDS, for study of type 2 DM[4]) have demonstrated that control of hyperglycemia reduces the risk or development of diabetic microvascular complications. However, the UKPDS suggested that the microvascular complications correlated with duration of the disease. Furthermore, neither study showed any clinically significant decrease in diabetic macrovascular complications with control of hyperglycemia. Because diabetic complications are correlated to the duration of disease and the intensity of hyperglycemia, the best chance of decreasing the socioeconomic burden of DM is to detect DM in the predisease phase to delay or prevent the development of DM. Over the last decade, several studies in Sweden and China suggested that lifestyle changes could prevent DM, but their conclusions were limited because of suboptimal study design.[5,6] Recently, 4 well-designed, randomized studies have demonstrated that the onset of type 2 DM can be delayed or prevented. The Finnish Diabetes Prevention Study Group enrolled 522 middle-aged (mean age, 55 years), obese (mean body mass index [BMI], 31 kg/m²) male and female subjects with impaired glucose tolerance (IGT). The study then randomized subjects to either a control group receiving brief dietary and exercise counseling or an intervention group participating in intense individualized counseling regarding a low-fat diet and weight reduction (7 visits with a dietitian in year 1) as well as exercise (supervised 30 minutes a day). After a mean follow-up of 3.2 years, the cumulative incidence of DM was significantly lower in the intervention group compared with the control group (23 vs 11%, respectively). This represents a 58% risk reduction in the intervention group. At the end of 2 years, the mean weight loss was 3.5 kg in the intervention group compared with 0.8 kg in the control group. In this study, 22 subjects with IGT had to be treated with aggressive lifestyle intervention for 1 year to prevent 1 case of DM.[7]

Another study, the Diabetes Prevention Program Group, enrolled 3234 obese subjects (mean BMI, 34 kg/m²) with IGT, aged 25 to 85 years (mean age, 51 years). Of the subjects, 68% were women, and 45% were members of minority groups. Subjects were assigned to one of the following 3 groups: (1) intensive lifestyle modification with a goal of reducing weight by 7%, following a low-fat diet, and exercising for 150 min/wk; (2) treatment with metformin hydrochloride (850 mg twice daily) and general information regarding diet and exercise; and (3) placebo pill twice a day plus general diet and exercise information. After an average follow-up of 2.8 years, the incidence of diabetes was 4.8, 7.8, and 11 cases per 100 person-years in the lifestyle, metformin, and placebo groups, respectively. The lifestyle group reduced the incidence of DM by 58%, whereas metformin therapy reduced it by 31%. In the lifestyle group, 50% of subjects achieved the weight reduction goal of 7% at 1 year but, by the end of the study, only 38% of this group maintained their 7% goal. In the lifestyle group, 74% of subjects achieved the goal of 150 min/wk of moderately intense exercise at the end of 2 months, but the percentage dropped to 58% by the end of the study. Lifestyle intervention was effective in both men and women, all ages, and all ethnic groups. Metformin was relatively ineffective in prevention of DM in older individuals (age, >60 years) and less overweight subjects (BMI, <30 kg/m²). However, metformin was as effective as lifestyle modification in younger individuals (aged 24 to 44 years) and heavier subjects (BMI, >35 kg/m²).[8,9]

In the Troglitazone in Prevention of Diabetes Study, 235 Hispanic women with a previous history of gestational DM were randomized to a placebo or troglitazone (later taken off the market because of liver toxicity). After a median follow-up of 30 months, the incidence of type 2 DM was 12.3% vs 5.4% in the placebo vs troglitazone group, respectively. Troglitazone had a 56% relative reduction in development of type 2 DM. The preventive effect of troglitazone was still present after an 8-month washout period. This suggests that troglitazone may afford some protection to the b-cell, helping to prevent rather than just delay the onset of DM.[9] The Stop-NIDDM (non–insulin-dependent DM) Trial randomized 1429 individuals with IGT (mean age of 55 years and mean BMI of 31 kg/m²) to placebo or a-glucosidase inhibitor (acarbose).[10] After a 3.3-year mean follow-up, there was a 25% decreased relative risk of type 2 DM. Of note, 31% of the acarbose group and 19% of the placebo group discontinued treatment early. Acarbose often produced flatulence and diarrhea.

SCREENING AND PREVENTION OF TYPE 2 DIABETES

With the knowledge that type 2 DM can be prevented, strategies can be developed to provide cost-effective screening programs using reliable and convenient tests. These strategies should consider estimates that disturbances in insulin secretion and/or action may start more than 10 years before the clinical diagnosis of type 2 DM.[11] Also, at the time of diagnosis of type 2 DM, 20% of these newly diagnosed diabetic individuals already have retinopathy, and 10% have nephropathy and neuropathy. Criteria for the diagnosis of diabetes are outlined in Table 62-1.

Current screening tests for type 2 DM include fasting plasma glucose (FPG), random glucose, and oral glucose tolerance test (OGTT). In 1997, the Expert Committee of the American Diabetes Association lowered the threshold for diagnosis of DM from an FPG level of 140 mg/dL (7.8 mmol/L) to 126 mg/dL (7.0 mmol/L). The change was made to eliminate a perceived discrepancy between the threshold cutoffs of the 2-hour plasma glucose after a 75-g oral glucose load and the FPG in diagnosing type 2 DM. The committee revised criteria for diagnosis of DM, advising that diagnosis of DM could be made on the basis of 2 fasting glucose values greater than 125 mg/dL (6.9 mmol/L) or 2 random glucose values over 200 mg/dL (11.1 mmol/L). This committee also released a new term, *impaired fasting glucose* (IFG), for individuals with fasting glucose between 110 mg/dL (6.1 mmol/L) and 125 mg/dL (6.9 mmol/L), paralleling the implications associated with IGT. Individuals with IGT do not have diabetic microvascular complications but are at increased risk of macrovascular disease and DM. The rate of progression from IGT to overt DM varies between different populations from 36 to 87 per 1000 person-years.[12] Since the OGTT has poor reproducibility and is inconvenient and expensive, the test generally is not performed in nonpregnant individuals for diagnosis of type 2 DM unless for research purposes.

Measurement of glycosylated hemoglobin (Hb A_{1C}) has been mentioned as a possible screening test for type 2 DM. In a 6-year prospective study in 381 high-risk nondiabetic Pima Indians, Hb A_{1C} appeared to be a better predictor for risk of type 2 DM than OGTT was. During this study, DM developed in 38% of individuals with an abnormal OGTT, in 50% with elevated Hb A_{1C} levels, and 69% with abnormality of both OGTT and Hb A_{1C} values. However, the International Expert Committee

T ABLE   62-1

Criteria for Diagnosis of Diabetes*

Normoglycemia	IFG or IGT	Diabetes†
FPG <110 mg/dL (<6.1 mmol/L); 2-h PG‡ <140 mg/dL (<7.8 mmol/L)	IFG: FPG 110–125 mg/dL (6.1–6.9 mmol/L) IGT: 2-h PG‡ 140–199 mg/dL (7.8–11.0 mmol/L)	FPG ≥126 mg/dL (≥7.0 mmol/L); 2-h PG‡ ≥200 mg/dL (≥11.1 mmol/L); or symptoms of diabetes and casual plasma glucose concentration ≥200 mg/dL (≥11.1 mmol/L)

*IFG indicates impaired fasting glucose; IGT, impaired glucose tolerance; FPG, fasting plasma glucose; and PG, plasma glucose. From *Diabetes Care.* 2003;26(suppl 1):S21–S24.[17] Reprinted with permission from the American Diabetes Association.

†A diagnosis of diabetes must be confirmed, on a subsequent day, by measurement of FPG, 2-hour PG, or random plasma glucose (if symptoms are present). The FPG test is greatly preferred because of ease of administration, convenience, acceptability to patients, and lower cost. Fasting is defined as no energy intake for at least 8 hours.

‡This test requires the use of a glucose load containing the equivalent of 75 g of anhydrous glucose dissolved in water. 2-hour PG, 2-hour postload glucose.

advised not to use Hb A_{1C} for screening because of lack of standardization and the imperfect correlation between Hb A_{1C} and FPG.[13] Fasting plasma proinsulin and the plasma insulin response during the first 30 minutes of an OGTT have been shown to predict diabetes but are not widely used for screening because of cost and availability.

Gestational DM is often thought of as a subgroup of type 2 DM. Approximately 7% of all pregnancies are complicated by gestational DM. However, the prevalence of gestational DM can vary depending on the population studied and tests used for diagnosis. Pregnant women can be classified by high risk, average risk, or low risk depending on age, weight, past medical history, family history, and ethnicity. The low-risk group includes pregnant females younger than 25 years with normal pre-pregnant weight; not belonging to a high-risk ethnic group; not having any first-degree relatives with DM; and not having any personal history of previous glucose intolerance or poor obstetric outcomes, hypertension, or hyperlipidemia. This low-risk group does not require glucose testing. Pregnant women at high risk are those with marked obesity and a personal history of gestational DM and/or strong family history of DM. These women should be tested as early as possible and, if they have a normal baseline FPG level, again at 24 to 28 weeks gestation with a serum glucose test 1 hour after a 50-g oral glucose challenge. A glucose value greater than 140 mg/dL (7.8 mmol/L) identifies up to 80% of individuals with gestational DM and should have confirmatory testing with a 100-g OGTT. Normal values for the 3-hour OGTT with 100 g of glucose are:[14]

Fasting	<95 mg/dL (<5.3 mmol/L)
2 h	<180 mg/dL (<10.0 mmol/L)
3 h	<140 mg/dL (<7.8 mmol/L)

If the test result is abnormal, the patient will need institution of therapeutic counseling or treatment, or both. Women with gestational DM should be reevaluated with an OGTT 6 to 8 weeks after delivery. Pregnant women at average risk merely should be screened for gestational DM with a plasma glucose test 1 hour after a 50-g oral glucose load at 24 to 28 weeks of gestation.[14] Women with a history of gestational DM should be screened yearly for DM with an FPG test. In addition, offspring of women with gestational DM have increased risk of obesity, glucose intolerance, and DM in adolescence and young adulthood.

The US Preventive Services Task Force and the American Diabetes Association have formulated recommendations for screening adults for type 2 diabetes.[15,16] Insufficient evidence exists to demonstrate that community screening is cost-effective in reducing morbidity or mortality associated with DM in presumably healthy individuals. Although the main benefit of community screening may be to raise public awareness of DM and its complications, less costly methods may be more appro-

priate.[17] The Expert Committee of the American Diabetes Association advises that screening for type 2 DM with an FPG test should start at age 45 years in presumptively healthy patients and be repeated at 3-year intervals unless there is a change in risk factors. Screening should be started earlier in adulthood and then yearly in the presence of any of the following risk factors:[12,17]

1. Obesity, defined as ideal body weight greater than 120%, BMI over 25 kg/m², waist-to-hip ratio greater than 0.95 in men or more than 0.85 in women, and waist circumference greater than 102 cm (44 in) in men or more than 88 cm (34 in) in women.[18]

2. Family history of DM in a first-degree relative. (Lifetime risk of type 2 DM is 70% to 80% for the offspring of 2 parents or a monozygotic twin with type 2 DM and 30% to 40% with having a dizygotic twin or any other first-degree relative with type 2 DM.)[19]

3. Habitual physical inactivity.

4. Belonging to a high-risk race or ethnic group: African American, Hispanic, Native American, or Asian American.

5. History of gestational DM or delivering a baby weighing more than 4 kg (9 lb) at term.

6. Being an offspring of a mother with gestational DM.

7. History of having a low birth weight (<3 kg [6.6 lb]), particularly in males.[20]

8. Irregular menses with intervals greater than 40 days, particularly when associated with hirsutism and relative infertility, which is often secondary to the polycystic ovarian syndrome.[21]

9. Presence of coronary and/or peripheral vascular disease.

10. Elevated markers of inflammation (ultra sensitive-C-reactive protein and interleukin-6) in women.[22]

11. Hypertension (blood pressure >140/90 mm Hg).

12. Triglyceride levels greater than 150 mg/dL (1.69 mmol/L) and/or low HDL-C (<35 mg/dL [0.91 mmol/L] in men and <45 mg/dL [1.16 mmol/L] in women.)

The above risk factors pertain to adults. With the increasing incidence of type 2 DM in children and adolescents, screening should be considered in young persons when they have excess body weight (BMI) greater than the 85th percentile for age and weight, body weight for height greater than the 85th percentile, or weight greater than 120% of ideal body weight and any 2 of the following risks:

1. Family history of type 2 DM in first- and second-degree relatives.

2. Member of a high-risk race and/or ethnic group.

3. Signs of insulin resistance or conditions associated with insulin resistance such as acanthosis nigricans.

Children fulfilling the above high-risk criteria should start screening for type 2 DM every 2 years beginning at age 10 years or at the onset of puberty if it occurs at an earlier age.[17]

Nondiabetic medications have been found to decrease the incidence of type 2 DM in the Pravachol in the West of Scotland Cardiovascular Disease Prevention Study [23] and the Ramipril in the Heart Outcome Prevention Evaluation (HOPE).[24] The mechanism of how these medications may delay or prevent type 2 DM is not known.

Primary prevention of DM depends on several factors:

- increasing public awareness of the importance of good eating habits, regular aerobic exercise, and attaining and maintaining ideal body weight

- increasing astuteness of physicians, dentists, and other health workers in identifying risks for the prediabetic state

- promoting appropriate screening, counseling, and treatment to individuals as needed

Clinical studies have shown that improved glycemic control benefits individuals with either type 1 or type 2 DM. Every 1% reduction in Hb A_{1C} level is estimated to reduce by 40% the risk of microvascular complications, including eye, kidney, or nerve function. Therefore, diabetic patients are advised to control blood glucose levels such that Hb A_{1C} is less than 7% or, even better if possible, closer to the normal level of less than 6%, without hypoglycemic adverse effects.

Blood pressure control also can reduce cardiovascular complications up to 33% to 50% and diabetic microvascular disease up to 33%.[2] For every 10-mm Hg reduction in systolic blood pressure, diabetic complications are estimated to be reduced by 12%. Therefore, diabetic patients are advised to optimally maintain blood pressure at less than 130/80 mm Hg.[2] Control of cholesterol and triglyceride levels can reduce cardiovascular complication levels up to 20% to 50%. Therefore, lipid control in diabetic patients should maintain goals of HDL-C over 45 mg/dL (1.16 mmol/L) in males and greater than 55 mg/dL (1.42 mmol/L) in females, and for both males and females low-density lipoprotein cholesterol (LDL-C) levels should be under 100 mg/dL (2.59 mmol/L) and triglyceride levels under 150 mg/dL (3.88 mmol/L).[2]

Diagnosis and treatment of diabetic eye disease with laser treatment can reduce severe visual loss up to 60% and blindness up to 90%. Only approximately 60% of individuals with diabetes undergo annual dilated eye examination.[2] Yearly comprehensive eye examinations should be undertaken by diabetic patients.

Comprehensive foot care can reduce the risk of amputation by 45% to 85%. Daily patient self-care of feet and periodic professional foot care are crucial for individuals with peripheral vascular disease and/or diabetic peripheral neuropathy.[2]

Diagnosis and treatment of early diabetic kidney disease can reduce the development of renal failure by 30% to 70%.[2] Optimizing blood pressure control to levels under 130/80 mm Hg and use of angiotensin-converting enzyme inhibitors help to preserve renal function.

Individuals with diabetes can develop a diabetic cardiomyopathy characterized by diastolic and/or systolic left ventricular dysfunction, often secondary to metabolic alterations, interstitial fibrosis, myocellular hypertrophy, microvascular disease, and autonomic dysfunction. Unfortunately, these subtle changes usually will not be detected with a standard treadmill exercise (stress) test but can be detected with an echocardiogram exercise test or pharmacologic stress testing. This testing should be considered in a diabetic patient with cardiovascular symptoms, hypertension, peripheral neuropathy, or peripheral vascular disease. As prevention of cardiovascular disease, persons with diabetes, IGT, or IFT are advised to consider taking 1 buffered baby aspirin (81 mg) daily with food unless they have active peptic ulcer disease, bleeding tendencies, aspirin sensitivity, or another contraindication.

Every year 10,000 to 30,000 diabetic individuals die of complications associated with influenza or pneumonia. Diabetic patients are 3 times more likely to die of these complications than are nondiabetic persons. Diabetic adults should receive pneumococcal vaccination at any age and 1 subsequent booster 5 years later as well as influenza vaccinations annually. Table 62-2 summarizes preventive management recommendations in diabetic patients.

PREVENTION OF TYPE 1 DIABETES

Type 1 DM is the most common metabolic disease affecting children and adolescents. In the United States, 0.19% of the population under age 20 years has diabetes, and approximately 13,000 new cases of type 1 DM occur each year in this age group.[25] The prevalence of type 1 DM in Finland is 1 in 200 at age 18 years, the highest prevalence in the world.[26] Before the discovery of insulin in 1922, type 1 DM was, fortunately, a rare disorder. Since the middle of the last century, however, there has been a linear increase in the incidence of type 1 DM.[26] This increase has far outpaced the rise that might be expected by an increase of type 1 DM susceptibility genes in the population due to survival of individuals with this type of DM and their ability to reproduce.[26] The rising incidence is most marked among children younger than 4 years.[27,28] In Denmark the overall incidence rate of type 1 DM rose from 14.03 per 100,000 person-years in 1976 to 19.4 in 2000.[27] The alarming increase of type 1 DM, combined with the new pandemic of type 2 DM in children

TABLE 62-2

Follow-Up Preventive Management Goals for Type 2 Diabetes*

Checkpoints	Goal	Frequency of Check
Blood pressure, with patient sitting and standing	<130/80 mm Hg	Every visit
Body weight		Every visit
Cardiovascular examination		Every visit
Foot examination		Every visit
Sensorineural examination (pinprick and vibration)		Every 6–12 mo
Deep tendon reflexes		Every 6–12 mo
Eye examination (dilated)		Yearly
Hb A$_{1C}$	<7% (<0.07)	Every 3–4 mo
HDL-C	Males >45 mg/dL (>1.16 mmol/L) Females >55 mg/dL (>1.42 mmol/L)	Yearly
LDL-C	<100 mg/dL (<2.59 mmol/L)	Yearly
Triglycerides	<150 mg/dL (<3.88 mmol/L)	Yearly
Spot urinary albumin-creatinine ratio	<30 mg/g	Yearly
Serum creatinine	<1.4 mg/dL (<123.8 μmol/L)	Yearly
Electrocardiogram		Every 1–2 y
Stress echocardiogram		Consider every 3–4 y
Diabetic education	Annual refresher	As needed
Nutritional counseling	Annual refresher	As needed
Exercise counseling	Annual refresher	As needed
Self-monitoring of blood glucose levels	Before meals <120 mg/dL (<6.7 mmol/L) 2 h Postprandial <140 mg/dL (<7.8 mmol/L)	As needed

*Hb 1AC indicates glycosylated hemoglobin; HDL-C, high-density lipoprotein cholesterol; and LDL-C, low-density lipoprotein cholesterol.

and adolescents, will make diabetes and its consequences a major public problem in the next 50 years.[29,30]

The development of type 1 DM probably involves environmental triggers that activate autoimmune mechanisms in genetically susceptible individuals, causing the demise of pancreatic islet B cells. Predisposition is mediated by a number of genes that interact in a complex manner with each other and the environment.[31] The HLA-DQA and DQB genes located on the short arm of chromosome 6 provide the strongest genetic influence on the development of type 1 DM. DQA*0501/DQB*0201 and DQ*0301/DQB*0201 are the most common type 1 DM–prone haplotypes, whereas DQA*0102/DQB*0602 is protective and makes the development of type 1 DM unlikely, even when islet cell antibodies are present.[32] The incidence of type 1 DM varies greatly between ethnic groups, probably reflecting differences in the prevalence of type 1 DM susceptibility genes within the groups.[33]

If the pool of susceptible individuals in the population has remained nearly constant over the past 50 years, the rising incidence of childhood type 1 DM strongly suggests that something has changed in the environment to which children are exposed.[25] Some of the postulated

changes include infectious agents such as enteroviruses and *Streptomyces*.[30] Other proposed changes include early exposure to cow's milk or increased levels of nitrates in drinking water.[34] Careful surveillance of childhood immunizations, and the timing of the immunizations, strongly suggests that childhood immunizations are probably not one of these environmental risk factors.[35] An alternative hypothesis is that some protective factor has been lost from the environment. The hygiene hypothesis postulates that early exposure to infectious agents is required for normal immune development. In the absence of such exposure, deleterious autoimmune diseases may develop later. However, there is little evidence to support this as a cause of type 1 DM.[26]

Once a genetically susceptible child has been exposed to a triggering environmental factor, an indolent cell-mediated autoimmune destruction of pancreatic islet B cells begins. This indolent phase can last from weeks to years; generally the younger the individual, the shorter the duration. During this time, humoral islet cell antibodies can be detected in the blood as markers of this autoimmune attack. These islet cell antibodies have been specifically identified as antibodies to glutamic acid decarboxylase-65, tyrosine phosphatase–like protein 1A-2A, and insulin. The presence of 1 or more of these antibodies is one way of identifying individuals at risk before the actual onset of clinical type 1 DM.

The way the B cell stores and secretes insulin also changes before the development of type 1 DM. In response to a rapid intravenous infusion of glucose, the B cell should immediately release stored insulin (first-phase insulin response). Several minutes later, newly synthesized insulin is secreted to maintain normal glucose levels. Loss of the first-phase insulin response in children with islet cell antibodies places these individuals at a very high risk of type 1 DM developing within the next 5 years.[36]

Because of the autoimmune nature of type 1 DM, various immunosuppressive agents have been given to children with a recent onset of type 1 DM. The list of failed therapies is large and includes, among others, cyclosporin, azathioprine, FK506, levamisole, BCG vaccination, and even oral insulin. It is now believed that any immunomodulating therapy would have to be initiated early during the indolent phase to have any hope of preserving B cell mass and function. With this in mind, 2 large-scale studies are nearing completion.[37] The Diabetes Prevention Trial—Type 1 (DPT-1), sponsored by the National Institutes of Health (NIH), studied both subcutaneous and oral insulin treatment in first-degree relatives of individuals with type 1 DM. Those subjects who had both islet cell antibodies and absent first-phase insulin response were randomized to a subcutaneous insulin treatment group or an observation group. This study showed, after a median follow-up of 3.7 years, that type 1 DM had developed in approximately 40% of the subjects in both groups. Thus, there appears to be no protective effect of starting subcutaneous insulin therapy before the onset of clinical type 1 DM.[38] Those subjects who had islet cell antibodies but normal first-phase insulin response were randomized to receive either oral insulin or placebo. Results of this study have not yet been released. The European Nicotinamide Diabetes Intervention Trial (ENDIT) also studied first-degree relatives of individuals with type 1 DM. Subjects with positive islet cell antibodies were randomized to receive nicotinamide or placebo. The mechanism whereby nicotinamide might prevent the progression of autoimmune B-cell destruction is not well understood.[37] Results of this trial also have not yet been released.

Identifying individuals who might be at risk of type 1 DM has no current practical utility because no intervention has yet been found that can effectively and safely alter the progression of the autoimmune destruction of pancreatic B cells once it has started. Testing for islet cell antibodies can be helpful when a clinician wants to determine whether an obese child who is serendipitously found to have hyperglycemia has early type 1 DM or type 2 DM, since the treatment strategy will be different for each.

The NIH also has initiated the Type 1 Diabetes Trial Net. This multicenter study will coordinate the ongoing screening of relatives of individuals with type 1 DM for islet cell antibodies, and other determinations of risk of type 1 DM, such as genotyping. This study also will coordinate trials of new immunomodulating therapies in the hope of identifying one that will alter the indolent autoimmune destruction of the pancreatic B cells and prevent the development of clinical type 1 DM.

Some of the immunomodulating therapies that may be studied in the future include DAB-IL-2 (a diphtheria toxin conjugated to part of the interleukin-2 molecule), monoclonal antibodies against intercellular adhesion molecules, DiaPep227 (a peptide derived from 60-kd heat shock protein), and anti-CD3 monoclonal antibodies.[39]

REFERENCES

1. King H, Aubert RE, Herman W. The global burden of diabetes—1995 through 2025: prevalence, numerical estimate and projections. *Diabetes Care.* 1998;21:1414–1431.

2. National Institute of Diabetes and Digestive and Kidney Diseases. *National Diabetes Statistics Fact Sheet: General Information and National Estimates on Diabetes in the United States, 2000.* Bethesda, Md: US Department of Health and Human Services; 2002.

3. The Diabetes Control and Complications Trial Research Group. The effect of intensive treatment of diabetes on the development and progression of long-term complications in insulin-dependent diabetes mellitus. *N Engl J Med.* 1993;329:977–986.

4. United Kingdom Prospective Diabetes Study (UKPDS) Group. Intensive blood-glucose control with sulphonylureas or insulin compared with conventional treatment and risk of complications in patients with type 2 diabetes (UKPDS33). *Lancet.* 1998;352:837.

5. Eriksson KF, Lindgarde F. Prevention of type 2 (non-insulin dependent) diabetes mellitus by diet and physical exercise: the 6-year Malmo feasibility study. *Diabetologia.* 1991;34:891–898.

6. Pan XP, Li GW, Hu YG, et al. Effects of diet and exercise in preventing NIDDM in people with impaired glucose tolerances: the Da Qing IGT and Diabetes Study. *Diabetes Care.* 1997;20:537–544.

7. Tuomilehto J, Lindstrom J, Eriksson JG, et al. Prevention of type 2 diabetes mellitus by changes in lifestyle among subjects with impaired glucose tolerance. *N Engl J Med.* 2001;344:1343–1350.

8. Diabetes Prevention Research Group. Reduction in evidence of type 2 diabetes with lifestyle intervention or metformin. *N Engl J Med.* 2002;346:393–403.

9. American Diabetes Association. Clinical practice recommendations 2003: the prevention or delay of type 2 diabetes. *Diabetes Care.* 2003;26(suppl 1):S62–S69.

10. Chiasson Jl, Josse KG, Gomis R, et al, for the Stop-NIDDM Trial Research Group. Acarbose for prevention of type 2 diabetes mellitus: the STOP-NIDDM randomized trial. *Lancet.* 2002;359:2072–2077.

11. Ramlo-Halsted BA, Edelman SV. The natural history of diabetes mellitus: implications for clinical practice. *Primary Care.* 1999;26:771–789.

12. McCulloch DK, Robertson RP. Prediction and prevention of type 2 diabetes mellitus. *UpToDate.* May 2002.

13. Barr RG, Nathan DM, Meigs JB, et al. Tests of glycemia for the diagnosis of type 2 diabetes mellitus. *Ann Intern Med.* 2002;137: 263–272.

14. American Diabetes Association. Practice recommendations 2003: gestational diabetes mellitus. *Diabetes Care.* 2003;26(suppl 1):S103.

15. Harris R, Donahue K, Rathore S, et al. Screening adults for type 2 diabetes: a review of the evidence for the U.S. Preventive Services Task Force. *Ann Intern Med.* 2003;138:215–229.

16. US Preventive Service Task Force. Screening for type 2 diabetes mellitus in adults: recommendations and rationale. *Ann Intern Med.* 2003;138:212–214.

17. American Diabetes Association. Clinical practice recommendations 2003: screening for type 2 Diabetes. *Diabetes Care.* 2003;26(suppl 1):S21–S27.

18. Janssen I, Katzmarzyk PT, Ross R. Body mass index, waist circumference, and health risk. *Arch Intern Med.* 2002;162:2074–2079.

19. Florez J, Altshuler D. The inherited basis of type 2 diabetes: current knowledge and future prospects. *Endocrinol Grands.* 2002;1(9).

20. Forsen T, Eriksson J, Tuomilehto J, Osmond C, Barker D. The fetal and childhood growth of persons who develop type 2 diabetes mellitus. *Ann Intern Med.* 2000;133:176–182.

21. Solomon CG, Hu FB, Dunaif A, et al. Long or highly irregular menstrual cycles as a marker for risk of type 2 diabetes mellitus. *JAMA.* 2001;286:2421–2426.

22. Pradhan AD, Manson JE, Rifai N, Buring JE, Ridker PM. C-reactive protein, interleukin 6 and risk of developing type 2 diabetes mellitus. *JAMA.* 2001;386:327–334.

23. Freeman DJ, Norrie J, Sattar N, et al. Provastalin and the development of diabetes mellitus: evidence for protective treatment effect in the West of Scotland Coronary Prevention Study. *Circulation.* 2001;103:357–362.

24. Yusuf S, Sleight P, Pogue J, Bosch J, Davies R, Dagenais G, for the Heart Outcomes Prevention Study Investigators. Effects of an angiotensin-converting enzyme inhibitor, ramipril, on cardiovascular events in high-risk patients. *N Engl J Med.* 2000;342:145–153.

25. National Institute of Diabetes and Digestive and Kidney Diseases. General information and national estimates on diabetes in the United States, 2000. Available at: www.niddk.nih.gov/health/diabetes/pubs/dmstats/dmstats.htm. Accessed January 7, 2003.

26. Gale EAM. The rise of childhood type 1 diabetes in the 20th century. *Diabetes.* 2002;51:3353–3361.

27. Svensson J, Carstensen B, Molbak AG, et al, for the Danish Study Group of Diabetes in Childhood. Increased risk of childhood type 1 diabetes in children born after 1985. *Diabetes Care.* 2002;25:2197–2201.

28. Charkaluk ML, Czernichow P, Levy-Marchal C. Incidence data of childhood-onset type 1 diabetes in France during 1988–1997: the case for a shift toward younger age at onset. *Pediatr Res.* 2002;53:859–862.

29. Fagot-Campagna A, Pettitt DJ, Engelgau MM, et al. Type 2 diabetes among North American children and adolescents: an epidemiologic review and a public health perspective. *J Pediatr.* 2000;136:664–672.

30. Zimet P, Alberti KGMM, Shaw J. Global and societal implication of the diabetes epidemic. *Nature.* 2001;414:782–787.

31. Atkinson MA, Maclaren NK. The pathogenesis of insulin-dependent diabetes mellitus. *N Engl J Med.* 1994;331:1428–1436.

32. Owerbach D, Gunn S, Ty G, Wible L, Gabbay KH. Oligonucleotide probes for HLA-DQA and DQB genes define susceptibility to type 1 (insulin-dependent) diabetes mellitus. *Diabetologia.* 1988;31:751–757.

33. Bennett PH, Rewers MJ, Knowler WC. Epidemiology of diabetes mellitus. In: Porte D Jr, Sherwin RS, Baron A, eds. *Ellenberg & Rifkin's Diabetes Mellitus.* 6th ed. New York, NY: McGraw-Hill; 2003:281.

34. McCulloch DK. Pathogenesis of type 1 diabetes mellitus. Available at: www.uptodateonline.com/application/topic/print.asp?file+diabetes/5832. Accessed January 7, 2003.

35. Destefano F, Mullooly J, Okoro C, et al, for the Vaccine Safety Datalink Team. Childhood vaccinations, vaccination timing, and risk of type 2 diabetes mellitus. *Pediatrics.* 2001;108:1–5.

36. Ginsberg-Fellner F, Witt ME, Franklin BH, et al. Triad of markers for identifying children at high risk of developing insulin-dependent diabetes mellitus. *JAMA.* 1985;254:1469–1472.

37. Schatz DA, Rogers DG, Brouhard BH. Prevention of insulin-dependent diabetes mellitus: an overview of three trials. *Cleve Clin J Med.* 1996;63:270–274.

38. Diabetes Prevention Trial—Type1 Diabetes Study Group. Effects of insulin in relatives of patients with type 1 diabetes mellitus. *N Engl J Med.* 2002;346:1685–1691.

39. McCulloch DK. Prevention of type 1 diabetes mellitus. Available at: www.uptodateonline.com/application/topic/print.asp?file=diabetes/925. Accessed January 7, 2003.

RESOURCES

American Association of Diabetic Educators, 100 W Monroe St, Suite 400, Chicago, IL 60603; 800 338-3633.
Web site: www.aadenet.org.

American Diabetes Association, 1701 North Beauregard St, Alexandria, VA 22311; 800 342-2383.
Web site: www.diabetes.org.

Division of Diabetes Translation, National Center for Chronic Disease Prevention and Health Promotion, Centers for Disease Control and Prevention, 4770 Buford Hwy NE, Mailstop K-10, Atlanta, GA 30341; 770 488-5000.
Web site: www.cdc.gov/diabetes.

Juvenile Diabetes Research Foundation International, 120 Wall St, New York, NY 10005; 800 533-2873.
Web site: www.jdrf.org.

National Diabetes Education Program.
Web site: www.ndep.nih.gov.

National Diabetes Information Clearinghouse.
E-mail: nidc@info.niddk.nih.gov.

chapter 63

Thyroid Disease

Anne M. Rosenberg, MD, and Vahab Fatourechi, MD

INTRODUCTION

Clinical preventive medicine is used in various thyroid disorders. An example of primary prevention is iodine supplementation of salt to prevent thyroid disorders caused by iodine deficiency. An example of secondary prevention is the early detection of thyroid cancer in patients with a history of radiation exposure. Tertiary prevention would include prescribing the appropriate dose of thyroid replacement in hypothyroid patients to avoid complications from iatrogenic hypothyroidism or hyperthyroidism. Several preventive measures in the specialty of thyroid disease will be discussed in this chapter.

PREVENTION OF IODINE DEFICIENCY AND IODINE DEFICIENCY THYROID DISORDERS

Iodine is an element present in small amounts in the human body (15 to 20 mg). The recommended daily dietary allowance for iodine by the World Health Organization (WHO) is 90 μg for preschool children 0 to 59 months, 120 μg for children 6 to 12 years old, 150 μg for children older than 12 years and adults, and 200 μg for pregnant and lactating women.[1] The only known role of iodine is for the synthesis of thyroid hormones triiodothyronine (T_3) and thyroxine (T_4). Therefore, iodine deficiency may lead to impaired thyroid hormone production.[2]

Thyroid hormones T_3 and T_4 are required for prenatal and postnatal brain development. Therefore, the greatest impact of iodine deficiency on cognition occurs during gestation and early postnatal life. If the physiological requirements for iodine are not met, a variety of clinical complications may occur, such as goiter, hypothyroidism, endemic cretinism, decreased fertility, increased perinatal death, and infant mortality (Table 63-1).[2,3] Collectively, these complications are known as iodine deficiency disorders (IDDs). Iodine deficiency is the most important risk factor for development of goiter and for intellectual deficiency worldwide.[4,5]

Iodine deficiency disorders are preventable with adequate dietary intake of iodine. The iodine content in most foods is generally low, with the highest content found in

TABLE 63-1

Spectrum of Iodine Deficiency Disorders*

Fetus
Abortions
Stillbirths
Increased perinatal and infant mortality
Endemic cretinism
Neurologic cretinism
Mental deficiency
Deaf-mutism
Spastic diplegia
Squint
Myxedematous cretinism
Mental deficiency
Hypothyroidism
Dwarfism
Neonate
Goiter
Neonatal hypothyroidism
Infant, child
Goiter
Adolescent
Juvenile hypothyroidism
Impaired mental and physical development
Adult
Goiter
Hypothyroidism
Endemic mental retardation
Decreased fertility rate

*From the World Health Organization.[3]

fish and smaller amounts found in milk, eggs, and meat.[6] The importance of IDDs was addressed at the World Summit for Children at the United Nations in 1990 when the goal of elimination of IDDs by the year 2000 was endorsed. The main strategy employed to reach this goal was universal iodination of all salt ingested by humans and livestock.[7] Iodized salt has been used in the United States since 1924, and 90% of households in the Americas have access to iodized salt. However, IDDs continue to occur because of various socioeconomic, cultural, and political limitations to iodine supplementation programs.[2] In fact, only 27% of European households have access to iodized salt.[1]

Iodine nutrition in the United States was analyzed based on data from the National Health and Nutrition Examination Surveys (NHANES) I (1971–1974) and III (1988–1994).[4] The urinary iodine (UI) concentration is the most useful tool to monitor iodine nutritional status. The median UI concentrations should be greater than 10 μg/dL, and less than 20% of the population should have UI below 5 μg/dL. Overall, the UI concentrations in the United States indicate adequate iodine intake. However, the median UI concentrations for the US population fell from 32.0 μg/dL between 1971 and 1974 to 14.5 μg/dL in 1988 to 1994 (P<.0001). Additionally, there was a 4.5-fold increase in the number of people with low UI concentrations (<5 μg/dL) during this same period. This downward trend in iodine status will require close monitoring in the future to avoid the reappearance of iodine deficiency in the United States.

PREVENTABLE RISK FACTORS FOR GOITER

The WHO has defined criteria for the classification of goiter by palpation. A grade 0 goiter is one that is not palpable or visible by physical examination. A grade 1 goiter is palpable but not visible when the neck is in the normal position. A goiter is classified as grade 2 if there is swelling in the neck that is clearly visible when the neck is in normal position and is consistent with an enlarged thyroid when the neck is palpated.[1]

Iodine deficiency is the most important risk factor for goiter, underscoring the importance of population-based iodine supplementation programs to eradicate iodine deficiency. However, a goiter does not always indicate iodine deficiency. Thyroid volume tends to increase up to the age of 40 years and then decreases. The prevalence of goiter is 2 to 10 times higher in women. Parity is a known risk factor for goiter, as pregnancy may increase thyroid volume in iodine-deficient areas. However, this only partially explains the sexual difference in goiter prevalence.[5] Women are also predisposed to goiter and thyroid dysfunction because of genetic and hormonal immunologic factors.

Goitrogens in food have been studied in certain geographic areas. Natural goitrogens were first discovered in vegetables from the *Cruciferae* family. These vegetables contain thioglucosides that, when digested, have antithyroid properties. Another group of naturally occurring goitrogens are the cyanoglucosides, which are found in foods such as cassava, maize, bamboo shoots, sweet potatoes, and lima beans. After digestion, cyanoglucosides release thiocyanate, which is a powerful inhibitor of thyroid iodide transport and at high levels can compete with iodide inorganification.[2]

PREVENTION AND EARLY DETECTION OF THYROID CANCER

The annual incidence of follicular cell–derived thyroid cancer ranges between 2.0 and 3.8 cases per 100,000 in women and 1.2 to 1.6 cases per 100,000 in men. Women of childbearing age are at the highest risk.[8] Because of its favorable prognosis, thyroid cancer is responsible for less than 1% of all cancer-related deaths in the United States. Overall, few modifiable lifestyle factors greatly increase the risk of thyroid cancer.

Several studies have shown that thyroid cancer is 2 to 4 times more frequent in females than males.[8] This difference is negligible before puberty and subsequent to female menopause, which suggests that the etiology of thyroid cancer may be related to reproductive function and female sex hormones. Observational studies have provided limited support for this hypothesis. However, it remains unclear how sex hormones influence thyroid oncogenesis.

Risk Factors for Thyroid Cancer

Dietary habits may have an impact on the risk of thyroid cancer. Individuals with high consumption of butter, cheese,[9] or refined cereals[10] may have an increased risk of follicular cell–derived thyroid cancer. Increased consumption of fish may have a protective effect in areas with current or remote iodine deficiency.[11] Consumption of fruits and vegetables may reduce the risk of thyroid cancer.[8,12]

Most studies demonstrate that the histopathological types of cancer differ in iodine-deficient areas and iodine-sufficient areas. The latter have a predominance of more differentiated forms of thyroid cancer, particularly papillary cancer. Iodine-deficient areas have a predominance of follicular and anaplastic thyroid cancers, which have a worse prognosis than papillary cancer.[13-15]

Several studies have demonstrated that cigarette smokers have a decreased risk of thyroid cancer compared with nonsmokers. The decreased risk exhibits a dose-response effect, and current smokers appear to be at a lower risk than past smokers.[16-18] A recent cohort study did not reproduce the previously observed negative effect of cigarette use on thyroid cancer risk.[19]

Occupational exposure to radiation from diagnostic X-ray equipment may increase the risk of follicular cell–derived thyroid cancer. However, this increased risk may reflect earlier detection of cancers in health care workers because of their ready access to health care.[8,20] Careers in wood processing, pulp and papermaking or exposure to silica may also increase the risk of papillary thyroid cancer.[21]

Radiation exposure, particularly as a child, is a well-established risk factor for the development of thyroid nodules and increased risk of a thyroid nodule being malignant. Up to 40% of clinically palpable thyroid nodules discovered in survivors of childhood therapeutic radiation are reported to be malignant.[22] In contrast, 5% of thyroid nodules in the general population of adults are likely to be malignant. Carcinomas that develop in association with radiation exposure are nearly all well-differentiated papillary or papillary-follicular carcinomas. It is extremely rare to develop anaplastic carcinoma as a result of radiation exposure.[2] There is a linear relationship between radiation dose and risk of thyroid cancer in children.[23] The risk decreases with age, as there is little apparent increased risk for patients exposed to radiation after 20 years of age. When interviewing a patient with a history of neck irradiation, it is essential to obtain history regarding the amount of radiation, site of radiation, and age at which the patient received radiation.

Surveillance for Thyroid Cancer After Radiation Exposure

Thyroid malignancies that develop after childhood therapeutic radiation therapy may not become evident for several years after the exposure, making lifelong clinical surveillance a necessity.[22] The optimal mode of surveillance is an area of controversy. Thyroid ultrasound is clearly a more sensitive screening modality than physical examination or thyroid scanning. Ultrasound is able to detect small lesions that would be undetectable by physical examination. However, the increased sensitivity of ultrasound may give rise to unnecessary additional studies and surgeries on clinically insignificant nodules.[24] A second flaw of ultrasound is operator dependence. There can be great interoperator variation in the assessment of thyroid nodules by ultrasound. Annual neck palpation and, according to some experts, periodic ultrasound examinations are advised in patients with a history of radiation exposure.

Once a thyroid nodule has been detected, regardless of the method, fine-needle aspiration biopsy (FNAB) is not only necessary but also a cost-effective, minimally invasive, safe, and clinically efficient test to determine whether the nodule is benign or malignant.[25] In the general population, the mean sensitivity of FNAB to detect thyroid malignancy is 82% (65% to 98%) and its specificity is 92% (72% to 100%). However, sensitivity may be slightly lower in patients who have received radiation therapy.[26] The 2 major limitations of FNAB for detection of thyroid malignancy are an inadequate sample and a nondiagnostic specimen, which occurs in up to 20% of cases.

Fortunately, external beam radiation is no longer used for treatment of benign disease, such as enlargement of the tonsils, adenoids, thymus, and lymph nodes as well as acne, pertussis, tinea capitis, and asthma. However, external beam radiotherapy for treatment of malignant diseases such as Hodgkin disease and laryngeal cancer persists. Children exposed to external beam radiotherapy are at increased risk of thyroid cancer, whereas patients receiving high-dose external beam irradiation in adulthood usually develop hypothyroidism rather than malignancy. Lifelong surveillance is needed in all patients receiving external beam radiotherapy at any age.

Prevention of Thyroid Cancer After Radiation Exposure

More than 200,000 people died of immediate complications of the atomic bomb explosions in Hiroshima and Nagasaki in 1945. The long-term survivors of the bombing have been followed up to assess long-term health risks of radiation exposure. The risk of thyroid cancer was greatest in children younger than 10 years of age at the time of the bombing. People older than 40 years at the time of exposure do not show any increased risk to thyroid cancer.[8] Atomic bomb testing in the Marshall Islands in 1954 and the Chernobyl nuclear reactor accident in 1986 also resulted in many people being exposed to iodine 131 (^{131}I). Follow-up of people in these exposed areas confirmed the increased risk of thyroid cancer in children.[1,8,27-29] Adults had a greater than expected number of thyroid nodules and thyroid cancer in the Marshall Islands. However, there was exposure to other isotopes of iodine and gamma radiation.

Potassium iodide (KI) is the cornerstone of preventive therapy after known exposure to radioactive iodine. When ingested around the time of exposure, KI saturates the thyroid, thereby inhibiting the uptake of radioactive iodine. Prevention is key because there is no agent, except thyrotropin, that will accelerate the elimination of radioactivity once concentrated within the thyroid gland. The radioactivity persists for weeks, and the concentrations decrease slowly.[30] If taken in the correct dose promptly after exposure, KI can prevent the effects of radiation on the thyroid.[31] The US Food and Drug Administration (FDA) recommends KI administration at various levels of radioactive iodine exposure (Table 63-2[31,32]). The FDA maintains that, when given correctly, KI is a safe and effective means to prevent radioactive iodine uptake by the thyroid gland in the event of a radiation emergency, thereby decreasing the risk of thyroid cancer.

T A B L E   63-2

Guidelines for Potassium Iodide Administration*

Patient	Exposure Gy (rad)	KI Dose (mg)
Adult >40 y	>5 (500)	130
Adults 18–40 y	≥0.1 (10)	130
Pregnant or lactating women	≥0.05 (5)	130
Adolescents 12–17 y[†]	≥0.05 (5)	65
Children 4–11 y	≥0.05 (5)	62
Children 1 mo through 3 y	≥0.05 (5)	32
Birth through 1 mo of age	≥0.05 (5)	16

*From the American Academy of Pediatrics[32] and the Food and Drug Administration.[33]

[†]Adolescents weighing more than 70 kg should receive the adult dose.

The possible adverse effects of KI prophylaxis include iodine-induced hyperthyroidism or hypothyroidism and nonthyroidal adverse effects. Potassium iodide prophylaxis in adults is recommended at higher levels of radioactive exposure than in children. This is because, first, adults are more likely to have underlying thyroid disease, which increases the possibility of adverse effects from KI use. Secondly, adults are less likely to experience an increased risk of thyroid cancer after radiation exposure, thereby decreasing the expected benefit of KI prophylaxis.[30]

Possible nonthyroidal adverse effects of KI include allergic and anaphylactic responses to iodine that may include fever, edema, shortness of breath, and rash. These effects are rare, and a strong correlation between iodine and these symptoms has not been clearly demonstrated.

MULTIPLE ENDOCRINE NEOPLASIA TYPE 2

Multiple endocrine neoplasia type 2 (MEN2) is an autosomal dominant syndrome with 3 variants: MEN2A, MEN2B, and familial medullary thyroid carcinoma. The first variant, MEN2A, is a syndrome of medullary thyroid carcinoma (MTC), pheochromocytoma, and parathyroid adenoma. Familial MTC is characterized by MTC only. The third variant, MEN2B, is characterized by the presence of MTC, pheochromocytoma, mucosal and intestinal ganglioneuromatosis, and skeletal deformity. Parathyroid adenomas seen in MEN2A are not present in MEN2B.[33]

All 3 variants of MEN2 show a high prevalence of MTC such that this carcinoma eventually will develop in 90% of carriers. Medullary thyroid carcinoma is a rare calcitonin-producing tumor of the parafollicular cells, or C cells, of the thyroid, which can be lethal. Surgical treatment is the only chance for a cure, so early detection and/or prophylactic thyroidectomy is the goal in high-risk patients. Traditionally, all first-degree relatives of patients with known MEN2 were screened annually for pheochromocytoma, thyroid carcinoma, and hyperparathyroidism from the age of 6 years to 35 years. This was accomplished by measuring pentagastrin-stimulated calcitonin levels, 24-hour urinary excretion of catecholamines, and serum levels of calcium and parathyroid hormone. Many patients underwent prophylactic thyroidectomy before the age of 6 years.[33]

This rigorous screening and aggressive surgical approach is rarely necessary now that the genetic mutation responsible for MEN2 has been identified. Nearly all variants of MEN2 are caused by a germline mutation in the rearranged during transfection (*RET*) gene, which has been localized to chromosome 10q11.2.[34] This mutation has been identified in more than 90% of families with MEN2. Testing for this mutation by the polymerase chain reaction provides a way to confirm a clinically suspected diagnosis or to screen asymptomatic family members of an affected individual known to have the *RET* proto-oncogene mutation.[33] All first-degree relatives of an affected person should be screened for the mutation before the age of 6 years. If the test result is positive, this DNA-based testing is 100% accurate in families with known mutations. If the test result is negative in families with known mutations, the patient may be assured that he or she does not have MEN2 and that it will not develop later in life. In the minority of families with MEN2 but no known *RET* mutation, further genetic testing would not be helpful.

Patients with the mutation should undergo annual screening for MTC, pheochromocytoma, and hyperparathyroidism from the age of 6 years to 35 years. These patients should be offered prophylactic thyroidectomy, since they will likely have either C-cell hyperplasia or occult medullary cancer.

PREVENTIVE MEASURES IN GRAVES OPHTHALMOPATHY

Hyperthyroidism caused by Graves disease is the result of thyrotropin receptor–stimulating antibodies. The exact cause of Graves ophthalmopathy (GO) is not known, making primary prevention difficult. In Olmsted County, Minnesota, the incidence of GO is 16 cases per 100,000 population per year for females and 2.9 cases per 100,000 population per year for males.[35] There is a bimodal distribution in both sexes, with a higher mean age at onset in men. There is a peak incidence in the age groups 40 to 44 years and 60 to 64 years in women and 45 to 49 years and 65 to 69 years in men.[35] Thyroid eye disease is generally bilateral (85% to 95% of cases) but may be unilateral (5% to 15% of cases).[36] Pooled data from 842 patients showed that eye disease was present before hyperthyroidism in 20% of cases and after hyperthyroidism in 41% of cases.

Many studies have shown that smoking is strongly associated with both the development and the severity of GO. A case-control study of 100 subjects showed an odds ratio of 7.7 (95% CI, 4.3 to 14.7) for GO in smokers vs nonsmokers.[37] Smoking not only increases the risk of GO developing but also decreases the response to treatment of GO. A study of smokers and nonsmokers with GO treated with steroids and orbital radiation showed significantly more improvement in the clinical activity score of the nonsmokers compared with the smokers.[38] Smokers are also less likely to respond favorably to the antithyroid medications carbimazole or propylthiouracil.[39] Unfortunately, the standard advice given to patients regarding the risk of GO with smoking did not result in smoking cessation in a recent study by Karadimas et al.[40] Given the abundant data on the adverse effects of smoking on GO, smoking cessation should be considered primary prevention for the development of GO. All patients with Graves disease with or without GO should be strongly advised against tobacco use.

According to a nonrandomized trial, treatment of Graves disease with radioactive iodine may cause progression of GO in 15% of patients. Progression of GO after radioiodine treatment may be prevented if glucocorticoids are given concomitantly.[41] At Mayo Clinic in Rochester, Minnesota, the need for repeated radioactive iodine therapies is avoided by giving an initial large dose and treating hypothyroidism early.

PREVENTION OF SUBCLINICAL AND CLINICAL HYPOTHYROIDISM

The reference range for peripheral thyroid hormone levels is relatively wide. The individual variation in peripheral thyroid hormone levels is much narrower than the laboratory reference range and varies little in serial measurements in the same person over a 12-month period.[42] Thus, free thyroxine in one person may be decreased greatly in mild thyroid failure and reach below that person's usual range but still be in the normal laboratory reference range. Fortunately, because of the feedback mechanism, the thyrotropin response to variation in thyroid hormone levels is exquisitely sensitive. A log-linear elevation of serum thyrotropin levels will be noted despite peripheral hormone levels being in the normal laboratory reference range. This condition, a normal free thyroxine level and elevated thyrotropin level, is called subclinical hypothyroidism or, more appropriately, mild thyroid failure.

When questioned thoroughly, patients will often describe mild symptoms of hypothyroidism when the thyrotropin level is above 10 μIU/L.[43] Most patients with serum thyrotropin levels between 5 and 10 mIU/L have either no symptoms or symptoms that may not be relieved by thyroxine therapy.

In areas with sufficient iodine intake, the most common cause of spontaneous hypothyroidism is autoimmune thyroid disease, occurring in 1% to 2% of the population. It has been suggested that increased dietary iodine may increase the prevalence of autoimmune thyroid disease, including Hashimoto thyroiditis, while decreasing endemic goiter, which is a more serious epidemiologic problem.

Spontaneous hypothyroidism increases with age and is 10 times more common in women than in men.[44] People at high risk of the development of subclinical hypothyroidism include patients with type 1 diabetes, a history of neck irradiation, treated hyperthyroidism, postpartum thyroiditis, and patients receiving certain medications, including amiodarone, lithium, or interferon-α. A cross-sectional multicenter study determined that patients with human immunodeficiency virus (HIV) are also at greater risk of hypothyroidism. Any HIV-infected male patients with low CD4 counts and those receiving the reverse transcriptase inhibitor stavudine are at particularly high risk compared with the general population.[45]

Treatment of Subclinical Hypothyroidism

The arguments in favor of treating subclinical hypothyroidism include prevention of progression to overt hypothyroidism, improvement of serum lipid levels, and treatment of mild symptoms of hypothyroidism. The Whickham Survey evaluated the progression to overt hypothyroidism in 2800 adults between 1972 and 1974.[43] After 20 years of follow-up, women who had elevated serum levels of thyrotropin and antithyroid antibodies were 38 times more likely to have hypothyroidism develop than were women with normal serum thyrotropin levels and no detectable antithyroid antibodies.[43]

Studies have demonstrated an association between subclinical hypothyroidism and elevated low-density lipoprotein cholesterol, low high-density lipoprotein cholesterol, and elevated lipoprotein (a) levels. Treatment of subclinical hypothyroidism with thyroxine has been shown to lower total serum cholesterol levels by 0.2 to 0.4 mmol/L and low-density lipoprotein cholesterol levels by about 0.2 mmol/L. The estimated reduction in cardiovascular mortality is 9% to 31%.[44] This benefit on serum lipids applies primarily to those patients with a serum thyrotropin level above 10 μIU/L. More data on the benefits in patients with lower levels of thyrotropin are needed.

Overt hypothyroidism is a risk factor for coronary heart disease because of associated metabolic abnormalities. The atherogenic aspects of subclinical hypothyroidism are less clear. In the population-based Whickham cohort study, 20-year follow-up did not demonstrate increased mortality due to cardiovascular causes in the group with subclinical hypothyroidism at baseline compared with normal persons.[44] However, in a recent case-control study from Rotterdam, Holland,[46] subclinical hypothyroidism in women with a mean age of 69 years was associated with a greater age-adjusted prevalence of aortic atherosclerosis (odds ratio, 1.7) and myocardial infarction (odds ratio, 2.3). These increased odds persisted after adjustment for body mass index, systolic and diastolic blood pressure, tobacco abuse, total cholesterol, and high-density lipoprotein levels.

Possible atherogenic factors other then hyperlipidemia in mild thyroid failure have been suggested, including increased homocysteine and lipoprotein (a) levels. It is now clear that although homocysteine levels are elevated in overt hypothyroidism, they are not elevated in subclinical hypothyroid patients.[47] Evidence that subclinical hypothyroidism increases lipoprotein (a) is also insufficient.[48] Recently, an elevated C-reactive protein level was demonstrated in subclinical hypothyroidism, and this raises the possibility of an apparent association with an inflammatory process.[47]

Of the several prospective, placebo-controlled trials on treatment of subclinical hypothyroidism, few have shown significant clinical benefit on symptoms. Some patients who were treated have experienced improved mood and memory. Women with ovulatory dysfunction may experience fertility with correction of their subclinical hypothyroidism. Although weight gain often is attributed to mild thyroid failure, treatment with thyroxine is unlikely to result in weight loss.[43]

There is uniform agreement on treatment of mild thyroid failure if the thyrotropin is above 10 μIU/L. For lower thyrotropin levels, therapy is controversial. Carefully designed studies are needed to settle this controversy, as it will affect management of millions of patients who have mild thyroid failure. The strongest argument for treatment is prevention of overt hypothyroidism, particularly if antithyroid antibodies are positive and there is a progressive increase of thyrotropin. The information obtained in the Whickham Survey is used, in part, at Mayo Clinic Rochester in the clinical decision of when or if to initiate thyroxine therapy. Analysis of 450 patients treated at our institution between January 1, 1995, and December 31, 1996, revealed that thyroxine therapy was prescribed for 39% of patients with mildly elevated thyrotropin levels (between 5.1 and 10.0 μIU/L).[49] The strongest predictors for initiation of thyroxine therapy were thyrotropin level, free thyroxine level, and thyroid microsomal antibody status.[49]

Screening for Hypothyroidism

When to screen for mild thyroid dysfunction is an area of controversy. The American Thyroid Association recommends screening both women and men at the age of 35 years and every 5 years thereafter.[50] The American College of Physicians recommends screening women over the age of 50 years.[51] If the screening thyrotropin test is performed and the level is found to be greater than 10.0 μIU/L, most endocrinologists would advocate thyroxine therapy.[49] A starting dosage of thyroxine of 0.05 to 0.075 mg daily is typically sufficient to normalize the serum thyrotropin level. Patients with coronary disease should be started at a dosage of 0.0125 to 0.025 mg daily. The serum thyrotropin level should be measured every 6 weeks after therapy is initiated and after any dose change. Once a stable dose of thyroxine is reached, annual measurements of serum thyrotropin levels are recommended.[43]

SUMMARY

Primary, secondary, and tertiary prevention of thyroid disease encompasses a number of health problems. Primary prevention of thyroid disease in the form of iodine supplementation of salt has been extremely successful in the United States. The role of secondary and tertiary prevention of thyroid disease will, hopefully, be clarified further in the years to come. This will include early detection and treatment of patients at risk of clinical and subclinical hypothyroidism, thyroid cancer, Graves eye disease, and genetic syndromes such as MEN2.

REFERENCES

1. World Health Organization (WHO)/United Nations Children's Fund (UNICEF)/International Council for Control of Iodine Deficiency Disorders (ICCIDD). *Assessment of Iodine Deficiency Disorders and Monitoring Their Elimination: A Guide for Programme Managers.* 2nd ed. Geneva, Switzerland: WHO; 2001:1–124. Publication WHO/NHD 01.1. Available at: www.who.int/reproductive-health/docs/iodine_deficiency.pdf. Accessed November 17, 2003.

2. Werner SC, Ingbar SH, Braverman LE, Utiger RD. *Werner & Ingbar's The Thyroid: A Fundamental and Clinical Text.* 8th ed. Philadelphia, Pa: Lippincott Williams & Wilkins; 2000.

3. WHO/UNICEF/ICCIDD. *Progress Towards the Elimination of Iodine Deficiency Disorders (IDD).* Geneva, Swizterland: WHO; 1999:1–33. Publication WHO/NHD 99.4.

4. Hollowell JG, Staehling NW, Hannon WH, et al. Iodine nutrition in the United States: trends and public health implications: iodine excretion data from National Health and Nutrition Examination Surveys I and III (1971–1974 and 1988–1994) [comment]. *J Clin Endocrinol Metab.* 1998;83:3401–3408.

5. Knudsen N, Laurberg P, Perrild H, Bulow I, Ovesen L, Jorgensen T. Risk factors for goiter and thyroid nodules. *Thyroid.* 2002;12:879–888.

6. Koutras DA, Papapetrou PD, Yataganas X, Malamos B. Dietary sources of iodine in areas with and without iodine-deficiency goiter. *Am J Clin Nutr.* 1970;23:870–874.

7. Francois D, Burgi H, Chen ZP, Dunn JT. World status of monitoring iodine deficiency disorders control programs. *Thyroid.* 2002;12:915–924.

8. Nagataki S, Nystrom E. Epidemiology and primary prevention of thyroid cancer. *Thyroid.* 2002;12:889–896.

9. Galanti MR, Hansson L, Bergstrom R, et al. Diet and the risk of papillary and follicular thyroid carcinoma: a population-based case-control study in Sweden and Norway. *Cancer Causes Control.* 1997;8:205–214.

10. Chatenoud L, La Vecchia C, Franceschi S, et al. Refined-cereal intake and risk of selected cancers in Italy. *Am J Clin Nutr.* 1999;70:1107–1110.

11. Bosetti C, Kolonel L, Negri E, et al. A pooled analysis of case-control studies of thyroid cancer. VI. Fish and shellfish consumption. *Cancer Causes Control.* 2001;12:375–382.

12. Bosetti C, Negri E, Kolonel L, et al. A pooled analysis of case-control studies of thyroid cancer. VII. Cruciferous and other vegetables (international). *Cancer Causes Control.* 2002;13:765–775.

13. Pettersson B, Coleman MP, Ron E, Adami HO. Iodine supplementation in Sweden and regional trends in thyroid cancer incidence by histopathologic type. *Int J Cancer.* 1996;65:13–19.

14. Lind P, Langsteger W, Molnar M, Gallowitsch HJ, Mikosch P, Gomez I. Epidemiology of thyroid diseases in iodine sufficiency. *Thyroid.* 1998;8:1179–1183.

15. Lind P, Kumnig G, Heinisch M, et al. Iodine supplementation in Austria: methods and results. *Thyroid.* 2002;12:903–907.

16. Galanti MR, Hansson L, Lund E, et al. Reproductive history and cigarette smoking as risk factors for thyroid cancer in women: a population-based case-control study. *Cancer Epidemiol Biomarkers Prevention.* 1996;5:425–431.

17. Kreiger N, Parkes R. Cigarette smoking and the risk of thyroid cancer. *Eur J Cancer.* 2000;36:1969–1973.

18. Rossing MA, Cushing KL, Voigt LF, Wicklund KG, Daling JR. Risk of papillary thyroid cancer in women in relation to smoking and alcohol consumption. *Epidemiology.* 2000;11:49–54.

19. Iribarren C, Haselkorn T, Tekawa IS, Friedman GD. Cohort study of thyroid cancer in a San Francisco Bay area population. *Int J Cancer.* 2001;93:745–750.

20. Sigurdson AJ, Doody MM, Rao RS, et al. Cancer incidence in the US radiologic technologists health study, 1983–1998. *Cancer.* 2003;97:3080–3089.

21. Fincham SM, Ugnat AM, Hill GB, Kreiger N, Mao Y, for Canadian Cancer Registries Epidemiology Research Group. Is occupation a risk factor for thyroid cancer? *J Occup Environ Med.* 2000;42:318–322.

22. Acharya S, Sarafoglou K, LaQuaglia M, et al. Thyroid neoplasms after therapeutic radiation for malignancies during childhood or adolescence. *Cancer.* 2003;97:2397–2403.

23. Ron E, Lubin JH, Shore RE, et al. Thyroid cancer after exposure to external radiation: a pooled analysis of seven studies. *Radiation Res.* 1995;141:259–277.

24. Schneider AB, Bekerman C, Leland J, et al. Thyroid nodules in the follow-up of irradiated individuals: comparison of thyroid ultrasound with scanning and palpation. *J Clin Endocrinol Metab.* 1997;82:4020–4027.

25. Gharib H, Goellner JR. Fine-needle aspiration biopsy of the thyroid: an appraisal [comment]. *Ann Intern Med.* 1993;118:282–289.

26. Kikuchi S, Perrier ND, Ituarte PH, et al. Accuracy of fine-needle aspiration cytology in patients with radiation-induced thyroid neoplasms. *Br J Surg.* 2003;90:755–758.

27. Rubino C, Cailleux AF, De Vathaire F, Schlumberger M. Thyroid cancer after radiation exposure. *Eur J Cancer.* 2002;38:645–647.

28. Shibata Y, Yamashita S, Masyakin VB, Panasyuk GD, Nagataki S. 15 years after Chernobyl: new evidence of thyroid cancer. *Lancet.* 2001;358:1965–1966.

29. Moysich KB, Menezes RJ, Michalek AM. Chernobyl-related ionising radiation exposure and cancer risk: an epidemiological review [comment]. *Lancet Oncol.* 2002;3:269–279.

30. Verger P, Aurengo A, Geoffroy B, Le Guen B. Iodine kinetics and effectiveness of stable iodine prophylaxis after intake of radioactive iodine: a review. *Thyroid.* 2001;11:353–360.

31. American Academy of Pediatrics Committee on Environmental Health. Radiation disasters and children. *Pediatrics.* 2003;111:1455–1466.

32. US Food and Drug Administration, Center for Drug Evaluation and Research. *Guidance Document: Potassium Iodide as a Thyroid Blocking Agent in Radiation Emergencies.* Available at: www.fda.gov/cder/guidance/4825fnl.htm. Accessed October 24, 2003.

33. Eng C. Seminars in medicine of the Beth Israel Hospital, Boston. The RET proto-oncogene in multiple endocrine neoplasia type 2 and Hirschsprung's disease. *N Engl J Med.* 1996;335:943–951.

34. Brandi ML, Gagel RF, Angeli A, et al. Guidelines for diagnosis and therapy of MEN type 1 and type 2 [comment]. *J Clin Endocrinol Metab.* 2001;86:5658–5671.

35. Bartley GB. The epidemiologic characteristics and clinical course of ophthalmopathy associated with autoimmune thyroid disease in Olmsted County, Minnesota. *Trans Am Ophthalmol Soc.* 1994;92:477–588.

36. Wiersinga WM, Bartalena L. Epidemiology and prevention of Graves' ophthalmopathy. *Thyroid.* 2002;12:855–860.

37. Prummel MF, Wiersinga WM. Smoking and risk of Graves' disease [comment]. *JAMA.* 1993;269:479–482.

38. Eckstein A, Quadbeck B, Mueller G, et al. Impact of smoking on the response to treatment of thyroid associated ophthalmopathy. *Br J Ophthalmol.* 2003;87:773–776.

39. Chowdhury TA, Dyer PH. Clinical, biochemical and immunological characteristics of relapsers and non-relapsers of thyrotoxicosis treated with anti-thyroid drugs. *J Intern Med.* 1998;244:293–297.

40. Karadimas P, Bouzas EA, Mastorakos G. Advice against smoking is not effective in patients with Graves' ophthalmopathy. *Acta Med Austriaca.* 2003;30:59–60.

41. Bartalena L, Marcocci C, Bogazzi F, et al. Relation between therapy for hyperthyroidism and the course of Graves' ophthalmopathy [comment]. *N Engl J Med.* 1998;338:73–78.

42. Andersen S, Pedersen KM, Bruun NH, Laurberg P. Narrow individual variations in serum T(4) and T(3) in normal subjects: a clue to the understanding of subclinical thyroid disease. *J Clin Endocrinol Metab.* 2002;87:1068–1072.

43. Cooper DS. Clinical practice. Subclinical hypothyroidism [comment]. *N Engl J Med.* 2001;345:260–265.

44. Vanderpump MP, Tunbridge WM. Epidemiology and prevention of clinical and subclinical hypothyroidism. *Thyroid.* 2002;12:839–847.

45. Beltran S, Lescure FX, Desailloud R, et al. Increased prevalence of hypothyroidism among human immunodeficiency virus-infected patients: a need for screening. *Clin Infect Dis.* 2003;37:579–583.

46. Hak AE, Pols HA, Visser TJ, Drexhage HA, Hofman A, Witteman JC. Subclinical hypothyroidism is an independent risk factor for atherosclerosis and myocardial infarction in elderly women: the Rotterdam Study. *Ann Intern Med.* 2000;132:270–278.

47. Christ-Crain M, Meier C, Guglielmetti M, et al. Elevated C-reactive protein and homocysteine values: cardiovascular risk factors in hypothyroidism? A cross-sectional and a double-blind, placebo-controlled trial. *Atherosclerosis.* 2003;166:379–386.

48. Caraccio N, Ferrannini E, Monzani F. Lipoprotein profile in subclinical hypothyroidism: response to levothyroxine replacement, a randomized placebo-controlled study. *J Clin Endocrinol Metab.* 2002;87:1533–1538.

49. Fatourechi V, Lankarani M, Schryver PG, Vanness DJ, Long KH, Klee GG. Factors influencing clinical decisions to initiate thyroxine therapy for patients with mildly increased serum thyrotropin (5.1–10.0 mIU/L). *Mayo Clin Proc.* 2003;78:554–560.

50. Ladenson PW, Singer PA, Ain KB, et al. American Thyroid Association guidelines for detection of thyroid dysfunction [comment; erratum appears in *Arch Intern Med.* 2001;161:284]. *Arch Intern Med.* 2000;160:1573–1575.

51. Helfand M, Redfern CC. Clinical guideline, part 2. Screening for thyroid disease: an update. American College of Physicians [comment; erratum appears in *Ann Intern Med.* 1999;130:246]. *Ann Intern Med.* 1998;129:144–158.

RESOURCES

The American Thyroid Association
Web site: www.thyroid.org.

Werner SC, Ingbar SH, Braverman LE, Utiger RD. Werner & Ingbar's the thyroid: a fundamental and clinical text. 8th ed. Philadelphia. Lippincott Williams & Wilkins, 2000. *Thyroid.* October 2002;12;10.

chapter 64

Preventable Dementia

José G. Merino, MD, MPhil, and Vladimir Hachinski, MD, DSc, FRCPC

INTRODUCTION

Almost 10% of people older than 65 years and 35% of those over 85 years have dementia;[1] mild cognitive impairment is twice as common. Every year 750,000 people in the United States and Canada develop cognitive impairment, and 50% will become demented in the next 5 years.[2] Alzheimer disease (AD) and vascular dementia (VaD), the most common subtypes of dementia in the Western hemisphere, have been considered diagnoses of exclusion, but recent evidence suggests that this dichotomy is artificial.[3] Neuronal loss, neurofibrillary tangles, and neuritic plaques are the hallmarks of AD, whereas vascular damage defines VaD. However, the brains of elderly individuals often have coexisting Alzheimer-type and vascular pathology,[4] and the effect of these processes on cognition are additive[5] or even multiplicative.[6] Large population-based epidemiologic studies that began in the 1980s and early 1990s have shown that vascular risk factors contribute to the clinical and pathological presentation of AD, and results of experimental and pathological studies support this view.[7] Vascular dementia and AD have risk factors in common.[7-9] In addition, AD and VaD share etiologic pathways.[8] The border between AD and VaD has become blurred as shared pathophysiological processes have been identified.[9]

In 1992 Hachinski[10] proposed a conceptual system for thinking about VaD that focuses on primary (brain-at-risk stage), secondary (predementia stage), and tertiary prevention in patients at risk of VaD. The awareness that vascular disease plays a major role in the genesis and expression of AD means that preventive strategies can have a greater impact than initially envisioned. Furthermore, recent epidemiologic data suggest that dietary factors, social engagement, participation in recreational and physical activities, and cognitive stimulation influence the risk of cognitive decline later in life.[11,12] This new knowledge opens new opportunities for prevention.

Given the potential to prevent or modify the course of cognitive decline, primary care physicians, psychiatrists, and neurologists must shift their focus from diagnosing dementia to identifying individuals at risk for or with mild cognitive and behavioral changes. Epidemiologic and therapeutic studies now focus on people with mild cognitive impairment,[13] and the broad concept of vascular cognitive impairment helps us identify subjects at risk of dementia (whether AD or VaD) in whom vascular risk factors have an etiopathogenic role.[14]

Prevention of dementia requires interventions at different levels.[15] Some risk factors can be addressed only at a societal level (eg, providing universal access to education and preventing head trauma by mandating the use of helmets for motorcycle riders and seat belts for passengers in automobiles). Other risk factors need individual management (eg, lowering blood pressure, using anticoagulants for patients with atrial fibrillation). The prevention of cardiac and cerebral vascular disease has a major impact on the prevalence of dementia, and the data from epidemiologic studies and clinical trials highlight the importance of pharmacologic and lifestyle preventive strategies for cognition. While high-quality observational studies suggest the association between several modifiable risk factors and dementia, the data supporting specific interventions are scarce. The reader should beware of making management decisions based on mechanistic and observational data. There are many examples in the literature of conclusions drawn from these studies that were not confirmed by the results of clinical trials, such as the unexpected deleterious effect of combined hormone replacement therapy (HRT) reported by the Women's Health Initiative.[16]

MANAGEMENT OF VASCULAR RISK FACTORS

Stroke

Dementia is common in patients with cerebrovascular disease. One fourth to one third of patients with stroke meet operationalized criteria for dementia 3 to 6 months after the vascular event,[17] and up to 60% have impairment in at least one cognitive domain.[18] Compared with people without cerebrovascular disease, stroke-affected patients have a 2-fold to 10-fold higher risk of dementia developing, even after several years, particularly when multiple infarcts are present. In the general population, silent or unrecognized brain infarcts double the risk of dementia developing in the subsequent 3 years,[19] perhaps because they are a marker of high risk of additional infarcts.

Cognitive decline in patients with cerebrovascular disease is due to the stroke itself when a large volume of brain is affected by ischemia or hemorrhage or when the lesion, because of its strategic location, interrupts brain circuits that are critical for cognition.[20] However, vascular lesions commonly coexist with Alzheimer-type disease,[4] leading to a mixed state, perhaps the most common cause of dementia.[7] The effect of these pathological processes is additive.[5,21] For example, in an autopsy study, nuns who had Alzheimer-type disease and cerebral infarcts had more severe cognitive impairment and a higher prevalence of dementia than did sisters with isolated AD.[5] Similarly, investigators of the Consortium to Establish a Registry for Alzheimer Disease (CERAD) found that the overall severity of dementia was greater, and the performance on tests of language and cognitive function worse, in patients with plaques, tangles, and cerebral infarcts than in those with isolated neurodegenerative changes.[21]

Clearly, interventions that reduce the incidence of stroke will reduce the burden of cognitive impairment and dementia. Primary prevention strategies for stroke are aimed at a high-risk population: middle-aged and elderly individuals who do not have cerebrovascular disease ("brain-at-risk" stage).[14] These include lifestyle changes (eg, healthy diet, an active lifestyle, smoking cessation) and aggressive management of risk factors, including hypertension, nonvalvular atrial fibrillation, and hypercholesterolemia.[22] Secondary prevention, on the other hand, is aimed at those who had a stroke yet are not demented ("predementia" stage).[14,22] The risk of recurrent stroke can be lowered with the use of antiplatelet agents and the vigorous treatment of hypertension, atrial fibrillation, and symptomatic high-grade carotid artery stenosis. Results from the Perindopril Protection Against Recurrent Stroke Study (PROGRESS)[23] suggest that preventing recurrent stroke reduces the incidence of dementia and cognitive decline.[24] Although several studies show that 3-hydroxy-3-methylglutaryl coenzyme A (HMG-CoA) reductase inhibitors may reduce the risk of stroke by 30%,[25] trials to test their effectiveness in the secondary prevention of stroke have not been completed. Clinical trials are under way to test the effectiveness of multivitamin supplementation to reduce homocysteine levels for stroke prevention. This strategy has led to reduced rates of restenosis and myocardial infarction after coronary angioplasty.[26] Recent reviews and practice guidelines more completely review stroke prevention.[22,27,28]

Hypertension

Hypertension affects 50 million Americans and is the greatest risk factor for stroke and heart failure as well as a major risk factor for heart disease, VaD, and AD.[7,8] The brains of nondemented hypertensive individuals have more senile plaques and neurofibrillary tangles, lower weight, and more radiographic white-matter changes than those of people with normal blood pressure. Cross-sectional studies looking at the relationship between hypertension and dementia have been inconclusive. High[29,30] and low blood pressure[31] were associated with cognitive impairment and dementia in some studies, whereas others did not find any association.[32,33] The association is more consistent in longitudinal studies published in the last decade.[34-36] For example, in a longitudinal population-based study in Göteborg, Sweden, the risk of dementia developing between the ages of 80 and 85 years was higher in individuals who had elevated systolic and diastolic blood pressure 10 to 15 years previously, despite the fact the hypotension immediately preceded the onset of dementia.[36] The authors concluded that small vessel disease and white-matter lesions mediate the association. In Hiroshima, Japan, patients who had high blood pressure 25 to 30 years previously were 30% more likely to have vascular dementia at the time of the cognitive examination.[37] Hypertension in middle age was a significant predictor of cognitive decline and reduced brain volume 20 to 30 years later in several studies,[34,35,38] but the adverse cognitive effect of hypertension was evident within 4 years in a study in Nantes, France.[39] Higher pulse pressure may also be a risk factor for dementia in general and AD in particular.[40]

Several studies examined the effect of antihypertensive treatment on the risk of dementia. The Systolic Hypertension in Elderly Prevention (SHEP)[41,42] and the Medical Research Council[43] trials did not find a significant difference in the incidence of cognitive decline between participants in the active (low-dose diuretic or β-blocker) or placebo treatment arms, despite reductions in blood pressure, which averaged 11.5/4.1 mm Hg and 10.6/5.6 mm Hg, respectively. A reanalysis of the SHEP data, however, suggests that the effect of differential dropout by placebo-treated patients may have obscured the appraisal of the protective effect of treatment.[44] In the Systolic Hypertension in Europe (Sys-Eur) trial, treatment of isolated systolic hypertension (systolic blood pressure, 160 to 219 mm Hg; diastolic blood pressure, <95 mm Hg) with the calcium channel blocker nitrendipine, with or without enalapril and/or hydrochlorothiazide, reduced incident dementia by 50%, from 7.7 to 3.8 cases per 1000 patient-years, compared with placebo.[45] In a subsequent analysis after 4 years of follow-up, the treatment effect remained the same[46] and was highly statistically significant. The authors inferred that treatment of 1000 patients for 5 years could prevent 20 cases of dementia. The between-group difference in blood pressure during the whole follow-up period averaged only 7/3 mm Hg, raising the possibility that calcium channel blockers may have a neuroprotective effect beyond blood pressure reduction.[46] In the PROGRESS trial, the use of an angiotensin-converting enzyme inhibitor, perindopril, and a diuretic, indapamide, reduced the risk of stroke and other major vascular events by 43% in individuals with cerebrovascular disease, whether or not they were hypertensive.[23] Treatment with both drugs led to a greater reduction in blood pressure and was more effective than the use of perindopril alone.[23] In this study, dementia and cognitive decline were prespecified end points.[24] The relative risk reduction of dementia with treatment was 12%, but this result was not statistically significant. However, the composite outcome of "dementia with recurrent stroke" was reduced by approximately one third, the overall risk of cognitive decline was reduced by about one fifth, and the risk of the composite outcome "cognitive decline with recurrent stroke" was reduced by about one half. Since the incidence of dementia and cognitive impairment was low, the numbers needed to treat, even for the significant outcomes described above, are high.[24] The results were independent of the effects of treatment on mortality and were similar in hypertensive and normotensive subjects. These effects may be due to fewer recurrent strokes in the treated patients.[23]

These studies highlight the need for aggressive treatment of all hypertensive patients. To determine whether strategies should be different in those at higher risk of dementia, we need trials that are sufficiently powered to assess the effect of treatment on cognitive outcomes. Until they are completed, blood pressure must be managed according to the guidelines of the Seventh Report of the Joint National Committee on Prevention, Detection, Evaluation and Treatment of High Blood Pressure.[47] The goal of treatment is to lower blood pressure to less than 140/90 mm Hg for most persons (130/80 mm Hg for those with diabetes and chronic kidney disease) with the use of pharmacologic and lifestyle interventions.

Cholesterol

There are biological reasons why lipid metabolism abnormalities are associated with dementia. The apolipoprotein (APOE) gene codes for a cholesterol transport protein (apoE), and the presence of the ε4 allele is associated with increased plasma cholesterol, low-density lipoprotein cholesterol (LDL-C) levels, atherosclerosis, and cardiovascular disease. It is also a well-established risk factor for AD and VaD. Animals fed a high-cholesterol diet have greater β-amyloid (Aβ) deposition in the hippocampus, and the brains of subjects with AD have higher levels of LDL-C, apolipoprotein B, and Aβ, and lower levels of high-density lipoprotein cholesterol (HDL-C)

than do controls. Cholesterol directly affects Aβ secretion. Depletion of membrane cholesterol may lead to cleavage of the amyloid precursor protein to nonamyloidogenic proteins instead of Aβ. Simvastatin and lovastatin reduce intracellular and extracellular levels of Aβ 42 and Aβ 40 in primary culture of hippocampal and mixed cortical neurons, and guinea pigs treated with simvastatin showed a reduction of cerebral Aβ levels.[48]

Observational studies examining the association between cholesterol and AD have yielded conflicting results.[49,50] Among male survivors of the Finnish cohort of the Seven Countries Study, high serum total cholesterol level at 40 to 59 years predicted AD in later life.[51] In another prospective cohort, high LDL and total cholesterol levels were associated with cognitive impairment,[52] and in a longitudinal study in Kuopio, Finland, midlife elevated serum cholesterol levels were a risk factor for incident AD 21 years later.[53] On the other hand, there was no association between average cholesterol level at visits 1 to 15, or total cholesterol level at visit 20, and risk of incident AD among 1026 subjects from the original Framingham cohort who were alive at examination cycle 20.[54] Differences in study design, the inclusion of prevalent dementia cases, varying case definitions of dementia, and use of fasting rather than nonfasting cholesterol level can possibly explain these differences.[54]

A growing body of epidemiologic evidence suggests that lowering serum cholesterol may retard the pathogenesis of AD.[55] In a cross-sectional analysis of 3 independent hospital databases, patients receiving lovastatin or pravastatin exhibited a 69.9% reduction in the prevalence of AD. Simvastatin had only a weak effect.[56] In a nested case-control study with information from 368 general practices, people aged 50 years or older who were prescribed statins had a substantially lower risk of dementia than those who did not receive these drugs, independent of lipid levels or exposure to nonstatin lipid-lowering agents.[57] Cross-sectional and case-control studies are subject to indication bias, as physicians may be more likely to prescribe statins to younger, healthier, better-educated patients from a higher socioeconomic level, all factors associated with a lower risk of dementia.[52] However, the protective effect of statins has been noted in some prospective studies. Women enrolled in the Heart Estrogen/Progestin Replacement Study who were receiving statins were less likely to have cognitive impairment after 4 years of follow-up,[52] independent of their baseline lipid levels. In the Canadian Study of Health and Aging, the odds ratio for all types of dementia in those aged less than 80 years who were receiving statins was 0.26 after stratifying by age and adjusting for sex, educational level, and self-rated health.[58] The effect was not seen with nonstatin lipid-lowering drugs.

The ongoing Prospective Study of Pravastatin in the Elderly at Risk (PROSPER) will examine the efficacy of statins in slowing cognitive decline and dementia.[59]

Follow-up studies of AD and dementia in patients enrolled in statin trials will also furnish important data to guide treatment recommendations.[56] Until these data are available, patients with hyperlipidemia should be treated according to the National Cholesterol Education Program guidelines.

Homocysteine

A high level of total homocysteine, or h(e), is a risk factor for cardiovascular[60] and cerebrovascular disease[61,62] and is a marker for low concentration of the vitamins that are its main determinants, folate and vitamin B_{12}.[63] Homocysteine may be directly neurotoxic, as it causes DNA damage and apoptosis, and may cause endothelial injury. Through these mechanisms, it may lead to stroke, VaD, and AD. Dietary, lifestyle, genetic, renal, and clinical factors affect h(e) concentration.[62]

Case-control studies suggest a link between low vitamin B12 levels and dementia[6,64] and high h(e) levels and VaD and AD.[65] Hyperhomocysteinemia also is associated with poor performance in neuropsychological tests measuring specific cognitive functions.[66,67] Prospective studies have consistently shown an association between hyperhomocysteinemia and dementia or cognitive decline. In the Kungsholmen Project, individuals aged 75 years or more who had normal cognition but low concentration of folate or vitamin B12 at baseline had 3 times the risk of AD than did subjects with normal levels of those vitamins.[68] In a small cohort of healthy elderly persons, hyperhomocysteinemia at baseline was independently associated with lower cognitive test scores 5 years later, and, in a separate study, patients with h(e) concentration greater than 11.1 mmol/L had a more rapid progression of AD over the next 3 years than did those with h(e) below this cutoff.[69] In a study from the Framingham study's cohort, dementia developed in 111 of 1092 participants. Hyperhomocysteinemia 8 years before the onset of dementia was a strong, independent risk factor for the development of dementia and AD.[70]

Although data from observational studies are compelling, clinical trials are needed to prove an association and to guide treatment decisions. Currently, 2 trials are examining the effectiveness of vitamin supplementation for stroke prevention; if the findings are positive, the use of vitamins will have an impact on stroke-related dementia. In addition, the Alzheimer's Disease Cooperative Study (ADCS) is planning a multicenter trial testing the effectiveness of treatment with B vitamins to slow the progression of disease in patients with AD. A trial involving patients with mild cognitive impairment is needed. Although we acknowledge that this is a controversial issue, we currently screen our patients for hyperhomocysteinemia and, if found, begin treatment with vitamin B12 (250 µg/d), folic acid (1 mg/d), and vitamin B6 (25 mg/d).

OTHER PHARMACOLOGICAL INTERVENTIONS

Oxidative Stress and Antioxidant Vitamins

Oxidation and inflammation play a role in the development of AD. β-Amyloid is toxic to neuronal cell cultures through mechanisms involving free radicals. However, the relationship between antioxidant vitamin intake and risk of dementia is not well understood, since cross-sectional and observational studies have yielded conflicting results. Some recent large observational cohort studies found a lower risk of AD in patients taking antioxidants. In the Rotterdam Study, a high intake of vitamin C or vitamin E was associated with a lower risk of AD.[71] Among participants in the Chicago Health and Aging Project, those in the highest quintiles of vitamin E intake had one third the risk of incident AD of those in the lowest quintile. The effect was noted, however, only among individuals without the *APOE* ε4 allele.[72] On the other hand, in the Washington Heights-Inwood Columbia Aging Project, the intake of carotenes, vitamin C, or vitamin E (total, dietary, or supplemental) was not related to a decreased risk of AD.[73] The discrepancies may be due to age of the cohort, follow-up, and measurement imprecision of the dietary variables.[73] Results from the Nurses' Health Study suggest that verbal fluency scores were consistently higher in the subjects taking vitamins E and C than in those who took vitamin C or E alone.[74] Since early changes in verbal fluency may predict subsequent dementia, the results are intriguing. Recently the ADCS completed a clinical trial of vitamin E (2000 IU/d) and selegiline (10 mg/d) supplementation in patients with moderate AD to determine whether treatment could slow cognitive decline. Treatment with vitamin E, selegiline, or both significantly reduced the risk of reaching a primary end point (institutionalization, loss of basic activities of daily living, severe dementia, or death). Compared with the placebo group, the vitamin E group had a favorable hazard ratio and a prolonged time to event for all end points.[75] These results suggest that vitamin E may slow the progression of the disease. As a result, the ADCS began a multicenter, randomized, double-blind, placebo-controlled, parallel-group clinical trial to determine whether vitamin E can prevent or delay a clinical diagnosis of AD among patients with mild cognitive impairment over 3 years, and a trial of vitamin E and selenium to prevent dementia has been added to the ongoing Selenium and Vitamin E Chemoprevention Trial.

Many physicians, including ourselves, currently use vitamin E in high doses (2000 IU/d) in patients with mild cognitive impairment and mild to moderate dementia. It has few side effects, as demonstrated in multiple trials of vitamin E in coronary artery disease. However, in one study vitamin E was associated with increased triglycerides level,[76] and in another increased levels of plasma triglycerides, LDL-C, and total cholesterol;[77] thus, we advise caution in patients with lipid abnormalities. In addition, there was a nonsignificant increase in ischemic stroke with vitamin E supplementation in the Alpha-Tocopherol Beta Carotene Study.[78] Recently the US Preventive Services Task Force (USPSTF) concluded that there is insufficient evidence to recommend for or against the use of supplements of vitamins A, C, or E; multivitamins with folic acid; or antioxidant combinations for the prevention of cancer or cardiovascular disease, but they did not comment on their use for dementia prevention.[79]

Hormone Replacement Therapy

Estrogens affect the brain at the cellular, metabolic, and neurotransmitter level. Prospective and case-control studies have found that women who take estrogen have a 50% lower risk of AD,[80-82] and a meta-analysis of observational studies suggests that HRT is associated with a decreased risk of dementia.[83] There have been several trials of HRT to prevent or slow the progression of cognitive decline, but the number of patients enrolled was low, and the quality of the studies was variable. Two recent Cochrane meta-analyses concluded that there is only limited evidence to support the use of HRT to preserve cognitive function in healthy postmenopausal women,[84] and that the data did not support their use in women with AD.[85] A trial of 120 women with mild to moderate AD with a history of hysterectomy that was published after the meta-analyses did not find a difference in cognitive function after 1 year of follow-up between placebo and high-dose (1.25 mg/d) or low-dose (0.625 mg/d) estrogen.[86]

The Women's Health Initiative is conducting a trial of treatment with 0.625 mg/d of conjugated estrogen, with or without 2.5 mg of medroxyprogesterone acetate, to prevent adverse outcomes in postmenopausal women. The combined treatment arm was stopped prematurely in July 2002 because the overall risks outweighed the benefits.[87] Combined HRT had deleterious effects on the nervous system. After 4 years of follow-up, 61 of 4532 women aged 65 years or older were demented; 40 in the combined arm and 21 in the placebo group.[16] Women receiving the combination therapy had a greater likelihood of declining more than 2 SDs on the modified Mini Mental State Examination than women receiving placebo.[88] In addition, the combined therapy was associated with a twofold higher risk of stroke,[16] and vascular dementia developed in 5 patients in the treatment arm but only 1 in the control group.[89] Based on these results, combined therapy should not be recommended for the prevention of any adverse outcome, including dementia.[90] The effect of estrogens alone is still under evaluation.

Nonsteroidal Anti-Inflammatory Drugs

Inflammation contributes to neuronal damage in AD. Animal and epidemiologic studies suggest that nonsteroidal anti-inflammatory drugs (NSAIDs) may prevent AD.[91] In a meta-analysis of 9 studies published between 1996 and 2002, the pooled risk ratio of AD among NSAID users was 0.72; the effect was dependent on duration of use and was strongest for those who took the drugs for more than 24 months.[91] A trial of NSAIDs for the prevention of AD is under way (176). A recent multicenter, randomized, double-blind, placebo-controlled, parallel-group trial showed that nonselective (naproxen) or selective (rofecoxib) cyclooxygenase (COX-2) inhibitors did not prevent progression of mild and moderate AD.[92] Adverse events (including fatigue, dizziness, dry mouth, and hypertension) were more common in the treatment groups,[92] and patients in each of the treatment groups had almost twice as many serious events (death, stroke, gastrointestinal bleeding, subdural hematoma, and myocardial infarction) as those treated with placebo. Given the risks and lack of benefit, treatment of patients with these agents for the prevention of development or progression of dementia cannot be recommended until further data are available.

Ginkgo biloba

Ginkgo biloba, an extract of the leaves of the maidenhair tree, has been used for centuries to enhance cognition. Its beneficial properties are ascribed to its effects on blood clotting and viscosity, vascular tone, neurotransmitter metabolism, and oxidative stress. The active components of *G biloba* include flavonoids, terpenoids, and terpene lactones (ginkgolides and bilobalides); the latter can be found only in *G biloba.* Several trials evaluated the effectiveness of ginkgo in preventing and treating dementia, and overall they were positive.[93,94] However, only 4 high-quality trials were identified in a semiquantitative analysis of the literature in 1998. There was a small but significant effect of treatment with *G biloba* (120 to 240 mg/d) on objective measures of cognitive function in patients with AD, but the authors of that study did not make any treatment recommendations.[93] The Cochrane collaboration found 33 clinical trials that studied ginkgo in patients with AD or VaD, many with major methodologic flaws.[94] The Cochrane authors feel that the evidence for cognitive improvement with ginkgo is promising, but they conclude that a large trial using modern methods is needed to provide robust estimates of the size and mechanisms of any treatment effects.[94] A trial published after the Cochrane meta-analysis did not find ginkgo more effective than placebo for enhancing memory in healthy elderly people.[95] A 6-year trial of *G biloba* (240 mg/d) for the prevention of dementia among community-dwelling elderly individuals began enrolling patients in 2003. It is sponsored by the National Institutes of Health.

Ginkgo biloba is well tolerated, and the side effects are mild, transient, and reversible (gastrointestinal distress, headache, and nausea). In the studies included in the Cochrane meta-analysis, the side effects profile was similar in the placebo and the active groups.[94] A few instances of bleeding have been reported, and the extract can interact with anticoagulants. Seizures have occurred in children taking ginkgo. [95] The usual dose is 120 mg/d (in 3 doses), but trials have used 120 to 320 mg/d. The clinical effects are evident after 4 weeks of treatment.

LIFESTYLE MODIFICATION

Nutrition

A higher intake of calories (energy) and fat may be associated with a higher risk of AD, particularly in individuals carrying the apoE allele.[96] A high intake of fat, saturated fat, and cholesterol doubled the risk of dementia in the Rotterdam Study, and high linoleic acid intake was associated with cognitive impairment in the Zutphen Elderly Study.[97] In a cohort from Chicago, the intake of saturated or *trans*-unsaturated fats also increases the risk of AD, those in the highest fifth of intake had twice the risk of AD over 2.3 years.[98] On the other hand, long-chain *n*-3 polyunsaturated fatty acids and docosahexaenoic acid can reduce this risk.[12] Cross-cultural epidemiologic studies show the protective effect of fish consumption,[99] and in several longitudinal studies fish consumption halves the risk of cognitive decline.[12,97,100,101]

These findings are consistent with studies that show that a diet rich in saturated fats increases cerebral Aβ deposition in mouse, rabbit, and monkey models of AD,[102] and polyunsaturated fats can decrease the risk. Omega-3 polyunsaturated fatty acids may enhance the stability of atherosclerotic plaques, lower serum cholesterol levels, and alter membrane stability and influence *APP* cleavage.[99] They also increase transcription of transthyretin and Aβ scavenger in the hippocampus of old rats. In addition, fish consumption may lower the risk of dementia by reducing the risk of stroke. Women[103] and men[104] who eat fish regularly have a lower risk of stroke than people who do not.

A diet based on grains, vegetables, and fruit; regular fish consumption; and limited amounts of saturated fat from meat and dairy products is associated with better cardiovascular health and may reduce the risk of dementia through various pathways. In combination with an active lifestyle, it leads to optimal weight control and prevention of hypertension and diabetes.

Alcohol

Several case-control studies nested in large population cohorts show that moderate alcohol consumption is associated with a 50% decreased risk of dementia.[105-109] People who drink moderate amounts of alcohol have higher psychomotor speed and cognitive flexibility,[110] and better cognitive status, than those who abstain or who drink heavily.[111,112] Some studies have noted the inverse association between moderate alcohol use and dementia regardless of type of alcohol (wine, beer, or spirits),[107-109,111,112] whereas others found that only wine was protective.[105,106] On the other hand, heavy alcohol intake, particularly when sustained over time, is associated with cognitive decline and dementia,[106,109] and alcohol abuse leads to neuronal loss and brain atrophy, particularly in the frontal association cortex. The reasons for the protective effect of alcohol are not well understood. In most cohort and case-control studies, low to moderate alcohol consumption decreases the risk of ischemic stroke, and this may partially explain the link. Due to the effect of alcohol on acetylcholine release and prostaglandin metabolism, particularly with wine, the antioxidant effects of flavonoid (also found in fruits and vegetables) have also been implicated.[113] In addition, a higher social economic status of wine drinkers may partially explain the health benefits associated with wine intake.[114]

Clinicians are faced with the question of what to do with these data. Middle-aged and elderly drinkers can be encouraged to continue to drink if they do so in moderation, but the data do not warrant a recommendation for teetotalers to start drinking. Further research into the biological mechanisms that underlie the association between alcohol intake and dementia is needed to extend the benefits noted in clinical studies to the general population.

Coffee and Cigarettes

Caffeine has neuroprotective effects in animal models of ischemia and hypoxia, and it may be protective against dementia. In the Canadian Study of Health and Aging, people who drank coffee had a lower risk of AD than in people who did not,[115] and in a case-control study, regular caffeine intake from any source over the preceding 20 years was associated with lower prevalence of AD, independent of other habits, medical disorders, and potential risk factors for AD.[116]

Smoking, independent of its cardiovascular effects, increases the risk of AD.[117,118] Among individuals 45 to 70 years old, smoking is associated with reduced cognitive flexibility and psychomotor speed.[110] All smokers must be encouraged to stop.

Activity

Physical, cognitive, and social activities can help prevent or slow cognitive decline. Participation in cognitively demanding leisure activities in late life may provide protection against dementia,[11,119-123] and reduced involvement in these activities is associated with a greater risk of cognitive decline.[124] In the recent prospective Bronx Aging Study, a high level of participation in leisure activities at baseline lowered the risk of dementia after 21 years of follow-up.[11] In a longitudinal study spanning 12 years, Bassuk and colleagues[125] evaluated the degree of social engagement of 2812 elderly persons living in the community. They relied on these indicators of social engagement: (1) presence of a spouse, (2) monthly visual contact with at least 3 relatives or close friend, (3) yearly phone contact with 10 relatives or friends, (4) regular attendance (at least once month) at religious services, and (5) regular participation in recreational activities. Subjects with higher level of social disengagement had a greater degree of cognitive impairment; the odds of experiencing cognitive decline were approximately twice as great in the most disengaged persons than in the most socially engaged respondents, after adjusting for sociodemographic and health factors.[125]

Studies of the effect of physical activity have been less consistent. Animal studies show that exercise has effects on calcium metabolism and dopamine that may improve some symptoms of AD.[126,127] Exercise may have beneficial effects on cerebrovascular and cardiovascular risk factors and, thus, affect risk of AD and VaD. However, some epidemiologic studies have found a protective effect of exercise and some have not. In the Canadian Study of Health and Aging, regular physical activity was associated with decreased risk of AD,[115] and in one prospective study, strenuous, but not moderate, daily activities were associated with less cognitive decline in a healthy older cohort.[128] Cognitively normal women aged 65 years or older who walked regularly were less likely to develop cognitive decline.[129] On the other hand, in the Bronx Aging Study physical activity (other than dancing) did not confer any protection.[11] Several trials have failed to show a benefit of exercise intervention,[130,131] whereas others have found improved cognitive function with physical activity.[130,132-134]

Engagement in leisure activities may result in functionally more efficient cognitive networks and a cognitive reserve that delays the onset of the clinical manifestations of dementia.[135] Alternatively, it may strengthen existing synaptic connections, which promote plastic changes in the brain that circumvent the pathologic changes underlying symptoms of dementia.[136] In addition, it may lead to better cardiovascular health. However, the association between social engagement, participation in leisure activities, physical activity, and dementia does not prove causality. Inactivity and social isolation may be risk factors for development of the disease, a reflection of very early subclinical effects, or both. Physical activity may be a marker for "wellness," and people who do not feel well are less likely to exercise. Nevertheless, the data support recommendations for participation in cognitive activities that parallel the exercise recommendations for patients with cardiovascular disease.[11] Given the potential benefits and the lack of side effects, all patients with mild cognitive impairment or mild to moderate dementia should be encouraged to exercise regularly and to participate in cognitively challenging and social activities.

IMMUNOTHERAPY

In young transgenic mice, immunization with the Aβ 42 peptide prevents the development of Alzheimer-type disease, whereas treatment of older animals in whom these changes are well established markedly reduces the extent and progression of the disease.[137] Immunization also has a positive effect on behavior[138] and memory.[139,140] These findings led to clinical trials in humans. In a phase 1 study in 104 patients, active immunization with Aβ 42 was safe and well tolerated, and led to the formation of Aβ 42 antibodies in 25% of patients.[141] In 2001, more than 300 patients were enrolled in a double-blind, placebo-controlled trial in 30 centers in Europe and the United States. They were 50 to 85 years old and had mild to moderate probable AD. The trial, which was scheduled to run for 2 years, was terminated prematurely in January 2002 after 4 patients were found to have meningoencephalitis with subacute cognitive decline, extensive radiological white-matter changes, and abnormal cerebrospinal fluid. Subsequently, another 14 patients (6% of the sample) became ill (1 died); all were in the active treatment arm.[141] Vaccination induced formation of antibodies with a high degree of selectivity for the pathogenic target structure,[142] but the risk of meningoencephalitis did not correlate with antibody titers.[141] In a subset of patients from the Aβ vaccine trial, those who generated Aβ antibodies showed slower decline of cognitive functions and activities of daily living, compared with individuals in whom the antibodies did not develop.[143] Autopsy results from the patient who died showed that the inflammatory reaction was T-cell mediated and that the immune response against the Aβ peptide led clearance of amyloid plaques in the cortex but not in blood vessels.[144]

Although the results of the clinical trial preclude further testing of this drug, they show that an immunotherapy may help prevent or slow the development of AD. Alternative strategies to provide antibodies to Aβ are currently under study.[145] Potential strategies include passive immunization with anti-Aβ antibodies, manipulation of Aβ antigen to remove problematic T-cell epitopes while preserving B-cell response, development of antibodies against specific residues of the Aβ peptide,[146] and creation of a high-affinity Aβ sink that sequesters Aβ into the periphery with antibodies or other Aβ-binding compounds.[147]

SUMMARY

The data discussed above raise the possibility that for many people the onset and progression of dementia can be prevented or delayed. The implications at the individual and societal level are immense. The task ahead is to identify all modifiable risk factors through careful analysis of basic science discoveries and epidemiologic studies that have solid methodological bases, and to test possible interventions with well-designed clinical trials.

REFERENCES

1. Lobo A, Launer LJ, Fratiglioni L, et al, for Neurologic Diseases in the Elderly Research Group. Prevalence of dementia and major subtypes in Europe: a collaborative study of population-based cohorts. *Neurology.* 2000;54(suppl 5):S4–S9.

2. Petersen RC, Doody R, Kurz A, et al. Current concepts in mild cognitive impairment. *Arch Neurol.* 2001;58:1985–1992.

3. Roman GC. Vascular dementia may be the most common form of dementia in the elderly. *J Neurol Sci.* 2002;203–204:7–10.

4. Pathological correlates of late-onset dementia in a multicentre, community-based population in England and Wales: Neuropathology Group of the Medical Research Council Cognitive Function and Ageing Study (MRC CFAS). *Lancet.* 2001;357:169–175.

5. Snowdon DA, Greiner LH, Mortimer JA, Riley KP, Greiner PA, Markesbery WR. Brain infarction and the clinical expression of Alzheimer disease: the Nun Study. *JAMA.* 1997;277:813–817.

6. Hachinski V. Multi-infarct dementia. *Neurol Clin.* 1983;1:27–36.

7. Breteler MM. Vascular risk factors for Alzheimer's disease: an epidemiologic perspective. *Neurobiol Aging.* 2000;21:153–160.

8. Skoog I. Status of risk factors for vascular dementia. *Neuroepidemiology.* 1998;17:2–9.

9. de la Torre JC. Alzheimer disease as a vascular disorder: nosological evidence. *Stroke.* 2002;33:1152–1162.

10. Hachinski V. Preventable senility: a call for action against the vascular dementias. *Lancet.* 1992;340:645–648.

11. Verghese J, Lipton RB, Katz MJ, et al. Leisure activities and the risk of dementia in the elderly. *N Engl J Med.* 2003;348:2508–2516.

12. Morris MC, Evans DA, Bienias JLTCC, et al. Consumption of fish and n-3 fatty acids and risk of incident Alzheimer disease. *Arch Neurol.* 2003;60:940–946.

13. DeCarli C. Mild cognitive impairment: prevalence, prognosis, aetiology, and treatment. *Lancet Neurol.* 2003;2:15–21.

14. Bowler JV, Steenhuis R, Hachinski V. Conceptual background to vascular cognitive impairment. *Alzheimer Dis Assoc Disord.* 1999;13(suppl 3):S30–S37.

15. Cooper B. Thinking preventively about dementia: a review. *Int J Geriatr Psychiatry.* 2002;17:895–906.

16. Shumaker SA, Legault C, Thal L, et al. Estrogen plus progestin and the incidence of dementia and mild cognitive impairment in postmenopausal women: the Women's Health Initiative Memory Study: a randomized controlled trial. *JAMA.* 2003;289:2651–2662.

17. Tatemichi TK, Desmond DW, Mayeux R, et al. Dementia after stroke: baseline frequency, risks, and clinical features in a hospitalized cohort. *Neurology.* 1992;42:1185–1193.

18. Pohjasvaara T, Erkinjuntti T, Ylikoski R, Hietanen M, Vataja R, Kaste M. Clinical determinants of poststroke dementia. *Stroke.* 1998;29:75–81.

19. Vermeer SE, Prins ND, den Heijer T, Hofman A, Koudstaal PJ, Breteler MM. Silent brain infarcts and the risk of dementia and cognitive decline. *N Engl J Med.* 2003;348:1215–1222.

20. Tatemichi TK, Desmond DW, Prohovnik I. Strategic infarcts in vascular dementia: a clinical and brain imaging experience. *Arzneimittelforsch.* 1995;45:371–385.

21. Heyman A, Fillenbaum GG, Welsh-Bohmer KA, et al. Cerebral infarcts in patients with autopsy-proven Alzheimer's disease: CERAD, part XVIII. Consortium to Establish a Registry for Alzheimer's Disease. *Neurology.* 1998;51:159–162.

22. Straus SE, Majumdar SR, McAlister FA. New evidence for stroke prevention: scientific review. *JAMA.* 2002;288:1388–1395.

23. Randomised trial of a perindopril-based blood-pressure-lowering regimen among 6,105 individuals with previous stroke or transient ischaemic attack. *Lancet.* 2001;358:1033–1041.

24. Tzourio C, Anderson C, Chapman N, et al. Effects of blood pressure lowering with perindopril and indapamide therapy on dementia and cognitive decline in patients with cerebrovascular disease. *Arch Intern Med.* 2003;163:1069–1075.

25. Vaughan CJ. Prevention of stroke and dementia with statins: effects beyond lipid lowering. *Am J Cardiol.* 2003;91:23B–29B.

26. Schnyder G, Roffi M, Pin R, et al. Decreased rate of coronary restenosis after lowering of plasma homocysteine levels. *N Engl J Med.* 2001;345:1593–1600.

27. Wolf PA, Clagett GP, Easton JD, et al. Preventing ischemic stroke in patients with prior stroke and transient ischemic attack: a statement for healthcare professionals from the Stroke Council of the American Heart Association. *Stroke.* 1999;30:1991–1994.

28. Albers GW, Amarenco P, Easton JD, Sacco RL, Teal P. Antithrombotic and thrombolytic therapy for ischemic stroke. *Chest.* 2001;119(suppl):300S–320S.

29. Cacciatore F, Abete P, Ferrara N, et al, for Osservatorio Geriatrico Campano Group. The role of blood pressure in cognitive impairment in an elderly population. *J Hypertens.* 1997;15:135–142.

30. Starr JM, Whalley LJ, Inch S, Shering PA. Blood pressure and cognitive function in healthy old people. *J Am Geriatr Soc.* 1993;41:753–756.

31. Guo Z, Viitanen M, Fratiglioni L, Winblad B. Low blood pressure and dementia in elderly people: the Kungsholmen project. *BMJ.* 1996;312:805–808.

32. Farmer ME, White LR, Abbott RD, et al. Blood pressure and cognitive performance: the Framingham Study. *Am J Epidemiol.* 1987;126:1103–1114.

33. Scherr PA, Hebert LE, Smith LA, Evans DA. Relation of blood pressure to cognitive function in the elderly. *Am J Epidemiol.* 1991;134:1303–1315.

34. Swan GE, DeCarli C, Miller BL, et al. Association of midlife blood pressure to late-life cognitive decline and brain morphology. *Neurology.* 1998;51:986–993.

35. Kilander L, Nyman H, Boberg M, Hansson L, Lithell H. Hypertension is related to cognitive impairment: a 20-year follow-up of 999 men. *Hypertension.* 1998;31:780–786.

36. Skoog I, Lernfelt B, Landahl S, et al. 15-year longitudinal study of blood pressure and dementia. *Lancet.* 1996;347:1141–1145.

37. Yamada M, Kasagi F, Sasaki H, Masunari N, Mimori Y, Suzuki G. Association between dementia and midlife risk factors: the Radiation Effects Research Foundation Adult Health Study. *J Am Geriatr Soc.* 2003;51:410–414.

38. Launer LJ, Masaki K, Petrovitch H, Foley D, Havlik RJ. The association between midlife blood pressure levels and late-life cognitive function: the Honolulu-Asia Aging Study. *JAMA.* 1995;274:1846–1851.

39. Tzourio C, Dufouil C, Ducimetiere P, Alperovitch A, for Epidemiology of Vascular Aging Study Group. Cognitive decline in individuals with high blood pressure: a longitudinal study in the elderly. *Neurology.* 1999;53:1948–1952.

40. Qiu C, Winblad B, Viitanen M, Fratiglioni L. Pulse pressure and risk of Alzheimer disease in persons aged 75 years and older: a community-based, longitudinal study. *Stroke.* 2003;34:594–599.

41. SHEP Cooperative Research Group. Prevention of stroke by antihypertensive drug treatment in older persons with isolated systolic hypertension: final results of the Systolic Hypertension in the Elderly Program (SHEP). *JAMA.* 1991;265:3255–3264.

42. Applegate WB, Pressel S, Wittes J, et al. Impact of the treatment of isolated systolic hypertension on behavioral variables. Results from the systolic hypertension in the elderly program. *Arch Intern Med.* 1994;154:2154–2160.

43. Prencipe M, Ferretti C, Casini AR, Santini M, Giubilei F, Culasso F. Stroke, disability, and dementia: results of a population survey. *Stroke.* 1997;28:531–536.

44. Di Bari M, Pahor M, Franse LV, et al. Dementia and disability outcomes in large hypertension trials: lessons learned from the systolic hypertension in the elderly program (SHEP) trial. *Am J Epidemiol.* 2001;153:72–78.

45. Forette F, Seux ML, Staessen JA, et al. Prevention of dementia in randomised double-blind placebo-controlled Systolic Hypertension in Europe (Syst-Eur) trial. *Lancet.* 1998;352:1347–1351.

46. Forette F, Seux ML, Staessen JA, et al. The prevention of dementia with antihypertensive treatment: new evidence from the Systolic Hypertension in Europe (Syst-Eur) study. *Arch Intern Med.* 2002;162:2046–2052.

47. Chobanian AV, Bakris GL, Black HR, et al. The Seventh Report of the Joint National Committee on Prevention, Detection, Evaluation, and Treatment of High Blood Pressure: the JNC 7 report. *JAMA.* 2003;289:2560–2572.

48. Fassbender K, Simons M, Bergmann C, et al. Simvastatin strongly reduces levels of Alzheimer's disease beta-amyloid peptides Abeta 42 and Abeta 40 in vitro and in vivo. *Proc Natl Acad Sci U S A.* 2001;98:5856–5861.

49. Hofman A, Ott A, Breteler MM, et al. Atherosclerosis, apolipoprotein E, and prevalence of dementia and Alzheimer's disease in the Rotterdam Study. *Lancet.* 1997;349:151–154.

50. Romas SN, Tang MX, Berglund L, Mayeux R. APOE genotype, plasma lipids, lipoproteins, and AD in community elderly. *Neurology.* 1999;53:517–521.

51. Notkola IL, Sulkava R, Pekkanen J, et al. Serum total cholesterol, apolipoprotein E epsilon 4 allele, and Alzheimer's disease. *Neuroepidemiology.* 1998;17:14–20.

52. Yaffe K, Barrett-Connor E, Lin F, Grady D. Serum lipoprotein levels, statin use, and cognitive function in older women. *Arch Neurol.* 2002;59:378–384.

53. Kivipelto M, Helkala EL, Hanninen T, et al. Midlife vascular risk factors and late-life mild cognitive impairment: a population-based study. *Neurology.* 2001;56:1683–1689.

54. Tan ZS, Seshadri S, Beiser A, et al. Plasma total cholesterol level as a risk factor for Alzheimer disease: the Framingham Study. *Arch Intern Med.* 2003;163:1053–1057.

55. Scott HD, Laake K. Statins for the prevention of Alzheimer's disease. *Cochrane Database Syst Rev.* 2001;CD003160.

56. Wolozin B, Kellman W, Ruosseau P, Celesia GG, Siegel G. Decreased prevalence of Alzheimer disease associated with 3-hydroxy-3-methylglutaryl coenzyme A reductase inhibitors. *Arch Neurol.* 2000;57:1439–1443.

57. Jick H, Zornberg GL, Jick SS, Seshadri S, Drachman DA. Statins and the risk of dementia. *Lancet.* 2000;356:1627–1631.

58. Rockwood K, Kirkland S, Hogan DB, et al. Use of lipid-lowering agents, indication bias, and the risk of dementia in community-dwelling elderly people. *Arch Neurol.* 2002;59:223–227.

59. Shepherd J, Blauw GJ, Murphy MB, et al, for PROSPER Study Group. The design of a prospective study of Pravastatin in the Elderly at Risk (PROSPER). *Am J Cardiol.* 1999;84:1192–1197.

60. Danesh J, Lewington S. Plasma homocysteine and coronary heart disease: systematic review of published epidemiological studies. *J Cardiovasc Risk.* 1998;5:229–232.

61. Perry IJ, Refsum H, Morris RW, Ebrahim SB, Ueland PM, Shaper AG. Prospective study of serum total homocysteine concentration and risk of stroke in middle-aged British men. *Lancet.* 1995;346:1395–1398.

62. Eikelboom JW, Hankey GJ, Anand SS, Lofthouse E, Staples N, Baker RI. Association between high homocyst(e)ine and ischemic stroke due to large- and small-artery disease but not other etiologic subtypes of ischemic stroke. *Stroke.* 2000;31:1069–1075.

63. Cunha UG, Rocha FL, Peixoto JM, Motta MF, Barbosa MT. Vitamin B12 deficiency and dementia. *Int Psychogeriatr.* 1995;7:85–88.

64. Teunisse S, Bollen AE, van Gool WA, Walstra GJ. Dementia and subnormal levels of vitamin B12: effects of replacement therapy on dementia. *J Neurol.* 1996;243:522–529.

65. Nilsson K, Gustafson L, Faldt R, et al. Hyperhomo-cysteinaemia—a common finding in a psychogeriatric population. *Eur J Clin Invest.* 1996;26:853–859.

66. Duthie SJ, Whalley LJ, Collins AR, Leaper S, Berger K, Deary IJ. Homocysteine, B vitamin status, and cognitive function in the elderly. *Am J Clin Nutr.* 2002;75:908–913.

67. Ravaglia G, Forti P, Maioli F, et al. Homocysteine and cognitive function in healthy elderly community dwellers in Italy. *Am J Clin Nutr.* 2003;77:668–673.

68. Wang HX, Wahlin A, Basun H, Fastbom J, Winblad B, Fratiglioni L. Vitamin B(12) and folate in relation to the development of Alzheimer's disease. *Neurology.* 2001;56:1188–1194.

69. Clarke R, Smith AD, Jobst KA, Refsum H, Sutton L, Ueland PM. Folate, vitamin B12, and serum total homocysteine levels in confirmed Alzheimer disease. *Arch Neurol.* 1998;55:1449–1455.

70. Seshadri S, Beiser A, Selhub J, et al. Plasma homocysteine as a risk factor for dementia and Alzheimer's disease. *N Engl J Med.* 2002;346:476–483.

71. Engelhart MJ, Geerlings MI, Ruitenberg A, et al. Dietary intake of antioxidants and risk of Alzheimer disease. *JAMA.* 2002;287:3223–3229.

72. Morris MC, Evans DA, Bienias JL, et al. Dietary intake of antioxidant nutrients and the risk of incident Alzheimer disease in a biracial community study. *JAMA.* 2002;287:3230–3237.

73. Luchsinger JA, Tang MX, Shea S, Mayeux R. Antioxidant vitamin intake and risk of Alzheimer disease. *Arch Neurol.* 2003;60:203–208.

74. Grodstein F, Chen J, Willett WC. High-dose antioxidant supplements and cognitive function in community-dwelling elderly women. *Am J Clin Nutr.* 2003;77:975–984.

75. Sano M, Ernesto C, Thomas RG, et al. A controlled trial of selegiline, alpha-tocopherol, or both as treatment for Alzheimer's disease: the Alzheimer's Disease Cooperative Study. *N Engl J Med.* 1997;336:1216–1222.

76. Redlich CA, Chung JS, Cullen MR, Blaner WS, Van Bennekum AM, Berglund L. Effect of long-term beta-carotene and vitamin A on serum cholesterol and triglyceride levels among participants in the Carotene and Retinol Efficacy Trial (CARET). *Atherosclerosis.* 1999;145:425–432.

77. MRC/BHF Heart Protection Study of antioxidant vitamin supplementation in 20,536 high-risk individuals: a randomised placebo-controlled trial. *Lancet.* 2002;360:23–33.

78. Alpha-Tocopherol, Beta Carotene Cancer Prevention Study Group. The effect of vitamin E and beta carotene on the incidence of lung cancer and other cancers in male smokers. *N Engl J Med.* 1994;330:1029–1035.

79. Morris CD, Carson S. Routine vitamin supplementation to prevent cardiovascular disease: a summary of the evidence for the U.S. Preventive Services Task Force. *Ann Intern Med.* 2003;139:56–70.

80. Tang MX, Jacobs D, Stern Y, et al. Effect of oestrogen during menopause on risk and age at onset of Alzheimer's disease. *Lancet.* 1996;348:429–432.

81. Kawas C, Resnick S, Morrison A, et al. A prospective study of estrogen replacement therapy and the risk of developing Alzheimer's disease: the Baltimore Longitudinal Study of Aging. *Neurology.* 1997;48:1517–1521.

82. Zandi PP, Carlson MC, Plassman BL, et al. Hormone replacement therapy and incidence of Alzheimer disease in older women: the Cache County Study. *JAMA.* 2002;288:2123–2129.

83. LeBlanc ES, Janowsky J, Chan BK, Nelson HD. Hormone replacement therapy and cognition: systematic review and meta-analysis. *JAMA.* 2001;285:1489–1499.

84. Hogervorst E, Yaffe K, Richards M, Huppert F. Hormone replacement therapy for cognitive function in postmenopausal women. *Cochrane Database Syst Rev.* 2002;(3):CD003122.

85. Hogervorst E, Yaffe K, Richards M, Huppert F. Hormone replacement therapy to maintain cognitive function in women with dementia. *Cochrane Database Syst Rev.* 2002;(3):CD003799.

86. Mulnard RA, Cotman CW, Kawas C, et al. Estrogen replacement therapy for treatment of mild to moderate Alzheimer disease: a randomized controlled trial. Alzheimer's Disease Cooperative Study. *JAMA.* 2000;283:1007–1015.

87. Rossouw JE, Anderson GL, Prentice RL, et al. Risks and benefits of estrogen plus progestin in healthy postmenopausal women: principal results from the Women's Health Initiative randomized controlled trial. *JAMA.* 2002;288:321–333.

88. Rapp SR, Espeland MA, Shumaker SA, et al. Effect of estrogen plus progestin on global cognitive function in postmenopausal women: the Women's Health Initiative Memory Study: a randomized controlled trial. *JAMA.* 2003;289:2663–2672.

89. Wassertheil-Smoller S, Hendrix SL, Limacher M, et al. Effect of estrogen plus progestin on stroke in postmenopausal women: the Women's Health Initiative: a randomized trial. *JAMA*. 2003;289:2673–2684.

90. Yaffe K. Hormone therapy and the brain: déja vu all over again? *JAMA*. 2003;289:2717–2719.

91. Etminan M, Gill S, Samii A. Effect of non-steroidal anti-inflammatory drugs on risk of Alzheimer's disease: systematic review and meta-analysis of observational studies. *BMJ*. 2003;327:128.

92. Aisen PS, Schafer KA, Grundman M, et al. Effects of rofecoxib or naproxen vs placebo on Alzheimer disease progression: a randomized controlled trial. *JAMA*. 2003;289:2819–2826.

93. Oken BS, Storzbach DM, Kaye JA. The efficacy of *Ginkgo biloba* on cognitive function in Alzheimer disease. *Arch Neurol*. 1998;55:1409–1415.

94. Ernst E. Usage of complementary therapies in rheumatology: a systematic review. *Clin Rheumatol*. 1998;17:301–305.

95. Birks J, Grimley EV, Van Dongen M. Ginkgo biloba for cognitive impairment and dementia. *Cochrane Database Syst Rev*. 2002;(4):CD003120.

96. Luchsinger JA, Tang MX, Shea S, Mayeux R. Caloric intake and the risk of Alzheimer disease. *Arch Neurol*. 2002;59:1258–1263.

97. Kalmijn S. Fatty acid intake and the risk of dementia and cognitive decline: a review of clinical and epidemiological studies. *J Nutr Health Aging*. 2000;4:202–207.

98. Morris MC, Evans DA, Bienias JL, et al. Dietary fats and the risk of incident Alzheimer disease. *Arch Neurol*. 2003;60:194–200.

99. Friedland RP. Fish consumption and the risk of Alzheimer disease: is it time to make dietary recommendations? *Arch Neurol*. 2003;60:923–924.

100. Kalmijn S, Launer LJ, Ott A, Witteman JC, Hofman A, Breteler MM. Dietary fat intake and the risk of incident dementia in the Rotterdam Study. *Ann Neurol*. 1997;42:776–782.

101. Barberger-Gateau P, Letenneur L, Deschamps V, Peres K, Dartigues JF, Renaud S. Fish, meat, and risk of dementia: cohort study. *BMJ*. 2002;325:932–933.

102. Sparks DL, Martin TA, Gross DR, Hunsaker JC III. Link between heart disease, cholesterol, and Alzheimer's disease: a review. *Microsc Res Tech*. 2000;50:287–290.

103. Iso H, Rexrode KM, Stampfer MJ, et al. Intake of fish and omega-3 fatty acids and risk of stroke in women. *JAMA*. 2001;285:304–312.

104. He K, Rimm EB, Merchant A, et al. Fish consumption and risk of stroke in men. *JAMA*. 2002;288:3130–3136.

105. Orgogozo JM, Dartigues JF, Lafont S, et al. Wine consumption and dementia in the elderly: a prospective community study in the Bordeaux area. *Rev Neurol Paris*. 1997;153:185–192.

106. Truelsen T, Thudium D, Gronbaek M. Amount and type of alcohol and risk of dementia: the Copenhagen City Heart Study. *Neurology*. 2002;59:1313–1319.

107. Ruitenberg A, van Swieten JC, Witteman JC, et al. Alcohol consumption and risk of dementia: the Rotterdam Study. *Lancet*. 2002;359:281–286.

108. Huang W, Qiu C, Winblad B, Fratiglioni L. Alcohol consumption and incidence of dementia in a community sample aged 75 years and older. *J Clin Epidemiol*. 2002;55:959–964.

109. Mukamal KJ, Kuller LH, Fitzpatrick AL, Longstreth WT Jr, Mittleman MA, Siscovick DS. Prospective study of alcohol consumption and risk of dementia in older adults. *JAMA*. 2003;289:1405–1413.

110. Kalmijn S, van Boxtel MP, Verschuren MW, Jolles J, Launer LJ. Cigarette smoking and alcohol consumption in relation to cognitive performance in middle age. *Am J Epidemiol*. 2002;156:936–944.

111. Launer LJ, Feskens EJ, Kalmijn S, Kromhout D. Smoking, drinking, and thinking: the Zutphen Elderly Study. *Am J Epidemiol*. 1996;143:219–227.

112. Galanis DJ, Joseph C, Masaki KH, Petrovitch H, Ross GW, White L. A longitudinal study of drinking and cognitive performance in elderly Japanese American men: the Honolulu-Asia Aging Study. *Am J Public Health*. 2000;90:1254–1259.

113. Mukamal KJ, Longstreth WT Jr, Mittleman MA, Crum RM, Siscovick DS. Alcohol consumption and subclinical findings on magnetic resonance imaging of the brain in older adults: the Cardiovascular Health Study. *Stroke*. 2001;32:1939–1946.

114. Mortensen EL, Jensen HH, Sanders SA, Reinisch JM. Better psychological functioning and higher social status may largely explain the apparent health benefits of wine: a study of wine and beer drinking in young Danish adults. *Arch Intern Med*. 2001;161:1844–1848.

115. Lindsay J, Laurin D, Verreault R, et al. Risk factors for Alzheimer's disease: a prospective analysis from the Canadian Study of Health and Aging. *Am J Epidemiol*. 2002;156:445–453.

116. Maia L, de Mendonca A. Does caffeine intake protect from Alzheimer's disease? *Eur J Neurol*. 2002;9:377–382.

117. Ott A, Slooter AJ, Hofman A, et al. Smoking and risk of dementia and Alzheimer's disease in a population-based cohort study: the Rotterdam Study. *Lancet*. 1998;351:1840–1843.

118. Merchant C, Tang MX, Albert S, Manly J, Stern Y, Mayeux R. The influence of smoking on the risk of Alzheimer's disease. *Neurology*. 1999;52:1408–1412.

119. Fabrigoule C, Letenneur L, Dartigues JF, Zarrouk M, Commenges D, Barberger-Gateau P. Social and leisure activities and risk of dementia: a prospective longitudinal study. *J Am Geriatr Soc.* 1995;43:485–490.

120. Laurin D, Verreault R, Lindsay J, MacPherson K, Rockwood K. Physical activity and risk of cognitive impairment and dementia in elderly persons. *Arch Neurol.* 2001;58:498–504.

121. Wilson RS, Bennett DA, Bienias JL, et al. Cognitive activity and incident AD in a population-based sample of older persons. *Neurology.* 2002;59:1910–1914.

122. Wilson RS, Mendes De Leon CF, et al. Participation in cognitively stimulating activities and risk of incident Alzheimer disease. *JAMA.* 2002;287:742–748.

123. Wang HX, Karp A, Winblad B, Fratiglioni L. Late-life engagement in social and leisure activities is associated with a decreased risk of dementia: a longitudinal study from the Kungsholmen project. *Am J Epidemiol.* 2002;155:1081–1087.

124. Friedland RP, Fritsch T, Smyth KA, et al. Patients with Alzheimer's disease have reduced activities in midlife compared with healthy control-group members. *Proc Natl Acad Sci U S A.* 2001;98:3440–3445.

125. Bassuk SS, Glass TA, Berkman LF. Social disengagement and incident cognitive decline in community-dwelling elderly persons. *Ann Intern Med.* 1999;131:165–173.

126. van Praag H, Christie BR, Sejnowski TJ, Gage FH. Running enhances neurogenesis, learning, and long-term potentiation in mice. *Proc Natl Acad Sci U S A.* 1999;96:13427–13431.

127. Sutoo D, Akiyama K. Regulation of brain function by exercise. *Neurobiol Dis.* 2003;13:1–14.

128. Albert MS, Jones K, Savage CR, et al. Predictors of cognitive change in older persons: MacArthur studies of successful aging. *Psychol Aging.* 1995;10:578–589.

129. Yaffe K, Cauley J, Sands L, Browner W. Apolipoprotein E phenotype and cognitive decline in a prospective study of elderly community women. *Arch Neurol.* 1997;54:1110–1114.

130. Pierce TW, Madden DJ, Siegel WC, Blumenthal JA. Effects of aerobic exercise on cognitive and psychosocial functioning in patients with mild hypertension. *Health Psychol.* 1993;12:286–291.

131. Madden DJ, Blumenthal JA, Allen PA, Emery CF. Improving aerobic capacity in healthy older adults does not necessarily lead to improved cognitive performance. *Psychol Aging.* 1989;4:307–320.

132. Dustman RE, Ruhling RO, Russell EM, et al. Aerobic exercise training and improved neuropsychological function of older individuals. *Neurobiol Aging.* 1984;5:35–42.

133. Williams P, Lord SR. Effects of group exercise on cognitive functioning and mood in older women. *Aust N Z J Public Health.* 1997;21:45–52.

134. Kramer AF, Hahn S, Cohen NJ, et al. Ageing, fitness and neurocognitive function. *Nature.* 1999;400:418–419.

135. Scarmeas N, Stern Y. Cognitive reserve and lifestyle. *J Clin Exp Neuropsychol.* 2003;25:625–633.

136. Coyle JT. Use it or lose it: do effortful mental activities protect against dementia? *N Engl J Med.* 2003;348:2489–2490.

137. Schenk D, Barbour R, Dunn W, et al. Immunization with amyloid-beta attenuates Alzheimer-disease-like pathology in the PDAPP mouse. *Nature.* 1999;400:173–177.

138. Janus C, Pearson J, McLaurin J, et al. A beta peptide immunization reduces behavioural impairment and plaques in a model of Alzheimer's disease. *Nature.* 2000;408:979–982.

139. Morgan D, Diamond DM, Gottschall PE, et al. A beta peptide vaccination prevents memory loss in an animal model of Alzheimer's disease. *Nature.* 2000;408:982–985.

140. Dodart JC, Bales KR, Gannon KS, et al. Immunization reverses memory deficits without reducing brain Abeta burden in Alzheimer's disease model. *Nat Neurosci.* 2002;5:452–457.

141. Orgogozo JM, Gilman S, Dartigues JF, et al. Subacute meningoencephalitis in a subset of patients with AD after Abeta42 immunization. *Neurology.* 2003;61:46–54.

142. Hock C, Konietzko U, Papassotiropoulos A, et al. Generation of antibodies specific for beta-amyloid by vaccination of patients with Alzheimer disease. *Nat Med.* 2002;8:1270–1275.

143. Hock C, Konietzko U, Streffer JR, et al. Antibodies against beta-amyloid slow cognitive decline in Alzheimer's disease. *Neuron.* 2003;38:547–554.

144. Nicoll JA, Wilkinson D, Holmes C, Steart P, Markham H, Weller RO. Neuropathology of human Alzheimer disease after immunization with amyloid-beta peptide: a case report. *Nat Med.* 2003;9:448–452.

145. Dodel RC, Hampel H, Du Y. Immunotherapy for Alzheimer's disease. *Lancet Neurol.* 2003;2:215–220.

146. McLaurin J, Cecal R, Kierstead ME, et al. Therapeutically effective antibodies against amyloid-beta peptide target amyloid-beta residues 4-10 and inhibit cytotoxicity and fibrillogenesis. *Nat Med.* 2002;8:1263–1269.

147. Mathews PM, Nixon RA. Setback for an Alzheimer's disease vaccine: lessons learned. *Neurology.* 2003;61:7–8.

RESOURCES

Alzheimer's Association
Web site: www.alz.org

National Institutes of Health
Web site: www.nih.gov

National Institute on Aging
Alzheimer's Disease Education and Referral Center
Web site: www.alzheimers.org/index.html

These codes were selected for this appendix from *CPT 2004 Professional Edition* for their application to preventive medicine.

EVALUATION AND MANAGEMENT

Preventive Medicine Services

The following codes are used to report the preventive medicine evaluation and management of infants, children, adolescents and adults.

The extent and focus of die services will largely depend on the age of the patient.

If an abnormality/ies is encountered or a preexisting problem is addressed in the process of performing diis preventive medicine evaluation and management service, and if the problem/abnormality is significant enough to require additional work to perform the key components of a problem-oriented E/M service, then the appropriate Office/Outpatient code 99201–99215 should also be reported. Modifier '–25' should be added to die Office/Outpatient code to indicate that a significant, separately identifiable Evaluation and Management service was provided by the same physician on the same day as the preventive medicine service. The appropriate preventive medicine service is additionally reported.

An insignificant or trivial problem/abnormality that is encountered in the process of performing the preventive medicine evaluation and management service and which does not require additional work and the performance of the key components of a problem-oriented E/M service should not be reported.

The "comprehensive" nature of the Preventive Medicine Services codes 99381–99397 reflects an age and gender appropriate history/exam and is NOT synonymous with the "comprehensive" examination required in Evaluation and Management codes 99201–99350.

Codes 99381–99397 include counseling/anticipatory guidance/risk factor reduction interventions which are provided at the time of the initial or periodic comprehensive preventive medicine examination. (Refer to codes 99401–99412 for reporting diose counseling/anticipatory guidance/risk factor reduction interventions that are provided at an encounter separate from the preventive medicine examination.)

Immunizations and ancillary studies involving laboratory, radiology, other procedures, or screening tests identified with a specific CPT code are reported separately. For immunizations, see 90471–90474 and 90476–90749.

New patient

99381 Initial comprehensive preventive medicine evaluation and management of an individual including an age and gender appropriate history, examination, counseling/anticipatory guidance/risk factor reduction interventions, and the ordering of appropriate immunization(s), laboratory/diagnostic procedures, new patient; infant (age under 1 year)

> ➔ *CPT Assistant* Winter 91:11, Spring 92:24, Summer 92:1. Spring 93:14,34, Spring 95:1, Aug 97:1, Jul 98:9, Nov 98:3–4, May 02:1; *CPT Changes: An Insider's View 2002*

99382 early childhood (age 1 through 4 years)

> ➔ *CPT Assistant* Winter 91:11, Spring 92:24, Summer 92:1, Spring 93:14,34. Spring 95:1, Aug 97:1, Jul 98:9, Nov 98:3–4, May 02:1

99383 late childhood (age 5 through 11 years)

> ➔ *CPT Assistant* Winter 91:11, Spring 92:24, Summer 92:1, Spring 93:14,34, Spring 95:1, Aug 97:1, Jul 98:9, Nov 98:3–4, May 02:1

⊘= Modifier '-51' Exempt   ▶◀ or ▶ ◀= New or Revised Text   ✚= Add-on Code   ➔ = Reference Material   ▲= Revised Code   ●= New Code

99384   adolescent (age 12 through 17 years)
> ➲ *CPT Assistant* Winter 91:11, Spring 92:24, Summer 92:1, Spring 93:14,34, Spring 95:1, Aug 97:1, Jul 98:9, Nov 98:3–4, May 02:1

99385   18–39 years
> ➲ *CPT Assistant* Winter 91:11, Spring 92:24, Summer 92:1, Spring 93:14,34, Spring 95:1, Aug 97:1, Jul 98:9, Nov 98:3–4, May 02:1

99386   40–64 years
> ➲ *CPT Assistant* Winter 91:11, Spring 92:24, Summer 92:1, Spring 93:14,34, Spring 95:1, Aug 97:1, Jul 98:9, Nov 98:3–4, May 02:1

99387   65 years and over
> ➲ *CPT Assistant* Winter 91:11, Spring 92:24, Summer 92:1, Spring 93:14, 34, Spring 95:1, Aug 97:1, Jul 98:9, Nov 98:3–4, May 02:1

Established patient

99391   Periodic comprehensive preventive medicine revaluation and management of an individual including an age and gender appropriate history, examination, counseling/anticipatory guidance/risk factor reduction interventions, and the ordering of appropriate immunization(s), laboratory/diagnostic procedures, established patient; infant (age under 1 year)
> ➲ *CPT Assistant* Winter 91:11, Spring 92:24, Summer 92:1, Spring 93:14, 34, Spring 95:1, Aug 97:1, Jul 98:9, Nov 98:3–4, May 02:1;
> *CPT Changes: An Insider's View 2002*

99392   early childhood (age 1 through 4 years)
> ➲ *CPT Assistant* Winter 91:11, Spring 92:24, Summer 92:1, Spring 93:14,34, Spring 95:1, Aug 97:1, Jul 98:9, Nov 98:3–4, May 02:1

99393   late childhood (age 5 through 11 years)
> ➲ *CPT Assistant* Winter 91:11, Spring 92:24, Summer 92:1, Spring 93:14,34, Spring 95:1, Aug 97:1, Jul 98:9, Nov 98:3–4, May 02:1

99394   adolescent (age 12 through 17 years)
> ➲ *CPT Assistant* Winter 91:11, Spring 92:24, Summer 92:1, Spring 93:14,34, Spring 95:1, Aug 97:1, Jul 98:9, Nov 98:3–4, May 02:1

99395   18–39 years
> ➲ *CPT Assistant* Winter 91:11, Spring 92:24, Summer 92:1, Spring 93:14,34, Spring 95:1, Aug 97:1, Jul 98:9, Nov 98:3–4, May 02:1

99396   40–64 years
> ➲ *CPT Assistant* Winter 91:11, Spring 92:24, Summer 92:1, Spring 93:14,34, Spring 95:1, Aug 97:1, Jul 98:9, Nov 98:3–4, May 02:1

99397   65 years and over
> ➲ *CPT Assistant* Winter 91.11, Spring 92:24, Summer 92:1, Spring 93:14,34, Spring 95:1, Aug 97:1, Jul 98:9, Nov 98:3–4, May 02:1

Counseling and/or Risk Factor Reduction Intervention

New or established patient

These codes are used to report services provided to individuals at a separate encounter for the purpose of promoting health and preventing illness or injury.

Preventive medicine counseling and risk factor reduction interventions provided as a separate encounter will vary with age and should address such issues as family problems, diet and exercise, substance abuse, sexual practices, injury prevention, dental health, and diagnostic and laboratory test results available at the time of the encounter.

These codes are not to be used to report counseling and risk factor reduction interventions provided to patients with symptoms or established illness. For counseling individual patients with symptoms or established illness, use the appropriate office, hospital or consultation or other evaluation and management codes. For counseling groups of patients with symptoms or established illness, use 99078.

Preventive medicine, individual counseling

99401   Preventive medicine counseling and/or risk factor reduction intervention(s) provided to an individual (separate procedure); approximately 15 minutes
> ➲ *CPT Assistant* Aug 97:1, Jan 98:12

99402   approximately 30 minutes
> ➲ *CPT Assistant* Aug 97:1

99403   approximately 45 minutes
> ➲ *CPT Assistant* Aug 97:1

99404   approximately 60 minutes
> ➲ *CPT Assistant* Aug 97:1

Preventive medicine, group counseling

99411   Preventive medicine counseling and/or risk factor reduction intervention(s) provided to individuals in a group setting (separate procedure); approximately 30 minutes
➜ *CPT Assistant* Aug 97:1

99412   approximately 60 minutes
➜ *CPT Assistant* Aug 97:1, Jan 98:12

Other preventive medicine services

99420   Administration and interpretation of health risk assessment instrument (eg, health hazard appraisal)

99429   Unlisted preventive medicine service

MEDICINE

Immunization Administration for Vaccines/Toxoids

Codes 90471–90474 must be reported in addition to the vaccine and toxoid code(s) 90476–90749.

If a significant separately identifiable Evaluation and Management service (eg, office or other outpatient services, preventive medicine services) is performed, the appropriate E/M service code should be reported in addition to the vaccine and toxoid administration codes.

90471   Immunization administration (includes percutaneous, intradermal, subcutaneous, intramuscular and jet injections); one vaccine (single or combination vaccine/toxoid)
➜ *CPT Assistant* Nov 98:31, Jan 99:1, Apr 99:10, Nov 99:47–48, Nov 00:10, Feb 01:4, Jul 01:1, Nov 02:11; *CPT Changes: An Insider's View 2002*

✛ 90472   each additional vaccine (single or combination vaccine/toxoid) (List separately in addition to code for primary procedure)
➜ *CPT Assistant* Nov 98:31, Jan 99:1, Apr 99:10, Nov 99:47–48 Nov 00:10, Feb 01:4, Jul 01:1, Nov 02:11; *CPT Changes: An Insider's View 2000*

(Use 90472 in conjunction with code 90471)

(For administration of immune globulins, use 90780–90784, and see 90281–90399)

(For intravesical administration of BCG vaccine, use 51720, and see 90586)

90473   Immunization administration by intranasal or oral route; one vaccine (single or combination vaccine/toxoid)
➜ *CPT Assistant* Nov 02:11; *CPT Changes: An Insider's View 2002*

✛ 90474   each additional vaccine (single or combination vaccine/toxoid) (List separately in addition to code for primary procedure)
➜ *CPT Assistant* Nov 02:11; *CPT Changes: An Insider's View 2002*

(Use 90474 in conjunction with code 90473)

Vaccines/Toxoids

Codes 90476–90748 identify the vaccine product only. To report die administration of a vaccine/toxoid, the vaccine/toxoid product codes 90476–90749 must be used in addition to an immunization administration code(s) 90471, 90472. Do not append the modifier '–51' to the vaccine/toxoid product codes 90476–90749.

If a significantly separately identifiable Evaluation and Management service (eg, office or other outpatient services, preventive medicine services) is performed, the appropriate E/M service code should be reported in addition to the vaccine and toxoid administration codes.

To meet the reporting requirements of immunization registries, vaccine distribution programs, and reporting systems (eg, Vaccine Adverse Event Reporting System) the exact vaccine product administered needs to be reported. Multiple codes for a particular vaccine are provided in C/Twhen the schedule (number of doses or timing) differs for two or more products of the same vaccine type (eg, hepatitis A, Hib) or the vaccine product is available in more than one chemical formulation, dosage, or route of administration.

Separate codes are available for combination vaccines (eg, DTP-Hib, DtaP-Hib, HepB-Hib). It is inappropriate to code each component of a combination vaccine separately. If a specific vaccine code is not available, the unlisted procedure code should be reported, until a new code becomes available.

(For immune globulins, see codes 90281–90399, and 90780–90784 for administration of immune globulins)
➜ *CPT Assistant* Nov 99:48

⊘ **90476**   Adenovirus vaccine, type 4, live, for oral use
➜ *CPT Assistant* Nov 98:31–33, Jan 99:1, Sep 99:10

⊘ **90477**   Adenovirus vaccine, type 7, live, for oral use
➜ *CPT Assistant* Nov 98:31–33, Jan 99:1

⊘= Modifier '–51' Exempt   ▶◀ or ▶ ◀ = New or Revised Text   ✛= Add-on Code   ➜ = Reference Material   ▲= Revised Code   ●= New Code

⊘ **90581** Anthrax vaccine, for subcutaneous use
➔ *CPT Assistant* Nov 98:31–33, Jan 99:1

⊘ **90585** Bacillus Calmette-Guerin vaccine (BCG) for tuberculosis, live, for percutaneous use
➔ *CPT Assistant* Nov 98:31–33, Jan 99:1

⊘ **90586** Bacillus Calmette-Guerin vaccine (BCG) for bladder cancer, live, for intravesical use
➔ *CPT Assistant* Nov 98:31–33, Jan 99:1, Nov 02:11

⊘ **90632** Hepatitis A vaccine, adult dosage, for intramuscular use
➔ *CPT Assistant* Nov 98:31–33, Jan 99:1

⊘ **90633** Hepatitis A vaccine, pediatric/adolescent dosage-2 dose schedule, for intramuscular use
➔ *CPT Assistant* Nov 98:31–33, Jan 99:1

⊘ **90634** Hepatitis A vaccine, pediatric/adolescent dosage-3 dose schedule, for intramuscular use
➔ *CPT Assistant* Nov 98:31–33, Jan 99:1

⊘ **90636** Hepatitis A and hepatitis B vaccine (HepA-HepB), adult dosage, for intramuscular use
➔ *CPT Assistant* Nov 98:31–33, Jan 99:1

⊘ **90645** Hemophilus influenza b vaccine (Hib), HbOC conjugate (4 dose schedule), for intramuscular use
➔ *CPT Assistant* Nov 98:31–33, Jan 99:1

⊘ **90646** Hemophilus influenza b vaccine (Hib), PRP-D conjugate, for booster use only, intramuscular use
➔ *CPT Assistant* 98:31–33, Jan 99:1

⊘ **90647** Hemophilus influenza b vaccine (Hib), PRP-OMP conjugate (3 dose schedule), for intramuscular use
➔ *CPT Assistant* Nov 98:31–33, Jan 99:1

⊘ **90648** Hemophilus influenza b vaccine (Hib), PRP-T conjugate (4 dose schedule), for intramuscular use
➔ *CPT Assistant* Nov 98:31–33, Jan 99:1

⊘ ● **90655** Influenza virus vaccine, split virus, preservative free, for children 6–35 months of age, for intramuscular use
➔ *CPT Changes: An Insider's View 2004*

⊘ ▲ **90657** Influenza virus vaccine, split virus, for children 6–35 months of age, for intramuscular use
➔ *CPT Assistant* Nov 98:31–33, Jan 99:1, Feb 02:10; *CPT Changes: An Insider's View 2004*

⊘ ▲ **90658** Influenza virus vaccine, split virus, for use in individuals 3 years of age and above, for intramuscular use
➔ *CPT Assistant* 98:31–33, Jan 99:1; *CPT Changes: An Insider's View 2004*

▶ **90659** has been deleted. (To report influenza virus vaccine, split virus, see 90657 or 90658) ◀

⊘ **90660** Influenza virus vaccine, live, for intranasal use
➔ *CPT Assistant* Nov 98:31–33, Jan 99:1

⊘ **90665** Lyme disease vaccine, adult dosage, for intramuscular use
➔ *CPT Assistant* Nov 98:31–33, Jan 99:1

⊘ **90669** Pneumococcal conjugate vaccine, polyvalent, for children under five years, for intramuscular use
➔ *CPT Assistant* Nov 98:31–33, Jan 99:1, Jun 00:10; *CPT Changes: An Insider's View 2001*

⊘ **90675** Rabies vaccine, for intramuscular use
➔ *CPT Assistant* Nov 98:31–33, Jan 99:1

⊘ **90676** Rabies vaccine, for intradermal use
➔ *CPT Assistant* Nov 98:31–33, Jan 99:1

⊘ **90680** Rotavirus vaccine, tetravalent, live, for oral use
➔ *CPT Assistant* Nov 98:31–33, Jan 99:1

⊘ **90690** Typhoid vaccine, live, oral
➔ *CPT Assistant* Nov 98:31–33, Jan 99:1

⊘ **90691** Typhoid vaccine, Vi capsular polysaccharide (ViCPs), for intramuscular use
➔ *CPT Assistant* Nov 98:31–33, Jan 99:1

⊘ **90692** Typhoid vaccine, heat- and phenol-inactivated (H-P), for subcutaneous or intradermal use
➔ *CPT Assistant* Nov 98:31–33, Jan 99:1

⊘ ▲ **90693** Typhoid vaccine, acetone-killed, dried (AKD), for subcutaneous use (U.S. military)
➔ *CPT Assistant* Nov 98:31–33, Jan 99:1; *CPT Changes: An Insider's View 2004*

⊘ ● **90698** Diphtheria, tetanus toxoids, acellular pertussis vaccine, haemophilus influenza Type B, and poliovirus vaccine, inactivated (DTaP - Hib - IPV), for intramuscular use

⊘ **90700** Diphtheria, tetanus toxoids, and acellular pertussis vaccine (DTaP), for intramuscular use
➔ *CPT Assistant* Jan 96:5, Nov 98:31–33, Jan 99:1

⊘ = Modifier '-51' Exempt   ▶◀ or ▶ ◀ = New or Revised Text   ✚ = Add-on Code   ➔ = Reference Material   ▲ = Revised Code   ● = New Code

⊘ **90701**   Diphtheria, tetanus toxoids, and whole cell pertussis vaccine (DTP), for intramuscular use
➔ *CPT Assistant* Jan 96:6, Nov 98:31–33, Jan 99:1

⊘ **90702**   Diphtheria and tetanus toxoids (DT) adsorbed for use in individuals younger than seven years, for intramuscular use
➔ *CPT Assistant* Jan 96:6, Nov 98:31–33, Jan 99:1, Sep 99:10, June 00:10; *CPT Changes: An Insider's View 2001*

⊘▲ **90703**   Tetanus toxoid adsorbed, for intramuscular use
➔ *CPT Assistant* Jan 96:6, Nov 98:31–33, Jan 99:1, Sep 99:10; *CPT Changes: An Insider's View 2004*

⊘▲ **90704**   Mumps virus vaccine, live, for subcutaneous use
➔ *CPT Assistant* Nov 98:31–33, Jan 99:1; *CPT Changes: An Insider's View 2004*

⊘▲ **90705**   Measles virus vaccine, live, for subcutaneous use
➔ *CPT Assistant* Nov 98:31–33, Jan 99:1; *CPT Changes: An Insider's View 2004*

⊘▲ **90706**   Rubella virus vaccine, live, for subcutaneous use
➔ *CPT Assistant* Nov 98:31–33, Jan 99:1; *CPT Changes: An Insider's View 2004*

⊘▲ **90707**   Measles, mumps and rubella virus vaccine (MMR), live, for subcutaneous use
➔ *CPT Assistant* Jan 96:6. May 96:10, Apr 97:10, Nov 98:31–33, Jan 99:1; *CPT Changes: An Insider's View 2004*

⊘▲ **90708**   Measles and rubella virus vaccine, live, for subcutaneous use
➔ *CPT Assistant* Nov 98:31–33, Jan 99:1; *CPT Changes: An Insider's View 2004*

⊘ **90710**   Measles, mumps, rubella, and varicella vaccine (MMRV), live, for subcutaneous use
➔ *CPT Assistant* May 96:10, Apr 97:10, Nov 98:31–33, Jan 99:1

⊘ **90712**   Poliovirus vaccine, (any type(s)) (OPV), live, for oral use
➔ *CPT Assistant* Jan 96:6, Nov 98:31–33, Jan 99:1

⊘ **90713**   Poliovirus vaccine, inactivated, (IPV), for subcutaneous use
➔ *CPT Assistant* Nov 98:31–33, Jan 99:1

⊘● **90715**   Tetanus, diphtheria toxoids and acellular pertussis vaccine (TdaP), for use in individuals seven years or older, for intramuscular use

⊘ **90716**   Varicella virus vaccine, live, for subcutaneous use
➔ *CPT Assistant* Jan 96:6, May 96:10, Apr 97:10, Nov 98:31–33, Jan 99:1

90717   Yellow fever vaccine, live, for subcutaneous use
➔ *CPT Assistant* Nov 98:31–33, Jan 99:1

⊘▲ **90718**   Tetanus and diphtheria toxoids (Td) adsorbed for use in individuals seven years or older, for intramuscular use
➔ *CPT Assistant* Mg 96:10, Nov 98:31–33, Jan 99:1, Jun 00:10; *CPT Changes: An Insider's View 2001, 2004*

⊘ **90719**   Diphtheria toxoid, for intramuscular use
➔ *CPT Assistant* Nov 98:31–33, Jan 99:1, Sep 99:10

⊘ **90720**   Diphtheria, tetanus toxoids, and whole cell pertussis vaccine and Hemophilus influenza B vaccine (DTP-Hib), for intramuscular use
➔ *CPT Assistant* Jan 96:5, Nov 98:31–33, Jan 99:1

⊘ **90721**   Diphtheria, tetanus toxoids, and acellular pertussis vaccine and Hemophilus influenza B vaccine (DtaP-Hib), for intramuscular use
➔ *CPT Assistant* Jan 96:5, Nov 98:31–33, Jan 99:1; *CPT Changes: An Insider's View 2000*

⊘ **90723**   Diphtheria, tetanus toxoids, acellular pertussis vaccine, Hepatitis B, and poliovirus vaccine, inactivated (DtaP-HepB-IPV), for intramuscular use
➔ *CPT Changes: An Insider's View 2001*

⊘ **90725**   Cholera vaccine for injectable use
➔ *CPT Assistant* Nov 98:31–33, Jan 99:1

⊘▲ **90727**   Plague vaccine, for intramuscular use
➔ *CPT Assistant* Nov 98:31–33, Jan 99:1; *CPT Changes: An Insider's View 2004*

⊘ **90732**   Pneumococcal polysaccharide vaccine, 23-valent, adult or immunosuppressed patient dosage, for use in individuals 2 years or older, for subcutaneous or intramuscular use
➔ *CPT Assistant* Nov 98:31–33, Jan 99:1; *CPT Changes: An Insider's View 2002*

⊘= Modifier '–51' Exempt   ▶◀ or ▶ ◀= New or Revised Text   ✚= Add-on Code   ➔ = Reference Material   ▲= Revised Code   ●= New Code

⊘ ▲ **90733**   Meningococcal polysaccharide vaccine
(any group(s)), for subcutaneous use
➔ *CPT Assistant* Nov 98:31–33, Jan 99:1,
Dec 99:7; *CPT Changes: An Insider's
View 2001, 2004*

⊘ ● **90734**   Meningococcal conjugate vaccine,
serogroups A, C, Y and W-135 (tetravalent),
for intramuscular use

⊘ **90735**   Japanese encephalitis virus vaccine, for
subcutaneous use
➔ *CPT Assistant* Nov 98:31–33, Jan 99:1

⊘ **90740**   Hepatitis B vaccine, dialysis or
immunosuppressed patient dosage
(3 dose schedule), for intramuscular use
➔ *CPT Assistant* Apr 01:10: *CPT Changes:
An Insider's View 2001*

⊘ **90743**   Hepatitis B vaccine, adolescent (2 dose
schedule), for intramuscular use
➔ *CPT Changes: An Insider's View 2001*

⊘ **90744**   Hepatitis B vaccine, pediatric/adolescent
dosage (3 dose schedule), for
intramuscular use
➔ *CPT Assistant* Jan 96:5, Jun 97:10, Nov
98:31–33, Jan 99:1, Nov 99:48–49, Jun
00:10: *CPT Changes: An Insider's View
2000, 2001*

⊘ **90746**   Hepatitis B vaccine, adult dosage, for
intramuscular use
➔ *CPT Assistant* Jan 96:5, Nov 98:31–33,
Jan 99:1

⊘ **90747**   Hepatitis B vaccine, dialysis or
immunosuppressed patient dosage (4 dose
schedule), for intramuscular use
➔ *CPT Assistant* Jan 96:5, Jun 97:10,
Nov 98:31–33, Jan 99:1, Apr 01:10,
Jun 00:10; *CPT Changes: An Insider's
View 2001*

⊘ **90748**   Hepatitis B and Hemophilus influenza b
vaccine (HepB-Hib), for intramuscular use
➔ *CPT Assistant* Nov 97:37, Nov
98:31–33, Jan 99:1, Sep 99:10

⊘ **90749**   Unlisted vaccine/toxoid
➔ *CPT Assistant* Jan 96:6, Nov 98:31–33,
Jan 99:1, Nov 02:11

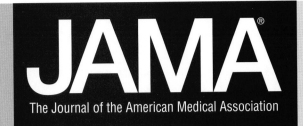
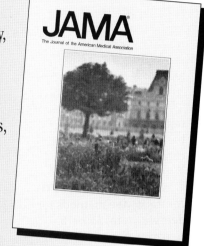
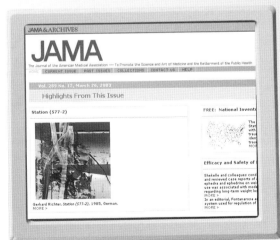
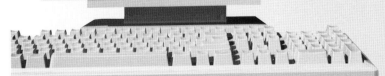

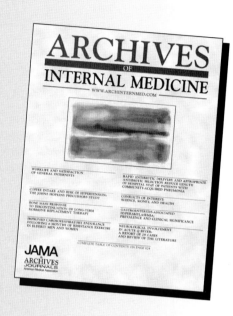
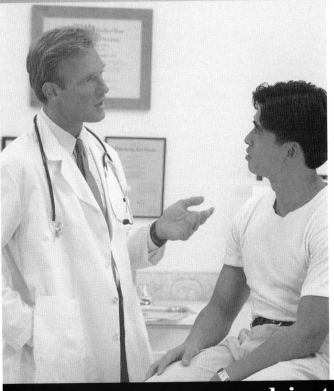

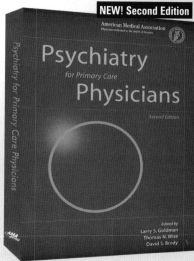
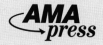
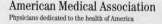